ERCP

ELSEVIER

1600 John F. Kennedy Blvd.
Ste 1800
Philadelphia, PA 19103-2899

ERCP: THIRD EDITION

ISBN: 978-0-323-48109-0

Notices

Knowledge and best practice in this field are constantly changing. As new research and experience broaden our understanding, changes in research methods, professional practices, or medical treatment may become necessary.

Practitioners and researchers must always rely on their own experience and knowledge in evaluating and using any information, methods, compounds, or experiments described herein. In using such information or methods, they should be mindful of their own safety and the safety of others, including parties for whom they have a professional responsibility.

With respect to any drug or pharmaceutical products identified, readers are advised to check the most current information provided (i) on procedures featured or (ii) by the manufacturer of each product to be administered, to verify the recommended dose or formula, the method and duration of administration, and contraindications. It is the responsibility of practitioners, relying on their own experience and knowledge of their patients, to make diagnoses, to determine dosages and the best treatment for each individual patient, and to take all appropriate safety precautions.

To the fullest extent of the law, neither the Publisher nor the authors, contributors, or editors assume any liability for any injury and/or damage to persons or property as a matter of products liability, negligence, or otherwise or from any use or operation of any methods, products, instructions, or ideas contained in the material herein.

Previous editions copyrighted 2013 and 2008.

ISBN: 978-0-323-48109-0

Content Strategist: Nancy Anastasi Duffy
Senior Content Development Specialist: Ann Anderson
Publishing Services Manager: Catherine Albright Jackson
Senior Project Manager: Doug Turner
Designer: Brian Salisbury

Printed in China

Last digit is the print number: 9   8   7   6   5   4   3   2   1

Working together
to grow libraries in
developing countries

www.elsevier.com • www.bookaid.org

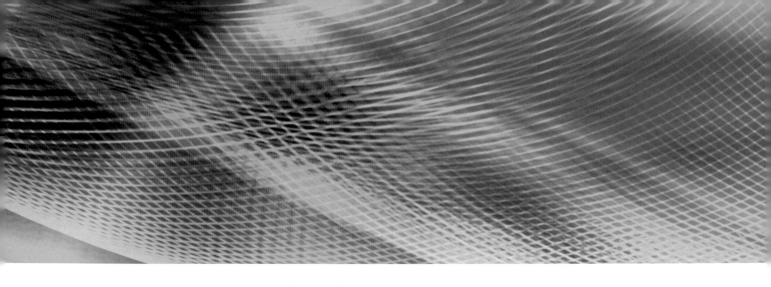

ERCP

Third Edition

Todd H. Baron, MD, FASGE

Professor of Medicine
Division of Gastroenterology and Hepatology
University of North Carolina School of Medicine
Chapel Hill, North Carolina

Richard A. Kozarek, MD, FASGE

Executive Director
Digestive Disease Institute
Department of Gastroenterology
Virginia Mason Medical Center
Seattle, Washington

David L. Carr-Locke, MD, FRCP, FASGE, FACG

Clinical Director
Center for Advanced Digestive Care
Division of Gastroenterology and Hepatology
Weill Cornell Medicine
Cornell University
New York, New York

ELSEVIER

The third edition of *ERCP* is dedicated to our patients… as well as to our families, who have endured our long days at work only to watch in exasperation as we spent our evenings and weekends finessing verbiage, adding images and references, and cajoling tardy chapter authors: it's finally your turn! At least until we plan the fourth edition.

CONTRIBUTORS

Douglas G. Adler, MD, FACG, AGAF, FASGE
Professor of Medicine
Director of Therapeutic Endoscopy
Director of GI Fellowship Program
Gastroenterology and Hepatology
University of Utah School of Medicine
Huntsman Cancer Center
Salt Lake City, Utah

Sushil K. Ahlawat, MD, FACP, FASGE, AGAF
Associate Professor of Medicine
Director of Endoscopy
Program Director, Gastroenterology and
    Hepatology Fellowship
Program Director, Advanced Endoscopy
    Fellowship
Division of Gastroenterology and
    Hepatology
Rutgers New Jersey Medical School
Newark, New Jersey

Jawad Ahmad, MD, FRCP, FAASLD
Professor of Medicine
Division of Liver Diseases
Icahn School of Medicine at Mount Sinai
New York, New York

Firas H. Al-Kawas, MD
Professor of Medicine
Division of Gastroenterology and
    Hepatology
Johns Hopkins University
Baltimore, Maryland
Director of Johns Hopkins Endoscopy
    Program
Sibley Memorial Hospital
Washington, District of Columbia

Michelle A. Anderson, MD
Associate Professor of Medicine
Taubman Center
University of Michigan
Ann Arbor, Michigan

Everson Luiz de Almeida Artifon, MD, PhD, FASGE
Coordinator of Pancreatic Biliary
    Endoscopy Unit
GI Endoscopy Service
Hospital de Clinicas of the University of Sao
    Paulo
Associate Professor of Surgery
University of Sao Paulo
Sao Paulo, Brazil

João Guilherme Guerra de Andrade Lima Cabral, MD
Endoscopist
Advanced Endoscopy Unit
A.C. Camargo Cancer Center
São Paulo, Brazil

John Baillie, MD
Professor of Medicine
Chief of Endoscopy
Virginia Commonwealth University School
    of Medicine
Richmond, Virginia

Rupa Banerjee, MD, DTM
Consultant Gastroenterologist
Asian Institute of Gastroenterology
Hyderabad, India

Todd H. Baron, MD, FASGE
Professor of Medicine
Division of Gastroenterology and
    Hepatology
University of North Carolina School of
    Medicine
Chapel Hill, North Carolina

Omer Basar, MD
Gastrointestinal Unit
Pancreas Biliary Center
Massachusetts General Hospital
Boston, Massachusetts
Professor of Medicine
Department of Gastroenterology
Hacettepe University Medical School
Ankara, Turkey

Petros C. Benias, MD
Director of Endoscopic Surgery
Division of Gastroenterology
Northwell Health System
Hofstra Zucker School of Medicine
Manhasset, New York

Ivo Boškoski, MD, PhD
Digestive Endoscopy Unit
Cattolic University of Rome
Rome, Italy

Michael J. Bourke, MBBS, FRACP
Clinical Professor of Medicine
Director of Endoscopy
Gastroenterology and Hepatology
Westmead Hospital
Sydney, Australia

Brian C. Brauer, MD
Associate Professor of Medicine
University of Colorado School of Medicine
Aurora, Colorado

William R. Brugge, MD
Professor of Medicine
Harvard Medical School
Director of Gastrointestinal Unit
Pancreas Biliary Center
Massachusetts General Hospital
Boston, Massachusetts

Jonathan M. Buscaglia, MD
Associate Professor and Division Chief
Gastroenterology and Hepatology
Stony Brook University School of Medicine
Stony Brook, New York

David L. Carr-Locke, MD, FRCP, FASGE, FACG
Clinical Director
Center for Advanced Digestive Care
Division of Gastroenterology and
    Hepatology
Weill Cornell Medicine
Cornell University
New York, New York

Prabhleen Chahal, MD
Physician
Department of Gastroenterology and
    Hepatology
Cleveland Clinic
Cleveland, Ohio

Sujievvan Chandran, MBBS, FRACP
Therapeutic Endoscopy Fellow
Gastroenterology
St. Michaels's Hospital
Toronto, Ontario, Canada

Yen-I Chen, MD
Assistant Professor of Medicine
Division of Gastroenterology and
    Hepatology
McGill University Health Center
Montreal, Quebec, Canada

Anthony J. Choi, MD
Resident Physician
Department of Medicine
Weill Cornell Medicine
Cornell University
New York, New York

Jonah Cohen, MD
Clinical Fellow in Advanced Endoscopy
Division of Gastroenterology
Beth Israel Deaconess Medical Center
Boston, Massachusetts

Guido Costamagna, MD, FACG
Digestive Endoscopy Unit
Catholic University
Gemelli University Hospital
Rome, Italy
Chair of Digestive Endoscopy
USIAS Strasbourg University
Strasbourg, France

Gregory A. Coté, MD
Associate Professor of Medicine
Division of Gastroenterology and
  Hepatology
Department of Medicine
Medical University of South Carolina
Charleston, South Carolina

Peter Cotton, MD, FRCS, FRCP
Professor of Medicine
Digestive Disease Center
Medical University of South Carolina
Charleston, South Carolina

Koushik K. Das, MD
Assistant Professor of Medicine
Division of Gastroenterology
Washington University School of Medicine
St. Louis, Missouri

Jacques Devière, MD, PhD
Professor of Medicine
Head
Department of Gastroenterology,
  Hepatology, and Digestive Oncology
CUB Erasme
Université Libre de Bruxelles
Brussels, Belgium

Steven A. Edmundowicz, MD
Professor of Medicine
University of Colorado School of Medicine
Aurora, Colorado

Ihab I. El Hajj, MD, MPH
Assistant Professor of Medicine
Division of Gastroenterology and
  Hepatology
Indiana University
Indianapolis, Indiana

Douglas O. Faigel, MD, FACG, FASGE, AGAF
Professor of Medicine
Department of Gastroenterology and
  Hepatology
Mayo Clinic
Scottsdale, Arizona

Pietro Familiari, MD, PhD
Fondazione Policlinico Gemelli
Digestive Endoscopy Unit
Rome, Italy

Paul Fockens, MD, PhD, FASGE
Professor and Chair
Gastroenterology and Hepatology
Academic Medical Center
Amsterdam, Netherland

Evan L. Fogel, MD
Professor of Medicine
Division of Gastroenterology and
  Hepatology
Indiana University School of Medicine
Indianapolis, Indiana

Victor L. Fox, MD
Associate Professor of Pediatrics
Harvard Medical School
Director of GI Procedure and Endoscopy
  Unit
Division of Gastroenterology, Hepatology,
  and Nutrition
Boston Children's Hospital
Boston, Massachusetts

Martin L. Freeman, MD
Professor of Medicine
Division of Gastroenterology, Hepatology,
  and Nutrition
University of Minnesota
Minneapolis, Minnesota

S. Ian Gan, MD
Department of Gastroenterology
Virginia Mason Medical Center
Seattle, Washington

Andres Gelrud, MD, MMSc, FASGE
Director
Pancreatic Disease Center
Miami Cancer Institute
Miami, Florida

Gregory G. Ginsberg, MD
Professor of Medicine
Department of Medicine
Division of Gastroenterology
Hospital of the University of Pennsylvania
Philadelphia, Pennsylvania

Michael Gluck, MD
Past Chief of Medicine
Department of Gastroenterology
Virginia Mason Medical Center
Seattle, Washington

Khean-Lee Goh, MBBS, FRCP, MD
Professor
Gastroenterology and Medicine
University of Malaya
Kuala Lumpur, Malaysia

Robert H. Hawes
Professor of Medicine
University of Central Florida College of
  Medicine
Medical Director
Florida Hospital Institute for Minimally
  Invasive Therapy
Center for Interventional Endoscopy
Florida Hospital Orlando
Orlando, Florida

Jennifer T. Higa, MD
Advanced Endoscopy Fellow
Department of Gastroenterology
Virginia Mason Medical Center
Seattle, Washington

Jordan D. Holmes, MD
Gastroenterologist
Iowa Digestive Disease Center
Clive, Iowa

Shayan Irani, MBBS, MD
Department of Gastroenterology
Virginia Mason Medical Center
Seattle, Washington

Takao Itoi, MD, PhD, FASGE, FACG
Professor and Chair
Department of Gastroenterology and
  Hepatology
Tokyo Medical University
Tokyo, Japan

Priya A. Jamidar, MD
Professor of Medicine
Director of Endoscopy
Section of Digestive Diseases
Yale University
New Haven, Connecticut

Michel Kahaleh, MD
Professor of Medicine
Division of Gastroenterology and
  Hepatology
Department of Medicine
Weill Cornell Medicine
Cornell University
New York, New York

Anthony N. Kalloo, MD
The Moses and Helen Golden Paulson
    Professor of Gastroenterology
Director of Division of Gastroenterology
    and Hepatology
The Johns Hopkins Hospital
Baltimore, Maryland

Mouen A. Khashab, MD
Director of Therapeutic Endoscopy
Associate Professor of Medicine
Department of Gastroenterology and
    Hepatology
The Johns Hopkins Hospital
Baltimore, Maryland

Michael L. Kochman, MD
Wilmott Family Professor of Medicine
Division of Gastroenterology
Department of Medicine
Perelman School of Medicine
University of Pennsylvania
Philadelphia, Pennsylvania

Tadashi Kodama, MD, PhD
Advisor
Department of Gastroenterology
Iwasaki Hospital
Mitoyo City, Kagawa, Japan

Andrew Korman, MD
Division of Gastroenterology and
    Hepatology
Saint Peter's University Hospital
New Brunswick, New Jersey

Paul Kortan, MD, FRCPC, FASGE, AGAF
Department of Medicine
St. Michael's Hospital
University of Toronto
Toronto, Ontario, Canada

Tatsuya Koshitani, MD, PhD
Director of Department of Gastroenterology
Japan Community Healthcare Organization
Kobe Central Hospital
Kobe City, Hyogo, Japan

Richard A. Kozarek, MD, FASGE
Executive Director
Digestive Disease Institute
Department of Gastroenterology
Virginia Mason Medical Center
Seattle, Washington

Michael Larsen, MD
Gastroenterologist
Digestive Disease Institute
Virginia Mason Medical Center
Seattle, Washington

James Y.W. Lau, MD
Chairman and Yao Ling Sun Professor of
    Surgery
The Chinese University of Hong Kong
Shatin, Hong Kong, China

Ryan Law, DO
Clinical Lecturer
Division of Gastroenterology
University of Michigan
Ann Arbor, Michigan

Glen Lehman, MD
Professor of Medicine
Division of Gastroenterology
Department of Medicine
Indiana University
Indianapolis, Indiana

**Joseph W. Leung, MD, FRCP, FACP,
MACG, FASGE**
Mr. and Mrs. C.W. Law Professor of
    Medicine
Division of Gastroenterology and
    Hepatology
University of California Davis School of
    Medicine
Sacramento, California
Section Chief of Gastroenterology
Veterans Affairs Northern California Health
    Care System
Mather, California

Dario Ligresti, MD
Endoscopy Service
Department of Diagnostic and Therapeutic
    Services
IRCCS ISMETT (Instituto Mediterraneo per
    i Trapianti e Terapie ad Alta
    Specializzazione)
Palermo, Italy

Eugene Lin, MD
Attending Radiologist
Virginia Mason Medical Center
Seattle, Washington

Simon K. Lo, MD, FACP
Director of Endoscopy
Head of Pancreatic Diseases Program
Division of Digestive Diseases and
    Hepatology
Cedars-Sinai Medical Center
Clinical Professor of Medicine
David Geffen School of Medicine at UCLA
Los Angeles, California

Michael X. Ma, MBBS, FRACP
Advanced Endoscopy Fellow
Gastroenterology and Hepatology
Westmead Hospital
Sydney, Australia

John T. Maple, DO
Associate Professor of Medicine
Division of Digestive Diseases and Nutrition
University of Oklahoma
Oklahoma City, Oklahoma

Alberto Mariani, MD
Pancreato-Biliary Endoscopy and
    Endosonography Division
Pancreas Translational and Clinical Research
    Center
San Raffaele Scientific Institute
Vita Salute San Raffaele University
Via Olgettina
Milan, Italy

Gary May, MD, FRCPC, FASGE
Division of Gastroenterology
Department of Medicine
The Center of Advanced Therapeutic
    Endoscopy and Endoscopic Oncology
St. Michael's Hospital
University of Toronto Faculty of Medicine
Toronto, Ontario, Canada

Lee McHenry, MD
Professor of Medicine
Division of Gastroenterology
Department of Medicine
Indiana University
Indianapolis, Indiana

Meir Mizrahi, MD
Director of Advanced Endoscopy
Internal Medicine
Division of Gastroenterology
University of South Alabama College of
    Medicine
Mobile, Alabama

Rawad Mounzer, MD
Assistant Professor of Medicine
Digestive Institute
Banner-University Medical Center
University of Arizona
Phoenix, Arizona

**Thiruvengadam Muniraj, MD, PhD,
MRCP(UK)**
Assistant Professor of Medicine
Director of Yale Center for Pancreatitis
Section of Digestive Diseases
Yale University School of Medicine
New Haven, Connecticut

Horst Neuhaus, MD
Professor of Medicine
Chief of the Department of Internal
   Medicine
Evangelisches Krankenhaus Düsseldorf
Düsseldorf, Germany

Ian D. Norton, MBBS, PhD
Associate Professor
Department of Gastroenterology
Royal North Shore Hospital
Sydney, Australia

Manuel Perez-Miranda, MD, PhD
Head of Gastroenterology and Hepatology
Hospital Universitario Rio Hortega
Associate Professor of Medicine
Valladolid University Medical School
Valladolid, Spain

Bret T. Petersen, MD
Professor of Medicine
Department of Gastroenterology and
   Hepatology
Mayo Clinic
Rochester, Minnesota

Douglas Pleskow, MD
Associate Clinical Professor
Department of Medicine
Harvard Medical School
Chief of Clinical Gastroenterology
Beth Israel Deaconess Medical Center
Boston, Massachusetts

Tugrul Purnak, MD
Associate Professor of Medicine
Gastroenterology and Hepatology
Hacettepe University Medical School
Ankara, Turkey

G. Venkat Rao, MS, MAMS, FRCS
Director and Chief of Gastrointestinal and
   Minimally Invasive Surgery
Asian Institute of Gastroenterology
Hyderabad, India

Anthony Razzak, MD
Gastroenterologist
Oregon Clinic
Portland, Oregon

D. Nageshwar Reddy, MBBS, MD, DM
Director and Chief Gastroenterologist
Asian Institute of Gastroenterology
Hyderabad, India

Andrew S. Ross, MD
Section Head of Gastroenterology
Medical Director
Therapeutic Endoscopy Center of Excellence
Virginia Mason Medical Center
Seattle, Washington

Alexander M. Sarkisian, MD
Resident Physician
Internal Medicine
Tulane University School of Medicine
New Orleans, Louisiana

Beth Schueler, PhD
Professor of Medical Physics
Department of Radiology
Mayo Clinic
Rochester, Minnesota

Dong Wan Seo, MD, PhD
Professor
Gastroenterology
University of Ulsan College of Medicine
Asan Medical Center
Seoul, South Korea

Raj J. Shah, MD, FASGE, AGAF
Professor of Medicine
Division of Gastroenterology
University of Colorado School of Medicine
Director of Pancreaticobiliary Endoscopy
Division of Gastroenterology
University of Colorado Anschutz Medical
   Campus
Aurora, Colorado

Reem Z. Sharaiha, MD, MSc
Assistant Professor of Medicine
Division of Gastroenterology and
   Hepatology
Weill Cornell Medicine
Cornell University
New York City, New York

Stuart Sherman, MD
Professor of Medicine and Radiology
Glen Lehman Professor in Gastroenterology
Division of Gastroenterology and
   Hepatology
Indiana University
Indianapolis, Indiana

**Chan Sup Shim, MD, PhD, FASGE,
AGAF**
Professor
Department of Gastroenterology
Kunkuk University Medical Center
Seoul, South Korea

Ajaypal Singh, MD
Director of Advanced Endoscopy
Rush University Medical Center
Chicago, Illinois

Adam Slivka, MD, PhD
Professor of Medicine
Associate Chief of Clinical Services
Division of Gastroenterology, Hepatology,
   and Nutrition
University of Pittsburgh School of Medicine
Pittsburgh, Pennsylvania

Sanjeev Solomon, MD
Howard University Hospital
Washington, District of Columbia

Tae Jun Song, MD, PhD
Associate Professor
Gastroenterology
University of Ulsan College of Medicine
Asan Medical Center
Seoul, South Korea

Indu Srinivasan, MD
Advanced Endoscopy Fellow
Maricopa Integrated Health System
Chandler, Arizona

Joseph J.Y. Sung, MD, PhD
President and Vice Chancellor
Mok Hing Yiu Professor of Medicine
The Chinese University of Hong Kong
Shatin, Hong Kong, China

Ilaria Tarantino, MD
Endoscopy Service
Department of Diagnostic and Therapeutic
   Services
IRCCS ISMETT (Instituto Mediterraneo per
   i Trapianti e Terapie ad Alta
   Specializzazione)
Palermo, Italy

Paul R. Tarnasky, MD
Physician
Methodist Dallas Medical Center
Dallas, Texas

Pier Alberto Testoni, MD, FASGE
Director of Division of Gastroenterology
   and GI Endoscopy
San Raffaele Scientific Institute
Vita Salute San Raffaele University
Via Olgettina
Milan, Italy

Catherine D. Tobin, MD
Associate Professor of Anesthesiology
Department of Anesthesia
Medical University of South Carolina
Charleston, South Carolina

Mark Topazian, MD
Professor of Medicine
Department of Gastroenterology and
  Hepatology
Mayo Clinic
Rochester, Minnesota

Sachin Wani, MD
Associate Professor of Medicine
Division of Gastroenterology and
  Hepatology
University of Colorado Anschutz Medical
  Campus
Aurora, Colorado

John C.T. Wong, MD
Clinical Professional Consultant
Institute of Digestive Disease
The Chinese University of Hong Kong
Shatin, Hong Kong, China

Andrew W. Yen, MD, MAS, FACG, FASGE
Associate Chief of Gastroenterology
Veterans Affairs Northern California Health
  Care System
Mather, California
Assistant Clinical Professor of Medicine
Division of Gastroenterology and
  Hepatology
University of California Davis School of
  Medicine
Sacramento, California

FOREWORD

What a difference 10 years makes. Since the first edition of *ERCP* published in 2008, it seems like there has been a cosmic shift in the practice of gastrointestinal medicine and endoscopy. Diagnostic ERCP has given way to continued improvements in computed tomography and magnetic resonance imaging, as well as to endoscopic ultrasound (EUS), which provides information not only about the diameter, contents, and contours of the pancreaticobiliary ducts but also about the pancreatic and liver parenchyma, contiguous organs, relevant vasculature, and lymph nodes. Additionally, EUS has been shown to have improved sensitivity for the diagnosis of pancreatic malignancy compared with brushing or biopsy done at time of ERCP. Moreover, as technology and EUS experience have expanded, therapeutic procedures previously relegated to ERCP (or interventional radiology) are increasingly being done with an echoendoscope: gallbladder and bile duct access for cholecystoduodenal, hepatobiliary, and choledochoduodenal stenting; endoscopic anastomosis of obstructed afferent limbs; gastroenterostomy for bypass of malignant duodenal obstruction; PD imaging and duct decompression in difficult-to-access anatomy; and imaging and treatment of pancreatic fluid collections, many of which were previously imaged and variably treated with ERCP. The barbarians are at the gate!

Or are they? ERCP with sphincterotomy and/or balloon dilation remains the treatment of choice for choledocholithiasis and for many cases of pancreatic stones. Moreover, it maintains primacy for the treatment of benign pancreaticobiliary strictures and most malignancies causing obstructive jaundice. In contrast, therapeutic EUS has evolved to allow access in complex postoperative anatomy, duodenal obstruction, or after failed ERCP. In fact, we are the barbarians who often employ both echoendoscopes and duodenoscopes in the same patient under a single anesthesia to stage a patient with malignant obstructive jaundice, obtain a definitive tissue diagnosis, and render appropriate palliative therapy. Alternatively, we may use EUS to access the pancreaticobiliary tree as part of a rendezvous procedure to improve the success rate of ERCP. The third edition of this text acknowledges the expanded role that EUS has come to play in patients previously undergoing diagnostic or therapeutic ERCP alone. Utilizing one procedure without access to the other is a disservice to our patients and encourages the overuse of one of the (potentially) more dangerous therapeutic endoscopic procedures we perform.

What a difference 10 years makes. Look for the new chapters, including one on endoscope disinfection. This should not come as a surprise to anyone as both the lay press and medical literature have been awash in cases of antibiotic resistant bacterial infections, which can be traced back to duodenoscopes contaminated with the same organism. What else is new in the third edition of *ERCP*? Almost everything: new images, updated videos, and multiple chapters that incorporate EUS and place it into the perspective of modern ERCP practice. However, there is much that has not changed in the current edition of this text. Most notably we have retained the world's premier clinicians and endoscopic researchers to share their ERCP experience, their wisdom, and their cautions to us all.

ACKNOWLEDGMENT

The Editors thank our medical colleagues and support staff for their outstanding contributions to our patients' care and the authors of this textbook for their new or updated contributions.

Todd H. Baron, MD, FASGE
Richard A. Kozarek, MD, FASGE
David L. Carr-Locke, MD, FRCP, FASGE, FACG

CONTENTS

VIDEO CONTENTS

1

Approaching 50 Years: The History of ERCP

Lee McHenry and Glen Lehman

Endoscopic retrograde cholangiopancreatography (ERCP) has been a remarkable technological advance that has evolved over its nearly 50 years in the field of gastrointestinal endoscopy and has redefined the medical and surgical approach to patients with pancreatic and biliary tract diseases. Since its inception in 1968, the medical community has witnessed significant achievements by the pioneers in endoscopy who incrementally advanced ERCP techniques from their infancy to maturity. The infancy focused on diagnoses, the adolescence on therapies of common biliary tract diseases such as bile duct stones and malignant strictures, the early adulthood on therapy for diseases of the pancreas and prevention of pancreatitis, and now the mature adulthood focuses on continued refinement of techniques to make ERCP safer and more effective. The pioneers in the ERCP field are numerous and have played significant roles in developing new techniques and novel instrumentation, spearheaded innovative techniques to reduce adverse events, and effectively trained future generations of endoscopists to safely perform ERCP. We are now approaching a 50-year milestone, and as we look back, we can recall a journey in ERCP that has been enjoyable, exciting, and replete with enthusiastic innovation, and in the end has benefitted many patients (Box 1.1). It would encompass an entire book to incorporate all of the important contributions made by the many ERCP endoscopists over the past 50 years. We apologize in advance to individuals who have advanced the field and are not mentioned in this brief summary of the history of ERCP.

ERCP IN ITS INFANCY: 1968 TO 1980

In the 1920s, bile duct imaging was performed by surgeons Evarts Graham and Warren Cole with the use of intravenously administered iodinated phenolphthalein that was selectively excreted into the bile and recorded radiographically. Oral cholecystography and percutaneous skinny "Chiba" needle cholangiography were additionally developed to improve the visualization of the bile duct.[1,2] What defied the clinician was a nonoperative technique to image the pancreatic duct. In 1965 two innovative radiologists, Rabinov and Simon,[3] fashioned a bendable catheter that was inserted through a per oral basket catheter. The medial duodenal wall was "blindly scratched" with the tip of the catheter and the first pancreatogram was successfully obtained nonoperatively. In eight attempts, an interpretable pancreatogram was obtained in two patients. The gastrointestinal endoscopist now entered the arena. In 1968 William McCune and his surgical colleagues at George Washington University were credited with the first report of endoscopic cannulation of the ampulla of Vater in living patients.[4] McCune used an Eder fiberoptic

duodenoscope (Eder Instrument Company, Chicago, IL), which had both a forward and side lens and an endotracheal-type cuff placed on the scope just beyond the lens. The balloon was inflated and deflated to enable adequate focal length for mucosal visualization. McCune taped a small-diameter plastic tube that served as a tract to the endoscope that could house a bendable cannula. The cannula was advanced to the major duodenal papilla under endoscopic guidance. In his report of 50 patients, McCune's duodenal intubation success rate was only 50%, with only 25% pancreatic duct opacification. As stated in his discussion: "Anyone who looks through one of these instruments has to have 2 personality characteristics. First, he has to be honest, and second, must have an undying, blind, day and night, uncompromising persistence." ERCP was now born, and it slowly grew to an established technique as a result of the honesty and persistence of the pioneers of endoscopy.

In March 1969 in Japan, Oi (Fig. 1.1) and colleagues—in close collaboration with Machida (Machida Endoscope, Ltd., Tokyo, Japan) and Olympus corporations (Olympus Optical Co., Ltd., Tokyo, Japan)—developed a side-viewing fiberoptic duodenoscope with a channel and an elevator lever to enable manipulation of the cannula. Initially, Oi visualized the ampulla in about half of 105 cases.[4] In a subsequent report, Oi cannulated the papilla in 41 of 53 patients (77%) without significant morbidity.[5] By 1972, Jack Vennes and Steven Silvis of the University of Minnesota published the experience in their first 80 attempts at cannulation of the bile and pancreatic ducts, paving the way for acceptability in the American endoscopic wilderness[6] (Table 1.1).[7,8] Over the next 5 years, pioneers such as Safrany, Cotton, Geenen, Siegel, Classen, and Demling and the Japanese groups embraced this new technique and reported on the successes (cannulation rates of >90%) (Fig. 1.2), the shortcomings (e.g., post-ERPC pancreatitis [PEP]), the nuances (variety of cannula types, cannulation angles), and the practical application of ERCP in our understanding of biliary and pancreatic disorders.[9–15] But what could we as endoscopists do with this new-found knowledge?

Simultaneously in 1973, in separate regions on the globe, ERCP investigators conceived the concept of a therapeutic application of ERCP. The sphincter of the intact papilla served as a barrier to reflux of duodenal contents into the bile and pancreatic duct and was an impediment to removal of stones from the bile duct. Independently, Demling and Classen in Erlangen, Germany, and Kawai in Kyoto, Japan, developed similar techniques to split the sphincter. Demling and Classen developed a high-frequency diathermy snare, the Demling-Classen probe consisting of a Teflon catheter with a thin steel wire that could be protruded to create a "bowstring" that would sever the papillary muscle (Fig. 1.3).[15–17]

BOX 1.1 History of ERCP: Five Decades, Decade by Decade

1970s: Diagnosis and Therapy
- Locating the ampulla
- Biliary and pancreatic duct cannulation
- Interpretation of cholangiography and pancreatography, identifying pathology
- First reports of biliary sphincterotomy
- Developing the instruments: balloon extraction of bile duct stones and stent placement

1980s: Slowly Shifting from Surgery to Endoscopic Management of Pancreaticobiliary Disorders
- Refinement of accessories, improvements in radiographic imaging
- Reporting adverse events of sphincterotomy
- Biliary stent placement for obstructive jaundice and shift from palliative surgery
- Introduction of the teaching head: "seeing is believing"
- Acceptance of ERCP by the medical community
  - Management of CBD stones shifts from surgery to endoscopy
- ERCP training gets its start for physicians and ERCP nurses
  - Basic threshold numbers for competence

1990s: Training and Expanding Our Therapies
- More emphasis on advanced training
- Endoscopic photography and videography: sharing images with others
  - Referring MDs, patients, and industry
  - Comparison of one procedure to another
  - Teaching and training
- "Theater presentations" of ERCP
- Therapies for pancreatic disorders: chronic pancreatitis, pseudocysts, and necrosis
- Era of laparoscopic cholecystectomy and bile duct injuries

- Safer sphincterotomy: monofilament wires and computer-regulated blended current
- Self-expandable metallic stents
- Complementary pancreaticobiliary techniques developed
  - Endoscopic ultrasonography (EUS) and magnetic resonance cholangiopancreatography (MRCP)

2000s: Prevention, Pulverizing, and Peculiar Pancreas Diseases
- Pancreatic stents and post-ERCP pancreatitis prevention
- Improved techniques for extraction of "large" bile duct stones are implemented
  - Papillary balloon dilation
  - Single-operator system for intraductal lithotripsy
- Intraductal papillary mucinous neoplasm (IPMN) and autoimmune pancreatitis (AIP) recognized
- "Hands-on" courses
- EUS and ERCP therapeutic interface

2010s: Refinements of ERCP Techniques and New Treatments
- Pharmacologic agents (rectal NSAIDs) for post-ERCP prevention
- Revised recommendations for sphincter of Oddi dysfunction diagnosis and therapy
- ERCP scope infections are revisited and rigorous cleaning processes of ERCP scopes are revised
- Novel ERCP treatments for cholangiocarcinoma, including photodynamic therapy and radiofrequency ablation, are introduced
- Charge-coupled device (CCD) imaging improves intraductal cholangioscopy and pancreatoscopy

---

TABLE 1.1 ERCP in Its Infancy: Cannulation Rates Around 1972

Group	Total	Overall Success (%)*	Selective Success Pancreatic (%)	Selective Success Biliary (%)
Ogoshi	283	88		
Oi	310	81		
Kasugai	270	74		
Cremer	144	76	68	63
Cotton	132	83	78	73
Classen	541	86		
Safrany	145	94		
Vennes	80	75		

*Generally defined as entry into either duct.
From Cotton PB. Progress report: cannulation of the papilla of Vater by endoscopy and retrograde pancreatography (ERCP). *Gut* 1972;13:1014–1025.

Canine experiments ensued and demonstrated that a papillotomy could be performed safely without bleeding or perforation. An added benefit of the Demling-Classen probe was that contrast dye could be instilled while the catheter was in place. In Japan, Kawai developed a papillotomy device consisting of two separate 2-mm-long diathermy knives that protruded from the catheter tip and could be used to incise the papillary sphincter, similar to the present-day needle knife technique.[15] This device was particularly useful in patients with impacted stones at the papilla. The Erlangen probe, because of a perceived reduction in the risk of perforation, was more accepted in the West, and sphincterotomy as a technique was born. The initial concern of postsphincterotomy scarring was postulated, but the incidence was found to be infrequent. The first

therapeutic application during ERCP, with incumbent well-chronicled risks, was gradually adopted by endoscopists around the world. Bile duct stones were accurately diagnosed at the time of cholangiography, biliary sphincterotomy was performed, and the stones were left in the bile duct to pass on their own. This clinical problem needed a solution, and as is true with the many endoscopic techniques, the fundamental elements for major endoscopic technological advances were borrowed heavily from other fields (i.e., urology: basket, stent, and balloon technology; radiology: catheter and guidewire technology; cardiology: catheters and metallic stents). To solve the clinical problem of removing stones from the bile duct, in 1975 Zimmon and colleagues[18] in New York reported removal of bile duct stones with balloon-tipped catheters, a technique that further expanded the endoscopist's therapeutic armamentarium. Long, flexible balloon-tipped catheters, basket catheters, stone-grasping forceps, and endoscopic laser or ultrasound stone disintegrators were miniaturized to fit through the endoscope working channel, and removal of bile duct stones no longer required surgical laparotomy and open choledochotomy.

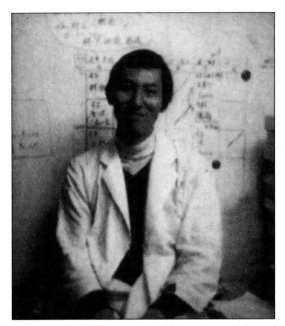

FIG 1.1 One year after Dr. William McCune successfully performed the first ERCP at George Washington University, in Japan Dr. Itaru Oi, with his chief, Dr. Takemoto, performed endoscopic cholangiopancreatogram (ECPG), as it was called, with a Machida scope in 1969.[5] The method used was almost the same as Dr. McCune's method of using a prolonged gastrofiberscope. In close collaboration with the Machida and Olympus corporations, Oi developed a side-viewing fiberoptic duodenoscope with a channel and an elevator lever to enable manipulation of the cannula. (Photo courtesy Dr. Peter Cotton, Medical University of South Carolina.)

The 1970s were an exciting time for ERCP, but many physicians (gastroenterologists and surgeons) were appropriately concerned about the dangers of the procedure, particularly PEP, bleeding, and biliary sepsis. In 1976, Bilbao and colleagues[19] surveyed 402 U.S. owners of side-viewing duodenoscopes who had collectively performed 10,435 ERCPs. The procedure failed in 30%, adverse events occurred in 3%, and death occurred in 0.2%. Pancreatitis was associated with injection into the pancreatic duct and sepsis with injection into an obstructed bile duct. Inexperience led to a fourfold increase in failures (62%) and twice the rate of adverse events (7%). ERCP was the riskiest procedure for the endoscopist, yet was gradually embraced, and the physicians who had the willingness and ability to perform ERCP forged ahead. In looking back in ERCP history over the past 5 decades, the gastroenterology community was aware of the high incidence and potentially severe adverse events associated with ERCP; however, the absolute requirement of advanced training and expertise before subjecting patients to this potentially lethal procedure was understated, minimized, and inadequately addressed. These should serve as reminders and lessons for the future as new endoscopic procedures are introduced.

Malignant bile duct obstruction posed a problem to the ERCP physician in the 1970s. Endoscopic cannulation of the bile duct introduced bacteria-laden contrast dye into an obstructed biliary tree, and endoscopic sphincterotomy alone would not provide adequate biliary drainage except in the most distal bile duct or ampullary cancers. Percutaneous transhepatic methods for biliary drainage were commonly employed preoperatively in patients with deep jaundice or for palliation, and the first report of a percutaneous transhepatic cholangiography (PTC)-guided internal bile duct prosthesis was reported by Burcharth et al. in 1979.[20] In 1980, the ERCP groups in England (Laurence and Cotton[21]) and Germany (Soehendra and Reynders-Frederix[22]) reported the early cases of internal decompression of malignant biliary obstruction by ERCP-directed biliary endoprosthesis placement (Fig. 1.4). The initial methods relied on "borrowed" technology and reported the uses of a 7-Fr nasobiliary drain fashioned from an angiographic catheter and a "pigtail" stent cut from a 7-Fr Teflon catheter. Over the next 30 years, with the aid of industry and ingenuity, biliary endoprosthesis design continued to advance from the back table of the craftsman/endoscopist to the precision engineering of multisized polyethylene stents and

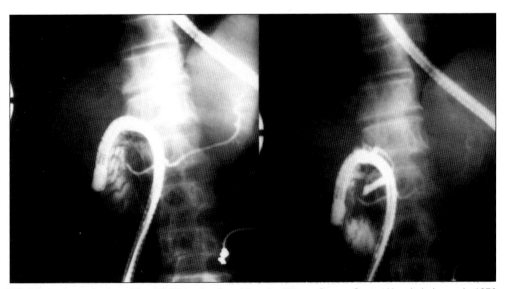

FIG 1.2 In the early days: First ERCP by Dr. Ogoshi at the Niigata Cancer Center Hospital, Japan, in 1970. Radiographs showing complete pancreatography (left) and the distal bile duct (right). Note the long scope position to obtain pancreatography. (Photo courtesy Dr. Peter Cotton, Medical University of South Carolina.)

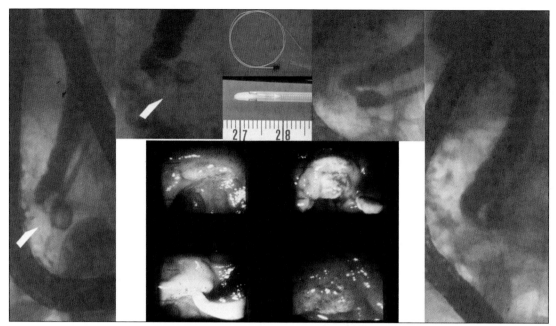

FIG 1.3 The endoscopic and fluoroscopic images from the first sphincterotomy performed by Drs. Nakajima and Kawai in Kyoto, Japan, in 1974. *Clockwise from left:* The fluoroscopic images on the left show the distal bile duct calculus *(arrow)* with upstream filling of the bile duct. The catheter was used for cannulation and sphincterotomy. On the right, the cholangiogram and pancreatogram revealing bile duct clear of filling defect. In the bottom middle is the limited field of view of the duodenal papilla on the left and the papilla after sphincterotomy on the right. (Photo courtesy Dr. Peter Cotton, Medical University of South Carolina.)

self-expandable metallic stents. Effective palliation of malignant biliary obstruction was wrestled from the surgeon and radiologist, and planted for good into the endoscopist's hands.

THE SECOND DECADE: 1980 TO 1990

Over the next 10 years from 1980 to 1990, medicine witnessed an explosion in the number of ERCPs performed throughout the world. However, this explosion did not occur in a vacuum and was fueled by burgeoning technology in other medical disciplines such as radiology, anesthesia, pathology, and surgery. In 1979, the Nobel Prize in Medicine was awarded jointly to Godfrey N. Hounsfield (U.K.) and Allan McLeod Cormack (Tufts University, Medford/Somerville, MA) for independently inventing the computerized axial tomography (CAT) scanner. Assessment of the patient with pancreatobiliary disease was transformed from physical examination, ultrasound, and plain radiographs, and their inherent limitations to precise computed tomography (CT) characterization and localization of the problem at hand. Improved perioperative management and anesthesia care made the ERCP procedure more acceptable to patients. Pathologic interpretation of endoscopic biopsies and cytologic assessment of brushings continued to improve, with increased number of specimens and physician experience allowing tissue diagnosis to be made nonoperatively. The surgeon's role evolved from exploration for diagnosis with its inherent morbidity and mortality to a more focused therapeutic operation that would lead to improved patient outcomes.

Industry played a major role in the close collaboration with endoscopists in designing improved versions of ERCP accessories, including cannulas, sphincterotomes, and endoscopic stents, which led to improved therapeutics and improved patient outcomes. Companies such as Wilson-Cook (now Cook Endoscopy, Winston-Salem, NC), Olympus (Center Valley, PA, and Tokyo, Japan), Bard (now ConMed, Utica, NY), and Microvasive (now Boston-Scientific, Marlborough, MA) and many others forged tight, long-lasting relationships with the pioneers in ERCP, which accelerated innovation in the field (Fig. 1.5). Both ERCP endoscopists and patients benefited from increased cannulation rates, improved sphincterotomies, and reliable prostheses. The domain of bile duct stones and palliation of malignancies shifted from surgeons to endoscopists. One of the recurring themes in endoscopic advances is the importance of close collaboration of engineers and clinicians to attempt to solve clinical problems.

Fiberoptic endoscopy was the platform for the ERCP gastroenterologist in the 1970s and posed a challenge for performance of and training and reporting in ERCP. Documenting endoscopic findings was limited in quality, as the camera head attachment was bulky and, when affixed, precluded real-time visualization of the endoscopy image. To share the endoscopy experience, a teaching head apparatus would connect to the endoscope to allow a second observer (an ERCP trainee or procedural nurse) to visualize the endoscopic image. The major drawbacks were halving of the light transmitted through the fibers to the eyepiece, allowing only one observer on the teaching head, and limiting the nurse to the use of only one hand to perform important functions such as wire advancement while holding the teaching head with the other hand. The first videoendoscope had a small television camera in the tip of the endoscope (charge-coupled device [CCD]) and was connected to a computer capable of transforming electronic signals into a recognizable image. Sivak and Fleischer[23] in the United States and Classen and Phillip[24] in Germany reported on their first experiences in 1984. Videoendoscopy had transformed the ERCP experience for the performing physician, the trainees, and the ERCP nurses to a more dynamic, less solitary experience and launched ERCP training to a new level.

THE THIRD DECADE: 1990 TO 2000

In the decade of 1990 to 2000, several breakthrough technologies in radiology, endoscopy, and surgery were introduced that would impact

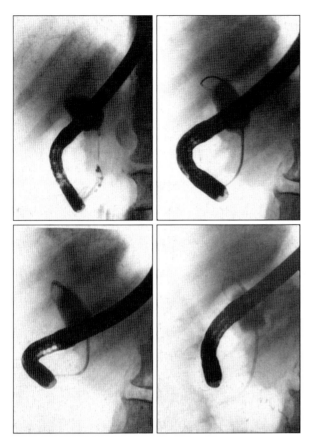

FIG 1.4 ERCP-directed bile duct drainage using biliary stents was introduced by Soehendra and Reynders-Frederix from Hamburg, Germany, in 1979, adding to the armamentarium of therapeutic ERCP. The team used a 20-cm-long, 7-Fr radioopaque angiographic catheter with 12 side holes inserted over a guidewire with a single pigtail that allowed it to be fixed inside the bile duct. (Photo courtesy Dr. Peter Cotton, Medical University of South Carolina.)

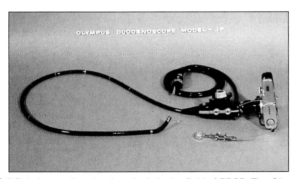

FIG 1.5 Industry played a pivotal role in the field of ERCP. The Olympus duodenoscope model JF (pictured here with camera attached) was introduced in 1971. The JF duodenoscope was fiberoptic, had a 65-degree view angle, and was fitted with an elevator. The channel size was <2 mm diameter, limiting the size of catheters that could be used and making suctioning around the catheter problematic. (Photo courtesy Dr. David Barlow, Olympus Corporation.)

the field of pancreaticobiliary disease and the ERCP endoscopist. These technologies blossomed and ultimately transformed the indications for ERCP from a diagnostic/therapeutic procedure to a predominately therapeutic one.[25] This transformation was driven in part by the introduction of magnetic resonance imaging (MRI)/magnetic resonance cholangiopancreatography (MRCP) to image noninvasively the bile and pancreatic ducts.[26,27] Endoscopic ultrasonography (EUS), originally described in 1980 by DiMagno et al.,[28] was introduced with the radial scanning echoendoscope, which became a staple for clinical care in the late 1980s. Linear endosonography followed in 1994 and had the added advantage of diagnostic fine-needle aspiration. Laparoscopic cholecystectomy was first performed in 1987 by Mouret (unpublished) and reported in 1989 in Europe by Dubois et al.[29] and Perissat et al.[30] and in the United States by Reddick and Olsen.[31] Laparoscopic cholecystectomy transformed the practice of ERCP, with more reliance on endoscopists to remove bile duct stones preoperatively or postoperatively.[32]

ERCP IN THE NEW MILLENNIUM

In the fourth and fifth decades, ERCP as an endoscopic procedure was widely available and practiced by many gastroenterologists in nearly every hospital with more than a 50-bed capacity. In the earlier decades of ERCP, the technique was adopted initially based on logic and began to grow based on cannulation success and eventually therapeutic success. There were few prospective, controlled, randomized, outcome-based studies in the early years, in part because of the excitement and enthusiasm of innovation and the lack of funding (and applications for funding) for endoscopic studies. The growth of ERCP decade by decade was in part attributable to the continued refinement of techniques and introduction of new innovations. In the new millennium, the "science of ERCP" has now become the focus. Prospective scientific studies have flourished since the year 2000, including studies evaluating the role of ERCP in gallstone pancreatitis,[33] malignant biliary obstruction (preoperative endoscopic drainage followed by pancreaticoduodenectomy compared with primary pancreaticoduodenectomy alone),[34] and sphincter of Oddi dysfunction (National Institutes Health–sponsored EPISOD trial) comparing sham therapy to manometrically directed sphincterotomy),[35] and studies using pancreatic stents and pharmacologic agents to prevent PEP.[36] Comparative trials evaluating novel therapies for cholangiocarcinoma, including photodynamic therapy (PDT) and radiofrequency ablation (RFA), emerged.

With the benefit of hindsight, in the 5-decade history of ERCP we could pose the following: What were the shortcomings of the incorporation of this technology into standard clinical practice? The risks of ERCP were underrecognized and underreported, particularly with respect to pancreatitis and perforation.[37] An attempt to stratify patients at the greatest risk for PEP was not addressed until the fourth decade by Freeman and colleagues in 2001.[38] Informed consent for ERCP was cursory, and in many instances, full disclosure of the potential risks and severity of adverse events was not provided to patients. Self-training was the norm in the first decade of ERCP, but advanced training became more readily available in the 1980s and 1990s. The endoscopy societies were lax in guiding ERCP training programs and community hospitals in the number of ERCPs necessary to attain a base level of competence. The Gastroenterology Core Curriculum of the Gastroenterology Leadership Council (joint effort of the American Association for the Study of Liver Diseases [AASLD], American College of Gastroenterology [ACG], American Gastroenterological Association [AGA], and American Society for Gastrointestinal Endoscopy [ASGE]) in 1996 did not recommend a specific number of ERCPs necessary to assess competence. An early ASGE guideline recommended 100 ERCP procedures (75 diagnostic and 25 therapeutic) as the minimum number of ERCPs before one could assess competency. The threshold still remains unclear, with the suggestion that at least 180 procedures are necessary.[39] Yearly ERCP volume by the endoscopist practicing ERCP has not been established to guide credentialing agencies.

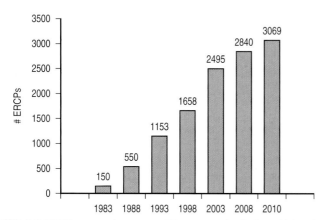

ERCP CASES OVER 25 YEARS
INDIANA UNIVERSITY GI DIVISION

FIG 1.6 ERCP case volume over 25 years at the Indiana University Division of Gastroenterology.

A "shift" of high-risk, complicated ERCP procedures to referral centers is reflected in the growing number of ERCPs performed at our institution over the past 15 years (Fig. 1.6). Hands-on training opportunities for practicing gastroenterologists to improve ERCP skills are scarce, and real-life simulators for ERCP are still not available.

THE FUTURE OF ERCP

As we look back at the history of ERCP, we can take time to speculate about ERCP in the future. Capsule cameras and remote-guided cameras may complement or replace handheld gastroscopy, enteroscopy, and colonoscopy, but we foresee that endoscopic cannulation of the pancreaticobiliary system will remain the standard. Improvements with CCDs, even smaller-diameter choledochoscopes, and pancreatoscopes are eagerly awaited and should soon become a practical reality. However, optimal view, steerability, and durability remain as challenges. Hands-free manipulation of endoscopes, similar to robotic-assisted surgery, is anticipated with the advantages of reduced endoscopist fatigue, improved ability to train endoscopists, and more refined movement of accessories. Pancreaticobiliary tumor diagnosis and tissue sampling will undoubtedly improve with advances in intraductal endoscopy. Endoscopic pancreatic cancer screening of high-risk groups may become a reality. Pancreatitis management may benefit from a more defined endoscopic role. Dissolution of intraductal pancreatic stones may be possible with the aid of endoscopically placed catheters. Studies of pancreatic juice may provide predictors of recurrent pancreatitis, pancreatic cancer risk, and response to chemotherapy. Continued effort is needed to make ERCP safer and more effective. Advanced training programs must continue to ensure that ERCP endoscopists are adequately trained and skilled in the performance of this procedure.

The complete reference list for this chapter can be found online at www.expertconsult.com.

KEY POINTS

- In the early years of ERCP in the 1970s, pioneers such as McCune, Oi, Classen, Kawai, Cotton, Vennes, Silvis, Geenen and others established a new technology.
- Close collaboration was vital between the endoscopist and industry to design new instrumentation, leading to higher cannulation rates, improved sphincterotomy, more effective drainage techniques, and improved outcomes.
- The early adopters of ERCP were self-taught, and subsequent trainees were schooled using the apprentice model. Training accelerated with introduction of videoendoscopy. Minimum qualifications for ERCP competency were poorly defined.
- In the new millennium, ERCP endoscopists have emphasized scientific rigor with several prospective, outcome-based studies. Newer techniques such as prophylactic pancreatic stent placement were adopted to make ERCP safer in high-risk patients.

2

The ERCP Room

Brian C. Brauer and Steven A. Edmundowicz

The ERCP room can range from very basic to state-of-the-art. Whereas smaller institutions with low ERCP volumes often perform ERCP in the radiology department or operating room, most centers with a larger ERCP volumes perform ERCP in dedicated rooms within the endoscopy unit. The basic ERCP room requires a quality fluoroscopy unit with still-image capability in addition to standard endoscopic equipment. Major innovations in the field of interventional endoscopy have led to the development of multipurpose interventional rooms with the ability to combine endoscopic ultrasonography (EUS), cholangioscopy, pancreatoscopy, confocal endomicroscopy, and other interventions in combination with ERCP. A well-designed ERCP room is needed to accommodate this expansion in the procedural intensity of ERCP. In addition, changes in the patient population have led to the necessity to be able to perform ERCP on morbidly obese patients and those with altered anatomy using deep enteroscopy instruments. Many centers have moved to have anesthesia support for all ERCPs. The cumulative effect of these changes in the practice of ERCP has led to significant changes in the design of the typical ERCP room with the incorporation of new technology to benefit the patient, physician, and staff.

EVOLUTION OF THE ERCP ROOM

The basic intent of ERCP has not changed. Endoscopic visualization of the ampulla and cannulation of the desired ductal system with high-quality radiographic imaging guiding the appropriate therapy is still the goal. In the great majority of cases the basic equipment is all that is needed to remove a stone or place a stent across uncomplicated strictures. What has changed is the potential complexity of ERCP, especially at tertiary referral centers. The need for high-quality radiographic imaging of focal pathology in larger patients has led to modified digital fluoroscopy equipment with improved resolution, reduced radiation exposure, and the ability to function continuously for long procedures without overheating. In addition, wider tables (>30 inches) capable of accommodating larger, heavier patients (≥450 lbs.) and space for anesthesia to assist in these procedures have become essential. Additional room space is also needed to accommodate larger beds and stretchers to allow for bariatric patients (Fig. 2.1). The use of a mobile or fixed C-arm system is often employed to improve visualization of the biliary tree by allowing the plane of examination to be altered to profile the bifurcation and selected ductal systems. Additional space for supplemental equipment for cholangioscopy, EUS, laser lithotripsy, electrohydraulic lithotripsy, deep enteroscopy, and other adjuvant techniques has increased the size of the typical advanced ERCP room. Space for anesthesia equipment has further increased the need for additional space at the patient's head. All this, in combination with the need to accommodate morbidly obese patients and store a large variety of devices in close proximity to the patient, has increased the size of well-designed, advanced interventional endoscopy rooms to greater than 500 square feet.

STAFFING FOR THE ERCP PROCEDURE

Staffing for ERCP procedures varies across the world. Typically, a physician and a minimum of two additional assistants are necessary. The first assistant (nurse or technician) stands immediately adjacent to the physician and operates devices such as guidewires and accessories. A sedation nurse or member of the anesthesia staff is positioned at the patient's head and administers sedation or anesthesia while monitoring the patient throughout the procedure. Often, a second assistant (nurse or technician) assists in preparing devices for use and documents specifics of the procedure. In some settings a radiology technician is also needed to operate the radiographic equipment. In many centers, a trainee is often present. This creates a close working environment for the procedure with at least three individuals clustered around the patient's head. A well-designed workspace makes this proximity tolerable and efficient.

ROOM LAYOUT

The key to successful room design is early collaboration with all the disciplines that will be involved in performance and delivery of ERCP so that the room is functional and beneficial to all parties. Collaborative input from ERCP physicians, the endoscopy nursing team and technicians, anesthesia team, patient advocates, radiologists and technicians, radiation safety technicians, the ergonomics consultant, and the construction or design team can result in major design evolution to allow the final design to be optimized for the work group. The layout of a typical tertiary-level ERCP room is depicted in Fig. 2.2. The ERCP room can be divided into multiple work areas. The epicenter of the ERCP room is the fluoroscopy table. The physician stands adjacent to the patient's head while performing ERCP. In this room design the physician also has direct access to the radiographic equipment controls that allow movement of the fixed C-arm or table to obtain the optimum radiographic imaging. The first assistant's workspace is immediately to the right of the physician. Space for a trainee is preferably located immediately to the physician's left side. Adjacent to the first assistant's work space is a preparation area for a second assistant with a countertop or movable table to prepare devices. This space should be immediately adjacent to the in-room storage of the most often used devices. Directly above the patient's head is space for the sedation nurse or anesthesia team member. This space also includes room for all necessary medications, monitoring equipment, and resuscitative equipment. When using anesthesia, often there are two carts: the anesthesia machine at the patient's head, and a secondary cart for medication and equipment storage, which must be within easy reach of the anesthesia provider. An optimal room design will allow ample space for these pieces of equipment, and easy access to all spaces during the procedure. Ideally, adequate additional space for radiograph review and report generation should be available. This space may be behind a protective lead glass screen or in another space altogether. In some configurations, a separate control room space for

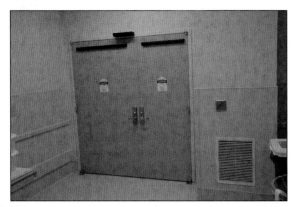

FIG 2.1 Large-capacity room door and extra space around the radiography table allow for transfer of large patients. There is easy access to the back of the table to facilitate movement of sedated patient after the procedure.

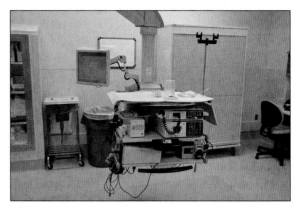

FIG 2.3 The endoscopic equipment boom allows easy access to the endoscope processor, the light source, and other key equipment, including the electrosurgical generator, CO_2 insufflator, and water irrigator. The boom keeps wires and electrical cords organized and off the floor.

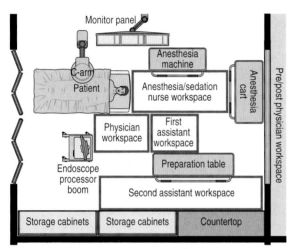

FIG 2.2 Drawing of a modern interventional endoscopy room with workspace for the endoscopist, first assistant, anesthesia or sedation nurse, and second assistant. The drawing also depicts the endoscopist preprocedure and postprocedure work area, suspended bank of monitors, and endoscopic equipment boom.

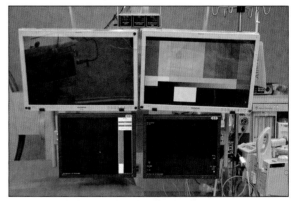

FIG 2.4 Adjustable monitor boom that can be adjusted to a height suitable for the endoscopist and assistants. The upper monitors can display inputs from a variety of sources.

the radiographic equipment may be necessary; alternatively, if required, a radiation technologist may be in the room.

The physician should have immediate access to all the endoscopic and radiographic controls that are necessary to complete ERCP. The use of ceiling booms greatly facilitates the placement of processors and devices in close proximity to the physician and assistant with minimal cords or tubing on the floor of the procedure room (Fig. 2.3). The boom can be used to house the endoscope processor and light source, electrocautery unit, and other ancillary equipment such as a CO_2 insufflator, water irrigation system, EUS equipment (if compact), and other devices. The typical room design has the endoscopic and radiographic monitors directly across from the physician to allow a direct line of sight (Fig. 2.4). The monitors should be adjustable in height to accommodate physicians of various heights and be freely mobile during patient positioning and procedure preparation. An ancillary monitor to display additional images or information such as choledochoscopy, manometry, EUS, or even patient vital signs greatly facilitates the completion of procedures without awkward head angulation. Rooms with video integration systems allow multiple video sources to be displayed on the monitor array in the patient room. This can be

particularly helpful if viewing an imaging study (computed tomography and magnetic resonance imaging) is necessary during the procedure. The monitors should be in the line of sight of the first assistant as well to allow coordinated device manipulation with endoscopic and/or fluoroscopic guidance. There should be ample space for ancillary devices (EUS processors, choledochoscopy devices, etc.) to be placed in the room in close proximity to the physician. In larger centers with multiple ERCP rooms, infrequently used equipment may be placed on carts that can be moved from room to room. In the overall layout of the room, there should be sufficient space for patients to be moved on large stretchers or beds. Mobile ceiling-mounted booms greatly facilitate patient movement. For improved efficiency, a portal for endoscope cleaning should be considered to allow rapid movement of used endoscopes to the cleaning room to facilitate room turnover. If this is not available, appropriate containers for rapid and safe transport of used endoscopes should be kept in the ERCP suite adjacent to the endoscope reprocessor (Fig. 2.5).

RADIOLOGIC IMAGING EQUIPMENT

The selection of a radiologic system is one of the most important and expensive decisions to be made during ERCP room design or upgrade. Most hospital systems have purchasing agreements and alignments with specific vendors, and all major manufacturers of radiology and fluoroscopy rooms have a unit that can be well adapted to ERCP. There are

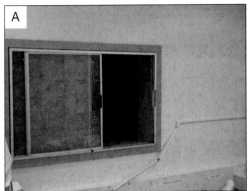
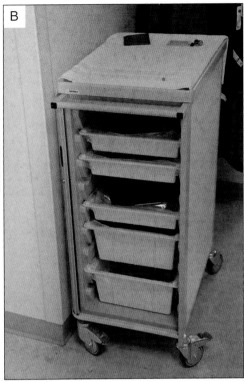

FIG 2.5 **(A)** Portal to cleaning and cold sterilization area. **(B)** Trays are then covered, and following scope use, these trays are used to immediately transfer contaminated equipment back to the reprocessing area.

TABLE 2.1 Available Fluoroscopy Units

Company	C-arm	Fixed Unit	Flat Detector	Website
Philips	Y	Y	Y	usa.philips.com
Seimens	Y	Y	Y	usa.healthcare.seimens.com
Omega	N	Y	Y	omegamedicalimaging.com
GE	Y	Y	Fixed unit only	www3.gehealthcare.com
Toshiba	N	Y	Y	medical.toshiba.com

also dedicated ERCP systems and portable digital C-arm systems. A review of the principles of radiographic imaging and different imaging systems is found in Chapter 3. The transition to digital imaging systems in the last decade has greatly simplified image processing and storage while essentially eliminating the need for in-room radiologic support. The selection of a radiologic system is dependent on many factors, including case volume, type, and patient mix. For low-volume, relatively simple ERCP cases, many available systems are adequate. For high-volume, complex case work (American Society for Gastrointestinal Endoscopy [ASGE] grade of difficulty type 2 or 3 cases),[1] a high-end dedicated fixed C-arm is often best. High-end fixed rooms have sufficient power and imaging systems to optimally image obese patients and complex strictures and allow visualization of devices and guidewires in situations where mobile units are inadequate. In addition, pulse rates may be adjusted for more rapid image acquisition during difficult maneuvers while still avoiding continuous fluoroscopy. Digital flat panel detectors provide improved image quality, have durability over traditional analog image intensifiers, and allow magnification of the image without increasing radiation dose. They are available on most fixed fluoroscopy systems and many portable C-arm platforms, but at a substantially increased cost. A list of available fluoroscopy units is provided in Table 2.1. In addition, the radiation generation and cooling properties of fixed units allow for prolonged procedure times without overheating or image degradation. Investment in a fixed fluoroscopy room also allows the room design to include dedicated shielding and radiation protection for the staff. The addition of a radiation-attenuating drape around the image detector has been shown to significantly decrease the radiation dose to staff during ERCP.[2] The use of ceiling-mounted and table-mounted shielding can greatly reduce radiation scatter and staff exposure (Fig. 2.6a). Portable shields on wheels may also be integrated to provide additional shielding (Fig. 2.6b). Building codes and hospital safety mandates may also require shielding of the walls and doors of the suite.

ROOM INTEGRATION SYSTEMS

Video integration systems have evolved to give the operator control over the numerous video inputs used in a state-of-the-art interventional room. Several manufacturers sell integrated units that can be customized for a specific room or unit layout. In a well-designed integration system, video inputs from multiple sources can be placed on the main imaging display in the room (Fig. 2.7). The typical integration system has multiple inputs for EUS, choledochoscopy, or any other video signal to be placed

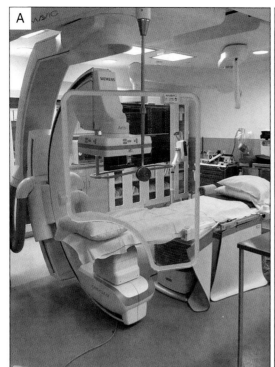
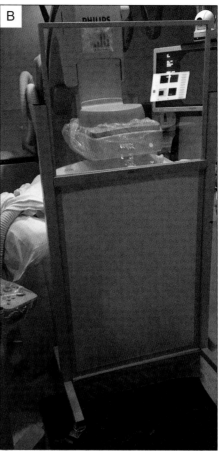

FIG 2.6 (A) Ceiling-mounted lead shielding that can be positioned to shield those close to the radiation source. **(B)** Rolling shield on wheels that can be used in units without ceiling-mounted shielding.

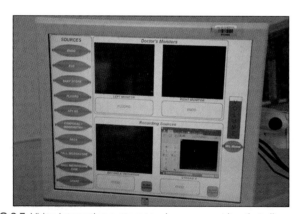

FIG 2.7 Video integration system touch screen monitor that allows any video input to be placed on one of four video monitors in direct view of the endoscopist and assistant.

into the system for recording and display on the in-room monitors, and can be controlled by the physician or assistant directly from the room. More sophisticated systems may allow for inputs from the hospital radiology imaging system and electronic medical record (EMR) so that radiology images from diagnostic studies, as well as text, images, and other information from the EMR, can be displayed in the procedure room. Some integration systems allow for recording and editing of inputs to create compilation recordings or for broadcasting of multiple inputs to a local or even distant conference room. When planning a

video integration system, it is important to have the flexibility to add new inputs to the system as new technology becomes available.

ENDOSCOPIST WORK AREA

Intraprocedure

The endoscopist workspace during the procedure should be ergonomically designed to be comfortable, shielded from radiation, and efficient.[3,4] A soft floor surface or cushioned mat will help prevent operator fatigue that results from prolonged standing.[5] The main room video monitors should be directly in front of the endoscopist at eye level to reduce the need for head rotation and to minimize neck strain.[6] The monitors should be adjustable in height and positioned to simultaneously visualize endoscopy and fluoroscopy without the need for significant head movement (eye shifting only) (Fig. 2.8).

The floor of the endoscopist workspace can become crowded with pedals needed to operate the radiology equipment, electrocautery units, irrigators, electrohydraulic lithotripsy units, and lasers. Having a set orientation for the different activation pedals can be helpful and easily integrated into the staff room setup procedure.

PREPROCEDURE AND POSTPROCEDURE WORK AREA

An extensive amount of preparation is necessary before and after performance of interventional endoscopic procedures (see Chapter 10); a well-designed ERCP suite provides a comfortable and convenient

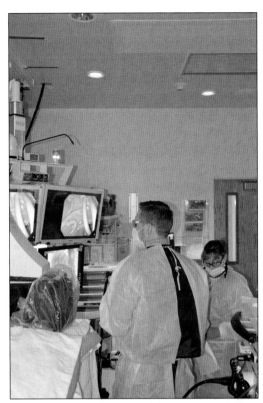

FIG 2.8 Adjustable boom positioned so that it is in direct line of sight for endoscopist.

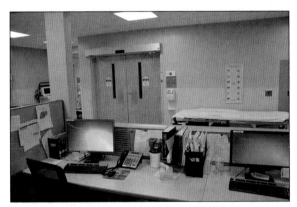

FIG 2.9 Separate physician workspace adjacent to ERCP suite.

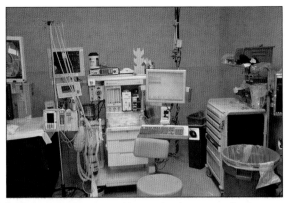

FIG 2.10 Anesthesia space with anesthesia cart, medication cart, and space for anesthesia provider to sit or stand.

and access to the opposite side of the fluoroscopy table. In addition, a bariatric patient lift may be required if a high volume of bariatric procedures are performed.

The anesthesia or sedation work area is located at the head of the bed and allows direct access to the patient's airway. There is significant institutional variability to sedation and anesthesia approaches for ERCP. The approaches range from general anesthesia with airway intubation to deep sedation. Anesthesia issues related to ERCP are covered in detail in Chapter 6. The anesthesia or sedation space contains room for a medication cart, airway equipment, and monitors to include CO_2 capnography and pulse oximetry (Fig. 2.10). Many units have smaller-sized anesthesia machines available for the ERCP room that allow administration of general anesthetics and high-flow (100%) O_2. Airway management equipment, including nasal airways, masks, and bag valve masks for ventilation, endotracheal tubes, laryngoscopes, and other intubation tools, should be readily available. In some centers a sedation nurse monitors the patient's airway and provides intravenous moderate sedation.

NURSING AND TECHNICIAN WORK AREA

The workspace necessary for those individuals assisting the endoscopist is critical to the success of the ERCP room. This workspace requires ample room for device preparation, exchange, and equipment and accessories. This can be accomplished with a countertop or a movable table that can be placed in position next to the endoscopist to allow device preparation. This area should be immediately adjacent to the in-room storage space for the devices and accessories that may be needed during an interventional procedure. The storage space is ideally protected against splash contamination using glass doors or rolling panels (Fig. 2.11). The in-room storage space should allow for a small number of each type of accessory needed for all procedures, and a larger storage area should be located remotely in the endoscopy facility for additional devices from which the in-room supply can be restocked. Barcode scanners, dedicated chips containing specific information about device and par levels, and even commercial inventory management vendors may be used to maintain adequate and predictable inventory. Direct inventory systems that are placed in the rooms and charge supplies as they are used are also available and function in a similar manner to medication-dispensing systems.

Space for additional equipment such as EUS and choledochoscopy systems has become vital for complex interventional procedures. These systems often need to be in close proximity to the patient's head and occupy a portion of the first assistant's space. Ample room size to allow

workspace for record review, EMR access, radiograph review, report generation, and phone or electronic communication (Fig. 2.9). This workspace is ideally located adjacent to the procedure space to allow easy communication during the preprocedure and postprocedure period.

ANESTHESIA/SEDATION WORK AREA

The obesity epidemic has led many centers to modify their approach to room design. The use of fixed fluoroscopy systems with wider tables (30 inches plus) and increased weight limits (≥450 lbs.) has become the norm. Access to the radiography table with larger stretchers and beds has required room designs with additional space. Transferring the sedated or recovering patient from the fluoroscopy table to the stretcher or bed can be challenging and should be facilitated with sliding boards

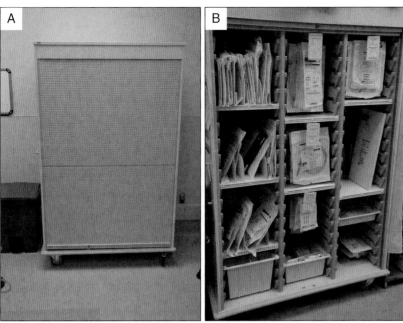
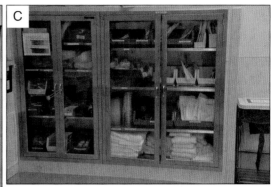

FIG 2.11 (A) Cabinet with rolling door for supply storage in ERPC suite. **(B)** Same cabinet in panel A with rolling door opened. **(C)** Built-in glass cabinets for supply storage in ERCP suite.

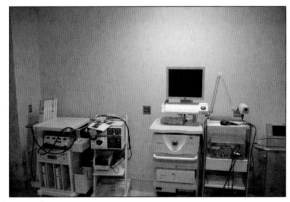

FIG 2.12 Dedicated storage adjacent to ERCP suite. Large equipment is kept in a designated location where it can easily be found.

movement around this equipment to facilitate device passage, specimen handling, and other duties is key to successful room design and use. Ancillary equipment must be stored close to the ERCP room so that it can be accessed relatively quickly (Fig. 2.12).

ERGONOMICS

Room ergonomics that benefit the staff are also essential. Cushioned flooring, easy visualization of monitors at eye level, protective radiation shielding, and chairs for sitting during long cases are all beneficial and help prevent work-related fatigue and injury. Lightweight lead, appropriately fitted for the individual, can greatly reduce fatigue and muscle strain and is an important investment for any high-volume unit. Several manufacturers also offer real-time dose management systems that can help tailor exposure to both the patient and the staff and help guide shielding and radiation practices (RightDose [Siemens AG, Muenchen, Germany]; DoseWise Portal [Philips North America, Andover, MA]; RaySafe X2 [Unfors Raysafe, Inc., Cleveland, OH]).

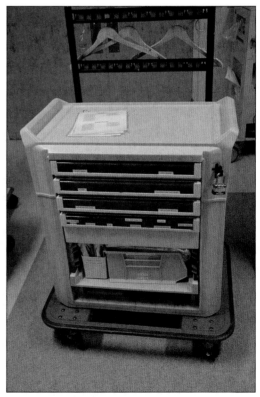

FIG 2.13 Portable ERCP accessory cart. Commonly used devices can be kept in this cart and inventoried in the same manner as a procedure room. This cart has been adapted to allow lead aprons to be hung from the back for easy transport.

Room design that creates close proximity of key items (devices, specimen repository, endoscope cleaning site) reduces the number of steps and fatigue.

MISCELLANEOUS ISSUES

Even with a high-volume dedicated interventional room with anesthesia support, occasional ERCPs will need to be done in an operating room, bedside in the intensive care unit (ICU), and in interventional radiology suites and other remote locations. The ERCP room layout can be achieved in these areas with mobile endoscopy carts, monitors, and a travel equipment cart that holds essential ERCP equipment (Fig. 2.13). This allows replication of the space and roles defined in the typical room in almost any location. When performing procedures in the operating room, using a room equipped for laparoscopic procedures is beneficial. The video for endoscopic and fluoroscopic view monitors can be transmitted to the monitors normally used for laparoscopic image visualization, thus placing the image in a more ergonomically correct position for the endoscopist and staff. The travel equipment cart can also be used for additional device storage and supplement the in-room storage when periods of increased device use occur.

The complete reference list for this chapter can be found online at www.expertconsult.com.

3

Radiologic Issues and Radiation Safety During ERCP

Eugene Lin and Beth Schueler

The scope and practice of endoscopic retrograde cholangiopancreatography (ERCP) has evolved over the past 2 decades. First, with the advances in magnetic resonance cholangiopancreatography (MRCP; see Chapter 34) in both academic and private settings alike, nearly all ERCP is therapeutic.[1,2] Increased complexity and emerging capabilities of therapeutic ERCP often lead to longer procedure times and the potential for increased radiation exposure to patients, endoscopists, nurses, and other personnel involved in the procedure. Coupled with the emergence of endoscopic ultrasonography (EUS) for diagnostic and therapeutic applications (see Chapters 32 to 34), more than ever the shift in practice patterns heightens the importance of communication between the endoscopist and radiologist in order to provide the patient with the best possible and most consistent interpretation of images acquired during ERCP, and with physicists to ensure patient safety.[3] This chapter focuses not only on techniques of image acquisition during ERCP using examples of pathology (discussed in depth elsewhere in the book) to demonstrate imaging principles but also on essential radiation safety considerations for patients and personnel during the procedure.

Before the ERCP procedure, review of other imaging studies (computed tomography [CT], magnetic resonance imaging [MRI], or ultrasonography) is often helpful to plan and expedite the case. Depending on the planned procedure, particularly when drainage is anticipated, it is important to recognize that imaging information varies with the modality being used. Distal common bile duct (CBD) stones are difficult to visualize in a nondilated system by transabdominal sonography, but are well depicted on MRCP. The complexity of pancreatic collections is better identified with MRI compared with CT, and although both are comparable for early assessment of necrosis and inflammation in acute pancreatitis, MRI, even without benefit of intravenous contrast enhancement, has advantages over CT in detecting biliary lithiasis (Fig. 3.1) and pancreatic hemorrhage (Fig. 3.2).[4] If therapeutic endoscopic interventions are intended, availability of the pancreaticobiliary surgeon or interventional radiologist for treatment of potential adverse events or participation in combined procedures is desirable. In our practice, discussion during multidisciplinary conferences or evaluation of the patient with pancreatic pathology in multidisciplinary clinics is beneficial for diagnostic and therapeutic planning. The patient's history of medical allergies, including to contrast material, should be ascertained during the consent process.

FLUOROSCOPIC IMAGING SYSTEMS

Real-time image guidance for ERCP is most commonly provided by fluoroscopy. The basic components of a fluoroscopic system include an x-ray tube, generator, image receptor, and video system for image display and recording (Fig. 3.3). Modern fluoroscopy systems incorporate multiple operational modes and configurations. Therefore it is important that physicians using fluoroscopy have adequate knowledge of its appropriate use.

An x-ray tube produces the primary beam with adjustment of x-ray energy (tube potential, or kVp) and beam intensity (tube current, or mA) provided by generator. An important operational feature of fluoroscopic systems is automatic exposure control (AEC). As patient attenuation changes when the primary beam is panned across the body, x-ray beam energy and intensity must be adjusted to maintain consistent quality in the displayed fluoroscopic image. With AEC, these adjustments are made continuously during imaging without operator intervention. X-ray tube heat can build up quickly during procedures involving long fluoroscopy exposure and acquisition of multiple images. When heat loading limits are reached, fluoroscopic equipment will typically terminate operation or exclude selection of high-dose imaging modes to allow for cooling to occur.

On the exit port of the x-ray tube, a collimator is used to define the shape of the x-ray beam. The collimator automatically limits the x-ray beam to the image receptor field of view (FOV) as changes are made in the magnification mode selection or source-to-image distance. Additionally, the operator can further limit the exposed area by manually moving collimator blades closer to the area of clinical interest.

Fluoroscopy can be performed with continuous x-ray generation or x-ray pulses with frame rates ranging from 30 frames per second (fps) to 1 fps or below. One advantage of pulsing is an improvement in temporal resolution. Motion blur occurring within each image is reduced because of the shorter acquisition time, making pulsed fluoroscopy useful for examining moving structures. In addition, pulsing with low pulse rates can reduce radiation dose. When fluoroscopic imaging is stopped, last-image-hold allows for display of the last image on the monitor for continued study and review. Fluoroscopy loop recording is available on some models to store and review short video clips. Higher-dose image acquisition can consist of a single exposure or a series of exposures at frame rates ranging from 30 to 1 fps or below. Methods for image recording include capture of fluoroscopic video, which can be stored and reviewed with captured endoscopic video, and output of acquired images for review and long-term archive.

Two different types of image receptors are currently available on fluoroscopy systems: image intensifiers and flat panel detectors. Image intensifiers produce a circular image by converting x-rays into light with electronic intensification. A video camera is used to capture the output image and display it on a monitor. Image intensifiers are available with input surface diameters ranging from 10 to 40 cm, with selection of one or more magnification modes. To maintain consistent output image quality as the FOV is decreased, the x-ray exposure rate is increased, resulting in higher patient dose rates when smaller FOVs are used.

Flat panel detectors are solid-state detectors that produce a digital electronic signal. Fluoroscopy flat panels are available in square or rectangular formats with sizes ranging from 17×17 cm to 40×40 cm.

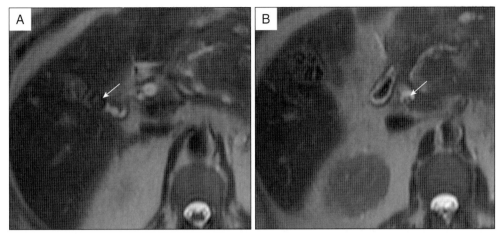

FIG 3.1 MRCP cholelithiasis. **A,** Dark filling defects in the gallbladder *(arrow)* and **B,** distal common bile duct *(arrow)* are easily seen within a nondilated system on heavily T2-weighted axial MRCP images. MRCP, magnetic resonance cholangiopancreatography.

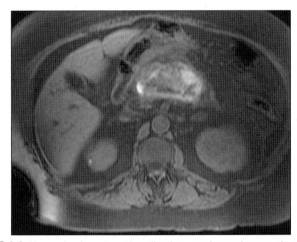

FIG 3.2 Hemorrhagic pancreatic collection unenhanced magnetic resonance imaging.

Selection of magnification modes is also possible. In contrast to image intensifiers, which produce an image in which the peripheral area has decreased magnification (pincushion distortion) and reduced brightness level (vignetting), flat panel detectors are distortion-free with uniform image brightness.

Before display of the image, modern fluoroscopic systems apply digital image processing techniques to enhance image appearance. Processing options include gray-scale processing, edge enhancement, and temporal frame averaging. Gray-scale processing adjusts displayed image contrast and brightness to accentuate contrast in a desired density range. This may also mitigate the appearance of flare, which is a bright area in an image where the signal has become saturated, reducing or completely eliminating contrast. Flare is particularly apparent in image intensifier systems, which have reduced dynamic range compared with flat panel detectors. Edge enhancement increases the sharpness of small objects and boundaries between areas of differing density. For temporal frame averaging, the current video frame is averaged with one or more previous video frames to decrease the appearance of image noise. Objects moving in the image may appear blurred when this technique is applied, or multiple ghost images of a high-contrast moving object may be seen if the object is moving rapidly. Adjustment of image processing parameter settings to optimize image quality for the clinical application and user preference is a critical step in equipment configuration.

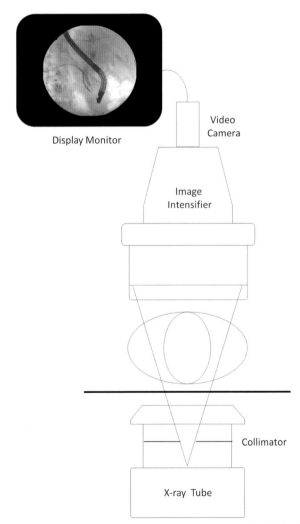

FIG 3.3 Components of a fluoroscopic system. (Author sketch.)

Most fluoroscopy systems include a display of patient dose (required for equipment manufactured in the United States since 2006). The dose parameter displayed is the entrance skin air kerma with units of milligray (mGy). During fluoroscopy, the air kerma rate is displayed, and after fluoroscopy, the patient's cumulative air kerma is shown. Typical air kerma rates for an average-sized adult abdomen range from 20 to 60 mGy/min. Regulatory requirements limit the maximum air kerma rate to 88 mGy/min in the normal mode. Fluoroscopy equipment may include high-level control mode, which can be activated to allow for higher exposure levels, up to 176 mGy/min. For ERCP procedures, Buls et al.[5] reported a median cumulative entrance air kerma of 271 mGy (maximum 1180 mGy).

These basic fluoroscopic equipment components are available in several different configurations to meet the requirements of specific diagnostic and interventional applications. One common stationary fluoroscopy configuration used for ERCP has an incorporated patient table with an undertable x-ray tube and image receptor above the patient. Another stationary configuration employed for ERCP fluoroscopy has a reverse design with an overtable x-ray tube and the image receptor located under the table. Mobile fluoroscopy units are also frequently used. In a mobile fluoroscopy system, the x-ray tube and image receptor are mounted on a C-arm positioner that allows for angulation of the image chain around the patient. It should be noted that a radiolucent procedure table is needed for this fluoroscopy imaging configuration. A mobile C-arm can also be moved between procedure rooms for a more flexible clinical workflow. More recently, stationary multiple-purpose fluoroscopy systems have been introduced that incorporate a tilting C-arm positioner with a right side–mounted table for easy ERCP access. These units offer the advantage of C-arm angulation with table-side control. Consideration of the x-ray source is important when shielding the patient is necessary, such as during ERCP in pregnant patients (see Chapter 30).

RADIATION DOSE MANAGEMENT IN FLUOROSCOPIC PROCEDURES

The endoscopist has control over multiple parameters that can be adjusted to alter patient radiation dose during a fluoroscopic procedure. Though the risk of radiation injury is low, deterministic effects (including skin burns and cataract formation) and stochastic effects (increased risk of cancer) are possible. Deterministic injuries occur only after the radiation dose to the tissue exceeds a given threshold dose. For fluoroscopic procedures, patient skin injury may occur. A threshold dose of 2000 mGy results in transient erythema, with more severe effects (including epilation and desquamation) resulting from higher dose levels. Although a single ERCP procedure is not likely to reach the threshold dose level for skin injury, if patients have had fluoroscopic exposure in the same anatomic area in the past 60 days, the total skin dose should be evaluated and actions taken to minimize dose to that entry area should be considered if needed. Additional information on radiation injury can be found in several recommended reviews.[6–8] Because of the potential of radiation injury, care must be taken to minimize radiation exposure when performing procedures where fluoroscopy is used. Dose optimization requires attention to several basic principles summarized below.

Limiting fluoroscopy time is the most direct dose reduction technique. Fluoroscopy should never be activated unless the operator is looking at the image display. Short taps of fluoroscopy are generally sufficient for observation instead of continuous operation. Last-image-hold or fluoroscopy loop recording is useful for consultation and review without the need for additional fluoroscopic exposure. Last-image-hold may also be stored for image archive as an alternative to an additional acquired image. Note that reducing exposure time will also limit x-ray tube heat buildup, which will minimize procedure delays required for tube cooling.

Low dose rate fluoroscopy modes should be used whenever possible. A pulsed fluoroscopy mode with a low frame rate is generally the best selection for dose reduction. Fluoroscopy systems should be configured to default to a low dose setting, allowing the operator to increase the dose rate if needed to achieve adequate image quality for the task. The use of high-level control fluoroscopy should be limited.

The location of the patient relative to the x-ray tube and image receptor also affects radiation dose levels. X-ray beam intensity is inversely proportional to the inverse square of the distance from the x-ray tube. Therefore, when C-arm positioners are used, the patient should be positioned as far as possible from the x-ray tube. Because the exposure rate can be very high at the exit port of the x-ray tube assembly, a spacer cone should be installed on C-arm positioners to keep the x-ray tube a safe distance from patient anatomy. Moreover, reducing the source–to–image receptor distance by positioning the image receptor as close as possible to the patient exit surface will also reduce patient dose. For example, when using a stationary undertable x-ray tube fluoroscopy system, the operator should lower the image receptor to near the patient's body when possible.

Collimator blades should be manually adjusted to include only the area of interest in the exposure field. This action reduces patient dose by reducing the exposed volume of tissue. Tight collimation will improve image quality by reducing flare, especially when imaging near the lung fields or near the edge of the body. Another detriment to image quality is caused by scattered x-rays. When primary beam x-rays interact in patient tissue, some of the x-rays are scattered and are emitted from the body in all directions. When these scattered x-rays strike the image receptor, they increase signal intensity throughout the image, masking the shadow of patient attenuation formed by transmitted x-rays. As a result, image contrast is reduced. Because a larger volume of exposed tissue produces more scattered radiation, collimation results in increased image contrast.

Magnification modes are useful to improve visualization of image detail during fluoroscopy by increasing both spatial resolution and image contrast. However, as the magnification is increased, the dose rate must be increased to maintain image quality. Therefore magnification modes should be used sparingly, when subtle pathology dictates.

Be aware that patient dose rates are higher for larger patients. As patient thickness increases, the patient entrance dose rate is approximately doubled with every additional 3 cm of tissue up to the maximum dose rate. The added tissue also results in increased scatter radiation. This scatter radiation, along with the increased x-ray beam energy needed for adequate penetration, results in reduced image contrast, making fluoroscopy of obese patients problematic.

The displayed patient cumulative radiation dose should be monitored throughout the procedure. Postprocedure, the final dose value should be recorded in the patient's medical record. This information is necessary for monitoring dose administered to patients receiving multiple procedures over time. Monitoring and recording of radiation dose also helps endoscopists maintain awareness of potential radiation harms. Similarly, monitoring of personnel radiation exposure is essential to ensure worker safety. Specific protocols for monitoring will vary by facility as determined by the facility radiation safety officer. Radiation monitoring may use a single dosimeter worn at the collar level outside a protective apron or two dosimeters, one worn at the collar and the other worn under a protective apron. For accurate estimation and reliable tracking of occupational dose, dosimeters should be worn and exchanged consistently. The recommended annual dose limit for personnel is 50 mSv whole body and 150 mSv to the lens of the eye.[9]

The primary x-ray beam is the major source of radiation exposure for the patient. Scattered x-rays emanating from the exposed patient tissue are the major source of radiation exposure for personnel in the room during fluoroscopy. Scatter dose rates are typically 1 to 10 mGy/h adjacent to the irradiated patient volume and decrease in intensity in proportion to the inverse square of the distance from that volume. As the patient entrance dose rate increases, the scatter dose rate increases

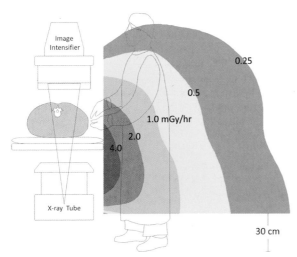

FIG 3.4 Scatter radiation isodose plot for a C-arm fluoroscopy system with undertable x-ray tube and overtable image receptor. (Adapted from Schueler BA, Vrieze TJ, Bjarnason H, et al. An investigation of operator exposure in interventional radiology. *RadioGraphics.* 2006;26:1533–1541.)

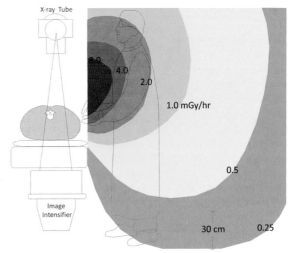

FIG 3.5 Scatter radiation isodose plot for an overtable x-ray tube fluoroscopy system. (Author sketch.)

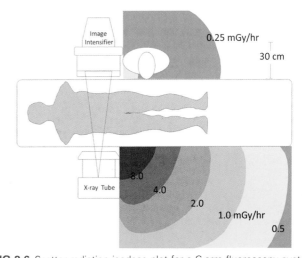

FIG 3.6 Scatter radiation isodose plot for a C-arm fluoroscopy system in a lateral projection. (From Schueler BA. Operator shielding: how and why. *Tech Vasc Interv Radiol.* 2010;13:167–171.)

proportionally. Therefore implementation of the patient dose reduction techniques above will also result in decreased scatter levels.

Fig. 3.4 shows a representative scatter isodose plot for a C-arm fluoroscopy configuration with the x-ray tube positioned under the table. Note that radiation intensity is concentrated in the area below the procedure table near the x-ray tube. Although x-ray tube leakage results in a small amount of radiation released from the sides of the x-ray tube, scattered radiation levels are substantially higher. This distribution is caused by higher levels of scattered x-rays produced at the primary x-ray beam patient input port. Forward scattered x-rays from the first few centimeters of tissue depth are heavily attenuated by the rest of the patient tissue, resulting in lower radiation levels in the region back near the image receptor. The intensity of scatter radiation for an overtable x-ray tube fluoroscopy system is shown in Fig. 3.5 and a lateral projection is shown in Fig. 3.6.

OCCUPATIONAL IONIZING RADIATION EXPOSURE

To minimize occupational exposure, personnel should be aware of the locations in the procedure room where scattered radiation levels are highest so that they can avoid these areas. In a controlled, phantom study of radiation doses to personnel during ERCP, Johnlin et al.[10] described that largest doses are received by the person at the head of the table, generally the nurse who monitors the patient and administers drugs. The next highest dose is received by the endoscopist, who stands at the right-hand corner of the fluoro table, and the lowest dose is received by the assistant who stands alongside the endoscopist when the assistant is positioned at the level of the patient's abdomen. However, often the assistant is located to the right of the technician. The low dose received by the assistant at the patient's abdomen is explained by the use of vertically oriented lead drapes (when present) that attach to the fluoro tower and diminish the amount of scatter radiation. Whenever possible, it is best to create distance from the exposed area of the patient, as the scatter levels fall off rapidly with distance. For C-arm fluoroscopy systems, the x-ray tube should be placed under the patient table. When the C-arm is angled or positioned horizontally, personnel should stand nearest the image receptor where scatter levels are lower. Note that, for stationary overtable x-ray tube fluoroscopy systems, the highest scatter

radiation intensity will be directed toward the operator's upper body and head. As a result, additional personnel protection measures may be needed if overtable x-ray tube fluoroscopy systems are used routinely.

Various types of radiation shielding devices have been developed to lower radiation exposure for personnel during fluoroscopy procedures. These devices include apparel, such as aprons, thyroid shields, and leaded eyewear. Also, mobile shields can be mounted on the floor, ceiling, or procedure table. In general, shields should be used whenever possible to keep personnel exposure as low as reasonably achievable, without lengthening the procedure or compromising patient safety.

All personnel in a procedure room during fluoroscopy must wear a protective garment unless they are positioned completely behind a radiation shield. Radiation protective apparel is available in 0.25- to 1-mm lead-equivalent thickness. In most areas, regulations require that protective apparel with a thickness of at least 0.5-mm lead-equivalent be used, which attenuates more than 90% of scattered x-rays that strike it. Different designs are available, including aprons with front coverage only, aprons that wrap around the body, and two-piece garments with vest and kilt. If there is potential for personnel to have their backs to the patient during the procedure, a wraparound or vest-and-kilt garment should be worn. Whatever design is selected, it is important to ensure that the garment fits properly with adequate coverage at the neckline and armholes. Because of the heavy weight of protective aprons constructed from lead, lightweight lead composite or lead-free models are now available. Aprons made from these materials, including barium, tungsten, tin, and antimony, provide the same attenuation as an equivalent thickness of lead at approximately 30% of the weight.[11]

Thyroid shields are typically an optional radiation protection tool. They are recommended for personnel who receive collar radiation monitor readings more than 4 mSv per month.[9] Weight and inconvenience to the wearer are relatively minimal, and so thyroid protection is also commonly used by workers receiving lower exposure levels. It should be noted that the use of thyroid shields becomes less critical for personnel over 40 years of age because the risk of radiation-induced thyroid cancer is significantly reduced with age.

Until recently, it has been generally accepted that radiation-induced cataracts do not form below a threshold lens dose of 2 to 5 Gy for fractionated exposure. This threshold provided the basis for the maximum permissible dose of 150 mSv per year for the lens. However, new data on the radiosensitivity of the eye indicate that the absence of a threshold dose, and current dose limit recommendations are currently being reassessed.[9] Therefore careful attention to radiation protection of the eye is warranted to minimize cataract risk. This is particularly important for physicians who routinely perform fluoroscopy procedures with overtable x-ray tube systems. Protective shielding to reduce radiation exposure to the eye from scatter includes leaded eyewear and ceiling-suspended shields.

It is important that all personnel present in the procedure room during fluoroscopy have a general knowledge of safe operating procedures in a radiation environment. Those performing the procedure should also be thoroughly familiar with the particular fluoroscopic equipment being used and general fluoroscopic dose reduction and image quality optimization principles. Appropriate education in radiation protection is the best way to avoid unnecessary exposure to patients and personnel.

CREATING AND VIEWING IMAGES

During the ERCP procedure, the orientation of the fluoroscopic image on the image intensifier tower may be viewed in a number of ways. Depending on the clinical circumstances, fluoroscopy rooms may be shared by radiology and gastroenterology personnel. In that case, some endoscopists prefer to view the fluoroscopic images in the anatomic position as they are obtained, that is, with the prone patient's left side on the right side of the image intensifier screen and the cephalad portion projecting at the bottom of the screen. The "head" of the ERCP table equals the "foot" of the x-ray fluoro table; in this scenario, what you see is what you get. Alternatively, some endoscopists prefer to flip the image so that the anatomy appears upright and in the classic anatomic position on the image intensifier. With this scenario, when the fluoro tower is moved, one must remember this inverse relation to achieve the desired location of the x-ray beam in the patient's body. The orientation of the image on the tower may easily be changed during the examination.

Our ERCPs take place in dedicated digital fluoroscopy rooms within an endoscopy suite located in our hospital. The images acquired in the endoscopy fluoro rooms are transmitted to and archived within the Department of Radiology pictorial archive and communication system (PACS), and the digital images are available throughout the hospital and clinics of our medical center once they are transmitted to the PACS. During most ERCPs, the patient is generally positioned in either a prone or a left lateral decubitus (LLD) position, depending on the

endoscopist preference. Increasingly, ERCP is performed in the supine position because of anesthesia support and airway management. Changes in patient position are key to visualization of both normal ducts and duct pathology. In this chapter, the patient position is described relative to the tabletop rather than the image intensifier; for example, left anterior oblique (LAO) refers to prone patient with left side angled down against the tabletop and right side angled up.

Also, with conventional radiographic film screen combinations, the exposure creates a "white duct on black background" image. With digital images, the "black on white" images that appear similar to the fluoroscopic image can be filmed or viewed as such, or converted to a standard "white on black" appearance on PACS or film, if preferred. In our opinion, free air, particularly retroperitoneal (Fig. 3.7), is easier to detect with "white on black" images, as are small stones (Fig. 3.8), but to our knowledge there has been no formal, controlled perception study to support this theory.

Contrast preferences also vary among endoscopists. Some prefer to dilute contrast to half strength when looking for bile duct stones. Others use full-strength contrast injected slowly while looking stringently for filling defects, or employ the technique of chasing the initial contrast injection with saline to achieve lesser opacity through which stones may become more evident. Still others use full-strength contrast with the argument that the bile in a potentially obstructed or dilated system will dilute the contrast enough to preclude having to do so proactively; this approach produces varying results in dilution of contrast and may minimize the volume of contrast injection (Fig. 3.9).

The sequence of images obtained during ERCP should tell the story of the examination, whether diagnostic or therapeutic. Initially, a scout radiograph reveals any residual contrast from recent imaging studies, calcifications, tubes, drains, or stents already in place, and any other material that may obscure the region of interest during contrast injection (Fig. 3.10). Most gallstones are radiolucent and will not be seen on the scout radiograph; however, pancreatic stones are frequently seen. Once contrast is administered, radiopaque stones in either ductal system may be obscured because the stones become isodense with the surrounding contrast. The diagnostic images should include early filling as well as full duct opacification and generally are acquired with a 9- or 6-inch image intensifier FOV mode. These overview images of the bile or pancreatic ducts should be supplemented with spot radiographs of abnormal or suspicious findings. The spot images may be obtained at different degrees of magnification (6- or 4.5-inch mode) for emphasis. Delayed films often are critical for assessing biliary drainage (Fig. 3.11) or lack thereof, or stent location and expansion (Fig. 3.12). A final film obtained with a large image intensifier FOV (12 or 15 inches) is helpful to evaluate potential retroperitoneal or intraperitoneal air (see Fig. 3.7).

For calculation of actual duct size with digital or standard radiographic images, knowledge of the endoscope caliber enables a simple proportion to be created to determine the exact magnification for each image. In a hypothetical example, if an 11.5-mm-caliber endoscope is used during an ERCP in which there is biliary dilation above a strictured region, the exact degree of duct dilation may be calculated by measuring the dilated portion of the duct as well as the endoscope on the image. The following simple proportion is then set up:

$$\frac{\text{Measured caliber of scope on film}}{11.5\,\text{mm (actual scope caliber)}} = \frac{\text{Measured caliber of dilated duct}}{X\,\text{mm}}$$

Solving for X alleviates the need to calculate pixel correction measurements (for digitally acquired spot images) or to estimate magnification on standard radiographic spot images. This is also important when calculating the length from the papilla to a stricture in order to select

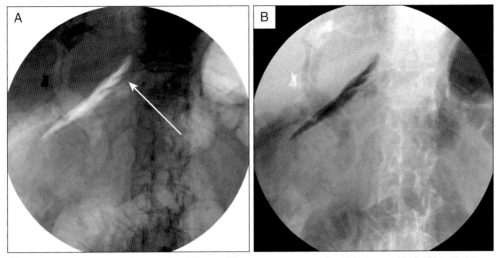

FIG 3.7 Intraperitoneal air *(arrow)* after biliary sphincterotomy comparing "black on white" **(A)** to "white on black" **(B)** image presentation.

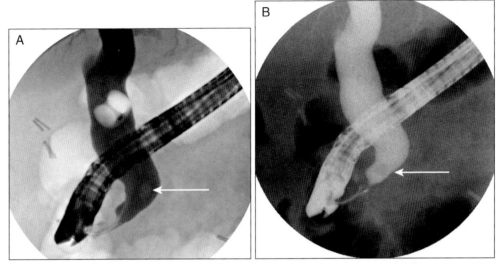

FIG 3.8 Small distal common bile duct stone *(arrow)* in dilated system comparing "black on white" **(A)** to "white on black" **(B)** image presentation.

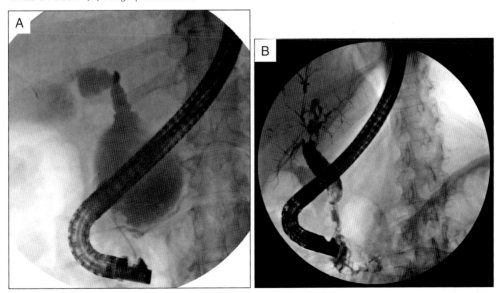

FIG 3.9 Two different patients with nondiluted contrast injection beyond focal strictures: varying stone visualization. **A,** Spot radiograph demonstrating adequate visualization of multiple small faceted gallstones in a dilated type 1 choledochal cyst. **B,** Spot radiograph demonstrating larger stones in a less dilated midcommon duct in a patient with a distal stricture caused by focal autoimmune pancreatitis (AIP). Note also focal central intrahepatic duct strictures from the AIP.

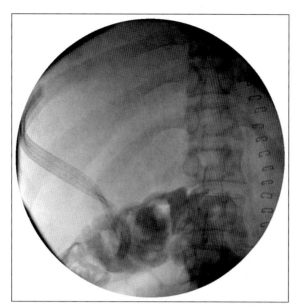

FIG 3.10 Scout radiograph in a patient about to undergo ERCP to evaluate posttraumatic (gunshot wound) bile leak. The radiopaque oral contrast from abdominal computed tomography performed 12 hours earlier is located in the hepatic flexure of the colon, potentially interfering with visualization of extravasated contrast.

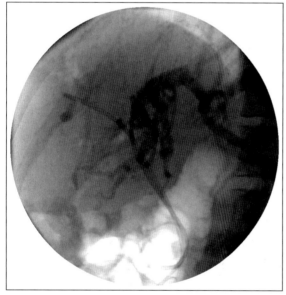

FIG 3.11 Successful placement of biliary stent, with adequate drainage. Note plastic biliary stents in right and left intrahepatic ducts, with partial emptying of contrast and presence of pneumobilia indicating patency.

the appropriate-length stent, although the use of a ruled catheter or wire withdrawal may be more accurate for selecting stents than use of x-ray film measurements.[12] If a new or different-sized endoscope is used for a particular procedure, this information should be communicated to the radiologist to ensure accuracy of measurements.

BILE DUCT EVALUATION

The distal portion of the CBD is opacified by injection of the major papilla at the ampulla of Vater. The normal caliber of the injected extra

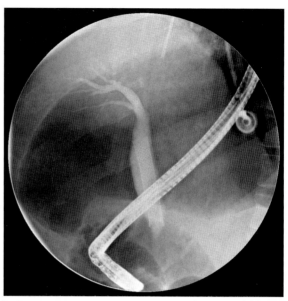

FIG 3.12 Drainage film showing suboptimal bile duct stent placement and no biliary drainage. The distal end of the stent is located above the level of neoplastic stricture in the pancreatic head.

hepatic bile duct ranges from 3 to 9 mm, with the larger normal caliber more typically seen in older individuals[13–16] and in patients who have undergone cholecystectomy,[16–20] although the wider caliber does not significantly increase in the postoperative period.[13] This is opposed to the relatively smaller upper limits of normal for duct caliber as measured by cross-sectional imaging such as ultrasonography or CT, where there is not active injection occurring to distend the duct,[17–20] yet the same trends in larger normal calibers in older and postcholecystectomy patients are seen.[16,19,20] Variability of insertion of the cystic duct leads to different degrees of obliquity required for adequate visualization. In the case of a long common channel between the CBD and cystic duct, the best position to identify entrance of the cystic duct or potential cystic duct stones is typically LAO. The best position to identify the confluence of right and left hepatic ducts, particularly important in the evaluation of hilar tumors (Fig. 3.13), is right anterior oblique (RAO). With the patient prone or in LLD position, there is preferential opacification of the left intrahepatic ducts because of gravity. Placing the patient in a right decubitus position or supine position helps opacify the right-sided ducts. The posterior segmental branches may be best seen with the patient supine as these branches are dependent. In some patients, particularly in the prone position, it is necessary to tilt the head of the table down to opacify the right intrahepatic ducts, and other endoscopic measures such as proximal common hepatic duct injection or balloon occlusion injection may help opacify all of the intrahepatic ducts (IHDs) concurrently (Fig. 3.14). If there is complete opacification of the intrahepatic duct system and the cystic duct and gallbladder do not fill despite changing the patient's position, cystic duct obstruction should be suspected.[21] Changing the patient's position (Fig. 3.15) in attempts to visualize all intrahepatic ducts is especially critical in patients with strictures near the confluence, as is injecting near the stricture (Fig. 3.16). Inadequate filling may result in overestimation of strictures, and the "shouldered" feature of malignant strictures may not be ideally demonstrated without adequate duct filling (Fig. 3.17). Likewise, the characteristics of benign strictures are better delineated with adequate duct filling. Rapid or unexpected washout of the contrast during injection of the biliary system in the liver should raise awareness that the anatomy being evaluated indicates abnormal ducts or is not

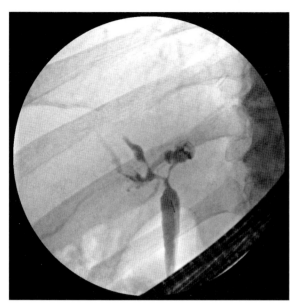

FIG 3.13 Klatskin tumor, best seen in right anterior oblique projection.

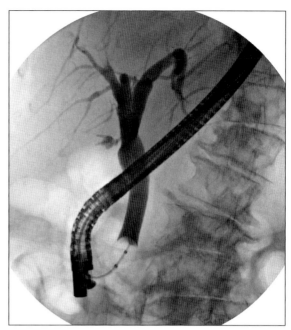

FIG 3.14 The entire intrahepatic duct system is opacified during injection using balloon occlusion technique.

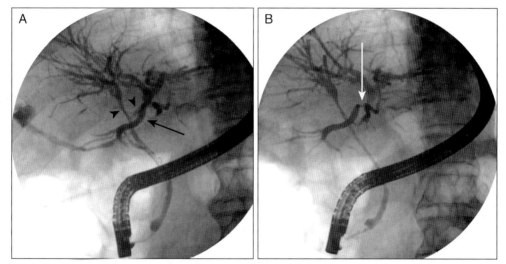

FIG 3.15 Hilar strictures caused by lymphoma. **A,** The long, relatively smooth stricture (*arrowheads*) of the main left and right bile ducts in the hilum is well seen on the prone image. There is also dilation of the posterior segmental branch duct (*arrow*) that drains aberrantly into the left duct. **B,** With the patient obliqued, the strictured region (*arrow*) of the aberrant duct is now evident.

ductal (i.e., vascular) (Fig. 3.18). Changing the patient's position may also help correctly identify the source of bile leak if aberrant or overlapping ductal structures are present. When contrast is seen opacifying a nearby drain (Fig. 3.19), continued injection while changing the obliquity of the patient should be pursued in order to uncover the site of extravasation. As in the case of injecting near a stricture to better characterize its extent and character, injecting near the site of a bile leak or obstructing lesion, or using balloon occlusion techniques (Fig. 3.20), is important to fully understand the pathology. In the case of the endoscope obscuring portions of the bile duct (generally this occurs in the suprapancreatic portion of the extrahepatic duct) (Fig. 3.21), attempts to change endoscope position to allow direct visualization of the duct may be necessary; these include rotation of the fluoroscopy.

For long bile duct strictures, obtaining orthogonal view spot images may help characterize the stricture and demonstrate extrinsic effect. The same is true for intrahepatic bile duct abnormalities produced by hepatic parenchymal disease such as polycystic liver disease or cirrhosis. Drainage films may be facilitated by tilting the head of the table up for several minutes before image exposure. A final image may indicate stent malfunction or malposition that necessitates further manipulation (see Fig. 3.12).

PANCREATIC DUCT EVALUATION

The pancreas is oriented with the head and tail located relatively more posteriorly within the patient compared with the neck and body region.

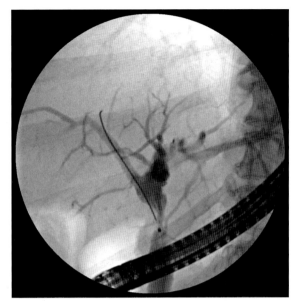

FIG 3.16 Maximizing luminal caliber by injecting at site of stricture. This extrinsic compression of the proximal common hepatic duct just below the porta, caused by lymph node metastases from breast carcinoma, is best depicted with injection at the level of the stricture.

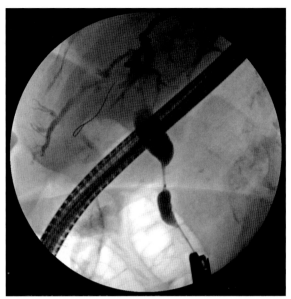

FIG 3.17 Malignant stricture in superior pancreatic head.

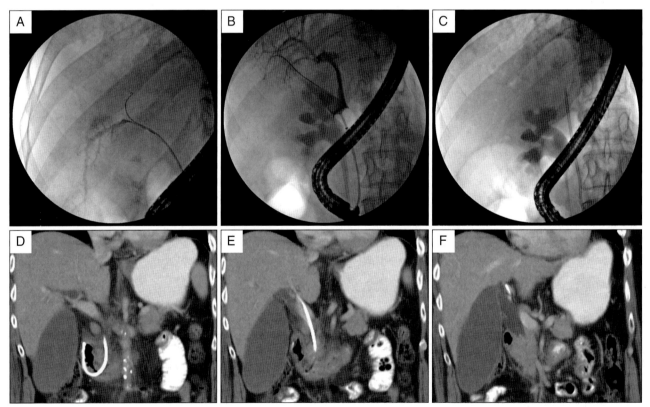

FIG 3.18 Perforation of bile duct into portal vein. **A–C,** Spot radiographs during ERCP demonstrate successive injections into right segmental portal vein branches and stent placement. There was no evidence of bleeding during the procedure, and the aberrant location of the cephalad portion of the stent was not immediately apparent. **D–F,** Contrast-enhanced coronal reformatted computed tomography images reveal the distal end of the stent in the duodenum (on **A**) and the proximal end outside the extrahepatic bile duct.

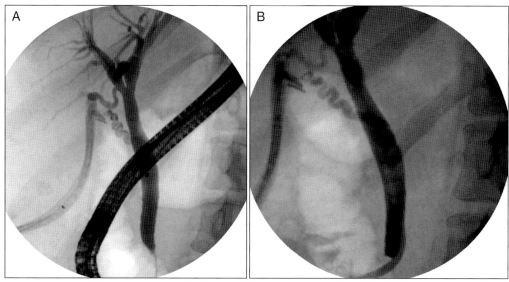

FIG 3.19 Postcholecystectomy bile leak. **A,** Prone image during filling of the common and intrahepatic ducts reveals contrast within the drain in the right upper quadrant. Both the stapled end of the cystic duct and an aberrant right branch overlie the drain. No early film was obtained to determine the site of the leak; however, with the patient obliqued slightly in **B,** contrast appeared to extravasate from the aberrant duct rather than the cystic duct stump. Note air bubbles in distal common bile duct after stent placement in **B.**

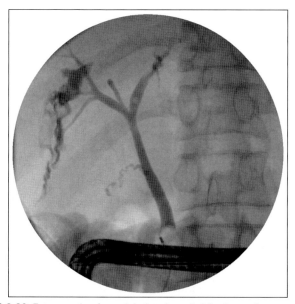

FIG 3.20 Extravasation from right intrahepatic bile ducts after gunshot wound. Balloon occlusion ensures adequate pressure to opacify the injury.

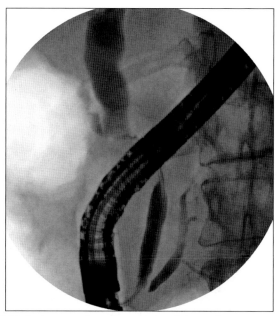

FIG 3.21 Endoscope obscuring majority of the malignant stricture of the common bile duct in a patient with pancreatic adenocarcinoma involving the superior head region. Note adjacent stricture of the main pancreatic duct.

Thus, with injection at the level of the papilla, contrast must travel against gravity, or posteriorly in the patient, to reach the tail region when the patient is prone on the fluoroscopic table. Changing the patient to the supine position will often allow more prompt visualization of the duct in the pancreatic tail. The main pancreatic duct is approximately 20 cm long and variable in caliber.[21] In general, the caliber of the duct is greatest in the downstream or head region next to the papilla, tapering continually toward the upstream or tail region. Normal caliber of the injected pancreatic duct in general is 4 mm in the head, 3 mm in the body, and 2 mm in the tail,[21,22] though larger diameters are considered normal in advanced age.[23] If the patient has a pronounced anterior to posterior curve of the pancreas within the abdomen (readily noted

with CT or MRI axial images), combined RAO and LAO images, rather than direct anteroposterior prone or supine images, may best lay out the duct for complete visualization. Because the normal pancreatic duct drains rapidly, image acquisition during active contrast injection at a rate of two to three images per second may avoid repeated injections and allow complete visualization of all portions, including pathologic regions of the duct. This may be critical in that repeated pancreatic injections have been shown to increase risk for post-ERCP pancreatitis.[24–26] As for bile duct leaks, placement of the catheter adjacent to the site of a peripancreatic collection (depicted on preprocedure cross-sectional imaging) helps identify extravasation (Fig. 3.22). With pancreatic endotherapy, determination of ductal communication affects therapeutic options (transpapillary or transmural approach), and ductal injection following successful pseudocyst or walled-off necrosis helps determine which patients have a disconnected duct (Fig. 3.23).

GENERAL IMAGING CONSIDERATIONS

In general, it is the focal change in caliber of either the bile duct or the pancreatic duct that indicates pathology and warrants further image acquisition. If the catheter is placed farther into the duct up to the location of a suspected stricture or filling defect, the interpreting physician can be relatively certain that the affected area is visualized adequately (see Figs. 3.13 and 3.16). Although most often not intentionally produced, when acinarization occurs distal to or downstream from a stricture (Fig. 3.24), one may be sure that the diminished caliber or obstruction of the duct is not caused by technical factors. It is also important to remember that when contrast passes through a strictured region to fill

a more dilated proximal duct segment, there will be dilution of the contrast and sometimes layering of the contrast,[3] making estimation of the length of stricture or the degree of upstream dilation potentially inaccurate. Likewise, to show that a biliary or pancreatic leak has sealed, injection of contrast near the site of prior extravasation during follow-up studies is helpful to exclude technical factors such as underfilling of the affected duct that may produce false-negative results. If extravasation occurs from either the pancreatic duct or the bile duct, the size of the cavity is typically underestimated on ERCP because of the relative limited volume of contrast injected and dependent passage of contrast, and better assessed with cross-sectional imaging (Fig. 3.25).

The evaluation of the filling defects within either duct may be difficult without good communication between the endoscopist and radiologist. Amorphous stasis stones may produce filling defects similar to blood clots or soft intraductal masses (Fig. 3.26), but will be very different in presentation during the procedure. Distinguishing between air bubbles that tend to be round or oval and small gallstones or pancreatic concretions that tend to be angular or faceted (Fig. 3.27) but may also be round generally can be accomplished by changing patient position.[27,28] With the head of the table tilted up, gallstones will proceed downward within the duct system (gravity), and air bubbles will rise upward. Air bubbles are to be expected after sphincterotomy. When a large amount of air enters the duct, identification of stones may be difficult, if not impossible (see Fig. 3.26). In the case of precut (access) sphincterotomy, there will be no initial injection to clearly document the presence of stones before the introduction of air into the duct system. Paying particular attention to the shape and movement of intraductal filling defects may help distinguish between the two, even in this circumstance. When filling defects are removed without documentation of their presence on the images, there is no way for an accurate interpretation to occur after the fact. Because the most common indication for endoscopic retrograde cholangiography remains biliary obstruction[21] and for endoscopic sphincterotomy continues to be choledocholithiasis, documentation of stones on images obtained before stone removal and/or communication of real-time endoscopic findings help ensure consistent reporting. In addition, the performance of sphincterotomy should be communicated as the sphincterotome may simply be used to cannulate the major papilla in patients with a difficult entry angle.[29] The radiologist cannot assume that a sphincterotomy has occurred because the

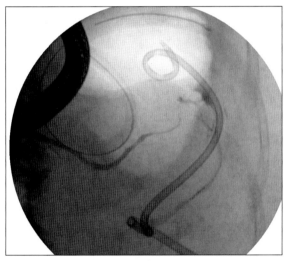

FIG 3.22 Injection into the pancreatic duct in the body or tail region reveals extravasation into the left upper quadrant in the region of a postoperative peripancreatic collection (seen on computed tomography, not shown) after debulking for ovarian carcinoma.

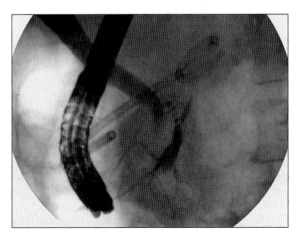

FIG 3.23 Injection into the pancreatic duct after transduodenal collection drainage reveals abrupt termination of the duct in the neck region, without communication with the collection cavity or upstream duct. (Same patient as in Fig. 3.32.)

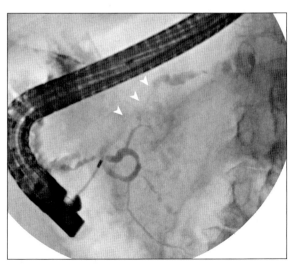

FIG 3.24 Acinarization during pancreatic duct injection. With injection under pressure, there is acinarization of contrast and filling of the tight malignant stricture *(arrowheads)* in the pancreatic neck region, accompanied by upstream dilation in a patient with pancreatic adenocarcinoma.

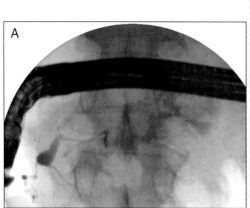

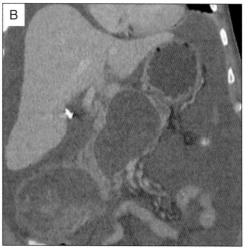

FIG 3.25 Extravasation because of pancreatic duct disruption in severe acute pancreatitis. **A,** Injection into the main pancreatic duct reveals extravasation into an amorphous cavity overlying the vertebral column and left paramedian upper quadrant. **B,** Coronal reformatted computed tomography image demonstrates the extent of the pancreatic collection, underestimated by the limited degree of extravasation during pancreatic duct injection.

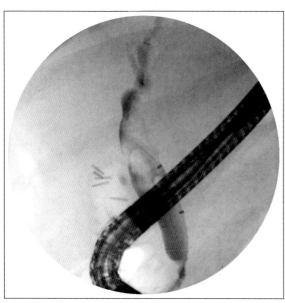

FIG 3.26 Large intraductal adenoma. The large, amorphous filling defect in the midcommon duct near the cystic duct remnant insertion is nonspecific with respect to etiology. If a clot, hemobilia should be apparent endoscopically; if a stasis stone, it would break up with balloon dragging and basket retrieval.

instrument is documented on an image. Because there is a higher risk of perforation when sphincterotomy is performed,[30] the presence of retroperitoneal air should be sought more stringently in these patients on a final postprocedure spot or overhead radiograph.

In the case of minor papilla injection or therapeutic maneuver (minor papillotomy and/or stent placement), the long scope position (Fig. 3.28) typically employed to access the more proximally located minor papilla may be a hint to the interpreting radiologist that the duct of Santorini has been injected, even if the major papilla and typical features of pancreas divisum are not documented elsewhere in the procedure. For the most effective reporting, this information should be communicated by the endoscopist.

Some therapeutic maneuver images speak for themselves, such as biopsy (Fig. 3.29), stone extraction (Fig. 3.30), or stent placement (see Fig. 3.11), as long as an image is obtained to document the event. When an endoscopic drainage has occurred (Fig. 3.31), although the spot radiographs may demonstrate wires beyond the confines of the stomach and transluminal stents are left in place (as during pancreatic drainage procedures), the details of the drainage are not captured on images and therefore must be described in the endoscopy report. After drainage, follow-up ERCP to assess ductal integrity is often complemented by secretin MRCP when findings of disconnected duct are present (Fig. 3.32, same patient as Fig. 3.23), and the interpreting radiologist should be familiar with the limitations, strengths, and complementary information provided by both modalities. For newer procedures such as fiducial marker insertion for radiation therapy (Fig. 3.33), it is helpful to discuss goals so that the radiologist can adequately evaluate radiographic confirmation of procedure outcome such as marker placement. In other circumstances, such as in patients with sphincter of Oddi dyskinesia, both the bile and the pancreatic ducts may be morphologically normal, and the diagnosis cannot be made on the basis of images alone. Communication of manometric measurements, if acquired, and clinical factors in these patients is critical to an accurate interpretation of the radiographs. Finally, the endoscopist should always be aware, particularly during interventions, of the findings of contrast intravasation into the duodenal wall, or extravasation into the retroperitoneum (Fig. 3.34), both of which may be the harbinger of perforation or other adverse events. As opposed to contrast collecting within a periampullary diverticulum (Fig. 3.35), which readily moves into the duodenal lumen proper as patient position is changed, intravasated or extravasated contrast remains stationary in the periampullary or periductal tissues.

In summary, the modern-day practice of ERCP involves a large percentage of therapeutic procedures. Planning ideally involves a multidisciplinary review of available cross-sectional imaging and discussion of contributory imaging tests and therapy options. Present-day practice constraints frequently do not permit the radiologist to be in the endofluoroscopy suite concurrently with the endoscopist; therefore prompt case-specific communication is critical to the rendering of adequate radiologic reporting and concurrence with endoscopic findings. Some centers are equipped with interdepartmental intercoms and video

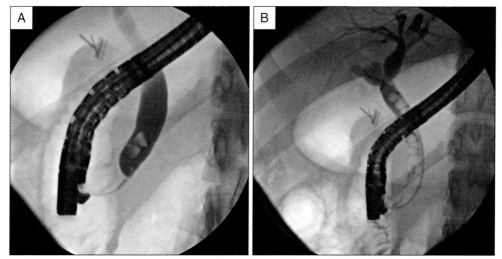

FIG 3.27 Gallstones versus air bubbles. **A,** Triangular filling defects in the distal common bile duct are indicative of faceted stones. **B,** Once air is introduced into the bile duct with sphincterotomy, numerous rounded filling defects are highly consistent with air bubbles, which could mask round stones if present.

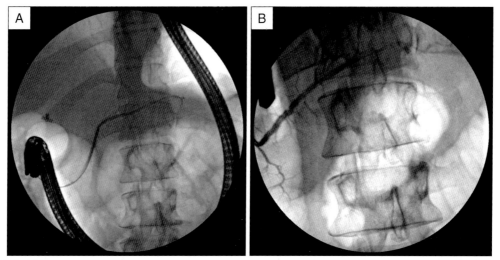

FIG 3.28 Long scope position during injection of minor papilla. **A,** Early filling reveals a normal-caliber dorsal duct with evidence of abnormal side branches on further injection **(B).**

monitors to allow real-time discussion between the endoscopist and radiologist while they are physically located in different rooms. In the case of more remote (both spatial and temporal) endoscopy–radiology cooperation, voice recognition dictation systems that allow immediate reporting, digital medical record archiving, and hospital system–wide accessibility to documents enable rapid reporting of ERCP but cannot replace real-time communication. If real-time information exchange is not feasible, then careful documentation of normal or abnormal structures as well as image documentation of endotherapeutic maneuvers during ERCP are necessary to ensure optimal patient care.

It is also important to realize that some centers are moving away from radiologist-interpreted images and the entire interpretation falls upon the endoscopist. This can avoid communication difficulties between endoscopist and radiologist, as well as interpretation in discrepancies between endoscopist and radiologist. There is now a CPT code (74328), "endoscopic catheterization of the biliary (or pancreatic) ductal system, radiologic supervision and interpretation," that can be incorporated into the procedural billing. However, the radiologist cannot also bill

for interpretation of the same images. In this situation, the images are passed through the PACS, often without any commentary from the radiologist.

ADDITIONAL CANCER RISKS FROM MEDICAL RADIATION

Medical radiation now comprises close to 50% of per capita radiation dose, compared with 15% in the early 1980s.[31] This has primarily been because of a substantial increase in the use of CT over this time period. It has been estimated that 29,000 future cancers (approximately 2% of the cancers diagnosed annually in the United States) could be related to CT performed in the United States in 2007.[32] For this reason, there has been increased emphasis on the additional cancer risks associated with medical radiation. The radiation dose is the amount of energy absorbed in the body from radiation exposure. The absorbed dose is expressed in grays (Gy): energy deposition of 1 J/kg of tissue is the equivalent of 1 Gy. As different types of radiation will have different biological effects, the dose equivalent is often used instead of absorbed dose. This is the product of the absorbed dose and a radiation weighting factor and is expressed in sieverts (Sv). In medical imaging, 1 Gy is equivalent to 1 Sv, as the weighting factor for x-rays and gamma rays is 1. Radiation doses in medical imaging are typically expressed in millisieverts (mSv). For reference, the average yearly background radiation dose (primarily from radon gas in the home) is around 3 mSv, and the average U.S. per capita dose from medical sources is also around 3 mSv.[33] Ionizing radiation is an established carcinogen. The relevant carcinogenic effect is stochastic: increasing with dose, with no threshold, but the severity of the outcome is not related to dose. This can be contrasted to deterministic effects such as radiation-induced dermatitis, which occur above a threshold, and the risk and severity of adverse outcome are dose related. Most of the evidence on radiation-induced cancer risk comes from 4 groups: Japanese atomic bomb survivors, medically exposed populations, occupationally exposed groups, and environmentally exposed groups.[34] By far the most robust data come from study of the Japanese atomic bomb survivors. The Life Span Study of the Hiroshima and Nagasaki bombings was a cohort study of more than 105,000 survivors.[35] From the Life Span Study, the lifetime risk of cancer per mSv of whole-body radiation dose is 0.005% per mSv. Thus, if a patient receives a dose of 5 mSv during endoscopic retrograde cholangiogram (ERCP), the additional cancer risk would be 0.025% (5 × 0.005%). This assumes a linear no-threshold risk model for cancer risk, where dose response at low levels occurs in a generally linear pattern with no threshold. However, some researchers[36] believe that a linear relationship may not hold at very low doses; for example, cells can repair low levels of radiation damage. Therefore radiation risk estimates based on data from atomic bomb survivors may represent the worst-case scenario.

One useful way to express radiation risk is to compare it to activities of daily life. For example, doses in the range of 1 to 10 mSv (this includes

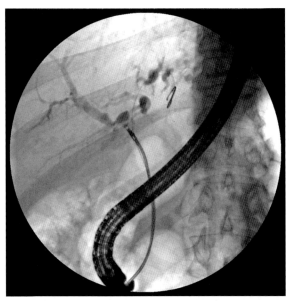

FIG 3.29 Endoscopic biopsy of hilar cholangiocarcinoma.

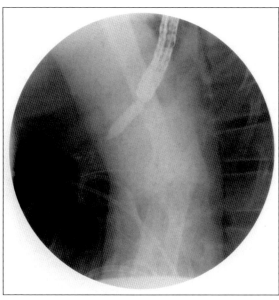

FIG 3.31 Transgastric drainage of pancreatic fluid collection. Lateral view demonstrates the endoscope in place in the gastric lumen, the wire in the pancreatic collection inferiorly, and balloon dilation of the transgastric tract. Note the patient's arm obscuring detail.

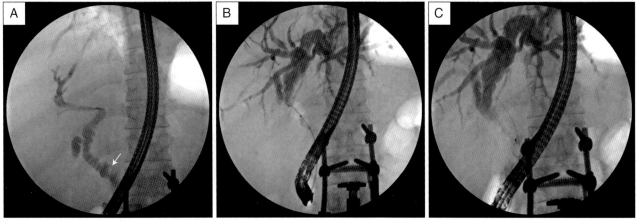

FIG 3.30 Cholelithiasis and stone retrieval. **A,** Injection into the distal common bile duct reveals an angular filling defect *(arrow)* as well as a corrugated appearance of the duct wall, a finding seen in cholangitis. **B,** Balloon dragging of the duct and **C,** basket retrieval of the stone were performed after sphincterotomy.

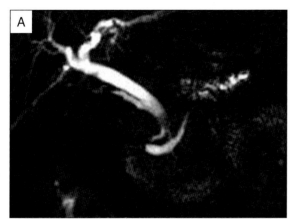

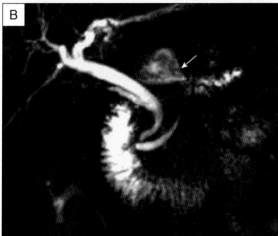

FIG 3.32 Magnetic resonance pancreatogram in disconnected duct syndrome (same patient as in Fig. 3.23). **A,** Although the endoscopic injection terminated at the site of duct disruption, the duct upstream to the site of obstruction is well depicted on magnetic resonance cholangiopancreatography. **B,** Secretin injection may reveal persistent function and extravasation from the functioning upstream duct; in this case a patent fistula to the site of prior transduodenal drainage *(arrow)* was opacified after secretin administration.

most ERCP procedures) carry a risk of death comparable to driving 2000 miles.[37] Medical radiation doses can be conceptually divided into three tiers.[38] There is clear evidence of radiation-induced cancer risk above 100 mSv, but few patients will fall into this category. Between 10 and 100 mSv, the risk is more controversial because of limited statistical power. An international multidisciplinary group of experts[39] has concluded that the lowest dose of x-ray or gamma radiation for which there is a good evidence of increased human cancer risk is 10 to 50 mSv for an acute exposure, and 50 to 100 mSv for protracted exposure, while also recognizing the uncertainty of these estimates. This is a dose range that is relevant to medical imaging, as certain CT examinations (such as multiphasic contrast-enhanced studies of the liver and pancreas), nuclear cardiology examinations, and complex procedures involving extended fluoroscopy time fall into this range. Below 10 mSv, which is a dose range relevant to radiography, most fluoroscopy, most nuclear medicine studies, and many CT studies, no direct epidemiologic data support increased cancer risk. However, this does not mean that there is no risk, as even large epidemiologic studies would not have the statistical power to detect risk, at present, at low radiation doses. The medical practitioner is responsible for ensuring that a radiologic procedure provides adequate images for diagnosis and treatment while keeping the radiation dose as low as reasonably achievable (ALARA). This includes proper setup and maintenance of imaging equipment, as well as procedures and protocols to produce the clinically required information while keeping radiation dose as low as possible. This is a joint effort involving medical practitioners, radiologic technologists, medical physicists, and manufacturers.

Although the additional cancer risk of indicated imaging examinations is very small compared with the natural incidence of cancer mortality, this risk may be clinically relevant compared with benefits that are very low or not established. For example, the excess cancer risk of a whole-body screening CT (as well as possible follow-up studies generated by the initial screening) may be clinically relevant compared with the uncertain benefit, particularly when taking into account additional risks of false-positive results and overdiagnosis. Published evidence-based appropriateness criteria,[40] perhaps integrated with clinical decision support systems, can be helpful in choosing appropriate studies. One role of the radiologist is to aid in choosing the most suitable imaging study.

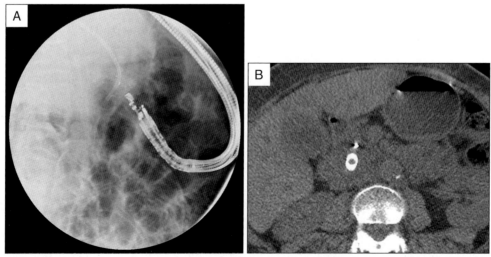

FIG 3.33 Endoscopic placement of fiducial markers for radiation therapy. **A,** ERCP spot radiograph demonstrates delivery of radiopaque fiducials (generally made of carbon or gold) into the borders of the pancreatic neoplasm for treatment planning. **B,** Unenhanced axial computed tomography image demonstrating the small marker anterior to the stent in the pancreatic head.

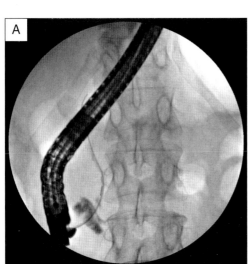

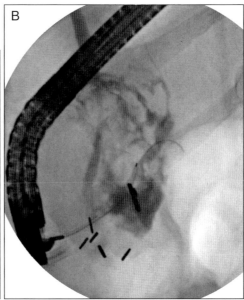

FIG 3.34 Extravasation in two different patients. **A,** Intramural duodenal intravasation after cannulation with the sphincterotome (same patient as in Fig. 3.18). **B,** Intrapancreatic extravasation during attempted deeper pancreatic duct cannulation. Both demonstrate nonanatomic heterogeneous contrast collections that did not change.

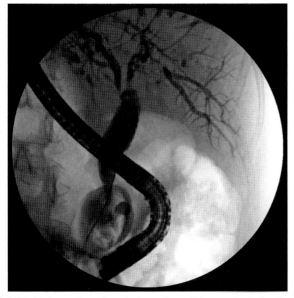

FIG 3.35 Periampullary diverticulum. Smoothly marginated collection of contrast in the region of the ampulla contains air and debris; the diverticulum would also have been evident during the procedure. (Same patient as in Fig. 3.9, *B*).

TABLE 3.1　Additional Cancer Risks of Common Imaging Studies

Examination	Effective Dose (mSv)	Additional Cancer Risk
Abdomen x-ray 50 y/o M	0.7	1 in 28,246
Abdomen x-ray 50 y/o F	0.7	I in 21,133
ERCP 35 y/o M	4	1 in 3,273
ERCP 35 y/o F	4	1 in 2,221
ERCP 65 y/o M	4	1 in 7,468
ERCP 65 y/o F	4	1 in 6,159
CT abdomen/pelvis 35 y/o M	14	1 in 935
CT abdomen/pelvis 35 y/o F	14	1 in 635
CT abdomen/pelvis 65 y/o M	14	1 in 2,134
CT abdomen/pelvis 65 y/o F	14	1 in 1,760

Radiation dose and additional cancer risk values obtained from http://www.xrayrisk.com/ (accessed May 24, 2016); original radiation dose values from Mettler et al.[43]

In addition, alternative procedures, such as magnetic resonance imaging and ultrasonography, which do not use ionizing radiation, should always be considered. For example, the American College of Radiology[41] recommends magnetic resonance cholangiography rather than CT for the follow-up of incidentally detected pancreatic cysts, because of the lack of ionizing radiation.

Other factors to take into account when using medical radiation are the age, health status, and sex of the patients. Epidemiologic studies have shown the minimum latency for development of solid tumors after radiation exposure is 10 years or longer. Radiation exposure is associated with a lifelong elevation of the natural age-specific risk for solid tumors.[35] Thus, younger patients are at a substantially higher risk from radiation as they usually have more remaining years of life during which a radiation-induced cancer might develop. Young children are at additional risk because they are also inherently more radiosensitive, perhaps 3 to 4 times more sensitive than adults.[37] Conversely, given the lag period of 10 years or longer for solid tumor development, radiation dose may be of minimal or no concern in some very ill patients or very elderly patients.

Women have a higher risk of radiation-induced carcinogenesis than men, approximately 1.5 times. The increased risk is greatest for chest examinations, because of the additional risk of breast cancer and high lung cancer coefficients,[32,42] but is also present for abdominal and pelvic examinations.

As an example of these effects, in Table 3.1, the estimated additional cancer risk of an ERCP in a 35-year-old woman is 1 in 2221, compared with 1 in 7468 in a 65-year-old man.

The complete reference list for this chapter can be found online at www.expertconsult.com.

4

Endoscopes, Guidewires, and Accessories

Sushil K. Ahlawat and Firas H. Al-Kawas

Endoscopic retrograde cholangiopancreatography (ERCP) has become the preferred technique for the management of patients with a variety of benign and malignant pancreaticobiliary disorders. Procedural success and safety depend to a large extent on proper patient selection for the appropriate indication, proceduralist skills, and an organized and functional ERCP unit. In addition to a dedicated ERCP room and a fluoroscopy unit, essential equipment for ERCP includes a duodenoscope and a variety of ancillary devices and accessories. A growing range of ERCP accessories have been developed to support the increasing demands and complexity of therapeutic ERCP. This chapter describes current and emerging accessories that are available to use during diagnostic and therapeutic ERCP.

ENDOSCOPES

Side-Viewing Endoscopes

Modern duodenoscopes are side-viewing video endoscopes equipped with an elevator. They are routinely used for diagnostic and therapeutic ERCP procedures. The elevator facilitates cannulation of the papilla and placement of accessories (Fig. 4.1), whereas the large-diameter working channels of therapeutic duodenoscopes (4.2 and 4.8 mm) allow passage of large-bore (10 to 11.5 Fr) accessories. The improved technology has allowed most current ERCP endoscopes to have a large "therapeutic" channel without increasing the size of the insertion tube—similar to what was formerly referred to as "diagnostic" ERCP scopes. Smaller outer shafts of 7.4-mm-diameter pediatric duodenoscopes with a 2.2-mm channel are available for use in neonates (see Chapter 29). Unfortunately, the small working channel of such pediatric endoscopes limits their use to mostly diagnostic purposes and limited therapeutics such as stone extraction, while requiring smaller, dedicated accessories. In general, the standard adult duodenoscope can be used in most children aged above 2 years. A jumbo-sized duodenoscope (5.5-mm channel) was previously available as a "mother/baby" scope system to allow passage of a cholangioscope (see Chapter 27). However, this system was difficult to manipulate and is now rarely used.

Forward-Viewing Endoscopes

Upper endoscopes, colonoscopes, and enteroscopes are used in patients with surgically altered anatomy (e.g., hepaticojejunostomy, gastrectomy with Roux-en-Y anatomy) (see Chapter 31). Conventional forward-viewing endoscopes do not have an elevator and are limited with respect to control of accessories during cannulation or therapy. In addition, visualization of the ampulla may be limited. When using a colonoscope, "long" length accessories may be needed, as not all standard biliary accessories are of adequate length.

Balloon-Assisted Enteroscopes

Single-balloon (Olympus America Inc., Lehigh Valley, PA) and double-balloon (Fujinon, Tokyo, Japan) enteroscopes enable deep intubation of the small bowel. These endoscopes have a specialized disposable overtube with an inflatable balloon that anchors the endoscope in place during shortening maneuvers. Double-balloon enteroscopes have a second balloon on the endoscope insertion tube. Balloon-assisted enteroscopes enable diagnostic and therapeutic ERCP in most patients with surgically altered anatomy.[1,2] However, there are few available accessories for therapeutic interventions because these enteroscopes have long lengths (200 cm) and small-diameter working channels. A "short" double-balloon enteroscope (Fujinon, Tokyo, Japan) with a 2.8-mm working channel and a 152-cm working length allows standard biliary accessories of ≤7-Fr diameter to be used.[3,4] More recently, this same endoscope has become available with a 3.2-mm working channel. However, the combination of a forward view and the lack of an elevator limits the success rate in patients with intact papilla for enteroscopy-assisted procedures. Recently the American Society for Gastrointestinal Endoscopy (ASGE) published a detailed report on devices and techniques used for ERCP in the surgically altered gastrointestinal (GI) tract.[5]

Echoendoscopes

Curvilinear echoendoscopes (GF-UC180 or GF-UCT180; Olympus America Inc., Lehigh Valley, PA, and Pentax, Montvale, NJ) have been used successfully to obtain access to biliary or pancreatic ducts in patients with failed ERCP and those with inaccessible papillae (see Chapters 32 and 33).[6] Therapeutic curvilinear echoendoscopes (Pentax and Olympus America Inc.) with 3.8-mm working channel allow passage of standard ERCP accessories for transmural access and drainage of pancreatic fluid collections with ability to place large-diameter (10 Fr) plastic stents or self-expandable metal stents that have large-diameter delivery systems. A 19-gauge or 22-gauge fine-needle aspiration needle or cautery device (Cystotome [Cook Endoscopy, Winston-Salem, NC], standard needle knife) can be used for puncture and entry at the defined location under real-time ultrasound guidance (see Chapter 56). The Cystotome (Fig. 4.2) is an electrocautery system that incorporates an inner wire with a large-diameter needle-knife tip on a 5-Fr inner catheter, and a 10-Fr outer catheter equipped with a diathermy ring at its distal tip. The proximal end of this device includes a handle with connectors for active cords for each of the two cautery components and a fitting to provide for injection of contrast. The Cystotome is discussed in more detail in Chapter 32. Recently, fully covered lumen-apposing self-expanding metal stents (LAMS) (Fig. 4.3) have been introduced and appear to be safe and effective for draining a variety of pancreatic fluid collections (see Chapter 56), such as pancreatic pseudocysts and walled-off pancreatic necrosis. Advantages of LAMS over other stents include single-step deployment, short length, large diameter, and ability to perform direct endoscopic necrosectomy while limiting stent migration.[7,8]

ACCESSORIES

Accessories are devices or pharmacologic agents that assist in the endoscopist's accomplishment of diagnostic and therapeutic procedures.

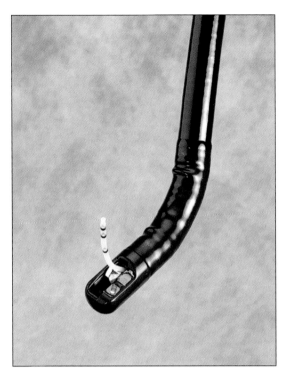

FIG 4.1 A 4.2-mm channel duodenoscope. (Courtesy Pentax Medical, Montvale, NJ.)

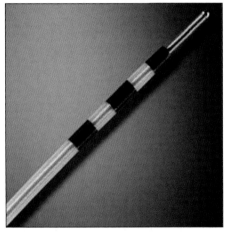

FIG 4.2 Cystotome. (Courtesy Cook Endoscopy, Winston-Salem, NC.)

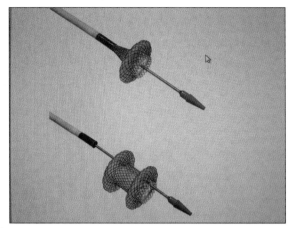

FIG 4.3 Axios stent. (Lumen-apposing self-expandable metal stent; courtesy Boston Scientific, Natick, MA.)

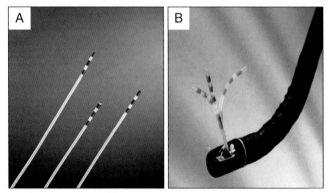

FIG 4.4 **A,** ERCP cannulas. **B,** Swing-tip ERCP cannula. (**A,** Courtesy Cook Endoscopy, Winston-Salem, NC; **B,** Courtesy Olympus America Inc., Center Valley, PA.)

Cannulation of the desired duct is a prerequisite to successful diagnostic and therapeutic ERCP. A variety of devices are currently available to gain duct access.[9] In particular, the use of sphincterotomes/guidewires and precut sphincterotomes has increased the ability to achieve deep cannulation of the desired duct.

Standard Cannulation Catheters

Standard ERCP cannulas are 5-Fr to 7-Fr catheters, with straight, tapered, or rounded tips that accept guidewires up to 0.035-inch diameters (Fig. 4.4, A). Use of double-lumen or triple-lumen devices or attachment of a side-arm adaptor allows contrast injection without need for removal of the guidewire. The use of tapered-tip (4.5 Fr to 4 Fr to 3.5 Fr) or ultratapered-tip (5 Fr to 4 Fr to 3 Fr) catheters may improve ductal access. However, these tapered-tip cannulas often accommodate only smaller-caliber guidewires (0.018 to 0.025 inches). There are no published studies that directly compare cannulation success rates between standard and tapered catheters, and the latter carry a higher risk of submucosal injection.

Standard cannulas with or without guidewires are limited in their ability to vary the angle of approach to the papilla. The swing-tip catheter (Olympus America Inc.) (Fig. 4.4, B) overcomes the limitations of conventional catheters and offers the endoscopist the ability to bend the cannula tip in either the up–down or left–right directions, thereby facilitating biliary cannulation or selective entry into the right or left hepatic ducts.

The Cremer needle-tip catheter (Cook Endoscopy) is 1.8 mm in diameter and has a metal needle tip that facilitates minor papilla cannulation (Fig. 4.5, A and B).

The standard pancreaticobiliary manometry catheter is a water-perfused 5-Fr catheter with a tip diameter of 3.5 Fr and is used during sphincter of Oddi manometry studies (Fig. 4.6, A) (see Chapter 16). A variety of catheter types can also be used. Some manometry catheters have a longer "nose" to help maintain catheter position. The standard catheter has three side ports spaced 2 mm apart for simultaneous pressure measurement. The Lehman manometry catheter (Cook Endoscopy) sacrifices one port for aspiration of water from the pancreatic duct during infusion to prevent overfilling; this reduces the risk of post-ERCP pancreatitis (PEP). Standard water-perfused motility recording systems used for esophageal manometry are utilized for sphincter of Oddi manometry. More recently, a compact water perfusion pump has become

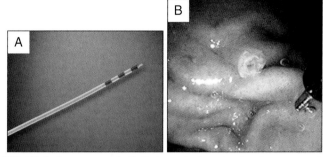

FIG 4.5 A, Cremer cannula. **B,** Endoscopic view showing Cremer cannula and minor papilla. (**A,** Courtesy Cook Endoscopy, Winston-Salem, NC.)

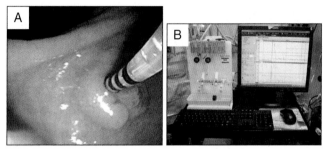

FIG 4.6 A, Endoscopic view showing motility catheter. **B,** Manometry tracing sphincter of Oddi motility recording system.

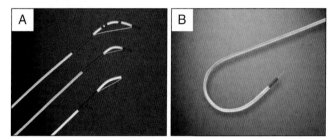

FIG 4.7 A, Standard and precut sphincterotome. **B,** Needle-knife sphincterotome. (Courtesy Cook Endoscopy, Winston-Salem, NC.)

available (Mui Scientific, Mississauga, Canada) (Fig. 4.6, *B*). A microtransducer catheter that does not require water perfusion is also available. This catheter appears to be associated with a lower risk of PEP. A detailed discussion on currently available sphincter of Oddi manometry devices can be found in technology status evaluation report by the ASGE[10] and in Chapter 16.

Sphincterotomes

Pull-type (Erlangen) sphincterotomes were designed for biliary sphincterotomy. They consist of a Teflon catheter containing a continuous wire loop with 20 to 30 mm of exposed wire exiting at a variable distance from the tip (Fig. 4.7, *A*). Early precut sphincterotomes were pull type, and the cutting wire extended to the tip (Fig. 4.7, *A*). The other end of the wire is insulated and connected to an electrosurgical unit. Over the last decade or so, endoscopists have recognized the need to angle the catheter upward to selectively enter the bile duct. Subsequently, prospective randomized trials comparing standard catheters with sphincterotomes have shown a cannulation rate of 84% to 97% with sphincterotomes compared with 62% to 67% with standard catheters (see Chapter 17). In addition, because sphincterotomy is performed in a large percentage of ERCPs, sphincterotomes have become the primary biliary cannulation

device during ERCP in patients with native anatomy and an intact papilla.

Sphincterotomes are available with single, double, and triple lumens; nearly all units have moved to the use of triple-lumen devices. Double-lumen sphincterotomes allow for either injection of contrast or introduction of a guidewire and facilitate cannulation and therapeutic interventions. Contrast can be injected either by removing the guidewire or by leaving the wire in and using a side arm adaptor (e.g., Tuohy-Borst Adapter; Cook Medical). Triple-lumen sphincterotomes allow injection of contrast without the need for removing the wire because there is an additional port. Unfortunately, because of the small size of the injection lumen, the contrast infuses slowly and with much resistance, making it difficult for the assistant because of the force required during injection. Contrast injection is facilitated by the use of a small syringe and by dilution of contrast, as full-strength contrast is more viscous. A sphincterotome is available that incorporates a combination of cutting and balloon stone extraction (Stonetome; Boston Scientific, Marlborough, MA); however, the addition of a balloon increases the catheter diameter and tip size, which may make cannulation more difficult.

When sphincterotomy is performed, a variety of generator currents can be used: cutting, autocut, coagulation, or blended. Limited data suggest that the use of a pure cutting current is associated with a lower risk of PEP, whereas the use of an autocut mode is associated with a lower risk of intraprocedural bleeding and eliminated the "zipper cut" phenomenon during sphincterotomy. When performing pancreatic sphincterotomy, pure cutting current is often used to reduce the risk of pancreatic duct injury and subsequent stenosis (see Chapter 11).

Rotatable sphincterotomes are designed to rotate the tip so that one can alter the desired trajectory of cannulation, which may be useful in improving cannulation, especially in patients with unusually oriented or distorted papillae or in patients with Billroth II–type anatomy. Rotatable sphincterotomes may also help orient the cutting wire during sphincterotomy. However, no published data are available to show this advantage. A wire-guided sphincterotome with a cutting wire oriented in the opposite direction relative to standard sphincterotome is available for use in Billroth II–type anatomy (Cook Endoscopy). In addition, a sphincterotome with an S-shaped tip is also useful in patients with surgically altered anatomy.

Guidewires are used with a standard catheter or sphincterotome to achieve deep cannulation of the bile and pancreatic ducts. Wire-guided cannulation is associated with increased cannulation success rates and a lower risk of PEP.[11] A randomized controlled trial found no difference in cannulation success and adverse event rates between 5-Fr and 4-Fr sphincterotomes.[12] For further information on biliary cannulation, see Chapter 14.

Access Sphincterotomes

Precut or "access" sphincterotomy refers to a variety of endoscopic techniques used to gain access to the bile or pancreatic duct after conventional methods of cannulation have failed (see Chapter 15). Needle-knife and precut sphincterotomes are the two most commonly used devices to gain access into the bile duct. The needle-knife sphincterotome was first described by Huibregtse in 1981 and is essentially a bare electrocautery wire that protrudes 4 to 5 mm from the end of a Teflon catheter (Fig. 4.7, *B*). Several publications discuss the use of this device. Additional versions include additional lumens for guidewire passage or contrast injection (double lumen) and both wire and contrast injection (triple lumen). The precut sphincterotome was first reported by Soehendra and the Hamburg group in 1996 (Fig. 4.7, *A*). This sphincterotome allows "papillary roof incision."[13] A double-lumen version is also available. It has the advantage of having separate lumens for contrast and guidewire. Biliary sphincterotomy can be immediately completed by using the same instrument and is facilitated by having a preloaded hydrophilic-tip wire. A new needle-knife sphincterotome has an insulated tip to prevent energy dispersion from the tip of the incising needle.[14] The coated-tip needle knife is believed to prevent unintentional deep cuts or perforations because it enables users to keep the sphincterotome tight in the papillary orifice. The optimal device for precut sphincterotomy is unknown because there are limited data comparing different precut techniques and devices.[15]

Guidewires

Guidewires are the cornerstone of diagnostic and therapeutic ERCP. During ERCP, guidewires are used for cannulation and for achieving and maintaining access and placing and exchanging devices. Guidewires are useful for cannulation, essential for passage of accessories, and useful to guide sphincterotomy, and are required for traversing strictures, stricture dilation, cytologic tissue sampling, and stent placement.

Ideal guidewire characteristics for gaining access to the duct of interest and traversing stricture are different from those for advancement and exchange of accessories. Guidewires with slippery and flexible leading tips and shafts are generally used for cannulation and to gain access through tight biliary and pancreatic strictures, but may be difficult to keep in place during exchange. On the other hand, stiff and taut guidewires are best used for advancement of devices such as biliary stents or dilators. Stiff and taut wires also minimize lateral deviation and facilitate forward axial transmission of forces. Friction can aid in maintaining wire tension but hinders both wire and device movement. A variety of guidewires are currently available (Table 4.1) and these vary in material, length, diameter, and design to optimize performance.[16]

In general, three guidewire designs are available for ERCP applications: (1) Monofilament wires are designed for rigidity and made of stainless steel. (2) Coiled wires are stiff and flexible and have an inner monofilament core and an outer spiral coil made of stainless steel. Inner core and outer spiral coil design provide stiffness and flexibility, respectively. Most coiled wires are coated with Teflon (DuPont, Washington, DE) to minimize resistance and to optimize traversing tortuous biliary strictures because of combined stiffness and flexibility. (3) Coated or sheathed wires have a monofilament core made of stainless steel or nitinol and an outer sheath made of Teflon, polyurethane, or another lubricious polymer. The outer sheath material improves radiopacity, slipperiness, and electrical insulation properties. Flexibility of coated wire tips depends on the taper of the inner core. Many wires have a platinum-tipped core to improve fluoroscopic visualization. The configuration of the guidewire can be straight or angled (J-shaped) (Fig. 4.8, A). Some wires have graduated or continuous markings for visual endoscopic measurement or movement detection. Most wires are only minimally steerable in the radial direction.

Guidewires are advanced under fluoroscopic monitoring through a catheter or sphincterotome, which imparts stiffness and direction. Guidewire passage is easier after flushing water through dry or contrast-filled devices by minimizing friction, because contrast is "sticky." Moistening hydrophilic portions of a guidewire prevents drying and sticking of the wire to the accessories. Maintenance of wire position is critical for safe and effective use of over-the-wire accessories, such as dilators and stents. The risk of wire displacement can be minimized by using guidewires that have graduated or continuous markings or movement detection, printed distance markers, and movement guides (Fig. 4.8, B). In addition, fixation of the proximal end (outside the patient)

TABLE 4.1 Currently Available Guidewires for ERCP Applications

Wire Type/Name (Manufacturer)	Diameter (in)	Length (cm)	Core Material	Sheath Material	Tip Material
Monofilament					
Axcess 21 (CE)	0.021	480	Nitinol	None	Platinum
Amplatz (BS)	0.038	260	SS	None	Platinum
Coiled					
Standard Wires (CE)	0.018, 0.021, 0.025	480	SS	Stainless coil, 0.035 Teflon painted	Stainless tapered core coil
Coated					
Tracer Metro Direct (CE)	0.021, 0.025, 0.035	260, 480	Nitinol	Teflon	Platinum, hydrophilic
Delta (CE)	0.025, 0.035	260	Nitinol	Polyurethane	Hydrophilic
Acrobat (CE)	0.025, 0.035	260, 450	Nitinol	Polytetrafluoroethylene	Hydrophilic
Tracer Metro (CE)	0.035, 0.035	260, 480	Nitinol	Teflon	Platinum, hydrophilic
Roadrunner (CE)	0.018	480	Nitinol	Teflon	Platinum
Jagwire* (BS)	0.038, 0.035, 0.025	260, 450	Nitinol	Teflon	Tungsten, hydrophilic
Hydra Jagwire (BS)	0.035	260, 450	Nitinol	Endoglide coating	Tungsten, hydrophilic
NovaGold (BS)	0.018	260, 480	Triton alloy	Hydrophilic	Straight, shapable
NaviPro (BS)	0.018, 0.025, 0.035	260	Nitinol	Polyurethane	Platinum hydrophilic coating on entire length
Pathfinder (BS)	0.018	450	Nitinol	Endoglide	Platinum, hydrophilic
VisiGlide (O)	0.025	450, 270	Superelastic alloy	Fluorine	Hydrophilic
LinearGuideV (O)	0.035	270, 450	Nitinol	Polytetrafluoroethylene	Hydrophilic
X wire* (CM)	0.035, 0.025	260, 450	Nitinol	Hydrophilic	Nitinol

BS, Boston Scientific, Marlborough, MA; *CE,* Cook Endoscopy, Winston-Salem, NC; *CM,* ConMed, Utica, NY; *O,* Olympus America Inc., Lehigh Valley, PA; *SS,* stainless steel.
*Available in a stiff version.
Adapted with permission from Cortas GA, Mehta SN, Abraham NS, et al. Selective cannulation of the common bile duct: a prospective randomized trial comparing standard catheters with sphincterotomes. *Gastrointest Endosc.* 1999;50:775–779.

using short-wire system locking devices can also decrease the risk of wire dislodgement.

Guidewire types include conventional, hydrophilic, and "hybrid," with diameters ranging from 0.018 to 0.035 inches and lengths most often ranging from 260 to 480 cm, and are summarized in Table 4.1. Wire lengths longer than 400 cm (up to 600 cm) are used for "long-length" exchange of longer accessories used with 200-cm endoscopes during altered anatomy ERCP. It is recommended that coated wires approved for use during electrocautery applications are used during sphincterotomy.

Data are limited regarding the relative efficacy of specific wires for ERCP applications. Clinical experience suggests that coated and hydrophilic wires improve ERCP success rates in negotiating difficult papillae or strictures. Completely hydrophilic wires (Glidewire; Olympus Corporation, and Terumo, Tokyo, Japan) are slippery and highly torqueable, allowing difficult strictures to be traversed, but can make catheter exchange difficult, leading to inadvertent displacement from ducts or strictures. Combination (hybrid) wires—such as Jagwire, Hydra Jagwire (Boston Scientific); FX, X (ConMed, Utica, NY); VisiGlide (Olympus America Inc.); and Metro (Cook Endoscopy)—provide a combination of a slippery tip with a nonslippery, stiffer shaft (Fig. 4.8, *A*). As mentioned earlier, recent data suggest that biliary cannulation using a guidewire through a sphincterotome lowers the risk of PEP, presumably because of less trauma to the papilla and limited pancreatic injection.[11] Teflon-coated wires are least expensive, but rarely used. Hybrid wires are more user-friendly but more expensive. A useful and detailed review of guidewires can be found in a recent ASGE technology assessment report.[16]

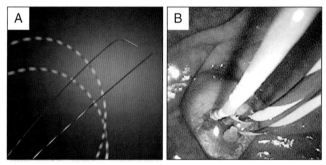

FIG 4.8 A, Straight and angled-tip guidewires. **B,** Endoscopic view showing the markings on the guidewires. (**A,** Courtesy Boston Scientific, Natick, MA.)

Wire Safety

Perforation and failed device placement are the two main wire-related risks in the pancreas or biliary tree during ERCP. Applying excessive force from below a stricture or at an acute angle can result in wire-related perforation. Loss of wire tension or access from a stricture while using rigid devices such as biliary dilators can also result in perforation. Wire-guided sphincterotomy over standard Teflon-coated guidewires can transmit electrical current from the cutting wire to the bile duct. Intact, coated wires are effectively insulated against transmission of short circuits or induced currents. All damaged wires are potential sources of current conduction.

Exchange Assistance Devices (Short-Wire ERCP Systems)

Multiple devices are frequently required for successful therapeutic ERCP. Frequently, an exchange or series of exchanges over a previously placed guidewire is required to introduce subsequent devices. Several exchange assistance devices have been developed by different manufacturers to facilitate exchange of over-the-wire accessories in order to reduce reliance on the assistant, and to minimize guidewire loss. These devices employ the use of short-length (260 cm) guidewires and may increase efficiency while reducing fluoroscopy time. Potential problems with exchange assistance devices include a restriction in the choice of accessories, difficulty in reusing the same accessory during the procedure, and cost. A detailed discussion on currently available short-wire systems can be found in a recent ASGE technology status evaluation report.[17] It is worth noting that completely hydrophilic short wires can be exchanged using a hydraulic technique through standard, nonmonorail catheters.[18]

Rapid Exchange Biliary System

The Rapid Exchange (RX) Biliary System (Boston Scientific) is a monorail design that provides the endoscopist with control over the guidewire during wire advancement and subsequent exchanges. The system is composed of three integral units: a guidewire locking device (Fig. 4.9, *A*), a specially designed RX catheter, and a 260-cm-long guidewire. A locking device secures the position of the guidewire during exchange of over-the-wire accessories, advancement of accessories, and manipulation. The locking device can accommodate multiple guidewires that can be secured at any time and thus allows for multiple therapeutic interventions. Cannulas and sphincterotomes have a distal open channel (beginning 5 cm from the tip and extending proximally 30 cm) that allows the guidewire to exit at this point rather than at the hub of the

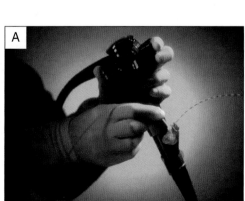
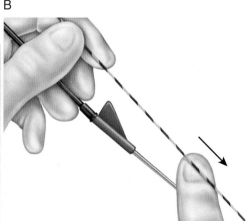
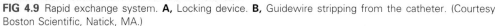

FIG 4.9 Rapid exchange system. **A,** Locking device. **B,** Guidewire stripping from the catheter. (Courtesy Boston Scientific, Natick, MA.)

endoscope. Once cannulation is achieved, the wire is separated from the catheter (Fig. 4.9, *B*) and is secured in the guidewire locking device at the biopsy port. A variety of RX accessories are available to use with this system.

Potential benefits of RX Biliary System include shorter total procedural and postcannulation times and a reduction in use of fluoroscopy. However, its cost is higher than that of standard long-length equipment and may limit the choice of accessories. Cost–benefit studies using the RX Biliary System are not available.

Fusion System

This short-wire system is made by Cook Endoscopy. The name "Fusion" is derived from the ability of the system to be used as either a long-wire or a short-wire system. It consists of double-lumen and triple-lumen catheters and a triple-lumen sphincterotome. The design of this system facilitates the exchange of accessories without removing the guidewire or exchanging the initially placed catheter/sphincterotome over the full length of the guidewire.

The main difference between this system and the conventional design is that a side hole is placed 6 cm from the tip of the catheter (or any accessories from this line of products except the stent introducer system, in which the side hole is placed 2.5 cm from the tip) (Fig. 4.10, *A*). The guidewire is 185 cm long and most accessories are 220 cm long. To provide proper control of these much shorter accessories and guidewire, the system uses a special disposable biopsy valve with a locking mechanism to anchor the guidewire while performing exchanges (Fig. 4.10, *B*).

A major advantage of the Fusion system lies in the ability to place multiple stents without removing the guidewire. With this system, the guidewire can remain within the bile duct and an "intraductal exchange" can be performed. This facilitates deployment of subsequent stents without concerns about losing access across a stricture and saves time because there is no need to recannulate the duct and/or traverse a stricture, and there is no need for wire exchange. Another advantage of the short-wire system is the ability to remove a 10-Fr stent that has

not been deployed. In situations where intervention requires the use of standard-length or conventional accessories, a standard-length guidewire can be inserted through the end of the catheter or sphincterotome after removing the inner nylon stylet, and exchange can be performed in the usual manner. Controlled data regarding efficiency with the Fusion system are not available.

V-System

The Olympus V-system integrates Olympus endoscopes and endotherapy devices, though the V-scope can be used with any other devices and accessories. This design offers the option of guidewire manipulation by the physician or by the assistant and allows easier exchange of "long-length" catheters using a short guidewire. The V-endoscope has an increased elevator angle and V-groove that allows the endoscopist to "lock" the wire at the level of the elevator when it is closed. This endoscope design may also enhance selective biliary cannulation capability. The V-system features a C-hook, V-markings, and V-sheath for device control in addition to the V-groove on the elevator of the duodenoscope (Fig. 4.11, *A*).

The C-hook attaches the device to the endoscope just below the biopsy port (Fig. 4.11, *B*) and allows a choice of control of the device by the physician or the assistant. V-markings are present on the proximal portion of all V-system devices. When the V-marking on the accessory device reaches the biopsy port of the endoscope, the tip of the catheter has reached the endoscope elevator V-groove indicating that raising the elevator at that point would lock the guidewire in the V-groove. The V-sheath design allows the guidewire sheath and the injection/handle sheath to be separated, offering the choice of control by the endoscopist or the assistant. The V-scope and V-system accessories can also be used with long-length and short-length 0.035-inch and smaller guidewires and with ERCP accessories from other device manufacturers. Initial evaluation using this system (V-scope) has shown improved reliability of guidewire fixation; however, limited data exist on efficiency of catheter/guidewire exchanges. In addition, completely hydrophilic wires (e.g., Terumo) are not always held in place with the V-scope.

Currently available short-wire systems are easy to learn and provide physicians with direct control of the guidewire and the accessory. Potential advantages include faster device exchanges, less fluoroscopy time, and the ability to perform therapeutic ERCP with less experienced assistants. The use of some exchange assistance devices may limit the choice of accessories. Currently, controlled data to support these advantages are lacking. The effect of short-wire systems on cannulation success and adverse event rates remains unknown.

ACCESSORIES

Drainage Devices

Drainage devices include stents and nasobiliary drains. Stents are used for a variety of purposes and are available in various materials and

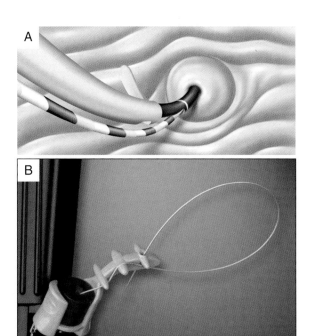

FIG 4.10 Fusion system. **A,** Fusion catheter. **B,** Biopsy valve with locking mechanism. (Courtesy Cook Endoscopy, Winston-Salem, NC.)

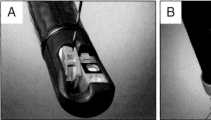
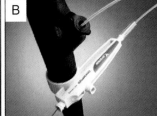

FIG 4.11 V-system. **A,** V-scope tip. **B,** Hook. (Courtesy Olympus America Inc., Center Valley, PA.)

configurations. Nasobiliary and nasopancreatic drains are infrequently used in the United States and are discussed in Chapter 22.

Plastic Stents

Plastic stents are made of polyethylene or Teflon and are available in varying sizes, shapes, and lengths for biliary and pancreatic pathologies. A pusher tube is used to place plastic stents over a guidewire with or without an inner guiding catheter. Delivery systems are available for plastic stents that combine the pushing and guiding catheters. The standard stent delivery system for 10-Fr stents comprises a 0.035-inch guidewire (480 cm), a 260-cm-long 6-Fr radiopaque Teflon inner guiding catheter with a tapered tip to facilitate passage across strictures, and a pusher tube. Some guiding catheters have two metal rings (placed 7 cm apart) at the distal end that help measure stricture length. The pusher tube is made of Teflon (8, 10, or 11.5 Fr according to stent diameter) and used for advancing the stent.

Most plastic stents are made of radiopaque polyethylene and are available in various diameters (3 to 11.5 Fr), lengths, and configurations. In general, stents of 3 to 7 Fr do not have inner guiding catheters as part of the stent delivery system; however, one company (Boston Scientific) has an inner guiding catheter available for all stents ≥7 Fr in diameter when the Advanix biliary stent is used with NaviFlex RX Delivery System. Straight "Amsterdam-type" stents are predominantly used for biliary drainage (Fig. 4.12, A). Based on Poiseuille's law there is a clear relationship between stent diameter and duration of stent patency (Fig. 4.13).[19] A straight configuration also appears to improve stent patency. Attempts to improve stent patency by eliminating side holes, changing stent material, or coating the inner surface with a hydrophilic substance have been largely unsuccessful. The addition of an antireflux valve or use of different coating on the stent surface to prolong stent patency has shown some promise in prolonging patency.[20,21] Double-pigtail configurations (see Fig. 4.12, A) help anchor the stent to prevent proximal and distal migration. These stents are frequently used in patients with difficult bile duct stones because the ducts are usually dilated in caliber and there is an absence of underlying stricture that would otherwise prevent migration. They are also used in some patients with hilar strictures where the rate of stent migration is high.

Single-pigtail stents (Fig. 4.12, B) are made from a variety of materials and are frequently used in the pancreatic duct to prevent inward (proximal) migration, because the pigtail is located proximally (external to the papilla when placed). Limited data suggest that smaller-diameter stents (3 to 4 Fr) cause less ductal damage when placed into normal pancreatic ducts.[22] Elimination of side holes and flaps and the use of shorter stents may prolong patency when used long-term and promote spontaneous migration of prophylactic pancreatic stents.[23,24] Stents with running channels (star-shape), an inner lumen only the size of a

guidewire, and without side holes (GI Supply, Camp Hill, PA) are designed to prolong patency but limited data are available to support this concept.

Plastic stent delivery catheters that are compatible with short-wire ERCP systems are available. One randomized controlled trial showed significant reduction in the time needed for device exchange and for stent insertion compared with traditional long-wire devices.[25] As mentioned previously, the Fusion system (Cook Endoscopy) allows for intraductal exchange, which facilitates insertion of multiple side-by-side stents.[26]

Stents can be removed using snares, baskets, and foreign body forceps (see Chapter 24). Large-bore (10 Fr) stents can be removed through the channel of a therapeutic endoscope with a standard polypectomy snare. Smaller stents (3-Fr to 5-Fr pancreatic stents) can also be removed via the working channel of the endoscope using a foreign body forceps (e.g., rat tooth forceps) or standard biopsy forceps. The Soehendra stent retriever (Cook Endoscopy) consists of a screw-tipped wire-guided device that allows stent removal while maintaining guidewire position (Fig. 4.14, A). It is also available with an extended-tip design to facilitate cannulation. In patients with difficult strictures, maintaining wire access can also be accomplished by passing a guidewire through the stent lumen and passing a standard polypectomy snare over the wire.

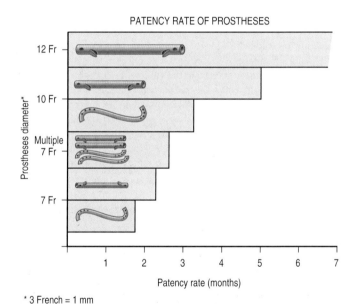

FIG 4.13 Relationship between stent diameter and the duration of functional patency. (Adapted with permission from Siegel JH, Pullano W, Kodsi B, et al. Optimal palliation of malignant bile duct obstruction: experience with endoscopic 12 French prostheses. *Endoscopy.* 1988;20:137–141.)

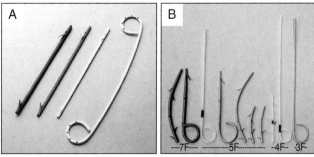

FIG 4.12 **A,** Straight and double-pigtail stents. **B,** Single-pigtail stents. (**A,** Courtesy Olympus America Inc., Center Valley, PA; **B,** Courtesy Cook Endoscopy, Winston-Salem, NC.)

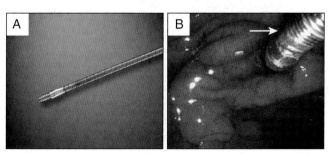

FIG 4.14 **A,** Stent retriever. **B,** Endoscopic view showing stent retrieval *(arrow).* (**A,** Courtesy Cook Endoscopy, Winston-Salem, NC.)

TABLE 4.2   Self-Expandable Biliary Metal Stents

	Wallflex (BS)	Wallstent* (BS)	Viabil (GM)	X-Suit NIR (Olympus)	Bonastent (EC)	Zilver* (CE)
Material	Platinol	Elgiloy	Nitinol	Nitinol	Nitinol	Nitinol
Length (cm)	4/6/8/10	4/6/8/10	4/6/8/10	4/6/8/10	5/7/8/9/10	4/6/8
Deployed diameter (mm)	8/10	8/10	8/10	8,10	8/10	6, 8, 10
Stent foreshortening	Yes	Yes	No	No	No	No
Introducer diameter (Fr)	8.5	8	8.5	7.5	7	6, 7.5, 6

BS, Boston Scientific, Marlborough, MA; *CE,* Cook Endoscopy, Winston-Salem, NC; *EC,* Endochoice, Alpharetta, GA; *GM,* GoreMedical, Flagstaff, AZ.
*According to the manufacturer, magnetic resonance imaging compatible.

Self-Expandable Metal Stents

Self-expandable metal stents (SEMS) were introduced to prolong stent patency over plastic stents. SEMS expand to diameters of 8 to 10 mm and are available as bare (uncovered), partially, or fully covered. Uncovered SEMS do not occlude from bacterial biofilm (see Chapter 23). In the United States, available uncovered SEMS with an open mesh design include the Wallstent/Wallflex (Boston Scientific), the Evolution and Zilver stent (Cook Endoscopy), Flexxus (ConMed), Alimaxx-B (Merit Medical Endotek, South Jordan, UT), and *Olympus X-Suit* NIR (Table 4.2; Fig. 4.15, *A* and *B*). Recently, TaeWoong Medical (Seoul, South Korea) introduced an uncovered biliary SEMS (Niti-S) in the U.S. market. Most SEMS are made of stainless steel or nitinol, a nickel–titanium alloy that provides a high degree of flexibility and is kink resistant. However, nitinol is less radiopaque than stainless steel, and additional radiopaque (gold or platinum) markers are added to the stents to improve radiopacity in order to facilitate proper positioning during deployment. Stents are available in 8-mm and 10-mm diameters. Uncovered 8-mm stents are preferred by some for side-by-side stent placement in patients with unresectable malignant hilar obstruction (Fig. 4.15) (see Chapter 40). Partially or fully covered SEMS are also available. Examples include the Wallstent/Wallflex (Boston Scientific) and Viabil (Gore Medical, Flagstaff, AZ) stents. Partially covered Wallstent/Wallflex stents have a polymer (Permalune) coating on the inside of the stent except for the proximal and distal 5 mm. This membrane is designed to prevent tumor ingrowth and prolong stent patency. The Wallflex stent (Boston Scientific) is also available in a fully covered version composed of a type of nitinol (Platinol) and with rounded, less traumatic ends than the Wallstent. The fully covered version has a distal lasso that facilitates repositioning or removal of SEMS. Viabil stents are covered with expanded polytetrafluoroethylene and fluorinated ethylene propylene (ePTFE/FEP) and are available with or without fenestrations designed to be positioned over the cystic duct to prevent cholecystitis. Fully covered SEMS and, to a lesser extent, partially covered SEMS can be removed using a snare or a foreign body retrieval forceps (Fig. 4.16) for a duration well beyond placement. Fully covered SEMS are increasingly used to treat benign pancreaticobiliary disorders though only one is approved in the United States for benign disease, and FDA approved it specifically for management of distal common bile duct strictures caused by chronic pancreatitis for up to 12 months (Wallflex RMV; Boston Scientific).

The delivery system for preloaded SEMS varies in design (see Table 4.2). The stents are collapsed and constrained on a 6-Fr or 6.5-Fr introducer catheter by an 8-Fr or 8.5-Fr overlying plastic sheath. Introducer systems as small as 6-Fr diameter are available. The entire system is advanced over the guidewire through the endoscope channel and passed under fluoroscopic guidance across the stricture using radiopaque markers. The Wallstent/Wallflex delivery system allows recapture and repositioning of the stent before reaching the 80% marker.

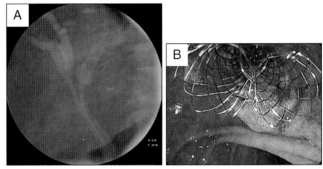

FIG 4.15 Self-expandable dual-metal stents for hilar stricture. **A,** Endoscopic view of the stents. **B,** Fluoroscopic image of the stents.

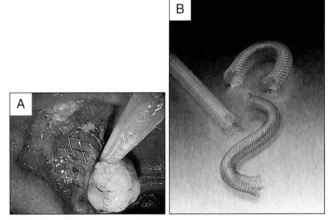

FIG 4.16 **A,** Fully covered self-expandable stent removed with a snare. **B,** Wallflex fully covered stent. (Courtesy Boston Scientific, Natick, MA.)

A major limitation of uncovered SEMS is embedding into the surrounding tissue, which prevents removal within a short period of time after placement; SEMS are costly compared with plastic stents, though may be overall cost-effective in patient management, particularly for malignant disease because they reduce the need for reintervention.

Nasobiliary and Pancreatic Drainage Catheters

Nasobiliary drainage catheters (see Chapter 22) are used for temporary drainage of the biliary tree and are available as 250-cm-long 5-Fr, 7-Fr, and 10-Fr diameter catheters with 5 to 9 side holes that facilitate drainage. Multiple tip configurations are available (pigtail, straight, flaps). Nasopancreatic drainage catheters are 5 Fr in diameter and may be used to drain the main pancreatic duct after pancreatic sphincterotomy or to irrigate and drain pancreatic fluid collections. Nasobiliary and nasopancreatic tubes are placed over a 0.035-inch guidewire. A nasal transfer tube is needed for rerouting the tube from the mouth to the nose after the endoscope is withdrawn from the patient. A connecting tube is needed to attach the catheter to a bag when gravity drainage is used.

Tissue Sampling Devices

Brush cytology devices are available as single-lumen or multiple-lumen systems. When a single-lumen cytology system is used, cell loss is inevitable because the brush is pulled back through the entire length of the catheter. In the event that single-lumen cytology brushes are used, it is useful to aspirate bile from the catheter to collect any dislodged cells within the catheter to improve the diagnostic yield. Double-lumen cytology brush systems are preferable (Fig. 4.17, A) and allow the guidewire and brush to pass through two separate lumens so that access is not lost. In addition, this design minimizes cell loss by eliminating the need to pull back the brush through the entire length of the catheter. Dedicated biliary biopsy forceps (Olympus America Inc.) are useful for selectively obtaining biopsy specimens from the bile duct under fluoroscopy (Fig. 4.17, B), although standard forceps as used for upper endoscopy can also be used. Pediatric forceps are more flexible and easier to pass through the side-viewing endoscope.

Stricture and Papilla Dilation Devices

In general, pancreaticobiliary dilation can be accomplished using balloons (Fig. 4.18, A) or bougies (Fig. 4.18, B). Balloon dilators are made of noncompliant polyethylene and are available in 4-mm, 6-mm, 8-mm, and 10-mm diameters and 2-cm to 4-cm lengths. The balloons are passed over a guidewire through the accessory channel of the endoscope. A radiopaque band proximal to the taper indicates the point of maximal dilation. Papillary dilation using large-diameter balloons (12 to 20 mm) is reported to be safe and effective for treatment of choledocholithiasis when combined with biliary sphincterotomy (see Chapters 18 and 19).[27,28] For this indication, esophageal/pylorus/colon balloons 5.5 cm in length and 12 to 20 mm in diameters are currently used because biliary dilation balloons of this diameter are not available (Fig. 4.19). Recently, a sphincterotome with an embedded dilation balloon has been

introduced (Stone Master V; Olympus America Inc.). This sphincterotome incorporates a 12-mm to 18-mm dilation balloon (Fig. 4.20) and is designed specifically for combined sphincterotomy/balloon dilation for removal of large stones to avoid the need for mechanical lithotripsy.

Soehendra dilators (Cook Endoscopy) are standard-shaped, tapered bougies that are available in 6-Fr to 11.5-Fr diameters and passed over a guidewire. The 10-Fr and 11.5-Fr dilators require the use of a large endoscope accessory channel.

Threaded-tip Soehendra stent retrievers have also been used to dilate very tight pancreaticobiliary strictures that otherwise only allow passage of a guidewire. The wire-guided screw-tipped device is used to negotiate high-grade strictures (Fig. 4.14, A and B). A modified device is now commercially available as a dilator (Cook Endoscopy). For pancreaticobiliary stricture dilation, there are no well-controlled published comparisons of techniques or devices.

Stone Extraction Accessories

Accessories useful for stone extraction include double-lumen or triple-lumen balloon catheters, wire baskets, and mechanical lithotriptors (see Chapter 19). The stone extraction balloon (Fig. 4.21, A) consists of a 5-Fr to 6.8-Fr double-lumen or triple-lumen catheter with a soft, compliant balloon located at the tip (8-mm to 18-mm diameter when inflated). Multisize stone extraction balloons are currently available. Before insertion into the endoscope it is useful to ensure that the balloon inflates correctly. The balloon catheter can be inserted over a guidewire or freehand directly into the desired duct without guidewire. The Stonetome (Boston Scientific) is a double-lumen sphincterotome with an 11.5-mm-diameter extraction balloon mounted on the tip.

Stones can also be removed using wire baskets (Fig. 4.21, B), which are available in a variety of sizes and configurations.[29] The basket is shaped such that the wires open like a trap to engage the stones. Basket

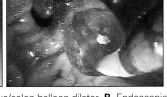
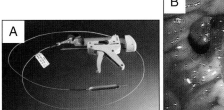

FIG 4.19 **A,** CRE esophageal/pylorus/colon balloon dilator. **B,** Endoscopic view showing CRE balloon dilation of ampulla. (**A,** Courtesy Boston Scientific, Natick, MA.)

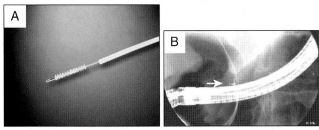

FIG 4.17 **A,** Cytobrush. **B,** Fluoroscopic image showing biliary biopsy forceps *(arrow).* (**A,** Courtesy Cook Endoscopy, Winston-Salem, NC.)

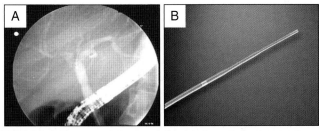

FIG 4.18 **A,** Fluoroscopic image of dilator balloon. **B,** Soehendra dilator. (Courtesy Cook Endoscopy, Winston-Salem, NC.)

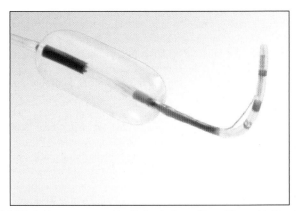

FIG 4.20 Sphincterotome with dilation balloon, Stone Master V. (Courtesy Olympus America Inc., Center Valley, PA.)

function varies depending on the number of wires. Newer design baskets can be advanced over a guidewire allowing the basket to reach difficult areas (Trapezoid basket [Boston Scientific] and Flower basket [Olympus America Inc.]). The Trapezoid basket has a handle designed to allow mechanical lithotripsy to be performed and has an emergency release feature to prevent basket entrapment. There are no published data demonstrating superiority of one extraction balloon or basket device over another.

Mechanical Lithotriptors

Lithotripsy wire baskets facilitate removal of large (≥1.5 cm) bile duct stones by crushing the stones before extraction. The original Soehendra

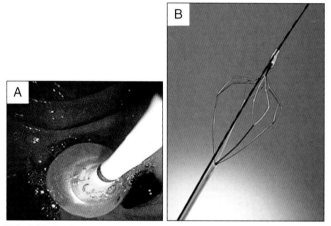

FIG 4.21 A, Endoscopic view of stone extractor balloon. **B,** Stone extractor basket. (Courtesy Olympus America Inc., Center Valley, PA.)

external lithotriptor (Cook Endoscopy) does not pass through the endoscope channel and requires cutting the handle of the basket and removing the endoscope before stone fragmentation. This device consists of a 14-Fr metal sheath and a self-locking crank handle (Fig. 4.22, *A*). The lithotriptor can be used with most standard stone extraction baskets to break the stone, or as a rescue device in the event the basket with entrapped stone becomes affected at the ampulla. Indeed, the latter situation is when external lithotripters are most often utilized.

Another mechanical lithotriptor is a preassembled through-the-scope (TTS) lithotripsy basket that can be inserted through a therapeutic duodenoscope (Fig. 4.22, *B to D*) (BML lithotripsy baskets; Olympus Medical Inc.). The most recent version allows TTS, over-the-wire passage.[30] This device is available in disposable and reusable versions. A single-piece disposable mechanical lithotriptor with the basket, metal sheath, and crank handle is also available (Monolith; Boston Scientific). Details and specifications of commercially available mechanical lithotriptors are published in a recent ASGE technology review.[30]

Cholangiopancreatoscopy

Duodenoscope-assisted cholangiopancreatoscopy (Fig. 4.23, *A* and *B*) allows for the direct visualization of the biliary and pancreatic ducts (see Chapters 26 and 27). In the past, a dedicated mother–daughter system was required. Currently, a variety of electronic and fiberoptic miniscopes are available that can be passed through a 4.2-mm channel therapeutic duodenoscope for direct visualization of the biliary and pancreatic duct. These instruments are now available in diameters of 10 mm or less. They have a small working channel (1.2 mm) that allows passage of small-diameter forceps and fibers for tissue acquisition and for the application of laser and electrohydraulic lithotripsy. Currently available cholangioscope systems are from Pentax, Olympus, and Boston

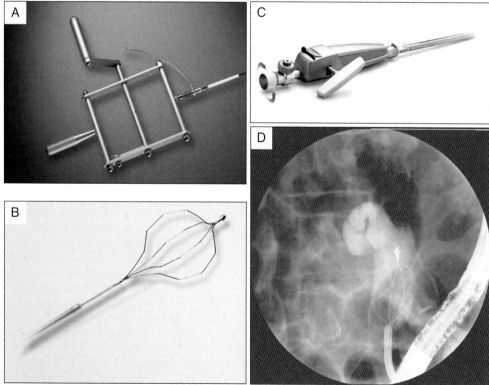

FIG 4.22 A, Soehendra mechanical lithotriptor handle. **B,** Through-the-scope mechanical lithotriptor basket. **C,** Through-the-scope mechanical lithotriptor handle. **D,** Fluoroscopic image of mechanical lithotriptor. (**A,** Courtesy Cook Endoscopy, Winston-Salem, NC; **B** and **C,** Courtesy Olympus America Inc., Center Valley, PA.)

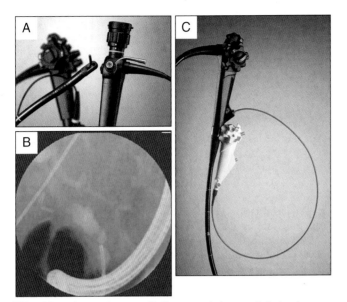

FIG 4.23 A, Cholangioscope. **B,** Fluoroscopic image of cholangioscope. **C,** SpyScope. (**A,** Courtesy Pentax Medical, Montvale, NJ; **C,** Courtesy Boston Scientific, Natick, MA.)

Scientific.[31] Limitations include the fragility of these devices, the small working channel, and the need for two endoscopists except for the Boston Scientific system. The latter is now available in digital form (SpyGlass DS), and with markedly improved optics over its fiberoptic predecessor. The Pentax cholangioscope remains fiberoptic. The Olympus videocholangioscope has become available in the United States. Although it is reusable, it remains relatively fragile and endoscope repair is costly.

The Boston Scientific system (SpyGlass) has four-way tip deflection, a dedicated irrigation channel, and a longer and smaller diameter allowing access to the proximal biliary tree (Fig. 4.23, *C*). Digital imaging version of the SpyGlass (SpyGlass DS; Boston Scientific) was introduced recently. SpyGlass DS has a much better image quality, easier setup, and usability compared with the fiberoptic version (now called SpyGlass Legacy). Biopsy forceps and lithotripsy probes are available that can be used for tissue sampling and stone fragmentation, respectively, by passing through the channel of the SpyScope (Fig. 4.24, *A* to *C*). These devices are discussed in more detail in Chapters 26 and 27.

Ultraslim upper endoscopes with an outer diameter of 5 to 5.4 mm and a working channel of 2 mm are available (Olympus and Pentax) and can be used for direct access into the bile or pancreatic duct after sphincterotomy or sphincteroplasty. This is referred to as direct peroral cholangioscopy (or pancreatoscopy when used in the pancreatic duct). In one report, the use of an intraductal balloon catheter with a detachable handle facilitated the introduction of a small-caliber endoscope into the biliary tree.[32] Unfortunately, air embolization was reported and the dedicated catheter was withdrawn from the market. If direct cholangioscopy is to be used, carbon dioxide should be used for insufflation to minimize the risk of embolization.

Intraductal Ultrasound Probes

Increased availability of high-frequency ultrasound probes has made it possible for experts to use these devices for evaluation of biliary strictures and to detect small stones and sludge. Endoscopic ultrasound probes are introduced freehand or over-the-wire (Fig. 4.25) through the working channel of the duodenoscope, allowing for "real-time" evaluation of biliary strictures and surrounding vascular structures. Limited data suggest that these probes can enhance the ability to

distinguish between benign and malignant biliary strictures (see Chapter 41). Patient selection, operator experience, and cost continue to be limiting factors to widespread use of this technology.

PROBE-BASED CONFOCAL LASER ENDOMICROSCOPY

Confocal laser endomicroscopy is a relatively new endoscopic imaging technique that enables the endoscopist to obtain in vivo histologic assessment. The probe-based system (Cholangioflex miniprobe by Mauna Kea Technologies, Paris, France) can be passed through the biopsy channel of cholangioscope or inside a catheter and enables real-time microscopic visualization of pancreaticobiliary strictures (Fig. 4.26).[33] Recently, consensus criteria have been developed for confocal laser to determine malignancy in biliary strictures (see Fig. 4.26).[34,35]

OTHER ACCESSORIES

Pharmacologic and chemical agents are not considered accessories in the classic definition. However, intravenous injection of secretin with or without the use of methylene blue sprayed on the papilla has been used to facilitate cannulation of the pancreatic duct, especially in patients with pancreas divisum (Fig. 4.27) (see Chapter 21). These agents are also helpful in identifying the pancreatic duct opening after biliary sphincterotomy or endoscopic ampullectomy. Glucagon and hyoscyamine often are used to relax motility and have been found to be of similar efficacy, but there are no placebo-controlled trials.

Radiographic Contrast Media Used in ERCP

High-osmolality and low-osmolality contrast media agents are used for pancreatography and cholangiography. Low-osmolality agents are considered safer than high-osmolality agents but this has not been confirmed in clinical studies. The risk of serious adverse reactions is related to the amount of contrast systemically absorbed. The rise in serum iodine concentration associated with contrast administration during ERCP is one-hundredth that seen with intravenous administration. Data on adverse reactions to contrast media used in ERCP are very limited and there is no evidence-based standard of practice for prophylaxis against contrast reactions during ERCP in patients who have experienced such reactions with intravenous administration. An ASGE guideline recommends preprocedural intravenous administration of prophylactic agents and/or use of low-osmolality contrast media during ERCP for patients considered at high risk for contrast media reactions.[36]

The Use of Carbon Dioxide in ERCP

Gas embolization is a rare but serious ERCP-related adverse event.[37] Reported risk factors for embolization during ERCP include cholangioscopy, sphincterotomy, metallic stent placement, prior biliary surgery, transhepatic portosystemic shunts, preexisting transhepatic drainage catheters, and transmural endoscopic necrosectomy.[38,39] It is reasonable to use CO_2 insufflation during ERCP instead of room air because of the rapid tissue absorption of CO_2 compared with room air, which minimizes risk of gas embolization. Although CO_2 embolization has been reported, it appears to be well tolerated and therefore CO_2 is preferred for insufflation during ERCP. Additional benefits of CO_2 insufflation during ERCP are less postprocedural distension and abdominal pain compared with air insufflation.[38] However, standard endoscopic systems marketed by all major manufacturers support air insufflation. Commercial CO_2 insufflators are available that can be integrated with currently available endoscopes. The ASGE published a technical review in reference to use of CO_2 in GI endoscopy.[39]

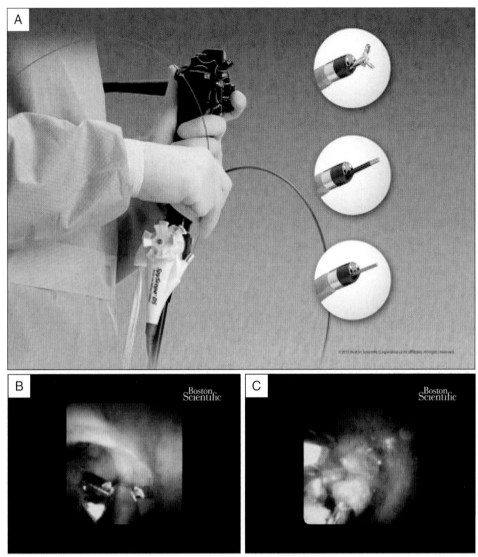

FIG 4.24 **A,** SpyGlass DS. **B,** SpyBite forceps. **C,** Lithotripsy probe. (**A,** Courtesy Boston Scientific, Natick, MA; **B,** Courtesy Boston Scientific, Natick, MA; **C,** Courtesy Boston Scientific, Natick, MA.)

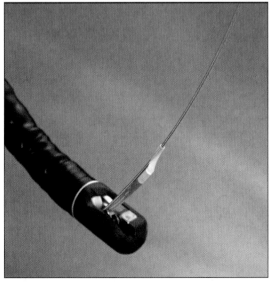

FIG 4.25 Intraductal ultrasound probe. (Courtesy Olympus America Inc., Center Valley, PA.)

Accessories for Use in Patients With Altered Anatomy

Standard accessories are designed for use with a duodenoscope and are usually 200 to 260 cm in length. However, in patients with surgically altered anatomy, such as Roux-en-Y gastroenteric and bilioenteric anastomoses, a standard ERCP duodenoscope may not be able to reach the ampulla, or biliary anastomosis, and the use of a longer endoscope such as a pediatric or adult colonoscope or enteroscope may be needed. Some accessories such as balloons, sphincterotomes, and push catheters are available in longer versions for this purpose (Cook Endoscopy and Olympus America Inc.). In addition, "reverse" sphincterotomes are available for use in patients with Billroth II–type anatomy. In most patients with Billroth II–type anatomy, however, sphincterotomy can be performed using standard accessories such as a needle knife (see Chapter 31). The endoscopist should ensure that appropriate accessories for an individual patient are available before initiating ERCP when long endoscopes are required.

Single-Use Versus Reusable Accessories

The choice between single-use, disposable, and reusable ERCP accessories depends on various medical and economic factors. Additionally, liability

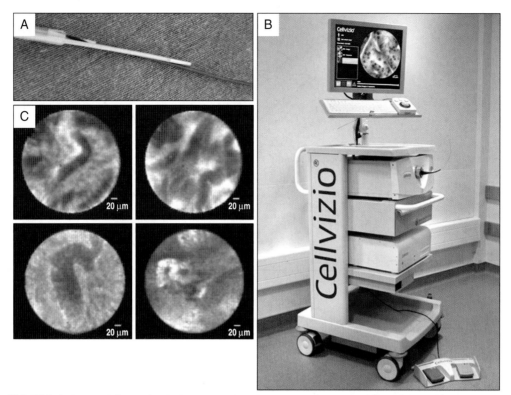

FIG 4.26 A, Cholangioflex probe. **B,** Probe-based confocal endomicroscopy system. **C,** Typical probe-based confocal laser endomicroscopy findings in biliary cancer. (**B,** Courtesy Mauna Kea Tech, Paris; **C,** Reprinted with permission from Wallace M, Lauwers GY, Chen Y, et al. Miami classification for probe-based confocal laser endomicroscopy. *Endoscopy.* 2011;43:882–891.)

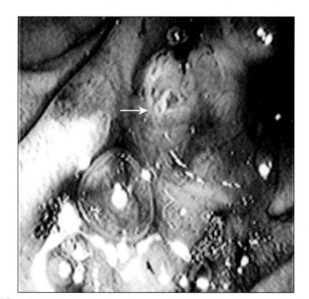

FIG 4.27 Endoscopic view showing identification of pancreatic duct orifice using methylene blue spray *(arrow).*

issues may result from reusing single-use devices. In several studies in which reuse of ERCP accessories was evaluated, a reusable sphincterotome could be safely and efficiently used. A disposable sphincterotome was cost-effective (compared with reprocessing) after 2.2 uses, and a reusable sphincterotome after 7.9 uses. According to a recent ASGE guideline on disposable endoscopic accessories, the selection of reusable or disposable devices must be based on local purchase costs, reprocessing costs and abilities, storage and disposable facilities, and personal preferences.[40]

Storage of Accessories

A specialized ERCP room with a fluoroscopy unit offers the advantage of a better floor plan, organization, and ready access to stored accessories required (see Chapter 2). The room is organized to facilitate equipment such as an endoscope/processor, monitors, echoendoscopes, cholangioscopes, and the fluoroscopy unit. The fluoroscopy and endoscopy monitors should be placed side-by-side at eye level to avoid the need for repeated turning of the head, which is ergonomically unsound and can displace the endoscope position. The dedicated ERCP room should be large enough to house and store accessories in locations that are properly labeled and easily accessible to the assistant during a procedure, which increases procedural efficiency.

ROLE OF THE U.S. FOOD AND DRUG ADMINISTRATION IN DEVICE EVALUATION AND MONITORING

The Center for Devices and Radiological Health (CDRH) is the component of the Food and Drug Administration (FDA) responsible for regulating medical devices. The CDRH reviews manufacturing processes, distribution, labeling, product evaluation, clinical investigation, premarket review, and postmarket performance review of medical devices. ERCP accessories are considered moderate-risk devices. The MedWatch program allows users, including patients and health care professionals, to report device-related adverse events to the FDA. Currently all reports are investigated and the results of the investigations are collected on the

Manufacturer and User Device Experience (MAUDE) database. The searchable database is available for public access. The role of the FDA in device evaluation and monitoring is discussed at length in a recent technology evaluation report by the ASGE.[41]

RADIATION EXPOSURE

ERCP relies on the use of fluoroscopy, but the risks associated with radiation exposure to patients and to personnel during the procedure are not well documented (see Chapter 3). A prospective study suggested that personnel as well as patients may be exposed to radiation doses that equate to an estimated additional lifetime fatal cancer risk of 1 in 3500 to 7000.[42] Radiation exposure to personnel is proportionally related to the distance from the beam and the duration of fluoroscopy. Higher voltage and lower current for fluoroscopy is used to minimize radiation exposure to personnel. Various other strategies that are used to minimize radiation exposure include protective lead shielding, the use of digital imaging, and an "undercouch" x-ray emitter tube. Radiation dose falls off exponentially as the distance from the source increases. Therefore the operator should be vigilant in avoiding prolonged use of fluoroscopy and, if possible, stand at a distance from the radiation source. Exposure to patients, particularly those at high risk, such as young patients and pregnant women (discussed further in Chapters 3, 29, and 30), can be minimized by shielding the pelvic area with a lead-lined apron. In addition, obtaining "held" digital fluoroscopic images in lieu of "hard-copy" images can further reduce exposure. Lower radiation exposure has been reported with single-frame fluoroscopy.[43] A recent study showed that fluoroscopy time is shorter when ERCP is performed by endoscopists with increasing experience both in years and in number of procedures.[44,45] Wire-guided biliary cannulation and choledochoscopy without the use of fluoroscopy are safe and effective in avoiding or minimizing radiation exposure in pregnant patients undergoing ERCP for symptomatic choledocholithiasis.[46] Ongoing quality assurance programs should be instituted with hospital radiation safety officers to monitor fluoroscopy use during ERCP.

The natural history of an endoscopic device involves an initial learning curve followed by rapid adoption and then a relatively slow phase of stability followed by incremental innovation (Fig. 4.28).[47] ERCP

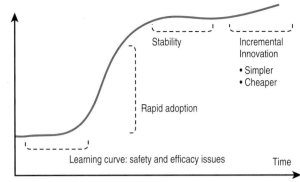

FIG 4.28 The natural history of an endoscopic device. (Reprinted with permission from Pasricha PJ. The future of therapeutic endoscopy. *Clin Gastroenterol Hepatol.* 2004;2:286–289.)

accessories have also followed this natural history. Major advances have been made over the last decade. In general, however, many "new" accessories are in fact evolutions of old ones as a result of innovations by endoscopists in collaboration with product engineers and specialists. In addition, several products developed for other intraluminal interventions (e.g., vascular, cardiac, and urologic diseases) have similar applications in ERCP. Guidewires and expandable metal stents are examples. Subsequently, some "new" accessories are applications or modifications of available products. This means that many products are approved using 510(k) premarket notification to the FDA. Many products may not have rigorous premarketing evaluation and their use may be based on word-of-mouth, personal experience, or, at best, case series. Major limitations continue to be cost compared with reimbursement and the lack of cost-effectiveness and premarketing studies. The FDA MedWatch program allows reporting of problems with medical devices, and health care professionals should make an effort to report such problems so that systemic problems can be discovered. Postmarket monitoring is imperative to ensure patient safety and clinical outcomes.

The complete reference list for this chapter can be found online at www.expertconsult.com.

5

Duodenoscope Reprocessing

Jennifer T. Higa, Michael Gluck, and Andrew S. Ross

An increasing amount of evidence suggests that Food and Drug Administration (FDA)–recommended measures for duodenoscope reprocessing are insufficient to guarantee against transmission of infection. As a result, improved techniques for endoscope reprocessing have attracted interest from many research groups. Reported outbreaks of endoscope-transmitted multidrug-resistant organisms (MDRO) emerged out of Europe and the United States in 2012 despite full compliance with reprocessing measures. Endoscopy-related infections are an established, although rare, risk. However, investigations into these recent outbreaks imputed infectious transmission to bioburden retained near the duodenoscope's cantilevered elevator mechanism. In spite of the connate risk associated with these devices and the difficulty of resolving what is, most likely, a multifactorial set of contamination conditions, ERCP remains a critical diagnostic and therapeutic platform that is, as yet, irreplaceable for the minimally invasive treatment of pancreaticobiliary disease. In this chapter, we review the historical context of such outbreaks, the federally mandated measures that followed, technical challenges inherent to duodenoscope reprocessing, and areas of ongoing research.

BACKGROUND

The pathogenic transmission potential for duodenoscopes has been a well-documented problem since the inception of ERCP, primarily because of the cantilevered elevator mechanism that confers the endoscope's utility within the pancreaticobiliary system.[1] This innately complex endoscope is difficult to clean, with a design precluding autoclave-based heat sterilization or high-temperature steam treatment. Although manufacturers are required to demonstrate that endorsed protocols result in a 6-$\log_{10}$ reduction in mycobacterium, which serves as a "surrogate marker for elimination of the risk of scope-to-person transmission of infectious agents,"[2] such accelerated failure testing may be insufficient, as multiple recent outbreaks have occurred in spite of adherence to published protocol standards. Overall rates of endoscope-transmitted infections remain very low, with one retrospective study reporting 1.8 nosocomial infections per 1 million procedures performed,[3] although this is considered an underestimate. Historical accounts of endoscope-transmitted infections are notable for unifying threads of reprocessing errors or noncompliance with manufacturer processing protocols[4–6] and failures of automated endoscope reprocessors. Also noted are issues with failures by personnel to comply with recommended strict manual reprocessing measures.[7,8]

HISTORY OF MDRO IN ENDOSCOPY

The early North American outbreaks of ERCP-related carbapenem-resistant Enterobacteriaceae (CRE) were attributed to breaches in protocol of high-level disinfection (HLD) and insufficient manual cleaning.[9,10] Endoscopy-related infections are neither novel nor unanticipated but rather an unfortunate reflection of the endoscope's complex design, heavy utilization, and intolerance to high-temperature sterilization. The organisms associated with nosocomial infections are primarily enteric gram-negative bacteria, though there have been transmitted cases of hepatitis B (1983) and hepatitis C viruses (1997).[11,12] Additionally, some bacterial species are prone to forming biofilms, a feature that further complicates the HLD process.

In 2012, serial outbreaks of CRE and other MDRO infections emerged despite proper reprocessing techniques and compliance with manufacturer recommendations. The incidences of MDRO infections were likely underreported because of difficulty in identifying outbreaks, given that many of the U.S.-based cases were characterized by unique antibiotic resistance patterns and clonality of bacteria found only by using polymerase chain reaction (PCR).[13] Outbreak sites were typically large, well-resourced medical centers with higher-volume endoscopy centers. Furthermore, county and state health departments assisted certain large urban centers with their investigations into outbreaks of clonally related MDRO (e.g., Seattle and Los Angeles). It is plausible that smaller sites without sophisticated resources would not have detected even a small series of patients infected.

Investigators from Erasmus hospital in the Netherlands were among the first to report this phenomenon, describing infections from a VIM-2–producing *Pseudomonas aeruginosa* after the introduction of the TJF-Q180V duodenoscope developed by Olympus Corporation in 2010.[14] Thirty patients were infected, with 22 of these cases singularly attributed to a newly introduced duodenoscope. After an exhaustive investigation, including dissection of the new endoscope using electron microscopy, the culprit duodenoscope was withdrawn from use and rates of infectious adverse events returned to baseline.

Subsequently, multiple medical centers published serial cases of patients infected with MDRO, including CRE, with a total of 19 U.S.-based outbreaks reported to date.[15] Outbreaks occurred in high-volume ERCP centers without identifiable lapses in reprocessing. The hospitals typically confirmed clonal relatedness of the organism using PCR, verifying that the likely mechanism of infection originated from a common source,[16–18] and culprit endoscopes were usually identified in each outbreak. To date, outbreaks have been documented with endoscopes produced by each of the three major manufacturers of commercially available duodenoscopes—namely, Olympus, Fujifilm, and Pentax.[14,19]

In 2012, a Seattle-based high-volume endoscopy center discovered a carbapenem-susceptible *Escherichia coli* with a unique resistance mechanism (hyperproduction of AmpC/HAC plus a porin mutation) during participation in a voluntary, statewide surveillance initiative.[20] Between October 2012 and November 2013, 1149 ERCPs were performed, and 32 cases of infection were reported. A collaborative investigation was undertaken between the medical center, city, and state public health departments and the Centers for Disease Control and Prevention. In 7 of the 32 cases "acute case deaths" occurred, defined as death occurring within the same hospital admission and within 30 days of isolate collection. Significantly higher rates of malignancy were noted among those deceased ($p = 0.01$), and carbapenem-resistant strains of AmpC *E. coli* had a greater mortality risk than did infection with carbapenem-susceptible strains ($p = 0.004$).[20] The institutional investigation revealed negative environmental cultures, with cleaning practices exceeding manufacturer's reprocessing guidelines. Two duodenoscopes were identified as vectors for the AmpC-producing *E. coli,* and using pulsed-field gel electrophoresis, clonality was confirmed identifying the pathogen's origins from the suspect devices. All duodenoscopes were submitted for manufacturer's inspection, and four of the eight endoscopes were found to have critical damage, although all were without any sign of operational defects. Such reports of occult mechanical defects are the reason to consider routine endoscopic maintenance and servicing, because critical damages may harbor infectious nidi.

As the result of these findings, the medical center implemented an overhaul of the endoscope reprocessing area and instituted a culture and quarantine process for all duodenoscopes, necessitating the purchase of 20 additional duodenoscopes. Ergonomic changes to scope reprocessing facilities were enacted to minimize worker fatigue and error, and other infection prevention measures—such as provider staff education, skill task alignment (periprocedural handling of endoscope by skilled technicians only), and routine endoscope maintenance checks—were mandated. Separate informed consent forms for duodenoscope use were implemented to increase patient awareness of procedural risks associated with duodenoscope use. All patients undergoing ERCP underwent screening bile and perianal cultures for MDRO. In total, instituting a method of culture and quarantine with HLD, making procedural changes, and adding a 1.0 full-time equivalent microbiology laboratory employee were achieved at a cost of $1 million to meet high ERCP volumes.[21]

After introducing the per-procedure culture and quarantine process, the Seattle-based center evaluated culture data from >2500 swab cultures collected from duodenoscopes. Twenty-nine tested positive for pathogenic bacteria (*Acinetobacter, Enterococcus, E. coli, Enterobacter, Pseudomonas* sp.); however, no subsequent infections were detected. Culture results were stratified into two classes of high-concern and low-concern organisms with requisite repeat reprocessing until negative for high-concern organisms. High-concern organisms were defined by Centers for Disease Control and Prevention (CDC) surveillance protocols[22] as noncontaminant, pathogenic microbes such as *Staphylococcus aureus, Streptococcus viridans, Enterococcus,* and other pathogenic enteric gram-negative organisms. In contrast, low-concern organisms carry a lower pathogenic potential and, when cultured from endoscopes, are usually regarded as contaminants. Endoscopes were not used until culture results returned. As previously discussed, these modifications required additional resources allocated to the microbiology laboratory, endoscopy staff training, and an increase in the number of duodenoscopes available for rotation. Despite the thorough overhaul of institutional, engineering, and personnel controls, an HLD defect rate was defined at 1.9% based on initial year testing.[21] The 20-month aggregate HLD rate (36 total positive cultures) for high-concern organisms ultimately yielded an HLD defect rate of 1.3%.[23]

HIGH-LEVEL DISINFECTION AND REPROCESSING

Endoscopy unit directors and infection prevention teams have had a long-standing focus on optimizing endoscope reprocessing to mitigate procedural risk. In 1968 the Spaulding classification deemed flexible endoscopes semicritical instruments, requiring that they meet the standards of HLD with demonstrated 6-$\log_{10}$ reduction in bioburden to minimize risk of transmission of infectious pathogens.[24] As estimates of bioburden after endoscope use (blood and lumenal secretions) range

from 10^5 to 10^{10} CFU/mL after clinical use,[25,26] the current HLD process focuses on volumetric reduction in bioburden by immediate postprocedure flushing and manual cleaning before automatic endoscope reprocessing (AER). However, it should be noted that HLD is defined as the elimination of >99% of pathogenic organisms, but not all; the previously mentioned MDRO outbreaks occurred in spite of compliance with manufacturer's reprocessing recommendations designed under HLD standards. Moreover, the 1.3% defect rate for HLD at the Seattle center demonstrates a nonzero risk of introducing pathogens during endoscopic procedures and in fact approaches a 2-$\log_{10}$ reduction.[23,27] Because of these realities, current standards for reprocessing and disinfection under HLD must be examined to determine whether risk mitigation strategies may be improved.

For this reason, some centers have opted for programs aimed at complete sterilization of endoscopes, though this approach represents unique challenges.[28] Endoscopes are heat sensitive, precluding conventional steam sterilization, and therefore low-temperature sterilization techniques must be used to preserve functionality of the equipment. Currently FDA-approved low-temperature methods include gas sterilization using ethylene oxide (EtO) and liquid chemical sterilization using peracetic acid.[29] AER protocols exist for EtO, glutaraldehyde, peracetic acid, hydrogen peroxide, chlorine dioxide, and the like, but are burdened by unique caveats. EtO sterilization systems have been implemented by some endoscopy centers in response to recent outbreaks; however, EtO is a significant occupational hazard with documented carcinogenic, teratogenic, and neurotoxic effects.[30] Peracetic acid–based sterilization is limited by cumbersome protocols and methods that have yet to be validated for duodenoscope use. Additionally, limited data exist on long-term efficacy and the sterilization defect rates using these agents. Recently one center reported a duodenoscope reprocessing failure rate of 1.2% after positive surveillance culture, and notably there was one positive surveillance culture for a CRE *Klebsiella pneumoniae* after 592 EtO sterilization cycles.[31] Although no patients were infected and the duodenoscope had no mechanical defects, the lingering question remains whether this finding represents a true defect rate in EtO sterilization versus incidental contamination or insufficient reduction of bioburden from the preceding HLD.

More recently developed biocides may offer sterilization methods with better utility but remain in nascent stages of clinical use. These include electrolyzed acid and superoxidized water, which are inexpensive, nontoxic, and nonirritating to biologic tissues, making them safer for reprocessing staff.[26,32] Work is being done to evaluate low-temperature liquid sterilization protocols using the FDA-approved peracetic acid–based system; encouraging results have been seen in early trials by using a "fractional cycle" of 50% sterilant exposure time in efforts to improve usability. If proven efficacious, the potential advantages of peracetic acid over EtO sterilization include decreased processing time, formal validation for use in duodenoscopes, lower risk of equipment damage, and decreased toxicity risk to staff.[33] Biocides, like hydrogen peroxide plasma or ozone gas, are potential options for the future, but these have yet to receive FDA approval for use on duodenoscopes, these are expensive to implement, and instrument tolerance has yet to be determined.

The technical challenge of sterilization is an important aspect of reprocessing, but procedural elements may be just as critical. A recent review highlighted the issue of residual disinfectants persisting in endoscope channels, potentially masking the presence of microbes and obscuring accurate postprocessing contamination assessments.[13] To prevent this, the incorporation of biocide neutralizer before obtaining surveillance cultures may be a necessary component of reprocessing protocols. One study using narrow-lumen tubing inoculated with enteric bacteria (thereby mimicking the long working channel of a duodenoscope) demonstrated a lackluster efficacy (39.7% and 35%, respectively) of gas sterilization using EtO gas or hydrogen peroxide gas plasma alone without any preceding HLD,[34] supporting the need for stringent manual cleaning with HLD before sterilization.[35]

Adenosine triphosphate (ATP), hemoglobin, carbohydrates, and other nonbiotic residual tissue markers have been proposed for testing reprocessing efficacy and vetting sterilization techniques. This too may be inadequate, as adequate cleaning does not guarantee sterility.[36–38] At present, trials using ATP bioluminescence have demonstrated poor correlation with culture results, and multiple reports of high false-negative rates using this modality limit its utility as a standalone surveillance method[22]; however, some internal guidelines recommend consideration for use.[39] Overall ATP bioluminescence and other biomarkers remain inappropriate as sole reprocessing quality indicators but may have potential as an adjunct quality metric pending availability of validated reprocessing measures.

REACTION FROM REGULATORY BODIES

After the Erasmus and Chicago outbreaks,[14,16] the CDC alerted the FDA to the evolving association between duodenoscopes and CRE/MDRO infections occurring despite adherence to manufacturer endoscope care instructions (Fig. 5.1).[40] Subsequently, the CDC engaged with professional gastroenterology societies, the FDA, and field experts in early 2014 to address the need for industry guidance in the face of these critical issues. The FDA propagated regulatory discussions with industry groups, prompting updated reprocessing instructions and expert panel recommendations.[41]

Inquiries by U.S.-based, high-volume ERCP centers into the trend of scope-related infections started as early as December 2012. Although multiple high-volume ERCP centers had filed reports with the FDA as early as January 2013 about MDRO infections related to ERCP, these centers were working in isolation from each other. Mass media was instrumental in catalyzing responses from government and industry authorities and continues to report on the evolving process between federal regulatory bodies, the medical community, and duodenoscope manufacturers Olympus, Pentax, and Fujifilm.[42,43] In March 2015, the CDC published an "Interim Duodenoscope Surveillance Protocol,"[22] proposing measures for sampling and culture surveillance intended for adaptive use by endoscopy centers, followed shortly thereafter by a validated manual reprocessing guideline from Olympus Corporation.[44]

Small-bristled brushes specifically designed for improved manual reprocessing of the 160 and 180 series duodenoscopes were mandated, as well as the recommendation by Olympus of more vigorous flushing to address the elevator mechanism recess. In May 2015, the FDA convened a public forum; the "Gastroenterology and Urology Devices Panel of the Medical Devices Advisory Committee Meeting" intended to seek scientific and expert opinion on reprocessing strategies that were reflected in the August 4, 2015, keystone FDA publication, "Supplemental Measures to Enhance Duodenoscope Reprocessing."[45] In conjunction with strict adherence to manufacturers' reprocessing instructions, the updated supplemental measures suggest, but do not mandate, the following: microbiologic culturing, EtO sterilization, liquid chemical sterilant processing system, and (empiric) repeat HLD. In January 2016, the Olympus Corporation announced the recall and intended retrofit of the forceps elevator mechanism on all TJF-Q180V duodenoscopes.[46]

STRATEGIES FOR RISK REDUCTION

ERCP remains an essential diagnostic and treatment modality in the face of high-risk surgical alternatives. What operational strategies do we currently have to reduce the risk of infectious transmission? Elimination of biofilm formation is a proven mitigating factor to decrease risk of infection transmission and is used as one justification for endoscope and equipment surveillance.[47] The CDC currently recommends surveilling duodenoscopes with postreprocessing cultures after 60 procedures; however, this recommendation and frequency of culturing have not been validated. Many iterations of the per-procedure culture and quarantine have evolved—bespoke protocols suited to each institution's needs and resources.[48] Surveillance practices have evolved as well, with attempted streamlining by CDC guidelines. However, many recommendations from governing bodies are formed from expert opinion, reflecting pragmatism rather than established evidence-based practice. Careful attention should be paid to reprocessing efforts and their integrity. One group evaluating the efficacy of HLD at a single center endorsed assessments of germicidal activity of the glutaraldehyde component of the HLD using test strips for every five AER cycles plus scheduled servicing of the AER machinery every 3 to 6 months.[49]

Many publications emerged questioning the feasibility of implementing the stringent and complex protocols mandated by CDC guidelines.

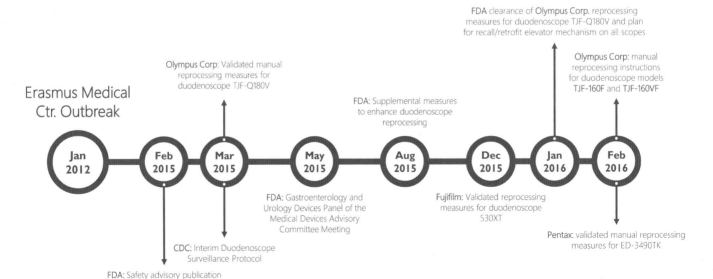

FIG 5.1 Timeline of safety and advisory publications.

To address these issues, one group proposed a novel and user-friendly alternative protocol to the CDC protocol in order to improve detection of duodenoscope carriage of pathogenic organisms.[50] Using a modified ESGE protocol (MEP), the authors demonstrated a 64.1% recovery rate of gram-negative organisms compared with 32.9% using the CDC protocol. For gram-positive organisms, there were equivalent recovery rates of 60% from both MEP and CDC protocols, showing that equivalent or improved rates of recovery of pathogenic organisms are possible using more easily implemented, less-complex protocols. Furthermore, differences in recovery rates were of greatest significance for *P. aeruginosa* (80.3% MEP vs 46.2% CDC, $p = 0.04$) and *K. pneumoniae* (66.0% MEP vs 32.1% CDC, $p = 0.001$) at 100 CFU/scope, whereas recovery rates for *E. coli* approached significance, suggesting that these protocols are particularly suitable for eliminating microorganisms associated with endoscopic infection risk and that currently recommended methods for surveillance can be refined to improve usability without compromising recovery of a wide range of pathogenic organisms.

Interpreting culture results is also important for refining reprocessing measures, and specific results offer some insight into reprocessing steps where breakdowns may be occurring. A quality assurance publication from the ESGE-ESGENA (2007) provides interpretative guidance for endoscope surveillance culture results: Enterobacteriaceae (insufficient HLD), *P. aeruginosa* (insufficient final rinse/drying before storage), *Staphylococci* sp. (endoscope recontamination), *Legionella* sp. or atypical Mycobacteria (contamination of water systems, washer-disinfector apparatus), and so forth.[39,51] Furthermore, despite efforts to refine the surveillance process,[50] there remains an as-yet-undefined correlate between endoscope culture positivity and degree of infectivity. Thus an informed consent specifically created for instances when an endoscope with elevator mechanism is to be used is an opportunity for full procedural disclosure and a chance to admit inability to completely mitigate risk within the current standard of care. Further work is being done to evaluate patients at higher risk for such endoscope-related infections. A recent retrospective analysis of all CRE cases at one high-volume center found that significant patient risk factors associated with CRE transmission from a contaminated duodenoscope include antibiotic exposure, active inpatient status, cholangiocarcinoma, and biliary stent placement.[52]

Culture and quarantine programs have been criticized as cost-prohibitive and lacking technical feasibility for use in smaller-volume centers.[53] One recent cost analysis of competing strategies—culture and quarantine versus FDA reprocessing guidelines versus EtO sterilization versus surgical laparoscopy (i.e., halting ERCP completely)—demonstrated that for symptomatic common bile duct stones, the FDA reprocessing procedures were the least expensive, citing a $69 duodenoscope reprocessing strategy cost (vs culture and quarantine $400 vs EtO sterilization $1044).[54] The surgical alternative of laparoscopic cholecystectomy with bile duct exploration for CBD stones was the least effective and most costly of all strategies. ERCP with EtO sterilization for CBD stones exceeded $50.5 million per additional QALY gained compared with culture and quarantine at >$4.2 million per additional quality-adjusted life year (QALY) gained. Furthermore, early data suggest that EtO sterilization is imperfect as well, with one center publishing 1/645 (0.16%) rate of endoscope-positive cultures for their EtO-based reprocessing.[31] Although the positively cultured endoscope became negative after repeat sterilization, these results suggest a need for surveillance despite adherence to rigorous sterilization protocols. One recent review summarized advantages and disadvantages of HLD versus sterilization and other enhancements for endoscope reprocessing.[48] The numerous unvetted options leave most centers operating without clear guidance or easily implementable strategies.

Once outbreaks are confirmed, a root-cause analysis and institutional evaluation of the reprocessing and surveillance protocols should be undertaken. Outbreaks should be carefully investigated to assure compliance with safety measures. It is important to remember that negative surveillance cultures do not absolve the endoscope as the source of infection. Furthermore, manufacturer evaluation of the endoscope should be undertaken even in the absence of obvious dysfunction.[21]

POTENTIAL SOLUTIONS

Advancements in endoscope (re-)design and sterilization techniques are needed to assure greater safety for patients undergoing ERCP/therapeutic endoscopic ultrasonography. Although medical centers with reported MDRO/CRE infections are predominantly high-volume ERCP centers, patients of small-volume centers remain at a stochastically elevated risk, perhaps even higher than those receiving care in a center equipped with the resources to implement an aggressive culture and quarantine program.

We propose the following considerations for endoscopy centers looking to enact compliance with CDC recommendations and minimize risk. All levels of staff and administration should be involved in the process to evaluate and improve reprocessing measures, be it prophylactic or after an outbreak. Staff training and competency must be prioritized with consideration given to direct observation and feedback by outside organizations to vet reprocessing measures. There is substantial merit in offering staff certification in flexible endoscope reprocessing as well. Other measures to consider for implementation include skill task alignment, ergonomic workspace optimization, and a feedback process for all levels of staff to report system problems in a nonthreatening manner.

An obvious long-term solution is a design change eliminating the current elevator mechanism. However, there are no impending solutions at this time and such a change is likely many years from feasibility. Interim solutions include enhanced cleaning methods, quality metrics and redundancy built into the reprocessing procedures, exhaustive informed consent, and routine maintenance of endoscopes. Other potential solutions include modifications to the duodenoscope that improve tolerance for high-temperature sterilization, validation and FDA approval for alternative low-temperature gas or liquid chemical sterilization protocols, increasing disposable endoscope components, and adjunctive tools for reprocessing. Based on previously published data, a double-cycle HLD process would produce a 1-log reduction of persistent infections[21]; however, this is not a zero-risk solution and therefore not a good long-term option. One recent publication from a single high-volume endoscopy center described their protocol including double-reprocessing with manual cleaning and HLD for all elevator mechanism–based endoscopes, with EtO sterilization for any positive-culture duodenoscopes (i.e., two consecutive positive cultures for any microorganism and empirically for patient-carriers of CRE).[55] During the study period, 329 duodenoscopes were randomly selected for culture and quarantine, rather than performed for each procedural encounter. They described a 9.1% culture rate ($n = 30$), with only two of those being potentially pathogenic organisms (0.6%). A recent report from a 21-site health system providing 30 days of surveillance data found that 201 of 4032 (5%) specimens cultured positive for any microbes, and 0.6% cultured positive for enteric bacterial pathogens (without any MDRO), despite adhering to manufacturer-recommended HLD practices.[56] These results suggest an ongoing need to refine HLD practices and guidelines.

CONCLUSIONS

Existing manufacturer-recommended HLD protocols are inadequate to guarantee pathogen-free instruments. However, optimizing these measures remains the most judicious strategy to allow ongoing delivery of ERCP, a platform that remains necessary and considerably lower risk compared with other treatment alternatives. At high-volume ERCP centers, patients are referred for complex procedural care that is often life-saving, palliative, or surgery-sparing. Halting the practice of ERCP is not a reasonable option to mitigate infection risk.

The issues of adequate duodenoscope reprocessing, appropriate surveillance, and outbreak protocols will remain relevant because the problems are likely related to the inherent complexity and resulting deficiencies in the design of the duodenoscope and inadequacies in the HLD process. What is the proper recourse for lower-volume centers where this plan may not be feasible for financial or logistical reasons? Portions of the changes implemented at high-volume centers may be tailored to smaller practices until improved duodenoscope designs arrive. Still needed are a validated manufacturer-recommended schedule for routine duodenoscope maintenance and reprocessing protocols that can be implemented in the vast majority of endoscopy units (with reasonable equipment and operational costs). The ideal program would balance safety for both patients and technicians while providing early indicators of endoscope contamination so that they can be rectified before patient use. These changes will undoubtedly take time and effort, plus demonstrable and quantifiable evidence of improvement to regain and rebuild patient and professional trust.

The complete reference list for this chapter can be found online at www.expertconsult.com.

6

Sedation in ERCP

Catherine D. Tobin and Gregory A. Coté

Unlike routine endoscopic procedures, endoscopic retrograde cholangiopancreatography (ERCP) combines several unique challenges. Despite defined indications, the complexity and length of each procedure are often difficult to predict because of unforeseen challenges with cannulation and subsequent therapy. Patients are usually in the prone position to maintain a stable, short endoscope position. In addition, the prone position and overlying fluoroscopy unit make airway monitoring and interventions difficult, particularly with an acute decline in the patient's respiratory status. Furthermore, many indications for ERCP are associated with a functional or mechanical gastric outlet obstruction, increasing the risk for periprocedural aspiration. Finally, the obesity epidemic and the rising prevalence of overt and subclinical obstructive sleep apnea (OSA) result in a high-risk patient population for sedation-related adverse events (AEs). For these reasons, the endoscopist must be meticulous in assessing preprocedure risk to determine the optimal approach to sedation for ERCP. This chapter will discuss (1) the approaches to sedation during ERCP, including the rationales for anesthesia-administered sedation and empirical endotracheal intubation; (2) risk assessment for sedation-related AEs; and (3) methods for attenuating this risk.

DEFINING THE CONTINUUM OF SEDATION

Sedation is typically characterized using the American Society of Anesthesiologists (ASA) Continuum of Sedation, which defines four discrete levels of sedation (Table 6.1).[1] Depth is most frequently defined by patient responsiveness to voice, light tactile stimulation, and painful stimulation during the procedure. However, the corresponding cardiopulmonary sequelae of this degree of awareness do not directly translate into the probability of sedation-related AEs. In moderate (also known as "conscious") sedation, patients may be sleeping but will have purposeful response to tactile stimuli, yet may not respond to voice. In patients who are deeply sedated, this response occurs only after repeated or painful stimuli. Patients who do not respond to painful stimuli even if they are breathing on their own are by definition under general anesthesia. *Monitored anesthesia care* (MAC) is a term often used when talking about sedation. MAC does not describe the level of sedation; it just means that a trained anesthesia provider was involved in the care and the administration of drugs. In reality, a patient's level of sedation rarely meets only one of these definitions during the course of endoscopy, and these levels actually represent a continuum. The amount of sedation administered to achieve moderate sedation often inadvertently leads to deep sedation.[2] Similarly, patients who are targeted for deep sedation often meet criteria for general anesthesia.

Many patients undergoing ERCP often require deep sedation, as opposed to the light or moderate sedation that is usually adequate for colonoscopy or esophagogastroduodenoscopy. ERCP procedures are typically longer in duration and require less spontaneous patient movement to achieve technical success. In a study serially assessing sedation depth during ERCP, 85% of patients met criteria for deep sedation during a segment of the procedure.[2] Consequently, the ASA recommends that the sedation provider be adequately trained in rescue maneuvers commensurate with one level of sedation *higher* than the intended target. Therefore patients targeted for deep sedation should be managed by a provider who is trained in the administration of general anesthesia.[3] This would include management in bag mask ventilation, laryngeal mask airway placement, and endotracheal intubation. The Centers for Medicaid & Medicare Services (CMS) have endorsed this recommendation, releasing a clarification letter to their policy on hospital anesthesia services in 2010 after the major gastrointestinal (GI) societies in the United States made a concerted effort to endorse nonanesthesiologist-administered propofol for low-risk patients undergoing standard endoscopy.[4,5]

The current options for sedation in ERCP can be simplified into two categories: endoscopist-administered sedation and anesthesiologist-administered sedation. Computerized sedation systems that incorporate real-time patient feedback have been evaluated for standard endoscopic procedures but have not been investigated for patients undergoing ERCP.[6] Because propofol can be administered only by anesthesia providers in the United States, endoscopist-administered sedation implies moderate sedation using conventional agents such as the combination of a benzodiazepine (e.g., midazolam) and an opiate (e.g., fentanyl or meperidine). Of note, benzodiazepine can be reversed by flumazenil and opioids by naloxone in the event of oversedation. Anesthesiologists may choose between general anesthesia with endotracheal intubation at the onset of the procedure and general anesthesia with use of a nasal cannula and having the patient breathe spontaneously during the procedure. In the latter scenario, patients are typically sedated using a propofol-based regimen, with a goal of achieving deep sedation or general anesthesia. Endoscopists increasingly prefer anesthesia-administered sedation for all endoscopic procedures. The growing role of propofol in endoscopic practice is reflected in epidemiologic data demonstrating a consistent increase in anesthesia-administered sedation.[7,8] The overuse of anesthesia services for colonoscopy is under increased scrutiny.[9] With a greater emphasis on cost-effectiveness in health care, judicious use of anesthesia will mandate an improved preprocedure risk assessment; this is particularly important in ERCP, where the potential for sedation-related complications is highest.

Initially approved for the induction and maintenance of anesthesia, propofol (2,6-diisopropylphenol) has become an increasingly popular sedative for endoscopic procedures because of its rapid onset of action (30 to 45 seconds) and short duration of effect (4 to 8 minutes).[10,11] In the United States, propofol is currently restricted to anesthesiologists and some emergency medicine physicians because of its relative potency, lack of an antagonist, and potential for rapid change in the depth of sedation from moderate sedation to general anesthesia. Nevertheless, in a meta-analysis of 12 trials of propofol sedation during routine

TABLE 6.1 ASA Continuum of Sedation[1]

	Minimal Sedation/ Anxiolysis	Moderate Sedation/Analgesia ("Conscious" Sedation)	Deep Sedation/Analgesia	General Anesthesia
Responsiveness	Normal response to verbal stimulation	Purposeful response to verbal or light tactile stimulation	Purposeful response after repeated or painful stimulation*	Unarousable even with painful stimulus
Airway	Unaffected	No intervention required	Intervention may be required	Intervention often required
Spontaneous ventilation	Unaffected	Adequate	May be inadequate	Frequently inadequate
Cardiovascular function	Unaffected	Usually maintained	Usually maintained	May be impaired

ASA, American Society of Anesthesiologists.

*Reflex withdrawal from a painful stimulus is *not* considered a purposeful response.

Because sedation is a continuum, it is not always possible to predict how an individual patient will respond. Hence, practitioners intending to produce a given level of sedation should be able to rescue patients whose level of sedation becomes deeper than initially intended. Individuals administering moderate sedation/analgesia ("conscious" sedation) should be able to rescue patients who enter a state of deep sedation/ analgesia, whereas those administering deep sedation/analgesia should be able to rescue patients who enter a state of general anesthesia. Rescue of a patient from a deeper level of sedation than intended is an intervention by a practitioner proficient in airway management and advanced life support. The qualified practitioner corrects adverse physiologic consequences of the deeper-than-intended level of sedation (e.g., hypoventilation, hypoxia, and hypotension) and returns the patient to the originally intended level of sedation. It is not appropriate to continue a procedure at an unintended level of sedation (adapted from ASA guidelines with approval).[1]

TABLE 6.2 ASA Physical Status Classification System[17]

Class	Definition
1	A normal healthy patient (i.e., healthy, nonsmoking, no or minimal alcohol use)
2	A patient with mild systemic disease (examples include [but are not limited to] current smoker, social alcohol drinker, pregnancy, obesity [30 < BMI < 40], well-controlled DM or HTN, mild lung disease)
3	A patient with severe systemic disease (examples include [but are not limited to] poorly controlled DM or HTN, COPD, morbid obesity [BMI ≥40], active hepatitis, alcohol dependence or abuse, implanted pacemaker, moderate reduction of ejection fraction, ESRD undergoing regularly scheduled dialysis, premature infant PCA <60 weeks, and history [>3 months] of MI, CVA, TIA, or CAD/stents)
4	A patient with severe systemic disease that is a constant threat to life (examples include [but are not limited to] recent (<3 months) MI, CVA, TIA, or CAD/stents; ongoing cardiac ischemia or severe valve dysfunction; severe reduction of ejection fraction; sepsis; DIC; ARD or ESRD; and not undergoing regularly scheduled dialysis)
5	A moribund patient who is not expected to survive without the operation (examples include [but are not limited to] ruptured abdominal/thoracic aneurysm, massive trauma, intracranial bleed with mass effect, ischemic bowel in the face of significant cardiac pathology, or multiple organ/system dysfunction)
6	A declared brain-dead patient whose organs are being removed for donor purposes

ARD, Acute renal disease; *ASA*, American Society of Anesthesiologists; *BMI*, body mass index; *CAD*, coronary artery disease; *COPD*, chronic obstructive lung disease; *CVA*, cerebral vascular accident; *DIC*, disseminated intravascular coagulation; *DM*, diabetes mellitus; *ESRD*, end-stage renal disease; *HTN*, hypertension; *MI*, myocardial ischemia; *PCA*, postconceptual age; *TIA*, transient ischemia attack.

An addition of "E" denotes emergency surgery. An "E" is noted after the ASA number (e.g., ASA 3E). (An emergency is defined as existing when delay in treatment of the patient would lead to a significant increase in the threat to life or body part.)

endoscopy, endoscopic ultrasonography (EUS), and ERCP, the overall rate of cardiopulmonary AEs was lower than that of standard combination opiate–benzodiazepine regimens.[12]

There are several unique characteristics of ERCP compared with other endoscopic procedures that may accentuate the benefits of propofol. Specifically, ERCPs tend to be longer in duration and require sustained patient cooperation in order to achieve technical success.[13] Longer procedures require higher cumulative doses of benzodiazepines and opiates to maintain moderate sedation, which translates into longer recovery times.

DEFINING SEDATION-RELATED COMPLICATIONS (ADVERSE EVENTS)

Adverse events (AEs) specifically related to sedation are usually classified in the literature by objective criteria such as oxygen desaturation, aspiration, laryngospasm, apnea, hypotension, arrhythmia, myocardial ischemia, and need for airway rescue maneuvers or reversal agents. Mortality data related to sedation in endoscopy are sparse, particularly in ERCP. The risk of death is probably close to 0.03% for patients undergoing standard endoscopy using conventional sedation regimens.[14] Fewer studies track the frequency of airway rescue maneuvers, such as a chin lift, nasal trumpet insertion, and transient positive pressure (i.e., bag-mask) ventilation.[15] These may be performed as a preventive maneuver in anticipation of hypoxemia or apnea and reflect the importance of having a sedation provider experienced in airway rescue. Rates of conversion from nasal cannula to endotracheal intubation during administration of intravenous propofol during ERCP are less defined, although a study of 528 patients undergoing ERCP with MAC reported a 3% incidence of unplanned endotracheal intubation.[16] In a cohort study that included all endoscopic procedures performed during a 5-year period, patients with a higher ASA class[17] (Table 6.2) and those undergoing ERCP were more likely to require reversal agents such as flumazenil or naloxone.[18]

RISK ASSESSMENT

A thorough preprocedure assessment of patient risk before ERCP can be challenging, particularly for patients with urgent or emergent indications. ASA guidelines acknowledge the dearth of publications confirming the value of the preprocedure assessment in reducing sedation-related AEs, but expert consultants strongly agree that this is a vital precursor for all procedures requiring sedation. Identifying risk factors for sedation-related complications should help the endoscopist determine the need for an anesthesiologist. The endoscopist should always conduct a focused history to assess for significant organ dysfunction (with a particular emphasis on the cardiopulmonary system), cervical spine disease, OSA, fasting interval, and prior substance abuse. Because more than 30% of Americans are overweight or obese, the incidence of subclinical sleep apnea may be 10% or greater.[19,20] A bedside assessment for OSA risk, such as the STOP-BANG instrument, can identify patients who are at higher risk for needing active airway management during the procedure.[21,22] In this questionnaire, the patient is asked about snoring (S), feeling tired (T), observed apnea (O), high blood pressure (P), body mass index >35 kg/m^2 (B), age above 50 years (A), neck circumference >16 inches (N), and male gender (G). The physical assessment should include a routine examination of the heart and lungs along with a dedicated examination of the airway, head, and neck. Particular features that portend a more complex airway include a macrognathia, trismus, short chin–sternal notch distance, and large uvula. The Mallampati score (0 to 4)[23] is a validated bedside tool to assess airway risk. A summary of selected features associated with sedation-related AEs and difficult airway assessments to evaluate on preprocedure history and physical examination is in Table 6.3.[15] Although vague, the ASA physical status classification system is another bedside tool to gauge risk, with scores of 3 or greater being associated with a higher probability of sedation-related complications (see Table 6.2).[8] One must consider that when a patient is at higher risk for sedation-related complications, use of the anesthesia team may be needed because of endotracheal intubation or airway management.

In addition to patient factors, the endoscopist should also consider the indication for ERCP and estimated procedure length when choosing the optimal sedation strategy. Although anticipating the complexity of ERCP is often challenging, specific indications such as stent removal and stent exchange in a patient with prior sphincterotomy are almost always of short duration; these patients may not be critically ill and often undergo the procedure in the ambulatory setting. In these cases, the threshold to use anesthesia assistance or adjunct medications to supplement a standard combination regimen is much lower. Situations that may be advisable to incorporate the anesthesia team include end-stage liver disease patients with cirrhosis and massive ascites, patients on high-dose chronic opioids, high preprocedure baseline pain, and sepsis. These patients may be at risk for aspiration, airway obstruction, hypotension requiring vasopressors, or higher dose opioids than normal. For drainage of a large pancreatic fluid collection (e.g., pseudocyst), we prefer to perform empiric endotracheal intubation because of the anticipated influx of pancreatic juice into the stomach.

ANESTHESIOLOGIST-ADMINISTERED SEDATION

With an estimated 1 death per 200,000 to 300,000 anesthetics administered, the safety profile of general anesthesia is excellent[24]; however, there are limited data regarding the safety of anesthesiologist-administered sedation specifically during ERCP.[13,16,25,26] For patients in the prone position undergoing ERCP, some anesthesiologists are reluctant to deliver MAC by intravenous sedation without a secured airway because it is difficult to maintain a patent airway, to monitor respirations, and to gain access to the airway in an emergency. Although monitoring chest wall excursions is more difficult in ERCP with the overlying fluoroscopy equipment, the prone position is not an independent predictor of sedation-related complications and in fact may confer some protection against aspiration versus patients who are supine.[15,27] There is a perceived higher risk of aspiration when the patient is supine as opposed to prone when not intubated endotracheally. The left lateral decubitus position may confer less risk of aspiration than supine, but this confounds the acquisition of fluoroscopic images. Airway obstruction occurs less often in the prone position than in the supine position because the tongue rests off the hard palate. When administered by an experienced provider, anesthesiologist-administered intravenous propofol without an endotracheal tube has a favorable safety profile for sedation during ERCP and other advanced endoscopic procedures.[15,16] Lastly, the experience of and consistent staffing with the same anesthesia providers minimizes the risk of hypoxemia during deep sedation and reduces facility costs as a result of room efficiency.[28]

The decision to perform empiric endotracheal intubation before commencing ERCP is made on a case-by-case basis. Endotracheal intubation is preferred for patients at high risk for aspiration, airway obstruction, and oxygen desaturation. Patients with OSA and obesity should be intubated because of a high likelihood of desaturation from upper airway obstruction. Risk factors for aspiration include patients with delayed gastric emptying and patients with gastric outlet obstruction; examples would include patients using opioids, late-term pregnancy, diabetic gastroparesis, obesity, and nonfasting state (Table 6.4). Fasting recommendations are guidelines and do not assure complete gastric emptying. Certain disease states, such as diabetic and nondiabetic

TABLE 6.3 Factors Associated With Sedation-Related Complications

History	Physical Examination	Scoring Instruments
Previous problems with sedation/anesthesia	Short neck with limited neck extension	ASA Physical Status Classification system
Cardiac disease (e.g., aortic stenosis)	Decreased hyoid-mental distance (<3 cm in adults)	Mallampati score
Pulmonary disease	Trismus	Body-mass index
Obstructive sleep apnea (consider use of a bedside screening instrument)	Macroglossia	STOP-BANG (bedside tool to assess risk of Obstructive Sleep Apnea)
Difficulties with positive-pressure ventilation or endotracheal intubation	Tonsillar hypertrophy	
Advanced rheumatologic disease	Micrognathia	
Advanced osteoarthritic cervical spine disease	Obesity	
	Edentulous	
	Full beard	

ASA, American Society of Anesthesiologists.

TABLE 6.4   Fasting Guidelines Recommended by ASA[29]

Meal	Minimum Fasting Time (hr)	Examples
Clear liquids	2	Black coffee, tea, apple juice, nonpulp juice
Breast milk	4	
Infant formula	6	
Nonhuman milk	6	
Light meal	6	Dry toast and clear liquid

ASA, American Society of Anesthesiologists.

TABLE 6.5   Modified Observer's Assessment of Alertness/Sedation (MOAA/S)[44]

Score	Definition	Correlation With ASA Continuum of Sedation
5	Responsive and alert	Minimal sedation
4	Lethargic, but responsive to normal verbal command	Moderate sedation
3	Responsive to loud verbal command	
2	Responsive to shaking only	Deep sedation
1	Unresponsive to shaking	

ASA, American Society of Anesthesiologists.

gastroparesis, may delay emptying, and one should consider extending the recommended timelines.[29]

Other considerations for empiric endotracheal intubation include patients who have recently undergone surgery, severe pain at baseline, and anticipated very long or high-risk procedure. Finally, certain pulmonary conditions that often mandate empiric endotracheal intubation include patients with a home oxygen requirement and pulmonary hypertension of any etiology, the latter to avoid hypercarbia, which would worsen the pulmonary vascular resistance. Cardiac conditions such as presence of coronary stents, history of myocardial ischemia, and cardiomyopathy do not mandate empiric endotracheal intubation, unless the patient is at risk for hypoxemia for reasons outlined earlier. A laryngeal mask airway could minimize the risk of upper airway obstruction but does not mitigate the risk of aspiration.[30]

NONANESTHESIOLOGIST (ENDOSCOPIST)–ADMINISTERED SEDATION

In most facilities, ASA practice guidelines for sedation administered by nonanesthesiologists are used as the standard for local practices such as preprocedure evaluation and duration of fasting.[1] The ASA periodically releases guidelines for institutions that are responsible for granting privileges to administer sedation.[3,31] Endoscopist-directed sedation in ERCP generally refers to the use of a combination of benzodiazepines and opiates targeted for moderate sedation. Advantages of this combination include the ability to administer reversal agents in the event of a sedation-related AE, amnestic effect, and sustained analgesia during the postprocedure recovery period (typically several hours). In cases where these agents cannot provide adequate depth or duration of sedation to complete the procedure, the addition of antihistamines (e.g., diphenhydramine or promethazine) and droperidol, among others, may be used.[32–34] Use of antihistamines increases the likelihood of requiring reversal agents by potentiating the risk of apnea. Although still used in some endoscopy units, droperidol has fallen out of favor because of QT interval prolongation and potential for ventricular arrhythmia. That being said, conventional agents are limited by their slower onset of action compared with propofol-based regimens, difficulty in titration during prolonged ERCP, and limited efficacy. This is compounded by a higher risk of AEs among patients using opiate medications before the procedure, which is particularly common in patients undergoing ERCP. This is because of obstructive pathology of the pancreatobiliary tree (e.g., stones, tumors) causing pain at the time of clinical presentation. ERCP technical success rate is significantly higher when patients are sedated using general anesthesia compared with moderate sedation regimens as a result of improved sedation.[13] Hence, there is a growing trend in the use of propofol-based sedation in ERCP.

MONITORING

The ASA and Joint Commission standards require a qualified individual, other than the person performing the procedure, be present to monitor the patient throughout the procedure.[1,35] For patients targeted for moderate sedation, the individual administering sedation may execute focused, interruptible tasks during the procedure; when deep sedation is intended, the individual must have no other responsibilities and be trained in the administration of general anesthesia.

Standard monitoring equipment for all patients should include continuous pulse oximetry, 3-lead or 5-lead electrocardiography, and a noninvasive blood pressure cuff.[36] In addition, capnography is now recommended by the ASA for all patients targeted for moderate sedation or greater. Carbon dioxide monitoring via a transcutaneous electrode[37] or capnography[38,39] has been studied in ERCP in an effort to recognize hypopnea or apnea before the onset of hypoxemia. Capnography represents end-tidal carbon dioxide ($ETCO_2$) and is a real-time monitor of every inhalation and exhalation. Normal $ETCO_2$ is 35 to 45 mm Hg, and watching the curve is more important than the number when it is used to monitor sedation. If apnea or airway obstruction develops, $ETCO_2$ will drop immediately, yet pulse oximetry may take minutes to reflect hypoxemia caused by apnea/hypopnea. Therefore, when using capnography, one can react faster to address the etiology of airway problems before they have permanent and dangerous outcomes. A meta-analysis of five studies that included a variety of procedures, including endoscopy, found that the use of capnography increased the detection rate of respiratory depression.[40] Capnography reduces the incidence of severe hypoxemia or apnea in patients using a propofol-based regimen or a standard combination of benzodiazepine and opiate. In healthy individuals, the benefit of capnography during standard endoscopic procedures in healthy individuals using moderate sedation is questionable.[41,42] Still, economic models based on existing data suggest that it may be cost-effective.[43] Given the complexities of sedation specific to ERCP, universal use of capnography should be strongly considered.

A quantitative measure of sedation depth is the Modified Observer's Assessment of Alertness/Sedation (MOAA/S) score (Table 6.5).[44] This scale from 1 to 5 reflects patient responsiveness alone, and no studies to date have evaluated the impact of frequent measurements (e.g., every 2 minutes) of the MOAA/S score on sedation-related outcomes. Because frequent assessments of patient alertness are already compulsory in ERCP, the utility of MOAA/S is probably limited to research as a tool for quickly measuring sedation depth but not as an instrument for titrating sedation per se. Nevertheless, this is a reminder of the importance of frequent interval assessments throughout the procedure to

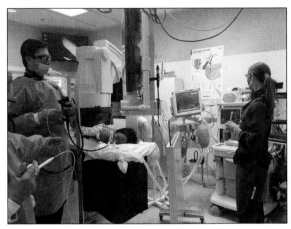

FIG 6.1 Example of room configuration. Note lead shield and aprons worn by staff, patient monitor, and emergency bag-mask ventilation device all in clear site. The anesthesia provider is in close proximity to the patient's airway and monitors.

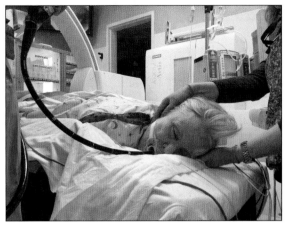

FIG 6.2 Jaw thrust in the prone position. This image depicts an anesthesia provider performing a jaw thrust on a patient undergoing ERCP in the prone position. The patient is receiving oxygen through a nasal cannula, which is also being used to monitor end-tidal CO_2.

recognize imminent sedation-related complications before the onset of a severe AE.

Automated responsiveness monitors (ARMs) are useful for patients targeted for monitored sedation, where responsiveness should be preserved throughout the procedure. An ARM is a computer-generated auditory or tactile stimulus that requires the patient to react (e.g., press a button) within a defined interval.[45] This technology is effective in computerized titration of propofol in standard endoscopy and reduces the frequency of sedation-related complications compared with standard combination regimens.[6,46–48] Computerized titration of sedation in ERCP has not been studied; because patients are more frequently targeted to deep sedation, the utility of ARMs may be limited. However, further study is needed in ERCP and other interventional endoscopic procedures.

ROOM SETUP AND CONSIDERATIONS FOR SAFETY

The room setup and configuration are extremely important (Fig. 6.1). The person administering sedation needs to be able to see the patient monitor and patient simultaneously. A jaw thrust maneuver is often required while continuing to monitor vital signs (Fig. 6.2). It is important to also have a bag valve mask within arm's reach. Furthermore, a stretcher needs to be close by in the event of an emergency requiring the patient to be repositioned supine, such as for endotracheal intubation in the setting of refractory airway obstruction or cardiopulmonary arrest.

Radiation protection for the person administering sedation should be emphasized (see Chapter 3). It is important to wear personal protective equipment, including a lead apron, thyroid shield, and glasses. If possible, the person administering sedation should try to position himself or herself behind a radiation shield.

CONCLUSIONS

ERCP is an increasingly complex therapeutic procedure that is performed on patients with high baseline morbidity. Sedation in ERCP should be individualized because the risk of sedation-related complications depends on a variety of patient-specific and procedure-specific factors. There is a trend toward greater utilization of anesthesiology-administered sedation in ERCP and all endoscopy in the United States, although systemic pressure to control health care costs may obligate endoscopists to have a higher threshold for anesthesia-administered sedation in the future. Future research and policy are expected to expand the use of propofol-based sedation regimens in all endoscopic procedures, perhaps enhanced by automated response monitors. Although these changes are expected to primarily affect standard endoscopic procedures initially, physicians performing ERCP should still be intimately familiar with this procedure's unique sedation risk profile. No matter the approach to sedation in ERCP, preprocedure recognition of high-risk patients and comfort with airway rescue maneuvers are paramount.

The complete reference list for this chapter can be found online at www.expertconsult.com.

7

Indications for and Contraindications to ERCP

Sanjeev Solomon and John Baillie

The appropriate use of endoscopic retrograde cholangiopancreatography (ERCP), as well as avoidance of this procedure when it is contraindicated or when there are alternative diagnostic procedures, is a quality issue for gastrointestinal (GI) endoscopists. The Standards of Practice guidelines of the American Society for Gastrointestinal Endoscopy (ASGE) are widely regarded as the standard of care for GI endoscopists in the United States and have been widely adopted in other countries. Over the years, the Standards of Practice and Training Committees of ASGE, and a Joint ASGE/American College of Gastroenterology (ACG) Taskforce on Quality in Endoscopy have produced position statements that address issues relating to ERCP. These were recently revised and include "The Role of ERCP in Benign Diseases of the Biliary Tract" (2015)[1] and "Quality Indicators for ERCP" (2015).[2] This review will serve to outline what has been proposed in the past as well as to highlight what has changed in the practice of ERCP because the most recent ASGE guidelines were promulgated.

It should be stated clearly that even when an ERCP is indicated, not all ERCP endoscopists are competent to perform the procedure, especially when procedures are more complicated (ASGE grade of difficulty 3 and 4). Competence is a difficult attribute to define[3] and is beyond the scope of this review (see Chapter 9). A 1996 prospective study of ERCP training, in which the senior author of this chapter participated, found that at least 180 to 200 supervised procedures were necessary for trainees to achieve minimum acceptable competence, defined as 80% success in ERCP skills such as selective cannulation and biliary sphincterotomy.[4] However, few experienced ERCP teachers believe that 200 procedures constitute anywhere near adequate training. Since 1996, ERCP practice has become overwhelmingly therapeutic; competence in ERCP now requires skill at placing pancreatic duct (PD) stents for prophylaxis against post-ERCP pancreatitis (PEP), needle-knife papillotomy (NKP), and papillectomy. A 2007 study from the United Kingdom found that only 66% of trainees achieved competence after performing 200 procedures.[5] The authors concluded that "quality [of ERCP] suffers [in the United Kingdom] because there are too many trainees in too many low-volume ERCP centers." This problem is not unique to Britain; there are many low-volume centers in the United States that claim to provide credentialable ERCP training. A Mayo Clinic study that evaluated the learning curve of a single trainee found that it took between 350 and 400 supervised procedures for the trainee to achieve consistent success at cannulation (≥80%)[6]; this rose to 96% after a further 300 procedures. In our opinion, this is a more realistic estimate of what it takes to develop expertise in ERCP. The following discussion of indications and contraindication assumes that the endoscopist has appropriate supervised training and experience in the necessary techniques and familiarity with the equipment required to perform them.

INDICATIONS FOR AND CONTRAINDICATIONS TO ERCP

An understanding of indications and contraindications for any procedure is part of being a well-trained endoscopist, a fact recognized in the 2002 ASGE guidelines on Methods of Granting Hospital Privileges for Performing Endoscopy.[7] The list of attributes indicating satisfactory training in ERCP included "a thorough understanding of the indications, contraindications, individual risk factors and benefit-risk considerations for the individual patient." There are very few indications for purely diagnostic ERCP in modern practice. Therefore there is no role for the solely diagnostic ERCP endoscopist. As the technical demands of ERCP have increased, so have the range and complexity of tasks that the ERCP endoscopist is expected to master. All ERCP endoscopists need to know how to perform safe and effective biliary sphincterotomy, remove bile duct stones, dilate biliary strictures, place plastic and expandable metal biliary stents, and provide PEP prophylaxis with small-caliber PD stents. In the "old days," many ERCP endoscopists avoided pancreatic intervention altogether. However, now that the benefits of PD stenting as prophylaxis against PEP have become clear from multiple published studies,[8,9] the ability to place a PD stent is a necessary part of the modern ERCP endoscopist's skill set.

The authors of the 2015 ASGE/ACG Taskforce for Quality in Endoscopy publication "Quality Indicators for ERCP"[2] identified the level of confidence of each recommendation based on the available literature (Box 7.1). Laudable as this effort appears, solid evidence was frequently missing in support of what we consider important parts of the preparation for, performance of, and follow-up after ERCP (Table 7.1).

Another way of looking at such evidence is the GRADE system, such as the one that the 2015 ASGE Practice Guideline "The role of ERCP in Benign Diseases of the Biliary Tract"[1] offered: high-quality evidence (4+), moderate-quality evidence (3+), low-quality evidence (2+), and very low-quality evidence (1+) (see also Box 7.1).

The ASGE offered the following position statements on ERCP:
- We recommend that diagnostic ERCP not be undertaken for the evaluation of pancreaticobiliary-type pain in the absence of objective abnormalities on other pancreaticobiliary imaging or laboratory studies (3+).
- We recommend that routine ERCP before laparoscopic cholecystectomy not be performed in the absence of objective signs of biliary obstruction or stone (3+).
- We recommend that ERCP in patients with acute biliary pancreatitis be limited to those with concomitant cholangitis or biliary obstruction (4+).

BOX 7.1 Grades of Recommendation

1A. Clear. Randomized trials without important limitations. Strong recommendation; can be applied to most clinical settings. [Clear benefit]

1B. Clear. Randomized trials with important limitations (inconsistent results, nonfatal methodological flaws). Strong recommendation; likely to apply to most practice settings. [Clear benefit]

1C+. Clear. Overwhelming evidence from observational studies. Strong recommendation; can apply to most practice settings in most situations. [Clear benefit]

1C. Clear. Observational studies. Intermediate-strength recommendation; may change when stronger evidence is available. [Clear benefit]

2A. Unclear. Randomized trials without important limitations. Intermediate-strength recommendation; best action may differ depending on circumstances or patient or societal values. [Unclear benefit]

2B. Unclear. Randomized trials with important limitations (inconsistent results, nonfatal methodological flaws). Weak recommendation; alternative approaches may be better under some circumstances. [Unclear benefit]

2C. Unclear. Observational studies. Very weak recommendation; alternative approaches likely to be better under some circumstances. [Unclear benefit]

3. Unclear. Expert opinion only. Weak recommendation; likely to change as data become available. [Unclear benefit]

From Chutkan RK, Ahmad AS, Cohen J, et al. ERCP core curriculum. *Gastrointest Endosc.* 2006;63:361–376.

TABLE 7.1 Summary of Proposed Quality Indicators for ERCP

Quality Indicator	Grade of Recommendation
1. Appropriate indication	1C+
2. Informed consent	1C
3. Appropriate antibiotics	2B
4. Trained and credentialed ERCP endoscopist	3
5. Annual number of ERCPs recorded	1C
6. Cannulation rates of desired duct	1C
7. Cannulation rates of desired duct—native anatomy	1C
8. Fluoroscopy/radiation dose recorded	2C
9. Extraction of common bile duct stones	1C
10. Biliary stent placement	1C
11. Complete documentation	3
12. Adverse event rates/hospital transfers	3
13. PEP rates	1C
14. Perforation rates	2C
15. Hemorrhage rates	1C
16. Delayed adverse events	3

PEP, Post-ERCP pancreatitis.

- We recommend ERCP with dilation and stent placement for benign biliary strictures (3+).
- We recommend that ERCP be undertaken as first-line therapy for postoperative biliary leaks (4+).
- We suggest that cholangioscopy be considered as an adjunctive technique for the management of difficult bile duct stones not amenable to removal after sphincterotomy with or without balloon dilation or mechanical lithotripsy (2+).
- We suggest that cholangioscopy with directed biopsy be considered as an adjunctive technique for the characterization of biliary strictures (2+).

BOX 7.2 Indications for ERCP

A. The jaundiced patient suspected of having biliary obstruction (appropriate therapeutic maneuvers should be performed during the procedure)

B. The patient without jaundice whose clinical and biochemical or imaging data suggest pancreatic duct or biliary tract disease

C. Evaluation of signs or symptoms suggesting pancreatic malignancy when results of direct imaging (e.g., endoscopic ultrasonography, ultrasonography, computed tomography, magnetic resonance imaging) are equivocal or normal

D. Evaluation of pancreatitis of unknown etiology

E. Preoperative evaluation of the patient with chronic pancreatitis and/or pseudocyst

F. Evaluation of the sphincter of Oddi by manometry

G. ERCP with or without sphincter of Oddi manometry is not recommended in patients with suspected type III sphincter of Oddi dysfunction (editor's revision as a consequence of the EPISOD trial[20])

H. Endoscopic sphincterotomy:
  H1. Choledocholithiasis
  H2. Papillary stenosis or sphincter of Oddi dysfunction type I and II
  H3. To facilitate placement of biliary stents or dilation of biliary strictures
  H4. Sump syndrome
  H5. Choledochocele involving the major papilla
  H6. Ampullary carcinoma in patients who are not candidates for surgery
  H7. Facilitate access to the pancreatic duct

I. Stent placement across benign or malignant strictures, fistulae, or postoperative bile leaks, or in high-risk patients with large unremovable common duct stones

J. Dilation of ductal strictures

K. Balloon dilation of the papilla

L. Nasobiliary drain placement

M. Pancreatic pseudocyst drainage in appropriate cases

N. Tissue sampling from pancreatic or bile ducts

O. Ampullectomy of adenomatous neoplasms of the major papilla

P. Therapy of disorders of the biliary and pancreatic ducts

Q. Facilitation of cholangioscopy and/or pancreatoscopy

- We recommend ERCP with sphincterotomy for patients with type I SOD (3+).
- We recommend against the performance of ERCP for the evaluation or treatment of type III SOD (4+).
- We recommend rectal indomethacin with or without a pancreatic stent for prophylaxis against post-ERCP pancreatitis when ERCP is performed in patients with suspected SOD (3+).

INDICATIONS FOR ERCP

The recommended indications for ERCP in the ASGE/ACG Joint Taskforce document "Quality indicators for ERCP"[2] are listed in Box 7.2 (A through Q). This alphabetic scale is unrelated to the quality of evidence scale (4+, 3+, 2+, and 1+) as just discussed. We added a few miscellaneous indications as an extra category, identified as R. Text added by us to clarify descriptions is in italics.

A. Jaundice thought to be the result of biliary obstruction

  Comment: ERCP is not always indicated in this setting. Patients who are candidates for resection of tumors causing biliary obstruction may not require preoperative biliary drainage. In the last decade, surgeons have claimed that preoperative ERCP and biliary stenting increase the risk of adverse events of surgery.[10,11] Some of the most vocal condemnation of endoscopic intervention arose from poorly done retrospective studies. Prospective data confirmed what most biliary and pancreatic surgeons already knew; that is, preoperative biliary drainage increases postoperative infections, presumably because of the introduction of bacteria into a sterile system (the biliary tree) via cannulas and other instruments, but does not increase mortality.[12,13] Experts now agree that the decision to preoperatively drain the biliary tree in a patient awaiting surgery for malignant jaundice should be made by consensus, with the active involvement of the surgeon, the ERCP endoscopist, and (if available) the interventional radiologist. Patients who are septic with cholangitis (which is rare in malignant jaundice) or have severe pruritus caused by biliary obstruction (despite antipruritic drugs) need their biliary trees drained if there is going to be significant delay in surgery (e.g., for preoperative chemo-irradiation)[14]; this can be done endoscopically (ERCP) or percutaneously (transhepatically). On the other hand, patients who are asymptomatic and who can be scheduled for their surgery within a week or so of presentation are probably better served by not having drainage. In the authors' experience, many surgeons prefer the convenience of having the biliary tree drained preoperatively and having an anatomic and cytologic (or histologic) diagnosis to discuss with the patient and his or her family. In the "old days," ERCP in a patient with presumed obstructive jaundice was often a "fishing trip," as the cause was uncertain. In the era of high-quality cross-sectional imaging such as helical computed tomography (CT), magnetic resonance cholangiopancreatography (MRCP), and endoscopic ultrasonography (EUS) (see Chapter 34), it is now rare for the diagnosis to be in doubt, although small tumors, small stones, and papillary stenosis continue to present diagnostic difficulty.

B. Clinical and biochemical or imaging data suggestive of pancreatic or biliary tract disease

Comment: Previously, minor elevations of liver enzymes or pancreatic enzymes were often used to justify ERCP. Without imaging evidence of biliary obstruction or pancreatitis, the yield of ERCP in these circumstances is low and makes it difficult to justify the potential risks. All patients with sphincter of Oddi dysfunction (SOD) type I and the majority of those with SOD type II should have transient elevation of serologic liver test levels that normalize between episodes.[15] Patients whose liver tests fail to normalize between attacks should not be classified as having SOD. They may have papillary stenosis, some other cause of subtle biliary structuring, or a chronic disorder affecting the liver parenchyma, such as fatty liver (steatosis). Similarly, persistent mild elevation of serum amylase and lipase in the absence of radiologic abnormality is unlikely to reflect pathology that will be revealed by ERCP. However, acute recurrent idiopathic pancreatitis does justify endoscopic imaging (see "D. Pancreatitis of unknown etiology" and Chapter 52). If biliary microlithiasis is suspected, EUS is less invasive and more sensitive for this diagnosis.[16] Increasingly, EUS is being used immediately before planned ERCP in low-yield, high-risk settings. If the EUS is negative, the ERCP can be avoided, sparing the patient the risk of a more invasive procedure.[17]

C. Signs or symptoms suggesting pancreatic malignancy when direct imaging results are equivocal or normal

Comment: It is difficult to know exactly what was intended here. If there is doubt about the presence or absence of a mass, usually in the head of the pancreas, or the significance of biliary and/or pancreatic ductal dilatation, EUS is probably the investigation of choice, ahead of ERCP. The imaging resolution of EUS is so good that a small stone or subtle stricture is more likely to be identified by EUS than by ERCP.

D. Pancreatitis of unknown etiology

Comment: By "pancreatitis," we believe that "acute pancreatitis" was intended. Patients with idiopathic acute recurrent pancreatitis (IARP) who have an intact gallbladder but have had negative imaging (e.g., transcutaneous ultrasonography, CT, magnetic resonance imaging [MRI]) for cholelithiasis and choledocholithiasis should have EUS to look for biliary sludge (microlithiasis) and small stones. EUS is frequently positive for these findings when repeated imaging by other means has been negative. Any patient with IARP should have inspection of the main duodenal papilla by duodenoscopy with a side-viewing instrument to look for obvious anatomic abnormalities, such as a choledochocele or an ampullary tumor. The anatomic abnormality of pancreas divisum (P. Div.) is now often recognized by MRCP or EUS (i.e., not requiring pancreatography through the minor duodenal papilla).[18] Minor papilla cannulation and contrast injection to confirm the diagnosis of P. Div. should be performed only if therapy (i.e., minor papillotomy) is planned, in the appropriate clinical setting (i.e., IARP without other explanation). If IARP is considered to be caused by pancreatic sphincter dysfunction, ideally the patient should be referred to a center where pancreatic manometry is available to confirm the diagnosis before treatment (i.e., pancreatic sphincterotomy). In current ERCP practice, however, many endoscopists proceed with empiric pancreatic sphincterotomy (usually done over a stent placed in the PD orifice) without prior manometry. Pancreatic sphincterotomy and PD stenting are not entirely benign interventions, risking perforation, PEP, stenosis of the opening, and focal "groove" pancreatitis across the length of the stent (from side branch occlusion). The risks and benefits of empiric pancreatic endotherapy should always be carefully weighed before proceeding.

E. Preoperative evaluation of chronic pancreatitis or pancreatic pseudocyst

Comment: The quality of modern CT scanning and MRI is so good that endoscopic retrograde pancreatography (ERP) may have little or nothing to add in the preoperative evaluation of chronic pancreatitis (CP). In addition, EUS allows aspiration for biochemical studies when the diagnosis is in doubt. However, fistulae from the pancreatic duct to adjacent structures or communicating with pseudocysts are still most accurately identified by ERP, when this is deemed necessary. Endoscopic pseudocyst decompression is increasingly being performed by EUS alone.[19] As a result, the opportunity to perform ERP to identify and stent (where possible) a communicating PD fistula during endoscopic pseudocyst drainage is becoming less common and reserved for patients with smaller pseudocysts that are not in optimal locations for EUS-guided drainage. There are no data yet available to indicate whether the lack of a retrograde pancreatogram adversely affects the outcome of EUS-guided pseudocyst decompression.

F. Sphincter of Oddi manometry (SOM) (see Chapter 16).

Comment: SOM remains one of the few indications for mainly diagnostic ERCP. However, some SOM procedures (i.e., those showing abnormally high pressures) will lead to therapeutic intervention, usually sphincterotomy, and all should include placement of a small-diameter PD stent to preclude or mitigate procedural pancreatitis.

G. Empirical biliary sphincterotomy without sphincter of Oddi manometry is not recommended in patients with suspected type III sphincter of Oddi dysfunction.

Comment: The EPISOD trial conducted in 2014 was a 2-arm parallel, randomized, double-blind, sham-controlled, multicenter study that confirmed that SOM and sphincterotomy do not benefit patients with type III SOD and are associated with significant rates of adverse events.[20] Indeed, it is anticipated that this diagnosis will be eliminated as an entity.

H. Endoscopic sphincterotomy (ES)

Comment: ES may be used in the primary management of certain conditions, such as papillary stenosis, and to facilitate other therapeutic interventions in the biliary tree.

H1. Choledocholithiasis

Comment: ERCP is used not only for access to recover bile duct stones, but also to access and retrieve stones in the cystic duct and gallbladder and to place nasocystic drains and stents.

H2. Papillary stenosis or sphincter of Oddi dysfunction (SOD) (see Chapter 47)

Comment: Only symptomatic patients should be investigated and treated.

H3. Facilitate biliary stent placement or dilation of biliary strictures.

Comment: Biliary and pancreatic duct stricture dilation is mentioned elsewhere. Balloon dilation of the biliary sphincter ("biliary sphincteroplasty," Chapter 18) is an alternative to sphincterotomy.[21] However, increasingly the two are being used in combination: a relatively small sphincterotomy is performed, followed by balloon dilation for removal of large stones.

H4. Sump syndrome

Comment: Sump syndrome is increasingly rare, as choledochoduo-denostomy has largely been abandoned in favor of hepaticoje-junostomy for biliary diversion.

H5. Choledochocele

Comment: Choledochoceles are often incised using a needle-knife papillotome, with the opening being extended as necessary using a standard "pull" papillotome.

H6. [Decompressing biliary obstruction in] Ampullary carcinoma in poor surgical candidates

Comment: Large sphincterotomies intended to open bile ducts obstructed by ampullary tumors carry a significant risk of bleeding. The preferred approach by many endoscopists today is to place a stent across the stenosis rather than perform sphincterotomy in this setting.

H7. Access to pancreatic duct

Comment: Access to the pancreatic duct for contact or mechanical lithotripsy of stones, and their extraction, or pancreatoscopy using miniscopes requires pancreatic sphincterotomy.

I. Stent placement across benign or malignant strictures, fistulae, or postoperative bile leaks, or alongside large nonextractable common bile duct stones

J. Dilation of ductal strictures

K. Balloon dilation of the papilla

L. Nasobiliary (and nasopancreatic) drain placement for acute cholangitis and to lavage pancreatic stone fragments following PD stone litho-tripsy, respectively

Comment: Nasobiliary drains are uncomfortable for patients, and their placement is an increasingly rare event in modern ERCP practice.

M. Pancreatic pseudocyst drainage in appropriate cases

Comment: Increasingly, pancreatic pseudocyst drainage is being performed using EUS alone, especially with the introduction of lumen-apposing, covered, self-expanding metal stents that allow for single-step deployment and the ability to perform endoscopic debridement with minimal stent migration.[22]

N. Tissue sampling from pancreatic or bile ducts

Comment: This does not always require endoscopic sphincterotomy, as brushes and other sampling devices can usually be advanced into the duct of interest without enlarging the opening.

O. Ampullectomy of adenomatous neoplasms of the major papilla

P. Pancreatic and biliary therapeutics

Comment: To include transpapillary stenting for PD strictures and leaks and removal of PD stones (see Chapters 54 and 55).

Q. Facilitation of cholangioscopy and/or pancreatoscopy

Comment: Cholangioscopy and pancreatoscopy are important procedures for evaluation of pancreaticobiliary disorders, including indeterminate strictures (see Chapter 41) and missed stones during ERCP.[23]

In addition to the above, we suggest adding the following indications:

R. Access to the bile duct to recover migrated stents, facilitate combined endoscopic-radiologic procedures, investigate (and occasionally treat) hemobilia, and remove parasites (see Chapter 49).

SPECIAL CASES

ERCP has been shown to be safe and effective in pregnancy[24] (see Chapter 30) and in children (see Chapter 29),[25] provided that the indications are appropriate and that the necessary precautions are taken (e.g., radiologic shielding of the fetus in pregnancy, sedation modified for use in children).

CONTRAINDICATIONS TO ERCP

A discussion of the contraindications to ERCP (Box 7.3) is intended to increase safety by reducing risk to the patient. There are numerous potential adverse events of ERCP, and many of them are serious and potentially life threatening (see Chapter 8).[26] These may be considered "relative" or "absolute," depending on the circumstances. To reflect the possibility that unusual or exceptional circumstances may render a normally contraindicated procedure appropriate, the authors of the 2012 ASGE guidelines on "Appropriate use of GI endoscopy"[27] were sparing in their use of the word *contraindicated*, preferring the phrase *generally not indicated* for all but the most dangerous circumstances, which they regarded as *generally contraindicated*. This phrasing offers some "wiggle room" for the endoscopist should litigation result from such an intervention, because it is generally inadvisable from a legal point of view to talk in absolutes (see Chapter 13). There are contraindications that apply to endoscopic procedures in general, and others that are specific to ERCP. From the 2012 ASGE Appropriate Use document:

GI endoscopy is generally not indicated:

- When the results will not contribute to a management choice
- For periodic follow-up of healed benign disease unless surveillance of a premalignant condition is warranted

GI endoscopy is generally contraindicated:

- When the risks to patient health or life are judged to outweigh the most favorable benefits of the procedure
- When adequate patient cooperation or consent cannot be obtained
- When a perforated viscus is known or suspected

ERCP is generally not indicated:

- In the evaluation of abdominal pain of obscure origin in the absence of objective findings that suggest biliary or pancreatic disease (magnetic resonance cholangiopancreatography and EUS are safe diagnostic procedures that can obviate ERCP)
- In the evaluation of suspected gallbladder disease without evidence of bile duct disease
- As further evaluation of proven pancreatic malignancy unless management will be altered

Professional organizations in other countries, such as Canada,[28] have offered more detailed lists of ERCP contraindications. For example:

BOX 7.3 Contraindications to ERCP

Section A
General
GI endoscopy is generally contraindicated:
- When the risks to patient health or life are judged to outweigh the most favorable benefits of the procedure
- When adequate patient cooperation or consent cannot be obtained
- When a perforated viscus is known or suspected

Specific
ERCP is generally not indicated:
- In the evaluation of abdominal pain of obscure origin in the absence of objective findings that suggest biliary or pancreatic disease
- In the evaluation of suspected gallbladder disease without evidence of bile duct disease
- As further evaluation of proven pancreatic malignancy unless management will be altered

ERCP is generally contraindicated when:
- A competent patient refuses to give his or her consent for the procedure
- The endoscopist is untrained or inadequately trained in ERCP
- There is a lack of required equipment and/or accessories

Section B
Additional Considerations That May Contraindicate ERCP
- A high-risk procedure such as biliary sphincterotomy in a patient who is fully anticoagulated with Coumadin or therapeutically dosed with clopidogrel (Plavix)
- When the patient has suffered a prior severe allergic reaction to ERCP contrast medium
- When the appropriate level of anesthesia is unavailable
- When anatomic conditions (pathology, surgical alteration) limit access to papilla
- When the patient is in the midst of an attack of acute pancreatitis

Section A recommendations from ASGE Standards of Practice Committee. Appropriate use of GI endoscopy. *Gastrointest Endosc.* 2012;75:1127–1131. Section B recommendations from non-ASGE sources, including Cockerham A. Canadian Association of Gastroenterology practice guideline for clinical competence in diagnostic and therapeutic endoscopic retrograde cholangiopancreatography. *Can J Gastroenterol.* 1997;11:535–538.

- When a competent patient refuses to give his or her consent for the procedure
- When the endoscopist is untrained or inadequately trained in ERCP
- When there is a lack of required equipment and/or accessories
- When a high-risk procedure (e.g., biliary sphincterotomy) is planned in a patient who is fully anticoagulated with Coumadin (now to include direct oral anticoagulants) or therapeutically dosed with clopidogrel (Plavix) (now to include other antiplatelet agents)
- When there is known or suspected perforation of the GI tract
- When the patient has suffered a prior severe allergic reaction to ERCP contrast medium
- When the appropriate level of anesthesia is unavailable
- When anatomic conditions limit access to papilla
- When the patient is in the midst of an attack of acute pancreatitis

Obviously, some of these contraindications need to be qualified. One of the most difficult issues for modern ERCP endoscopists is the ubiquitous use of antiplatelet agents such as clopidogrel (Plavix) and anticoagulants, especially Coumadin. A detailed discussion of the modification of anticoagulation for elective ERCP and the management of full antiplatelet therapy and anticoagulation in urgent cases is beyond the scope of this review (see Chapter 10). The recent ASGE Standards of Practice document "The management of antithrombotic agents for patients undergoing GI endoscopy"[29] should be required reading for every ERCP endoscopist. In the era of natural orifice transluminal endoscopic surgery (NOTES) procedures, even suspected or known perforation is not an absolute contraindication to endoscopy (e.g., closure of mucosal defects using clips after ampullectomy). Anatomic barriers to ERCP that may have defeated endoscopists in the past (e.g., accessing the duodenal papilla through a long Roux limb) are no longer considered contraindications to attempting procedures using appropriately modified instruments and accessories. The appropriateness of attempting ERCP in the setting of acute pancreatitis depends greatly on the severity of the disease, and relief of papillary obstruction during acute gallstone pancreatitis with biliary obstruction is, in fact, a good indication for the procedure.

The complete reference list for this chapter can be found online at www.expertconsult.com.

8

Adverse Events of ERCP: Prediction, Prevention, and Management

Indu Srinivasan and Martin L. Freeman

Endoscopic retrograde cholangiopancreatography (ERCP) has evolved from a diagnostic modality to a primarily therapeutic procedure for pancreatic and biliary disorders. ERCP alone or with associated biliary and pancreatic instrumentation and therapy can cause a variety of short-term adverse events, including pancreatitis, hemorrhage, perforation, and cardiopulmonary events (Box 8.1). These adverse events can range from minor, with one or two additional hospital days followed by full recovery, to severe and devastating, with permanent disability or death. Adverse events may cause not only significant morbidity to the patient but also significant anxiety and exposure to medical malpractice claims for the endoscopist.

Major advances in the approach to adverse events of ERCP have occurred in several areas: standardized consensus-based definitions of adverse events,[1] large-scale multicenter multivariate analyses that have allowed clearer identification of patient-related and technique-related risk factors for adverse events,[2–9] and introduction of new devices and techniques to minimize the risks of ERCP-related adverse events.

DEFINITIONS OF COMPLICATIONS, ADVERSE EVENTS, UNPLANNED EVENTS, AND OTHER NEGATIVE OUTCOMES

In 1991, standardized consensus definitions for complications of sphincterotomy were introduced,[1] and although they are widely used (Table 8.1), a consensus definition of adverse events for all endoscopic procedures, including ERCP, has been more recently adopted.[10] Severity is graded primarily on number of hospital days and type of intervention required to treat the complication. This classification allows uniform assessment of outcomes of ERCP and sphincterotomy in various settings. Beyond immediate complications, there is an increasing awareness of the entire spectrum of negative (as well as positive) outcomes, including technical failures, ineffectiveness of the procedure in resolving the presenting complaint, long-term sequelae, costs, extended hospitalization, and patient (dis)satisfaction. Accordingly, the terminology has evolved from *complications* to *adverse events,* and more recently to *unplanned events.* The term *adverse event* is used throughout this book. Adverse events must be viewed in the context of the entire clinical outcome: a successful procedure with a minor or even a moderate adverse event may sometimes be a preferable outcome to a failed procedure attempt without any obvious adverse event. Failure at ERCP usually leads to a repeated ERCP or to an alternative percutaneous or surgical procedure that may result in significant additional morbidity, hospitalization, and cost.

Video for this chapter can be found online at www.expertconsult.com.

ANALYSES OF ADVERSE EVENT RATES

Reported adverse event rates vary widely, even between prospective studies. In two large prospective studies, pancreatitis rates ranged between 0.74% for diagnostic and 1.4% for therapeutic ERCP, in one study,[7] compared with 5.1% (about 7 times higher) for diagnostic ERCP and 6.9% (5 times higher) for therapeutic ERCP in another prospective study.[3] Reasons for such variation include (1) definitions used; (2) thoroughness of detection; (3) patient-related factors; and (4) procedural variables, such as extent of therapy or use of prophylactic pancreatic stents or nonsteroidal antiinflammatory drugs (NSAIDs). For all of these reasons, it should not be assumed that a lower adverse event rate at one center necessarily reflects better quality of practice.

Most recent studies have used multivariate analysis as a tool to identify and quantify the effect of multiple potentially confounding risk factors, but these are not infallible as many potentially key risk factors were not examined in most studies, and some are overfitted (too many predictor variables for too few outcomes). Only a limited number of studies have included more than 1000 patients. Tables 8.2, 8.3, and 8.4 show summaries of risk factors for adverse events of ERCP and sphincterotomy based on published multivariate analyses.

OVERALL ADVERSE EVENTS OF ERCP AND SPHINCTEROTOMY

Most prospective series report an overall short-term adverse event rate for ERCP and/or sphincterotomy of about 5% to 10%.[2–9] Traditionally there has been a particularly high rate of adverse events for patients with known or suspected sphincter of Oddi dysfunction (up to 20% or more, primarily pancreatitis, with up to 4% severe adverse events) and a very low adverse event rate for routine bile duct stone extraction, especially in tandem with laparoscopic cholecystectomy (less than 5% in most series).[2] Sphincterotomy bleeding occurs primarily in patients with bile duct stones, whereas cholangitis occurs mostly in patients with malignant biliary obstruction.

Summaries of multivariate analyses of risk factors for overall adverse events of ERCP and sphincterotomy are shown in Table 8.2. Although relevant studies are heterogeneous and sometimes omit potentially key risk factors, several patterns emerge (see Table 8.2):

1. Indication of suspected sphincter of Oddi dysfunction was a significant risk factor whenever examined.
2. Technical factors, likely linked to the skill or experience of the endoscopist, were found to be significant risk factors for overall adverse events. These technical factors include difficult cannulation, use of precut or "access" papillotomy to gain bile duct entry, failure to achieve biliary drainage, and use of simultaneous or subsequent percutaneous biliary drainage for otherwise failed endoscopic cannulation. In turn, the ERCP case volume of endoscopists or medical

centers, when examined, has almost always been a significant factor in adverse events by both univariate and multivariate analyses.[2–9]

3. Death from ERCP is rare (less than 0.5%) but has most often been related to cardiopulmonary adverse events, highlighting the need for the endoscopist to pay attention to issues of safety during sedation and monitoring (see Chapter 6).

Notably, risk factors found not to be significant are the following: (1) older age or increased number of coexisting medical conditions—on the contrary, younger age generally increases the risk by both univariate and multivariate analyses; (2) smaller bile duct diameter, in contrast to previous observations; and (3) anatomic obstacles such as periampullary diverticulum or Billroth II gastrectomy, although these do increase technical difficulty for the endoscopist.[2–9]

PANCREATITIS

Pancreatitis is the most common adverse event of ERCP, with reported rates ranging from 1% to 40%, with a rate of about 5% being most typical.[2–9] In the consensus classification, pancreatitis is defined as a clinical syndrome consistent with pancreatitis (i.e., new or worsened abdominal pain) with an amylase at least three times normal more than 24 hours after the procedure, and requiring more than one night of hospitalization (see Table 8.1).[1] Some events are difficult to classify in the consensus definitions. Examples include postprocedural abdominal pain and elevation of amylase to just under three times normal, serum lipase more than three times normal with less than three times elevation of amylase, and dramatic enzyme elevations with minimal symptoms

---

BOX 8.1   Adverse Events of ERCP

- Pancreatitis
- Hemorrhage
- Perforation
- Cholangitis
- Cholecystitis
- Stent-related adverse events
- Cardiopulmonary adverse events
- Endoscope-transmitted infection
- Anesthesia-related adverse events
- Miscellaneous adverse events

TABLE 8.1   Consensus Definitions for the Major Adverse Events of ERCP

	Mild	Moderate	Severe
Pancreatitis	Clinical pancreastitis, amylase at least three times normal more than 24 hours after the procedure, requiring admission or prolongation of planned admission to 2 to 3 days	Pancreatitis requiring hospitalization of 4 to 10 days	Hospitalization for more than 10 days, pseudocyst, or intervention (percutaneous drainage or surgery)
Bleeding	Clinical (i.e., not just endoscopic) evidence of bleeding, hemoglobin drop <3 g, no transfusion	Transfusion (4 units or fewer), no angiographic intervention or surgery	Transfusion (5 units or more), or intervention (angiographic or surgical)
Perforation	Possible, or only very slight leak of fluid or contrast, treatable by fluids and suction for ≤3 days	Any definite perforation treated medically for 4 to 10 days	Medical treatment for more than 10 days, or intervention (percutaneous or surgical)
Infection (cholangitis)	>38°C for 24 to 48 hours	Febrile or septic illness requiring more than 3 days of hospital treatment or percutaneous intervention	Septic shock or surgery

Any intensive care unit admission after a procedure grades the adverse event as severe. Other rarer adverse events can be graded by length of needed hospitalization.

TABLE 8.2   Risk Factors for Overall Adverse Events of ERCP in Multivariate Analyses

Definite*	Maybe†	No‡
Suspected sphincter of Oddi dysfunction	Young age	Comorbid illness burden
Cirrhosis	Pancreatic contrast injection	Small CBD diameter
Difficult cannulation	Failed biliary drainage	Female sex
Precut sphincterotomy		Billroth II
Percutaneous biliary access	Trainee involvement	Periampullary diverticulum
Lower ERCP case volume		

CBD, Common bile duct.
*Significant by multivariate analysis in most studies.
†Significant by univariate analysis only in most studies.
‡Not significant by multivariate analysis in any study.

TABLE 8.3   Risk Factors for Post-ERCP Pancreatitis in Multivariate Analyses

Definite*	Maybe†	No‡
Suspected sphincter of Oddi dysfunction	Female sex	Small CBD diameter
Young age	Acinarization	Sphincter of Oddi manometry
Normal bilirubin	Absence of CBD stone	Biliary sphincterotomy
History of post-ERCP pancreatitis	Lower ERCP case volume	
Difficult or failed cannulation	Trainee involvement	
Pancreatic duct wire passage		
Pancreatic sphincterotomy (especially minor papilla)		
Balloon dilation of intact biliary sphincter		
Precut sphincterotomy		
Metallic biliary stent		

CBD, Common bile duct.
*Significant by multivariate analysis in most studies.
†Significant by univariate analysis only in most studies.
‡Not significant by multivariate analysis in any study.

TABLE 8.4   Risk Factors for Hemorrhage After Endoscopic Sphincterotomy in Multivariate Analyses

Definite*	Maybe†	No‡
Coagulopathy	Cirrhosis	Aspirin or NSAID
Anticoagulation <3 days after ES	Dilated CBD	Ampullary tumor
	CBD stone	Longer length
Cholangitis before ERCP	Periampullary	sphincterotomy
Bleeding during ES	diverticulum	Extension of prior ES
Lower ERCP case volume	Precut sphincterotomy	

CBD, Common bile duct; *ES,* endoscopic sphincterotomy; *NSAID,* nonsteroidal antiinflammatory drug.
*Significant by multivariate analysis in most studies.
†Significant by univariate analysis only in most studies.
‡Not significant by multivariate analysis in any study.

that are not clearly suggestive of clinical pancreatitis. There are many potential mechanisms of injury to the pancreas during ERCP and endoscopic sphincterotomy (ES): mechanical, chemical, hydrostatic, enzymatic, microbiologic, and thermal. Although the relative contribution of these mechanisms to post-ERCP is not known, recent multivariate analyses have helped to identify the clinical patient-related and procedure-related factors that are independently associated with pancreatitis. Recent trials have concentrated more on determining the methods of preventing post-ERCP pancreatitis (PEP). Risks and interventions for PEP have been described as the four P's: patient-related factors, procedural techniques, pancreatic stents, and pharmacologic agents.

Patient-Related Risk Factors for Post-ERCP Pancreatitis

The risk of PEP is determined at least as much by the characteristics of the patient as by endoscopic techniques or maneuvers (see Table 8.3). Patient-related predictors found to be significant in one or more major studies include younger age, indication of suspected sphincter of Oddi dysfunction, history of previous PEP, and absence of elevated serum bilirubin.[2–9] Women may have increased risk, but it is difficult to sort out the contribution of sphincter of Oddi dysfunction, a condition that occurs almost exclusively in women. In one meta-analysis, female gender was clearly a risk[11] and accounted for a majority of cases of severe or fatal PEP.[2,12]

Sphincter of Oddi dysfunction, most often suspected in women with postcholecystectomy abdominal pain (see Chapter 47), poses a formidable risk for pancreatitis after any kind of ERCP, whether diagnostic, manometric, or therapeutic. Suspicion of sphincter of Oddi dysfunction independently triples the risk of PEP to about 10% to 30%. The reason for heightened susceptibility in these patients remains unknown. Contrary to the widely held opinion that sphincter of Oddi manometry is the culprit, multivariate analyses show that empirical biliary sphincterotomy or even diagnostic ERCP has similarly high risk in this patient population.[3] With the widespread use of aspiration instead of conventional perfusion manometry catheters (see Chapter 16), the risk of manometry has probably been reduced to that of cannulation with any other ERCP accessory. Most previous studies linking manometry with risk have been from tertiary centers in which manometry was always performed in patients with suspected sphincter of Oddi dysfunction, thus losing the ability to separate the contribution of procedural risk from that of patient risk. Two studies specifically compared risk of PEP in patients having ERCP for suspected sphincter of Oddi dysfunction with and without sphincter of Oddi manometry and found no detectable independent effect of manometry on risk.[2,13] Absence of a stone in patients with suspected choledocholithiasis has been found to

be a potent single risk factor for PEP in patients suspected of having stones, thus fitting into the category of possible sphincter of Oddi dysfunction. These observations point out the danger of performing diagnostic ERCP to look for bile duct stones in women with recurrent postcholecystectomy pain, as there is generally a low probability of finding stones in such patients and a high risk of causing pancreatitis. It is an erroneous and potentially dangerous assumption that merely avoiding sphincter of Oddi manometry will significantly reduce risk. These risk factors have been revealed to be additive, thus highlighting the importance of not only identifying risk factors but also abstaining from performing ERCP in cases with marginal indication (see Chapter 7). Ironically, people who have these procedures performed for least indicated reasons have higher chances of PEP.

History of previous PEP has been found to be a potential risk factor (odds ratio [OR] is 2.0 to 5.4)[3,4] and warrants special caution. Advanced chronic pancreatitis, on the other hand, confers some immunity against PEP, perhaps because of atrophy and decreased enzymatic activity.[3] Pancreas divisum is a risk factor only if minor papilla cannulation is attempted.

Despite many early studies suggesting small bile duct diameter to be a risk factor for pancreatitis, most recent studies have shown no independent influence of duct size on risk; small duct diameter may have been a surrogate marker for sphincter of Oddi dysfunction in the earlier studies using only univariate analysis. ERCP for removal of bile duct stones has been found to be relatively safe with respect to pancreatitis rates (<4%) in multicenter studies regardless of bile duct diameter.[2] IPMN with a small pancreatic duct has also been found to be a risk factor for PEP.[14] This is most likely related to the inability of mucus to drain well after instrumentation, despite placement of a prophylactic pancreatic duct stent. Neither the presence of periampullary diverticula nor Billroth II gastrectomy has been found to influence risk of pancreatitis.[2]

A recent study[15] has also shown current smoking and chronic liver disease to be protective against PEP.

Technique-Related Risk Factors for Post-ERCP Pancreatitis

Technical factors have long been recognized as important in causing PEP. Papillary trauma induced by difficult cannulation has a negative effect that is independent of the number of pancreatic duct contrast injections, which is also a risk factor for PEP.[2–9,11] Pancreatitis occurred in one study after 2.5% of ERCPs in which there was no pancreatic duct contrast injection at all.[3] Acinarization of the pancreas, although undesirable, is probably less important than generally thought and has not been found to be significant in two recent studies.[3,4]

Overall, the risk of pancreatitis is generally similar for diagnostic and therapeutic ERCP.[2–9,11] Performance of biliary sphincterotomy does not appear to add a significant independent risk of pancreatitis to ERCP,[3,4] a finding that is contrary to widely held opinion. This is probably not because of the safety of sphincterotomy, but rather because of the risk of diagnostic ERCP. Pancreatic sphincterotomy of any kind,[3] including minor papilla sphincterotomy,[4] has been found to be a significant risk factor for pancreatitis, although the risk of severe pancreatitis has been very low (<1%), perhaps because pancreatic duct stents were placed in nearly all of these patients in these studies. In a recently published study,[16] placement of metallic stents was also found to be a risk factor, likely because of transpapillary positioning causing compression of the pancreatic orifice.

Precut or access papillotomy to gain entry to the common bile duct is controversial with respect to risk of pancreatitis and other adverse events. Use of this technique among endoscopists varies, with some employing it in less than 5% of cases and others in as many as 30% of cases.[17] There are many variations on precut technique: standard needle knife inserted at the papillary orifice and cutting upward; needle-knife "fistulotomy" starting the incision above the papillary orifice and then cutting either up or down; and use of a pull-type sphincterotome wedged either in the papillary orifice or into the pancreatic duct intentionally (see Chapter 15). Any of these techniques has the potential to lacerate and injure the pancreatic sphincter, and precut techniques have been uniformly associated with a higher risk of pancreatitis in multicenter studies involving endoscopists with varied experience, with precut sphincterotomy found significant as a univariate or multivariate risk factor for PEP and/or overall adverse events.[2,7] In contrast, many series from tertiary referral centers have found adverse event rates of precut sphincterotomy to be no different than those of standard sphincterotomy, suggesting that risk of precut sphincterotomy is highly operator dependent.[18] In one study, endoscopists performing more than one sphincterotomy a week averaged 90% immediate bile duct access after precutting, versus only 50% for lower volume endoscopists, a success rate that does not seem to justify the risk of adverse events.[2]

Comparative studies of precut and standard sphincterotomy are hard to interpret because indications and settings may be very different, with precut preferentially performed in lower risk situations such as obstructive jaundice and prominent papillae. In addition, increasing use of pancreatic stents in series from tertiary centers may have neutralized the otherwise higher risk of precut sphincterotomy.[7] Adverse events of precut sphincterotomy vary with the indication for the procedure, occurring in as many as 30% of patients with known or suspected sphincter of Oddi dysfunction in older studies in which pancreatic stents were not used.[2] Paradoxically, in patients with sphincter of Oddi dysfunction, needle-knife sphincterotomy over a pancreatic stent placed early in the procedure has been shown to be substantially safer than conventional pull-type sphincterotomy without a pancreatic stent.[19]

There has been controversy as to whether increased risk of precut sphincterotomy is attributable to the technique itself or the prolonged cannulation attempts that often precede its use. A meta-analysis of 6 randomized trials with 966 subjects examined this issue.[20] The meta-analysis included trials in which patients were assigned to early precut implementation or persistent attempts at standard cannulation. PEP was significantly less common in the precut group compared with the persistent attempts at cannulation group (3% vs 5%). However, the overall rate of adverse events, including pancreatitis, bleeding, cholangitis, and perforation, did not significantly differ (5% vs 6%). The relevance of these studies might be diminished by the fact that few involved use of pancreatic stents—which is now considered fairly standard—or included patients with high-risk indications such as sphincter of Oddi dysfunction.

Although it is widely thought that contrast injection into the pancreatic duct is a principal culprit in causing PEP, recent studies have revealed that guidewire passage into the pancreatic duct (without subsequent pancreatic stent placement) is one, if not the major, independent technique-related factor.[8,21,22] In the first study ever to assess the independent role of PD wire passage,[8] a comprehensive evaluation of all the risk factors in 3178 ERCPs was undertaken. Independent risk factors included female gender (OR: 1.84, $p = 0.002$), age ≤ 60 years (OR: 1.59, $p = 0.025$), cannulation time >10 min (OR: 1.76, $p = 0.012$), ≥ 1 pancreatic deep wire pass (OR: 2.77, $p < 0.001$), and needle-knife precut (OR: 4.34, $p < 0.001$). Interestingly, contrast injections were not independently significant. These findings have been borne out by every subsequent study that evaluated pancreatic guidewire passage as a risk.[21,23] In another study, "double-wire technique" to cannulate the common bile duct was also associated with increased risk.[22]

Risk of PEP escalates in patients with multiple risk factors.[3] The interactive effect of multiple risk factors is reflected in the profile of patients developing severe PEP. In one study predating widespread use of pancreatic stents, female patients with normal serum bilirubin had a 5% risk of pancreatitis; with addition of difficult cannulation, the risk rose to 16%; with further addition of suspected sphincter of Oddi dysfunction (i.e., no stone found), the risk rose to 42%.[3] In two different studies, nearly all of the patients who developed severe pancreatitis were young to middle-aged women with recurrent abdominal pain, a normal serum bilirubin, and no biliary obstructive pathology.[3,12] These observations emphasize the importance of tailoring the approach of ERCP to the individual patient.

One recent study has clearly shown that trainee participation adds independent risk of pancreatitis.[4] In contrast, most multicenter studies have failed to show a significant correlation between endoscopists' ERCP case volumes and pancreatitis rates.[2,3,7] It is possible that none of the participating endoscopists in those studies reached the threshold volume of ERCP above which pancreatitis rates would diminish (perhaps >250 to 500 cases per year). However, most American endoscopists average fewer than two ERCPs per week,[3] and the reported rates of pancreatitis from the highest volume tertiary referral centers in the United States are often relatively higher than those in private practices. All of these observations suggest that case mix is at least as important as expertise in determining risk of PEP.

Specific Techniques to Reduce Risk of Post-ERCP Pancreatitis

It stands to reason that the most expeditious method of cannulation will likely be the safest. Use of a papillotome or steerable catheter for biliary cannulation has been prospectively compared with a standard catheter in a number of randomized trials.[18] Although all showed significantly higher success with the sphincterotome, there was no difference in rates of pancreatitis or other adverse events. Another randomized trial did show significant reduction of pancreatitis risk when a guidewire was used in conjunction with a papillotome, as opposed to a papillotome alone.[18]

Guidewire cannulation, using wire probe instead of contrast injection, has been shown to lower PEP rates in a number of prospective randomized trials, with rates of 0% to 3% in wire cannulation compared with 4% to 12% using contrast injection. In reality, a combination of careful guidewire plus very minimal contrast injection may be optimal, but this has not been formally evaluated.

Pancreatic stent placement can reduce risk of PEP in a number of settings (Table 8.5) and is widely performed at many advanced centers for this purpose (Fig. 8.1). It acts by reducing the flow disruptions caused by injury and maintaining the flow of pancreatic secretions. Specific situations where placement of a pancreatic stent has been shown to reduce risk include biliary sphincterotomy for sphincter of Oddi dysfunction, suspected sphincter of Oddi dysfunction with normal manometry, pancreatic sphincterotomy, precut sphincterotomy, balloon dilation of the biliary sphincter, and endoscopic ampullectomy after pancreatic wire-assisted biliary cannulation, probably after difficult cannulation in general, and even after unselected ERCP in patients with "virgin papilla," excluding those with pancreas divisum or cancer.[24–33]

Three meta-analyses suggest that use of pancreatic stents in high-risk patients reduced rates of pancreatitis by about two-thirds, with virtual elimination of severe PEP.[19,25,26] Another recent meta-analysis[34] showed that PD stent placement reduced the risk of mild, moderate, and severe PEP in both high-risk and low-risk to mixed-risk patients. Although effective in high-risk cases, placement of pancreatic stents is usually unnecessary regardless of cannulation difficulty in older, jaundiced patients if they have pancreatic duct obstruction in the setting of pancreatic cancer.

Pancreatic stenting has some limitations as a strategy to reduce risk.[31] Many endoscopists and their assistants are unfamiliar with their

TABLE 8.5 Pancreatic Stents to Reduce Risk of Post-ERCP Pancreatitis

Setting	Benefit	Evidence
Biliary sphincterotomy for SOD	Yes	RCT
Suspected SOD with normal manometry	Yes	Retrospective case-control
Pancreatic sphincterotomy	Yes	RCT, retrospective case-control
Biliary balloon dilation for stone	Trend	Retrospective case-control
Precut (access) sphincterotomy	Yes	RCT
High-risk (difficult cannulation, etc.)	Yes	RCT × 3
Pancreatic guidewire-assisted cannulation	Yes	RCT
Pancreatic brush cytology	Trend	Retrospective case-control
Endoscopic ampullectomy	Yes/trend	RCT, retrospective case-control
All consecutive ERCP, unselected	Yes	RCT × 2
IPMN	No	Retrospective case-control

IPMN, Intraductal papillary mucinous neoplasm; *RCT,* randomized controlled trial; *SOD,* sphincter of Oddi.

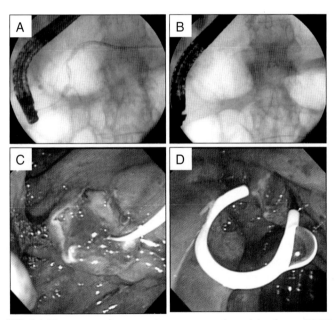

FIG 8.1 Placement of pancreatic stent to reduce risk of post-ERCP pancreatitis. **A,** A guidewire passed to body of pancreatic duct around genu. **B,** 4-Fr single-pigtail 9-cm-long unflanged pancreatic stent placed. **C,** Endoscopic view of guidewire in pancreatic duct after biliary sphincterotomy. **D,** 4-Fr single-pigtail pancreatic stent placed with drainage of pancreatic juice.

placement and may have a substantial failure rate, leaving the patient worse off than if no attempt was made.[28] Small-caliber wires (0.018 or 0.025 inches) are often optimal, and techniques for deep insertion of such guidewires may be unfamiliar to many endoscopists. Small tortuous ducts and ansa pancreaticus (360-degree alpha loop) may pose a challenge even for the most experienced endoscopist. A technique has been described that does not require deep wire passage but allows universal

success at placing stents in difficult anatomy[28]; a small-caliber nitinol-tipped wire can be knuckled inside the main pancreatic duct just beyond the sphincter and allow delivery of a small-caliber short stent.

Unfortunately, pancreatic stents may cause problems. They may be inadvertently advanced during placement, or subsequently migrate inside the pancreatic duct, especially stents of straight configuration without a pigtail on the duodenal end and those with dual inner flanges. This adverse event can largely be avoided by use of a single pigtail on the duodenal end that has a clear visual marker for deployment. A major concern about pancreatic stents is the potential to cause ductal or parenchymal injury or even perforation; ductal and parenchymal injury have been reported in up to 80% of patients with normal ducts using conventional 5-Fr or greater polyethylene stents, and sometimes leads to severe ductal stenosis with resulting relapsing pancreatitis.[35–38] Strategies to avoid this adverse event include use of smaller-caliber stents (3 or 4 Fr), which have been shown to be associated with lower rates of duct injury than conventional polyethylene 5-Fr stents,[37] and use of stents made of softer materials, which are now widely available. Pancreatic stents placed for prevention of PEP in normal ducts are designed to pass spontaneously. This should be documented by plain abdominal radiograph obtained approximately 2 weeks after placement. If they have not passed by then, they need to be removed.

Balloon dilation of the biliary sphincter has been introduced as an alternative to sphincterotomy for the extraction of bile duct stones (see Chapter 18). Although trials from outside the United States have shown adverse event rates to be equivalent to or less than for sphincterotomy, one US prospective study showed balloon dilation to markedly increased the risk of PEP, resulting in two deaths.[39] A meta-analysis of pooled studies also showed an increased risk of PEP after balloon dilation.[40] In general, balloon dilation of the intact biliary sphincter for extraction of bile duct stones is not recommended unless there is a relative con-traindication to sphincterotomy, such as coagulopathy or a need for early anticoagulation. When balloon dilation is performed under these circumstances, it should generally be accompanied by placement of a prophylactic pancreatic stent. If placement of a prophylactic pancreatic stent is not possible, NSAIDs should be administered. In contrast, balloon dilation performed after biliary sphincterotomy to facilitate large stone extraction appears to be safe (see Chapters 18 and 19) and may reduce the need for excessively large sphincterotomy and its associated risk of perforation or bleeding.[41]

Thermal injury is thought to play some role in causing pancreatitis after biliary and pancreatic sphincterotomy. A number of random-ized trials have compared the impact of pure cutting versus blended current, with mixed results but generally lower rates of pancreatitis using the pure cut current.[18,42] Automated current delivery systems programmed to deliver a specific tissue effect are now widely used. None of the available studies suggest a significant difference in rates of pancreatitis between these units compared with blended current, so it is not yet clear whether automated current delivery systems provide the same benefit for prevention of pancreatitis as do those using pure cut current.

Pharmacologic Agents

Many pharmacologic agents have been investigated as potential agents to reduce PEP, but results have generally been mixed or negative, until recently. In meta-analyses of randomized controlled trials, gabexate (a protease inhibitor) or somatostatin has been found to be marginally effective, but only if given over an extended infusion (up to 12 hours after ERCP), whereas shorter infusions (<4 hours) are generally inef-fective.[18] Neither of these agents is available in the United States, and the prolonged infusions severely limit the cost-effectiveness and practical-ity of these agents. More recently, rectal NSAIDs have attracted a great deal of attention and have been hailed as simple nontoxic solution to preventing PEP. Six randomized control trials[43-48] have been published in the past decade that have demonstrated that admission of rectal indomethacin reduced the incidence of PEP by 50% to 60%. Further meta-analyses have also confirmed the above findings and have resulted in rectal indomethacin being hailed as a panacea for prevention of PEP. More recently, in a single-center trial,[49] 449 patients were randomized to rectal indomethacin versus placebo. This trial failed to show any statistical difference between the groups. One of the reasons cited for this difference was that out of the six randomized controlled trials, only one was conducted in the United States, and that trial[43,50] consisted largely of patients with sphincter of Oddi type III, a now defunct indication for ERCP. In that study, administration of 100 mg of indomethacin via rectal suppository at the end of the ERCP resulted in a reduction in the rate of PEP from 17% in the control group to 9% in the treatment group. Of note is that most patients (80%) received a prophylactic pancreatic stent because of high risk of PEP. Thus the data so far on NSAIDs appear to be conflicting. Nonetheless, two very recent studies support the use of rectal NSAIDs, including for those who are considered to be at low risk for PEP.[51,52]

Prevention and Treatment of Post-ERCP Pancreatitis

The single most important way to avoid PEP is to avoid performing ERCP for marginal indications, especially in patients at higher risk of adverse events. Paradoxically, the risk is often higher and the potential benefit of therapy lower in marginally indicated ERCP than for patients with obstructive jaundice. ERCP should generally be avoided outside of specialized referral centers when the probability of finding stones or other obstructive pathology is low and other methods are available to assess stones (e.g., endoscopic ultrasonography, magnetic resonance cholangiopancreatography [MRCP]), or in situations in which the risk-benefit ratio of conventional diagnostic or biliary therapeutic ERCP is excessive (e.g., suspected sphincter of Oddi dysfunction). Alternative imaging techniques such as intraoperative laparoscopic cholangiography, MRCP, and endoscopic ultrasonography are safer alternatives for excluding obstructive biliary pathology. Patients who have negative evaluation by these alternative techniques, but who are still suspected to have a pancreatic or biliary cause for recurrent symptoms, are probably best served by referral to a tertiary ERCP center capable of advanced techniques for diagnosis, including endoscopic ultrasonography; advanced therapeutics, including pancreatic endotherapy; and with near-certain ability to place pancreatic stents.

Several studies have advocated the use of intravenous volume expansion through the use of normal saline before and continuing after the procedure. Although this may be effective, it can be difficult to institute such a protocol within endoscopy units, and there is a risk of volume overload.[53,54]

Once the decision has been made to proceed with ERCP, cannulation and sphincterotomy techniques should be tailored to the risk profile of that individual. In low-risk cases such as elderly patients with obstructive jaundice, manipulation is generally well tolerated, and whatever techniques are effective at gaining bile duct access and drainage are reasonable. In high-risk cases, manipulation should be minimized and placement of a pancreatic stent considered. Placement of pancreatic stents is recommended in most patients with suspected sphincter dysfunction, history of PEP, and difficult cannulation, or before precut sphincterotomy with unclear papillary anatomy or other risk factors. For pancreatic stent insertion, the size of the stent should be tailored to the caliber and course of the pancreatic duct, with small-caliber (3 to 5 Fr) pancreatic stents that are generally either short (2 to 3 cm) when 5-Fr stents are used or long (7 to 10 cm) when 3-Fr stents are used, and unflanged. Precut sphincterotomy in high-risk patients is

probably best performed by experts, early rather than late in the procedure, and after placement of a pancreatic stent in high-risk circumstances or unclear papillary anatomy.

As mentioned above with the publication of multiple randomized trials and meta-analyses, NSAIDs are now being raised as a "panacea" to prevent PEP. Their ease of administration and noninvasiveness, when combined with the lack of familiarity and technical skills to place a pancreatic duct guidewire and/or a pancreatic stent, even by some endoscopists at advanced centers, make them a popular choice. In addition, the European Society of Gastrointestinal Endoscopy now advocates the use of NSAIDs before every ERCP.[55] Despite this recommendation, there are limited data to suggest that NSAIDs are superior to pancreatic stents in preventing PEP. Although NSAIDs can be used in high-risk patients for PEP, the data do not show that their use completely eliminates the need for prophylactic pancreatic duct stents.[56]

Treatment of PEP is as for any other cause of acute pancreatitis. Early recognition of impending PEP can be facilitated by obtaining serum amylase or lipase within a few hours after the procedure in patients who are at high risk, and for those who have postprocedural abdominal pain. If serum amylase or lipase is normal, the probability of developing pancreatitis is very low and the patient can be considered for same-day discharge if other discharge criteria are met. On the other hand, if the pancreatic enzymes are significantly elevated (>3 times upper limits of normal), premature same-day discharge may be avoided and preemptive hospitalization for observation, fasting, and vigorous intravenous hydration initiated if the patient has symptoms suggestive of PEP. Severely ill patients should be hospitalized in the intensive care unit, with help obtained from other specialists in managing them.

"Salvage" ERCP with placement of a pancreatic stent soon after development of PEP with predictors of a severe course is a controversial but potential pathway for treatment of selected patients who either never received a pancreatic stent or in whom a pancreatic stent passed prematurely.[57]

HEMORRHAGE

Bleeding seen endoscopically during sphincterotomy is often reported as an adverse event; but of itself does not represent an adverse outcome to the patient unless there is clinically significant blood loss or a change in management. Some degree of bleeding, ranging from oozing to severe bleeding, is seen at the time of sphincterotomy in about 10% to 30% of cases. Clinically significant hemorrhage is defined in the consensus criteria (see Table 8.1) as clinical evidence of bleeding (e.g., melena or hematemesis) with or without an associated fall in hemoglobin or the requirement for secondary intervention such as endoscopy or blood transfusion. Clinically significant hemorrhage occurs in 0.1% to 2% of sphincterotomies.[2] Clinical presentation is generally delayed from 1 day to as many as 10 days after sphincterotomy.[2]

Risk Factors for Hemorrhage After Sphincterotomy

For clinically significant hemorrhage (see Table 8.4), risk factors include any degree of bleeding during the procedure; presence of any coagulopathy or thrombocytopenia (including hemodialysis-associated coagulation disorders); initiation of full anticoagulant therapy within 3 days after ES; and relatively low case volume on the part of the endoscopist (performance of not more than one sphincterotomy per week), which may reflect less precise control of the incision or less effective endoscopic control of bleeding once it has occurred.[2] Factors that do not appear to raise the risk of hemorrhage include using aspirin or NSAIDs, making a longer incision, or enlarging a previous sphincterotomy.[2] The effects of newer antiplatelet agents are unknown (see Chapter 10).

Methods to Prevent and Treat Hemorrhage

Bleeding after sphincterotomy can mostly be prevented by avoiding sphincterotomy in patients with risk factors such as coagulopathy. Balloon dilation of the biliary sphincterotomy can be substituted or added to sphincterotomy in higher-risk patients. Once sphincterotomy is undertaken, risk can be minimized by correcting any coagulopathies, by withholding anticoagulant medications for as many as 3 days afterward, and by using meticulous endoscopic technique. Prophylactic injection of the sphincterotomy site with epinephrine in patients with coagulopathy may reduce the risk of hemorrhage. Newer computerized tissue-effect electrocautery units have been shown to reduce the risk of immediate bleeding but have not as yet been shown to decrease the incidence of clinically significant hemorrhage, although such adverse events are increasingly rare.

Once hemorrhage occurs, either immediately during sphincterotomy or delayed, it generally can be controlled with endoscopic therapy with injection of dilute epinephrine via a sclerotherapy needle. Balloon tamponade using standard occlusion balloons may allow temporary control of bleeding and improve visualization of the bleeding site. Thermal therapy, such as bipolar coagulation or clipping, can follow (Fig. 8.2). Caution should be taken to avoid thermal injury or clip placement over the pancreatic sphincter, especially if the bleeding site is on the right-hand wall of the sphincterotomy incision. Care should be taken while deploying the clips through the duodenoscope, as the plastic sheath often becomes kinked while passing through the elevator. More recently, insertion of a fully covered self-expandable metal stent (SEMS) has been reported as a means to control postsphincterotomy bleeding. It was initially described in 2010[58] and in subsequent case series[59–61] as treatment of postsphincterotomy bleeding, especially in cases where other endoscopic methods fail. SEMS placement is promising, but there is no consensus among experts on the optimal stent diameter and the timing of stent removal. Stent migration also remains a concern. For now it is probably best reserved as a salvage therapy when traditional endoscopic methods fail. Rarely, angiography or surgery is required for refractory bleeding.

PERFORATION

Perforation may occur within the bowel wall by the endoscope, through extension of a sphincterotomy incision beyond the intramural portion of the bile or pancreatic duct with retroperitoneal leakage, or at any location because of extramural passage or migration of guidewires or stents (Figs. 8.3, 8.4, and 8.5). Perforation is now reported in less than 1% of ERCPs and sphincterotomies.[2–9] Risk factors for sphincterotomy perforation have been difficult to quantify because of the rarity of perforation. It is probable that bowel perforation is more common in

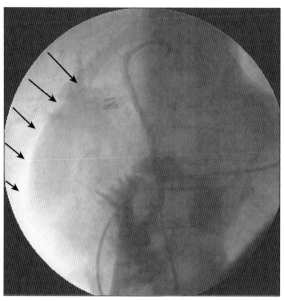

FIG 8.3 Fluoroscopic image after biliary sphincterotomy with large retroperitoneal perforation. A nasobiliary drain has been placed and a large amount of retroperitoneal air outlining the right kidney is apparent (arrows), with contrast tracking into retroperitoneum around the nasobiliary drain. As the leak was recognized immediately and was large and ongoing, this patient was managed with urgent operative intervention with oversew of the perforation but without duodenotomy and was discharged home 5 days later.

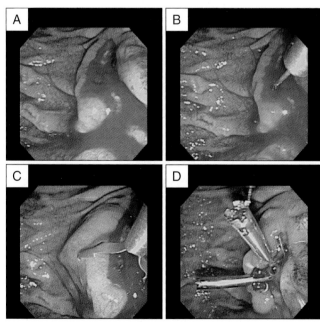

FIG 8.2 Endoscopic injection and clipping of sphincterotomy bleed. A, Bleeding from left edge of sphincterotomy. B, Injection of epinephrine. C, Positioning of endoscopic clip. D, Final placement of two clips on left edge of sphincterotomy with hemostasis.

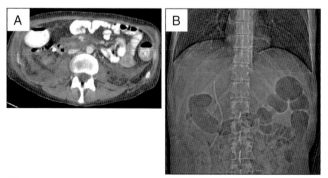

FIG 8.4 A, Distal migration of a biliary stent with perforation of the opposite wall of the duodenum. The stent was placed 5 days prior for hilar tumor obstruction. The patient presented with an acute abdomen. B, Computed tomography scan showing tip of stent and air in retroperitoneum anterior to the right kidney.

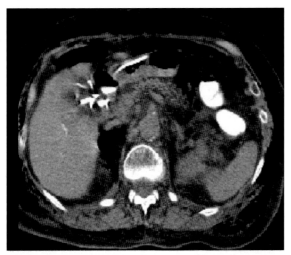

FIG 8.5 Computed tomography (CT) scan obtained immediately after biliary sphincterotomy perforation shows air in subcutaneous tissues (free intraperitoneal and retroperitoneal air). The patient developed crepitus during ERCP with sphincterotomy and lithotripsy for a large stone. A nasobiliary drain was placed. No contrast extravasation was demonstrated, either through nasobiliary drain or by CT, suggesting a favorable course for nonoperative management. This patient was treated with nasobiliary and nasogastric drainage and antibiotics and recovered fully without further intervention. (Courtesy Dr. Oliver Cass.)

patients with Billroth II or Roux-en-Y anatomy and that sphincterotomy perforation is more common after needle-knife precut techniques and in patients with suspected sphincter of Oddi dysfunction, all situations where control and extent of the required incision are uncertain.

Treatment of post-ERCP perforation varies with the type and severity of the leak and clinical manifestations. Bowel wall perforations must generally be treated surgically, whereas guidewire-related or stent-related perforations can usually be treated endoscopically by providing adequate ductal drainage.[62–64] Keys to avoiding perforation during sphincterotomy are to limit the length of cutting wire in contact with the tissue and to use stepwise incisions. If perforation is suspected during a sphincterotomy, careful fluoroscopy and injection of a small amount of contrast while pulling the catheter or papillotome through the incision over a guidewire will confirm or exclude extravasation and allow proactive treatment. Endoscopic clipping may be attempted in order to close a definite leak.[64] In most cases, a nasobiliary and/or nasopancreatic drain should be placed (depending on the sphincter cut) and the patient treated with nasogastric suction, intravenous antibiotics, strict fasting, surgical consultation, and in-hospital observation. The importance of early recognition and endoscopic drainage of suspected perforations is supported by the observation that nearly all patients with immediate recognition and endoscopic drainage did well with conservative management, in comparison with poor outcomes, including the need for surgery and some mortality in patients with delayed recognition.[63] Recently, placement of fully covered SEMS[65–67] for ERCP-related sphincterotomy perforations has been reported with success. The key to managing these injuries is to prevent leakage of bile into the peritoneum, and in such conditions SEMS can close the perforation appropriately. Once a perforation of any kind is suspected, a computed tomography scan of the abdomen should be obtained to assess for contrast leakage and any retroperitoneal or intraperitoneal air (see Fig. 8.5). If the leak is sizable and ongoing as suggested by ongoing contrast extravasation or if the patient's clinical condition deteriorates despite maximal intervention, including a fully covered SEMS, prompt drainage via a surgical or percutaneous approach is advisable (see Fig. 8.3).

CHOLANGITIS AND CHOLECYSTITIS

Cholangitis (ascending bile duct infection) and cholecystitis (gallbladder infection) are potential adverse events or sequelae of ERCP and sphincterotomy. Risk factors for cholangitis after ERCP and sphincterotomy consist primarily of failed or incomplete biliary drainage[2–9] and use of combined percutaneous-endoscopic procedures.[2] Other risk factors may include jaundice, especially because of malignancy, and operator inexperience.[2] Several studies have shown that prophylactic antibiotics can reduce the rate of bacteremia, but few studies have shown a reduction in clinical sepsis after ERCP, and a meta-analysis concluded that there was no clinical benefit to routine administration of antibiotics (see Chapter 10).[68] Thus the principal recommendation regarding prevention and treatment of cholangitis is to obtain successful and complete biliary drainage.

DUODENOSCOPE-ASSOCIATED BACTERIAL INFECTIONS

Iatrogenic infection is a well-documented complication of therapeutic endoscopy, which is beyond the scope of this chapter. Recently, severe and occasionally fatal duodenoscope-related infections have occurred in spite of compliance with device manufacturer–recommended protocols for high-level disinfection. Much effort has been devoted to identification of risk factors and elimination of this problem. Ongoing studies suggest that current protocols are likely inadequate to completely prevent endoscope-related transmission of infectious agents, but methods to solve this problem are under active investigation.[41] Chapter 5 is dedicated to duodenoscope reprocessing.

LONG-TERM ADVERSE EVENTS AND SEQUELAE

Recent studies have shown that if the gallbladder is left intact after sphincterotomy, both early and late cholecystitis occur more frequently than previously thought. Not surprisingly, both cholecystitis and recurrent bile duct stones are more common if the gallbladder left in situ contains stones. There is increasing concern about potential long-term sequelae of various components of endoscopic therapy, including endoscopic biliary and pancreatic sphincterotomy. These include recurrent stone formation, possibly resulting from sphincterotomy stenosis, or bacterobilia caused by duodenal-biliary reflux, or "sine-materia" cholangitis. Recurrent stones and other biliary problems may occur in 6% to 24% of patients undergoing long-term follow-up. Recurrent pancreatitis, presumably caused by thermal injury to the pancreatic sphincter, may occur after biliary sphincterotomy. The long-term effects of pancreatic sphincterotomy, increasingly performed in patients with and without chronic pancreatitis, are largely unknown.

OPERATOR EXPERIENCE AND ADVERSE EVENTS

The effect of endoscopic expertise on the outcome of ERCP is difficult to evaluate but is likely profound. Simple comparisons of adverse event rates of ERCP between centers can be misleading, because the case mix, intent of the procedure, and success rates at achieving biliary and pancreatic duct access vary widely. A number of studies have evaluated operator factors in adverse events of ERCP. Lower ERCP case volume, defined variably, was significantly associated with higher overall adverse event rates by univariate and multivariate analyses in all studies that have evaluated that risk factor. In one study, endoscopists who performed more than one sphincterotomy per week had somewhat lower rates of overall adverse events (8% vs 11%) but substantially lower rates of severe adverse events (0.9% vs 2.3%)[2]; in a multivariate model using only information available before ERCP, lower procedure volume was one of only three variables that predicted adverse events of sphincterotomy.[2] Lower case volume was significantly associated with higher rates of hemorrhage after sphincterotomy in two studies.[2,7] In contrast, lower ERCP case volume has not consistently been found to correlate with rates of PEP, suggesting the importance of case mix in determining this adverse event. In an Austrian multicenter study, endoscopists were considered high volume if they carried out more than 50 procedures a year. The data demonstrated that high-case-volume endoscopists had better diagnostic and therapeutic success (86.9% vs 80.3%) with fewer adverse events (10.2% vs 13.6%) than lower-case-volume endoscopists.[69] These data are similar to those of a previous Italian study in which the adverse event rates were higher (7.1% vs 2.0%) in centers with low volume (<200 per year).[7] In a multicenter study in the United States, endoscopists who carried out no more than one sphincterotomy per week had higher adverse event rates compared with their peers who carried out higher volumes of sphincterotomies each week.[2] These and other studies support the concept that a lower case volume affects outcomes adversely.[70,71] In contrast, another recent large multicenter study of assessment of risk factors for ERCP adverse events from the United Kingdom found no difference in overall adverse events between endoscopists with differing caseloads or hospital type.[9] The only difference found was a decrease in the risk of PEP when the procedure was carried out at a university hospital compared with a district hospital, interpreted to perhaps reflect the better support staff and environment available at university hospitals.

The available data probably underestimate the influence of operator experience on outcomes of ERCP, because high-case-volume endoscopists attempt higher-risk cases, and also have higher success rates at duct access. In one study, endoscopists averaging more than 100 ERCP cases per year had 96.5% success at bile duct access compared with 91.5% for lower-case-volume endoscopists.[3] In two other studies, rates of failure and adverse events for ERCP by higher-case-volume endoscopists were significantly lower than for those by lesser-case-volume endoscopists.[2,7] Failure to complete ERCP may have as much negative impact on patients as adverse events in terms of cost, need for further interventions, and extension of hospital stay.

BOX 8.2 Strategies to Reduce Adverse Events of ERCP

- Improved training, especially in placement of pancreatic stents for prevention of post-ERCP pancreatitis
- Education of endoscopists regarding risk factors
- Avoidance of marginally indicated ERCP
- Referral to advanced centers for complex or high-risk cases
- Fewer endoscopists performing more ERCPs
- Rectal nonsteroidal antiinflammatory agents

It is not known what minimum volume of cases is required to maintain proficiency, but probably in excess of 50 to 100 cases per year to sustain good outcomes for routine biliary therapy and 200 to 250 cases per year for advanced pancreatic techniques. A minority of endoscopists in the United States achieve such volumes of ERCP. The data suggest that outcomes will be optimal if fewer endoscopists perform more ERCPs. It is not feasible or palatable to suggest that all ERCPs be performed at advanced centers. Rather, adequate training and ongoing case volume should be prerequisites for performing ERCP in practice. Larger groups should funnel all of their ERCPs to a few dedicated individuals rather than dilute the experience, and smaller groups who are unable to sustain adequate volumes should consider contracting out their ERCP work to more experienced individuals. Endoscopists who perform limited numbers of complex ERCPs should be amenable to prompt referral to a specialized center for potentially complex cases, including difficult biliary problems, all pancreatic therapeutics, and most cases of suspected sphincter of Oddi dysfunction. The key is for each endoscopist to find the optimal balance between risk and benefit for the individual patient and his or her own individual expertise and experience (Box 8.2).

The complete reference list for this chapter can be found online at www.expertconsult.com.

9

ERCP Training

Rawad Mounzer and Sachin Wani

Endoscopic retrograde cholangiopancreatography (ERCP) continues to be one of the most technically challenging endoscopic procedures. Training in ERCP requires the mastery of a broad skill set for this procedure to be performed safely and effectively, given the higher rate and wider range of adverse events (post-ERCP pancreatitis, bleeding, and perforation) associated with ERCP in comparison to standard endoscopic procedures.[1–4] In addition to developing a high level of technical skill, training in ERCP also entails a thorough understanding of the indications, limitations, and inherent risks associated with ERCP and the alternative options of management (cognitive skills).[5] Over the past few decades, ERCP has evolved from a diagnostic to a predominantly therapeutic technique, with diagnostic ERCP having decreased 7-fold, whereas therapeutic ERCP has increased nearly 30-fold.[6] Additionally, there has been a trend toward increasing complexity of ERCP, which is routinely utilized to manage complex pancreaticobiliary diseases such as chronic pancreatitis, malignant jaundice, and postoperative biliary complications of liver transplantation. This shift from diagnostic to therapeutic ERCP has been driven predominantly by technological advancements in pancreaticobiliary imaging modalities, including magnetic resonance cholangiopancreatography (MRCP) and endoscopic ultrasonography (EUS), and the advent of novel ERCP devices allowing for more complex therapeutic interventions.[7,8] The higher risk profile of ERCP, coupled with the increasing sophistication of this technique and the need for additional interventions or repeat procedures after a failed ERCP (e.g., percutaneous transhepatic cholangiography, surgery, or repeat ERCP), underscores the importance of adequate training.[3,9] It is clear that ERCP is operator dependent and that additional training is required for the development of technical, cognitive, and integrative skills beyond those required for standard endoscopic procedures.[9] In this chapter, the authors highlight the current status of training and the shifting paradigm from procedure volume as a surrogate of competency to validated competency thresholds.[9]

TRAINING IN ERCP

Training in endoscopy entails both cognitive and technical elements that are required to safely and proficiently perform these procedures. Before embarking on learning ERCP, trainees are required to master standard upper endoscopy. This includes thorough visualization of the upper gastrointestinal tract, with proper identification of normal and abnormal findings, while minimizing patient discomfort and achieving proficiency in basic therapeutic techniques.[10] Understanding procedural indications, contraindications, risks, and limitations and learning how to interpret endoscopic findings (including interpretation of cholangiograms and pancreatograms) and incorporate them into medical and endoscopic management are an integral part of this process. Cognitive education through reading, reviewing videos and atlases, and attending lectures and conferences is combined with supervised hands-on

experience under the mentorship of expert endoscopists.[11] A core curriculum for training in ERCP by the American Society for Gastrointestinal Endoscopy (ASGE) has become the standard in the United States.[10]

The training process usually begins by observing a primary endoscopist perform ERCP and becoming acquainted with the unique endoscopic view of the duodenoscope and the function of the elevator. After this, the trainee traditionally will move on to attempt passing the duodenoscope. As with general endoscopy, one of the initial challenges is intubating the esophagus. Once in the esophagus, the duodenoscope is gently advanced until the gastric mucosa is visualized. The duodenoscope is then navigated along the greater curvature of the stomach and positioned in the antrum such that the pylorus is visualized in the "setting sun" position. The pylorus is then traversed and the duodenal sweep is negotiated. Once in the second part of the duodenum, the duodenoscope can be reduced to the "short" position, which usually brings the major papilla into view. In the "short" position, the duodenoscope can be seen in the classic "hockey stick" configuration under fluoroscopy. Attaining proficiency in the use of accessory devices and in the judicious and effective use of fluoroscopy is also crucial to performing safe and successful ERCP. This process involves performing supervised procedures, engaging in interactive observation with the primary endoscopist, and assisting the endoscopy nurse or technician in the handling of devices. In the early stages of their ERCP experience, it is reasonable for trainees to have hands-on experience in lower-risk cases, such as routine stent exchange or cannulation in the setting of prior sphincterotomy. Additionally, ERCP training should take place at a center fitted with all the basic equipment necessary to perform ERCP and where an adequate number of experienced trainers are present who have a track record of adequate case volume and effective endoscopic teaching. The key endpoints of training in ERCP are highlighted in Box 9.1. Trainees should maintain a procedure log of only those procedures during which hands-on experience occurred. This log should also include the indication, grade of difficulty (Table 9.1),[10] and specific endpoints achieved by the trainee. This will be helpful not only for credentialing purposes but also to allow for the assessment of competency.

CURRENT STATUS OF ERCP TRAINING

In the past, training in ERCP in the United States was a part of a traditional fellowship in gastroenterology for a limited subset of trainees.[12] The ASGE core curriculum for ERCP, however, currently requires a minimum of 12 months of dedicated training, which in most cases takes place in the form of an additional year of training.[10] During this time, trainees work toward developing their skill set with the goal of becoming capable of performing ERCP independently.[13]

At present, international societal thresholds for competence in ERCP are based on procedural volumes. The currently set thresholds are

BOX 9.1 Suggested Endpoints for ERCP Training

Technical Aspects

1. Esophageal intubation
2. Achieving the "short" position
3. Identification of the papilla
4. Selective deep cannulation of the duct of interest in cases with a native papilla
5. Advanced cannulation techniques (double-wire technique, placement of pancreatic duct stent, precut sphincterotomy)
6. Biliary and pancreatic sphincterotomy
7. Guidewire placement in the desired location
8. Stent removal and insertion
9. Stricture dilation and sampling
10. Stone extraction techniques (balloon extraction, use of baskets, and mechanical, electrohydraulic, or laser lithotripsy)
11. Recognition and management of adverse events (bleeding, perforation, pancreatitis, infections, cardiopulmonary events, hospitalization, and mortality)

Cognitive Aspects

1. Clear understanding of informed consent and procedure indications, contraindications, and alternatives
2. Appropriate use of fluoroscopy
3. Proficient use of real-time cholangiogram/pancreatogram interpretation and ability to identify the nature of pathology (stone, stricture, leak, etc.)
4. Logical plan based on cholangiogram/pancreatogram findings
5. Clear understanding of the techniques to reduce post-ERCP pancreatitis (rectal indomethacin, pancreatic duct stenting, intravenous fluids)
6. Clear understanding of the role of antibiotics and knowledge of anticoagulants

TABLE 9.1 ERCP Difficulty Grading Scale

Difficulty Grade	Biliary ERCP	Pancreatic ERCP
1	Diagnostic cholangiogram Brush cytology Standard sphincterotomy Stone extraction <10 mm Stricture dilation, stent placement, nasobiliary drain for extrahepatic stricture or bile leak	Diagnostic pancreatogram Brush cytology
2	Diagnostic cholangiogram in Billroth II anatomy Stone extraction >10 mm Stricture dilation, stent placement, nasobiliary drain for hilar disease or benign intrahepatic strictures	Diagnostic pancreatogram in Billroth II anatomy Cannulation of minor papilla
3	Sphincter of Oddi manometry Therapeutic ERCP in Billroth II anatomy Intrahepatic stone extraction Lithotripsy	Sphincter of Oddi manometry Pancreatoscopy Therapeutic ERCP Pseudocyst drainage

Adapted from ASGE Training Committee, Jorgensen J, Kubiliun N, et al. Endoscopic retrograde cholangiopancreatography (ERCP): core curriculum. *Gastrointest Endosc.* 2016;83:279–289.

extrapolated from limited data and expert opinion.[9,14] As per the Gastroenterology Core Curriculum, trainees are required to perform a minimum of 200 ERCPs, after which competency may be assessed. The ASGE ERCP core curriculum requires the same minimum procedural volume as the Gastroenterology Core Curriculum, with the caveat that at least half of these procedures are therapeutic.[10,14] The Canadian Association of Gastroenterology, similar to the Gastroenterological Society of Australia, requires at least 200 unassisted ERCPs, including 80 supervised procedures with independently performed sphincterotomies and the placement of a minimum of 60 biliary stents.[15,16] The British Society of Gastroenterology ERCP Working Party has also recently modified their guidelines, which now include key performance indicators for training programs. Trainees are required to participate in at least 300 ERCPs, with a target unselected cannulation rate of ≥80% during the last 50 cases. Additionally, trainees should also be able to appropriately select and consent patients, work within a multidisciplinary team, identify and manage procedural complications, and demonstrate the ability to perform level 1 and 2 procedures without verbal or physical assistance. These guidelines also suggest that trainees be mentored during the first 2 years of independent practice to ensure a safe and effective transition. After the completion of training, trainees are required to meet the minimum requirements for a competent ERCP practitioner within 2 years of mentored practice.[17]

These current guidelines lack validation with regard to competence and feasibility of training. Additionally, they do not account for the fact that trainees differ considerably in the rates at which they learn and develop endoscopic skills.[18–20] In fact, available data and expert opinion suggest that the majority of trainees are not competent at the above-defined thresholds and require double the number of proposed procedures to achieve competence in ERCP.[9] Thus, the number of procedures completed during training alone does not ensure competence and is a suboptimal marker of competence in ERCP.

Over the past 15 years, the number of advanced endoscopy fellowship programs (typically a 1-year training program of combined training in ERCP and EUS) has increased dramatically in the United States. These programs are currently not recognized by the Accreditation Council for Graduate Medical Education (ACGME).[12] Due to the lack of a fixed mandatory curriculum, there are limited data on the composition and outcomes of ERCP training among advanced endoscopy trainees completing these programs. Results from a recent prospective multicenter study evaluating competence among advanced endoscopy trainees showed that the median number of ERCPs performed per trainee was 350 (range 125 to 500) at the conclusion of training. The vast majority of procedures performed were for a biliary indication of grade 1 difficulty (77%), and a minority were performed for pancreatic indications (14%). The mean time allowed for cannulation was 5.7 minutes (standard deviation [SD] 4.8 minutes) in cases with a native papilla and 6.2 minutes (SD 5 minutes) in cases in which the trainee did not achieve cannulation. There was no change in the time allowed for native papilla cannulation during the 1-year training period. Trainees were also involved in a small proportion of cases requiring advanced cannulation techniques. At the end of training, the majority of trainees expressed comfort with performing ERCP independently (100%), cannulation (92%), sphincterotomy (85%), stone clearance (92%), and the placement of biliary (100%) and pancreatic stents (92%). Nearly half of the trainees planned to practice at an academic center and expected a majority of their practice to be in advanced endoscopy.[21]

LEARNING CURVES AND COMPETENCE IN ERCP

There are limited data on learning curves in ERCP among advanced endoscopy trainees.[9,19,20,22,23] As per the ASGE credentialing guidelines, "competence" is defined as "the minimal level of skill, knowledge, and/or expertise, derived through training and experience, required to safely and proficiently perform a task or procedure."[24] The Gastroenterology Core Curriculum, however, clearly points out that "endoscopic competence is difficult to define and quantify" and that its assessment remains "largely subjective."[25] Although the ASGE ERCP core curriculum sets a minimal procedural volume requirement, it highlights the variability of endoscopic skill acquisition among trainees and the need for objective measures of competence.[10,14] A success rate of ≥80% in "selectively and freely" cannulating the desired ductal system "reliably without assistance" in cases of normal anatomy is widely used as a surrogate for trainee competence in reported studies and is also suggested by existing guidelines and quality metrics. Others have suggested that a higher standard of successful cannulation (rate of 90%) is a more appropriate benchmark for competence and for those seeking independent practice after training.[5,10] Patients who have previously undergone a sphincterotomy, however, are frequently included in the denominator, and hence these data are of limited applicability.

If deep cannulation is to be used as a benchmark for competence in ERCP, learning curves describing cannulation in patients with native papillary anatomy are required. Data from recent studies further strengthen the value of using selective native papilla cannulation as the new benchmark for assessing successful cannulation during ERCP both in training and in independent practice.[9,23] Finally, the overall success of ERCP is dependent not only on successful cannulation but also on other technical maneuvers required to achieve complete procedural success, such as sphincterotomy, stone extraction, tissue sampling, and stent placement, in addition to relevant cognitive aspects (indication of the procedure and appropriate use and interpretation of fluoroscopy). Studies evaluating learning curves and competence in ERCP that address these relevant endpoints are limited.

In a landmark study performed in 1996, Jowell et al. suggested that at least 180 ERCPs were required before trainees could be considered competent. This study, however, was limited by the fact that only 3 of 17 total trainees attained the 180 ERCP threshold. Additionally, the grading system utilized in trainee assessment had not been previously validated and was extrapolated from a grading system used to evaluate competency in sigmoidoscopy.[22,26] Data have since emerged demonstrating significant variability in the achievement of competence among trainees. In a study by Verma et al. evaluating a single trainee during the fourth year of advanced endoscopy training, a ≥80% success rate of deep biliary cannulation in native papillae was achieved after 350 to 400 supervised ERCPs.[20] A subsequent study from the Netherlands prospectively evaluated 15 trainees during their final 2 years of training utilizing a self-assessment tool that incorporated both quality indicators and procedural degree of technical difficulty.[19,27,28] Although the common bile duct cannulation rate significantly increased from a baseline of 36% to 85% after 200 ERCPs ($p < 0.001$), the biliary cannulation rate of a native papilla was only 68% after 180 procedures. This further highlighted the need for assessing actual performance as opposed to minimal procedural volumes as a measure of competence.[19] In a study currently in abstract form, selective biliary cannulation was shown to improve during the initial 9 months of a 1-year training program, followed by the plateauing of performance and no change in the unintended rate of pancreatic duct cannulation during the training period.[29] Moreover, a recent meta-analysis of 9 studies including 137 trainees and 17,100 ERCPs revealed a wide range in procedural volumes needed to achieve competency in various technical elements of ERCP (overall competence 70 to 400, pancreatic duct cannulation 70 to 160, selective duct cannulation 79 to 300, common bile duct cannulation 160 to 400, native papilla deep bile duct cannulation 350 to 400).[23]

A recent prospective multicenter study by Wani et al. aimed to define learning curves and measure competence among trainees at advanced endoscopy training programs in the United States by utilizing a standardized evaluation tool and cumulative sum analysis. This tool incorporated the grade of procedural difficulty per the ASGE grading system and evaluated all relevant technical and cognitive aspects of ERCP (see Appendix 9.1).[9,14] Results of this study demonstrated substantial variability in the number of ERCPs performed during training and in the learning curves for the individual technical and cognitive aspects of ERCP. Although all trainees crossed the threshold for competence in overall cannulation, none of the trainees achieved competence in the cannulation of native papillae, underscoring the importance of using native papilla deep cannulation as the benchmark for assessing successful cannulation (Fig. 9.1).[9] It can be argued that the time allowed for a trainee to cannulate was limited, which is a true representation of current clinical training. It is also acknowledged that the proportion of trainees achieving competency could have increased if trainees were allowed more time. Although this study defined learning curves during ERCP training that encompassed all relevant technical and cognitive aspects in a prospective fashion using a standardized structured tool and strong statistical methodology, data regarding the impact of ongoing feedback based on learning curves during training remain limited. Similarly, competence can continue to improve after the completion of training, and trainees may achieve measures of competence during independent practice.

TOWARD COMPETENCY-BASED MEDICAL EDUCATION

The current status of ERCP training is limited by the lack of a clear definition of endoscopic competence and the ongoing use of volume-based thresholds as a surrogate marker for endoscopic skill level. Additionally, the currently set volume thresholds are founded on limited data, and the overall assessment by trainers remains highly subjective.[9,25] In an effort to base program accreditation on educational outcomes, the ACGME put forth the Next Accreditation System (NAS) in 2012, focusing heavily on competency-based medical education (CBME).[30] The NAS requires trainees of ACGME-accredited programs to receive competency-based training and achieve documented specialty-specific "educational milestones" to help ensure that they acquire the knowledge, skills, and attitudes necessary for safe and effective independent practice. In the setting of the NAS and an increasing emphasis on quality in health care, training programs in advanced endoscopy will need to incorporate CBME into their curricula.[9,31] In a nationwide survey of trainees and program directors of ACGME-accredited gastroenterology fellowship programs in the United States, 23% of the 94 participating programs lacked a formal endoscopy curriculum. Program directors reported procedural volumes and trainer-written evaluations as the primary measures of competence at the majority of these programs. Moreover, less than one-third of programs utilized skill assessment tools or specific quality metrics such as adenoma detection rates for the evaluation of competency.[32]

In an effort to standardize the evaluation of the cognitive and technical aspects of ERCP and more clearly define endoscopic competence, the use of a validated structured assessment tool is critical. The EUS and ERCP skills assessment tool (TEESAT) has been utilized in published and ongoing studies evaluating advanced endoscopy training in the United States[9,21,31] (see Fig. 9.1). This tool allows for documentation of the indication for the procedure, the grade of difficulty followed by the grading of trainees in basic ERCP maneuvers, and relevant technical and cognitive endpoints, with a clear distinction made between biliary and pancreatic indications. In addition, this tool assesses the time allowed for cannulation and trainee participation in advanced cannulation

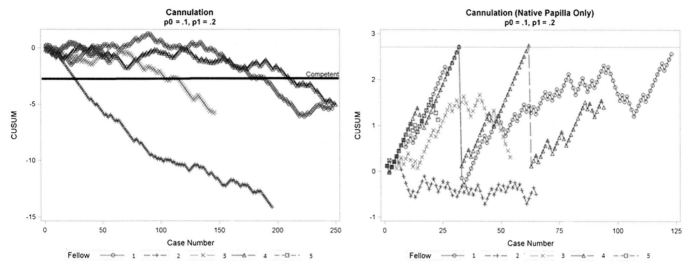

FIG 9.1 Learning curves of advanced endoscopy trainees using cumulative sum analysis for overall cannulation and native papilla cannulation, using acceptable and unacceptable failure rates of 10% and 20%, respectively. (Reprinted from Wani S, Hall M, Wang AY, et al. Variation in learning curves and competence for ERCP among advanced endoscopy trainees by using cumulative sum analysis. *Gastrointest Endosc.* 2016;83:711–719 e11.)

techniques. A 4-point scoring system is utilized with well-defined scoring anchors.

Recent studies have also described a novel and comprehensive data collection and reporting system that allows for the generation of learning curves on demand and the creation of a centralized database that enables program directors, trainers, and trainees to identify specific skill deficiencies in training and facilitate tailored and individualized remediation. This process allows for efficient data collection, interfacing, and analysis, and comparison of performance with peers nationwide (benchmarking).[9,33] Results from a recent large prospective multicenter study evaluating learning curves and competence in EUS and ERCP among 22 advanced endoscopy trainees using this comprehensive data collection and reporting system, and the validated tool (TEESAT) confirmed the substantial variability in achieving competence in ERCP among trainees. Overall technical and cognitive competence was achieved by 60% and 100% of participating trainees, respectively. Interestingly, competence in overall cannulation was achieved by 69% and sphincterotomy by 67% of trainees, with only 18% of trainees achieving competence in the cannulation of a native papilla.[33]

This work will facilitate advanced endoscopy training programs to evolve with the ACGME/NAS reporting requirements and establish reliable and generalizable learning curves (milestones) and competency benchmarks that national gastrointestinal societies and training programs can use to develop credentialing guidelines.[9] Ultimately, the implementation of CBME in medical subspecialties will require a paradigm shift in the evaluation of endoscopic training and in the definition of competence. Procedural volume thresholds can no longer be utilized as measures of competence, given the known variability in both trainee learning curves and procedural volumes at different institutions. Ensuring that trainees are capable of safely and proficiently performing ERCP independently at the conclusion of their training will require ongoing objective evaluations during the course of training to ensure that preset thresholds of technical and cognitive milestones are met.

ERCP TRAINING USING SIMULATION

Over the past few decades, several simulation modalities have been developed for ERCP training, including live animals, ex vivo organs, computer simulation, and mechanical models.[34–39] This work has largely been driven by the limited number of patients available for clinical training and the risks associated with ERCP.[34,40] A canine model of mongrel dogs was initially studied in 1974, and a swine model was subsequently proposed in 1990. The high expense and the fact that both canines and swine vary anatomically from humans in that they have separate biliary and pancreatic papillae have limited the widespread use of these models.[35,36] A baboon model was also evaluated in 1989. Although this provided similar anatomy to humans, it was also limited by expense and availability of primate training facilities.[35,41] In an attempt to develop a more cost-effective model with closer resemblance to humans, the Erlangen Endo-Trainer was designed in Germany. In this model, a porcine foregut, liver, gallbladder, and bile ducts are fitted into a human dummy torso, with small pebbles placed into the bile duct to mimic choledocholithiasis. The duodenal segment is positioned in a manner that allows the bile duct trajectory to more closely resemble that of humans. Fluoroscopy can then be utilized as an ERCP is performed with guidewire placement into the bile duct, followed by deep cannulation, sphincterotomy, stone extraction, and stent placement.[37]

More recently, a neo-papilla was developed using the left ventricle of a chicken heart to mimic the sphincter of Oddi. Porcine iliac or splenic arteries are sutured into the chicken heart to resemble the pancreatic and bile ducts, and this structure is then sutured into an explanted porcine duodenum. The ability to rotate the neo-papilla within the duodenum enables multiple sphincterotomies to be performed in uncut areas of the chicken heart. A mechanical simulator was then designed in 2007, which has a disposable papilla and video cameras placed in the ductal system to simulate fluoroscopy. This model allowed for training in selective cannulation, balloon dilation, brush cytology, and stent placement.[34] In a model developed for the simulation of cannulation and sphincterotomy, Itoi et al. utilized in vivo and ex vivo pig models in which mucosal blebs are created in the stomach or rectum by submucosal injections of hyaluronic acid solution with or without indigo carmine. The bulges that are formed resemble papillae, and a small incision is then made in the mucosal bleb using a needle knife to mimic the papillary orifice.[42]

Although there have been some promising results, data evaluating the impact of these simulators on ERCP training have been limited. In a study comparing live pigs to a computer-based simulation and the Erlangen model, the Erlangen model scored the highest in the majority of the realism indices, with computer simulation scoring significantly lower than both of the other models. The Erlangen model also scored highest in perceived usefulness for teaching basic ERCP and in ease of use. Computer simulation, however, was thought to be the easiest to incorporate into a fellowship program.[43] Similarly, in a study evaluating mechanical and computer simulation models in both trainers and trainees, the mechanical simulator significantly improved the understanding of ERCP, increased confidence in performing ERCP, and was deemed to be the more credible option for the supplementation of clinical training in comparison with computer simulation.[44] In a head-to-head comparison of the ERCP mechanical simulator to a pig explant among 22 endoscopists attending a training workshop, the mechanical simulator was found to confer a significantly higher degree of reported confidence among attendees after training. It was also thought to be a more useful modality for training in comparison to the explants.[40] Participants of a 2-day hands-on ERCP course utilizing live pigs reported increased confidence in complex interventions after completion of the course. This translated into a significant increase in the use of needle-knife precut sphincterotomy in clinical practice, supporting a role for simulators in continuing education.[45] There have been two studies evaluating the role of the ERCP mechanical simulator on trainee performance. In both studies, trainees in the early stages of training who participated in mechanical simulator practice were found to have higher success rates of biliary cannulation.[46,47]

Currently available data regarding ERCP simulation are promising and support a potential role for simulation as a supplement to formal mentored training with real cases. The ASGE, however, indicates that an objective benefit for simulation training in ERCP has not been clearly demonstrated. As such, simulation training alone is deemed insufficient to confer competence in ERCP and should be used only as an adjunct to clinical experience.[10]

MAINTENANCE OF ERCP SKILLS AND VOLUME FOR ERCP

Population-based studies have shown that the success rate of ERCP varies markedly between providers.[48] The case volume per endoscopist and center required to maintain ERCP skills and achieve optimal outcomes is unclear. As health care continues to shift from a volume-based to a value-based system, it will be increasingly important to deliver care that is efficient and effective. Understanding the factors associated with unsuccessful interventions, such as failed ERCP, will thus be of critical importance to both payers and patients. In most complex procedures there is a relationship between procedure volume and outcomes. This association in ERCP remains unclear, with only select studies showing an obvious increase in procedural success rate with increasing volume. Other studies, however, have not confirmed this relationship.[49,50]

In a large Austrian study, high case volume (>50 ERCPs per year) was shown to be associated with both higher procedural success rates and a decreased risk of adverse events.[51] A recent meta-analysis identified a significant relationship between higher endoscopist (odds ratio [OR] 1.6; 95% confidence interval [CI] 1.5 to 1.8; $p < 0.0001$) and center volume (OR 2.0; 95% CI 1.6 to 2.5; $p < 0.0001$) and overall procedural success. Furthermore, increasing endoscopist volume was also associated with a decrease in the rate of adverse events (OR 0.7; 95% CI 0.6 to 0.8; $p < 0.0001$).[52] Endoscopists with greater experience in ERCP also require shorter procedural fluoroscopy times, thus reducing radiation exposure to both patients and staff.[53] In a national US survey, endoscopists performing higher volumes of ERCP reported greater comfort and enjoyment with ERCP than physicians performing fewer cases.[54] Together,

these data highlight important variations in ERCP quality and safety and the potential role of regionalizing complex endoscopic care to centers and endoscopists with appropriate expertise.

Trainees also need to be aware of the potential for physician burnout associated with a career in interventional gastroenterology. A survey of self-reported stress levels among US gastroenterologists showed that interventional gastroenterologists worked more hours per week and were twice as likely to experience a major endoscopic adverse event within the prior year compared with noninterventional gastroenterologists.[54] Long hours and medical complications have been shown to be related to physician burnout.[55]

QUALITY MEASURES FOR TRAINEES

Given the currently changing health care landscape in the United States, the importance of measuring and monitoring quality in ERCP needs to be instilled early during training. With the endorsement of several gastroenterology quality measures by the National Quality Forum, quality measurement is the "new normal" in gastroenterology.[56] Unfortunately, available data suggest that trainees have limited knowledge of quality measures.[57] Training programs should promote a culture of continuous quality improvement among trainees and adopt formal approaches to educate trainees on defining and measuring the quality of care. Quality measures for ERCP were recently outlined by the ASGE/American College of Gastroenterology Task Force on Quality in Endoscopy.[5] The priority quality measures for ERCP include (1) frequency with which ERCP is performed for an appropriate indication and is documented, (2) rate of deep cannulation of the ducts of interest in patients with native papillae without surgically altered anatomy, (3) success rate of extraction of common bile duct stones <1 cm in patients with normal bile duct anatomy, (4) success rate of stent placement for biliary obstruction in patients with obstruction below the bifurcation and normal anatomy, and (5) rate of post-ERCP pancreatitis. Trainees should be engaged in formal educational programs on this topic and encouraged to monitor independent performance of ERCP with regard to these endpoints.

FUTURE DIRECTIONS

At the present time, data regarding ERCP performance among trainees during their initial few years of clinical practice are lacking. What has been shown, however, is that a great degree of variability exists in ERCP learning curves among trainees, which supports the notion that case volume alone does not guarantee competence in ERCP.[9] Additional studies are needed to assess the performance of trainees at the onset of independent practice to better characterize the adequacy of their training. Such data would shed light on the modifications that will need to be made to the current training structure to help ensure that trainees achieve competence at the time of completion of their formal training. Confirming the durability of a trainee's endoscopic proficiency once in independent clinical practice and the achievement of relevant quality metrics thresholds in ERCP (the definitive endpoint in endoscopic competency assessment) need to be addressed and confirmed in future studies.[5,58] As the majority of ERCPs in training are performed for biliary indications and are of ASGE grade 1 difficulty, strategies to increase trainee exposure to advanced ERCP techniques are warranted. Although available data confirm a significant relationship between increasing endoscopist and center volume and success, there is a need to standardize the definition of ERCP "success." Numerous definitions have been utilized in the literature, often based on data limitations rather than representing the most clinically useful endpoint. Several studies have utilized the need for percutaneous biliary drainage or an early repeat ERCP as a definition of failure, and cannulation of the duct of interest as a surrogate for procedural success. However, the most useful definition of success—an ERCP in which all intended therapeutic interventions occurred—is the most difficult to measure in administrative data sets and requires a detailed quality registry. As we move toward measuring ERCP success, trainees starting independent practice should ensure that they track this outcome—an outcome which is of central importance to the patient.

CONCLUSIONS

Training in ERCP remains closest to the apprenticeship model. Recent data, however, clearly demonstrate substantial variability in ERCP learning curves among trainees and indicate that general gestalt and specific volume thresholds during training do not ensure competence in ERCP. Given that methods for assessing competence during endoscopic training are in transition and given an increasing focus on CBME, emphasis needs to be shifted away from the number of procedures performed and directed toward well-defined and validated competency thresholds. Ensuring that all trainees achieve these thresholds and attain the skills necessary for safe and effective independent practice will ultimately improve the quality of patient care.

The complete reference list for this chapter can be found online at www.expertconsult.com.

The EUS and ERCP Skills Assessment Tool (TEESAT)

EUS

(Every 5th procedure; if 5th doesn't qualify,* then 6th)

☐ **Radial** ☐ **Linear** ☐ **Both**

Indication for EUS (mark all that apply):

☐ Pancreatic mass   ☐ Biliary dilation   ☐ Abdominal/mediastinal lymphadenopathy
☐ Possible subepithelial lesion ☐ Pancreatic cyst   ☐ Pancreatic duct dilation
☐ Luminal GI cancer staging   ☐ Mediastinal mass   ☐ Abdominal pain
☐ Rule out CBD stones   ☐ Rule out chronic pancreatitis ☐ Other: _____

ANCHORS

1 (superior) = achieves independently   **2 (advanced)** = achieves with minimal verbal instruction
3 (intermediate) = achieves with multiple verbal instruction or hands-on assistance
4 (novice) = unable to complete, requiring trainer to take over
N/T = not attempted for reasons other than trainee skill   **N/A** = not applicable

EUS: Technical Aspects
If possible, trainee to receive one minute per station prior to first verbal instruction.

Intubation	1	2	3	4	N/T	N/A
AP window	1	2	3	4	N/T	N/A
Body of pancreas	1	2	3	4	N/T	N/A
Tail of pancreas	1	2	3	4	N/T	N/A
Head/neck of pancreas	1	2	3	4	N/T	N/A
Uncinate	1	2	3	4	N/T	N/A
Ampulla	1	2	3	4	N/T	N/A
Gallbladder	1	2	3	4	N/T	N/A
CBD/CHD (trace CBD from hilum to ampulla)	1	2	3	4	N/T	N/A
Portosplenic confluence	1	2	3	4	N/T	N/A
Celiac axis	1	2	3	4	N/T	N/A

EUS: Technical Aspects

Achieve FNA	1	2	3	4	N/T	N/A
Achieve celiac plexus block/neurolysis	1	2	3	4	N/T	N/A

*Reasons for disqualification (e.g., obstructive esophageal mass, rectal EUS, intended limited exam [celiac plexus block/neurolysis])

ANCHORS

1 (superior) = achieves independently   **2 (advanced)** = achieves with minimal verbal instruction
3 (intermediate) = achieves with multiple verbal instruction or hands-on assistance
4 (novice) = unable to complete, requiring trainer to take over
N/T = not attempted for reasons other than trainee skill   **N/A** = not applicable

EUS: Cognitive Aspects

Identify lesion of interest or appropriately ruled out	1 2 3 4 N/T N/A
Appropriate TNM stage	1 2 3 4 N/T N/A
Characterize subepitheial lesion (wall layers)	1 2 3 4 N/T N/A
Appropriate differential diagnosis	1 2 3 4 N/T N/A
Appropriate management plan (FNA, refer to surgery, surveillance or no surveillance)	1 2 3 4 N/T N/A

Global Overall Assessment

Global Overall Assessment (subjective)			
1	**2**	**3**	**4**
Novice: Learning basic technical and cognitive aspects, requires significant assistance and coaching	Acquired basic technical and cognitive skills but requires limited hands-on assistance and/or significant coaching	Able to perform independently with limited coaching and/or requires additional time to complete	Competent to perform procedure independently

Immediate Postprocedure Complications

Procedure done in ambulatory setting?   ☐Yes   ☐No

Patient admitted postprocedure?   ☐Yes   ☐No
If yes,
☐Pain requiring hospitalization
☐Pancreatitis
      ☐Mild   ☐Moderate   ☐Severe
☐ Bleeding
      ☐Immediate   ☐Delayed
☐Perforation
☐Cardiopulmonary complications
☐Mortality
☐Other:_____

Recommendations for next procedure:

_____

_____

ERCP

(Every 5th procedure; if 5th doesn't qualify,* then 6th)

Indication for ERCP (mark all that apply):

Biliary
- ☐ Stent removal/change
- ☐ Suspected/established CBD stones
- ☐ Posttransplant stricture
- ☐ Stricture
  - ☐ Benign   ☐ Malignant   ☐ Indeterminate
  - ☐ Bismuth I ☐ Bismuth II   ☐ Bismuth III   ☐ Bismuth IV
- ☐ Bile leak
- ☐ Suspected sphincter of Oddi dysfunction
- ☐ Other:_____

Pancreatic
- ☐ Stricture
- ☐ Leak/fistula
- ☐ Recurrent acute pancreatitis
- ☐ Stent removal/change
- ☐ Suspected SOD
- ☐ Stone
- ☐ Minor papilla endotherapy
- ☐ Other:_____

ASGE ERCP Degree of Difficulty Grade
Biliary

Grade 1	Grade 2	Grade 3
☐ Diagnostic cholangiogram ☐ Biliary brush cytology ☐ Standard sphincterotomy ☐ +/- removal of stones <10 mm ☐ Stricture dilation/stent for benign extrahepatic stricture or bile leak	☐ Diagnostic cholangiogram with BII anatomy ☐ Removal of CBD stones >10 mm ☐ Stricture dilation/stent for hilar tumors or benign intrahepatic stricture or bile leak	☐ SOM ☐ Cholangioscopy ☐ Any therapy-altered anatomy ☐ Removal of intrahepatic stones with lithotripsy

Pancreatic

Grade 1	Grade 2	Grade 3
☐ Diagnostic pancreatogram ☐ Pancreatic cytology	☐ Diagnostic pancreatogram with BII anatomy ☐ Minor papilla cannulation	☐ SOM ☐ Pancreatoscopy ☐ Any therapy-altered anatomy ☐ All pancreatic therapy, including pseudocyst drainage

ANCHORS

1 (superior) = achieves independently   **2 (advanced)** = achieves with minimal verbal instruction
3 (intermediate) = achieves with multiple verbal instruction or hands-on assistance
4 (novice) = unable to complete, requiring trainer to take over
N/T = not attempted for reasons other than trainee skill   **N/A** = not applicable

Maneuvers (ALL ERCPs)

Intubation	1 2 3 4 N/T N/A	
Achieving the short position	1 2 3 4 N/T N/A	
Identifying the papilla	1 2 3 4 N/T N/A	
Native papilla?	☐ yes ☐ no	
Prior biliary sphincterotomy?	☐ yes ☐ no	
Prior pancreatic sphincterotomy?	☐ yes ☐ no	

*Reasons for disqualification (e.g., unable to perform due to medical instability or unable to reach papilla)

BILIARY ERCP
ANCHORS

1 (superior) = achieves independently   **2 (advanced)** = achieves with minimal verbal instruction
3 (intermediate) = achieves with multiple verbal instruction or hands-on assistance
4 (novice) = unable to complete, requiring trainer to take over
N/T = not attempted for reasons other than trainee skill   **N/A**= not applicable

Technical Aspects

Stent removal?	☐ yes ☐ no
Evaluate stent removal if performed by trainee:	1 2 3 4
Did trainee attempt cannulation?	☐ yes ☐ no
Time to attempt cannulation of first duct of interest for trainee (to start when cannulating device out of duodenoscope)? (in minutes)	
Cannulation achieved? (Achieved deep cannulation with contrast visualization)	☐ yes ☐ no
Evaluate cannulation if performed by trainee:	1 2 3 4
Inadvertent cannulation of pancreatic duct by trainee?	☐ yes ☐ no
Sphincterotomy performed during procedure?	☐ yes ☐ no
Evaluate sphincterotomy if performed by trainee:	1 2 3 4

Advanced Cannulation Techniques
(Double-wire, PD stent placement, precut sphinceteromy)

Double-wire used to cannulate bile duct	☐ yes ☐ no
Wire placed in pancreatic duct?	1 2 3 4 N/T N/A
Cannulation of CBD achieved?	☐ yes ☐ no
PD stent placed to facilitate BD cannulation?	☐ yes ☐ no
Wire placed in PD?	1 2 3 4 N/T N/A
PD stent placement?	1 2 3 4 N/T N/A
Cannulation of CBD achieved?	☐ yes ☐ no
Precut sphinceterotomy?	☐ yes ☐ no
Evaluate precut sphinceterotomy if performed by trainee:	1 2 3 4 N/T N/A

Technical Aspects

Wire placement in desired location in the bile duct? (e.g., desired liver segment, cystic duct)	☐ yes ☐ no
Evaluate wire placement if performed by trainee:	1 2 3 4 N/T N/A
Balloon sweep	1 2 3 4 N/T N/A
Use of basket	1 2 3 4 N/T N/A
Mechanical lithotripsy	1 2 3 4 N/T N/A
Stone clearance	1 2 3 4 N/T N/A
Stricture dilation	1 2 3 4 N/T N/A
Stent insertion	1 2 3 4 N/T N/A

Cognitive Aspects

Fellow demonstrated clear understanding of indication of procedure?	1 2 3 4 N/T N/A
Cholangiogram Appropriate use of fluoroscopy?	1 2 3 4 N/T N/A
Proficient use of real-time cholangiogram interpretation and ability to identity nature of pathology (stone, stricture, leak, etc.)?	1 2 3 4 N/T N/A
Logical plan based on cholangiogram findings?	1 2 3 4 N/T N/A
Fellow demonstrated clear understanding of appropriate use of rectal indomethacin?	1 2 3 4 N/T N/A

PANCREATIC ERCP
ANCHORS
1 (superior) = achieves independently   **2 (advanced)** = achieves with minimal verbal instruction
3 (intermediate) = achieves with multiple verbal instruction or hands-on assistance
4 (novice) = unable to complete, requiring trainer to take over
N/T = not attempted for reasons other than trainee skill   **N/A** = not applicable

Technical Aspects

Stent removal?	☐ yes ☐ no
Evaluate stent removal if performed by trainee:	1 2 3 4
Did trainee attempt cannulation?	☐ yes ☐ no
Time to attempt cannulation of first duct of interest for trainee (to start when cannulating device out of duodenoscope)? (in minutes)	
Cannulation achieved? (Achieved deep cannulation with contrast visualization)	☐ yes ☐ no
Evaluate cannulation if performed by trainee:	1 2 3 4
Sphincterotomy performed during procedure?	☐ yes ☐ no
Evaluate sphinceterotomy if performed by trainee:	1 2 3 4 N/T N/A
Balloon sweep	1 2 3 4 N/T N/A
Use of basket	1 2 3 4 N/T N/A
Stone clearance	1 2 3 4 N/T N/A
Stricture dilation	1 2 3 4 N/T N/A
Stent insertion?	☐ yes ☐ no
Evaluate stent insertion if performed by trainee:	1 2 3 4

Cognitive Aspects

Fellow demonstrated clear understanding of indication of procedure	1 2 3 4 N/T N/A
Pancreatogram Appropriate use of fluoroscopy	1 2 3 4 N/T N/A
Ability to identity nature of pathology (stone, stricture, leak, etc.)	1 2 3 4 N/T N/A
Logical plan based on pancreatogram findings	1 2 3 4 N/T N/A
Fellow demonstrated clear understanding of appropriate use of rectal indomethacin?	1 2 3 4 N/T N/A

Global Overall Assessment:

Global Overall Assessment (subjective)			
1	2	3	4
Novice: Learning basic technical and cognitive aspects, requires significant assistance and coaching	Acquired basic technical and cognitive skills but requires limited hands-on assistance and/or significant coaching	Able to perform independently with limited coaching and/or requires additional time to complete	Competent to perform procedure independently

Immediate Postprocedure Complications

Procedure done in ambulatory setting? ☐Yes ☐No

Patient admitted postprocedure? ☐Yes ☐No
If yes,
☐Pain requiring hospitalization
☐Pancreatitis
      ☐Mild   ☐Moderate   ☐Severe
☐Bleeding
      ☐Immediate   ☐Delayed
☐Perforation
☐Cardiopulmonary complications
☐Mortality
☐Other:_____

Recommendations for next procedure:

_____

_____

BII, Bismuth II; CBD, common bile duct; CHD, common hepatic duct; FNA, fine-needle aspiration; GI, gastrointestinal; SOD, sphincter of Oddi dysfunction; TNM, tumor-node-metastasis.

10

Preparation of the Patient for ERCP

John T. Maple

The planning required for successful endoscopic retrograde cholangio-pancreatography (ERCP) is more complex than that for routine endoscopic procedures and requires the synthesis of multiple variables. Preparation for ERCP involves preparing not just the patient, but also the endoscopist, the endoscopy team, the anesthesia team, and the necessary equipment. The purpose of this chapter is to review the most important preprocedural decisions and planning steps when ERCP is being considered, with the intent of maximizing the chances of a successful procedure. Other chapters in the first section of this textbook discuss some preparatory issues in detail, including Chapter 3 concerning radiologic issues and Chapter 6 concerning sedation issues; thus, these particular issues will be only briefly addressed herein. The flow of this chapter will be in a rough chronologic order of factors to consider as the procedure draws nearer.

SHOULD THIS PATIENT UNDERGO ERCP?

The refinement of alternative technologies, including magnetic resonance cholangiopancreatography (MRCP) and endoscopic ultrasonography (EUS), which provide similar (or better) diagnostic information about the pancreas and biliary tree, has essentially restricted the role of ERCP to a therapeutic one.[1-3] For this reason, critically questioning the strength of the indication for ERCP is the first step in planning. In answer to the question "Should this patient undergo ERCP?" the answer may range from "Yes" to "No" to "Not yet." In some cases, ERCP is clearly not indicated (e.g., simply as a diagnostic test for abdominal pain), whereas other cases may be more nuanced, such as when a reasonably healthy patient has new painless jaundice and a small mass in the head of the pancreas that appears surgically resectable. Additionally, the efficacy and safety of ERCP may be enhanced in some patients by delaying the ERCP, for example, to allow for an MRCP to provide a road map in a patient with a suspected hilar malignancy,[4] or to allow the correction of a coagulopathy before an elective ERCP.

WHEN, WHERE, AND WITH WHOM?

Once the decision has been made that an ERCP is indicated, the next decision points relate to urgency, locale, and the potential need for other physician assistance. The vast majority of ERCPs do not need to be conducted on an urgent basis. Patients with severe acute cholangitis not responding to antibiotics and fluid resuscitation represent the lone group for whom a truly urgent procedure is indicated.[5-7] However, there may be other instances in which a reasonably expedited ERCP is desirable, including patients with moderately severe acute cholangitis who are responding to conservative treatment.[8]

Patients who are critically ill, such as those receiving mechanical ventilation and vasopressors, may not be appropriate for transfer to the gastrointestinal (GI) laboratory or radiology department for ERCP.

In these instances, other options must often be explored, including performing the ERCP in a dedicated ICU procedure room or nearby operating room, in the patient's ICU room and bed with a portable C-arm fluoroscopy unit,[9] or in the patient's room without fluoroscopy (i.e., using bile aspiration to confirm location).[10] Many fluoroscopy tables have a weight limit of 350 lbs. (159 kg); some morbidly obese patients requiring ERCP may exceed these limits and must be cared for in an operating room with an appropriately rated table and portable fluoroscopy.[11]

Additional scheduling coordination will be necessary in ERCPs requiring a second physician for completion. Most commonly this may occur with "rendezvous" procedures, in which an interventional radiologist performs a percutaneous transhepatic cholangiogram and passes a wire antegrade across the major papilla into the duodenum to facilitate endoscopic retrograde cannulation.[12,13] Another instance of collaborative ERCP is laparoscopic-assisted ERCP for patients with prior Roux-en-Y gastric bypass, in which a laparoscopic gastrostomy is created into the excluded stomach and, during the same procedure, a duodenoscope is passed via the gastrostomy to perform ERCP (see Chapter 31 on surgically altered anatomy).[14,15]

EVALUATION OF THE PATIENT BEFORE ERCP
History and Physical

Clearly a thorough history and physical examination should be completed on all patients before ERCP. Comorbid medical conditions may affect ERCP decision making in a number of ways, including need for pre-anesthesia testing, method of sedation chosen, management of antithrombotic agents, and need for postprocedure inpatient observation. However, in some systems of care, the endoscopist performing the ERCP may not meet the patient until shortly before the scheduled procedure. This may occur in the hospital setting when a GI trainee or surgical service has evaluated an inpatient, or in the outpatient setting when a patient is referred by another gastroenterologist for ERCP. In some instances there are nuances to the case that may not be apparent on initial review but affect the appropriateness of the procedure. One example would be a minimally symptomatic elderly patient with advanced pancreatic malignancy and very poor functional status for whom hospice care may be more appropriate than biliary decompression. In patients who have had prior surgery involving the foregut or biliary tree, it is critical to have the best possible understanding of their anatomy before embarking on ERCP (Chapter 31). Many patients may be unable to provide a history more detailed than "stomach surgery," and even referring physicians may not appreciate the implications of various reconstructions as they relate to ERCP. As such, when postsurgical anatomy is uncertain, obtaining the operative notes for review or speaking with the surgeon for clarification is recommended. The nature of the surgically altered anatomy and the skill set of the endoscopist will influence whether to perform or refer the procedure, and certainly will also influence endoscope and device selection if the ERCP is undertaken.[16]

Laboratory Testing

The practice of routinely ordering laboratory tests before ERCP, irrespective of the specific clinical setting, is not recommended because of cost and low yield.[17] However, there are instances in which some preprocedure testing may be appropriate, tailored to the patient's specific clinical scenario and comorbidities. In patients with a known bleeding disorder, liver disease, malnutrition, or prolonged biliary obstruction, or in those receiving warfarin treatment, testing of the prothrombin time (PT) and international normalized ratio (INR) may be considered.[18,19] Routine measurement of the hematocrit and platelet count is not necessary, but may be appropriate in the setting of suspected anemia, perceived high risk for bleeding, myeloproliferative disorders, splenomegaly, or medications known to cause thrombocytopenia.[18,20,21] All women of childbearing age should be asked about the possibility of pregnancy, and pregnancy testing before the procedure may be considered in this patient subset.[22,23] A chemistry panel may be considered for patients with diabetes mellitus or chronic kidney disease, or in the setting of medications that may cause abnormalities of glucose, potassium, or renal function.[18,24] Finally, electrocardiography and chest radiography may be considered in older patients with cardiopulmonary comorbidities, but are not routinely necessary before ERCP.[18,21] A practice guideline from the American Society for Gastrointestinal Endoscopy (ASGE) covers the issue of laboratory testing before endoscopic procedures in more detail.[17]

Review of Imaging Studies

Although each patient will present with imaging studies of varying nature and quality, it is always useful to personally review available prior radiographic studies before ERCP. Anecdotally, it is not uncommon to detect potentially relevant findings not described in the radiologist's report, such as pancreas divisum or a subtly dilated pancreatic duct, on a computed tomography (CT) scan. Even reported findings may not be described in adequate detail; for example, a CT or magnetic resonance imaging (MRI) report may describe a malignant-appearing hilar stricture with intrahepatic biliary dilation but omit key findings such as apparent Bismuth classification or lobar atrophy that will be relevant to the patient's management.

PREPARING THE PATIENT: DAY(S) BEFORE ERCP

Management of Antithrombotic Agents

The central issue in the periendoscopic management of antithrombotic agents (e.g., aspirin, clopidogrel, warfarin) is balancing the risk for bleeding caused by the endoscopy against the risk for thromboembolic events caused by withholding these agents. The ASGE practice guideline titled "Management of antithrombotic agents for endoscopic procedures" provides a thorough review of the available relevant data on this topic.[25]

The risk for clinically relevant bleeding at ERCP is almost entirely derived from the performance of an endoscopic sphincterotomy (ES).[26–29] ERCP without ES poses very little risk for bleeding, even in the setting of antithrombotic agents, and as such, it is unnecessary to withhold these agents before ERCP without ES. The following paragraphs will discuss the management of antithrombotic agents when ERCP with ES is contemplated. A summary of commonly encountered antithrombotic agents and the suggested management of these agents before ERCP with ES are presented in Table 10.1.

Antiplatelet Agents

Aspirin. In a prospective trial that randomized patients undergoing ES to either a 100 mg indomethacin suppository (*n* = 289) or a placebo

TABLE 10.1 Management of Antithrombotic Medications Before Elective ERCP With Sphincterotomy

Drug Class	Agents	Suggested Management
Antiplatelet agents	Aspirin, dipyramidole, NSAIDs	Not necessary to hold for ES
	Thienopyridines (e.g., clopidogrel, ticlopidine)	Consider holding for 7 days*,†
Anticoagulants	Warfarin	Hold for 3 to 5 days‡
	Unfractionated heparin	Hold for 4 to 6 hours
	Low–molecular weight heparin	Hold for 12 to 24 hours
	Dabigatran	Hold for 1 to 2 days§
	Rivaroxaban	Hold for 24 hours
	Apixaban	Hold for 1 to 2 days
	Edoxaban	Hold for 24 hours§
	Fondaparinux	Hold for 2 to 4 days§

ES, Endoscopic sphincterotomy; *NSAIDs,* nonsteroidal antiinflammatory drugs.
*Avoid stopping thienopyridine until the minimum recommended treatment interval has been completed in patients with coronary stents.
†Sphincterotomy may be considered in patients on thienopyridine monotherapy; alternatively, stop the thienopyridine 1 week in advance and start aspirin.
‡Employ bridging therapy for high-risk conditions.
§Should be held longer in the setting of renal insufficiency.

suppository (*n* = 287) to evaluate post-ERCP pancreatitis (PEP) rates, 87 patients were taking aspirin (100 mg/day).[30] The rate of post-ES bleeding was not different between aspirin users (9/87, 10.3%) and nonusers (41/489, 8.4%, *p* = NS). Four retrospective case–control series found that patients who developed post-ES bleeding were not more likely to have used aspirin than control patients who did not develop bleeding after ES.[31–34] Similarly, aspirin was not found to be a risk factor for post-ES hemorrhage in a multivariate analysis of a large, prospective, multicenter trial of ES complications.[35] A retrospective cohort study examined 804 patients who underwent ES, including 124 patients actively taking aspirin, 116 patients who used aspirin but had stopped it 1 week before ES, and 564 patients who had never used aspirin.[36] The rate of post-ES bleeding was higher in the two aspirin groups (9.6%) than in the never users (3.9%, *p* = 0.01), but it was not different between those who had stopped aspirin for 1 week (9.5%) versus those actively taking aspirin (9.7%, *p* = NS). Also, the rate of post-ES bleeding across all groups in this series was unusually high, and thus these findings must be interpreted with some caution. Overall, the available data suggest that aspirin does not pose a significant risk for post-ES bleeding and that holding aspirin does not reduce the likelihood of post-ES bleeding.

Thienopyridines and dual-antiplatelet therapy. Data addressing the bleeding risk posed by ES in the setting of thienopyridine monotherapy (e.g., clopidogrel, ticlopidine) or dual-antiplatelet therapy (DAT; e.g., aspirin + clopidogrel) are very limited. In a post hoc analysis of a randomized controlled trial of indomethacin for PEP, post-ES bleeding was observed in 2/29 (6.9%) patients using clopidogrel and 48/547 (8.8%) patients not using clopidogrel (*p* = NS).[30] No post-ES bleeding was observed in 5 patients taking uninterrupted DAT in this study. Similarly, no bleeding was observed in a small retrospective case series of 8 patients taking uninterrupted DAT who underwent ES.[37] In a retrospective analysis of post-ES bleeding in 762 patients, no bleeding was observed in 24 patients who were either actively taking DAT or who had stopped DAT <7 days before ES.[34]

Patients are at significant risk for thrombosis after deployment of coronary stents, particularly in the first 30 days, and this likely represents the commonest indication for thienopyridine therapy.[38] In these patients, efforts should be made not to interrupt thienopyridine therapy until the minimum recommended treatment interval has been completed.[39] This might be accomplished by avoiding or delaying ES (e.g., placing a temporary biliary stent for a bile leak or bile duct stone). If ES delay is not appropriate, consideration could be given to holding the thienopyridine, yet continuing (or starting) aspirin to minimize thrombotic risk, or continuing thienopyridine monotherapy. However, the provider managing the antithrombotic agents and/or a physician who specializes in these agents (e.g., cardiologist) should be involved in decision making, especially when consideration is made for interrupting therapy.

Anticoagulants

Both coagulopathy before ES and resumption of full anticoagulation within 3 days after ES were found to be risk factors for post-ES bleeding in a prospective multicenter study.[35] In patients for whom reversal of coagulopathy is difficult or undesirable, alternatives to ES may be considered (e.g., balloon sphincteroplasty, stent placement). However, if ES is necessary, patients should have warfarin discontinued 3 to 5 days before ES. In patients at high risk for thrombosis, bridging therapy with unfractionated heparin (UFH) or low–molecular weight heparin (LMWH) may be appropriate once the INR is <2. High-risk conditions for thromboembolic events include complicated atrial fibrillation (e.g., atrial fibrillation associated with valvular heart disease or prosthetic valves), a mechanical valve in the mitral position, or a recently placed coronary stent, among others. A more complete enumeration of high-risk and low-risk conditions for thromboembolism can be found in the aforementioned ASGE guideline, "Management of antithrombotic agents for endoscopic procedures."[25] UFH should be held for 4 hours and LMWH held for 12 to 24 hours before ES.[40–42] Anticoagulation should be resumed as soon as is safely possible; in the absence of immediate bleeding complications, UFH should be reinitiated 2 to 6 hours post-ERCP and warfarin should be resumed within 24 hours of the procedure.

Dabigatran etexilate (a direct thrombin inhibitor) and rivaroxaban, apixaban, and edoxaban (direct factor Xa inhibitors) are oral anticoagulants that are used in the management of venous thromboembolic disease and for stroke prevention in patients with atrial fibrillation. Fondaparinux sodium is a subcutaneously administered factor Xa inhibitor that is FDA-approved for postsurgical venous thromboembolism prophylaxis, as well as treatment for acute deep venous thrombosis and pulmonary embolism. There are no data regarding the safety of ERCP with ES in patients taking these agents, and best practices regarding preprocedural discontinuation must be derived from pharmacokinetic data and recommendations from the pharmaceutical manufacturers.

The package insert for dabigatran recommends discontinuation 1 to 2 days before a procedure if the estimated creatinine clearance (Cl_{cr}) is 50 mL/minute or greater, or 3 to 5 days before a procedure if Cl_{cr} is less than 50 mL/minute, based on the half-life (12 to 17 hours) and predominant renal clearance of the drug.[43] The manufacturer of apixaban recommends discontinuation ≥48 hours before procedures with a moderate to high risk of clinically significant bleeding, and discontinuation ≥24 hours before procedures with a low risk of bleeding, or where bleeding could be easily controlled.[44] The half-life of apixaban is approximately 12 hours, and no change in dosing or discontinuation is recommended for patients with renal or hepatic impairment. Edoxaban has a half-life of 10 to 14 hours, and its manufacturer recommends

discontinuation at least 24 hours before invasive procedures.[45] Renal excretion is the primary clearance mechanism for edoxaban, and dose modifications are recommended if the Cl_{cr} is less than 50 mL/minute. As such, a longer period of discontinuation before ERCP should be considered in these patients. Although rivaroxaban has a somewhat shorter half-life (5 to 9 hours), holding the drug for at least 24 hours before ERCP is recommended.[46,47] Fondaparinux has a much longer half-life (17 to 21 hours) than LMWHs, and the manufacturer's insert warns that its anticoagulant effects may persist for 2 to 4 days in patients with normal renal function (i.e., at least 3 to 5 half-lives), and potentially even longer in patients with renal impairment.[48]

Duration of Fasting

Patients should be instructed to avoid solid food for 6 to 8 hours and clear liquids for 1 to 2 hours before ERCP in order to maximize safety (i.e., reduce risk for aspiration) and to improve endoscopic visualization.[49–51] In patients with known delay in gastric emptying or those in whom gastric outlet obstruction is suspected, a longer duration of fasting and/or passage of a nasogastric sump tube may be appropriate before the procedure.

METHOD OF SEDATION, PROPER PERSONNEL, AND PATIENT MONITORING

Selecting Sedation for ERCP

ERCP may be safely and successfully performed using moderate sedation (e.g., midazolam and meperidine), deep sedation (e.g., propofol), or general anesthesia. Factors influencing the method for anesthesia delivery include patient factors (age, body habitus, comorbidities), procedure factors (complexity, duration, risk), and availability and expertise of anesthesia providers. Chapter 6 ("Sedation in ERCP") of this textbook explores ERCP sedation in detail; however, a few salient points bear mentioning in relation to planning/preparation for ERCP sedation.

Two large prospective cohort studies of patients undergoing ERCP with monitored anesthesia care (MAC; typically comprising propofol +/− low-dose midazolam and narcotic) identified increased body mass index (BMI) and an American Society of Anesthesiologists (ASA) class of 3 or higher as risk factors for sedation-related complications (SRCs).[52,53] The most common SRCs in this setting are respiratory (e.g., hypoxemia), and may require airway maneuvers (AMs) such as chin lift, nasal airway placement, or endotracheal intubation. Another prospective cohort study demonstrated that advancing degrees of obesity were associated with incrementally higher risks for SRCs and need for AMs during ERCP with MAC; patients with a BMI >35 were at greatest risk, and required AMs in 27% of cases.[54] Obstructive sleep apnea (OSA) frequently complicates obesity, and may portend an even higher risk for SRCs and AMs. In a prospective study that used a validated screening tool for OSA (the STOP-BANG assessment) in patients undergoing ERCP with MAC, 20% of patients who were at high risk for OSA required AMs, whereas only 6% of low-risk patients required AMs.[55] Thus, as patients with an ASA score of 3 or more, increased BMI (>30), or known or predicted OSA are at higher risk for SRCs during ERCP, consideration should be given to a sedation plan that involves a provider solely responsible for airway management of these patient subsets.

A large retrospective study of patients undergoing ERCP with midazolam and meperidine confirmed that patients using chronic narcotics or benzodiazepines required higher doses of sedation; however, this subset was not associated with a higher risk for SRCs.[56] In this study, age >80, higher doses of meperidine, and the adjunctive use of promethazine were risk factors for the need for reversal agents. The immediate availability of flumazenil and naloxone should be confirmed before commencing any ERCP in which intravenous narcotics and benzodiazepines are used.

Proper Personnel

Staffing requirements for performing endoscopy (including ERCP) are not specifically mandated by the Joint Commission on Accreditation of Healthcare Organizations. Rather, the requirement is that "a sufficient number of qualified staff (in addition to the individual performing the procedure) are present to evaluate the patient, to provide the sedation and/or anesthesia, to help with the procedure, and to monitor and recover the patient."[57] If moderate sedation is employed, a registered nurse is needed to give intravenous (IV) medications and monitor the patient, and a second assistant provides technical assistance with devices to the endoscopist. If an anesthesia provider is employed, only a technical assistant is needed. However, in some ERCPs requiring multiple and/or complex devices, efficiency may be improved if two technical assistants are available. Depending on the type of fluoroscopy unit used, a radiologic technician may be necessary or simply helpful to operate the fluoroscopy unit. The Joint Commission mandates that "individuals administering moderate or deep sedation and anesthesia are qualified and have credentials to manage patients at whatever level of sedation or anesthesia is achieved."[57] However, each institution determines what qualifications and credentials are appropriate; many require Advanced Cardiovascular Life Support certification, but this is not uniformly so. A statement from the ASGE Standards of Practice Committee on "Minimum Staffing Requirements for the Performance of GI Endoscopy" discusses these issues in more detail.[58]

Proper Monitoring and Intervention Equipment

An ASA practice guideline for "Sedation and Analgesia by Non-Anesthesiologists" provides an overview of the recommended monitoring approach and associated equipment for moderate and deep sedation.[51] Routine monitoring of the patient's level of consciousness (e.g., response to voice), assessment of pulmonary ventilation, continuous oximetry, and periodic monitoring of heart rate and blood pressure are recommended for all patients undergoing moderate or deep sedation. For patients undergoing deep sedation, continuous ECG monitoring and capnography are also recommended. A trial of 263 patients undergoing ERCP with moderate sedation randomized the patients to either standard monitoring or the addition of a microstream capnography-based ventilation monitoring system.[59] The patients assigned to capnography experienced significantly fewer hypoxemic and apneic events than patients assigned to standard monitoring. Given these findings, and given the difficulties of manually assessing ventilation by chest rise in a darkened ERCP suite, capnography assessment should be considered for all patients undergoing ERCP with either deep or moderate sedation. Electroencephalography-guided sedation including bispectral index monitoring has been associated with more effective propofol titration and lower propofol dose requirements in patients undergoing ERCP,[60,61] but no reduction in the incidence of respiratory depression, and use of these techniques is not routinely recommended at this time. Patients undergoing ERCP who are pregnant should have fetal heart tones checked before and after sedation, and continuous fetal monitoring may be considered in cases of potential fetal viability.[22,23,62]

The ASA recommends the immediate availability of appropriate emergency equipment in units where moderate or deep sedation is administered.[51] This includes basic supplies for establishing a patent airway (e.g., oxygen source, suction source, nasal and oral airways, bag-valve masks), supplies for advanced airway management (e.g., laryngoscope handles and blades, endotracheal tubes), and supplies for starting an intravenous line (e.g., catheters, tubing, fluid). Ready access to a defibrillator is recommended for any patient with cardiovascular disease undergoing moderate or deep sedation. The availability of resuscitation equipment is also a Joint Commission requirement in units where moderate or deep sedation is being administered, and in practice, all of these items are typically grouped together on a "crash cart."[57]

PREPARING THE ENDOSCOPY TEAM

It is prudent to briefly discuss the indication and anticipated findings and maneuvers for each ERCP with the endoscopy team members before the case, to allow for best preparation and minimization of delays during the case. This might include the selection of specific accessories, preparation of alternative endoscopes (e.g., cholangioscope or balloon enteroscope), or even simply ensuring the ready availability of a pancreatic duct stent for a patient at high risk for PEP. Most GI labs will have glucagon readily available to aid in diminishing duodenal peristalsis. Further, the cholecystokinin agonist sincalide may be valuable in locating the major papilla in selected cases (e.g., intradiverticular papilla or duodenal mucosal congestion/edema),[63] and secretin is frequently helpful in pinpointing the os of the minor papilla.[64] As these latter two agents may not be routinely kept in the GI laboratory, anticipating their need before the case will avoid intraprocedural delay. Contrast diluted with saline may aid in stone visualization in patients with suspected choledocholithiasis, and this can be prepared by the GI technician beforehand. Though no conclusive benefit has been shown from the addition of antimicrobials (e.g., gentamicin) to contrast in the reduction of infectious adverse events, some practitioners may elect to prepare contrast in this manner for selected cases with complex or multifocal biliary strictures.[65,66] The use of carbon dioxide (CO_2) as the insufflating gas in ERCP has been associated with less postprocedure pain than cases performed with air,[67,68] and may be particularly desirable in cases that are anticipated to be longer in duration or associated with higher risk for perforation. If CO_2 supplies are available yet not routinely used, the GI technician can outfit the endoscopic light source with a CO_2 tank, regulator, and tubing before the case.

PREPARING THE PATIENT: THE DAY OF THE ERCP

Informed Consent

Given the enhanced risk profile of ERCP compared with other endoscopic procedures, a quality and thorough informed consent discussion is of particular importance. Ideally this discussion should occur before the day of the procedure; patients in a gown on a gurney with an intravenous line may feel a sense of pressure or inevitability in regard to the procedure. However, logistic practicalities frequently necessitate obtaining written consent on the day of the ERCP. The discussion should not be rushed, and the consenting physician must keep an open mind to potentially safer alternative approaches. The risks for each ERCP will be inherently different (particularly in regard to pancreatitis risk) based on patient-specific and procedure-specific factors. As such, the discussion of risks should be individualized. Further, endoscopists should ideally be aware of their own performance data in regard to cannulation rates and adverse event rates, rather than simply quoting published benchmarks. Medicolegal issues in ERCP, including informed consent, are also discussed in Chapter 13.

Periprocedural Antibiotics

The risk for infectious after ERCP approximates 1% in large prospective series, most commonly acute cholangitis.[27,28,35,69] The routine administration of preprocedural antibiotics was not shown to reduce the risk for ERCP-related cholangitis or septicemia in two meta-analyses of randomized controlled trials.[70,71] Similarly, a more recent Cochrane

Review that included additional trials ($n = 9$) reported a reduction in bacteremia, but not septicemia or cholangitis, with routine administration of prophylactic antibiotics at ERCP in a random-effects meta-analysis.[72] However, there are subsets of patients who appear to benefit from periprocedural antibiotics and, in some cases, continuation of antibiotics postprocedure. As incomplete biliary drainage appears to be the strongest predictor of post-ERCP cholangitis,[73,74] patients with complex biliary obstruction (e.g., hilar biliary obstruction, primary sclerosing cholangitis) in whom drainage is predicted to be incomplete should receive periprocedural antibiotics, and limited data suggest a benefit to continuing antibiotics for 5 to 7 days afterward in these patients as well.[75,76] The antibiotic chosen should provide good coverage against enteric gram-negative flora and enterococci. Although data are scant, practice guidelines based on expert opinion suggest periprocedural antibiotic administration for patients undergoing transmural pseudocyst drainage or ERCP in the presence of a pseudocyst with communication to the main pancreatic duct.[77] In a large single-center series comprising >11,000 patients over an 11-year time span, the authors sequentially changed their practice over several eras in regard to antibiotic administration at ERCP from initially nearly uniform (95%) to a selective policy (only those with predicted or actual incomplete drainage or immunosuppression) later on that involved 26% of patients.[78] The more selective policy was not associated with a higher rate of infections. In multivariable analysis, only patients who were status post–liver transplantation had an increased risk for infections. Clinical scenarios in which antibiotic prophylaxis is recommended for ERCP are summarized in Box 10.1.

Positioning the Patient and Preparing for Radiography

A variety of patient positions (e.g., prone, supine, oblique, or left lateral decubitus) are possible when performing ERCP. The position chosen will be influenced by patient factors (e.g., body habitus, presence of abdominal wounds or drains, neck mobility), anesthesia and airway considerations, and also the nature of the fluoroscopic imaging required. Left lateral and oblique imaging are generally sufficient for cases involving the extrahepatic bile duct, but are typically inadequate for cases requiring imaging of the pancreatic duct or biliary bifurcation. In these latter cases, either prone or supine positioning is optimal. However, a fluoroscopy system with a rotating C-arm can overcome many of the imaging limitations posed by patient positioning.

Two randomized controlled trials and one large retrospective case series have compared supine with prone positioning at ERCP. A single Italian center randomized 34 patients to either supine or prone positioning for ERCP with moderate sedation.[79] In this small study, a lower rate of successful cannulation (71% vs 100%, $p = 0.05$) and a higher rate of SRCs (41% vs 6%, $p = 0.04$) were observed in the group randomized to supine positioning. However, in a larger randomized controlled trial ($n = 120$, moderate sedation in all) performed at a tertiary referral center that also incorporated both trainees and experts, no differences

were observed in cannulation rates or adverse events between the prone and supine groups, irrespective of operator skill level.[80] Lastly, a retrospective series of 649 patients who underwent ERCP by a single expert endoscopist compared 506 prone examinations with 143 supine examinations; a mix of moderate sedation and general anesthesia was employed.[81] In this series, no differences in procedural success or adverse events were found between the prone and supine groups, despite a higher degree of procedural difficulty (i.e., Schutz and Abbott complexity grading[82]) in the supine group.

On a practical note, it is necessary to employ additional clockwise torque on the duodenoscope in supine patients to maintain a proper en face view of the major papilla. Although this may be achieved by rotating the shaft of the scope, it is more easily attained by the endoscopist standing with his or her back to the patient, which may necessitate adjustment of monitor placement in the room, often opposite of the usual placement, toward the head of the bed and facing toward the patient's feet. Variations in stance and hand position of the endoscopist for prone and supine patient positioning are shown in Fig. 10.1. Supine positioning for patients without a protected airway poses some risk for aspiration, but this can be significantly attenuated by frequent oropharyngeal suctioning and close airway supervision by the sedating nurse or anesthesia provider. In the experience of this author, supine positioning does slightly increase the technical difficulty of the examination because of the less favorable lie of the duodenoscope and the need for additional torque. Although almost all ERCPs can be completed with supine positioning, rare cases may arise in which supine position is associated with pronounced difficulty with endoscope positioning that is alleviated by changing to prone position.

Obtaining a routine scout film of the upper abdomen before commencing the ERCP is almost always advisable. Rarely, the scout film may obviate the need for the ERCP (e.g., in some patients returning for stent removal, when the scout film demonstrates spontaneous stent migration) or determine the need to delay the ERCP (e.g., prominent oral contrast from a prior CT study in the colon overlying and obscuring the area of interest). Scout films also provide visual information that can serve as a baseline reference after contrast is injected and assist in fluoroscopic interpretation when potentially confounding findings such as pancreatic calcifications, rib cartilage calcifications, surgical clips, or pneumobilia are present.

Efforts should be made to minimize fetal radiation exposure in pregnant patients undergoing ERCP. Wrapping the pelvis with a lead shield or apron before the procedure is one component in this process.[22,62] A more thorough discussion of ERCP in the pregnant patient can be found in Chapter 30.

Reviewing Intravenous Access and Allergies

The location, gauge, and proper function of intravenous access should be reassessed immediately before sedation in order to reduce the likelihood of losing access intraprocedurally. A second line should be started if there is concern regarding the adequacy of intravenous access. During the preprocedure patient verification ("time-out"), it is prudent to again review any patient medication allergies, particularly in regard to antibiotic agents and contrast media (CM). Systemic absorption of iodinated contrast administered at ERCP is frequent and well-documented (by urographic visualization on plain films or CT).[83,84] However, although adverse reactions to CM used in ERCP have been reported, they are exceedingly rare.[85] This is likely because of the fractionally smaller dose of iodine that reaches the systemic circulation in ERCP compared with direct intravenous administration of the same volume of CM.[86] For patients with a history of adverse reaction to IV CM, some endoscopists administer prophylactic regimens consisting of multiple doses of oral corticosteroids beginning 12 to 13 hours before the ERCP, and sometimes

---

BOX 10.1 Recommended Scenarios for Antibiotic Prophylaxis at ERCP

- Predicted incomplete biliary drainage (e.g., Klatskin tumor or primary sclerosing cholangitis)
- Actual incomplete biliary drainage*
- Immunosuppression, particularly post–liver transplantation
- Communicating pancreatic pseudocyst
- Transenteric pseudocyst drainage

*In this instance, antibiotics would be administered immediately after failed ERCP.

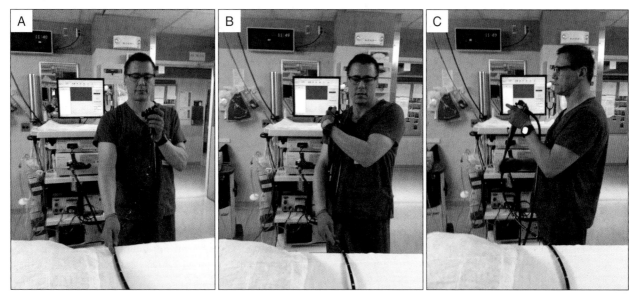

FIG 10.1 **A,** The patient is prone and the endoscopist is in a standard position. **B,** The patient is supine—note the exaggerated clockwise torque applied to the endoscope handle by the endoscopist's left hand. **C,** The patient is supine—the endoscopist is generating the same amount of clockwise torque by standing with his back to the patient.

also including an antihistamine.[85] Whether this practice is necessary or not remains uncertain. In a prospective series of 601 ERCPs, 80 patients reported prior reactions to intravenous CM.[87] No prophylactic medications were given to any patient, yet no adverse reactions to CM were observed in any of the patients. The decision of whether or not to administer prophylactic medications to a patient with a history of an adverse reaction to CM must be individualized, but providers should be vigilant in all cases and prepared to respond should any sign of a CM reaction develop.

The complete reference list for this chapter can be found online at www.expertconsult.com.

11

Principles of Electrosurgery

Petros C. Benias and David L. Carr-Locke

ELECTROSURGERY

Electrosurgery harnesses electricity with the intention of creating various thermal effects to achieve resection, incision, hemostasis, and devitalization of target tissues. The therapeutic basis of all electrosurgery is the production of thermal energy at the cellular level, typically as a result of a high-frequency alternating current created by an electrosurgery generator or unit.

Heat generated by this process is the result of resistance or impedance to the flow of electricity within the tissue. The electrical current must alternate (i.e., change direction between positive and negative) at a frequency of more than 100,000 times per second (100,000 Hz) to avoid the neuromuscular responses and shocks that occur with the typical 60-Hz household current. The process, however, should not be termed "electrocautery," as this is a misnomer referring merely to the ability to "burn" with electricity. "Electrosurgery" provides both cutting and coagulation, making it the ideal technology for producing therapeutic coagulation, resection, and tissue ablation throughout the gut. When the current density is sufficient within the targeted tissue, cellular water is rapidly heated, resulting in boiling and bursting of cellular membranes. When this energy is directed along a blade or wire, the result is electrosurgical cutting. At lower current densities, a less intense reaction results in tissue coagulation and desiccation without cutting.[1–4]

Electrosurgery has widespread use in multiple endoscopic applications, such as polypectomy, hemostasis, and tissue resection. The advent of flexible duodenoscopes and miniaturized electrosurgical tools allows electrosurgical applications to be applied to endoscopic retrograde cholangiopancreatography (ERCP), permitting sphincterotomy, tumor ablation, and intracorporeal stone destruction (lithotripsy). Present and future applications require a thorough understanding of electrosurgery.

A BRIEF HISTORY OF ELECTROSURGERY AND ERCP

Electrosurgery was first introduced in Europe in 1923 by ERBE Elektromedizin GmbH (Tübingen, Germany) and in the United States in 1926 by William Bovie and Harvey Cushing. In the 1960s and 1970s, electrosurgical units (ESUs) became an absolute mainstay in medical care, but without formal education regarding their use, many physicians experienced the catastrophic potential of an inadequately understood technology. It was not uncommon, for example, to experience return pad and alternate-site burns. Although burns can never be totally eliminated when using ESUs, the current "isolated systems" work with safety features in the generator to help prevent such injuries. They also have preprogrammed modes and microprocessors, allowing for intelligent control of the current.[4]

Electrosurgical technologies were first introduced to ERCP in 1974 when Kawai and Classen independently published case series of endoscopic sphincterotomy followed by stone extraction. Classen described the use of "a special high-frequency diathermy knife," essentially a miniaturized electrosurgical tool with cutting properties. The field was young, but the benefits of endoscopy with electrosurgical potential were immediate.[5]

ESUs have become more complex, but also more intelligent and arguably safer. For years it was difficult to account for all of the electrical variables and achieve consistently reproducible results. However, the introduction of regulated electrosurgery in the 1980s by the ERBE Company (ERBE Elektromedizin GmbH) was a significant advance. Modern ESUs now continuously monitor current and voltage, calculate parameters such as power and tissue resistance from these, and analyze these findings in milliseconds. Depending on the desired effect, these parameters are kept constant or modulated by the ESU. Electrosurgery, therefore, has become widespread and safe in its current form. The potential for danger, however, is still present and arises from a poor understanding of the technology, especially when the desired tissue effect is not achieved.[2,3]

BASICS OF ELECTRICITY AS APPLIED TO ELECTROSURGERY

Basics of Electricity

Basic laws of physics govern the behavior of electricity, and, as such, its behavior is predictable. There are four variables that can be used to describe a circuit and are entirely interdependent: resistance (R), voltage (V), current (I), and power (P). In its simplest form, a circuit must include a power source, a resistive element, and a path for the flow of current. Electrical *current* is defined as the flow of electrons, as measured in amperes or amps, through a circuit in response to an applied electromotive force termed *voltage*. *Resistance* or *impedance* represents the obstacle to the flow of current and is measured in ohms. The flow of current through a conductor is governed by Ohm's law, which ties together current (I), voltage (V), and resistance (R):

$$V = IR$$

It states simply that current increases as voltage increases for a constant resistance and that current decreases as resistance increases for a constant voltage. The relationship is predictable. Another simple relationship is represented by $P = VI = I^2R$, where P is the power generated in a circuit. *Power* is the transfer of energy and is measured in watts and rate per second as expressed in joules (watt-seconds). The ability of a current to do work is a result of the energy potential stored in a circuit, which is then dissipated at specific points, usually at the site of a resistor. In our human circuit, the tissue acts as the resistor and the power used is dissipated as thermal energy. The rise in temperature is governed by Joule's law:

$$Q = I^2 \times R \times t$$

where Q is the heat generated by a constant current (I) flowing through a conductor of electrical resistance (R) for a time (t). When electrosurgery is applied to a tissue, the effect, whether it is cutting or coagulation, depends directly on Q.[1]

The Electrosurgical Unit

In a typical monopolar endoscopic circuit, the electrosurgical generator serves as a voltage source. An active electrode, in this case a sphincterotome, conducts electrons to the patient. The patient acts as a resistive element. Electrons come back via the patient return electrode to the ESU. A power setting is present on the electrosurgical generator. This power is a representation of the amount of work the circuit will do at the point of contact. As noted above, because the power is set as a constant and the resistance is inherent to the human tissue, the generator will intelligently try to control the current and the voltage accordingly.[3,6]

Electrosurgery uses high-frequency alternating current, which may alternate polarity or direction up to 500,000 times a second. The cutting and coagulation effects that are desired in electrosurgery occur when the frequency is in the lower radiofrequency range of 300,000 to 1 million Hz. Modern ESUs contain microprocessors that not only control the frequency, voltage, and current but also calculate the impedance of the tissue in contact with the electrode. These ESUs have at least one selection that attempts to hold power constant as closely as possible to the selected watts over a broad range of impedances. As tissue desiccates and fulgurates, impedance increases and an ESU that can dynamically adjust for changing impedance within a tissue can also control for unwanted effects. For example, constant and consistent power during polypectomy helps reduce against snare entrapment as the snare begins to close and the current density increases. During sphincterotomy, as the wire shortens, the area of tissue contact may diminish and impedance rises as tissue desiccates; constant power allows for a controlled cut rather than a "zipper cut."

In addition, modern ESUs are "isolated" and keep current flow within the contained circuit to capture the current through the return plate. If the circuit is broken, no current will flow at any point within the system. An isolated ESU has a transformer that causes the current to return only to the generator and not use alternate pathways to return to its source. If this is not possible, the generator will shut down. An isolated ESU prevents alternate-site burns, but not patient return electrode burns.

Monopolar Versus Bipolar Circuits

Generators typically use one of two types of circuit—monopolar or bipolar. Monopolar circuits use the body between the active electrode and the grounding pad to complete the circuit back to the ESU (Fig. 11.1). Bipolar circuits are complete within the electrosurgical tool itself by containing both electrodes in close proximity. Both monopolar and bipolar circuits have specific uses and advantages in endoscopy.

In monopolar circuits, the return plate, dispersive pad, grounding pad, and neutral electrode are essential because they collect the electrosurgical energy from the patient and return it safely to the generator. Without a return plate, there is no circuit and the electrosurgical device will do no work. Additionally, the return plate, which is situated externally on the patient's skin, becomes an active part of the circuit, which in the past created potential for return-site burns. The energy returned, however, is of low current density, minimizing or eliminating this effect, but it can still potentially occur if the plate is poorly sited.

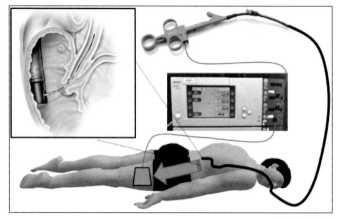

FIG 11.1 Typical monopolar circuit in which current flows from the electrosurgical unit (ESU) to a sphincterotome, through the patient's body to the return electrode (placed on the right thigh here), and back to the ESU.

The benefit of a monopolar device is its ability to achieve high levels of thermal effect with the versatility to cut and coagulate. Examples of the monopolar mode in endoscopy are polypectomy snares, sphincterotomes, needle knifes, ESD tools, and argon plasma coagulation. Although the bipolar mode does not require a grounding pad, the thermal effect is localized only to the tissue in direct contact with the device electrode. The advantage of this mode is the precise delivery of intense energy into a small space, such as in a bipolar hemostasis probe or electrohydraulic lithotripsy fiber.

Both types of circuits are similar, in that their result depends directly on the current density achieved by the tool at the site of the targeted tissue. Current density is the result of several variables but, in essence, represents the density of energy within a given electrical space. Given a constant amount of energy being generated, as when a sphincterotomy wire shortens or a snare closes, the current density increases. Current density is lower when spread over a greater volume of tissue, and the resulting effect will be slower heating. Energy spread over a ball tip or flat forceps jaw promotes coagulation by reducing the current density, as opposed to concentrating current along a snare or sphincterotome wire that promotes cutting.

Maximizing Safety

Safety has been dramatically improved with advent of microprocessor-controlled ESUs. The addition of preset modes makes the use of these ESUs simpler and allows for more uniform and reproducible outcomes. There are, however, safety concerns, especially with regard to the use of the return plate. The following are the most important safety rules:

1. All return plates have expiration dates, which should be obeyed. Plate adhesive has the potential to dry out, resulting in poor contact with the skin, a high current density at the return site, and a greater likelihood of thermal injury at the return site.
2. Return plates have well-designed shapes. These should not be modified, as the shape and area have been predetermined by the manufacturer and are specific to the ESU. One should also not interchange return pads of different manufacturers.
3. The return plate should be placed over well-perfused muscle tissue, preferably in close proximity to the target area. The skin must be clean, dry, and free of hair to avoid loss of contact between the plate and the skin. The electrode should not wrap around a limb. In endoscopy, a common area for return pad placement is the flank or just overlying the kidney on the latissimus dorsi muscle, if possible. Other alternative sites are the anterior thigh and upper arm, but both locations increase the circuit length.

4. The return plate should not be placed over bony protuberances, metal implants or prostheses, skin folds, scar tissue, hairy areas, any form of skin discoloration/injury, or limbs with a restricted blood supply; adjacent to ECG electrodes or pacemakers/implanted defibrillators; or onto pressure areas/points.
5. The patient plate should be of appropriate size for the patient's weight and should never be cut to size.
6. After removal of a patient plate, it cannot be reused and must be replaced by a new one.

Pacemakers

RF current has the potential to damage older pacemakers, but newer models are safe. The greatest potential for error occurs with the use of monopolar circuits. Care must be taken to place the return pad well away from the pacemaker. In contrast, implanted cardiac defibrillators (ICDs), which may be activated by short electrical bursts of the generator, may need to be deactivated by placement of a magnet on the skin surface directly over them. Removing the magnet allows immediate reactivation of the ICD after the procedure. This is safe to perform even by the endoscopy unit staff after proper training from cardiology personnel. Inadvertent firing of an active ICD is most dependent on voltage and application time, as well as the grounding pad position. Therefore it is best practice, even if the magnet is deactivated, to position the grounding pad on the lower half of the body and to limit electrical energy to short bursts of low power. Because some patients are pacemaker dependent, it is prudent to seek advice from the patient's cardiologist before "removing" the sensing function of a pacemaker or ICD.

Neuromuscular Stimulation

Neuromuscular stimulation can be caused by any number of faults within the circuit, including inadequate connections, poor insulation, and broken wire bundles underneath insulation or defective/broken adapters. Generator current is of radiofrequency and can produce this effect only if there is a break in the circuit allowing for demodulation of the current to below the 100-kHz threshold. The result can be as simple as muscular twitching, but particularly dangerous is the effect on the human myocardium, which can result in ventricular fibrillation and cardiac arrest. High-frequency current (>300 kHz) is used in electrosurgery because myocardial sensitivity decreases with increasing current frequencies. However, the risk of electrostatic losses increases with increasing frequencies, thus reducing the efficiency of current application and increasing the risk of burns to either the operator or the patient. Therefore high-frequency currents in the range of 300 to 1000 kHz are usually employed during electrosurgery.

Current Leaks

RF leakage currents are those that find alternate paths back to the ESU. These leakage currents take away from functional power that should be delivered to the operative site and can cause alternate-site burns to the patient or user. The accessory cables from the ESU should not be routed with other cables. They should be kept separated to avoid the phenomenon of capacitive coupling. This is a natural phenomenon that can be compounded when using electrosurgical accessories through endoscopes. Capacitive coupling or leakage from the active electrode within the endoscope channel to surrounding metal structures of the endoscope can occur. The escape of secondary currents can thus cause inadvertent burns away from the target site and loss of power at the active electrode. With older ESUs, it was not uncommon for the nonisolated endoscopist to be burned around the eyepiece of a fiberoptic endoscope (D.C.L., personal communication).

CLINICAL APPLICATIONS OF ELECTROSURGERY IN ERCP

Types of Current

There are two broad categories of current—cutting and coagulation—and there are various forms of blended or pulsed currents that allow for a variety of tissue effects. A pulsed or blended setting alternates cutting and coagulation currents according to user-defined intervals. This means that the cutting current is intermittent, with periods of interspersed coagulative current. This is different from a continuous cutting current, which is a perfect sinusoidal wave without disruptions.

Electrosurgical procedures lead to various tissue effects depending on the electrosurgical instrument, the energy transmitted to the biologic tissue, and the time of application. For a cutting effect, the electrical power has to be sufficient such that the tissue reaches 100°C quickly, whereas a coagulation current achieves its effect in the range of 50 to 80°C. A high current density creates a "microspark" phenomenon between the tool and the tissue that disrupts the tissue immediately. This extreme rapid heating results in cellular rupture, and the effect is perceived as "cutting," whereas coagulation currents devitalize and desiccate tissue slowly.

During coagulation, tissue is heated more slowly to desiccate and devitalize it. At temperatures beyond approximately 50°C, the tissue is irreversibly damaged (devitalized). Beyond 80°C, proteins are denatured (coagulated), and the tissue desiccates and shrinks. Longer application times result in higher desiccation of tissue. If the tissue is overheated as a result of long application times, a tissue carbonization effect occurs, with the potential of perforation. Modulated currents are critical to minimize excessive tissue injury while providing the necessary effect of cutting and coagulation. Detrimental effects are excessive sparking and carbonization. Modulation allows the device to produce high peak currents with calculated breaks. This prevents excessive carbonization and uncontrolled effects (e.g., rapid uncontrolled cutting) and reduces the risk of perforation.

Sphincterotomy

Sphincterotomes carry a monofilament or braided cutting wire (Fig. 11.2). Monofilament sphincterotomes may provide a more precise incision with less risk of heat injury at the sphincterotomy edges and the ampullary area, but, to our knowledge, a prospective randomized trial comparing the two devices has not been performed. Sphincterotomes may have one, two, or three independent lumens to accept the cutting wire, a guidewire, and contrast medium, respectively. Single-lumen sphincterotomes are rarely used as the guidewire has to be removed during sphincterotomy. Otherwise it would be in contact with the cutting wire, increasing the risk of a short circuit. Therefore multiple lumens are not only practical but also help with insulating the cutting component of the sphincterotome from the guidewire portion.

Another important factor is the power setting of the ESU and current selection. All of these affect initiation and propagation of the cut and can lead to adverse outcomes such as bleeding, perforation, and pancreatitis. Endoscopists can choose pure cutting current, coagulation current, or blended and/or pulsed current, which may be proprietary to the manufacturer. Cutting efficiency generally increases with power (30 to 60 W) and, if not controlled for, will also increase with shortening of the contact area of the wire. As the sphincterotomy is performed and the tissue is desiccated, impedance will increase. Microprocessor-controlled impedance feedback is now often built into ESUs, allowing for the endoscopist to simply choose a power setting while the ESU adjusts all other variables as the cut is being performed.

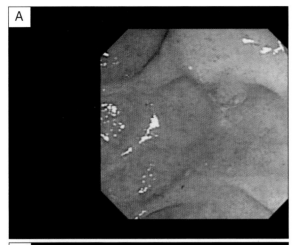

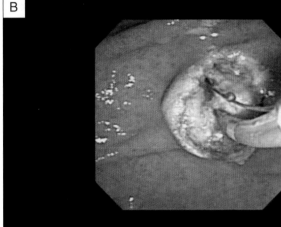

FIG 11.2 **A,** Intact papilla. **B,** Biliary sphincterotomy with sphincterotome in place, demonstrating coagulated cut edges and exposure of the intramural bile duct.

- If no effect is observed within 1 or 2 seconds after current application and the circuit is complete, it may be useful to reduce the length of wire in contact with the surrounding tissue. This increases the current density.
- Uncontrolled rapid cutting ("zipper effect") may develop as the length of wire in contact with the tissue decreases or when excessive mechanical force is applied with the sphincterotome, especially with older electrosurgical units that do not have microprocessor control. This increases the potential for perforation and bleeding.
- Factors associated with a higher effectiveness for cut initiation and propagation during biliary sphincterotomy include a smaller diameter of the electrode wire, a shorter length of wire in contact with the tissue, a higher force applied with the wire onto tissue, and higher power settings.

There have been many publications regarding the most effective and safest current to use for sphincterotomy. Heating from excessive coagulation is thought to favor the development of local edema that might obstruct pancreatic outflow and result in late stenosis caused by fibrosis.[7] A combination of current waveforms has been explored as a potential means to reduce postsphincterotomy pancreatitis (e.g., pure cut current for sphincterotomy initiation followed by blended current after having cut 3 to 5 mm of tissue). Pure cutting, however, has been consistently shown to result in an increased risk of postsphincterotomy bleeding. In a recent meta-analysis of four prospective randomized trials involving 804 patients,[8] the rate of pancreatitis after biliary sphincterotomy with pure cutting current was not significantly different from that with mixed current (3.8% vs 7.9%). Pure cutting current was associated with more episodes of postsphincterotomy bleeding, without an increase in morbidity or mortality, as most bleeding episodes were mild in nature

Box 11.1 presents a list of practical issues related to sphincterotomy.

Needle-Knife Access Papillotomy and Fistulotomy

Needle-knife access papillotomy (NKAP) (see Chapter 15) has facilitated biliary therapy by providing an alternative approach to access in failed biliary or pancreatic cannulation. Compared with standard endoscopic sphincterotomy, NKAP is usually a free-hand technique and is therefore operator dependent. In past series it has been shown to increase the risk of bleeding, pancreatitis, and perforation. However, large trials support its use and suggest that in experienced hands its rate of pancreatitis may be no different from that of traditional pull sphincterotomy.[9] The key to minimizing pancreatitis in these studies seems to be the decision to perform needle-knife access early, when it becomes obvious that traditional bile duct wire-guided access may fail.

Needle knives are monopolar devices that allow focused thermal energy along a very short and straight wire. The blend of current allows short bursts of cutting and coagulation, and typically the same settings as in sphincterotomy are used. The small surface of the needle knife, however, increases current density dramatically compared with a standard sphincterotome, and care needs to be taken, because uncontrolled zipper cuts or deep tissue injury may occur. It is best to perform needle-knife access over a pancreatic stent. If this is not possible, one can carefully start at the papillary orifice and work in the biliary direction, exposing layers of tissue until the biliary orifice or a stream of bile is identified. A variation of this technique is needle-knife fistulotomy. This can be safely performed when there is a large intraduodenal bile duct, as is the case when a stone is impacted at the level of the papilla. In this case a more direct approach can be taken to the distended intramural bile duct while cutting over or just above the stone to gain access to the duct under pressure.

Electrohydraulic Lithotripsy (see Chapters 19, 46, and 55)

Electrohydraulic lithotripsy (EHL) accomplishes its focused destruction of calculi by creating a high-voltage spark between two isolated electrodes (bipolar) located at the tip of a narrow probe (Fig. 11.3). The electric sparks are delivered in short pulses, which create an immediate expansion of the surrounding liquid. A spherical pressure wave is produced, generating sufficient pressure to fragment a stone. The waveform consists of a shock front, a compressive phase, and a tensile tail. The tensile phase can be thought of as a negative-pressure front, which produces cavitation and is crucial to fragmentation of calculi. Short pulses of high peak pressure provided by a low capacity and a high voltage have a greater effect on fragmentation than the corresponding broader shock waves of lower peak pressure carrying the same energy. Because the energy generated is indiscriminate, care must be taken to avoid injuring the bile duct wall. This is achieved by direct cholangioscopic visualization with the EHL probe passed through its working channel. Loss of effective lithotripsy can occur if there is loss of electrode integrity as a result of spark damage during use. Large studies have validated that EHL has a stone fragmentation rate of 96% and a stone clearance rate of 90%.[10,11]

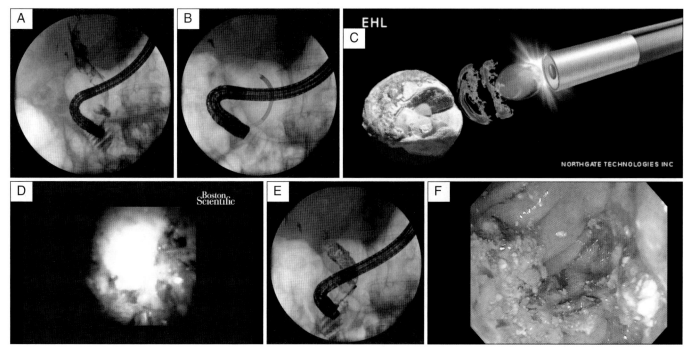

FIG 11.3 A, Initial ERCP showing multiple large stones. **B,** Cholangioscopy with electrohydraulic lithotripsy (EHL) probe. **C,** Diagram of EHL probe and shock waves causing stone fragmentation. **D,** Cholangioscopic view during EHL with the probe tip just visible at the 6 o'clock position. **E,** Bile duct now full of fragments. **F,** Appearance of fragments in the duodenum after basket extraction.

Papillectomy

Papillectomy (erroneously often termed "ampullectomy"; see Chapter 25) involves the same principles and risks as polypectomy because adenomatous tissue is present in both conditions (Fig. 11.4). In addition, the increased use of adjuvant thermal therapies (e.g., argon plasma coagulation) to achieve complete ablation of ampullary tumors or adenomas has the potential to increase adverse events. Pancreatic and biliary stenting, sphincterotomy, and the so-called smart currents confer lower morbidity.[12,13]

The snare is placed at the superior or inferior base of the tumor and thermal energy applied as the snare is closed. The correct balance between cutting and coagulation current is crucial. Early reports used a blended current similar to sphincterotomy. There are no head-to-head studies comparing the type of current and power settings. Common options include blended, pure cut, and ERBE Endocut, but no consensus has been reached. However, according to expert surveys it seems that 67% of biliary endoscopists prefer ERBE Endocut to blended current (17%).[14] Specifically, Endocut provides low power and continuous current followed by short bursts of cutting and coagulation.

Thermal injury to the biliary and pancreatic ducts also increases the risk of orifice stenosis. In a retrospective study, Catalano et al.[15] found that both acute pancreatitis and papillary stenosis occurred more frequently in patients in whom pancreatic stents were not placed (17% vs 3% for pancreatitis and 8% vs 3% for stenosis). Therefore pancreatic stent placement has become a routine practice when performing endoscopic papillectomy. Biliary stenosis, however, is less predictable. Given the adjunctive use of ablative techniques for tumors, it is reasonable to consider prophylactic biliary stenting.[16] Unlike endoscopic mucosal resection elsewhere in the gastrointestinal tract, papillectomy is not facilitated by injection of submucosal fluid tand may indeed be a hindrance.[17]

Pseudocyst Drainage and Necrosectomy

Endoscopic pseudocyst drainage has become common (see Chapter 56). Many techniques have been described and multiple devices have been created to produce an enterocystic stoma. The needle knife and a ring electrode, known as a "cystotome," are commonly used when cautery is applied, and both employ monopolar circuits to form a coagulated cut through the gastric or duodenal wall into the cyst cavity. Both devices produce a high current density at the point of contact, allowing for an easy track to be made through layers of the gastric or duodenal wall.

Most often the best window to achieve access for drainage is through the stomach, usually through the proximal posterior body or fundus. In this location the stomach wall can be quite thick, and this is also somewhat affected by the granulation tissue that makes up the wall of the pseudocyst. Classically, it is thought that the stomach wall and wall of the pseudocyst are one and the same; however, this is not always the case. There are multiple cases of wall separation, and if one inspects the wall carefully by endoscopic ultrasonography, intervening fat layers of incomplete adhesion can be seen. Therefore access should be chosen carefully and special consideration needs to be given to forming a secure and safe track. In order to do this, the tool and the type of current used should be considered.

The most frequently used tool is the needle knife, mostly owing to its widespread availability. Of note, the thin needle knife is not completely advanced from the sheath, because it may become distorted as it takes its path through the stomach wall and thus may not follow a straight line. After formation of a track, dilation can be performed to facilitate stent placement. Alternatively, a cystotome (6 to 10 Fr), a more robust device, does not suffer from these challenges. Often dilation is not necessary after using a cystotome, because the initial device and a self-expandable metal stent can be placed immediately afterward.

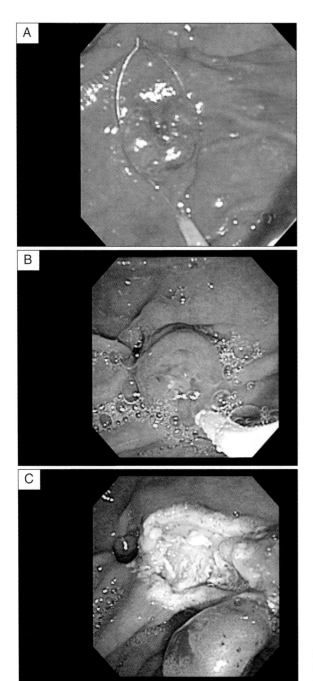

FIG 11.4 Sequence of papillectomy: **A,** snare placed over adenomatous papilla; **B,** snare closed just before papillectomy; **C,** appearance after papillectomy with the resected tumor lying at the bottom right.

There have been recent advances in pseudocyst drainage that allow for a simplified approach. The Axios (Boston Scientific Endoscopy, Marlborough, MA) system, especially the electrocautery-enhanced version, combines the benefits of a 10.5-Fr cystotome and lumen-apposing metal stent (LAMS) to access pseudocysts or walled-off necrosis in relatively few steps. Often this can be achieved without wire-guided access or the need for tract dilation.

Similar electrosurgical principles apply. In most cases the track is best formed with a blended current. Specific settings and application times have not been well studied or standardized. However, bleeding is somewhat negated by the expansive force of the LAMS. A short application period with pure cutting current may not result in an ideal coagulative effect on the tissue. Therefore it is our position that slow

advancement during entry should be undertaken so that the full coagulative effect can be delivered and minimize bleeding. There are currently no formal studies to guide this.

EUS Gallbladder Drainage

Gallbladder (GB) drainage with the LAMS has now been described in several series with success and safety. Using the electrocautery-enhanced Axios system, the GB can be safely drained to the stomach or duodenum. Long-term outcomes of creating such a fistula are as yet unknown, and it may complicate or prevent subsequent cholecystectomy. However, the initial technical and clinical success exceeds 95%.[18] Early results also suggest that this technique is equivalent to percutaneous GB drainage, and perhaps with superior long-term results owing to a reduced need

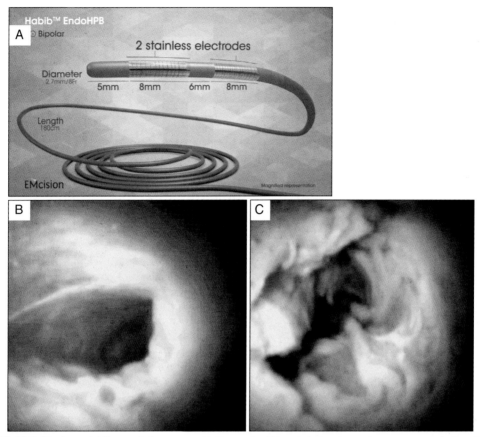

FIG 11.5 Bipolar endobiliary radiofrequency ablation probe **(A)** and cholangioscopic appearances before **(B)** and after **(C)** application of energy. (Courtesy Dr. Reem Sharaiha.)

for repeat interventions. In most cases the LAMS can be removed in 4 weeks, replaced with plastic stents, and/or used for definitive clearance of all GB stones.

Radiofrequency Ablation in the Bile Duct

Recent advances have allowed for the use of focused radiofrequency in segments of the biliary tree as an ablative technique (Fig. 11.5) (see Chapter 40). Radiofrequency ablation (RFA) produces carbonization of tissue and has been used for percutaneous and intraoperative delivery of heat energy, achieving localized tumor necrosis in primary and secondary hepatic cancers. An endobiliary probe that can treat malignant biliary strictures during an ERCP is now available. The Habib EndoHPB (EMcision UK, London, United Kingdom) catheter, which has US FDA and EU European Conformity approval, is the first probe to be used safely in humans. It uses bipolar RFA circuitry delivering energy at 400 kHz and at 7 to 10 W for 2 minutes, with a rest period of 1 minute during each session. Although randomized trials have not been performed, case series show excellent 90-day patency of the obstructed ducts after RFA and self-expandable metal stent placement.[19] In most cases stent placement could not be achieved without the application of RFA. The major limitation is that stricture length treated at each time is 25 mm, as this distance between the two ends of the circuit balances maximum current density and treatment effect. Thus longer strictures require several applications. Potential adverse events of RFA include extension of thermal injury into adjacent structures, difficulty reintroducing catheters into the bile duct after application, hemorrhage, and abscess formation.

Other potential applications of biliary RFA include the treatment of intraductal extension of ampullary lesions. In this situation, RFA alone or in combination with other ablative technologies (namely, argon plasma coagulation [APC]) seems to have excellent results, with >90% success long-term.[20] This type of ablative technology has promise but requires further study, especially in the neoadjuvant setting.

The complete reference list for this chapter can be found online at www.expertconsult.com.

12

Quality Issues and Measures in ERCP

Jordan D. Holmes and Douglas O. Faigel

Endoscopic retrograde cholangiopancreatography (ERCP) is a technically demanding procedure that requires considerable endoscopic skill. It is associated with the highest adverse event rates of any endoscopic procedure. It is important that endoscopists with competency in ERCP are granted privileges to perform the procedure. In response to this, the American Society for Gastrointestinal Endoscopy (ASGE) has proposed specific criteria for the training and granting of clinical privileges for ERCP.[1,2] Institutions are legally liable for negligent privileging.[3] In the era of evidence-based medicine, the need arises to establish a foundation for quality assurance related to ERCP. For this reason, the ASGE, along with the American College of Gastroenterology (ACG), has proposed specific quality indicators to allow for both measurement and improvement in ERCP. These indicators include both process and outcome measures. Process measures assess actual performance in the delivery of care compared with accepted standards. Outcome measures assess the results of care from the patient's perspective.

In this chapter, we will discuss the quality indicators that pertain to ERCP (Table 12.1).[1] These indicators are divided into preprocedure, intraprocedure, and postprocedure time frames.[4] The preprocedure period includes all patient contact up to the administration of sedation or anesthesia. The intraprocedure period is from the time of administration of sedation/anesthesia to endoscope withdrawal. The postprocedure period extends from completion of the procedure through patient follow-up. Each time period has specific indicators associated with it and is considered separately. Additionally there are indicators common to all endoscopic procedures that should be assessed (Box 12.1).

PREPROCEDURE QUALITY INDICATORS

The preprocedure period includes all contact between the patient and the endoscopy center staff (endoscopist, nurses, techs, schedulers, etc.) to the initiation of sedation or anesthesia. In addition to the specific ERCP indicators reviewed below, measures common to all endoscopic procedures may be assessed. These include documentation of a focused history and physical examination, risk stratification (American Society of Anesthesiologists [ASA] or Mallampati score), recording a sedation plan, timeliness of the performance of the procedure, addressing the use of anticoagulants or antiplatelet agents, and a preprocedure team pause (see Box 12.1).[4]

Appropriate Indication

One of the most important quality indicators for ERCP is an appropriate indication[5,6] (see Chapter 7). In the United States, lack of indication for ERCP is the most common reason for legal allegation[7,8] (see Chapter 13). Indications for ERCP vary[1,5,6] and include:
1. Obstructive jaundice
2. Clinical, biochemical, or imaging data suggestive of pancreatic or biliary tract disease

3. Clinical suspicion of pancreatic malignancy when direct imaging studies are normal or equivocal
4. Evaluation and treatment of idiopathic recurrent pancreatitis
5. Preoperative evaluation and treatment of chronic pancreatitis
6. Preoperative evaluation of pancreatic pseudocyst
7. Sphincter of Oddi manometry
8. Endoscopic sphincterotomy:
   a. Choledocholithiasis
   b. Papillary stenosis or sphincter of Oddi dysfunction causing disability
   c. Facilitation of biliary stent placement
   d. Facilitation of balloon dilatation
   e. Treatment of sump syndrome
   f. Treatment of symptomatic choledochocele
   g. Palliation of obstructive jaundice in poor surgical candidates with ampullary carcinoma
   h. To provide access to the main pancreatic duct
9. Stent placement for treatment of:
   a. Benign or malignant strictures
   b. Fistulas
   c. Postoperative leak
   d. Irretrievable large common bile duct stone(s)
10. Balloon dilatation of ductal stricture
11. Nasobiliary drain placement
12. Drainage of symptomatic and infected pancreatic fluid collections
13. Tissue sampling of pancreatic or bile ducts
14. Pancreatic therapeutics
15. Endoscopic papillectomy
16. Facilitation of cholangioscopy/pancreatoscopy

ERCP is generally *not* indicated in the following clinical scenarios[1,5,6]:
1. Abdominal pain without objective evidence of pancreaticobiliary disease. Objective evidence includes abnormal laboratory or imaging studies suggestive of pancreaticobiliary disease. The risk-benefit ratio is high in the absence of these objective findings. If ERCP is pursued for abdominal pain without objective evidence of pancreaticobiliary disease, it has been suggested that sphincter of Oddi manometry be performed (see Chapters 16 and 47).[9] A recent randomized controlled trial in type III sphincter of Oddi dysfunction found no benefit for sphincterotomy regardless of manometry findings.[10]
2. Routine ERCP before cholecystectomy. Preoperative ERCP before cholecystectomy should be performed in the setting of acute cholangitis or if the preprocedure likelihood for choledocholithiasis is high (e.g., abnormal imaging showing stones, persistently abnormal liver tests, biliary duct dilation).[11]
3. Routine ERCP for the relief of a malignant biliary obstruction in patients with resectable pancreaticobiliary malignancy. ERCP in this setting has been associated with higher preoperative and postoperative adverse events[12] compared with no ERCP, as confirmed in a recent

TABLE 12.1   Quality Indicators for ERCP

Quality Indicator	Measure Type
Appropriate indication*	Process
Informed consent	Process
Assessment of procedural difficulty	Process
Prophylactic antibiotics	Process
Endoscopist experience	Process
Native papilla cannulation rates*	Process
Use of precut	Process
Extraction of CBD stones*	Outcome
Biliary stent placement*	Outcome
Complete documentation	Process
Adverse event rates: pancreatitis,* perforation, cholangitis	Outcome
Fluoroscopy time and radiation dose	Process

CBD, Common bile duct.
*Priority quality indicators for ERCP.

BOX 12.1   Quality Indicators for All Endoscopic Procedures

Preprocedure
1. Proper indication
2. Informed consent
3. Preprocedure history and physical examination recorded
4. Risk stratification documented
5. Prophylactic antibiotics, when appropriate
6. Timeliness recorded
7. Sedation plan recorded
8. Anticoagulant and antiplatelet drug use recorded
9. Team pause

Intraprocedure
10. Photo documentation of major abnormalities
11. Patient monitoring
12. Medication documentation
13. Reversal agent use or need for airway management or resuscitation because of cardiopulmonary events

Postprocedure
14. Discharge criteria are met
15. Written discharge instructions provided
16. Pathology follow-up
17. Procedure report complete
18. Reporting of adverse events
19. Patient satisfaction surveyed
20. Communication with referring provider(s)
21. Plan for postprocedure resumption of anticoagulants

randomized prospective trial.[8] Nevertheless, ERCP should be considered in the setting of a malignant biliary obstruction in patients with intense pruritus, particularly if there is a delay in surgical resection, and to treat acute cholangitis.[12,13] The indication for the procedure should be documented in the medical record. If the ERCP is being performed for a nonstandard indication, this should be discussed with the patient in detail, well documented, and justified.[1]

Informed Consent

Given the high adverse event rate inherent with ERCP, informed consent must be obtained from the patient or legal guardian before the procedure, except in the setting of a life-threatening medical emergency.[1] The components of the informed consent process include the following: (1) voluntary consent, (2) rational decision-making capability of the patient or legal guardian, and (3) conveyance of "adequate information."[14] It is the physician's responsibility to disclose as much information as a *reasonable* patient would wish to know when making a decision. Determining "reasonable" is not a precise science, and the physician must simultaneously balance the need to avoid overwhelming the patient with providing pertinent risk information. The consent should address the most commonly encountered adverse events associated with ERCP and their expected rates. These include pancreatitis, infectious adverse events (cholangitis and cholecystitis, infection of pancreatic fluid collection), postsphincterotomy bleeding, perforation, and sedation-induced cardiopulmonary adverse reactions (see Chapter 8).[1] Although there are differing opinions as to whether patients must be informed of the potential need for surgery, a prolonged hospital stay, or death,[14] we cannot overemphasize the value of extensive patient education about ERCP and its potential adverse events. Disputes about the extent of the education and consent process are common in ERCP lawsuits (see Chapter 13).[7] Although state laws vary on who can legally obtain informed consent, most experts recommend that the endoscopist performing the procedure obtain the consent.[15,16] In a large prospective multicenter study describing the ERCP consent process in England, the majority of endoscopists (84%) obtained the consent themselves and 14% delegated this responsibility to another member of the team.[17]

The incidence of post-ERCP pancreatitis (PEP) typically ranges from 1% to 7% but can be higher in certain clinical situations.[1,18,19] Multiple studies have identified risk factors for PEP. These factors can be classified into patient-related and procedure-related factors based on prospective studies.[20–22] Patient-related factors include a history of PEP and known or suspected sphincter of Oddi dysfunction, age <60 years, female gender, absence of chronic pancreatitis, and normal serum bilirubin.[21,22] Procedure-related factors include more than one to two pancreatic contrast injections, moderate to difficult cannulation (defined variably but usually ≥10 attempts at cannulation), pancreatic sphincterotomy, precut sphincterotomy, minor papilla sphincterotomy, balloon sphincteroplasty without sphincterotomy, and trainee involvement. Although such factors should be addressed with the patient during the informed consent process,[21,22] the optimal degree of explanation (detail) of these factors is unknown and not standardized. However, patients should be informed that pancreatitis can be severe in a small percentage of cases and may require prolonged hospitalization.

Infectious complications are uncommon after ERCP. Acute cholangitis occurs in up to 1% of ERCPs.[23,24] Post-ERCP acute cholecystitis is seen in 0.2% to 0.5% of cases. Recently, carbapenem-resistant Enterobacteriaceae (CRE) has been transmitted person-to-person through exposure to duodenoscopes (see Chapter 5).[25] The complex design of the duodenoscope with the elevator assembly has been postulated to impede high-level disinfection, leading to transmission in several cases. One hospital changed its reprocessing to include ethylene oxide gas sterilization, without subsequent additional infections.[25] Other strategies for enhanced reprocessing have included a culture and sequester protocol (duodenoscopes are not returned to service until cultures return negative, usually 2 days later), and double reprocessing.[26,27] There have been and will likely continue to be updates to recommendations on duodenoscope reprocessing from endoscope manufacturers, with at least one manufacturer issuing a recall of duodenoscopes for a redesign of the elevator assembly.

Post-ERCP bleeding can occur after sphincterotomy, ampullectomy, or transmural drainage of pancreatic fluid collection. Postsphincterotomy bleeding occurs in 0.8% to 2% of cases,[28,29] and the possible need for transfusion, surgery, or radiologic embolization should be discussed. The patient's willingness to receive blood transfusion, if needed, should be discussed and documented.

ERCP-induced perforation can be related to the guidewire (periductal or ductal perforation), sphincterotomy (duodenal perforation), or endoscope induced at a site remote from the papilla.[30] Post-ERCP perforation occurs in 0.35% to 0.6% of cases,[20,28,29] and the potential need for surgery and prolonged hospital stay for this adverse event should be discussed. Death occurs after ERCP in 0.07% of cases.[29,31]

Assessment of the Difficulty of the Procedure

There is a wide range of complexity across any series of ERCP. With higher degrees of complexity, it is assumed that there will be lower success rates and higher adverse event rates.[20] To allow comparison among endoscopists, the ASGE Quality Committee proposed a grading system for ERCP.[32] The grading system was proposed based on surveying a large group of community and academic gastroenterologists in the United States, Canada, and Britain. The major limitation is that the grading complexity was formed by consensus rather than being evidence based. The proposed system for ERCP has four levels of complexity (Box 12.2). For all categories and contexts, one should increase one level (to a maximum of four) for any procedure done outside of normal working hours, procedure done on a child younger than 3 years, or procedure that had been previously unsuccessful.[32] It is expected that a competent endoscopist should achieve an 80%–90% success rate in all grade 1 ERCP cases.[1] Those with lower success rates should not

---

BOX 12.2   Proposed ERCP Levels of Complexity

1. Deep cannulation of duct of interest, main papilla, sampling
   Biliary stent removal/exchange
2. Biliary stone extraction <10 mm
   Treat biliary leaks
   Treat extrahepatic benign and malignant strictures
   Place prophylactic pancreatic stents
3. Biliary stone extraction >10 mm
   Minor papilla cannulation in divisum, and therapy
   Remove internally migrated biliary stents
   Intraductal imaging, biopsy, FNA
   Manage acute or recurrent pancreatitis
   Treat pancreatic strictures
   Remove pancreatic stones mobile and <5 mm
   Treat hilar tumors
   Treat benign biliary strictures, hilum and above
   Manage suspected sphincter of Oddi dysfunction (with or without manometry)
4. Remove internally migrated pancreatic stents
   Intraductal image-guided therapy (e.g., photodynamic therapy, electrohydraulic lithotripsy)
   Pancreatic stones impacted and/or >5 mm
   Intrahepatic stones
   Pseudocyst drainage, necrosectomy
   Ampullectomy
   ERCP after Whipple or Roux-en-Y bariatric surgery

FNA, Fine-needle aspiration.
Increase one level (to a maximum of four) for any procedure done outside of normal working hours, procedure done on a child younger than 3 years, or procedure that was previously unsuccessful.[30]

---

attempt more difficult ERCPs (i.e., grades 2 and 3).[33] The primary goal of general gastrointestinal (GI) fellowship programs that offer ERCP training is to train to competence in level 1 and 2 procedures (mainly standard biliary work). Postfellowship programs (i.e., advanced endoscopy fellowships) are needed to master more complex challenges at levels 3 and 4.[33] It has been recommended that the level of complexity of each ERCP procedure be graded and recorded.[33] We recommend using the more recent updated system.[32]

Prophylactic Antibiotics

Pre-ERCP antibiotics should be considered in patients with suspected biliary obstruction in whom there is a possibility of incomplete biliary drainage (see Chapter 10). Such patients include those with primary sclerosing cholangitis and hilar biliary strictures. If the biliary drainage is then incomplete, the antibiotics should be continued. Post–liver transplant patients who undergo therapeutic ERCP may benefit from prophylactic antibiotics and continuation postprocedurally for several days even if adequate drainage is achieved.[34,35] Prophylactic antibiotics should be administered to patients with biliary leak, pancreatic leak, pancreatic pseudocyst, and pancreatic necrosis.[34,36]

Endoscopist Experience

All endoscopic procedures require well-trained and competent endoscopists in order to provide optimal and safe patient care. ERCP carries greater risk, and experience level of the endoscopist becomes important. The endoscopist's case volume should be monitored as case volume has been shown to correlate with higher success rate and lower adverse events.[1]

INTRAPROCEDURE QUALITY INDICATORS

The intraprocedure time period starts with the administration of sedation and ends with the removal of the endoscope.[1] There are minimum performance elements that are essential to all sedated GI endoscopic procedures, including patient monitoring, documentation of administered medications, consideration of the need for sedation reversal or resuscitative efforts, and photo documentation of pertinent landmarks or pathologic findings (see Box 12.1).[4] In addition, the following quality indicators specific to ERCP should be considered[1]:

Cannulation Rates

Cannulation is pivotal to achieve the ultimate diagnostic and therapeutic goals of ERCP. Experts in ERCP achieve high cannulation rates of the desired duct with minimal adverse event rates. To achieve this high rate of cannulation, adequate training and continued experience in ERCP are required (see Chapter 9).[1,37]

Deep cannulation (see Chapters 14–16 and 21) is accomplished when the catheter's tip passes proximal to the papilla into the desired duct. This facilitates effective administration of contrast and hence visualization of the entire ductal system and permits the introduction of instruments to achieve therapeutic maneuvers.[1] Failed cannulation may lead to the need for repeat ERCPs, percutaneous transhepatic cholangiography (PTC), or surgery to achieve the goals of the intervention.[1]

The experienced ERCP endoscopist can achieve selective cannulation rates above 95%.[37,38] In the past, a cannulation rate of 80% was considered to represent the minimum threshold for competency.[39] However, a 90% cannulation rate is now considered an appropriate target for most endoscopists performing ERCP, and those endoscopists with less than 80% cannulation rate should consider undergoing further training or discontinue the performance of ERCP in their practice.[1] For purposes of quality measurement, failed cannulation should not include cases that were aborted because of inadequate sedation, prior abdominal surgery (including pancreaticoduodenectomy or Whipple operation, Billroth II anatomy, prior gastrojejunostomy, or hepaticojejunostomy), proximal duodenal obstruction, or high volume of retained gastric contents.[1]

Endoscopists should document whether deep cannulation was accomplished and specify the type of accessories that were used to achieve cannulation.[1] At least one or more fluoroscopic images should be included. The task force recommended photo documentation of any endoscopically identified abnormalities.[1]

If standard cannulation techniques fail, precut sphincterotomy can be performed (see Chapter 15). Precut sphincterotomy has been reported to increase the risk of post-ERCP adverse events, but this may correlate with experience and early adoption of this technique.[19,40–42] Most experienced endoscopists do not use precut techniques to achieve cannulation in more than 10% to 15% of cases.[43,44] Precut sphincterotomy should be considered as an alternative to standard cannulation techniques and is safe and effective in experienced hands.[44] It is important to note that half of ERCP lawsuits involving postsphincterotomy perforations were secondary to the use of precut.[7] Other endoscopic maneuvers are essential to achieve complete procedural success, including traversing of a stricture, stone extraction, and stent placement. Technical success for the most commonly performed procedures once cannulation is achieved should reach 85%.[1] Failed ERCP leads to a higher post-ERCP adverse event rate and the need to repeat ERCP or other interventional and imaging studies, which results in higher cost.[1]

Removal of Common Bile Duct Stones

One of the most common indications for ERCP is extraction of choledocholithiasis (see Chapter 46). Effective relief of biliary obstruction and clearance of the duct rapidly resolves acute cholangitis.[1]

Stones from the bile duct, including large stones greater than 2 cm in size, can be cleared by expert endoscopists in 95% to 99% of patients.[1,45] Nonetheless, competent ERCP endoscopists are expected to clear biliary stones less than 1 cm in diameter in at least 90% of cases using biliary sphincterotomy and retrieval balloons or baskets.[1,46] Large papillary balloon dilation with or without mechanical lithotripsy is useful in removing large or difficult stones when standard extraction techniques fail. Mechanical lithotripsy should increase the success rate to more than 90%.[1,46,47] Less than 10% of cases require advanced procedures such as electrohydraulic, laser, or extracorporeal shockwave lithotripsy.[1] Documentation regarding the removal of stones should include the location of the stone, the size, strictures (if present), postsurgical anatomy, and success.[1]

Stent Placement for Biliary Obstruction Below the Bifurcation

Indications for placement of biliary stents below the hepatic bifurcation include nonextractable bile duct stones, malignant biliary obstruction (pancreatic and ampullary cancer, metastatic disease to the head of the pancreas), and benign strictures (chronic pancreatitis, postbiliary surgery).[1] Placement of stents for strictures at or above the hepatic hilum is more technically challenging and less commonly performed, making it less useful as a quality measure.

Relief of biliary obstruction is essential in the setting of cholangitis and when contrast has been introduced into an obstructed biliary.[1] Competent endoscopists should be able to relieve nonhilar obstruction by placing stents in greater than 90% of cases.[1,48]

POSTPROCEDURE QUALITY INDICATORS

The postprocedure interval starts from the time the endoscope is withdrawn to patient discharge and completion of follow-up.[1] As with other endoscopic procedures, there are general postprocedure quality measures (see Box 12.1). These include documentation that discharge criteria have been met; provision of discharge instructions, including a plan for resumption of diet and medications such as anticoagulants; pathology follow-up; measurement of patient satisfaction; communication with other health care providers; measurement of adverse events; and preparation of a complete endoscopy report.[1,4] Specific elements and modifications have been proposed for ERCP.

Comprehensive Documentation

All endoscopic reports need to contain the following basic elements[49]:
A. Date of procedure
B. Patient identification data
C. Endoscopist(s)
D. Nurses and assistant(s)
E. Documentation of relevant patient history and physical examination
F. Documentation of informed consent
G. Procedure indication(s)
H. Type of endoscopic instrument used
I. Medications administered (type of sedation, antibiotics, antispasmodics)
J. Anatomic extent of examination
K. Limitations of examination, if any
L. Tissue or fluid samples obtained
M. Findings
N. Diagnostic impression
O. Types of therapeutic intervention and results
P. Adverse events, if any
Q. Disposition
R. Recommendations for subsequent care

ERCP reports should specifically describe the techniques and accessories used for cannulation and therapy and whether these were successful. The report should document all ducts cannulated and the extent of visualization on cholangiopancreatography. ERCP reports may be supplemented with representative radiographic images and endoscopic photographs, as appropriate.[1] Accurate documentation has medicolegal consequences. In addition, documentation of findings allows other clinicians involved in the patient's care to make appropriate management decisions.[1]

Adverse Event Rates

The rates of ERCP-associated pancreatitis, perforation, cholangitis, and bleeding should be measured (see Chapter 8).[1] Recording and measuring adverse event rates for invasive procedures is important. For ERCP, certain adverse events occur frequently enough to be used as specific quality measures. This is particularly true of PEP.

The reported rates of PEP in clinical practice are variable. Studies suggest that the rate of PEP ranges from 1% to 30% of procedures in academic centers.[50] This wide variation can be explained by the variable follow-up; definitions used for pancreatitis; and patient-related factors such as case heterogeneity, types of interventions, and the experience of the endoscopist.[50] For quality measurement purposes, PEP should be defined as typical abdominal pain occurring within 24 hours of the procedure associated with amylase or lipase elevations >3 times the upper limits of normal.[1] Rates of PE in all centers (community and academic) average 1% to 7%.[50] The endoscopist should disclose to the patient that PEP can be severe, resulting in prolonged hospitalization, need for surgery, and/or death.[1,50] Around half of ERCP lawsuits in the United States involve PEP.[7]

The expected rate of ERCP-induced perforation is less than 1% in patients with normal GI anatomy.[1] Perforations of the esophagus and stomach may occur as with any upper endoscopic procedure. Additionally, perforations unique to ERCP may occur. The Stapfer classification system describes iatrogenic perforations during ERCP according to their anatomic location and mechanism[51]:

1. Lateral or medial duodenal wall, endoscope related
2. Periampullary perforations, sphincterotomy related
3. Ductal or duodenal perforations caused by passage of instruments
4. Guidewire-related perforations with retroperitoneal gas on imaging

The Stapfer classification of perforations allows stratification of which patients can be managed conservatively or surgically based on a recently published algorithm, with Stapfer 2 perforations responding well to medical management.[30] Patients with surgically altered anatomy (e.g., Billroth II) are at higher risk for perforation within the afferent limb. Perforation encountered in this setting is intraperitoneal and may warrant surgical intervention[52] if endoscopic closure cannot be achieved.

Clinically significant postsphincterotomy bleeding occurs in less than 2% of cases.[40] Factors that increase this risk include coagulopathy, active cholangitis at the time of the procedure, institution of anticoagulants within 3 days after the procedure, and low endoscopist case volume (defined as fewer than one per week). The bleeding risk is higher when other therapeutic procedures such as papillectomy (see Chapter 25)[53] or transmural drainage of pancreatic fluid collection (see Chapter 56) are performed.[54] ERCP without sphincterotomy (e.g., pancreatic and biliary stent placement, balloon dilation, cytology) incurs almost no risk for clinical bleeding, even in patients with moderate thrombocytopenia and in those receiving therapeutic anticoagulation or antiplatelet agents.[1]

Cardiopulmonary events may be encountered during ERCP, some of which are related to sedation. The risk is associated with higher ASA class. Hence ASA class should be assessed and documented preprocedurally. Endoscopists should be prepared to manage adverse cardiopulmonary events.[1,55]

Patients should be monitored during the procedure to detect cardiopulmonary events. At many institutions, anesthesia support is routinely used for ERCP. Although the main responsibility of ensuring adequacy of sedation and cardiopulmonary function falls to the anesthesia provider, this does not abrogate the endoscopist's duty to conduct an adequate preprocedural assessment and to assist with any interventions if needed to manage adverse events. In some institutions, sedation is administered under the endoscopist's supervision using benzodiazepines and opioids with or without antihistamines, and in some units propofol.[56,57] It is advisable that the endoscopist and units adhere to established guidelines on monitoring and administration of sedation and anesthesia.[58,59]

Efforts should be made to contact the patient within 14 days postprocedure. This postprocedure contact is valuable in discussing pathology results and future treatment plans. Additionally, it allows identification of delayed adverse events. More data available on ERCP-related adverse events help in developing reliable outcome data in the future.[1]

Fluoroscopy Duration and Radiation Dose

The amount of radiation exposure may have detrimental effects on the patient and the staff (see Chapter 3). These risks include dermal injury, damage to vital organs, cataracts, carcinogenesis, and teratogenesis. The ALARA principle (As Low as Reasonably Achievable) has guided safety improvement efforts by radiologist and radiation therapists for decades.[60] Measuring and attempting to reduce the amount of radiation exposure has been a quality metric for other nonendoscopic fluoroscopic procedures[61] and is now routinely available with modern fluoroscopy equipment.[62] Reducing and recording fluoroscopy time along with radiation dose is a metric goal for every ERCP.[1,63,64] Measurements of radiation dosage include dose at reference point (Dose RP) and dose area product (DAP). Dose RP is a radiation dose delivered to a specific

point in space. This is usually along the central ray 15 cm from the isocenter. DAP is the product of the dose absorbed and the area irradiated. These measures more accurately reflect the amount of radiation the patient receives than fluoroscopy time alone.[62] There are multiple factors that influence radiation dose, including type of machine, radiation source distance, patient size, magnification, number of spot films, and oblique views. Radiation dosage is also higher in procedures applying therapy at or above the hepatic hilum.[62,65] A preliminary study suggested that recording and benchmarking fluoroscopy time decreases radiation exposure.[66] There are several ways to reduce radiation dose during ERCP. Principles include proper positioning of the patient relative to the source and imager, limiting fluoroscopy on time, avoiding magnified and oblique views, reducing the number of spot films, and using settings on the fluoroscopy machine that can decrease radiation dosages. Specific ALARA recommendations are in Box 12.3.

INITIATING QUALITY MEASUREMENTS

The purpose of quality measurement is to achieve quality improvement. The quality improvement cycle begins with identifying an area for improvement, measuring performance through quality metrics, intervening to improve performance, and remeasuring to ensure that improvement has been achieved. This concept is incorporated in the Plan-Do-Study-Act (PDSA) method, which employs cycles of planning (P), small-scale pilot testing (D), analysis of test results and lessons learned (S), followed by incorporation and maintenance of new processes into practice (A) versus repeated PDSA cycles.[59] The Define-Measure-Analyze-Improve-Control (DMAIC) method provides a similar structure for cyclic definition, testing, and reanalysis.

Given the large number of proposed quality indicators, initiating a quality improvement program can appear daunting. It is important to begin in small steps by first identifying a limited subset of areas to measure and improve. These can then be instituted in a time-limited (e.g., several months) quality improvement project. As processes are developed for quality measurement, reporting, and improvement, these projects may be lengthened and additional metrics incorporated.

Quality information may be used in several different ways depending on the measure and findings. In the case of an endoscopist performance measure (e.g., deep biliary cannulation rate), feedback to the endoscopist needs to be provided when underperformance is identified. Sharing the results may result in improvement if the endoscopist is receptive to feedback. A designated speaker, such as a physician in the practice, should meet with the underperforming employee to discuss the metrics and explore the reasons for underperformance. This encounter should not be confrontational but supportive and collaborative, focusing on patient care, to allow identification of strategies and implementation of a quality improvement project.

BOX 12.3   ALARA Principles

- Keep the patient away from the radiation source.
- Keep the detector close to the patient.
- Lower the exposure rate wear lead gown and protective eye wear.
- Use lowest-needed magnification.
- Use collimation.
- Limit fluoroscopy on time.
- Use fluorosave instead of acquisition images.
- Keep angulation to a minimum.
- Add 0.1-mm Cu filtration for all protocols.
- Step back during acquisition.
- Use personal protective equipment.
- Use lead shielding on the fluoroscopy unit.

Determining the degree of quality compliance—"How well are we doing?"—is greatly facilitated by external benchmarking. External benchmarking uses an independent and objective method to collect and analyze data from physicians within individual practices. This method uses evidence-based literature and standards to develop its measurement standards. For example, the GI Quality Improvement Consortium Ltd. (GIQuiC) is an educational and scientific 501(c)(3) organization established by physicians specializing in gastroenterology.[67] GIQuiC currently collects data primarily on colonoscopy, but it is anticipated that it will include ERCP. The ERCP Quality Network is a pilot project that collected quality data from over 100 physicians to create report cards and establish benchmarks[66]; it has already been used to reduce radiation exposure and examine practice differences between endoscopists with different experience levels.

Access to quality data remains a contentious issue. When used for quality assurance purposes, these data are not discoverable for use in allegations of medical malpractice. In some instances quality data have been made public. This public reporting is part of a general movement toward greater transparency. In some cases it is government mandated, as is the case for public reporting of hospital-acquired infections.[68] In other instances GI practices have chosen to publish their quality data on the internet[69] (Fig. 12.1).

Value-based purchasing programs have not yet included ERCP. Although more than half of health care maintenance organizations use pay for performance (P4P) incentives in their provider contracts,[70] no P4P programs have yet incorporated ERCP metrics. The 2010 Patient Protection and Affordable Care Act further codified federal value-based purchasing and P4P. This is primarily incorporated in the Centers for Medicare and Medicaid Services (CMS) Merit-Based Incentive Payment System (MIPS). MIPS came into being after the Medicare Access and CHIP Reauthorization Act of 2015 was passed. MIPS is a single program in which physicians will be measured on quality, resource use, clinical practice improvement, and meaningful use of the electronic health record. Although GI measures are available for MIPS, none are specific to ERCP.

Outcomes	MNGI	National data
Cannulation success: Bile duct	95.3%	95%
Adverse events: Total	5.0%	4% to 15%
Pancreatitis	3.97%	4.1% to 5.2%
Hemorrhage	0.74%	1% to 5%
Perforation	0.12%	1%
Infection	0.74%	2%
Patient satisfaction survey		
Patient visit rated excellent or very good*	95%	N/A

*Results are based on 484 completed patient surveys (60% response rate).

FIG 12.1 An example of public reporting of ERCP quality data on the internet. *MNGI,* Minnesota Gastroenterology, P.A. (From http://mngastro.advantagelabs.com/sites/mngastro.com/files/mngi_quality_outcomes_2008.pdf. Accessed December 12, 2011. Used by permission.)

CONCLUSIONS

The success of ERCP depends on achieving both high completion and low adverse event rates. Procedural competency is essential to ensuring ERCP quality. Patient outcome after ERCP can be improved through a constructive process of continuous quality improvement, leading to the performance of optimal ERCP techniques while improving safety. Hence, continuous quality improvement should be an integral part of ERCP programs. Institutions should select subsets of indicators that are appropriate to their individual needs. These indicators should be periodically reviewed and reassessed in a continuous quality improvement process.

The complete reference list for this chapter can be found online at www.expertconsult.com.

13

Medicolegal Issues in ERCP

Peter Cotton

Endoscopic retrograde cholangiopancreatography (ERCP) is one of the most dangerous procedures that gastroenterologists perform regularly; adverse events occur in at least 5% of cases, and lawsuits are common. However, the likelihood of being sued (as well as the success of a suit) can be greatly diminished if practitioners are aware of the reasons why suits are filed and act on that knowledge. There is substantial literature on the topic of medical malpractice in general and in gastroenterology specifically.[1,2] This chapter attempts to provide relevant information and practical guidance in the field of ERCP. The two most important key issues are practicing within the "standard of care" and exemplary communication with patients and family members before and after every single procedure.

Medicine is an imprecise science, influenced by the vagaries and unpredictable nature of biologic systems and the art of interpersonal relationships. Human illnesses are, from the outset, adverse outcomes of life, and it is often difficult for physicians to correct or mitigate illnesses. Furthermore, the techniques, tools, and technology available to aid in this task often have associated inadequacies or risks. Therefore restoring biologic function to its former healthy state is oftentimes incomplete, sometimes unsuccessful, and occasionally complicated by iatrogenic injury. Negative or adverse outcomes may include cognitive or technical failures, ineffective therapies, complications of therapy, high costs and extended hospitalizations, and missed work and life activities. Any or all of these may lead to patient dissatisfaction and a desire to assign blame and seek compensation.

It is in this environment of personal illness and fear, limited medical art and science, patient dissatisfaction, and legal avenues for redress that medicolegal issues arise. Physicians and insurance companies generally blame unrealistic patient expectations, avaricious trial lawyers, and inappropriately high jury awards for the increased number of lawsuits, which in turn lead to high malpractice insurance rates, diminished access to certain types of medical care, and the costly practice of defensive medicine. Alternatively, attorneys and some patients blame true medical negligence, high medical costs, inadequate policing of incompetent physicians, and poor financial management by insurance companies for the worsening medicolegal climate.

It is therefore appropriate for physicians to study medicolegal issues, especially in their specialty areas of practice, to optimize patient outcomes, limit patient harm and dissatisfaction, and to minimize the risk of malpractice litigation.

HOW OFTEN ARE GASTROENTEROLOGISTS SUED?

Gastroenterologists, like all physicians, have a reason to be concerned about malpractice litigation. Specialties vary in their exposure. Analysis of the Physician Insurers Association of America (PIAA) database from 1985 to 2005 showed that only 1.8% of claims concerned gastroenterologists[3] and that they ranked low on the scale of risk among specialties,

21st of 28.[4] However, a recent comprehensive review of claims and outcomes from a large liability insurer over 24 years showed that gastroenterologists ranked much higher (5th of 25 specialties).[5] No less than 12% faced a claim every year; this was less than most surgical specialties but, *surprisingly,* ahead of obstetrics and gynecology, and the authors calculate that by the age of 65 no less than 75% of physicians in the lowest risk specialties (and 99% in the highest) had faced a claim. It is reassuring that only 20% of claims result in a payment and that, contrary to popular belief, the risk for all specialties has reduced somewhat in the last decade.

It might be thought that the unfortunate rise in the risk rankings for gastroenterologists is attributable to the increasing invasiveness of their practice. Paradoxically, whereas an analysis published 20 years ago[6] found that errors in procedural performance were more common reasons for claims than cognitive errors, the reverse now appears to be the case.[3] Thus gastroenterologists not only need to take care to do their procedures well for appropriate indications but also must be mindful every day of the legal risk in diagnostic interviews, evaluations, medication prescriptions, injections, and vaccinations, as well as other forms of patient interactions, by themselves and their staff.

HOW COMMON ARE LAWSUITS INVOLVING ERCP?

Because ERCP is one of the most technically difficult procedures performed by gastrointestinal (GI) endoscopists and because complications, sometimes severe, are more common than with other endoscopic procedures, ERCP might be expected to account for a disproportionate number of claims against gastroenterologists. However, the relative risk of litigation arising from ERCP was actually less than that for other procedure types in the United States, at least when reported in 1995.[6] In a Canadian study, ERCP-related adverse events accounted for only about 6% of GI-related legal actions from 1990 to 1997.[7] This apparent discrepancy is probably attributable mainly to the huge difference in the relative number of procedures involved. By contrast, ERCP is the most common type of endoscopic procedure associated with lawsuits in Japan.[8] Hernandez et al. reported in 2013 that claim payments for ERCP suits were increasing in the United States.[9] A simple Google search for "ERCP lawsuits" provides plenty of interesting reading.

WHAT ARE THE KEY LEGAL PRINCIPLES?

The most common form of a medical malpractice action falls under the principles of tort law, a "civil wrong" rather than a criminal action. Such civil wrongs are generally compensated by monetary redress. To succeed in a medical malpractice action, the plaintiff must prove four basic legal elements by a preponderance of evidence (the fact at issue is more probable than not) rather than proving beyond a reasonable doubt, as in criminal actions.[6,9] The four basic elements that must be proven are:

1. The physician owed a duty of care to the patient.
2. The physician breached that duty by violating the applicable standard of care.
3. The breach of duty caused an injury.
4. The patient's injury is compensable (damages).

Duty

The physician's duty to the patient arises from the physician-patient relationship. The relationship is usually created through an office visit, hospital visit, or performance of a procedure, but may be created without an actual face-to-face meeting between the physician and the patient. For example, an appointment for an office visit or endoscopic procedure or the prescribing of a colon-cleansing agent before colonoscopy by a staff member can create a physician-patient relationship. Clearly defining a physician's duty or role in the management of an individual patient, thereby limiting the scope of the duty, can help to reduce subsequent liability. Once established, the physician-patient relationship continues until officially and appropriately terminated by the patient or physician. Failing to terminate in accordance with the relevant state's laws can lead to a claim of "abandonment."

Breach of Duty

Once the physician-patient relationship has been established, the duty of the physician is to practice within a reasonable standard of care (as described later). Failure to meet the standard of care constitutes negligence and is the central issue in most medical malpractice litigation.

Causation

To be successful in a medical malpractice suit, the plaintiff must prove that substandard care was the proximate (substantial rather than minor) cause of injury.

Injury

Further, to succeed, the plaintiff patient must establish that some type of physical or psychological injury occurred. Having shown that a breach of duty caused an injury, one or more of three types of damages might be awarded in the form of monetary payments. These include general damages for pain and suffering; special damages for past, present, and future medical expenses and loss of income, wages, and profits; and punitive damages for gross negligence, such as intentional harm, conscious indifference, or fraud. Punitive damages are rarely covered by malpractice insurance.

STANDARDS OF CARE AND GUIDELINES

Standard of care is a legal concept describing the duty that physicians must fulfill in their care of patients.[6] A failure to practice within the standard of care is a breach of that duty, one of the four central elements of a malpractice case. The standard of care is usually established through expert testimony, published data, and accepted practice guidelines. Of these, the most important in court is expert testimony. Expert testimony seeks to establish a standard of care reflecting the practice that is customary among competent gastroenterologists in good professional standing who are practicing with reasonable diligence and should reflect the current practice at the time of the injury. Simply stated, the standard of care is "average patient care." It is not defined as optimal or best medical practice exhibited by only a few noted experts in the field, but rather as what would be expected from a reasonable peer under the same circumstances. Defendants' lawyers sometimes suggest that the standard of care is somehow different, or less onerous, in their local community, as opposed to the situation in the ivory towers in which many experts live. This is a slippery slope, best avoided. The standard of care is national, not local.

However, because there are often many ways to manage a clinical problem, more than one standard of care may be applicable for evaluating or treating a condition. Practicing the "majority" standard, or the approach most commonly taken by most peers, is usually the most defensible method of practice. A less common approach, the "minority" standard, may be acceptable but should be explained in terms of why a strategy differing from the usual was employed.

Guidelines

Guidelines developed by specialty societies, federal agencies, or panels of experts may be useful in establishing standards of care. These guidelines are often widely available and provide consensus statements codifying professional custom that may then form the actual basis for a legal standard of care. The validity of such guidelines stems from the sponsoring organization's expertise and prestige, the nature and purpose of the guideline, conflicting views held by other authorities, and the direct applicability of the guideline to the case under consideration.

It might be tempting to assume that clinical guidelines would reduce malpractice risk by helping physicians understand a consensus of "good care," but in reality they are as likely to be used in malpractice litigation by plaintiffs as evidence that the physician failed to meet the standard of care. The American Society for Gastrointestinal Endoscopy (ASGE) guideline on the use of ERCP does leave room for flexibility.[11]

WHO MAY BE LIABLE? NOT ONLY THE ERCPIST

Although most medical malpractice actions are taken against individuals directly involved with an alleged wrongdoing, there is also a legal concept that allows liability to be extended beyond someone who directly caused an injury to persons on whose behalf that person may have acted. There are several circumstances in which vicarious liability may be invoked.[12] Respondeat superior is the legal principle that holds a master responsible for the wrongdoings of his or her servants. These "master-servant" definitions have evolved to include employer-employee relationships, corporate-agent relationships, and teacher-student relationships.[9,13,14] These relationships may apply to preceptors, proctors, administrators, or employers. Such a concept allows blame to be shared among doctors, trainees, nurses, and institutions and may provide additional financially responsible defendants, some with potentially greater resources than the original defendant, to share the liability for an injury. These relationships can be established directly by employment or ostensibly, meaning that under the circumstances it was reasonable for the patients to assume that the physician was employed by or somehow related to the hospital.

Employer Liability

A physician may be held responsible for an adverse outcome attributable to substandard service by office staff, such as violations in patient confidentiality, violations in sterile technique, or failure to provide appropriate training and supervision to ensure the proper functioning of office staff. This issue has become even more important recently with the increasing use of nonphysician providers in gastroenterology practices and ambulatory surgical centers.[15]

Preceptor

The concept of a preceptor as a teacher or instructor in the area of GI endoscopy is central to the training of young physicians new to the specialty and to practicing physicians acquiring new skills. Such a preceptor endoscopist might be found vicariously liable for current or future acts of his or her trainee. More to the point of ERCP, a supervising endoscopist might be held liable for part of the damages arising from a trainee learning the procedure, an experienced colleague acquiring new skills, or either in future misadventures. The degree of liability attributable to each of the principals would depend on many factors, including knowledge on the part of the patient that the procedure would be performed by a trainee, the experience of the trainee, and whether the trainee was performing the procedure within an appropriate standard of care such that the procedure was done for reasonable indications and with appropriate skill. With regard to future injuries after completion of training, liability would hinge on the appropriateness of training and the veracity of credentials.

The expert endoscopist should not train the unprepared novice endoscopist to take on complex difficult tasks before that trainee has the necessary training and experience to safely acquire these skills. Furthermore, training less-than-expert ERCP endoscopists for a technically difficult and seldom needed procedure exposes patients, endoscopists, and trainees to lawsuits, including lawsuits involving vicarious liability. These procedures should probably be conducted at advanced centers for complex or high-risk cases, and ERCP, particularly with advanced techniques, should be concentrated among fewer endoscopists who would thereby perform these procedures more frequently.

Proctor

A physician who observes and monitors another physician, particularly one seeking privileges, is known as a proctor. Proctors have no duty to the patient and therefore no liability because their role is simply to assess the capabilities of the physician being monitored. If the proctor becomes involved in the care of the patient, however, this could change. To avoid such entanglement, the proctor should not interfere with the proctored physician; should have a thorough understanding of proctoring and hospital endoscopy privileges; should not offer advice or interact with the patient; should report only to the hospital or regulatory committee; and in the event that he or she witnesses substandard medical care that is harmful to the patient, should consider contacting an appropriate superior, asking the proctored physician to discontinue the questionable actions, or, as a last resort, intervening with careful appropriate documentation.

Administrator

If a physician acts in an administrative capacity in an endoscopy unit or gastroenterology division, he or she has a duty to patients receiving care in that unit. Failure to develop policies and procedures that ensure a safe environment and comply with state and federal regulations may constitute vicarious liability or corporate negligence. Such responsibilities may include the acquisition and maintenance of endoscopic equipment, privileging, infection control, and workplace safety. Further, if the responsible director knew or should have known that an unskilled physician was practicing in the unit and did not take appropriate corrective actions, vicarious liability could exist.

Hospital Liability

Hospitals may be held responsible for the mistakes of a hospital-based physician employed by that institution or for inadequate oversight provided by endoscopy unit or gastroenterology division directors. They may also incur vicarious liability for improperly privileging physicians who are inadequately trained to perform a certain service.[13,16]

Summary of Vicarious Liability

The endoscopist may incur liability for the mistakes of individuals whom they supervise even if they themselves were unaware of the improper actions and even after their immediate supervisory role had ended. All of the aforementioned roles of preceptor, proctor, employer, and administrator should be approached with care and forethought. An understanding of potential vicarious liability may allow better risk management strategies to minimize exposure to liability.

INFORMED CONSENT

Medical malpractice actions most commonly involve the "tort of negligence," wherein a physician is felt to have practiced below the standard of care ("breach of duty"). There is, however, a common and independent cause of malpractice action involving the failure to obtain informed consent.[17–19] This is often a secondary allegation filed along with an allegation of practicing below the standard of care.

The ethical and legal requirement to obtain informed consent before a procedure comes from the concept of personal patient autonomy and is rooted in the theory of patient self-determination. Against such a backdrop, the courts have found that a person's right to self-determination warrants that a physician should obtain informed consent. The competent patient, after receiving appropriate disclosure of material risks of the procedure in question and understanding the risks, benefits, and alternative approaches, then makes a voluntary and uncoerced informed decision on whether to proceed.

Early on, the consent process operated under a provider-based standard (professional standard of disclosure) whereby the physician was expected to disclose information about the treatment that reasonable *physicians* believed relevant and that reasonable *physicians* generally disclosed to their patients in similar circumstances. More recently, however, courts have been moving toward a patient-based standard, which mandates that a treating physician disclose as much information as a reasonable *patient* would wish to know.

The essential elements of informed consent include:

1. The nature and character of the proposed procedure, preferably in nontechnical terms
2. The reason or indication for the procedure
3. The likely benefits of the procedure and its potential limitations
4. The material risks and complications of the procedure, including their relative incidences and severities
5. The alternatives to the procedure, including those that may be more or less hazardous than the one proposed, and the alternative of no treatment

The consent process should also include an assessment of the individual's competence to understand the information presented and the opportunity for patients to ask questions.

Obtaining informed consent is a process that includes more than placing a signature on a standardized consent form. It involves mutual communication and decision making as part of the physician-patient relationship. It can also be a risk management tool, transferring responsibility for risk to the patient, who has understood and accepted that even competently performed procedures can have adverse outcomes. This is an example of the very important emerging concept of patient engagement.

Material Risks

One essential element of disclosure is discussion of the specific risks and potential complications of the procedure. These risks should include procedure-specific material risks, those that a reasonable patient would want to know in order to make an appropriate decision. The four elements of risk that the physician needs to consider include:

1. The nature of the risk
2. The magnitude of the risk
3. The probability that the risk may occur
4. The timing of the risk, whether contemporaneous with the procedure, postprocedure, or delayed

Deciding what material should be disclosed is often not easy. One authoritative text on informed consent states: "The physician must walk a fine line between providing pertinent risk information and overwhelming the patient with frightening statistics. Providing too much extraneous information may be as likely to impair informed decision making as providing too little."[19] However, clearly the most serious risks must be reviewed.

Controversial Areas

The trend toward a patient-oriented standard of disclosure has allowed for a broader interpretation of the "material risks." What a "reasonable patient would wish to know" in making an appropriate decision might now argue for pertinent disclosure of the experience level and personal adverse event history of the specific physician, rather than national averages, as well as any pertinent economic interests of the physician. This question of the endoscopist's personal experience might be especially applicable to complicated endoscopic procedures such as ERCP. In a legal case involving difficult and risky brain surgery, a physician was found liable for not informing the patient regarding his or her lack of experience.[18] Although it is unclear where to draw the line, the physician must honestly set forth his or her experience or lack thereof if asked.

Exceptions to Informed Consent

Exceptions to the informed consent process are limited. These include:
1. Emergencies where the patient is incapacitated to a degree that consent cannot be obtained and delay would put the patient at risk
2. Legal mandate, whereby the court orders the patient to undergo medical therapy without the patient's consent
3. Incompetency, where the patient is unable to make a decision and that responsibility is given to the patient's legal guardian

Informed Refusal

This doctrine holds that a patient who refuses a procedure or treatment must do so in a well-informed way and that it is the physician's duty to ensure that such refusal is informed. This should be documented in a similar fashion.

Legal Consequences of Failing to Obtain Informed Consent

Failure to obtain informed consent is most often a secondary allegation attached to a charge of practicing below the standard of care. However, it can be an independent cause of malpractice action, alleging that even though the injury was not caused by substandard care, the patient would have refused the treatment or procedure if material risks had been known. The plaintiff would have to show, however, that a reasonable person in the same position would not have undergone the procedure knowing that a small risk of injury existed.

If there was absolutely no consent obtained for medical treatment, or if the treatment went well beyond the scope of consent, a charge of battery could be lodged. Although rare, a charge of battery is a criminal charge and is not covered by most malpractice insurance.

WHY DO ERCP LAWSUITS OCCUR?

It is obvious that most claims occur when something has gone badly wrong; that is, claims are usually made in response to serious adverse events such as pancreatitis and perforation. These are discussed in detail in Chapter 8. Adverse events occur after 5% to 15% of ERCPs, depending on the context.[20] Why do only a small proportion of those result in a suit? Some claims are entered simply in the hope of getting someone else to pay the huge hospital bills that are generated by severe adverse events but are easily dismissed if there is no evidence for malpractice.

The author, as a potential expert witness, has been contacted about more than 150 cases involving ERCP. The main issues remain the same as those we published on the first 59 cases[21] and an additional 20 later.[22] The two most common reasons why claims are pursued and often succeed are marginal indications and poor communication.

Marginal Indications

Most of these cases involved patients with some pain with or without minor abnormalities such as raised transaminases or a slightly dilated bile duct on an ultrasonography or computed tomography (CT) scan. Many had previously undergone cholecystectomy. The endoscopists usually claimed the need to rule out a stone or tumor but had failed to use or even discuss less invasive alternatives such as magnetic resonance cholangiopancreatography (MRCP) and endoscopic ultrasonography (EUS). In some such cases further injury was added to the insult by performing a speculative biliary sphincterotomy, even a precut.

Lawyers are familiar with the very clear recommendations of a seminal report from the National Institutes of Health from 2002.[23] The State of the Science conference on ERCP concluded strongly that ERCP should not be used for suspected sphincter of Oddi dysfunction (SOD), except at tertiary centers offering sphincter manometry. Defendants have claimed that "manometry is dangerous," but we now know that it is the type of patient who is at the highest risk (for pancreatitis), with or without manometry. This led many years ago to an editorial titled "ERCP is most dangerous for those who need it least."[24]

The whole concept of SOD is in flux after the recently published EPISOD study that showed that sphincterotomy was no better than sham treatment in patients with "SOD III."[25]

Poor Communication

It cannot be overstated that poor communication (before and after an adverse event) is the main reason why patients and family members seek legal recourse when things go wrong. It is often stated that "patients do not sue doctors they like." It is crucial to spend enough time to develop a rapport with patients and families and to develop mutual trust. The key elements of informed consent have already been emphasized. It is likely that most patients who have suffered adverse events after a procedure done for marginal indications would not have consented if they had been properly informed of the likely risk-benefit ratio. In most of the cases discussed above, the risk of pancreatitis was actually greater than the chance of finding something to treat.

Poor communication after an adverse event adds further insult to the injury. Patients who feel abandoned become angry and keen for revenge: "The b●●●●●d never came to see me after I came back to the emergency department or was transferred to a surgical wing." Advice on how to keep the confidence of the patient and family is given later.

There are other reasons why claims are made.

Poor Endoscopic Technique

Patients and families often assume that the doctor must have done something inappropriate in order for an adverse event to occur, despite what they were told in the consent process. Sadly, there are some obvious examples. In one case, a large biliary stent was placed in the pancreas by mistake, and the error was not discovered for days. There have been several cases in which pancreatic stents were inserted totally within the duct or migrated there later. Most can be removed by skilled endoscopists, but several patients have needed surgery. Failure to leave a temporary stent in the bile duct when a stone cannot be removed is difficult to defend. Precutting has long been a controversial topic.[26] Although obviously a useful technique in certain cases when biliary access is essential (when ERCP-treatable pathology is already established), it is too often used by inexperienced endoscopists who fail to achieve biliary cannulation in cases where there is no more than a suspicion of relevant disease. Precutting featured prominently in a review of ERCP-related deaths in Denmark.[27] Placement of a temporary pancreatic stent has been shown by many studies from expert centers to reduce the risk of post-ERCP pancreatitis in "high-risk cases" and is now common practice. However, whether it is now "standard of care" in the community is not clear. It is possible that attempts to place a stent by a less experienced endoscopist might be more dangerous than not doing so. That caveat does not apply to the use of preprocedure nonsteroidal antiinflammatory drug (NSAID) suppositories. Although shown to be helpful only in high-risk cases until now, many centers now use them in every case. Their use is easier to remember and has a negligible downside, and some of the "high-risk" designation is apparent only during the procedure (difficult cannulation, need for precut, etc.).

Sedation/Anesthesia Problems

Cardiopulmonary complications are not rare. Some patients are difficult to sedate, and oversedation can be disastrous. ERCP procedures are often prolonged (especially now that almost all are therapeutic), and monitoring may be more difficult in a darkened room. The trend, at least in the United States, is for all ERCP procedures to be done under anesthesia supervision, usually with propofol without endotracheal intubation. It is increasingly difficult to justify doing complex procedures using endoscopist-administered conscious/moderate sedation, especially for American Society of Anesthesiologists (ASA) class 3 and higher patients.

Poor Aftercare

Failure to appreciate, explain, and manage adverse events promptly can greatly aggravate the problem. Any situation may be made worse if the endoscopist who performed the ERCP is not available when the patient returns. The on-call physician may be less attuned to the possibilities and appropriate responses. Because it causes similar pain and is much less common, sphincterotomy-induced retroduodenal perforation is sometimes mismanaged as pancreatitis for many days, with disastrous consequences. In patients who develop severe pancreatitis, there is often a question about the adequacy of rehydration in the first few hours. Another common problem is failure to give antibiotics immediately after ERCP when undrained ducts have been contaminated.

Nosocomial Infection

There have been numerous outbreaks of nosocomial infection after ERCP.[20,28] This possibility should be considered when patients become seriously ill with organisms such as *Pseudomonas, Serratia, Escherichia coli,* or *Klebsiella*. Whereas prior outbreaks were usually attributed to inadequate scope reprocessing, studies of recent outbreaks of carbapenem-resistant Enterobacteriaceae (CRE) infections have raised broader concerns that are still being examined. ERCP endoscopists are at risk when these infections occur and thus must be familiar and comfortable with the local reprocessing procedures.

Delay in Performing ERCP

There have been cases in which patients with acute cholangitis have not been treated quickly enough, resulting in life-threatening sepsis.

HOW TO MINIMIZE THE RISK OF LITIGATION

Risk management is a process designed to identify reasons for poor patient outcomes and to suggest corrective actions to prevent both patient injury and malpractice risk. The formal process includes defining situations that place the patient and physician at risk, determining the likelihood and significance of these circumstances, applying risk

management strategies to individual cases, and developing preventive measures. These include proper training, rigorous privileging, understanding and avoiding adverse events and lawsuits, and dealing with lawsuits once filed.

The best defense against adverse outcomes and malpractice suits is good medical practice. Simply stated, it is important to "do the right thing, and to do it right." The first step in developing sound medical practice is attaining competence through proper training, details of which are given in Chapter 9.

Levels of Complexity in Training and Practice

It is important to realize that ERCP is not a single procedure. It simply describes a method for accessing the biliary and pancreatic ductal systems, within which there are a host of possible procedures. Different levels of procedural complexity were first proposed by Schutz and Abbot,[29] and a somewhat simplified three-tier system has been widely adopted. Grade 1 procedures are those biliary procedures that are often required at a community level (and sometimes urgently), such as stone extraction and management of low biliary strictures and leaks. Grade 2 cases are those of slightly greater complexity, such as large stones and minor papilla cannulation. Grade 3 cases are usually restricted to tertiary referral centers, such as most pancreatic therapies and sphincter manometry. This system was recently updated by a committee of the ASGE.[30]

It follows that endoscopists offering ERCP should restrict their practice as much as possible to the level of procedures for which they have been trained. This does not exclude the possibility of additional skills obtained through specific study. Endoscopists wishing to acquire new skills should not overestimate the need for these or overestimate their own skill level in seeking to acquire such techniques. Who is "experienced" enough to appropriately incorporate new or more advanced skills into one's practice and how is the training acquired? No rigid standards apply, but a reasonable guideline for experience and skill would be 3 years of experience beyond training, 95% technical success in gaining access to the desired duct, and a low personal adverse event rate compared with national averages. Further, there should be a compelling clinical need in one's practice and a persuasive lack of an alternative expert to refer to. Skills should be acquired in a formal training program or through a hands-on preceptorship with an experienced expert. It would not be wise to undertake a newly described but inadequately assessed technique or to engage in cases that are risky or difficult early in the endoscopist's experience. Ignoring these caveats will expose patients to adverse outcomes and endoscopists to malpractice litigation.

Ensuring continued competence at whatever level is an additional safeguard against adverse patient outcomes and malpractice litigation. Maintaining clinical and endoscopic skills in ERCP requires an ongoing effort. This effort includes staying current with the GI literature concerning ERCP, engaging in continuing medical education activities, and achieving familiarity with new endoscopic technologies. In addition, the endoscopist performing ERCP must also maintain an adequate case volume to maintain expert procedural skills. In general, studies have shown a correlation between higher case volumes and greater technical success.[20,25,31] Furthermore, higher ERCP volume has been associated with lower adverse event rates, especially with respect to severe adverse events. Also, there is probably an important effect of lifetime experience. The volume of procedures at the relevant center is also important, because a certain amount of ongoing activity is needed to maintain a team and the necessary equipment. The British Society of Gastroenterology has suggested that ERCP should be done only by endoscopists performing at least 75 procedures a year and in centers doing at least 200. It seems that less than half of endoscopists in the United States reach these thresholds[32] and that very few hospitals do more than 50 per year.[33] These startling facts led to a recent editorial titled "Are low-volume ERCPists a problem in the United States?"[34]

A good way for low-volume ERCP practitioners to avoid litigation is to stop doing the procedures.

How is competence ensured and documented? Privileging is the process by which an institution authorizes an individual to perform a specific procedure.[9] The privileging process should include a review of credentials provided by the training program or trainer and a review of the training experience and case load for each procedure for which privileges are requested. Ideally, an actual level of competency should be assured through proctoring, particularly for advanced procedures. Additionally, institutions should have guidelines on recredentialing and reprivileging that ensure continued competence in all procedures, but particularly the more complex, advanced procedures, such as ERCP. Hospitals have a duty to exercise due care in granting privileges to physicians, and they expose themselves to liability for granting specialized privileges to the poorly trained or inexperienced.[13,16] This vicarious liability extends not only to the hospital but also to individuals in administrative roles, such as the director of the endoscopy unit.

Peer review is intended to identify problems related to adverse outcomes, prevent their recurrence, and help in the reprivileging process. Ideally, this should be done in a nonthreatening manner but should be a formal process with a written record. Each physician should have a personal compilation of his or her own adverse events for comparison with peers. Patients have a right to know, in general terms, the physician's outcome profile.[35] Mechanisms for structured documentation of performance have been developed recently. The ERCP Quality Network was a voluntary pilot system for uploading data on ERCP cases and comparing practice and performance with others (benchmarking).[36] A similar tool for colonoscopy (GIQuiC) will be extended soon to include ERCP. Increasingly, anxious patients will demand data, not just bland reassurance, from their prospective interventionists. Credentialing committees should demand the data on which to make informed decisions.

Certification?

We all accept that it is necessary to pass a test to obtain a license to do certain dangerous things, for example, to drive a car, a truck, a train, or a plane. Why does that principle not apply to endoscopy, or at least to the more dangerous varieties, such as ERCP? Surgeons will point out that a surgical degree is all that is required for surgeons to perform any operation, but we are not swayed. We favor certification of ERCPists and the centers in which they work.

Recognizing Higher-Risk Situations

Because most suits result from bad outcomes, it is obviously helpful to appreciate the circumstances where the risk of complications is higher and to take all possible precautions. The well-trained endoscopist knows that there are some higher-risk patients and some higher-risk procedures and has the knowledge to approach them appropriately.

Higher-Risk Patients

This field has been reviewed in great detail recently by Romagnuolo and colleagues.[37,38] Cardiopulmonary adverse events are a common cause of death after ERCP.[20] The risk is increased by known disease in those organs, which is well reflected in the ASA score. One should not be hesitant to use an anesthesiologist for assistance, especially for patients with ASA scores of 3 or above. The endoscopist and key staff must be properly trained in life-support techniques. Postprocedure bleeding is more likely in patients with primary or secondary coagulopathy. Management of anticoagulant agents may require consultation with

the specialists who prescribed them. Infection may be more common in immunosuppressed patients (e.g., post–liver transplant). Pancreatitis is more likely to occur in healthy young patients and may be more severe in the obese. It probably is more common also in patients who have experienced it before. Patients who report previous reactions to intravenous contrast pose a dilemma. The risk of a severe reaction to ERCP contrast is extremely low but not nonexistent. It is wise to have a policy for this situation and to comply with this policy.

Higher-Risk Procedures

In general terms, the risk of ERCP procedures increases with their technical difficulty, as documented in the new complexity scales.[30] Endoscopists recognize the greater risks involved, for instance, in approaching ampullectomy or patients with sphincter dysfunction. However, there are also important technical details that apply to apparently simple cases. It is well known that postprocedure pancreatitis is more likely to occur with multiple pancreatic manipulations and injections. The use of temporary pancreatic stenting has been shown to reduce postprocedure pancreatitis in high-risk cases when done by experts, but it is not yet clear whether this should be recommended for routine practice, because the attempt to place the stent may itself be harmful. Precutting is a controversial topic, but there is little doubt that it increases the risk of both pancreatitis and perforation, at least in inexperienced hands. Troublesome bleeding is now rare after sphincterotomy, but attention to technique is important. Biliary sepsis may be induced if contrast is injected into ducts that cannot be drained. Immediate antibiotics are indicated, and alternative drainage methods may be needed. Intestinal perforation is a risk in patients with surgical biliary diversions.

The Context of the Procedure

Urgent procedures are often more dangerous, because the patients are acutely ill, and may increase when the procedure is performed in unfamiliar territory (e.g., in intensive care), with inadequate radiographic equipment, or without the usual ERCP-trained staff. It is a challenge for the facility and team to minimize these additional hazards.

Risk-Benefit

Clearly, the goal of both the patient and the endoscopist is to maximize the benefit and minimize the risk of the planned procedure. Some very risky things may be worth doing, for example, urgent stone extraction in a patient with acute cholangitis, because the patient may otherwise die. Conversely, as already emphasized, "speculative" ERCP with or without sphincterotomy in a fit patient with "pain only" clearly carries more risk than benefit. Thus scrupulous assessment of the likely risk-benefit ratio is crucial for both practitioner and patient.

Professional Behavior

A key component of sound medical practice is the interpersonal skill of the practitioner. This must be developed during training and polished once in practice. Effective communication with the patient and family and with other physicians and healthcare providers is a critical element of good healthcare and risk management. Conversely, patient dissatisfaction with a physician's interpersonal and communication skills can be a major factor in the decision to file a lawsuit.[39,40] Displaying a positive caring attitude and communicating honestly, beginning with the initial interview and extending to informed consent and beyond, are critical in forming a healthy physician-patient relationship. This good patient rapport greatly decreases the likelihood of lawsuits. It also helps define the role of the physician, limiting the physician duty and transferring some of the responsibility for an adverse event to the informed patient. A recent important trend in assuring that your patients' experience is positive is to survey them. Several specialty specific tools are available and effective.

Doing Informed Consent Right

There is no substitute for the essential personal, face-to-face interaction between the physician and (fully dressed) patient in an unhurried environment. There are some materials that may help in the process. Professional societies produce educational leaflets that can be distributed, and there is no shortage of websites that describe the procedure. If these are used or recommended, it is wise to review them carefully to ensure that they apply to local practice. Many centers prefer to produce their own. The leaflet in use at the Medical Center of South Carolina (MUSC) is shown in Fig. 13.1. On the reverse is a diagram of the relevant territory that can be used when describing the planned procedure. Note that this document gives some overall statistics of likely adverse events. The associated hospital consent form includes the statement, "I have received and reviewed the specially prepared information brochure, and have had the opportunity to ask questions."

Whenever possible, which should be almost always, the adjunctive materials should be provided before the day of the procedure so that they can be studied and digested at leisure with no element of duress.

There are now some interactive websites that add an intriguing new dimension to this process. The patient is sent a login and password along with his or her appointment. The procedure and key issues are described in lay terms. The innovation is that the sites are interactive. For instance, patients can decide how deeply to go into adverse events and write notes about questions that they need their doctor to answer when they meet. Most important, the systems document the length and extent of the patient's journey and can provide a printout for the records.

Documenting the Consent Process: "He Said, She Said"

Good documentation is an essential risk management tool and also a component of good medical care. The old adage, "If it isn't written down, it didn't happen," is often true in litigation. The extent of the consent interaction is often disputed in lawsuits: "I/Dad would never have agreed to the procedure if I/he had known that this could happen." Patients can always recall exactly what was said, or was not, but the endoscopist will not remember when challenged 2 to 5 years later and has to fall back on "what I always do and say," which is less convincing. The patient's signature on the consent form is inadequate evidence of a meaningful interaction. A verbatim written or dictated note is very helpful. The impressive comprehensive verbiage, which can now be generated by one click of a button on an electronic medical record (EMR), carries little authenticity.

A simple handwritten note affirming that discussions occurred regarding the nature of the procedure, the potential benefit, limitations, alternatives, risks (enumerating the major risks), sedation, and an opportunity for questions goes far in assuring that the physician has fulfilled this part of the duty to the patient and that the patient has participated in the decision-making process, thereby accepting some of the risk of the procedure. Some have advocated videotaping the consent process as an extreme method of documenting exactly what occurred.

Special Care Needed With "Open Access" and Urgent ERCP

Open access endoscopy is a legal minefield and carries risks especially relevant to screening colonoscopy. A duty to the patient exists as soon as the appointment is made. The patient may be requested by nonmedical staff to stop or change his or her medications before the procedure, with potential hazard, and, for colonoscopy, to go through arduous bowel preparation.

Most ERCP cases are done on an elective basis, with the opportunity for the patient and potential endoscopist to share an unhurried and meaningful discussion, preferably on a day before the planned procedure. However, some ERCPs are urgent and many are done at tertiary centers on a "same day" basis, that is, transfer from and directly back to another hospital. Such patients and their families usually know that the clinical situation is somewhat serious and that the treatment involves risk, but that does not absolve the endoscopist from ensuring that everyone understands what is planned and the possible consequences.

There have been cases where one member of a practice who does not perform ERCPs has recommended an ERCP to be done by a colleague. The appointment is scheduled by staff and the hurried colleague meets the patient on the radiographic table, with pressure to proceed without careful evaluation of the indication or an opportunity to develop a meaningful relationship with the patient.

Live Teaching Demonstrations

Live demonstrations by visiting experts became popular in the early days of endoscopy, and ERCP and undoubtedly played an important role in the education of many endoscopists. Witnessing a few serious adverse events during several such meetings led us to raise questions about their safety. In particular we worried about the problems that tired and potentially disoriented endoscopists might encounter with unfamiliar equipment and staff, working on patients whom they had not themselves selected or perhaps even met.[42] This polemic led to some useful guidelines by the American and European Endoscopy Societies, the most important of which is for the organizers of workshops to ensure that one of the local doctors is always in the procedure room and controlling the activities.[43,44] The discussion stimulated two studies of the relative risks of workshop procedures, in China and Holland, and the studies actually showed no increased risk of adverse events over daily practice.[45,46] Be that as it may, endoscopists invited to perform overseas should be aware of the issues and insist on meeting the patients and assisting staff beforehand. However, in this electronic age it is easier and probably safer for experts to beam their demonstrations from their own units.

Managing Adverse Events

ERCP is difficult and complex, and adverse events will occur even with good patient selection and good technique. The fact that an adverse event has occurred is not malpractice in and of itself; the failure to make a timely diagnosis could be, however. It is crucial to recognize the possibility of complications promptly and to be attentive to their signs and symptoms. Early diagnosis and treatment are vitally important.

Communication with the patient and family is crucial. A full explanation of the situation and the plan of treatment is necessary. Empathy, compassion, and honesty are essential. It is important for the patient and family members to recognize that you care, that you share their disappointment, and that you will work with them to rectify the situation. It is wise to refer back to the consent process; for example, "The x-ray confirms that there is a perforation; you recall that we discussed that possibility beforehand; I am sorry that it happened to you." Saying "sorry" shows that you care but does not imply any wrongdoing. Of course, it is important to avoid saying, "I must have cut too far," "I must have pushed too hard," and so on. Instituting such a "medical system error disclosure program" has been shown to reduce claims.[47]

During the treatment of adverse events, it is important to maintain contact with the patient and family so as not to engender feelings of abandonment and, further, to ensure that all necessary consultations are obtained expeditiously. Although often personally uncomfortable for the physician, such continued contact with the patient and family promotes good medical care, demonstrates compassion, and helps

ERCP stands for Endoscopic Retrograde Cholangiopancreatography

ERCP uses an endoscope which is a long narrow tube with a camera at the end. The doctor passes the endoscope through your mouth (under sedation/anesthesia) to get into the papilla of Vater, a small nipple in your upper intestine (duodenum). This papilla is the drainage hole for your bile duct and the pancreatic duct, which bring digestive juices from your liver, gallbladder and pancreas. X-rays are taken to show whether there any lesions such as stones, spasms or blockages. If the x-ray pictures do show a problem, the doctor may be able to treat it right away with instruments passed through the endoscope. The most common treatments are:

- **Sphincterotomy**. This involves making a small cut in the papilla of Vater to enlarge the opening to the bile duct and/or pancreatic duct. This is done to improve the drainage or to remove stones in the ducts. Removed stones are usually dropped in the intestine, and pass through quickly.

- **Stenting**. A stent is a small plastic tube which is left in a blocked or narrowed duct to improve drainage. The narrowing may need to be stretched (dilated) before the stent is placed. Some stents are designed to pass out into the intestine after a few weeks when they have done their work. Other stents have to be removed or changed after 3-4 months. There are also permanent stents made out of metal.

- Other treatments are used occasionally. Your doctor will explain these if necessary.

Limitations and risks? There are some drawbacks to ERCP. Discuss these with your doctor.

- The test and treatments are not perfect. Occasionally, important lesions may not be seen, and treatment attempts may be unsuccessful.

- Working on the pancreas and bile duct can cause complications, even in the best hands. Your doctor will explain these and answer your questions. The most common complication is

  - Pancreatitis (swelling and inflammation of the pancreas). This occurs in about one patient in twenty, and results in the need to stay in hospital for pain medications and IV fluids. This usually lasts for a few days, but can be much more serious.

  Other rare complications (less than 1 per 100) include, but are not limited to:

  - Heart and lung problems
  - Bleeding (after sphincterotomy).
  - Infection in the bile duct (cholangitis).
  - Perforation (a tear in the intestine).

  These may require surgery (about one case in 500), and prolonged stays in hospital. Fatal complications are very rare.

- The sedation medicines may make you sick. A tender lump may form where the IV was placed. Call your doctor if redness, pain or swelling appears to be spreading. You will receive a low dose of radiation from the x-rays.

Alternatives? There may be some different approaches to your problem. Discuss them with your doctor.

- Diagnoses can be made often by scans, such as CT and MRCP, or a test called Endoscopic Ultrasound (EUS). ERCP is usually done only when appropriate scans have failed to provide a diagnosis, or when they have shown something that is best treated by ERCP.
- Possible alternative treatments include surgical operations, or, in some cases, interventional radiology.

Address any questions to the Pancreato-biliary office at 843 8767230.

ERCP explanation pbc May 2011

FIG 13.1 The ERCP explanation sheet given to patients at the Medical Center of South Carolina.

manage legal risk. It may be worthwhile to ask whether there are other family members who are nurses or paralegals, for example, who would appreciate a phone call. One way to illustrate and operationalize your concern is to give your cell phone number to key family members. Finally, it is important to inform the insurance carrier about any major adverse event or significantly litigious situation.

WHEN YOU ARE SUED

The statistics suggest that most endoscopists are likely to be sued sometime in their career. It is a devastating experience, despite the fact that most cases are defended successfully. The severity of adverse patient outcomes is a more important predictor of plaintiff success in winning a malpractice claim than whether the physician was indeed negligent.[48] Sympathetic juries and judges often wish to reward a plaintiff who has been severely injured.

Physicians should become educated in the litigation process.[49] Obviously, if a lawsuit is filed, the physician's insurance carrier must be notified, and it is the responsibility of the physician to aid the insurance company in the defense of the case. Excellent advice on how to navigate and survive this experience has been given recently.[50,51]

Depositions generally benefit plaintiffs and are used as tools to gain information to help press cases against defendants. During deposition, physicians should be truthful but volunteer as little information as possible. Excessive elaboration can only harm the defendant. In deposition and at trial, demeanor is important. Arrogance, anger, or dismissive behavior will only reflect poorly upon the physician and engender sympathy for the plaintiff. It is also important to be well prepared for any type of testimony. Malpractice attorneys are usually intelligent and well versed. Physicians should be similarly knowledgeable and well prepared and should be deliberate in their testimony, pausing before every answer to ensure a proper and accurate response.

EXPERT TESTIMONY

The most common method for establishing the standard of care and subsequently a breach of duty is to rely on expert testimony from medical witnesses. They should be appropriately licensed and board certified and should have been practicing actively in the medical specialty area in question. The expert should receive reasonable compensation but not one based on the outcome of the case. The opinion of the medical expert should be unbiased and nonemotive, and as such it should not matter whether the expert is retained by the plaintiff or the defendant. Expert testimony requires a review of the medical record and an opinion regarding the patient's care. Such an opinion may be given in a variety of formats, including affidavit, deposition, or even testimony in court. The expert medical witness provides an important service to patients, physician colleagues, and the courts, provided that such opinions are thoughtful, accurate, and unbiased. Stimulated by some experts who failed to reach these standards, some professional societies have provided useful guidelines for this process.[52]

There are things to consider if you are asked to be such an expert. First, is your standing sufficient to ensure that your testimony can bear peer scrutiny? Second, it is necessary to do your homework assiduously. Read the records very carefully and write notes, not least because the process may stretch over several years. These notes are discoverable and so should be factual, not judgmental. Review the relevant literature, including your own writings on the topic, because the opposing team will try to catch you in a contradiction. They will have access to your prior legal depositions, and so your opinions should be consistent. When giving sworn testimony, it is wise to be deliberate and to refrain from trying to be funny. It is fine to say, "I don't know," when appropriate.

A SUMMARY OF RECOMMENDATIONS

1. Show patients and family members that you care, at all stages of the interaction.
2. Practice within your zone of comfort, which should be determined by the extent of your training and experience.
3. Know the standard of care, based on society guidelines and the current literature.
4. Avoid marginal indications, especially younger healthy patients with pain and little or no objective abnormalities.
5. Appreciate the patients and techniques that are associated with increased risk, and the methods for minimizing the risks.
6. Carefully assess the likely risk-benefit ratio for your proposed procedure.
7. Minimize pancreatic manipulations, and use precutting only when there is definite evidence for pathology that is treatable by ERCP methods.
8. Use pancreatic duct stents for high-risk patients if appropriately trained and experienced.
9. Give preprocedure NSAID suppositories, at least for patients at increased risk of pancreatitis (with the patient's consent).
10. Inform and consent patients carefully and personally, and document the process.
11. Assure yourself that your practice is as good as you think it is by measuring it. Survey your patients.
12. Employ good documentation of clinical events and decision making.
13. Be vigilant to assure early recognition and management of complications, communicate honestly with the patient and family, and maintain contact with them throughout the postcomplication period.

CONCLUSIONS

ERCP is a complex and difficult procedure with significant risks for adverse patient outcomes and for medical litigation. It is important for endoscopists performing ERCP to understand liability issues related to ERCP, including vicarious liability, and to understand the legal principles important in medical practice, including the elements of a malpractice case, standards of care, and informed consent. The endoscopist must realize that the deviations from a reasonable standard of care most likely to lead to ERCP-related medical litigation include procedural indications, procedural technique, post-ERCP care, and issues of informed consent. With this understanding, the endoscopist performing ERCP can formulate and adopt risk management strategies to improve patient safety, satisfaction, and outcomes while minimizing the risk of litigation. These strategies include practicing within a reasonable standard of care, focusing attention on the informed consent process and documentation, and understanding specific patient-related and technique-related risk factors for complications and lawsuits.

The most important single protection is to show the patient and family that you care about them, before and after the procedures, whatever the outcome might be.

ACKNOWLEDGMENTS

This chapter is an updated version of the chapter published in the second edition of this book, which was based on the version in the first edition coauthored by Jim Frakes and me. I am indebted to James W. Saxton, Esquire, CEO of Saxton and Stump LLC, for his helpful review of the manuscript.

The complete reference list for this chapter can be found online at wwww.expertconsult.com.

14

Cannulation of the Major Papilla

Michael J. Bourke and Michael X. Ma

Despite advances in imaging and device technology over the past decade, endoscopic retrograde cholangiopancreatography (ERCP) continues to be technically challenging and subject to adverse events and procedure failure. To some extent this is accounted for by the knowledge that among the most difficult aspects of the procedure is the very first step: selective biliary cannulation (SBC). Outside of expert high-volume centers, failed biliary cannulation occurs in up to 20% of cases.[1] Repeated and prolonged attempts at cannulation increase the risk of post-ERCP pancreatitis (PEP), delay definitive therapy, and necessitate alternative therapeutic techniques with inferior safety profiles.[2–5] Recent data have also shed light on appropriate requirements for trainee competency in cannulation (see Chapter 9). As expected, trainee technical success increases with experience, and competency in biliary cannulation is usually reached only after performing 350 to 400 ERCPs, a threshold substantially higher than previous estimates.[6,7]

In any patient with a given preprocedural risk profile (based on age, sex, and indication), cannulation technique and outcome is the primary determinant of adverse events in most ERCP procedures; it is obviously important in achieving success.[5] Preceding this and not to be overlooked, the first step in optimizing outcomes and minimizing ERCP adverse events is appropriate patient selection. This is done by avoiding diagnostic ERCP and using other, less hazardous imaging modalities—such as endoscopic ultrasonography or magnetic resonance cholangiopancreatography (MRCP)—when the pretest probability of the need for intervention at ERCP is low. Careful patient selection eliminates the awkward situation that may occur when conventional cannulation techniques fail and the probability of pathology is low. Then it should be decided whether to proceed with a more aggressive and potentially more hazardous ancillary technique (e.g., precut) to achieve SBC. Suddenly the risks of continuing the procedure may dramatically outweigh the clinical benefit of technical success. Therefore all possible cannulation scenarios must be envisaged before ERCP is undertaken, and the endoscopist must be comfortable with an array of techniques. Once under way, the risk profile of the patient and the intent of the procedure must be continuously factored into the approach. In an elderly patient with jaundice caused by obstructive biliary disease and no other anatomic or patient-related risk factors, time can be spent on different conventional access techniques to achieve SBC. Conversely, in younger patients with difficult cannulation or possible sphincter of Oddi dysfunction, early and repeated access to the pancreatic duct (PD) will dictate

a change in cannulation strategy and early placement of a pancreatic stent. However, sometimes the best decision during ERCP is to stop the procedure.[8]

The philosophy underpinning successful ERCP practice is precise cannulation technique with resultant swift and efficient, preferably single or minimal pass, SBC.

ESTABLISHING THE DUODENAL POSITION

Upon reaching the top of the second part of the duodenum, two options for achieving an "en face" position are available to the endoscopist:

1. The endoscope is gently advanced for 2 to 3 cm with slight counterclockwise torque, the left-right (LR) wheel is turned right, and then with clockwise torque of the shaft and gentle upward deflection of the big wheel, the instrument is withdrawn and the endoscopist has the sense of pulling oneself beneath the papilla. This is our preferred technique, and it minimizes endoscopic insertion length and patient discomfort. Caution should be taken in cases of stenotic or relatively fixed duodenal segments as it is possible to tear the duodenal wall during endoscope withdrawal, particularly if the LR wheel is locked.
2. Alternatively, one may pass the tip beyond the papilla to the distal second part and again perform full right positioning of the LR wheel and essentially repeat the endoscope withdrawal steps outlined in 1.

For occasions with a mobile second part of the duodenum (e.g., after hepatic lobectomy) or more inferiorly located papilla, technique 2 may be the only means to achieve a satisfactory position. Initially the papilla should be positioned in the center of the monitor for inspection, but because the catheter will emerge from the lower half of the right edge of the screen image, for optimal cannulation the papilla's monitor position should generally be slightly more superior and to the right. If the video screen is divided into four equal quadrants, then generally the optimal position sees the papilla located in the left lower corner of the right upper quadrant (Fig. 14.1).

For successful SBC, the duodenoscope position should be stable and the endoscopist must feel as though the scope tip is below or at least adjacent to the papilla (i.e., the papilla is easily positioned above the horizontal midpoint of the monitor). If the endoscope is above the papilla, cannulation will be difficult. Cannulation attempts should not commence until all efforts to achieve a satisfactory position have been exhausted. Occasionally a long scope position will be

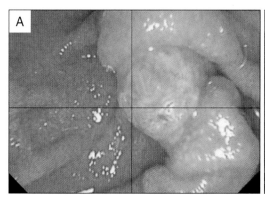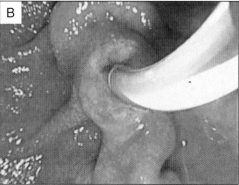

FIG 14.1 Optimal monitor position of papilla for cannulation. **A,** The papilla is not rotated on its long axis and the orifice draining bile is seen in the right lower corner of the left upper quadrant with bulge of the intramural segment seen running superiorly from this. **B,** A direct approach at 11 o'clock is appropriate.

necessary. This is achieved by pushing the instrument inferiorly with counterclockwise torque on the shaft toward the left-hand wall (as seen on the monitor). The insertion tube of the scope will bow along the greater curve of the stomach, with the tip of the endoscope dipping below the papilla, and then in approximately 80% of cases come back up adjacent to the papilla but in a more favorable infrapapillary orientation.

Movement of the up-down (UD) or large wheel will move the endoscope tip toward and away from the papilla, respectively. Small movements of the LR wheel move the endoscope above and below the papilla, with larger movements of this wheel moving the scope from side to side. The size, morphology, and orientation of the papilla; its relationship to the adjacent duodenum; and the anticipated direction of the intrapapillary and suprapapillary bile duct inform the cannulation approach. The presence of a peripapillary diverticulum may modify the approach (see section "Peripapillary Diverticulum"). The most common reason why an initially satisfactory duodenal position deteriorates is overdistension of the upper digestive tract, usually gastric. Aspirating gas and minimizing insufflation may remedy this situation, but on occasion it may be necessary to withdraw the endoscope into the stomach, remove air, and repeat the duodenal insertion phase. It is important to avoid gas insufflation during pauses in the procedure when full luminal insufflation is not necessary.

DEVICES AND EQUIPMENT FOR CANNULATION (SEE ALSO CHAPTER 4)

- Straight or angle-tipped hydrophilic guidewires: usually 0.035 inches, occasionally 0.025 or 0.021 inches; Jagwire or Dreamwire (Boston Scientific, Natick, MA), Tracer Metro and Acrobat wire (Cook Endoscopy, Winston-Salem, NC), or Visiglide wire (Olympus Corporation, Tokyo, Japan). When encountering difficult cannulation of the PD or for use through a 5-4-3 Fr cannula, a 0.018-inch platinum-tipped wire (Roadrunner; Cook Endoscopy) is useful. Many other varieties of specialty wires exist and may have particular advantages in niche situations.
- Triple-lumen sphincterotomes (STs) with 20-mm, 25-mm, or 30-mm cutting wire: CleverCut3V and CleverCut2V (Olympus Corporation); FusionOMNI with dometip, DASH ST, or Tri-Tome (Cook Endoscopy); or Autotome, Dreamtome, Hydratome, Jagtome, or TRUEtome RX (Boston Scientific, Natick, MA).
- Three-French or 5-Fr pancreatic stents: Zimmon or Geenen Sof-Flex (Cook Endoscopy), Advanix (Boston Scientific, Marlborough, MA), or Freeman-Aliperti (Hobbs Medical, Stafford Springs, CT).

- Microprocessor-controlled electrosurgical generator delivering alternating cycles of short pulse cutting with more prolonged coagulation current: ERBE VIO 300 (ERBE Elektromedizin GmbH, Tubingen, Germany) or Olympus ESG-100 (Olympus Corporation).
- Needle knives (Olympus Corporation, Cook Endoscopy, Boston Scientific).

CANNULATION TECHNIQUE

Most expert endoscopists opt to cannulate the naive papilla with an ST, given that almost all procedures are now therapeutic and, compared with a catheter, the ST orientation to the distal biliary tree is favorable and adjustable. High-quality comparative data are limited but indicate superior outcomes with an ST compared with a standard catheter.[9,10] The imprecise technique of impacting the ST into the papilla and injecting contrast should be avoided. This results in papillary trauma and often leads to PD opacification. In general, the preferred technique is to selectively insert the ST beyond the papilla and into the bile duct atraumatically. To comprehend the mechanics of biliary cannulation, a useful analogy is to imagine passing your hand up a shirt sleeve that is hanging over the back of a chair. The sleeve may be of variable length and caliber, draped over the chair at varying angles, and either floppy or more rigid. It is not possible to fix the sleeve in place, and so gentle manipulation is required and forceful manipulation with distortion of the sphincter mechanism is unlikely to be successful.

Guidewire or Contrast?

Traditional cannulation techniques relied on initial contrast opacification of the biliary tree. However, the contrast cannulation (CC) approach may result in inadvertent filling of the PD and progressive stepwise opacification of the body or tail from repeated injections to determine whether the cannulating device is in the biliary tree. The risk of PEP increases with the number of PD injections and extent of PD opacification.[3,5,11] In contrast, wire-guided cannulation (WGC) can enhance technical success while reducing the risk of PEP. A soft-tip hydrophilic guidewire may facilitate deep instrumentation of the bile duct, confirm duct selection without contrast injection, and in most cases totally avoid contrast opacification of the PD. In addition, gentle passage of the wire into the PD may not significantly increase the risk of PEP. A broad body of evidence now suggests that the wire-guided technique is the preferred approach.

A recent Cochrane systematic review and meta-analysis of 12 randomized controlled trials (RCTs) comprising 3450 patients assessed the effectiveness and safety of WGC and the conventional CC technique.[12]

The WGC technique, compared with CC, was associated with greater primary cannulation success (relative risk [RR] 1.07, 95% confidence interval [CI] 1.00 to 1.15), significantly reduced PEP (RR 0.51, 95% CI 0.32 to 0.82), less need for precut sphincterotomy (RR 0.75, 95% CI 0.60 to 0.95), and no increase in other ERCP-related adverse events. Ten studies comprising 1497 patients in the WGC technique and 1489 patients in the CC technique group were included in the main analysis for primary cannulation success rates. Significant heterogeneity among studies was noted ($p < 0.00001$, $I^2 = 83\%$). Unweighted pooled primary cannulation success rates were 83.6% for the WGC technique and 77.3% for the CC technique. The number needed to treat (NNT) was 18 (95% CI 9 to 625). In sensitivity analyses, the results remained statistically significant with both odds ratio (OR) (OR 1.50, 95% CI 1.05 to 2.14; $p = 0.03$) and a fixed-effect model (RR 1.08, 95% CI 1.04 to 1.12; $p < 0.00001$). Secondary cannulation success, defined by cannulation success after changing to the alternate technique, was reported in 4 of the 7 crossover studies comprising 100 patients in the WGC and 169 patients in the CC technique group. Unweighted pooled secondary cannulation rates were 34% after crossover to the CC technique and 49.7% after crossover to the WGC technique; however, there was no statistically significant difference in the cannulation success rates after crossover to either technique (RR 0.74, 95% CI 0.41 to 1.31; $p = 0.30$).

All 12 studies included in the main analysis reported PEP rates and included a total of 1784 patients in the WGC technique and 1666 in the CC technique group. Again, there was significant heterogeneity among the studies ($p = 0.04$, $I^2 = 45\%$). Unweighted pooled rates of PEP were 3.5% for the WGC technique and 6.7% for the CC technique. The WGC technique significantly reduced PEP compared with the CC technique based on ITT analysis (RR 0.51, 95% CI 0.32 to 0.82; $p = 0.005$) or per-protocol analysis (RR 0.51, 95% CI 0.32 to 0.83; $p = 0.007$). The NNT was 31 (95% CI 19 to 78). In sensitivity analyses, the results remained robust with either odds ratio or a fixed-effect model.

In all, the results indicate that the WGC technique significantly reduces PEP and enhances primary cannulation success. Although it is unlikely that in routine clinical practice biliary cannulation is performed with either technique in isolation, the results of the Cochrane review support use of the WGC technique as the most appropriate first-line primary cannulation technique.

Although the evidence is strong, some caveats are worth noting when interpreting the data. The significant heterogeneity among the included studies with respect to outcomes of cannulation success and PEP may be explained by differences in trial design, variability in blinding, use of prophylactic pancreatic stents, precut sphincterotomy, cannulation devices, operator experience, and involvement of trainees. Furthermore, the consensus definition of PEP developed in 1991[13] was not universally adopted, but it was used in most studies. Another potential limitation was the inclusion of five crossover studies, which may have diluted the effect of WGC for the prevention of PEP. Whether WGC is cost-effective relative to CC also remains to be proven. Nonetheless, a significant reduction in the risk of PEP with the WGC technique was found. The variability across the studies likely reflects real-world practices, and the narrow confidence intervals for the measured parameters suggest adequate precision of the results and therefore applicability to contemporary clinical practice.

At least three variations of the WGC technique exist, and their use does and should vary depending on the morphology of the papilla.[14]

1. Direct access with the ST: The ST is used to enter (drop or pop into) the biliary duct (BD) and then the wire is advanced, with its direction confirming SBC. This technique is used frequently by experienced biliary endoscopists and will swiftly succeed in more than 50% of cases. It is primarily used when the papilla is of normal size and position and a cannulation challenge is not anticipated. It may also work with a floppy papilla.

2. ST then wire: The ST is advanced 2 to 3 mm beyond the luminal aspect of the papilla in the biliary orientation and then the wire is gently advanced (either by the assistant [long wire] or by the endoscopist or the assistant [short wire]) to achieve SBC. This is useful in a floppy or mobile papilla or when technique 1 fails; this modification can be swiftly applied without withdrawing the ST. The ST can be used to straighten the intramural segment by drawing back on the impaled papilla and applying suction to encourage the papilla down onto the bowed ST.

3. Wire lead technique: The tip of the wire is positioned approximately 2 mm beyond the tip of the ST and the wire ST complex is then advanced in the biliary direction into the papilla. It may drop or pop into the BD as in technique 1, or the wire can be advanced as in technique 2 to achieve SBC. This technique is especially useful when the papilla is small and the tip of the ST is larger than the papilla. The wire acts as an introducer (Videos 14.1 and 14.2).

These techniques are all somewhat different, although they are unified by the goal of contrast-free SBC. Potentially they all have advantages and risks. For instance, a forcefully inserted guidewire may dissect intramurally within the papilla, creating a false passage. It is likely, although not yet proven, that a given technique may have advantages dependent on patient-related factors, particularly the morphology of the papilla. A large floppy papilla with a long intraduodenal segment of BD would be better suited to initial ST insertion beyond the orifice and then the intraduodenal segment straightened; SBC may subsequently occur with either wire or ST directly. Further trials of WGC more closely reporting on papillary morphology would be helpful.

Guidewire tip shape has also been postulated as a possible factor in cannulation success. Straight-tipped and angle-tipped guidewires have been used for WGC; however, there has been no clear evidence to suggest superiority of one type over the other.[15] Other tip shapes such as J-tip and loop-tip wires have also been studied in small RCTs, again without obvious benefit with respect to the success of biliary cannulation.[15,16] Comparison of wire caliber, in particular 0.025-inch with 0.035-inch wires, has not been shown to either significantly improve the success of biliary cannulation or reduce the incidence of PEP.[17–19] As such, a conventional 0.035-inch soft-tipped straight hydrophilic guidewire may be reasonably used routinely for WGC, although in select anatomic situations one of the other wires may be useful.

Avoidance of PEP is a primary objective of every ERCP procedure; however, at times it is unavoidable even in expert hands. Of paramount importance is attention to basic ERCP technique and careful attempts at cannulation. Two additional factors, pharmacologic prophylaxis and pancreatic stenting, likely also have a role in reduction of PEP risk. Overall, the available data suggest that rectal administration of nonsteroidal antiinflammatory drugs (NSAIDs) can reduce the incidence of PEP. Six meta-analyses published between 2009 and 2014 compared rectal NSAIDs versus placebo for prevention of PEP in high-risk and unselected patients.[20] All showed benefit of NSAIDs in reducing both the incidence and severity of pancreatitis, with NNT estimated to be between 11 and 17 to prevent one episode of pancreatitis. Whether rectal NSAIDs should be prescribed to all patients undergoing ERCP or reserved only for those at higher risk of PEP remains controversial. Two recent RCTs assessing outcomes from routine periprocedural administration of rectal indomethacin or placebo to consecutive average-risk patients found conflicting results with respect to prevention of PEP.[21,22] Rectal NSAIDs have also been indirectly compared with pancreatic stenting. A meta-analysis comparing rectal NSAIDs with pancreatic stenting found that rectal NSAIDs were superior for the prevention of PEP (OR 0.48, 95% CI 0.26 to 0.87).[23] Randomized controlled studies directly comparing rectal NSAIDs to pancreatic stenting, however, have not been completed, although at least one is currently under way.[24] Prevention of PEP and other adverse events of ERCP are discussed further in Chapter 8.

Papilla Assessment and Basic Technique

It is useful to ask the assistants to (quietly) prospectively record the number of separate attempts on the papilla and the total cannulation time from the first touch of the papilla. This information can aid in the decision as to when alternative or ancillary cannulation techniques should be considered or the procedure terminated. The number of attempts (and, as a corollary, total cannulation time) is an independent predictor of the risk of PEP, with the risk rising substantially after about 9 to 10 attempts (Fig. 14.2).[5,25] A cannulation attempt is defined as sustained contact between the cannulating device and the papilla for at least 5 seconds.

Once the duodenoscope is en face with the papilla, cannulation begins with careful inspection of this structure. Achieving an en face position may require adjustment of the LR or UD wheel, as the papilla may be obliquely oriented to the duodenal lumen. The location of the papillary orifice should be sought. It is usually in the 11 o'clock position,

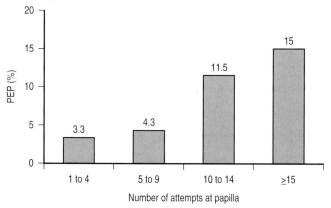

FIG 14.2 Rate of PEP according to number of attempts at cannulation of the papilla. Data derived from two prospective cannulation trials with comprehensive data collection (*n* = 732). As cannulation attempts increase, the risk of PEP escalates. *PEP,* Post-ERCP pancreatitis. (Redrawn from Bailey AA, Bourke MJ, Kaffes AJ, et al. Needle-knife sphincterotomy: factors predicting its use and the relationship with post-ERCP pancreatitis [with video]. *Gastrointest Endosc.* 2010;71:266–271.)

in the top left-hand corner of the papilla. Taking still images of the papilla and carefully evaluating the morphology before proceeding can be useful. An understanding of the three-dimensional anatomy in this area, especially the relationship of the bile duct to the PD, is important. Two particular aspects of the papilla need to be assessed:

- The face of the papilla: This can be compared with the face of a clock. As a reference point, the 12 o'clock position is aligned with the long axis of the papilla and is usually the most superior point on the face of the papilla. However, if duodenal anatomy is distorted (because of a diverticulum or neoplasm or as can be seen in older patients), the papilla may be rotated anywhere along its long axis (usually to the left), and the true 12 o'clock position may not be the most superior (cephalad) part of the papilla. In these cases, use the position of the long axis as the 12 o'clock reference point. In more than 95% of cases, the biliary orifice is located between 9 and 12 o'clock and often in the 11 o'clock position, as previously mentioned.
- The intramural segment of the BD: This is the portion of the BD located between the biliary orifice and the BD beyond the duodenal wall. It is variously referred to as the intramural, intraduodenal, or occasionally intrapapillary segment. We will use the term *intramural segment.* The BD often follows the same line as that suggested by the face of the papilla (see Fig. 14.1). However, the intramural segment may be of variable length, angulation, and rigidity and is largely dependent on the size of the papilla (Fig. 14.3). In some cases it can take a course quite different to the direction of initial ST entry into the papillary orifice (Fig. 14.4). Gentle passage of the guidewire and/or ST up the intramural segment is imperative for successful cannulation, as it is easily distorted by forceful attempts, particularly in papillae with a long intramural segment.

Taking a few moments to appreciate the anatomy of the papilla initially will greatly increase the likelihood of successful SBC. Often the first attempt has the highest chance of success as repeated contact with the papilla may result in edema and obscuration of the orifice. After careful inspection and assessment of the likely "biliary direction," cannulation should proceed generally with an ST that provides a favorable orientation to the distal BD. Note that a common mistake made by trainees is to direct the ST too horizontally (and can be recognized fluoroscopically), resulting in inadvertent cannulation of the PD or jamming against the septum. If the ST does not point in the appropriate direction, it can be "groomed" or with some devices rotated by twisting the handle. If the duodenal position of the endoscope is optimal, this should be an uncommon requirement.

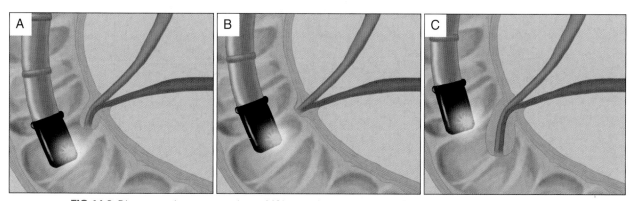

FIG 14.3 Diagrammatic representations of **(A)** normal-sized papilla and **(B)** small papilla and short intramural segment. Once the biliary sphincter is overcome, deep biliary cannulation is generally straightforward. **C,** Large and potentially floppy papilla: it may be difficult to get an en face position, achieve a good biliary orientation, or instrument the biliary tree deeply.

The ST is advanced and gently inserted into the top left corner in the 11 o'clock position. The goal is to place the tip of the ST in the superior aspect of the common channel above the septum (Fig. 14.5). If the biliary orifice can be clearly seen or if the papilla is small, it may be preferable to cannulate with the wire positioned 1 to 2 mm beyond the tip of the ST as described above (see Videos 14.1 and 14.2). Once the ST has advanced 1 or 2 mm beyond the edge of the mucosa of the papilla, the ST is bowed while opening the elevator to increase the vertical angulation and achieve a better approximation of the direction of the bile duct. Often at this moment, with some gentle pressure by moving the UD wheel downward, the ST will overcome the resistance of the sphincter and "pop" into the duct. Gently pulling back on the insertion tube of the endoscope will also help to "lift" the ST into the duct. The wire can then be gently advanced, the direction usually

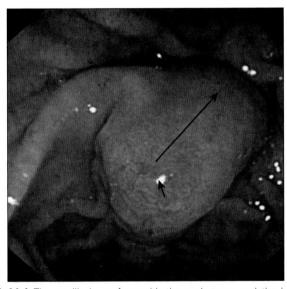

FIG 14.4 The papilla is en face with the endoscope and the biliary orifice is likely to be at 11 o'clock *(short arrow)*. However, the intramural segment *(long arrow)* runs backward to the right, and so for deep access it may be necessary to align the cannulating device with this axis once the papilla has been successfully engaged at the 11 o'clock position.

differentiating pancreatic system from biliary system. Caution is required at this point, as uncommonly PD and BD may run in parallel and the guidewire may pass out a side branch of the PD before it is apparent. Wire passage should be resistance-free. If the wire enters the pancreas, it is withdrawn into the ST while keeping the ST in place. The ST is then bowed further and very slowly withdrawn from the papilla. It is usually possible to gently move the ST back and forth (only 1 or 2 mm) without losing contact with the papilla and pick up the superior lip of the distal biliary tree, positioning the septum and PD beneath the ST. Slight adjustment of the duodenal position (LR or UD wheel) may be necessary to bring the axis of the ST in alignment with the axis of the intramural segment. The endoscopist may again have the sense that the ST has "dropped" into the common bile duct. If this occurs, then the ST tension is relaxed to relieve any distortion of the intramural segment, and the wire is once again gently advanced. If success has not been achieved after three or four attempts, it may be useful to define the anatomy by injecting a small pulse of contrast under fluoroscopic guidance. To minimize PD opacification, the authors prefer that the endoscopist, instead of the assistant, injects a small volume of full-strength contrast, which can be repeated until the anatomy of the distal segment is defined. A static radiographic image can be taken during the initial injection and the image fixed on a monitor adjacent to the active fluoroscopic image. This is then used to guide further wire cannulation attempts, including adjusting the direction of the wire to achieve the biliary direction. With this injection approach, PD opacification beyond the head of the gland is rarely encountered.

Sometimes the wire may be caught in the common channel or in the biliary sphincter (Fig. 14.6), forming a J-loop within the papilla as seen fluoroscopically. In this situation the endoscopist can slowly withdraw and then advance the ST (the ST and wire work as a single unit, with the relationship between them fixed), or the assistant or endoscopist may withdraw the wire into the ST and then readvance the wire. The aim of both techniques is to straighten the wire and reorient it to allow it to advance into the BD. Cannulation maneuvers used to select the BD and exclude the PD often distort the papilla (Fig. 14.7), potentially kinking the distal BD, and so even though the BD has been successfully cannulated, the guidewire will not advance and SBC may fail. Thus once the endoscopist has the sense that a good position has been achieved, it is useful to pull back a little on the ST, eliminating the distortion (while maintaining the preferred axis) and

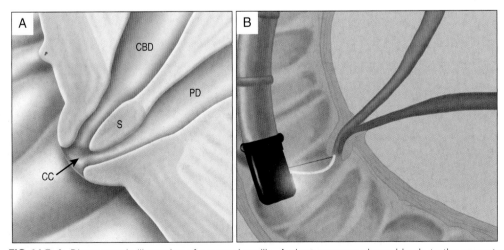

FIG 14.5 A, Diagrammatic illustration of a normal papilla. A short common channel leads to the separate ductal structures, which are separated by a short fibromuscular septum within the papilla. **B,** The sphincterotome is inserted into the tepapilla and adopted to the biliary direction. *CBD,* Common bile duct; *CC,* common channel; *PD,* pancreatic duct; *S,* septum.

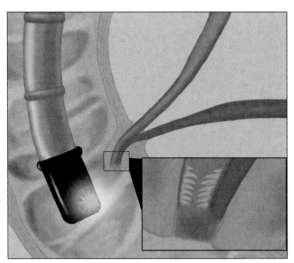

FIG 14.6 Schematic representation of the biliary sphincter mechanism that may entrap the tip of a guidewire.

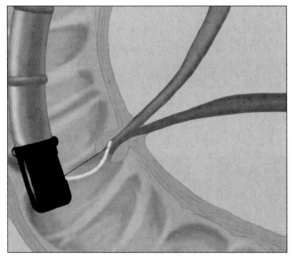

FIG 14.7 Selection of the biliary direction distorts the papilla. Once the bile duct has been selected, the distortion must be relieved to deeply instrument the duct.

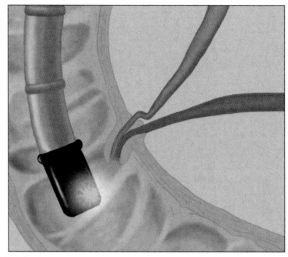

FIG 14.8 The bile duct takes an acute inferior angle upon crossing the duodenal wall before assuming the usual cephalad projection. Approximately 20% to 30% of bile ducts have this configuration. Once the catheter reaches this point, it may be helpful to temporarily pull the endoscope above the papilla to achieve a more favorable orientation to gain deep access.

reducing the tension on the papilla, and often the wire will easily advance into the BD. Sometimes a change in scope position may help, either pushing a little deeper or sometimes pulling back above the papilla, as possibly the ST is impacted superiorly in the intramural segment (see Fig. 14.7), or the BD may take an acute inferior angle (dip) where it transgresses the duodenal wall (Fig. 14.8). The general principle is to consider the sleeve analogy and the shape of the papilla, encourage the intramural segment to straighten, and minimize distortion.

If a skilled endoscopist has not achieved biliary cannulation after 5 minutes or more than 10 attempts at the papilla, success without an alternative strategy is unlikely (see section "Difficult Cannulation").[5,8]

Small Papilla

When the papilla is small, selective cannulation can be difficult and the 4-Fr to 5-Fr tip of the ST may be larger than the papilla itself. A wire lead cannulation technique can be very helpful in this situation. The wire is positioned 1 to 3 mm beyond the tip of the ST and, working with the wire ST complex as a single entity, the cannulation is undertaken

as described above. Sometimes an ultratapered cannula, such as 5-4-3 Fr, will enter an orifice resistant to guidewire cannulation.

Periampullary Diverticulum

If a periampullary diverticulum is present, the papilla is usually located on the lower rim of the diverticulum or just inside and generally somewhere between 4 and 8 o'clock when the diverticulum is viewed as a clock face. In approximately 10% of cases, the papilla may be buried within the diverticulum and make access difficult (Fig. 14.9). The intramural segment can often be readily visualized within the diverticulum beyond the papillary orifice (Fig. 14.10). This serves as a useful guide to determine the biliary direction and is also helpful to guide the direction of the sphincterotomy, if required. In contrast to the usual papillary anatomy, when there is a periampullary diverticulum, the biliary direction is often not as acutely angulated superiorly, but runs initially more directly horizontally (Fig. 14.11). Thus it is not necessary to angulate the guidewire or ST as acutely upward, and on occasion a standard catheter may be preferable for cannulation. Once a good position in relation to the papilla has been obtained, achieving SBC is generally quite easy, with the biliary sphincter seemingly more easily overcome than a conventional papilla. Cannulation should proceed in the usual manner; however, because of anatomic distortion from the diverticulum, the location of the BD and PD orifices may be aberrant rather than at the conventional 11 and 5 o'clock positions (although the relationship between the two ducts is usually preserved), and this should be borne in mind (Fig. 14.12). For a papilla situated deep inside a diverticulum or pointing in an unusual direction, special techniques may be required:

1. Often only the PD can be entered; however, a guidewire placed into the PD or pancreatic stent placement can be used to evert the papilla into the duodenal lumen, followed by ancillary cannulation techniques as described below (Fig. 14.13).[8,26]
2. Alternatively, one may evert the edge of the diverticulum by placing traction outside the edge with the ST and swiftly cannulating (Fig. 14.14). One may also use one cannula to hold the papilla in position and cannulate with a second cannula. Rarely, placement of a clip next to the diverticulum to retract the papilla into a suitable duodenal

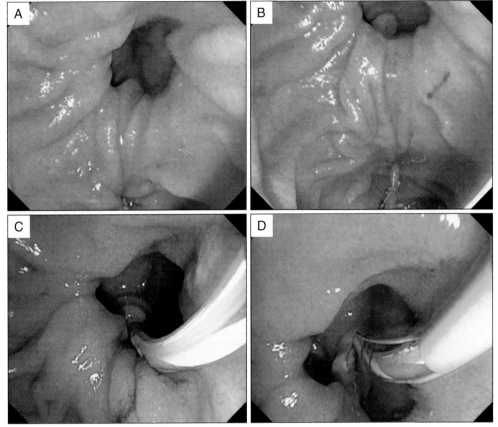

FIG 14.9 Papilla located deep within a diverticulum. **A** and **B,** The orifice is visible only just after downward traction of the infrapapillary mucosa using sphincterotome. **C,** Cannulation is completed after being exposed by the sphincterotome, followed by **(D)** sphincterotomy.

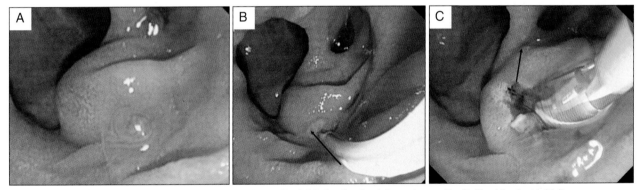

FIG 14.10 **A,** The intramural segment is readily visible leading back from the papilla. **B,** The bile duct initially takes a more horizontal course along the base of the diverticulum *(arrow).* **C,** It will be quite safe to cut along this line *(arrow).*

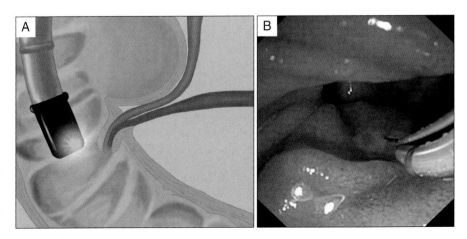

FIG 14.11 In the presence of a periampullary diverticulum, the bile duct is often not as acutely angulated superiorly, but runs initially more directly horizontally. A more horizontal approach is appropriate.

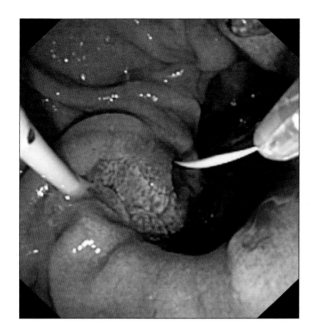

FIG 14.12 The papilla is located on the inside rim of a diverticulum and is rotated more than 90 degrees on its long axis because of the distortion of the usual anatomy created by the diverticulum.

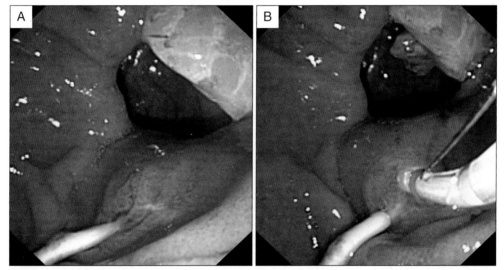

FIG 14.13 The papilla is located within a diverticulum. It has been everted by a pancreatic duct stent and then the bile duct can be cannulated above the stent.

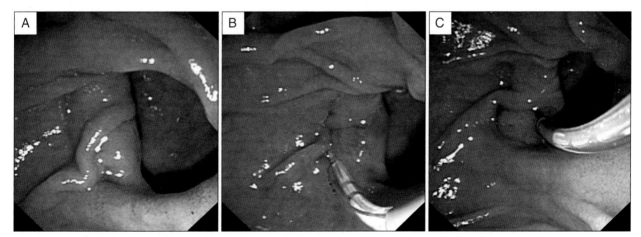

FIG 14.14 The papilla is located on the inside rim of a diverticulum. It is everted into the duodenal lumen by pushing on its outermost side and then swiftly cannulated.

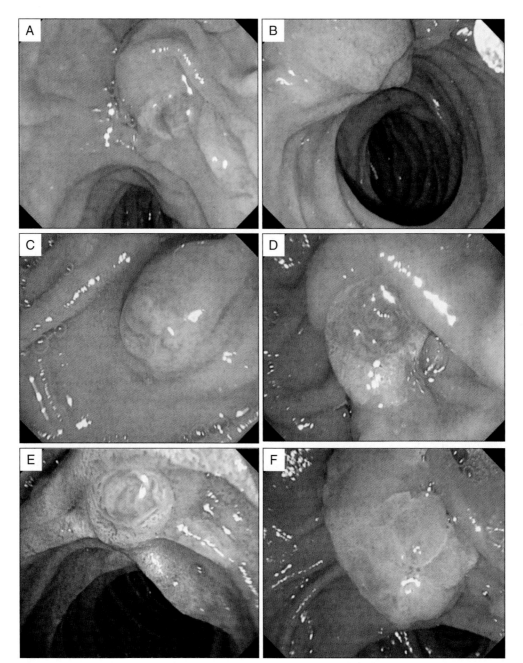

FIG 14.15 Images of different papilla morphologies and suggested approaches to cannulation. **A,** Floppy papilla/long intramural segment. Cannulation may be aided by aligning the sphincterotome with the direction of the intramural BD, placing the tip just within the orifice and advancing gently with the wire, thereby avoiding distortion of the papilla. **B,** Downward facing papilla. A long scope position may be helpful in achieving an en face view of the papilla. **C,** Left ward-facing papilla. Once the tip is placed in the orifice, align the sphincterotome with the intramural segment and gently advance with the wire. **D,** Papilla with protruding septum. The wire lead technique (see section "Repeated Cannulation of the Pancreatic Duct Without Biliary Access"), with wire placed in the 11 o'clock direction above the protruding septal tissue followed by advancing the wire/sphincterotome complex, may assist in selecting the BD. **E,** Papilla without a clear orifice. The orifice is most often in the 11 o'clock position in the left upper corner of the papilla. **F,** Papillary adenoma. Careful inspection to assess location of biliary orifice is required, and it may be in a more central position than expected because of spread of the adenoma. The tissue is friable and repeated attempts will cause bleeding, obscuring the orifice further. *BD,* Biliary duct.

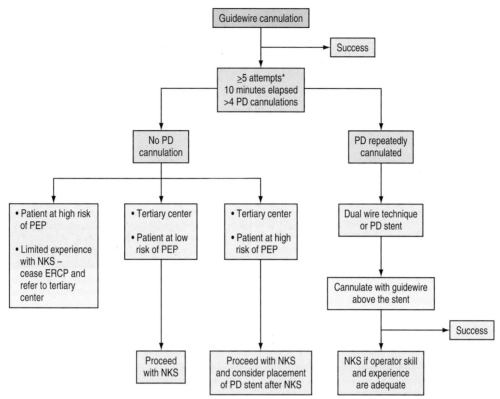

FIG 14.16 Algorithm for selective biliary cannulation during ERCP. *The number of attempts will vary depending on patient risk for PEP and operator experience. Placement of PD stent preferred to double-wire technique. *NKS,* Needle-knife sphincterotomy; *PD,* pancreatic duct; *PEP,* post-ERCP pancreatitis.

orientation may be useful. With large-mouthed diverticula, it may be possible to place the tip of the endoscope within the diverticulum and achieve an en face position. Care should be taken when maneuvering the scope in these circumstances to avoid perforation of the diverticulum.

Fig. 14.15 shows images of papillae with different morphologies and respective suggestions for cannulation.

DIFFICULT CANNULATION

The term *difficult cannulation* applies to a situation in which the papilla can be reached and positioned for cannulation but SBC proves to be a challenge. A consensus definition has not yet been agreed to, but all experienced biliary endoscopists are familiar with it, as it occurs in approximately 10% of routine procedures. Usually there is no obvious cause. A definition of difficult cannulation should take into account the time elapsed since the first touch of the papilla, the number of attempts on the papilla, and the number of inadvertent PD injections or wire cannulations. Based on the literature, 10 minutes, 5 attempts, and 4 PD cannulations are reasonable parameters.[14,20] Once one of the parameters is exceeded, then in general it is increasingly unlikely that a given technique, whether wire-guided or contrast-based, will succeed.[5] As time elapses, repeated attempts on the papilla enhance the risk of PEP and complete failure is imminent. All ERCP endoscopists must have a general strategy to both recognize and deal with this scenario. This may include simply stopping the procedure.[8] If the PD has been repeatedly instrumented, then placing a short PD stent to facilitate drainage before withdrawing the endoscope should be considered. Fig. 14.16 provides an overview of a useful cannulation algorithm.

Repeated Cannulation of the Pancreatic Duct Without Biliary Access

If the PD is repeatedly instrumented without selective biliary access being achieved, then alternative cannulation strategies should be considered. The decision to change strategy is best made early, particularly in patients at high risk of PEP (e.g., after four instrumentations of the PD), before the papilla is repeatedly traumatized and the pancreas extensively opacified. Repeated failed attempts at SBC and extensive PD opacification increase the risk of PEP.[2,11,20] Two strategies are preferred, and these may occur in sequence; both require the eventual placement of a PD stent. Placement of a PD stent in difficult cannulation reduces the risk of PEP.[27,28]

1. Dual wire (also termed *pancreatic wire*) technique: In an atraumatic fashion, a hydrophilic wire is placed into the PD to the distal body, if possible. The wire may have a manufacturer's preformed curve (J-tip) or be groomed as such by the endoscopist acutely angulating (fracturing) the soft hydrophilic portion 1 cm from the end. It may also be possible to create the loop within the PD by gently buckling the wire; care should be taken to avoid deep passage into a side branch. Having a J configuration to the leading edge of the guidewire facilitates easy passage beyond the genu and avoids side branch impaction, which can injure the pancreas. Once the wire is deeply anchored within the PD, it will often "straighten" the intramural segment of the bile duct. Using the shirt sleeve analogy, one can imagine that the distal portion of the sleeve is now more rigid and thus easier to pass a cannulation device through and beyond. The technique may also be used to position the face of the papilla more favorably, for example, if within a diverticulum. Leaving the wire in situ, the ST with an additional wire within it is then passed down

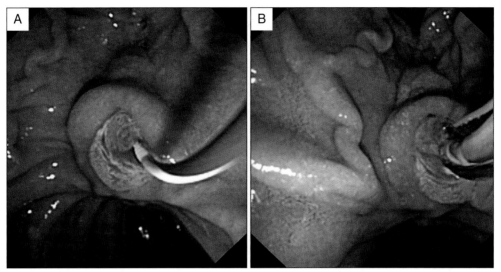

FIG 14.17 A wire is first placed into the pancreatic duct, and then the bile duct is cannulated with a wire lead technique or with the sphincterotome.

the working channel of the duodenoscope (a 4.2-mm channel is required for 0.035-inch wires). The ST is advanced until it is just in front of the papilla. It is bowed to approximate the biliary direction, and the hydrophilic guidewire is advanced in an 11 o'clock orientation to the pancreatic wire, which is at 5 o'clock (Fig. 14.17). One can either work with the ST and wire complex as a single unit, with the endoscopist directing the ST, or the assistant or endoscopist may advance the wire. In patients with small or tortuous PDs or an ansa loop, passing a wire to the tail can be impossible or at least highly traumatic. In those situations, use of a 0.018-inch or 0.021-inch guidewire with a J-tip can allow a knuckle to be created in the distal 2 to 3 cm of the PD and a sufficiently stable position for biliary access and eventual pancreatic stent placement.

2. Pancreatic stent placement with wire cannulation of the bile duct above the stent or needle-knife sphincterotomy (NKS) over the stent: If the above strategy does not work after 2 or 3 attempts, consider placing a short (2-cm to 5-cm) 5-Fr pancreatic stent (Zimmon or Geenen Sof-Flex stent; Cook Endoscopy) with the proximal tip of the stent not beyond the genu. Straight stents made of softer material are now available and may reduce the risk of duct injury. Three-French stents require a 0.018-inch or 0.021-inch guidewire and need to be positioned beyond the genu to avoid early migration. To minimize the risk of permanent duct injury, 5-Fr stents generally should not be passed beyond the genu. Spontaneous passage of the stent should be confirmed by a plain radiograph within 2 weeks. A convenient approach is to schedule the patient to undergo the radiography after a 6-hour fast so that same-day stent removal can be performed, if needed.

Once the stent is in situ, the pancreatic wire is withdrawn and a further attempt to cannulate above the pancreatic stent with the ST wire complex is made by a wire lead technique. This can be done by placing the inferior aspect of the tip of the ST on the top of the pancreatic stent and pushing down while orienting toward the 11 o'clock direction (Fig. 14.18). The ST is then bowed slightly to approximate the biliary direction, and either the wire may be gently advanced or, by pulling back slightly on the shaft of the endoscope, the ST may be "lifted" into the BD. If this fails, an NKS over the pancreatic stent may then be considered by appropriately trained and experienced biliary endoscopists. Alternatively, the procedure could be terminated, with a further attempt on another day or subsequent referral to a high-volume tertiary center. If an

appropriately skilled and experienced endoscopist has performed an adequate and appropriately directed NKS (see section "Needle-Knife Sphincterotomy"), then success will usually follow if the procedure is repeated after a few days. It is best to wait more than 48 hours to allow edema to resolve. Cannulation success rate after tertiary referral for all Schutz grades is 95% to 100%.[29,30]

Early use of the double-guide-wire technique (DGT) was assessed in a prospective multicenter RCT in 274 patients, finding no improvement in facilitation of SBC (RR 1.01, 95% CI 0.07 to 1.05, $p = 1.00$) or reduction in PEP (RR 1.17, 95% CI 0.71 to 1.94, $p = 0.53$) compared with repeated use of a single-wire technique.[31] Wire-guided cannulation over a pancreatic stent (WGC-PS) versus DGT in patients with difficult biliary cannulation was also compared in a recent retrospective study.[32] Successful cannulation was similar in both groups (WGC-PS 60/90 patients [66.7%] and DGT 61/87 patients [70.1%], $p = 0.632$), suggesting that both techniques may be equally effective as primary methods. The 26 patients with unsuccessful SBC using DGT followed on to receive WGC-PS, of which 14 cases were successful, with an overall reduction in need for a needle-knife (NK) precut technique. An overall lower rate of pancreatitis was recorded with WGC-PS than DGT (3.3% vs 10.3%, respectively), but this did not achieve statistical significance ($p = 0.077$). Overall these results support our preferred approach of placing a short 5-Fr pancreatic stent after repeated cannulation of the PD, in order to achieve SBC as well as aid PD drainage to lower the risk of PEP.

NEEDLE-KNIFE SPHINCTEROTOMY (SEE ALSO CHAPTER 15)

Needle-knife sphincterotomy (NKS) or precut (access) sphincterotomy is an advanced technique that divides the mucosa and submucosa of the papilla overlying the bile duct with the aim of exposing the biliary orifice. When performed by experienced endoscopists, it is an important and safe salvage technique to secure biliary access. An earlier four-center RCT provided the first contemporary evidence to support the use of early NK in difficult biliary cannulation.[33] In this study, patients were randomized to "early precut" by fistulotomy or "late access" after unsuccessful SBC by WGC for 10 minutes or 5 PD injections. In the late access group, a further 10 minutes of cannulation attempts continued. If SBC had still not been achieved, the endoscopist could choose whether

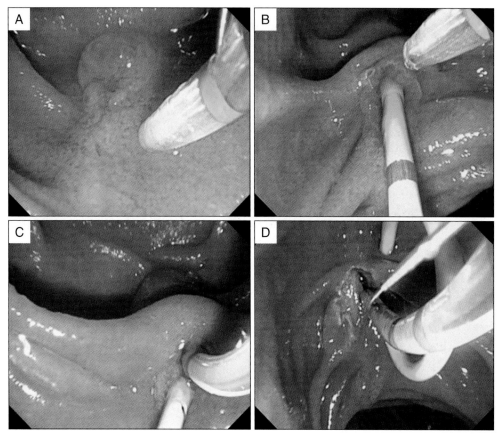

FIG 14.18 A minute papillary orifice has been cannulated and a 5-Fr pancreatic stent placed. The sphincterotome is then used to cannulate above the stent in the biliary direction.

to perform NKS or continue as before. The overall success of SBC was 85% after a single ERCP and 94% after a second procedure. PEP incidence was also markedly reduced, with early NKS at 2.6% versus 14.9% with late access ($p = 0.008$, OR 1.8, 95% CI 1.38 to 1.48). This was supported by results from a prospective RCT comparing early NKS with continued standard techniques for difficult cannulation, showing failure of early cannulation as a risk factor of PEP and that early use of NKS did not increase the risk of PEP.[34] The data were confirmed by a subsequent meta-analysis including studies by Manes et al.[33] and Swan et al.[34], along with three other RCTs comprising a total of 523 participants, showing that early NKS for difficult biliary access was associated with increased odds for primary cannulation success (RR 1.32, 95% CI 1.04 to 1.68). The overall incidence of PEP did not differ significantly between the early NKS and standard technique groups. However, subgroup analysis of studies involving only fully qualified biliary endoscopists (not fellows) showed significant reduction in PEP risk among patients receiving early NKS compared with standard technique (RR 0.29, 95% CI 0.10 to 0.86).[35] Although there are some methodological problems with some individual RCTs in the meta-analysis, the current evidence suggests that in experienced hands, early NKS may ameliorate the frequency and possibly the severity of PEP and enhance success. A caveat is that the technique must be undertaken only by an appropriately trained and experienced endoscopist.[36]

NKS Technique

The active or cutting segment of the NK should be no longer than 3 mm. Various knives have mechanisms that allow one to fix the amount of wire that extends beyond the catheter, although even if fixed this can still vary considerably with the action of the elevator compressing the catheter. It is therefore preferable that the maximal extension of the cutting wire beyond the catheter of the NK is limited to 2 to 3 mm (depending on the size of the papilla), so the tip of the NK catheter can be rested against the superior aspect of the papillary orifice so that the depth of the cut is easily controlled. The benefits of the pancreatic stent are threefold: protecting the pancreatic orifice during NKS, straightening the intramural segment to facilitate the cut, and optimizing biliary localization after completion of the NKS. The stent is usually at a 5 o'clock orientation to the biliary orifice. The cut is commenced at the top of the papillary orifice in the 12 o'clock position and extended upward in the 12 o'clock direction along the long axis of the papilla in 2-mm increments using short pulses of cutting current. The goal is to completely divide the majority of the papillary mound in a controlled, stepwise fashion in a single pass without excessive thermal injury. This technique unroofs the biliary orifice, rather than purposefully cutting into the distal bile duct, although this occasionally happens (Videos 14.3 and 14.4). Once the papilla is divided, the cleanly cut edges are then pushed back with the catheter of the NKS. The biliary orifice is usually seen as a small red dot or nipplelike structure, usually with the pancreatic stent in the 5 o'clock orientation to this (Fig. 14.19). Careful inspection while applying suction via the endoscope may allow bile flow to be seen, further aiding localization (Fig. 14.20). The bile duct can then be selectively cannulated with a guidewire passed through the ST (leading with the wire) or a 5-4-3 Fr cannula. If using the ST technique, then the wire and ST work as one, as in small papilla cannulation. Leading with the wire is important because a soft hydrophilic wire, if used carefully, will not dissect the divided tissue plains where a false passage can easily be created. In contrast, the blunt end of a catheter is often larger than the exposed biliary orifice and may traumatize

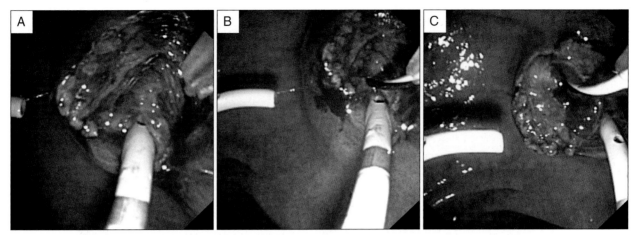

FIG 14.19 A needle-knife cut has been performed. Note the clean edges of the cut, which are then pushed back to reveal the biliary orifice appearing as a red punctum above the pancreatic stent **(A** and **B)**. The sphincterotomy is then completed in the conventional manner.

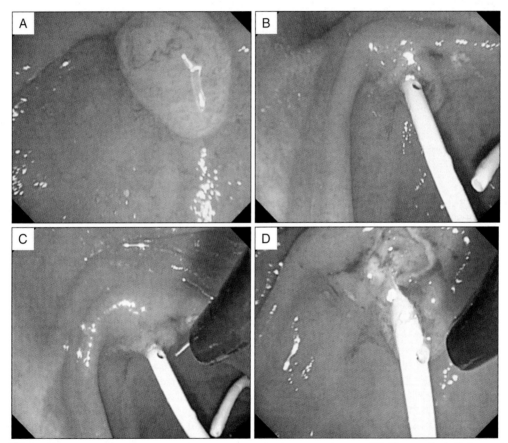

FIG 14.20 A naïve papilla **(A)** with a 5-Fr single-pigtail plastic pancreatic stent **(B)**. The needle knife is used to gain biliary access **(C)**. After papillotomy **(D)**, the biliary orifice is not obviously apparent; however, using the pancreatic stent as a guide to look for the orifice, one can see a small amount of bile draining from the 11 o'clock position just above the stent.

the exposed tissue plains. Blindly probing with a catheter or wire is not recommended; the latest generation of duodenoscopes has excellent imaging capability and the various structures can usually be identified and targeted with precision. SBC success is confirmed by resistance-free passage of the wire up toward the liver. The ST or catheter can then follow over the wire and the BD can be opacified. In general, it is preferable to avoid injection to define the anatomy when the catheter is still quite distal, as there is a significant risk of intramural extravasation within the divided tissue plains after NKS. After successful cannulation, the sphincterotomy should be completed in the conventional manner (Fig. 14.21). The pancreatic stent needs to be left in place for at least 72 hours and not be removed immediately.

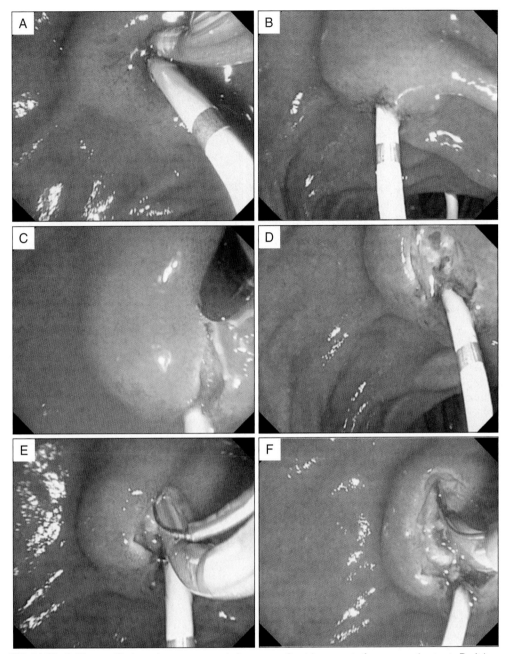

FIG 14.21 A, The papilla is resistant to cannulation even after placement of a pancreatic stent. **B,** A long intramural segment ideal for needle-knife technique. **C** and **D,** A needle-knife sphincterotomy is performed, exposing the biliary orifice, visible as a red punctum above the pancreatic stent, at the apex of the cut. **E** and **F,** Deep biliary cannulation is achieved and the sphincterotomy is completed.

CANNULATION OF THE PANCREATIC DUCT

Again considering the papilla as the face of a clock, the pancreatic orifice is located in the lower right quadrant and generally in the 5 o'clock position (see Fig. 14.5). In contrast to cannulation of the BD, cannulation of the ventral PD (duct of Wirsung) is usually performed in a short scope position with the endoscope level with or slightly above the papilla and slightly to the left. The catheter is oriented in a horizontal direction rather than upward.

Gentle atraumatic guidewire cannulation is preferable to the contrast injection method, as once success has been achieved, it confers the opportunity for a single slow continuous injection to achieve a complete pancreatogram. The resultant duct image is of superior quality (with minimal extravasated luminal contrast or unintentional side branch filling) and there is less hydrostatic distension of the PD from the single controlled injection and thus a lower risk of PEP. As a general rule, to reduce the risk of PEP, the number of attempts, the number of separate injections, and the total volume injected should be minimized.[37] Smaller-diameter guidewires (0.025 inches or smaller) are potentially useful for a PD that is resistant to 0.035-inch wire access. In patients who have undergone a complete biliary sphincterotomy, the pancreatic orifice is often readily identified as a separate opening on the right side of the divided papilla and inferior to the BD orifice. It can be located anywhere

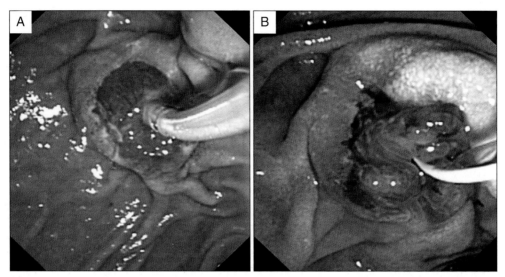

FIG 14.22 A, After biliary sphincterotomy, the pancreatic orifice can usually be found on the right edge of the divided papilla. **B,** If residual papillary structures such as mucosal fronds are present, they are often within the confines of these remnants.

along this right edge but generally is at the midpoint. It may be useful to look for residual papillary structures such as mucosal fronds, as the pancreatic orifice is often within the confines of these remnants (Fig. 14.22). Although most commonly used to facilitate cannulation of the minor papilla in patients with pancreas divisum, intravenous secretin can assist in localization and cannulation of the main PD as well.[37]

QUALITY AND ENHANCING OUTCOMES (SEE ALSO CHAPTER 12)

The challenge for all pancreaticobiliary services and their endoscopists is to provide the safest, most effective ERCP service possible. High-quality cannulation technique is the cornerstone upon which sound clinical practice is built. Agreed-upon cannulation protocols will serve as a useful baseline for building quality and safety initiatives. This framework can be modified in the context of the department's case mix, the skills of the proceduralists and assistants, and the other resources available. A high-volume, well-resourced tertiary referral center may appropriately undertake more aggressive and exhaustive cannulation procedures that would not be proper in a community hospital.

Prospective data collection, including cannulation parameters with scheduled clinical follow-up to identify and log adverse events, completes the feedback loop. Application of audit cycle methodology with regular morbidity analysis meetings can then be done to assess and interpret clinical results. With a thorough understanding of the entire procedure and its clinical consequences on both an individual and departmental level, incremental gains in safety and quality will be realized.

The complete reference list for this chapter can be found online at www.experconsult.com.

15

Access (Precut) Papillotomy

Sujievvan Chandran, Gary May, and Paul Kortan

The first and often most important step in endoscopic retrograde cholangiopancreatography (ERCP) is successful deep cannulation of the desired duct, most commonly the common bile duct (CBD). Although it remains the first step, cannulation of the CBD can be challenging even for the most experienced endoscopists. Yet obtaining deep access to the CBD is essential in order to undertake any diagnostic or therapeutic intervention. The need for diagnostic ERCP has become limited by improvements in computed tomography (CT) imaging and with the advent of magnetic resonance cholangiopancreatography (MRCP) and endoscopic ultrasonography (EUS), all of which can accurately identify and localize pancreaticobiliary pathology. This has limited diagnostic ERCP to assessment of sphincter of Oddi dysfunction (SOD) with manometry, tissue sampling from biliary or pancreatic lesions, and diagnostic cholangioscopy/pancreatoscopy, all of which require deep access to the duct in question.

Successful cannulation rates range between 90% and 95% in expert hands.[1] Failure to achieve deep biliary access therefore occurs in 5% to 10% of cases.[1] In instances of initial failure to gain deep biliary access, an alternative technique is required. The use of a needle-knife sphincterotome to undertake precut sphincterotomy was first described by Siegel in 1980.[2] Although the term *access papillotomy* more accurately describes the various techniques, we will use the more popularized term "precut" papillotomy in this chapter. This technique remains a challenge for many endoscopists and is often reserved for "experts," as it is often considered to be complex and associated with an escalation in the risk related to ERCP. Performing a precut is often an unplanned intervention, unlike traditional biliary sphincterotomy. Thus it is vital to understand the appropriate use and timing of precut.

This chapter focuses on techniques, accessories, outcomes, and adverse events of precut sphincterotomy. We will discuss the indications, contraindications, and evidence that support our recommendations. This chapter will not discuss the use of needle-knife sphincterotomy over a stent in special situations such as Billroth II anatomy or pancreas divisum, as this is covered in Chapters 21 and 31.

INDICATION FOR PRECUT PAPILLOTOMY

Biliary cannulation is one of the key components of ERCP (see Chapter 14), with success related to factors that include patient anatomy, endoscopist experience, and the availability of alternative accessory devices and alternative access techniques, such as percutaneous and EUS-guided approaches (see Chapter 32). Initial failure can occur even in the most experienced hands, and it is in these situations that alternative approaches are required. Precut papillotomy encompasses a variety of techniques, often reserved for the experienced endoscopist as a last resort, given the concerns about its risk profile as an independent risk factor for

Video for this chapter can be found online at www.expertconsult.com.

post-ERCP pancreatitis (PEP) in early studies.[3] However, when repeated instrumentation of the pancreatic duct occurs during attempted selective biliary cannulation, precut must be considered. It is important to change one's approach to cannulation rather than persisting with the same technique and/or accessory. Increasingly the recent literature points to the early adoption of an alternative technique that has not been shown to increase the risk of adverse events.[4] Early adoption of an alternative approach should be undertaken before traumatizing the ampulla and repeatedly passing guidewires and/or injecting contrast into the pancreatic duct. Before deciding to perform precut, two alternative techniques may be considered. It is our practice that if the pancreatic duct is selectively cannulated with a guidewire, a double-guidewire approach (DGT) is used, whereby a guidewire is advanced into the pancreatic duct and the catheter withdrawn. The sphincterotome or cannula preloaded with a second guidewire is advanced alongside the indwelling pancreatic duct wire to cannulate the bile duct. The pancreatic duct wire straightens the intraampullary portion of the distal bile duct to allow successful cannulation. If the DGT approach fails after several attempts, a small-caliber (3 or 5 Fr) pancreatic stent is placed and additional attempts to cannulate the bile duct above the stent are made. If deep cannulation is still not achieved, a precut papillotomy is performed.

The decision to proceed with a precut when standard techniques fail depends on several factors, which include the indication for ERCP, the expertise of the endoscopist, and the availability of alternative options for gaining biliary access (e.g., interventional radiology, EUS techniques). Marked variation exists in use of precut sphincterotomy, with reported rates between 1% and 38% of cases.[5,6] The initial success rates of precut sphincterotomy in the setting of difficult cannulation range from 70% to 90%, and the rates of cannulation at subsequent ERCP are nearly 100%.[5,6]

Alternative approaches after failed cannulation with standard techniques include stopping the procedure and reattempting cannulation at another session by the same endoscopist, or referring the patient to another, more experienced endoscopist at the same or a different center. Techniques such as percutaneous and EUS rendezvous techniques are alternatives for achieving deep biliary cannulation. However, in most situations in which standard biliary cannulation techniques have failed, a precut papillotomy is attempted before considering these alternative techniques. It is important that the endoscopist attempting a precut is experienced and comfortable with the technique. If not, it is best to abort the procedure and explore other options for gaining access (Box 15.1).

PRECUT ACCESSORIES

It is vital that appropriate equipment to perform a precut papillotomy is available for all ERCP procedures. The most commonly used accessory is the needle-knife sphincterotome. The key design feature is the retractable electrosurgical wire, which is controlled through the catheter handle. The wire is projected forward from the distal aspect of the catheter tip and its length can be adjusted. The wire is used to create an incision in the overlying mucosa via electrosurgical current and movement of the catheter via the elevator and/or the big wheel of the endoscope, which controls tip deflection. Needle-knife sphincterotomes are available in variable tip lengths (4 to 7 mm) and wire diameters and can be single, double, or triple lumen. The advantage of a double-lumen or triple-lumen configuration is that it allows a guidewire to be preloaded in the catheter to enable gentle wire probing of the incised area without having to exchange instruments. An insulated-tip needle knife designed to protect the papillary orifice also exists and has been found to be equivalent in terms of efficacy and safety to the more commonly used catheter; however, it is not yet widely available.[7] Another type of precut papillotome is the Erlangen-type sphincterotome, which has similarities to the standard traction sphincterotome. It has an ultrashort 5-mm-long monofilament cutting wire and a less-than-1-mm catheter tip distal to the wire.[8]

During precut, soft-tipped hydrophilic guidewires are essential to facilitating cannulation. We recommend the use of electrosurgical units with pulsed modes, which have a microprocessor-controlled generator in which the cutting and coagulation currents alternate and are automatically adjusted according to tissue resistance.[9] This allows for stepwise cutting and precise control of the incision direction, depth, and length. A 20-mL syringe filled with 1:20,000 epinephrine concentration can be used to irrigate the incision site through the wire or contrast port if bleeding occurs and obscures visualization.

TECHNIQUES

The principle of precut sphincterotomy to gain deep cannulation is to unroof the duodenal portion of the ampulla, thereby exposing the biliary orifice. In contrast, the purpose of traditional biliary sphincterotomy is to widen the biliary orifice for therapeutic purposes, such as stone extraction and stent placement. The precut was designed purely for biliary and occasionally pancreatic access (Box 15.2).

Before undertaking a precut sphincterotomy, it is vital that the three-dimensional anatomy of the ampullae of Vater is understood. The terminal portion of both the biliary and pancreatic ducts tapers before entering the medial wall of the duodenum. The ampullary segment itself consists of the pancreatic, biliary, and ampullary sphincters that envelop the tapering biliary and pancreatic ducts in order to control the flow of their secretions. The duodenal mucosa and submucosa overlay this ampullary segment. There are several anatomic variations of how the terminal portions of the biliary and pancreatic duct enter the medial duodenal wall. Most commonly, the ducts join to form a

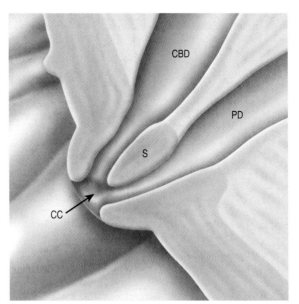

FIG 15.1 Papilla. *CBD,* Common bile duct; *CC,* common channel; *PD,* pancreatic duct; *S,* septum.

common channel of approximately 5 mm in length before entering the duodenum. In the majority of patients, the pancreatic duct enters the ampulla in a straight fashion at the 1 o'clock position, resulting in straightforward cannulation (Fig. 15.1). The bile duct runs more superficially and parallel to the duodenal wall, where it enters the ampullae at the 11 to 12 o'clock position. As the precut technique involves freehand cutting, it is imperative to understand this three-dimensional anatomy (Box 15.3).

Needle Knife From the Orifice

The most widely practiced precut method is the freehand needle-knife technique, in which the incision is made starting at the orifice and extending upward to the roof of the papilla (Fig. 15.2; Cases 15.1 and 15.2). Initially, a "sham" precut is performed with the needle retracted. A few practice maneuvers are performed to ensure that the incision will be performed in the intended direction (similar to practice swings in golf before striking the ball). The direction of the cut is the most critical aspect of the procedure and determines its success or failure.[10] Originally the technique was described by using an upward motion with the elevator.[11] It has been suggested by Howell that improved control and safety can be achieved by "loading" the needle knife through upward traction of the endoscope reference: Desilets DJ, Howell DA. Precut sphincterotomy: another perspective on efficacy and complications. Available at: www.uptodateonline. com. Accessed 11-1-2004. The length of the fully exposed needle is 4 to 7 mm, but we usually expose only 2 to 3 mm of the cutting wire. The tip of the needle is positioned at the upper lip or rim of the papillary orifice, current is applied, and a 2-mm to 5-mm incision is made on the papillary bulge. The length and depth of the incision depend on the size and configuration of the papilla and the length of the intraduodenal segment. We recommend that the incision be made in short increments, with repeated gentle strokes opening the papilla gradually, layer by layer.[10,11] When current is applied, the needle should be in continuous motion to avoid deeper thermal damage. Once the mucosa is separated, the mucosal edges should be pushed aside with the catheter to expose the sphincter muscle. Gentle suction often amplifies the sphincter and may promote bile drainage. The site is carefully examined, looking for nodularity of biliary epithelium, which usually appears as a pink or brownish nodule. The area is gently probed with the precut catheter and/or guidewire while the needle is retracted. It is very important that the incision is probed gently without contrast injection unless deep cannulation has been achieved endoscopically or

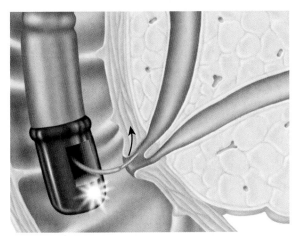

FIG 15.2 Needle-knife precut from the orifice.

fluoroscopically, because submucosal injection can compromise further cannulation attempts. We prefer to explore the precut site with a hydrophilic-tipped guidewire. Once deep access has been achieved, the sphincterotomy can be completed by changing to a standard sphincterotome. If cannulation is still not successful and the patient is stable, the procedure is aborted and a repeat attempt can be made 48 to 72 hours later. By that time the edema has subsided, and the biliary orifice is easily identified. The success rate for repeat attempts ranges from 80% to 100%.[12] However, depending on the clinical situation and especially if biliary drainage is urgent (e.g., severe cholangitis), placement of a percutaneous wire and/or drain or an EUS-guided approach may be required. The latter can be undertaken at the same procedure if expertise is available.

Needle Knife Above the Papillary Orifice (Fistulotomy)

As in many tertiary units, we prefer to perform a needle-knife fistulotomy, particularly when prior pancreatic duct stenting is not possible. This is also the preferred technique for cases of large-stone impaction at the papillary orifice. The advantage is avoidance of thermal injury to the pancreatic orifice, which theoretically reduces the risk of pancreatitis. This technique is most useful in patients with a dilated intraduodenal segment of the bile duct.[12] The fistulotomy variation can be performed upward (cutting toward the duodenal wall from above the papilla) or downward (cutting toward the papilla from the duodenal wall) depending on the anatomy of the papilla, location of the initial entry point (Fig. 15.3), and operator preference.[1,11] We perform the fistulotomy beginning 2 mm above the ampullary orifice and extend the cut upward toward the transverse fold. When the downward approach is chosen, the initial incision is made just below the transverse fold of the mound at the 11 to 12 o'clock position and extended downward until it stops just short of the papillary orifice.[6,11] The depth and direction of the incision are

---

CASE 15.1   Fistulotomy: Ampullary Tumor

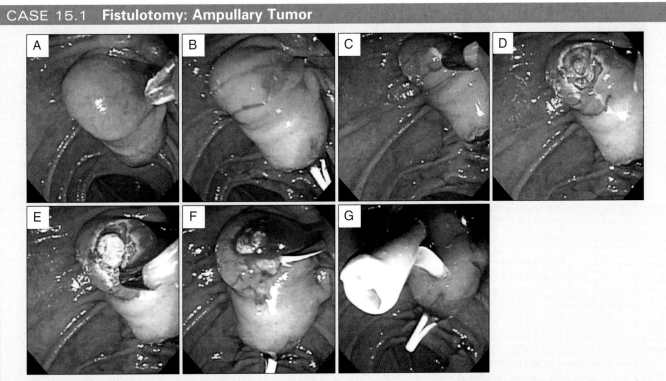

A, Large native papilla; **B,** pancreatic stent in place; **C,** fistulotomy with mucosal incision; **D,** biliary orifice; **E,** prolapsing papillary neoplasm; **F,** cannulation with wire; **G,** biliary and pancreatic stents in place.

CASE 15.2 Precut From Above the Orifice

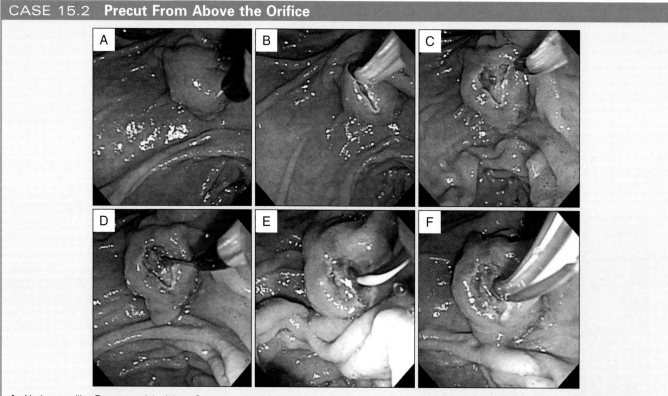

A, Native papilla; **B,** mucosal incision; **C,** exposed sphincter with biliary orifice; **D,** cannulation with wire; **E,** deep cannulation with wire; **F,** cannulation with catheter.

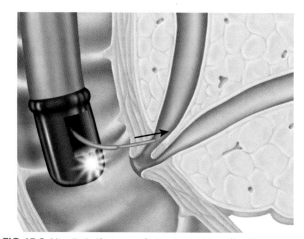

FIG 15.3 Needle-knife precut from above the orifice (fistulotomy).

again achieved through the combined movement of the endoscope, large wheel, and elevator. In individuals with small papillae, this may be the preferred method because the upper extent of the cut is predefined and it theoretically minimizes the risk of duodenal perforation. When performing these freehand techniques, it is important to avoid making the incision outside of the 11 to 12 o'clock corridor, which can result in retroperitoneal perforation. Clear visualization is essential, which if compromised by bleeding can be improved through the use of dilute epinephrine (1:20,000) irrigation through the injection port of the needle knife in order to achieve hemostasis and clear the field.[13] Submucosal injection of epinephrine, as is done to treat bleeding in other

situations, should be avoided because it results in distortion of the anatomy.

Data comparing the various precut techniques are limited. The first study, a prospective randomized trial, evaluated fistulotomy and precut involving the papillary orifice in 103 patients.[14] Although there was no significant difference in rates of successful biliary cannulation (91% with fistulotomy vs 89%), the fistulotomy technique resulted in a lower rate of pancreatitis (0% vs 7.59%, $p < 0.05$). The second study involved a retrospective cohort and assessed three variations of the precut technique: fistulotomy, precut from the ampullary orifice without pancreatic duct stenting, and precut with pancreatic duct stenting. Although there was no significant difference in cannulation rates, there was a trend toward lower rates of pancreatitis in the fistulotomy group (0%, 6%, and 3%, respectively).[15] The third study, again a retrospective design, assessed three strategies, precut from the papillary orifice, fistulotomy, and transpancreatic sphincterotomy, in 283 patients.[16] Again, although no significant differences were observed in cannulation rates, the overall adverse event profile and specifically the rates of PEP were lower in the fistulotomy group (3% fistulotomy, 21% precut from the orifice, 22% transpancreatic sphincterotomy).[16]

Needle Knife With an Insulated Tip

A Korean group reported using a needle knife with an insulated tip (Iso-Tome, MTW Endoskopie, Wesel, Germany) to prevent excessive conduction of electrocautery at the papillary orifice. Successful cannulation was achieved in 92% of patients; however, mild pancreatitis occurred in 20%.[17] A group from Hong Kong described a precut technique using an insulated angulotome. The device, in addition to possessing an insulated glass tip, has an angled needle to facilitate elevation of the papillary roof during cutting. Although involving a small group of

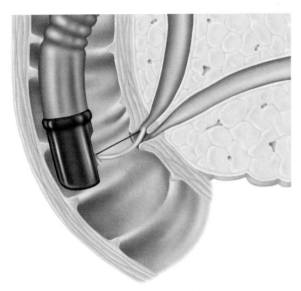

FIG 15.4 Short-nose precut sphincterotomy.

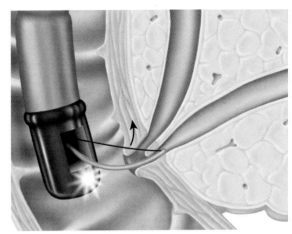

FIG 15.5 Transpancreatic sphincterotomy.

patients, successful cannulation was achieved in 100% of patients without adverse events.[18] Recently a Turkish group reported using a hybrid Iso-Tome with a completely round insulated tip, smaller than that used in prior studies. Patients were randomized to either the needle-knife or the Iso-Tome sphincterotomy group, with no significant differences observed in either cannulation or adverse event rates.[7]

Short-Nose Precut Sphincterotomy

Sohendra popularized an alternative precut sphincterotomy technique using a short-nose pull-type papillotome with a monofilament diathermy wire and a leading tip of only 1 mm (Fig. 15.4).[20] When this approach is used, the tip of the sphincterotome is inserted into the papillary orifice and directed to the 11 o'clock position to unroof the overlying ampullary mucosa and expose the biliary orifice. The incision extends over a length of approximately 5 mm. Using this approach, Binmoeller et al.[19] reported successful cannulation in 91% of 123 patients at the initial ERCP and 100% when attempted at a second procedure. The adverse event profile was not significantly different from conventional sphincterotomy, with a pancreatitis rate of 2.7%.[19] Another study from Germany randomized 291 patients with a variety of biliary disorders to group A, with a conventional wire-guided biliary cannulation (with precut being performed only when this failed), and group B, where precut was used up front to gain biliary access. The modified Erlangen-type sphincterotome with a 1-mm tip was used for precut. In group A, conventional cannulation failed in 42 patients; however, subsequent precut was successful in 41 of these patients, resulting in an overall success rate of 99.3%. In group B, primary precut was successful in 100% at the first attempt. There was no difference in the incidence of mild to moderate pancreatitis across the two groups (2.9% group A vs 2.1% group B).[20] The safety profile of this technique with the Erlangen-type sphincterotome was further supported in a more recent study, which retrospectively compared those who underwent conventional cannulation versus those who required precut. There was no significant difference in the adverse event rates between the two groups.[21] The advantages of the Erlangen pull-type precut sphincterotome over a needle knife include (1) the direction of the incision is more controllable and (2) the completion of the sphincterotomy can be performed with the same instrument. However, there is a potential increased risk of pancreatic duct trauma with the proximity of the sphincterotome wire to the pancreatic orifice.

Transpancreatic Sphincterotomy

Goff[22] described a technique whereby a standard traction sphincterotome is placed in the pancreatic orifice, followed by progressive small cuts toward the 11 o'clock position to unroof the common channel between the pancreatic and bile ducts (septotomy) (Fig. 15.5). Once the biliary orifice is exposed, biliary cannulation is then attempted. The success and pancreatitis rates were reported to be 96% and 1.96%, respectively, in this study.[22] This technique is similar to a conventional sphincterotomy and therefore technically easier than the other precut strategies. A number of other reports on wire-guided transpancreatic precut sphincterotomy have been published within the last decade, with successful biliary cannulation rates of 85% to 96% and PEP rates between 5% and 10.4%.[23–28] The emerging literature suggests that this technique has similar or higher biliary cannulation rates and an equivalent risk profile compared with freehand needle-knife sphincterotomy. In a recent randomized controlled trial (RCT) of 149 patients with difficult biliary cannulation, the cannulation rates were higher in the transpancreatic sphincterotomy group (95.9% vs 84.2%), with a shorter time to cannulation (193 vs 485 seconds) and no difference in risk profile compared with needle-knife sphincterotomy.[29] However, there are still concerns about this technique, as the long-term consequences of an unnecessary pancreatic sphincterotomy (which invariably occurs with this technique) are unclear.

Unconventional Techniques

Burdick described an intramural incision technique to obtain access to the bile duct in six patients in whom there was an inadvertent puncture of the intramural segment of the papilla with a guidewire sphincterotome.[29a] Performing an incision in this false channel may allow access to the bile duct. When a false complete or incomplete tract is formed while probing the papilla, the guidewire can be advanced into the duodenal lumen, usually at the upper margin of the papilla; the sphincterotome can be advanced through the same tract, bowed; and the intramural segment of the papilla is incised. This results in the splaying of the mucosa and frequent visualization of the biliary and pancreatic ductal openings. Four small studies exist evaluating this technique, with a reported success rate between 75% and 100% in the first attempt and close to 100% at the second attempt performed 1 to 4 weeks later.[30–33] Biliary access was more likely to be achieved with the Burdick technique (94.1% to 100%) compared with the needle-knife technique (91.5% to 94%) in two studies.[31,33] Adverse event rates were lower for the Burdick technique compared with needle-knife sphincterotomy (4.5% vs 8.5%). Variations of this technique have been described where the false tract is formed intentionally in difficult cannulation cases with similar success and adverse event rates.[31,32]

Artifon et al.[34] reported their experience with a technique of selective biliary cannulation using a novel needle puncture device followed by balloon dilatation of the tract for extraction of stones. The puncture technique was successful in 25 of 28 patients, allowing for completion of therapy. None of the patients developed pancreatitis.[34] Notably, the needle used for this technique, which is flexible and accepts a guidewire, is not widely available.

Use of Pancreatic Stents

Placement of transpapillary pancreatic stents (see Chapter 22) has markedly reduced pancreatitis rates in patients at high risk for PEP. These stents preserve drainage and, if placed before precut, are helpful with anatomic guidance to the bile duct. There is also a psychological component to having a pancreatic stent in place; seeing drainage of pancreatic fluid through the stent is reassuring for the endoscopist, who can concentrate on the precut rather than worrying about whether the patient will develop pancreatitis because of excessive manipulation.

Although there are extensive data regarding prophylactic pancreatic duct stenting in difficult biliary cannulation, there is a paucity specifically related to the precut setting (Fig. 15.6; Cases 15.3 and 15.4). A single-center randomized prospective study reported on 151 patients with failed free cannulation of the bile duct who subsequently went on to precut sphincterotomy. Of these patients, 93 had selective main pancreatic duct cannulation and subsequent pancreatic stent placement (5 to 7 F, 2 to 2.5 cm in length). Using the pancreatic stent as a guide, a needle-knife sphincterotome was used for biliary access. After access to the CBD and subsequent sphincterotomy, patients were randomized to immediate pancreatic stent removal or leaving the stent in place. The remaining 58 patients who did not undergo pancreatic stenting had a needle-knife precut sphincterotomy performed in a similar fashion. Both the frequency (4.3% vs 21.3%, $p = 0.027$) and severity (0% vs 12.8% moderate to severe pancreatitis, $p = 0.026$) of pancreatitis were lower in the group where the stents were left in place compared with immediate removal.[35] A retrospective cohort study involving 134 patients examined the adverse event rates of patients who underwent precut sphincterotomy without pancreatic stenting and those who underwent precut using the pancreatic stent as a guide. The pancreatic stent group had not only a lower rate of mild to moderate pancreatitis (6.1% vs 19.4%, $p = 0.028$) but also an improved biliary cannulation rate (96.9% vs 86.1%, $p = 0.0189$).[36]

The optimal stent length, diameter, and design for prophylactic pancreatic duct stenting remain controversial because of conflicting

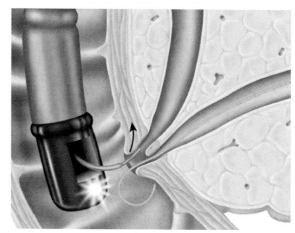

FIG 15.6 Needle-knife precut after placement of a pancreatic stent.

CASE 15.3   Impacted Stone

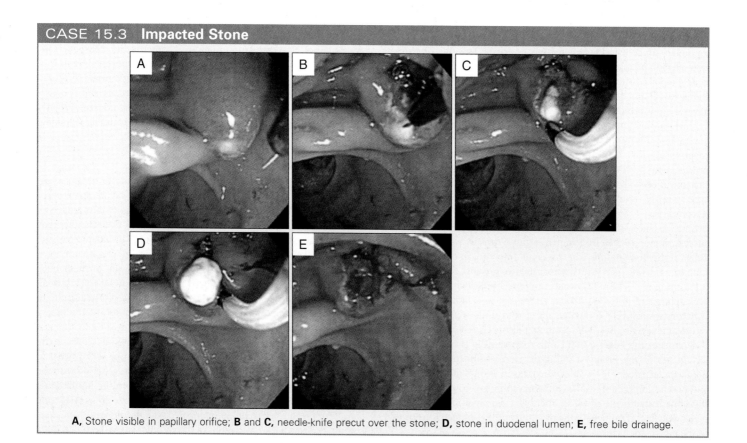

A, Stone visible in papillary orifice; **B** and **C,** needle-knife precut over the stone; **D,** stone in duodenal lumen; **E,** free bile drainage.

CASE 15.4   Precut Above Pancreatic Stent

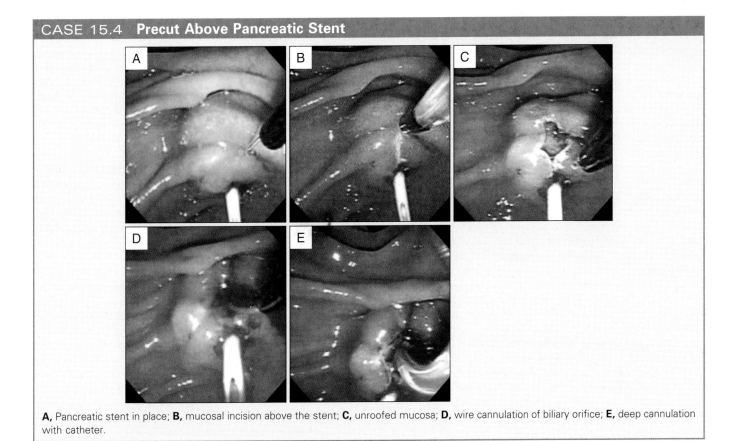

A, Pancreatic stent in place; **B,** mucosal incision above the stent; **C,** unroofed mucosa; **D,** wire cannulation of biliary orifice; **E,** deep cannulation with catheter.

data.[37–39] In our practice, pancreatic duct stents are placed when bile duct cannulation is difficult and repeated guidewire instrumentation occurs; even in the absence of pancreatic duct opacification, a short (3 to 5 cm) 5-Fr straight pancreatic duct stent with an external flange is placed before attempting a precut sphincterotomy. If pancreatic cannulation has not been achieved and pancreatic stent placement fails, then a technique that theoretically avoids thermal injury to the pancreatic orifice (e.g., fistulotomy) should be used.

ADVERSE EVENTS (SEE CHAPTER 8)

Traditionally, precut sphincterotomy was associated with an elevated risk of adverse events, especially pancreatitis. However, it was employed only as a salvage technique after multiple failed attempts at biliary cannulation with resultant ampullary trauma, in addition to unintentional pancreatic duct wire cannulation and/or contrast injection. Although the initial literature was controversial as it related to the documentation of a variable risk profile (2% to 34%), subsequent multiple meta-analyses support the use of early precut sphincterotomy in difficult biliary cannulation as it reduces the risk of pancreatitis.[4,6,40,41]

Pancreatitis

In 2003 Masci et al.[3] published a meta-analysis of risk factors for PEP. Data for precut were derived from seven studies involving 7622 patients. The incidence of PEP was 5.28% compared with 3.1% ($p < 0.001$) in patients who did not undergo precut. The second significant technical factor was repeated pancreatic duct injection. These two variables reflect difficult bile duct cannulation. Masci et al. stressed that the real risk of precut may be related to prolonged efforts at cannulation, but studies on timing of precut were lacking at that time.[3]

The concept of early precut sphincterotomy rather than persisting with standard cannulation techniques was described over 20 years ago, although the supporting literature validating such a strategy emerged only in 2005. These studies, which included one from our own institution, focused on the timing of needle-knife sphincterotomy in difficult biliary cannulation cases and confirmed that in experienced hands it was safe and effective.[42,43] Currently, although a consensus exists that precut should be performed in difficult biliary cannulation, there is not yet a globally accepted definition of difficult cannulation.

The definition of difficult cannulation should take into account the time from onset of initial cannulation, the number of attempts (touches) on the ampulla, the number of pancreatic wire passages, and the number of inadvertent pancreatic duct injections. The recent literature on early precut strategies defines difficult biliary cannulation as a procedure lasting longer than 5 minutes, 5 unsuccessful attempts at biliary cannulation, and unintentional pancreatic duct cannulation (range 1 to 3).[44,45] Once these parameters are exceeded, it is unlikely that the initial techniques will succeed, irrespective of whether wire-guided or contrast-based approaches are used. If more time is spent with repeated manipulation of the ampulla, the risk of pancreatitis increases and the likelihood of successful cannulation decreases.[46,47]

The recent literature on early precut sphincterotomy includes two trials and three meta-analyses. The most recent RCT by Mariani et al.[45] enrolled 375 patients with difficult biliary cannulation across 8 tertiary centers. Patients were randomized to early precut or repeated papillary cannulation, which, if failed, was followed by precut. There was no significant difference in biliary cannulation rates (90.8% in early precut group vs 92.6% in repeated cannulation). However, the rate of PEP was lower in the early precut group (5.4% vs 12.1%, OR 0.35, 95% CI 0.16 to 0.78). Importantly the incidence of PEP was lower in the early compared with the late precut group (5.4% vs 14.1%, OR 0.42, 95% CI 0.17 to 1.07).[45] These findings were supported by a recent single-center prospective cohort study by Lopes et al.,[44] in which 350 patients with difficult biliary cannulation were assigned to an early or late precut fistulotomy strategy. Cannulation and pancreatitis rates were similar across the two groups, but there was a trend of higher rates of PEP in the late precut group (8.6% vs 4.2%).[44] In a meta-analysis assessing the literature on early precut sphincterotomy, Sundaralingam et al.[4] analyzed data from 5 studies with a combined cohort of 532 patients. The overall cannulation and PEP rates did not differ significantly between early precut and persistent cannulation attempts; however, an increased success rate of primary cannulation was observed in the early precut group (RR 1.32, 95% CI 1.04 to 1.68). One subgroup analysis of studies excluding the involvement of fellows showed a significant reduction in the risk of PEP in the early precut group (RR 0.29, 95% CI 0.10 to 0.86).[4] The second meta-analysis, by Navaneethan et al.,[40] reviewed 7 RCTs with a combined cohort of 1039 patients. The overall cannulation rate was higher in the early precut group (OR 1.98, 95% CI 0.70 to 5.65), and there was no significant difference in adverse events, including PEP.[40] Finally, the third recent meta-analysis, by Choudhary et al.,[41] examined 7 RCTs and 7 nonrandomized trials separately with a total cohort of 4580 patients. There was no significant difference in biliary cannulation, and although there was a trend toward reduced PEP in the early precut group, this was not statistically significant (OR 0.58, 95% CI 0.32 to 1.05, $p = 0.07$).[41] The current literature therefore indicates that early precut sphincterotomy is not associated with an increased rate of adverse events over persistent attempts at standard cannulation and that, in experienced hands, early adoption of a precut strategy may reduce the risk of PEP.

Bleeding

The incidence of bleeding after precut varies according to the definition applied to bleeding. Rates may be as low as 1% to 2% or as high as 48% if minor intraprocedural bleeding is included in the latter. However, intraprocedural bleeding is almost always clinically insignificant.[48] The early literature indicated that precut sphincterotomy may be a significant risk factor for bleeding.[49] However, a recent meta-analysis suggests that there is no significant difference in bleeding rates between early precut sphincterotomy (0% to 6.5%) and conventional techniques (0% to 5.9%).[4,40,41] In a recent retrospective study, failure to achieve biliary access after precut sphincterotomy led to an increased risk of bleeding (15.2% vs 5.7%, $p = 0.001$) compared with a successful attempt.[50]

Most episodes of bleeding during precut stop spontaneously. As opposed to standard sphincterotomy, where injection of epinephrine is used for persistent bleeding, we avoid injecting epinephrine until deep biliary access is achieved, as mentioned earlier. The initial approach is to spray epinephrine on the bleeding area, which often results in hemostasis and completion of the precut.[13] Aggressive hemostatic techniques may obscure the anatomic landmarks and preclude successful cannulation after precut. In rare situations when significant bleeding occurs after precut, it may be best to abort the procedure and establish hemostasis.

Perforation

The risk of perforation after precut is between 0.1% and 0.8%, similar to standard sphincterotomy.[41,50] Retroperitoneal perforation may occur as a result of extending the precut beyond the intramural portion of the bile duct, cutting too deep, or precutting in an incorrect axis outside of the 11 to 12 o'clock corridor. The freehand nature of precut is highly operator dependent and requires more precision and care compared with standard sphincterotomy. Small perforations may not be apparent endoscopically but are recognized by retroperitoneal air on fluoroscopy or extravasation of contrast. Most small retroperitoneal perforations, if immediately recognized, can be managed conservatively by placement of a biliary stent (in some cases covered self-expandable metal stent).

A recent retrospective study involving 706 patients identified failed precut sphincterotomy as a significant risk factor for perforation.[41]

Failed Access and Cost

In the event of failed ERCP cannulation, studies indicate that 50% to 60% of patients undergo further therapeutic procedures, which may be radiologic, surgical, or repeat endoscopic. Our preferred approach is to perform a second ERCP in 48 to 72 hours unless the patient has an indication for immediate biliary drainage, such as severe cholangitis. From the point of view of the patient and health care provider, a successful procedure with a mild adverse event may be preferable to a failed procedure with no adverse event, because failure requires repeat or alternative invasive procedures, with their own morbidity and cost.

There is a paucity of data on the cost-effectiveness of precut techniques. Harewood and colleagues[51] published a cost-effectiveness analysis on alternative strategies for palliation of distal biliary obstruction after failed cannulation of the bile duct. This model simulated a patient with inoperable malignant distal bile duct obstruction in whom an initial attempt at biliary cannulation has failed and where a decision is made at the time of index ERCP whether to proceed with a precut or discontinue the procedure and obtain a percutaneous transhepatic cholangiography (PTC) in an attempt to place a metal biliary stent. They concluded that precut sphincterotomy followed by PTC, if necessary, is the most cost-effective approach for palliative biliary stent placement.[51] More recently there are emerging data to support EUS-guided biliary drainage as a viable technique in cases of failed access during ERCP, which can be performed during the same session. Artifon et al.[52] compared EUS-guided transluminal drainage and PTC in patients with distal biliary malignant obstruction and found no significant differences in technical success, adverse events, and hospital length of stay. However, a trend toward lower cost was observed in the EUS group.[52] More recently Khashab et al.[53] published a retrospective cohort study of 73 patients with distal malignant biliary obstruction in whom the ERCP attempt failed. These patients subsequently underwent either PTC or EUS-guided biliary drainage. Although the technical success rate was higher in the PTC arm (100% vs 86%), the adverse event rate, requirement for reintervention, and cost were lower in the EUS group.[53] Finally, the EUS approach allows biliary access during the index procedure, a strategy investigated by Gornals et al.,[54] who demonstrated this approach to be safe and cost-effective, where a saving of 658 euros/patient was observed.

The intent of precut sphincterotomy should always be to obtain access during the initial procedure. If the bile duct access is deferred, it may result in prolonged hospitalization, and if a second ERCP or PTC is required, this will be associated with significant cost. However, endoscopists must understand their limitations and know when further manipulation may result in a serious adverse event without a reasonable chance of success. Failure to cannulate is acceptable, but unreasonable persistence potentially resulting in very serious adverse events is not and would clearly add to the total cost of patient care.

The complete reference list for this chapter can be found online at www.expertconsult.com.

SUMMARY

Precut is a safe technique with a high degree of success, allowing for bile duct cannulation and therapy. However, there is probably no procedure in ERCP that requires more precise technique than precut. The choice of precut technique will depend on experience and personal preference. Most experienced endoscopists rely on the precut method in only 10% to 15% of cases. The ideal technique of precut is not known and is likely both operator dependent and patient dependent.

It is important that the endoscopist not use access techniques as a replacement for inadequate experience or poor cannulation technique.

The precut technique should be used by individuals with extensive experience in interventional ERCP. It should be limited to patients with a definite indication for deep CBD cannulation and should not be used to simply facilitate a diagnostic cannulation. Early precutting and pancreatic stenting in high-risk patients should be considered in difficult biliary cannulations. Precutting must be avoided for diagnostic purposes because other available modalities, including MRCP, EUS, and computed tomography, can provide the required diagnostic information.

16

Sphincter of Oddi Manometry

Tugrul Purnak and Evan L. Fogel

The sphincter of Oddi (SO) is a complex smooth muscle structure surrounding the terminal common bile duct, main pancreatic duct, and the common channel, when present (Fig. 16.1). The high-pressure zone generated by the sphincter ranges from 4 to 10 mm in length. The SO regulates the flow of bile and pancreatic exocrine juice and prevents duodenum-to-duct reflux (i.e., maintains a sterile intraductal environment).[1] The SO possesses a basal pressure and phasic contractile activities; the former appears to be the predominant mechanism regulating flow of pancreatobiliary secretions. Although phasic SO contractions may aid in regulating bile and pancreatic juice flow, their primary role appears to be maintaining a sterile intraductal milieu.

Sphincter of Oddi dysfunction (SOD) refers to an abnormality of SO contractility. It is a benign noncalculous obstruction to the flow of bile or pancreatic juice through the pancreatobiliary junction (i.e., the SO).[2] This may cause pancreaticobiliary-type pain, cholestasis, and/or recurrent pancreatitis.[1,3,4] The most definitive development in our understanding of the pressure dynamics of the SO came with the advent of sphincter of Oddi manometry (SOM). SOM is the only available method to measure SO motor activity directly.[5,6] SOM is considered by most authorities to be the most accurate means to evaluate patients for sphincter dysfunction.[7–9] Although SOM can be performed intraoperatively[10–12] and percutaneously,[13] it is most commonly performed endoscopically at the time of endoscopic retrograde cholangiopancreatography (ERCP). The use of manometry to detect motility disorders of the SO is similar to its use in other parts of the gastrointestinal tract. However, performance of SOM is more technically demanding and hazardous, with adverse event rates (in particular, pancreatitis) approaching 20% in several series. Its use therefore should be reserved for patients with clinically significant or disabling symptoms. Other noninvasive and provocative tests designed to diagnose SOD have therefore been evaluated.[1,3,14] Secretin-stimulated endoscopic ultrasonography[15] and magnetic resonance cholangiopancreatography (MRCP)[16–19] have low sensitivity and specificity for the diagnosis of SOD. Furthermore, nuclear cholescintigraphy, once advocated as an alternative noninvasive test of choice,[3] has led to disappointing results.[1,20,21] One needs to appreciate, however, that SOM is not likely an independent risk factor for post-ERCP pancreatitis when the aspirating manometry catheter is used (see section, "Equipment"). Questions remain as to whether the short-term observations (2-minute to 10-minute recordings per pull-through) reflect the "twenty-four-hour pathophysiology" of the sphincter.[3,22–28] Despite these problems and lingering doubts as to its clinical utility, SOM has gained more widespread application after 3 decades of evaluation.[1,3,29–31] In this chapter, we will discuss the technique of SOM, with an emphasis on the technical and cognitive skill sets required.

METHOD OF SOM

Sedation

SOM is usually performed at the time of ERCP. The initial step in performing SOM therefore is to administer adequate sedation that will result in a comfortable, cooperative, motionless patient. All drugs that relax the sphincter (anticholinergics, nitrates, calcium channel blockers, glucagon) or stimulate the sphincter (narcotics, cholinergic agents) should be avoided for at least 8 to 12 hours before manometry and during the manometric session. Early studies with midazolam and diazepam suggested that these benzodiazepines do not interfere with SO manometric parameters and therefore are acceptable sedatives for SOM.[32–36] Although one study did demonstrate a decrease in mean basal sphincter pressure in 4 of 18 patients (22%) receiving midazolam,[37] this result has not been duplicated to date. Opioids were initially avoided during SOM because of indirect evidence suggesting that these agents caused SO spasm.[38–44] However, two prospective studies[45,46] demonstrated that meperidine, at a dose of ≤1 mg/kg, does not affect the basal sphincter pressure but does alter phasic wave characteristics. Because the basal sphincter pressure generally is the only manometric criterion used to diagnose SOD and determine therapy, meperidine may be used to facilitate moderate sedation for manometry. Additionally, one study demonstrated that a low dose of fentanyl, administered topically, did not appear to affect the basal sphincter pressure.[47] Confirmatory data are awaited. Patients referred for SOM may take large doses of narcotics every day and frequently prove difficult to sedate at ERCP. Adjunctive agents for moderate sedation therefore have been sought. Our group demonstrated that droperidol did not significantly alter SOM results; concordance (normal vs abnormal basal sphincter pressure) was seen in 30 of 31 patients.[48] Wilcox and Linder,[49] on the other hand, suggested that droperidol did in fact influence SOM parameters. However, in their series of 55 patients, ERCP and SOM were carried out under general anesthesia in all but 10 patients. Indeed, an increasing recent trend has been to perform ERCP under general anesthesia or monitored anesthesia care (MAC). Although it has been suggested that SO motor function is not influenced by general anesthesia,[5] the effects of newer anesthetic agents are unknown, making interpretation of their results problematic. In one study, ketamine did not significantly alter SOM parameters, with concordance noted in 28 of 30 (93%) patients.[50] Limited experience with propofol suggests that this drug also does not affect the basal sphincter pressure,[51,52] but further study is required before routine use of ketamine or propofol for SOM is recommended. If glucagon must be used to achieve cannulation, a 15-minute waiting period is required to restore the sphincter to its basal condition.

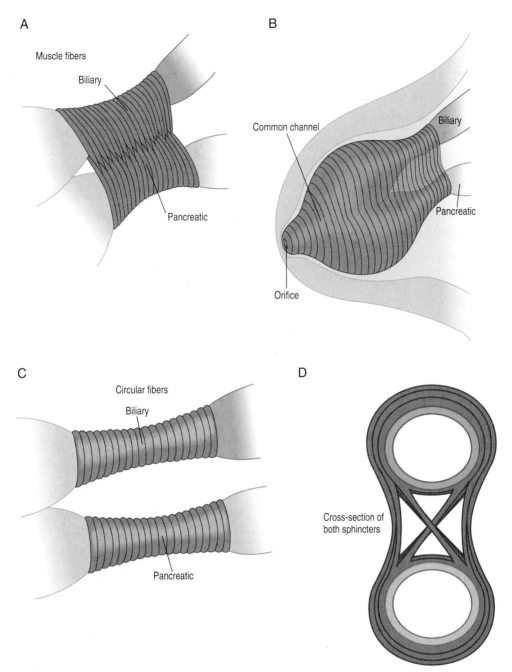

FIG 16.1 A–D, Schematic representation of the sphincter of Oddi, demonstrating the circular smooth muscle that surrounds the common channel, distal common bile duct, and pancreatic duct.

Equipment

Virtually all standards have been established with 5-Fr catheters; therefore these should be used. Triple-lumen catheters are state-of-the-art and are available from several manufacturers. Catheters with a long intraductal tip may help secure the catheter within the bile duct, but such a long nose is commonly a hindrance if pancreatic manometry is desired. A sleeve catheter is a perfused channel system that records pressure along its length, potentially limiting motion artifacts during the performance of SOM.[53] Limited data from Australia suggest that this sleeve method is comparable to standard SOM with triple-lumen catheters, possibly with lower pancreatitis rates.[9,54] Additionally, a guidewire-type manometer, similar to that used to measure arterial pressure in coronary angiography, was noted to be safe and easy to apply in 22 Japanese

patients.[55] Comparative data to standard techniques, however, are needed. Over-the-wire (monorail) catheters can be passed after first securing one's position within the duct with a guidewire. Whether this guidewire influences basal sphincter pressure has not been definitively elucidated (see section, "Technical Performance of SOM [Video 16.1]"). Some triple-lumen catheters will accommodate a 0.018-inch-diameter or 0.021-inch-diameter guidewire passed through the entire length of the catheter and can be used to facilitate cannulation or maintain position in the duct. Guidewire-tipped catheters are also being evaluated. Early experience with performance of SOM using perfusion systems demonstrated unacceptably high postprocedure pancreatitis rates.[56–60] Presumably, overdistension of small-caliber pancreatic ducts led to this adverse event. Aspiration catheters (Fig. 16.2), in which one recording port is sacrificed to permit both end-hole and side-hole aspiration of intraductal

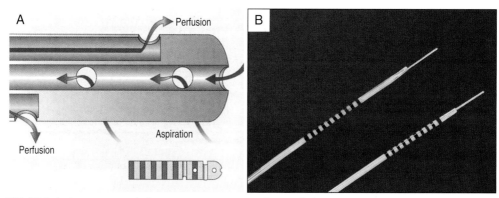

FIG 16.2 **A,** Long-nose and short-nose manometry catheters (Lehman manometry aspirating catheters). **B,** Schematic representation of a modified triple-lumen aspirating catheter.

juice and the perfusing fluid, are therefore highly recommended for pancreatic manometry. These catheters have been shown to reduce the frequency of post-SOM pancreatitis while accurately recording sphincter pressures.[9,58] Most centers prefer to perfuse the catheters at 0.25 mL/channel/minute using a low-compliance pump (Fig. 16.3). Lower perfusion rates will give accurate basal sphincter pressure measurements but will not give accurate phasic wave information. The perfusate generally is distilled water, although the use of physiologic saline needs further evaluation. The latter may crystallize in the capillary tubing of perfusion pumps and must be frequently irrigated. Solid-state catheters[59,61] and microtransducer manometry systems[62] are also available and used by some investigators in an attempt to avoid volume loading of the bilio-pancreatic system during perfusion manometry.[61,63] Preliminary data from a few centers demonstrate comparable SOM results to those achieved with perfusing catheters.[59,62] Draganov and colleagues[64] performed SOM using both the aspirating triple-lumen water-perfused catheter and solid-state catheter in 30 patients. There was complete agreement on the final results of SOM (normal/abnormal) between the two groups (accuracy 100%).

▶ Technical Performance of SOM (Video 16.1)

SOM requires selective cannulation of the bile duct and/or pancreatic duct. Maximal efficiency is achieved by combining ERCP and SOM in a single session. It is preferable to perform cholangiography and/or pancreatography before carrying out SOM, as certain findings (e.g., common bile duct stone) may preclude the need for SOM. This can be done simply by injecting contrast media through one of the perfusion ports. Alternatively, the duct entered can be identified by gently aspirating any port (Fig. 16.4). The appearance of yellow-colored fluid in the endoscopic view indicates entry into the bile duct. Clear, colorless aspirate indicates that the pancreatic duct has been entered. This technique may prove useful when attempting to access the bile duct after pancreatic SOM, as repeated pancreatic duct injections may increase post-ERCP pancreatitis rates.[65] If clear, colorless fluid is seen in the catheter, suggesting pancreatic duct entry, the catheter position is altered to achieve a more favorable angle for biliary cannulation. Blaut and colleagues[66] have shown that injection of contrast into the biliary tree before SOM does not significantly affect sphincter pressure characteristics. Similar evaluation of the pancreatic sphincter after contrast injection has not been reported. One must be certain that the catheter is not impacted against the wall of the duct in order to ensure accurate pressure measurements. On occasion, selective deep cannulation of the desired duct may be achieved only with a guidewire. However, stiffer-shafted nitinol-core guidewires within manometry catheters commonly increase basal biliary sphincter pressure measured at ERCP by 50% to 100%.[67]

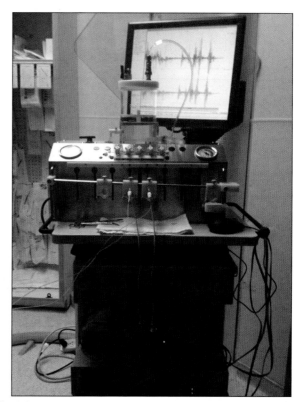

FIG 16.3 Photograph of a perfusion pump and accompanying monitor.

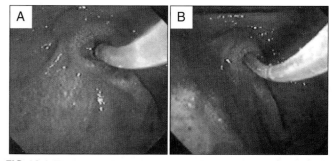

FIG 16.4 The duct entered during sphincter of Oddi manometry can be identified by aspirating the catheter. Clear fluid indicates pancreatic duct entry **(A)**, whereas yellow fluid signifies entry into the bile duct **(B)**.

Therefore, when wire-guided cannulation is performed, we recommend withdrawing the wire back into the catheter, outside of the duct and not traversing the sphincter, during performance of SOM. Alternatively, stiff guidewires need to be avoided or very soft-core guidewires can be used. Once deep cannulation is achieved and the patient acceptably sedated, the catheter is withdrawn across the sphincter at 1-mm to 2-mm intervals by standard station pull-through technique. Both the pancreatic and bile ducts may be studied, depending on the clinical scenario. Current data indicate that an abnormal basal sphincter pressure may be confined to one side of the sphincter in 35% to 65% of patients with abnormal manometry,[68–73] and thus one sphincter segment may be dysfunctional and the other normal. Raddawi and colleagues[70] reported that an abnormal basal sphincter pressure was more likely to be confined to the pancreatic duct segment in patients with pancreatitis and to the bile duct segment in patients with biliary-type pain and elevated liver function tests. However, more recently, a randomized trial demonstrated no additional benefit of dual pancreatic and biliary sphincterotomy compared with biliary sphincterotomy alone in patients with idiopathic recurrent pancreatitis and SOD.[74] Further discussion regarding the need to study one or both sphincter segments is discussed in Chapter 47.

Abnormalities of the basal sphincter pressure should ideally be observed for at least 30 seconds in each lead and be seen on two or more separate pull-throughs.[1,30,75] From a practical clinical standpoint, we perform one pull-through from each duct if the readings are clearly normal or abnormal. It is important that no kinking or impaction of the catheter occurs, which can cause spurious pressure rises or artifacts that might impair interpretation of the manometry tracing. During the pull-through, it is necessary to establish good communication between the endoscopist and the manometrist who is reading the tracing as it rolls off the recorder or appears on the computer screen. This permits optimal positioning of the catheter in order to achieve interpretable tracings. Alternatively, an electronic manometry system with a television screen can be mounted near the endoscopic image screen to allow the endoscopist to view the manometry tracing during endoscopy. This can be particularly helpful when vigorous duodenal motility is present, necessitating constant attention to catheter position in the duodenal lumen. Once the baseline study is completed, agents to relax or stimulate (e.g., cholecystokinin) the SO can be given and manometric and pain response monitored. The value of these provocative maneuvers for routine use needs further study before widespread application is recommended.

INTERPRETATION CRITERIA

Criteria for interpretation of a manometry tracing are relatively standard; however, they may vary somewhat from center to center. Some areas where there may be disagreement in interpretation include the required duration of basal sphincter pressure elevation, the number of leads in which basal pressure elevation is required, and the role of averaging pressures from the three (or two in an aspirating catheter) recording ports. Our recommended method for reading manometry tracings is first to define the "zero" duodenal baseline before and after the pull-through. Alternatively, intraduodenal pressure can be continuously recorded from a separate intraduodenal catheter attached to the endoscope. The highest basal pressure (defined as the pressure above the zero duodenal baseline; Fig. 16.5) that is sustained for at least 30 seconds is then identified. From the four lowest amplitude points in this zone, the mean of these readings is taken as the basal sphincter pressure for that lead for that pull-through. The basal sphincter pressures for all interpretable observations are then averaged; this is the final basal sphincter pressure. The amplitude of phasic wave contractions is

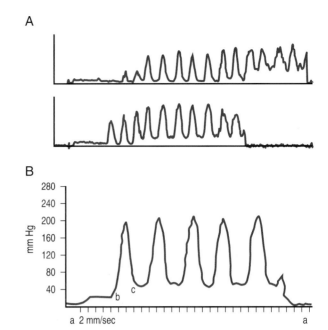

FIG 16.5 A, An abnormal station pull-through at sphincter of Oddi manometry. The study has been abbreviated to fit onto one page. **B,** Schematic representation of one lead of the above tracing. *(a)* Baseline duodenal zero reference, *(b)* intraductal (pancreatic) pressure of 20 mm Hg (abnormal), and *(c)* basal pancreatic sphincter pressure of 45 mm Hg (abnormal). Phasic waves are 155 to 175 mm Hg in amplitude and 6-second duration (normal).

measured from the beginning of the slope of the pressure increase from the basal pressure to the peak of the contraction wave. Four representative waves are taken for each lead and the mean pressure determined. The number of phasic waves per minute and the duration of phasic waves can also be determined. Most authorities use only basal sphincter pressure as an indicator of pathology of the SO. However, data from Johns Hopkins University[76] suggest that intrabiliary pressure, which is easier to measure than SO pressure, correlates with basal sphincter pressure. In this study, intrabiliary pressure was significantly higher in patients with SOD than in those with normal basal biliary sphincter pressure (20 vs 10 mm Hg; $p < 0.01$). In a similar study, the Milwaukee group[77] found that increased pancreatic duct pressure correlated with increased pancreatic basal sphincter pressure. Pancreatic duct pressure was significantly higher in SOD patients compared with those with normal SO motility (20 vs 11 mm Hg; $p < 0.001$). These studies await confirmation but support the theory that increased intrabiliary and/or intrapancreatic pressure is a cause of pain in patients with SOD.

The best study establishing normal values for SOM was reported by Guelrud and associates.[24] Fifty asymptomatic control patients underwent SOM, which was repeated on two occasions in 10 subjects. This study established normal values for intraductal pressure, basal sphincter pressure, and phasic wave parameters (Table 16.1). Moreover, the reproducibility of SOM was confirmed (see section, "Reproducibility of SOM"). A potential limitation of this study, however, was the exclusion of patients with difficult cannulation or failed deep cannulation. Potentially, patients with small-caliber ducts might prove difficult to cannulate with a 5-Fr catheter, leading to a high-pressure zone on a purely structural basis, unrelated to muscle contraction or spasm.[29] Despite this criticism, most authorities interchangeably use 35 or 40 mm Hg as the upper limit of normal for mean basal SO pressure. Such upper limits of normal values are mean values plus three standard

TABLE 16.1 **Suggested Standard for Abnormal Values for Endoscopic Sphincter of Oddi Manometry Obtained From 50 Volunteers Without Abdominal Symptoms**

Basal sphincter pressure*	>35 mm Hg
Basal ductal pressure	>13 mm Hg
Phasic Contractions	
Amplitude	>220 mm Hg
Duration	>8 seconds
Frequency	>10/minute

From Guelrud M, Mendoza S, Rossiter G, et al. Sphincter of Oddi manometry in healthy volunteers. *Dig Dis Sci.* 1990;35:38–46.
*Basal pressure determined by (1) reading the peak basal pressures (i.e., highest single leads as obtained using a triple-lumen catheter) and (2) obtaining the mean of these peak pressures from multiple station pull-throughs.
Values were obtained by adding 3 standard deviations to the mean (mean obtained by averaging the results on two to three station pull-throughs). Data combine pancreatic and biliary studies.

deviations. More studies are needed to determine whether 2 or 2.5 standard deviations above the mean would be more appropriate.

Interobserver variability for reading SOM is minimal when the observers are experienced in reading these tracings.[78]

REPRODUCIBILITY OF SOM

It has been questioned whether the short-term pressure recording obtained during SOM reflects the "twenty-four-hour pathophysiology" of the sphincter, as patients with SOD may have intermittent, episodic symptoms.[26] If the basal sphincter pressure does vary over time, performance of SOM on two separate occasions may lead to different results and affect therapy. Three studies have demonstrated reproducibility of biliary SOM in 34 of 36 symptomatic patients overall[23,25] and 10 of 10 healthy volunteers.[24] However, reproducibility of pancreatic SOM was found in only 58% (7/12) and 40% (12/30) of persistently symptomatic patients with previously normal SOM at two large referral centers.[22,26] Other studies have also shown that SO basal pressures are not constant,[79–81] perhaps because of the inherent physiological fluctuation of SO motor activity. Newer devices capable of portable, ambulatory, prolonged SOM would be of interest.

ADVERSE EVENTS OF SOM

Several studies have indicated that pancreatitis is the most common major adverse event after SOM. Historically, using standard perfused catheters, pancreatitis rates over 20% have been reported, especially after manometric evaluation of the pancreatic duct. Such high adverse event rates have limited more widespread use of SOM. Placement of a small-diameter, protective, temporary pancreatic duct stent has long been considered to be standard of care in these high-risk patients.[82–85] In addition, a multicenter randomized controlled trial demonstrated that rectal indomethacin (100 mg) was associated with a 46% relative risk reduction in pancreatitis rates post-ERCP in high-risk patients (16.9% placebo group vs 9.2% indomethacin group, $p = 0.005$), the majority of which were suspected/documented SOD.[86] However, a recent retrospective study in type 3 SOD patients comparing pancreatic stent placement alone with pancreatic stent placement plus 100 mg rectal indomethacin showed no difference between these two approaches with respect to incidence and severity of post-ERCP pancreatitis (incidence 23% vs 18%, $p = 0.39$).[87] Prospective studies to determine the optimal dose of indomethacin and to directly compare protective pancreatic stents to indomethacin alone are under way. A variety of other methods to decrease the incidence of postmanometry pancreatitis have been proposed. These include (1) using an aspiration catheter, (2) using gravity drainage of the pancreatic duct after manometry, (3) decreasing the perfusion rate to 0.05 to 0.10 mL/lumen/minute, (4) limiting pancreatic duct manometry time to less than 2 minutes (or avoidance of pancreatic manometry), and (5) using a microtransducer or solid-state (nonperfused) system. In a prospective randomized study, Sherman and colleagues[58] found that the aspirating catheter (a catheter that allows aspiration of the perfused fluid from end and side holes while accurately recording pressure from the two remaining side ports) reduced the frequency of pancreatic duct manometry–induced pancreatitis from 31% to 4% ($p = 0.01$). The reduction in pancreatitis with use of this catheter in the pancreatic duct and the very low incidence of pancreatitis after bile duct manometry lend support to the notion that increased pancreatic duct hydrostatic pressure is a major cause of this adverse event. Thus we routinely aspirate pancreatic juice and perfusate when we study the pancreatic duct by SOM.

SUMMARY

Mastery of the fundamentals of ERCP and appropriate training are necessary for the physician who evaluates patients with SOM. At a minimum, the endoscopist must be skilled in diagnostic ERCP, because performance of SOM cannot be accomplished without selective cannulation of the pancreatic duct and bile duct. The physician must be aware of the limitations of sedation imposed by manometry and familiar with the equipment needed to perform the procedure. Technical skills in manometric pressure recording techniques must be acquired, limiting the maneuvers that may lead to recording artifacts. Appropriate training in the interpretation of manometry tracings is essential for both the endoscopist and the manometrist. An expert panel has stated in their position paper that training should be obtained at a pancreatobiliary center that routinely performs SOM.[6] Although one group recently demonstrated that SOM could be performed in low numbers with results comparable to larger centers, all procedures were performed by a biliary endoscopist who performed more than 400 ERCPs per year.[75] There are no society guidelines recommending specific numbers of procedures that need to be performed during training; however, a minimum of 25 SOM studies performed during the course of a 3-year clinical gastroenterology fellowship or an advanced fourth-year fellowship seems reasonable. There is no substitute for practice and experience.

The complete reference list for this chapter can be found online at www.expertconsult.com.

17

Biliary Sphincterotomy

Horst Neuhaus

Diagnostic endoscopic retrograde cholangiopancreatography (ERCP) has been widely replaced by computed tomography (CT), magnetic resonance cholangiopancreatography (MRCP), and endoscopic ultrasonography (EUS) as noninvasive or less invasive imaging techniques. Indications for diagnostic ERCP should be limited to selected patients with indeterminate biliary strictures or filling defects for evaluation by tissue acquisition with or without cholangioscopic guidance. ERCP is mainly performed for therapeutic biliopancreatic interventions. Endoscopic sphincterotomy (EST) of the biliary sphincter is needed for most biliary interventions.

Since the introduction of EST in 1973, a variety of complementary methods have been developed, and they have become invaluable for minimally invasive therapy of biliary diseases and have gained worldwide acceptance. Prospective multicenter trials have defined the clinical, anatomic, and technical parameters of EST and its efficacy and safety. Outcomes after EST can be affected by ductal cannulation before EST, by its technique, by subsequent therapeutic interventions, and by endoscopist expertise.

DESCRIPTION OF THE TECHNIQUE

Premedication, duodenoscopy, and the approach to the papilla are the same as for diagnostic ERC, as discussed in Chapters 6 and 14. The use of a therapeutic channel endoscope (working diameter 4.2 mm) has become standard as it facilitates insertion of accessories and devices required for advanced interventions. The initial use of a sphincterotome for deep bile duct cannulation is recommended for several reasons. First, when it is anticipated that a sphincterotomy will be needed, exchange to a sphincterotome from a catheter is avoided. Second, it allows variable upward tip deflection in order to introduce the tip of the catheter into the biliary orifice; the tip deflection is then relaxed to achieve deep cannulation (see Chapter 14). Previous randomized controlled trials showed significantly higher success rates for primary cannulation with sphincterotomes compared with standard catheters, without significant differences in safety.[1,2] Recent meta-analyses demonstrated that guidewire-assisted cannulation increases the primary access rate and reduces the risk of post-ERCP pancreatitis (PEP) in comparison to the contrast-assisted cannulation approach.[3,4] A sphincterotome alone was used for both cannulation techniques in 7 of 12 analyzed trials.[4] These results suggest that wire-assisted cannulation with a sphincterotome is the best first-line technique for biliary access. There are few data comparing cannulation with different sphincterotomes.[5] Further details of cannulation of the major papilla are described in Chapter 14.

Instruments

The type of sphincterotome should be selected according to the individual anatomic situation and the preference of the endoscopist.

Sphincterotomes differ in the diameter and length of the tip, length and characteristics of the cutting wire, and shaft stiffness, which are described in detail in Chapter 4 and in a recent review.[5] Tapered devices, which require smaller wires (0.025-inch diameter or less), can be easier to insert into the papilla but are also more prone to cause tissue trauma and submucosal injection than those with a more blunted tip.

Modern sphincterotomes provide a lumen for insertion of a guidewire and an integrated hub for contrast injection. These devices allow for injection of contrast media without the need for guidewire removal. This approach can be very helpful in difficult cannulation for visualization of the ductal anatomy or in targeting ductal strictures with the wire under cholangiographic guidance. Sphincterotomes preloaded with a guidewire are convenient for the assistant and may accelerate the procedure (Fig. 17.1). Devices that allow the use of short guidewires are also helpful, because they reduce the length of over-the-wire exchange to a fraction of the total device length while locking the wire to reduce the risk of losing access. In addition, these short-wire systems offer the option of guidewire manipulation by the endoscopist, which can be advantageous depending on the expertise of the operator and the assistant. A short, 15-mm to 20-mm cutting wire can be precisely controlled, but it tends to orient the cutting direction toward the 2 o'clock position. Contact with the sphincter may be inadequate, thus making the cutting difficult in some situations. However, the advantage of short cutting wire over a 30-mm-long wire is the reduced risk of an uncontrolled large cut when inserted too deeply into the bile duct. In addition, the proximal part of a long cutting wire may come into contact with the elevator of the duodenoscope or overhanging duodenal folds; the former causes wire breakage when electrocautery current is applied. This problem can be overcome by use of a sphincterotome that is insulated on the proximal part of the cutting wire (Fig. 17.2). However, a recent prospective randomized controlled trial showed no significant difference between insulated and standard sphincterotome wires in terms of bleeding rates or other adverse events.[6] A thin monofilament wire provides a clean, sharp cut but may break more easily than a braided wire during application of electrocautery. On the other hand, braided wires are rarely used because they induce more thermal injury. There are no formal trials that compare the efficacy and safety of these different devices. As the endoscopists' experience grows, specific preferences develop for maintaining a limited array of accessories based on expertise, skill of assistants, and patient selection. The use of special sphincterotomes can be limited to particular cases. A device with a 4.0-Fr ultratapered tip is useful after failed cannulation using standard techniques in the setting of a small papilla, suspicion of a narrow ductal orifice, or difficulty in achieving proper cutting orientation. The latter problem can be overcome also by the use of a rotatable sphincterotome, which utilizes a specially designed handle that allows controlled tip rotation. Sphincterotomes with a tip length of more than 5 mm can occasionally be helpful when there is difficult access to the papillary orifice, as seen in patients with

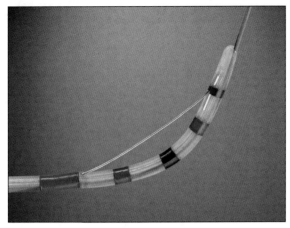

FIG 17.1 Smooth, tapered, rounded, polished tip of a sphincterotome with colored markers that allow for determination of the depth of insertion. A preloaded guidewire with a hydrophilic tip is helpful for selective cannulation. An integrated hub can be used for injection of contrast media without the need for guidewire removal.

a juxtapapillary duodenal diverticulum or altered surgical anatomy. Push-type or sigmoid-shaped sphincterotomes have been developed for EST in patients with Billroth II anatomy. A recently introduced sphincterotome combines the two steps of sphincterotomy and sphincteroplasty (balloon dilation) into one endoscopic device, which promises to simplify and accelerate the treatment of larger bile duct stones (Fig. 17.3). Malfunction of sphincterotomes infrequently occurs but can usually be managed without major adverse events.[5]

Procedure

The papilla is usually approached with the sphincterotome from a distance so that its precurved distal part can be seen exiting the endoscope. Alternatively the tip of the sphincterotome is gently introduced into the papillary orifice. A short, straight position of the duodenoscope facilitates precise control of the device. Subsequent bowing of the tip usually allows its insertion toward 11 o'clock into the opening of the common bile duct (Fig. 17.4, A, B). Straightening the tip and gently withdrawing the endoscope results in overcoming the sigmoid-type shape of the distal part of the common bile duct. A guidewire should then be gently passed in the direction of the bile duct under endoscopic and fluoroscopic guidance without contrast injection. For this approach, guidewires with a soft, preferably hydrophilic, tip should be used to reduce the risk of ductal injury (Fig. 17.5, A–E; Video 17.1). Trials

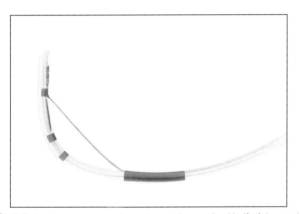

FIG 17.2 Sphincterotome with coating on the proximal half of the cutting wire.

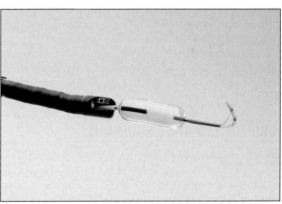

FIG 17.3 Sphincterotome with an integrated multisizing balloon that is adjustable to three controlled dilation diameters.

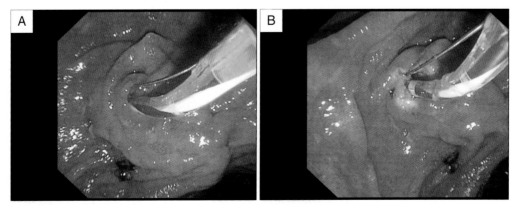

FIG 17.4 A, Approach to the papillary orifice with the tip of a slightly bowed sphincterotome to allow its insertion toward 11 o'clock into the opening of the common bile duct. The cutting wire is directed to 1 o'clock. **B,** Directing the cutting wire to 11 o'clock by pulling the sphincterotome back so that less than one-third of the wire is inside the papilla and slightly withdrawing the duodenoscope with rotation to the left side.

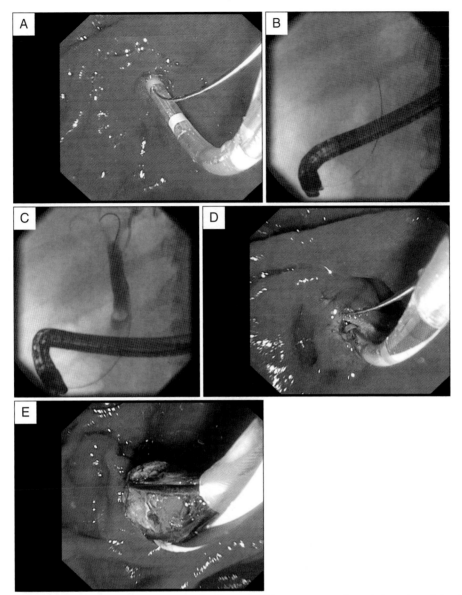

FIG 17.5 A, Close approach to the papilla with a bowed sphincterotome and gentle insertion of the tip of a hydrophilic wire toward the direction of the bile duct. **B,** Careful advancement of the wire under fluoroscopic control indicating the direction to the common bile duct. **C,** Advancement of the sphincterotome over the wire to the biliary confluence; contrast injection revealing a ductal stone below. **D,** After positioning the bent sphincterotome with a few millimeters of the cutting wire inside the papilla, cutting is directed to 11 o'clock alongside the roof of the papilla and away from a small duodenal diverticulum at the right lateral site. **E,** Extraction of the intact bile duct stone, extending force along the axis of the common bile duct; the guidewire is still in place to maintain biliary access; alternatively a basket catheter or a balloon can be inserted over the wire.

comparing different-diameter guidewires and straight or angle-tipped wires do not show significant differences in cannulation rates and incidence of PEP.[7,8] The unbowed sphincterotome can then be further advanced to achieve deep cannulation. Such a smooth, direct approach may fail and the procedure can become difficult and frustrating. Careful injection of contrast may allow visualization of the biliary anatomy for targeted guidance of the tip of the sphincterotome or insertion of a guidewire. However, repeated injections may induce edema of the papilla and increase the likelihood of PEP. Cannulation of the bile duct with a sphincterotome with or without use of a guidewire should succeed in approximately 90% of cases. Failures are mainly caused by difficult access to the papilla because of anatomic variation or previous

gastroduodenal surgery. Ampullary tumors or impacted stones creating a bulging papilla can also impair the approach to the papillary orifice or deep ductal cannulation. For these cases, lifting the roof of the papilla with the adjustable tip of the sphincterotome and using a hydrophilic guidewire are helpful in selective cannulation and controlled cutting.

When standard cannulation fails, a variety of additional techniques have been established. In case of unintended repeated cannulation of the main pancreatic duct, a guidewire with a hydrophilic tip can be inserted in the pancreas, which may facilitate straightening of an angulated course of a common channel or the distal part of the common bile duct (Fig. 17.6, *A–E*; Video 17.2). The wire can then be locked for removal and reinsertion of the sphincterotome alongside the pancreatic

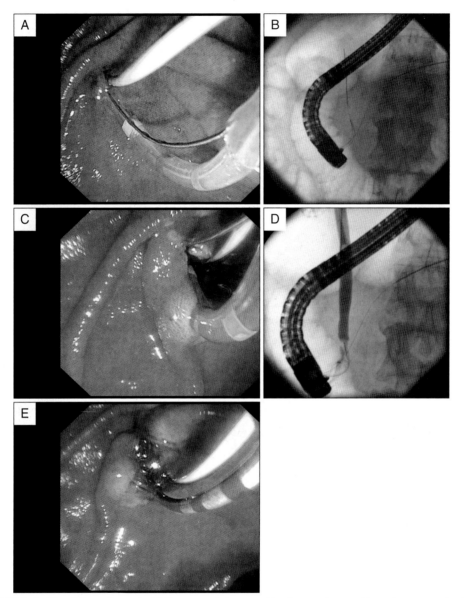

FIG 17.6 A, After failure of standard biliary cannulation, a guidewire was inserted into the pancreatic duct to prevent angulation of a common channel or the distal part of the common bile duct; the tip of the sphincterotome is redirected to 11 o'clock. **B,** Fluoroscopy showing the pancreatic duct wire in place and successful advancement of the second wire into the common bile duct followed by the sphincterotome. **C** and **D,** Endoscopic and fluoroscopic control of biliary sphincterotomy with only a short part of the cutting wire in the papilla. **E,** Biliary and pancreatic duct wires after endoscopic sphincterotomy, allowing further interventions and subsequent placement of a prophylactic pancreatic stent.

duct wire for further attempts to cannulate the bile duct (see Chapters 14 and 15). Alternatively, a 5-Fr pancreatic stent can be placed to facilitate biliary access (Fig. 17.7, *A–D*).

Precutting should be limited to cases in which there is difficult biliary cannulation and the absence of unintentional main pancreatic duct access or failure of pancreatic guidewire-assisted biliary cannulation.[9] There are three main types of precutting: needle-knife papillotomy over a pancreatic stent, or freehand without pancreatic stent placement; suprapapillary fistulotomy; and transpancreatic sphincterotomy. Details of these methods are described in Chapter 15. Precutting or persistent cannulation attempts present similar success and overall complication rates. The incidence of PEP does not increase or is even less frequent when early precut is performed.[9–13]

The appropriate use of these advanced techniques allows access to the biliary system in nearly all cases. A recent prospective cohort study of a single tertiary-care center demonstrated that the overall success of ERCP-guided cannulation was 99.4% of 518 patients in whom the ampulla was reached.[14] However, the risk of adverse events increases, in particular when "access" papillotomy is performed, which should therefore be limited to experienced endoscopists who achieve selective biliary cannulation with standard cannulation techniques in more than 80% of cases.[9]

After deep cannulation has been confirmed by contrast injection, a guidewire should be advanced to the proximal biliary system in order to secure ductal access for subsequent maneuvers and exchange of accessories. Short-wire technology allows fixation of the wire with the

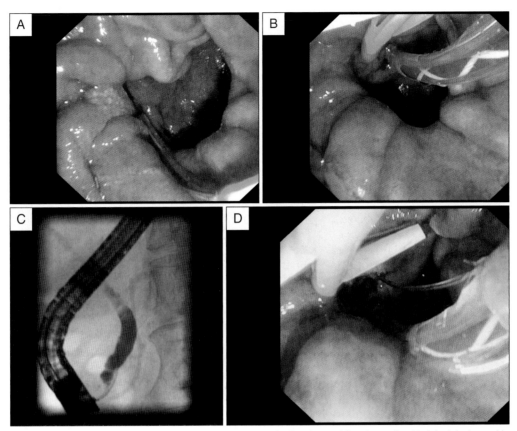

FIG 17.7 A, Exposing the papilla inside a duodenal diverticulum by pushing the wall at 7 o'clock below with the tip of a sphincterotome. **B,** The sphincterotome can be directed to the common bile duct after placement of a 5-Fr pancreatic stent. **C,** Fluoroscopy showing opacification of the common bile duct, revealing a ductal stone. **D,** Biliary endoscopic sphincterotomy within the diverticulum; alternatively balloon dilation would be justified in this difficult anatomy.

locking device attached to the duodenoscope. The tip of the sphincterotome is then slightly bowed so that it is in contact with the roof of the papilla. Stiff shaft guidewires deeply inserted into the biliary tree may limit bowing of the cutting wire. This infrequent problem can be overcome by withdrawing the guidewire until its flexible tip approaches the papilla, without losing biliary access. When performing the sphincterotomy, 5 mm or less of the cutting wire should be inside the papilla so that only a small amount of tissue will be cauterized. This approach enhances the incision and avoids a rapid, large incision ("zipper cut") that can occur when pure cutting current is used. The use of newer electrosurgical generators (see Chapter 11) has largely eliminated zipper cuts. Most sphincterotomes have endoscopically visible markers positioned at the distal part of the catheter, which allow one to determine the depth of insertion of the cutting wire into the bile duct. It is generally believed that orientation of the cutting wire between the 11 o'clock and 1 o'clock positions reduces the likelihood of bleeding and perforation. In spite of great efforts by accessory manufacturers to develop sphincterotomes with cutting wires that automatically cut along these directions, the devices may sometimes still orient in a 2 o'clock direction. In selective cases, a rotatable sphincterotome is helpful in achieving proper orientation. For appropriate cutting direction, the papilla has to be placed on the left side, preferably along the 11 o'clock position. This maneuver can be facilitated in difficult cases by rotating the left-right dial to the left while advancing the duodenoscope slightly into the "long" endoscope position (Fig. 17.8, *A–D*; Video 17.3). Alternatively the endoscope can be carefully withdrawn along with rotation to the left side (see Fig. 17.4, *B*).

The choice of electrosurgical current for EST is a source of controversy.[9,15,16] The combination of high cutting current with low coagulation current is most frequently used. Creation of edematous, extensively whitened or blackened tissue during EST is evidence of suboptimal cutting and may increase the risk of PEP or sphincter stenosis. Excessive cautery also occurs when an excessive amount of cutting wire is inside the papilla and/or contact of the wire with the tissue of the papillary roof is inadequate. Previous trials suggest that pure-cut electrocautery current is safer than blended current in terms of PEP without increasing the bleeding rate.[17,18] However, a recent meta-analysis of four randomized controlled trials showed that there was no significant difference between the rate of PEP when pure current was used and when blended current was used. Pure cutting current was associated with more episodes of bleeding.[19] When pure cutting current is used by less-experienced hands, there may be a higher risk of bleeding and perforation, especially when a longer part of the cutting wire is inside the papilla, which can lead to a fast, uncontrolled large cut (i.e., zipper cut). In a small trial, the combined technique of beginning the incision using cutting current and finishing using blended current was not associated with a decrease in the risk of PEP.[20] An alternative electrocautery option is the use of the Endocut mode (ERBE, Tübingen, Germany) or Pulsecut mode (Olympus, Tokyo, Japan) using electrosurgical generators, in which cutting and coagulation current are alternated in short bursts by intrinsic software (see Chapter 11). A potential advantage of this technology is a stepwise cutting action that allows precise control of the direction and length of the incision. This replaces the technique in which current is applied in short pulses controlled by foot pedal activation and is

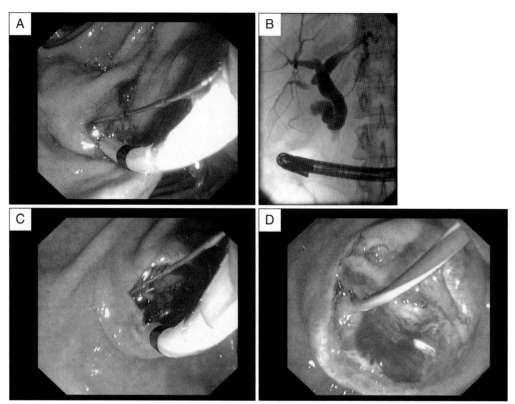

FIG 17.8 A, After tip insertion the cutting wire of the sphincterotome is bowing toward 3 o'clock. **B,** Fluoroscopy after rotation of the dial of the duodenoscope to the left while advancing the scope slightly toward the long scope position. **C,** Due to the maneuver shown in Figure 17.8B, the cutting wire is bowing toward 11 o'clock, allowing incision of the papilla in the optimal direction. **D,** The guidewire was left in place after complete sphincterotomy with exposure of the cut redish sphincter muscle.

recommended for pure-cut or conventional blended current to reduce the risk of a zipper cut. A large retrospective analysis suggested that microprocessor-controlled EST is associated with a significantly lower frequency of intraprocedural bleeding but had no impact on clinically evident bleeding.[21] On the other hand, a recent randomized controlled study of EST in 360 patients showed no significant difference between the Endocut mode and conventional blended cut mode in terms of success, adverse events, and procedural duration.[22]

The size of EST can vary and depends on the diameter of the distal portion of the common bile duct and the indication for sphincterotomy. During cutting, pressure on the papillary roof should be applied by upward lifting of the slightly bowed sphincterotome or by maneuvering the tip of the duodenoscope. EST should be continued only when the wire can be clearly seen and when it is directed between the 11 and 1 o'clock positions. Guidance and repositioning of the device should be mainly controlled with the tip and the shaft of the endoscope, which is maneuvered with the right hand of the operator like the handle of a knife. A small incision seems to be appropriate for stent placement in the setting of malignant biliary obstruction, whereas complete splitting of the sphincter should be attempted for treatment of bile duct stones and sphincter of Oddi dysfunction (SOD) to decrease the risk of recurrences and EST-related stenosis of the papilla. However, there are no data demonstrating a correlation between the length of cutting and the incidence of early or late adverse events of EST. Biliary sphincterotomy should be limited to the junction between the duodenal wall and the intraduodenal portion of the papilla of Vater, which is sometimes difficult to determine because there is no reliable endoscopic landmark. The incision is also complete if the inner lumen of the bile duct is completely visible or the bowed tip of the sphincterotome can be pulled through

the papilla without resistance. In view of modern techniques of lithotripsy and the option to combine EST with large-diameter sphincteroplasty, a large, potentially hazardous EST is not required. If a wide opening to the common bile duct is needed, it may be safer to perform a small to moderate-sized incision and then dilate the orifice with a balloon catheter rather than to increase the size by cutting (Video 17.4) (see Chapter 18). Compared with other indications, the risk of adverse events of EST is usually low in patients with a dilated common bile duct and in the presence of ductal stones, especially when the papilla is large and protruding because of an impacted stone.

Extension of a previous biliary sphincterotomy may be required for the treatment of recurrent bile duct stones or recurrence of symptoms after SOD. The technique of EST in this setting does not differ from when EST is performed initially. Data from anecdotal reports and small case series suggested that the incidence of bleeding was increased during a postsphincterotomy period of approximately 1 week because of a resultant increased vascularity. However, large prospective studies did not show extension of a previous EST to be an independent risk factor for hemorrhage.[23,24] Nevertheless, the risk of severe bleeding or duodenal perforation should be considered. Although it may not be related to previous EST, extension of the incision should be carefully performed in a stepwise manner. Sphincteroplasty could be a safer alternative, at least in cases with a difficult orientation and control of the cutting wire.[25]

EST in Patients With Difficult Anatomy

Juxtapapillary duodenal diverticula are found in 10% to 20% of patients undergoing ERCP.[26,27] Depending on the location of the papilla, cannulation of the bile duct can be difficult and may require special techniques, such as insertion of the tip of the endoscope into the diverticulum, use of a sphincterotome with a long nose, or pulling the papilla out of a diverticulum with biopsy forceps or a second catheter. Pancreatic duct stent placement and precut sphincterotomy or needle-knife fistulotomy are suitable alternative options to achieve cannulation.[9] After successful biliary access, it is strongly recommended to perform EST with a biliary guidewire in place. This facilitates cutting in the direction of the bile duct, which may otherwise be difficult to determine because of the altered anatomy. Moderate bending of the tip of the sphincterotome with a few millimeters of the cutting wire inside the papilla exposes the papillary roof to allow for a controlled incision. Any direction of the cutting wire toward the base of the diverticulum should be avoided (see Fig. 17.5, D). Data from a large retrospective analysis suggested that juxtapapillary duodenal diverticula is an independent risk factor for bleeding after EST.[26]

The approach to patients with postsurgical anatomy is discussed further in Chapter 31. Use of a duodenoscope in patients with Billroth II anatomy allows better visualization of the papillary roof and improves the maneuverability of accessories because of the availability of the elevator (Fig. 17.9, A). Precurved sphincterotomes should not be used for initial cannulation of the bile duct in these patients because they direct the tip of the catheter toward the pancreatic duct orifice. This is because the papilla is rotated 180 degrees compared with native anatomy. A straight, previously unused ERCP cannula and a straight guidewire with a hydrophilic tip aim in the direction of the bile duct and facilitate entry into the biliary orifice (see Fig. 17.9, B, C; Video 17.5). After successful placement of guidewire, a rotatable push-type or sigmoid-shaped sphincterotome can be used for EST. In spite of use of these special accessories, the correct direction of the cutting wire toward the desired 5 o'clock position (in this situation) can remain difficult because of the reversed anatomic orientation (see Fig. 17.9, D, E). It is usually easier to place a straight 7-Fr biliary stent and to sever the papillary roof with a needle-knife incision using the stent as a guide.[28] A combination of limited EST with a large papillary balloon dilation seems to be effective and safe in Billroth II patients for removal of bile duct stones (see Fig. 17.9, F; see Video 17.4).[29] A similar approach is required when performing EST in the setting of loop gastrojejunostomy (used for patients with duodenal or pyloric obstruction).

Reaching the papilla with a duodenoscope in patients with Roux-en-Y anatomy is usually not possible. The approach in these patients is to use a pediatric colonoscope or a balloon-assisted enteroscope.[30] However, therapeutic interventions are impaired because of the limited transmission of manipulations via the long insertion tube and the limited array of available accessories for these endoscopes based upon length and diameter of the working channel.

If the papilla is inaccessible because of altered anatomy or cannot be cannulated even after precut techniques, a rendezvous method should be considered. For a percutaneous route a transhepatic tract is established with placement of a 7-Fr catheter into the common bile duct. Thereafter, duodenoscopy is repeated. A percutaneously inserted 400-cm-long guidewire is antegradely passed through the papilla and grasped endoscopically with a snare passed through the endoscope. In cases where there is a long afferent loop, this technique allows one to pull the tip of the endoscope toward the papilla by applying tension on the guidewire simultaneously from the percutaneous portion of the wire and the wire exiting the endoscope. The sphincterotome is passed over the guidewire for subsequent EST. In selected cases, the sphincterotome can be percutaneously inserted for the performance of antegrade sphincterotomy under endoscopic retrograde visualization.[31] EUS-guided biliary drainage (Chapter 32) offers an effective and safe alternative to percutaneous procedures, with technical success rates ranging from 70% to 100% and adverse event rates of 3% to 77%.[32] Comparative studies of percutaneously assisted and EUS-guided procedures for

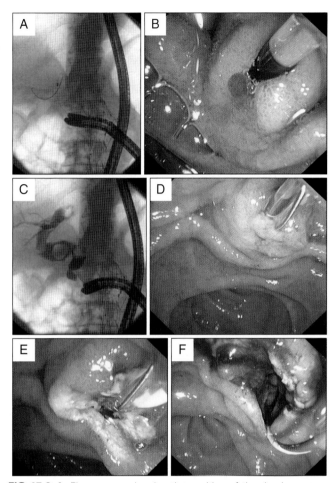

FIG 17.9 A, Fluoroscopy showing the position of the duodenoscope, with the tip in projection to the second part of the duodenum in a patient with a Billroth II anatomy. B, Cannulation of the common bile duct with a straight ERCP catheter directed to 5 o'clock. C, Retrograde cholangiography reveals a dilated common bile duct with several large stones. D, Successful insertion of a rotatable sphincterotome with a correct position of the cutting wire toward 5 o'clock. E, Opening of the biliary orifice after a limited sphincterotomy. F, Wide opening after additional sphincteroplasty, facilitating treatment and extraction of the large bile duct stones.

achieving biliary access after failed ERCP show conflicting results.[9] The selection of the appropriate method should be made with respect to local expertise and availability.

In rare cases, even rendezvous methods do not allow an endoscopic approach to the papilla. Antegrade sphincterotomy under percutaneous transhepatic cholangioscopic and fluoroscopic guidance can be performed, though this technique is potentially hazardous and should be restricted to centers with extensive expertise in percutaneous transhepatic interventions.

Alternatives to EST

Balloon sphincteroplasty is discussed in detail in Chapter 18. Compared with EST, endoscopic papillary balloon dilation (EPBD) offers the theoretical advantage of sphincter preservation, particularly in young patients with bile duct stones. In addition, it avoids postprocedural bleeding. Treatment of bile duct stones is considered the only indication for EPBD as an alternative to EST. Three recent meta-analyses demonstrated similar stone extraction rates for EST and EPBD.[33–35] Balloon dilation alone seems to require mechanical lithotripsy for stone removal more frequently than EST. There is no significant difference between either technique in overall rates of adverse events. However, EPBD is associated with a higher incidence of PEP and a lower rate of postprocedural bleeding compared with EST.[34,35] Because of the increased risk of pancreatitis in Western countries, recommendations are to limit EPBD without a concomitant EST except in selected patients, in particular those with coagulopathies or a difficult access to the papilla (e.g., Billroth II anatomy or a duodenal diverticulum).

Technical details of EPBD may also influence the clinical outcome. The procedure has not yet been standardized in terms of the inflation pressure, the duration of inflation, and the number of dilations. A recent meta-analysis and a randomized trial with a limited number of patients showed that papillary dilation for 5 minutes improves efficacy of stone extraction and reduces the risk of pancreatitis compared with conventional 1-minute EPBD.[33,36] However, further studies are needed to determine the optimal duration of EPBD.[37] Biliary sphincter function may be preserved with use of EPBD. It promises less duodenobiliary reflux, with the potential for reduced risk of cholangitis and formation of recurrent bile duct stones. A recent meta-analysis demonstrated lower long-term morbidity of EPBD compared with EST.[35] The incidence of stone recurrence after EPBD seems to be lower in patients with small stones in particular.[38]

Several meta-analyses and additional recent randomized controlled trials indicated that in contrast to the potential risks of EPBD alone, the combination of EST and EPBD is as effective and safe as EST alone, with significantly less need for mechanical lithotripsy in the treatment of bile duct stones.[39,40] Further details were recently reviewed in international consensus guidelines for EPBD and are discussed in Chapter 18 (see Video 17.4).[37]

INDICATIONS

Well-established indications for EST are common bile duct stones, acute cholangitis, severe acute biliary pancreatitis, palliation of ampullary malignancies, facilitation of biliary stent placement, and treatment of SOD types I and II (Box 17.1). Choledocholithiasis is still one of the major indications for biliary sphincterotomy in order to allow endoscopic stone extraction using basket or balloon catheters. The success rate of ductal clearance for standard procedures is approximately 90% depending on patient selection.[41,42] Adjunctive techniques for intracorporeal (intraductal) or extracorporeal lithotripsy further increase the clearance rates.[43] EST can be safely and effectively performed for the treatment of bile duct stones even in patients 90 years of age or older.[44,45] Previous restrictions of EST to elderly patients or those with previous

cholecystectomy are no longer valid. In a prospective US multicenter trial on EST, a group of 487 patients underwent sphincterotomy for bile duct stones within 30 days of laparoscopic cholecystectomy. Patients were significantly younger (on average 51 vs 64 years) and the common bile duct was smaller in diameter (8.7 vs 10.0 mm) compared with a group of 1113 patients with their gallbladder in situ or with previous cholecystectomy who underwent EST for the same indication. The adverse event rate of EST was significantly lower in the former group (4.9% vs 9.5%).[23] These results demonstrate that EST can be safely performed in young patients with bile duct stones shortly before, during, or after laparoscopic cholecystectomy. In this context, timing of EST should be coordinated between laparoscopic surgeons and endoscopists and often depends on local expertise and access to the required interventions. A recent systematic review and a meta-analysis of randomized controlled trials showed that intraoperative EST is as safe and effective as preoperative EST in patients with gallbladder and common bile duct stones and results in a significantly shorter hospital stay.[46,47] Preoperative EST for removal of bile duct stones followed by early laparoscopic cholecystectomy (within 72 hours) is associated with significantly fewer biliary events compared with a delayed operation after 6 to 8 weeks.[48]

Acute cholangitis caused by choledocholithiasis or ductal stenosis can be effectively treated by EST in conjunction with additional procedures such as removal of ductal stones or placement of drainage catheters or stents. Early EST has also been established in patients with severe acute biliary pancreatitis (see Chapter 50). A recent meta-analysis of 11 randomized controlled trials consisting of 1314 patients showed a significantly lower overall adverse event rate in patients who underwent EST compared with those who were treated conservatively (odds ratio 0.32).[49] There was a nonsignificant decrease in mortality for the ERCP group. In those with mild disease, a strong trend toward decreased complications in the ERCP group was seen. In a recent review it was stated that there is no role for early ERCP in patients with (predicted) mild biliary pancreatitis to improve outcome. However, regardless of pancreatitis severity, urgent EST is recommended in the presence of concomitant cholangitis.[50] A retrospective review of EST as a definitive treatment for gallstone pancreatitis in 101 high–surgical risk patients showed this approach to be a safe alternative to laparoscopic cholecystectomy to prevent further attacks of pancreatitis.[51]

Another potential indication for EST is biliary sphincterotomy as an initial therapeutic step before dilation and/or stent placement for treatment of biliary obstruction. However, sphincterotomy is not obligatory unless multiple large-bore stents are inserted, in particular for management of postoperative biliary strictures (see Chapter 43).[52] A small cut seems to be safe and is frequently performed to facilitate access to the biliary system for scheduled exchanges of plastic prostheses. A meta-analysis of three randomized controlled trials showed that EST reduced the incidence of PEP but caused a higher incidence of post-ERCP bleeding in patients with malignant biliary obstruction.[53] Another systematic review and meta-analysis did not show a significant difference when EST was used for stent placement for distal bile duct obstruction compared with no EST. However, this trial demonstrated a risk reduction in PEP when EST was performed before stenting for biliary leaks,[54] as had been shown in prior retrospective studies. A recent large randomized controlled trial showed no benefit of EST before implantation of self-expandable metal stents in patients with unresectable pancreatic cancer.[55] EST had no impact on the incidence of adverse events, stent patency, or patient survival times. The role of EST before placement of self-expandable metal stents (SEMS) for other indications remains to be determined.

Biliary sphincterotomy has become the method of choice for the treatment of patients with documented SOD (see Chapter 47). However, in a large randomized controlled multicenter trial, EST did not reduce

---

BOX 17.1 Indications for Biliary Endoscopic Sphincterotomy

- Common bile duct stones
- Facilitation of biliary stent placement (especially multiple stents) for malignant or benign common bile duct obstruction in selected cases
- Palliation of obstruction caused by malignant ampullary neoplasm as alternative to stent placement in selected cases
- Sphincter of Oddi dysfunction types 1 and 2, benign papillary stenosis
- Biliary leaks
- Miscellaneous conditions (choledochocele, sump syndrome, biliary parasites)
- Access for peroral choledochoscopy and/or ERCP-guided tissue acquisition
- Access for cannulation of the main pancreatic duct after failure of standard cannulation techniques

disability caused by pain compared with a sham procedure in patients with abdominal pain after cholecystectomy.[56] These conclusions apply to patients with SOD type III (see Chapter 47). Further studies of EST for type II SOD patients seem justified. Cannulation and cutting can be more difficult in patients with SOD compared with other indications for sphincterotomy because of small size of the papilla and a narrow orifice. Atraumatic cannulation of the papilla, careful manipulation of accessories, and precise control of the sphincterotomy incision while cutting over a guidewire are mandatory to minimize trauma to the tissue. For these reasons and because of the increased risks, only experienced endoscopists should perform EST for SOD. The increased risk of PEP can be significantly lowered by prophylactic placement of a 3-Fr or 5-Fr pancreatic stent.[57,58] Additionally, preprocedural rectal indomethacin should be considered to prevent pancreatitis in these patients.[59] However, the recent data question the efficacy of rectal nonsteroidal antiinflammatory drugs (NSAIDs) in unselected cohorts.[58]

The level of evidence is lower for a variety of other indications for EST, which are listed in Box 17.1. Most of these indications have been established on the basis of prospective uncontrolled trials or appropriate retrospective analyses. Randomized controlled trials are difficult to perform for many of these biliary disorders in particular because of low case volumes.

CONTRAINDICATIONS

Contraindications to ERCP and EST include an uncooperative or unstable patient, inability of the patient to provide informed consent, uncorrected coagulopathy, and passage of the endoscope through a newly created gastrointestinal anastomosis. Contrast hypersensitivity is not considered as a contraindication to EST, but prophylactic intravenous administration of corticosteroids may be considered. Preprocedure coagulation studies should be obtained in patients with known or suspected coagulopathy or bleeding disorders and must be corrected before sphincterotomy. The presence of Child's A cirrhosis and use of aspirin or other NSAIDs do not appear to be important predictors of bleeding.[23] However, antiplatelet drugs such as clopidogrel and ticlopidine should be interrupted for at least 7 days before elective sphincterotomy, depending on the individual clinical risks (see Chapters 7 and 10). EST using a pull sphincterotome should not be performed if proper positioning of the sphincterotome with its tip in the bile duct cannot be achieved. Cutting should be avoided if the position of the cutting wire cannot be seen or if the tip of the sphincterotome is bowing in the wrong direction because of difficult anatomy. If these problems cannot be resolved with changing the position of the device or other maneuvers, then balloon dilation of the biliary sphincter should be considered as an alternative to EST. The indication for EST should be reconsidered for the individual case if the level of evidence is fair or poor.

ADVERSE EVENTS AND THEIR MANAGEMENT (SEE CHAPTER 8)

A large prospective US multicenter trial reported a total adverse event rate of EST of 9.8% in 2347 patients (Table 17.1).[23] Acute pancreatitis was the most frequent major adverse event of EST and was seen in 5.4% of all cases. Hemorrhage, perforation, cholangitis, and cholecystitis occur less frequently and may be lower than previously reported. Another prospective multicenter trial of ERCP and related risk factors has been published, though in contrast to the study by Freeman et al., diagnostic procedures were also included.[23,60] The reported data do not allow a separate analysis of EST-related morbidity.[60]

Various risk factors, prophylactic measures, early recognition, and appropriate treatment should be considered to decrease the risks of EST. In an individual patient it may be difficult to determine whether complications were caused by EST, by bile duct cannulation, or by adjunctive therapeutic interventions.

EST-Related Post-ERCP Pancreatitis

Two definitions of PEP are currently used: the consensus definition and grading of severity of PEP according to Cotton et al. and the more recent revised Atlanta international consensus definition and classification of acute pancreatitis.[61–63] According to the Atlanta classification, the diagnosis of PEP requires two of the three following criteria: abdominal pain consistent with acute pancreatitis, serum lipase or amylase levels ≥3 times the upper limit of normal for the laboratory, and characteristic findings of acute pancreatitis on imaging. Pancreatitis is the most frequent adverse event after ERCP, with an incidence of 3.5% in unselected patients.[63] It is of mild or moderate severity in approximately 90% of patients. Definitive patient-related risk factors for PEP are suspected SOD, female gender, and previous pancreatitis. Precut sphincterotomy and pancreatic injection were analyzed as definitive procedure-related parameters that have been associated with an increased risk of PEP. EST-related risk factors that were identified in a multivariate analysis of the study by Freeman et al. are summarized in Table 17.2.[23] These parameters and preventive measures should be considered when patients are selected for EST in order to reduce the risk of PEP.

A variety of electrosurgical factors can influence the efficacy and safety of EST (see Chapter 11).[5,9,15] They include different waveforms and power settings of modern electrosurgical generators, but also the

---

TABLE 17.1   Complications of Biliary Endoscopic Sphincterotomy in 2347 Patients

Type of Complication	Incidence (%)	Severe Complications	Fatal Complications
Pancreatitis	5.4	0.4	<0.1
Hemorrhage	2.0	0.5	0.1
Perforation	0.3	0.2	<0.1
Cholangitis	1.0	0.1	<0.1
Cholecystitis	0.5	0.1	<0.1
Miscellaneous	1.1	0.3	0.2
Total	**9.8**	**1.6**	**0.4**

Data from Freeman ML, Nelson DB, Sherman S, et al. Complications of endoscopic biliary sphincterotomy. *N Engl J Med.* 1996;335:909–918.

TABLE 17.2   Risk Factors for EST-Related Pancreatitis

	Adjusted Odds Ratio* (95% CI)
Suspected SOD	5.1 (2.7 ± 9.2)
Precut EST	4.3 (1.7 ± 10.9)
Difficulty of cannulation	2.4 (1.1 ± 5.4)
Younger age	2.1 (1.4 ± 3.3)
Repeated pancreatic duct injection	1.4 (1.0 ± 1.8)

CI, Confidence interval; *EST,* endoscopic sphincterotomy; *SOD,* sphincter of Oddi dysfunction.
*Significant in a multivariate analysis.
Data from Freeman ML, Nelson DB, Sherman S, et al. Complications of endoscopic biliary sphincterotomy. *N Engl J Med.* 1996;335:909–918.

cutting wire contact length. The clinical relevance of these factors remains unclear. In view of conflicting results, the selection of electrosurgical current for biliary EST can be based primarily on endoscopist preference.

The impact of prophylactic pancreatic stent placement on the prevention of PEP was recently reviewed and evaluated in a meta-analysis.[64] The analysis of 10 randomized controlled trials showed that prophylactic pancreatic stents decreased the odds of PEP (odds ratio, 0.22; $p < 0.01$). The absolute risk difference was 13.3%. The number needed to treat was eight. Stents also decreased the level of hyperamylasemia. Similar findings were also noted from 10 nonrandomized studies. Although these data do not allow a separate analysis for EST, pancreatic stent placement is strongly recommended in patients undergoing EST with risk factors for PEP.[63]

Treatment of EST-related pancreatitis does not differ from the management of pancreatitis of other etiologies. Repeat ERCP should be considered in patients with residual bile duct stones, ongoing obstructive jaundice, or cholangitis.

EST-Related Hemorrhage

Clinically relevant hemorrhage can be defined as the presence of melena, hematochezia, or hematemesis associated with a hemoglobin decrease of at least 2 g/dL or the need for blood transfusion. The incidence of EST-related bleeding in prospective trials ranges from 0.8% to 2%.[23,65–67] In approximately half of the cases hemorrhage is delayed and occurs at 24 hours, though it can occur up to 1 week or more after EST. Risk factors for hemorrhage include coagulopathy before EST, therapeutic anticoagulation within 3 days after EST, cholangitis before EST, and bleeding during EST (Table 17.3). In addition, EST performed by endoscopists who perform fewer than approximately one EST per week is associated with a higher rate of bleeding compared with those performed by endoscopists with higher EST volumes.[23] A multivariate analysis of an Italian multicenter trial found precut procedures and obstruction of the papillary orifice as risk factors for EST-related hemorrhage.[59] The pattern of bleeding after EST during the procedure did not seem to predict the risk of delayed bleeding.[68] A recent retrospective analysis showed rebleeding in 22% of 35 patients after initial successful endoscopic hemostasis for delayed post-EST bleeding.[69] Malignant biliary stricture, serum bilirubin level of greater than 10 mg/dL, initial bleeding severity, and bleeding diathesis were significant predictors of rebleeding.

Oozing bleeding after EST frequently stops spontaneously and further therapeutic interventions can usually be performed without the need for hemostasis. However, ongoing hemorrhage or pulsatile bleeding,

TABLE 17.3   Risk Factors for EST-Related Hemorrhage[23]

	Adjusted Odds Ratio* (95% CI)
Anticoagulation ≤3 days after EST	5.1 (1.6 ± 16.7)
Coagulopathy before EST	3.3 (1.5 ± 7.2)
Cholangitis before EST	2.6 (1.4 ± 4.9)
Mean Case Volume of the Endoscopist	
≤1 EST/week	2.2 (1.1 ± 4.2)
Bleeding during EST	1.7 (1.2 ± 2.7)

EST, Endoscopic sphincterotomy; *SOD,* sphincter of Oddi dysfunction.
*Significant in a multivariate analysis.

which arises from an aberrant branch of the retroduodenal artery, requires endoscopic hemostasis. Repeated duodenal irrigation is mandatory for endoscopic localization of the bleeding site and to facilitate application of appropriate hemostatic interventions. The cutting wire of a sphincterotome can be used to apply pure coagulation to the apex of the bleeding site. Endoscopic injection of saline-epinephrine solution or fibrin glue at the proximal edge of the incision site is usually effective at achieving hemostasis in the setting of severe hemorrhage.[70] Multipolar or bipolar electrocoagulation is another option to treat hemorrhage, but should be carefully performed at an appropriate distance from the pancreatic orifice to prevent PEP; alternatively, pancreatic drainage can be secured with a pancreatic duct stent.[71–73] Placement of conventional endoclips through a side-viewing endoscope is technically difficult.[74] Bending of the tip and lifting of the elevator of the instrumentation channel should be minimized to allow release of the clips from the rigid applicator tip. Hemostasis can be also effectively achieved with cap-assisted endoclip application by use of forward-viewing endoscopes.[75] Placement of a biliary endoprosthesis or a nasobiliary drain should be considered if interventions for hemostasis cause obstruction of the common bile duct. In a small case series, covered SEMS allowed for hemostasis of uncontrolled post-EST bleeding.[76]

In rare cases endoscopic management of EST-related hemorrhage fails; angiographic transcatheter embolization or even laparotomy may be required, though the latter is associated with significant morbidity and mortality.[77]

EST-Related Perforation

Perforation of the bile duct or the pancreatic duct with the sphincterotome, guidewire, balloon, or other accessories can usually be managed by endoscopic or percutaneous placement of drainage catheters or stents into the bile duct and pancreatic duct. EST-related retroduodenal perforations are uncommon and mainly caused by "zipper cutting," which can be avoided by limited insertion of the cutting wire into the papilla and use of modern controlled-cut electrosurgical generators. Perforation occurs when EST is performed beyond the duodenal wall. Reported perforation rates for ERCP are between 0.3% to 0.6% and that related specifically to EST is 0.3%.[23,78] A univariate analysis of a recent retrospective trial indicated that EST, SOD, a dilated common bile duct, and biliary stricture dilation are risk factors for perforation.[78] Most cases are diagnosed intraprocedurally by the finding of free intraabdominal or retroperitoneal air on fluoroscopy, or postprocedurally on plain abdominal radiographs or CT scan. Clinical presentation is variable and can be mild. Perforation should be considered in cases of ongoing abdominal pain, signs of peritonitis, fever, leukocytosis, and an elevated C-reactive protein. Abdominal CT scan with luminal contrast into the duodenum is the method of choice for diagnosis and stratification for management. Conservative treatment with temporary parenteral nutrition and administration of antibiotics is appropriate if an ongoing leak is excluded. Otherwise an interdisciplinary approach should be employed.[79] A nasoduodenal tube and a nasobiliary or percutaneous transhepatic drain are useful to prevent gastric, pancreatic, and biliary fluid from entering into the retroperitoneal space. Closures of EST-related perforations of the duodenum or the bile duct can be attempted by placement of covered self-expanding biliary metal stents (Fig. 17.10, A–D).[80,81] Percutaneous drainage with large-bore tubes is indicated in cases of abscess formation in the retroperitoneum. Laparotomy is usually required when these measurements fail and/or there is evidence of sepsis or peritonitis.[82]

EST-Related Cholangitis

Prophylactic administration of antibiotics to prevent cholangitis is recommended for patients with incomplete biliary drainage, particularly

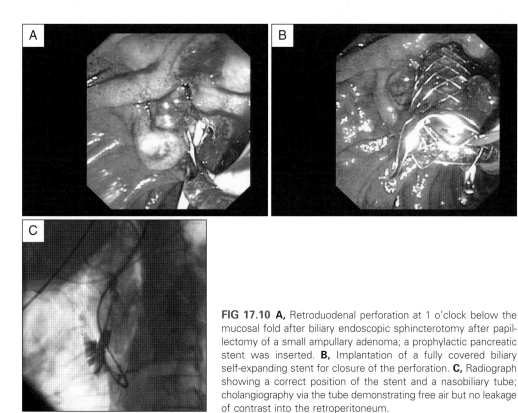

FIG 17.10 A, Retroduodenal perforation at 1 o'clock below the mucosal fold after biliary endoscopic sphincterotomy after papillectomy of a small ampullary adenoma; a prophylactic pancreatic stent was inserted. **B,** Implantation of a fully covered biliary self-expanding stent for closure of the perforation. **C,** Radiograph showing a correct position of the stent and a nasobiliary tube; cholangiography via the tube demonstrating free air but no leakage of contrast into the retroperitoneum.

for those patients with proximal stenoses caused by hilar tumors and for patients with primary sclerosing cholangitis (see Chapters 10 and 48). Nasobiliary catheters or endoprostheses should be placed when there is incomplete bile duct clearance after EST or adjunctive interventions for biliary stones. Repeated ERCP may be needed in cases of delayed cholangitis caused by biliary obstruction. Continuous bile duct irrigation via nasobiliary drains may be useful for management of selected patients with purulent cholangitis.

Long-Term Consequences of EST

Five studies comprising a large number of patients, with high follow-up rates and follow-up periods of more than 6 years after EST, have been previously reviewed.[33] The overall rate of late symptoms that can be attributed to EST ranges from 6% to 24%, with the rate being nearly 10% in three of the five trials. Common bile duct stones and papillary stenosis were the most common adverse events. Stones can usually be removed after extension of the previous EST or after balloon dilation. Papillary stenosis can be managed by extension of the sphincterotomy, with or without placement of biliary stents. A recent retrospective analysis showed that 16% of 80 patients developed ampullary restenosis during a median follow-up period of 16 months after EST. Repeat biliary EST was successful in 12/13 patients, with adverse events occurring in 3.[84] A Swedish population-based study showed an incidence of recurrent bile duct stones of 4.1% in 964 patients after EST for choledocholithiasis within a mean follow-up period of 8.9 years.[85] A 4-year extended follow-up of a randomized trial revealed recurrence of bile duct stones after endoscopic sphincteroplasty and sphincterotomy in 8% of 106 patients.[86] Cautery-induced distal bile duct strictures can be managed by balloon dilation and placement of one or more biliary stents.[87] Cholangitis caused by reflux of duodenal contents into the biliary system is rare but can occasionally require surgery for creation of a biliodigestive anastomosis. A correlation between the size of EST and these late complications cannot be determined from the current literature. Concerns about long-term biliary carcinogenic risks after sphincterotomy were not demonstrated in a large case-controlled Scandinavian study.[88]

The complete reference list for this chapter can be found online at www.expertconsult.com.

18

Balloon Dilation of the Native and Postsphincterotomy Papilla

Chan Sup Shim

Endoscopic sphincterotomy (EST; see Chapter 17) has become the procedure of choice for removal of stones from the bile duct, especially in postcholecystectomy patients.[1,2] The procedure is successful in 90% to 98% of patients, and 86% to 91% of all bile duct stones can be extracted using EST and balloon/basket extraction.[3–5]

In this chapter, we will discuss endoscopic balloon dilation with and without sphincterotomy. Small-diameter balloon dilation (≤10 mm) alone is performed in a different patient population (often young patients) for extraction of small stones, whereas large-diameter balloon dilation (≥12 mm), with or without EST, is performed for removal of large stones (often in elderly patients). Thus the risk profiles and techniques are markedly different.

Large stones, barrel-shaped stones, and tapering of the lower common bile duct (CBD) can make extraction difficult,[6] and in such cases other techniques, such as mechanical lithotripsy, are required. The success rate for removal of large, difficult stones using EST and mechanical lithotripsy is 79% to 98%.[7–11] However, EST is associated with adverse events such as bleeding, pancreatitis, and perforation (see Chapters 8 and 17),[12–14] and concerns about permanent damage to sphincter function have led to the proposal and investigation of alternatives to sphincterotomy.

Endoscopic papillary balloon dilation (EPBD) is an alternative to EST for removal of bile duct stones.[15–18] In an effort to avoid permanent destruction of the biliary sphincter, EPBD was suggested by early investigators, such as Staritz and Meyer zum Buschenfelde, who first reported it in 1983.[19] EPBD is performed to enlarge the opening of the bile duct at the level of the biliary sphincter. The main advantage is avoidance of cutting the biliary sphincter. Therefore acute adverse events such as bleeding and perforation should be less likely, with preservation of function of the biliary sphincter.[16]

The enthusiasm over the potential advantages of EPBD over EST for avoiding short-term adverse events of bleeding and perforation while preserving the biliary sphincter and possibly reducing the long-term sequelae of EST was soon dampened by reports of serious postprocedure pancreatitis (PEP).[20] Therefore EPBD was nearly abandoned as a treatment for bile duct stones, but its use was revived with the development of laparoscopic cholecystectomy. With several groups reporting favorable results using EPBD for stone extraction, conservation of the biliary sphincter regained popularity in the 1990s. In 1995 Mac Mathuna et al. reported good results with EPBD for treating bile duct stones in 100 consecutively treated patients.[15,16]

The results of subsequent randomized controlled trials comparing EST to EPBD are conflicting. Some authors have reported an increased incidence of PEP, whereas others have not, and an argument has been presented against EPBD and its failure to provide adequate access for extracting difficult (large or multiple) bile duct stones.[17,18,21] The final success rates for EST and EPBD are comparable; the reported success rates of stone removal are 81% to 99% for EPBD[15,17,18,21] and 85% to 98% for EST.[17,18] Randomized trials comparing EPBD to EST suggest that EPBD is at least as effective as EST in patients with small to moderate-sized bile duct stones.[16,17,21,22]

The lower rate of stone clearance, along with a higher usage of mechanical lithotripsy in EPBD, is most likely because EPBD does not enlarge the bile duct opening to the same extent as EST. Ersoz et al.[6] reported the use of large-balloon dilation after EST for removal of bile duct stones that were difficult to extract by conventional EST and extraction devices. Endoscopic papillary large-balloon dilation (EPLBD) has been introduced as an adjunctive tool to EST for removing large or difficult CBD stones. The concept is to combine the advantages of sphincterotomy with those of balloon dilation.

However, EPLBD is still not fully accepted as some endoscopists are concerned about potentially serious adverse events such as pancreatitis and bile duct perforation. However, recent data from various multicenter studies in both Eastern and Western countries[23–37] suggest that EPLBD with EST is safe and effective. Over the past 10 years, the technical methods and safety of EPLBD have been established and the indication has been expanded.

As an alternative method, EPLBD without a preceding EST was introduced as a simplified technique in 2009.[38–41] Several studies have reported that this technique is safe and effective in patients with large bile duct stones, without an increased risk of severe pancreatitis or bile duct perforation, though these studies have been limited to patients outside of the United States and Western countries.

EPLBD AFTER EST FOR REMOVAL OF LARGE STONES

To overcome the limitations of conventional EPBD, "large-balloon dilation after minimal biliary sphincterotomy" has been devised. Large-balloon dilation after minimal EST is effective for retrieving large biliary stones without the need for mechanical lithotripsy (Figs. 18.1 and 18.2). Although EST with a large incision may be effective in reducing the need for mechanical lithotripsy, a large incision has a higher risk of perforation and possibly a higher risk of bleeding than standard EST. EPLBD combined with EST—an innovative, novel method incorporating slow dilation of the papilla to a large diameter—can provide a larger opening than a large EST (see Fig. 18.1) and prevent perforation and bleeding. Subsequent retrieval of large or multiple bile duct stones is easy, safe, and effective (see Fig. 18.2).

TECHNIQUE OF LARGE-BALLOON DILATION OF POSTSPHINCTEROTOMY PAPILLA

Using a therapeutic duodenoscope (e.g., TJF 260V; Olympus Medical Systems, Tokyo, Japan), the endoscope is advanced to the duodenum.

Video for this chapter can be found online at www.expertconsult.com.

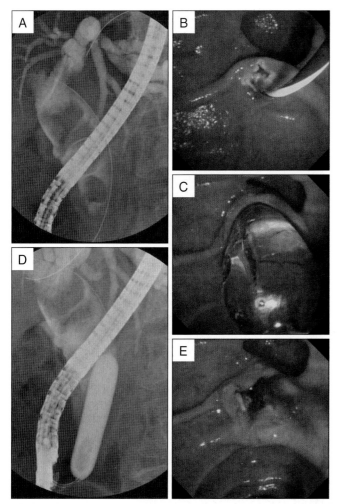

FIG 18.1 A case of large-balloon dilation after minimal EST in a patient with multiple large extrahepatic bile duct stones. **A,** Retrograde cholangiogram shows multiple large stones that completely fill the extrahepatic bile duct. **B–D,** After minimal EST, a large balloon is inflated up to 15 mm over the guidewire and through the sphincterotomized papilla. **E,** The papillary orifice is dilated fully and the bile duct mucosa is readily seen. *EST,* Endoscopic sphincterotomy.

It is important to use a duodenoscope with a large working channel (4.2 mm in diameter) for easier passage of large balloons. The difference from conventional EPBD is that EST is performed before balloon dilation. In most cases a major (complete) EST is not required and a minimal (<1/3 of the maximum possible length) EST is sufficient. This is because the purpose of EST is not to dilate the sphincter of Oddi (SO) but to direct SO dilation toward the biliary side and away from the pancreas. When using a large-diameter balloon to dilate the SO without EST, it is difficult to predict the direction in which the SO will be dilated. Therefore, by performing a minimal EST, the direction of papilla dilation can be predicted. Another reason for minimal EST is to prevent PEP by minimizing peripapillary edema that may occur after dilating the papilla.

After EST, a guidewire is inserted into the bile duct and a balloon catheter is guided over the wire. By definition, EPLBD involves balloons of 12 to 20 mm in diameter. Because the maximum diameter of standard biliary dilation balloons are only 10 mm in diameter, pyloric dilating balloons such as the CRE Wire Guided Balloon (Boston Scientific, Marlborough, MA) are needed (Fig. 18.3). Recently a combined sphincterotome with large-diameter balloon has become available (StoneMaster V; Olympus Medical Systems) so that EPLBD can be done with one device.

The diameter of the dilating balloon is determined by the size of the bile duct stone and of the bile duct proximal to the tapered distal biliary segment. EST with a small incision up to the pancreatic orifice is performed over a guidewire. Endoscopic papillary dilation is performed slowly with a large balloon (maximum 20 mm in diameter) to match the size of the bile duct.

Although the balloon diameter for EPLBD ranges from 12 to 20 mm, a balloon with a diameter of 15 mm or less is frequently used to prevent serious adverse events, even if the bile duct stones are larger than 15 mm in diameter. Therefore the diameter of the distal bile duct may be regarded as a more important factor when selecting the balloon rather than the size of bile duct stones because excessive balloon dilation beyond the diameter of the distal bile duct may increase the risk of perforation. A large-scale retrospective multicenter EPLBD study of 946 patients with large bile duct stones (>10 mm) noted that the diameter of the inflated balloon used was larger than that of the distal bile duct in 2 of 3 patients with fatal perforation.[42]

Dilation with large-diameter balloons is performed at the same session as EST. As mentioned, nonbiliary over-the-guidewire–type balloons intended for esophageal and pyloric dilation are used. The balloon catheters are passed over a guidewire and positioned across the biliary orifice; the middle portion of the balloon is gradually filled with diluted contrast medium under endoscopic and fluoroscopic guidance to maintain the correct position and to observe the gradual disappearance of the waist in the balloon, which is taken to indicate progressive dilation of the distal bile duct and biliary orifice.

During EPLBD, rapid and forcible inflation of the balloon across a tight distal bile duct stricture can lead to perforation and bleeding. Obvious bile duct strictures are easily visible on cholangiography, whereas obscure bile duct strictures are sometimes difficult to diagnose.

The balloon should always be inflated slowly and gradually, starting from a smaller diameter than the intended maximal target, in order to recognize obscure bile duct strictures, with attention paid to the balloon shape under fluoroscopy.[43]

If the central waist of the balloon does not disappear by 75% of maximal pressure prescribed for the particular balloon, the presence of an obscure stricture of the distal bile duct should be suspected and further balloon inflation should be halted to avoid perforation.[42]

Once the waist has disappeared, the balloon remains inflated in position for 20 to 45 seconds, after which it is deflated and removed. A standard stone basket or retrieval balloon catheter is then used to remove the stones. In some cases, the waist in the balloon does not disappear completely; in such cases, keeping the balloon inflated for more than 45 seconds may be useful. Stones are then retrieved from the bile duct with a retrieval balloon catheter or a stone basket. After stone retrieval, irrigation of the bile duct with normal saline may help remove any remaining stones or fragments.

A dilation time lasting less than 1 minute may actually induce bleeding, which may be attributable to insufficient compression time by the balloon. After dilating the papilla for 1 minute, the balloon catheter is removed and a basket is inserted to remove the stone. Dilation with a large-diameter balloon after EST can be especially useful for clearing bile duct stones in patients with a tapered distal bile duct. By using a larger balloon, the distal duct can be shaped into a near square, facilitating stone removal.

ADVERSE EVENTS OF EPLBD AFTER EST

Since 2003, there have been many reports on the outcomes and adverse events of EPLBD. Fortunately, most adverse events are mild and few

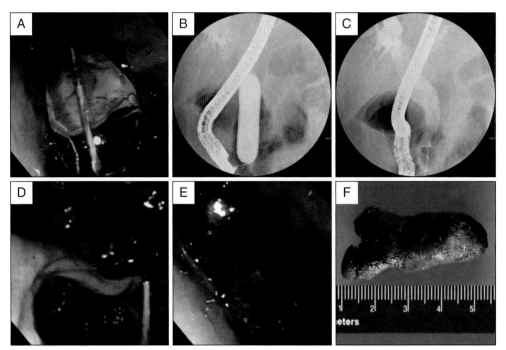

FIG 18.2 A huge stone is impacted at the bile duct bifurcation. After sphincterotomy, large-balloon dilation is performed up to 18 mm. **A** and **B,** Removal with a large basket catheter and mechanical lithotriptor fails, and retrieval of a large stone is attempted with a retrieval balloon catheter **(C)**. **D,** The stone is pulled out with a retrieval balloon catheter and extracted from the papilla. **E** and **F,** A huge stone (4.5 cm × 2.0 cm) is finally evacuated without crushing.

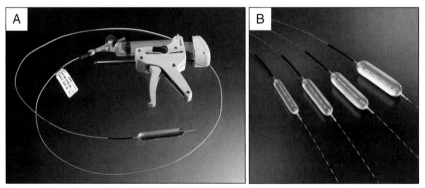

FIG 18.3 Dilating kit consisting of syringe/gauge assembly and inflation handle **(A)** and 6-mm to 8-mm, 8-mm to 10-mm, 12-mm to 15-mm, and 18-mm to 20-mm balloons **(B).**

serious adverse events have been reported, though there is a lack of large-scale multicenter randomized prospective studies.

A meta-analysis of randomized controlled trials that compared EPLBD and EST for retrieval of choledocholithiasis showed that EPLBD was associated with fewer overall adverse events than EST (5.8 vs 13.1%, OR 0.41, 95% CI 0.24 to 0.68, $p = 0.0007$).[44]

A summary of multiple published series using only dilation balloons of >10 mm after EST for removal of bile duct stones is shown in Table 18.1. Ten studies have been published as full papers in English,[6,24,27,29,30,34,45–47] whereas four studies are preliminary reports.[25,48–50] The reported stone removal success rates ranged from 73% to 100%, and the use of mechanical lithotripsy ranged from 1% to 33%. This wide range of lithotripsy use may be attributable to variable stone size and the diameter of dilation balloons used. The success rate of complete stone clearance in the first session in 1003 patients was 90.2% overall, and the use of mechanical lithotripsy was 11.6%.

The reported adverse event rate from published series has ranged from 1% to 23%, with a pancreatitis rate ranging from 0% to 5%. Analysis of all reported series showed a pooled adverse event rate of 10.9%, with a pooled pancreatitis rate of 2.6% (see Table 18.1). Most reported cases of pancreatitis were mild in severity. The pooled adverse event rate of this combined technique is similar to that after EST alone, with a mean overall adverse event rate of 8.2% and a pancreatitis rate of 1.9%.[38] However, two deaths from severe bleeding and perforation were reported,[25] which account for an overall mortality rate of 0.2% in 1003 patients.

Heo and colleagues from Korea[24] randomized 200 consecutive patients with bile duct stones in equal numbers to EST plus EPLBD (12-mm to 20-mm balloon diameter) or EST alone. There was no difference in the rate of PEP. In a multicenter study, Attasaranya et al. reported potential efficacy of EPLBD using large-diameter balloons (≥12 mm) after sphincterotomy in 107 patients with large CBD stones at five endoscopic

TABLE 18.1   Summary of Reported Series of EPLBD After EST for Removal of Extrahepatic Bile Duct Stones

Series	No. of Procedures	Balloon Size (mm)	Mean Largest Stone (mm)	% Success in First Session	% Use of Lithotripsy	ADVERSE EVENTS, n (%)				
						Overall	Pancreatitis	Bleeding	Perforation	Others
Ersoz et al.[6]	58	12–20	16/18[a]	83	7	9 (16)	2 (3)	5 (9)	0	2[b]
Minami et al.[66]	88	Up to 20	14 ± 3	99	1	5 (6)[c]	1 (1)	1 (1)	0	1[b]/1[d]
Heo et al.[24]	100	12–20	16.0 ± 0.7	97	8	5 (5)	4 (4)	0	0	1[b]
Maydeo and Bhandari[30]	62	12–15	16	92	5	5 (8.3)	0	5 (8.3)	0	0
Bang et al.[45]	22	10–15	10 (5–25)	72.7	9	1 (4.5)	1 (4.5)	0	0	0
Misra and Dwivedi[27]	50	15–20	NM (<15–25)	90	10	23 (46)	4 (8)	19 (38)	0	0
Attasaranya et al.[29]	107	12–18	13 (10–30)	95	27	6 (5.6)	0	2 (1.9)	1 (0.9)	1[e]/1[d]/1[d]
Kochhar et al.[46]	74	10–18	NM (10–15)	91.9	2.7	16 (21.6)	2 (2.7)	6 (8.1)	0	13[e]/1[d]
Kim et al.[34]	27	15–18	20.8 (≥15)	85	33	4 (15)	0	4 (15)	0	0
Kim et al.[47]	72	12–20	NM	87.5	17.9	6 (8.3)	5 (6.9)	0	0	1[b]
Yoo et al.[25]	166	15–20	16.1 ± 5.4	83	NM	11 (6.6)[f]	NM	1 (0.6)	1 (0.6)	NM
Park et al.[48]	70	15–20	NM (all >15)	100	16	13 (19)	3 (4)	10 (14)	0	0
Cho et al.[49]	69	NM	17.5/18.2[g]	91	NM	5 (7)	4 (6)	1 (1.4)	0	0
Cha et al.[50]	38	15–20	18.9 ± 5.3	95	3	1 (3)	0	1 (3)	0	0
Total	**1003**	**10–20**	—[h]	**90.2**	**11.6[i]**	**110 (10.9)**	**26 (2.6)[i]**	**55 (5.5)**	**2 (0.2)**	**24 (2.4)[i]**

EPLBD, Endoscopic papillary large-balloon dilation; *EST,* endoscopic sphincterotomy; *NM,* not mentioned.

[a]Median in two subgroups.
[b]Cholangitis or cholecystitis.
[c]Not including 10 patients who had hypotension after nitrate infusion (per protocol for prevention of procedure-related pancreatitis).
[d]Hypoxia, embedded broken basket, and intramural dissection.
[e]Abdominal pain.
[f]Two deaths from bleeding (1) and perforation (1).
[g]Mean in two subgroups with/without periampullary diverticulum.
[h]Cannot be calculated.
[i]Does not include Yoo et al.[25] and Cho et al.[49] series because of use of lithotripsy rate.
[j]Does not include Yoo et al.[25] series because pancreatitis and other adverse event rates not specified.

BOX 18.1   To Define Obvious or Occult Stricture of Bile Duct

- The balloon should be inflated slowly in gradual steps.
- Strong resistance and persistent waist during balloon inflation after applying 75% of the maximal inflation pressure. This should be used as the alarm sign.
- Further forcible inflation of the balloon can induce bile duct perforation.

retrograde cholangiopancreatography (ERCP) referral centers in the United States.[29] There were no reported cases of PEP. The absence of documented PEP in this study may be related to multiple factors. First, and perhaps most important, performing EPLBD after EST may decrease the risk of pancreatitis because the pancreatic orifice is separated from the biliary orifice after EST and the balloon dilation force will push the pressure away from the pancreatic duct. The significance of separated biliary and pancreatic orifices was reported by Mavrogiannis et al.,[51] showing that 81 patients with bile duct stones undergoing repeat EST had a significantly lower rate of pancreatitis than did 250 patients with initial EST (0% and 4.8%, respectively).

Second, this study included older patients with a mean age of 70.7 years, whereas the median age was 49 years in a prospective multicenter trial in the United States that showed a higher rate of pancreatitis after EPBD (small-diameter balloons and small stones).[34] Subgroup analyses in one recent meta-analysis comparing EST with EPBD for bile duct stones demonstrated that age <60 years was one of the factors associated with a higher rate of pancreatitis in patients treated with EPBD.[52] Age <60 years was also documented as one of the independent risk factors for ERCP pancreatitis in a prospective multicenter study.[53]

Third, pancreatography was infrequently done in this study (14%).[29] A small series showed that pancreatic contrast injection was the only single independent risk factor for pancreatitis in patients with bile duct stones treated with EPBD with a 6-mm to 8-mm balloon.[54] One recent study including 14,331 ERCPs in a single referral ERCP center showed that there was a significantly higher frequency of PEP when pancreatic duct injection was performed.[55]

Another hypothesis about the mechanism of pancreatitis after EPLBD has been suggested: the manipulation frequency of the Dormia basket and retrieval balloon catheter in EPLBD both with and without EST can be reduced because of a sufficiently widened ampullary orifice, resulting in less periampullary trauma and edema and a lower risk of pancreatitis. In contrast, the risk of injury to the ampullary orifice in EPBD by using small-diameter balloons may be increased because instruments for stone removal are passed through an inadequately widened ampullary orifice.

Bleeding occurs in 2% to 5% of patients undergoing EST to remove bile duct stones.[13,41] In contrast, no significant bleeding has been observed after endoscopic balloon dilation.[17,18] Misra and Dwivedi reported on EPLBD performed in India using 15-mm-diameter to 20-mm-diameter balloons in 50 patients after sphincterotomy.[27] Minor oozing bleeding was seen in 16 patients (32%), but oozing stopped spontaneously during the completion of the endoscopy. Major bleeding requiring surgery occurred in one patient. Ersoz et al.[6] reported three patients with moderate bleeding requiring blood transfusion and endoscopic therapy, which was thought to be attributed to EST, not balloon dilation. Although small-diameter balloon dilation alone is recommended by most experts as the treatment option for bile duct stones in patients with uncorrectable coagulopathy,[56–58] whether large-diameter balloon dilation after (concurrent or remote) EST is as safe as small-diameter balloon dilation alone in terms of bleeding requires additional study. In fact, one death with

bleeding has been reported,[48] and bleeding requiring endoscopic therapy was noted in 8.3% of patients in another preliminary study.[45] Use of large-diameter balloon dilation in patients with coagulopathy (even when using it alone in the setting of remote biliary sphincterotomy) should be undertaken cautiously.

In all six randomized controlled trials[24,29,30,34,59,60] and three of four meta-analyses[61–63] that were conducted to compare the clinical outcomes between EPLBD with EST and EST alone, the rate of bleeding was similar, whereas the remaining meta-analysis by Feng et al.[44] found that the rate of bleeding was significantly lower for EPLBD with EST than that for EST alone. However, EST incision length is considered as the major factor of post-EPLBD bleeding, although the large dilation may result in tearing of underlying vessels. In a systematic review of 32 EPLBD studies, the rate of bleeding was significantly higher for EPLBD with large EST than for EPLBD with limited EST (OR 3.33, $p < 0.001$) or without EST (OR 2.17, $p = 0.049$).[64] However, no significant difference in the bleeding rate was noted between EPLBD with limited EST and without EST ($p = 0.35$).

In a multivariate analysis, the presence of a distal CBD stricture was an independent predictor of perforation, and Park et al.[42] suggested that the presence of a distal CBD stricture should be considered a relative contraindication to EPLBD. In addition, they recommended gradual inflation, as well as caution, when a persistent waist at the distal CBD is identified after inflation to 75% of the manufacturer's recommended maximum inflation pressure[23,42,43] (Box 18.1).

If strong resistance is encountered during balloon inflation, additional pressure should not be applied. In such cases, converting to alternative stone retrieval methods or providing drainage, with plans for repeat ERCP, is recommended.[42] Large-balloon dilation should not be performed if the entire extrahepatic duct is small or normal in size. However, in all patients with large stones, the bile duct is dilated to at least the size of the stone.[42]

Even if there is no obvious distal CBD stricture or tapered distal CBD after a cholangiogram, any marked resistance during balloon inflation or a distinct waist or severe pain during balloon inflation (depending on degree of sedation) at any step should suggest a previously unrecognized stricture.

If there is a suspicion of distal bile duct stricture during ERCP, especially in patients with a tapered distal bile duct, one can consider withdrawing a large-diameter inflated stone retrieval balloon through the suspected site to unmask its existence.[64]

EPLBD WITHOUT PRECEDING SPHINCTEROTOMY (EST)

Recent studies[27,46] have shown that EST followed by large-balloon dilation or large-balloon dilation only[60] for the removal of large or difficult stones from the CBD has good efficacy and acceptable adverse event rates. Theoretically, EPLBD without EST is easier to manipulate than the combined method and is also more suitable for patients with concomitant large stones and bleeding tendency. Also, the main purpose of EPLBD for large bile duct stones is to preclude additional endoscopic procedures, such as endoscopic mechanical lithotripsy (EML), to simplify the process of stone extraction and reduce adverse events.

TECHNIQUE OF EPLBD WITHOUT SPHINCTEROTOMY

When the major papilla is accessed, the bile duct is cannulated as usual and cholangiography performed. The bile duct and stone diameters are measured during ERCP and corrected for magnification with the external diameter (13.5 mm) of the distal end of the duodenoscope

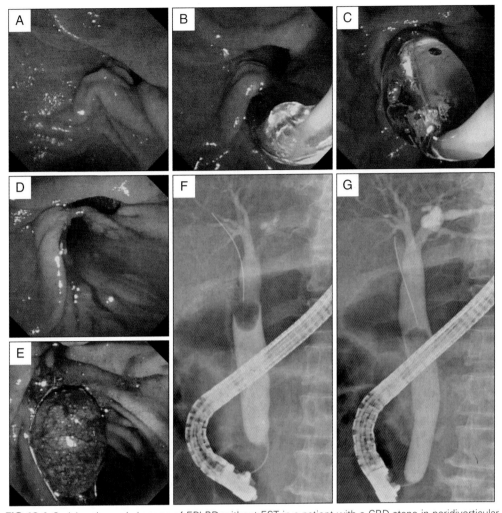

FIG 18.4 Serial endoscopic images of EPLBD without EST in a patient with a CBD stone in peridiverticular papilla. **A,** Balloon-tipped catheter is inserted into the CBD over the guidewire. The balloon is inflated. **A–C,** The balloon catheter is inflated without preceding EST over the guidewire up to 15 mm. **D,** After removing the balloon, the papillary orifice is widely opened. **E,** A large stone (15 mm in diameter) is extracted using a Dormia basket. **F** and **G,** Retrograde cholangiogram shows a large stone in the CBD and a fully inflated balloon across the papilla. *CBD,* Common bile duct; *EPLBD,* endoscopic papillary large-balloon dilation; *EST,* endoscopic sphincterotomy.

(e.g., TJF 260V; Olympus Medical Systems) as a reference. If the maximum transverse diameter of the largest stone and extrahepatic bile duct is ≥10 mm and ≥15 mm, respectively, a balloon catheter is used with a diameter larger than 15 mm and EPLBD is performed without a preceding EST. A 0.035-inch guidewire is passed through the diagnostic cannula into the bile duct. An over-the-wire hydrostatic balloon catheter used for esophageal and pyloric dilation (CRE balloon; Boston Scientific) is passed over the guidewire and placed across the ampulla. The balloon is then inflated gradually up to 15 mm or more with diluted contrast using an inflation device. The sphincter is considered to be adequately dilated if the waist of the balloon disappears completely on fluoroscopic examination. The fully expanded balloon is maintained in position for 30 to 60 seconds and then deflated and removed (Fig. 18.4). The bile duct stones are extracted with a Dormia basket and/or a retrieval balloon catheter. A mechanical lithotriptor can be used to crush the stones when stone extraction cannot be achieved by using a basket or retrieval balloon, even after EPLBD.

In a study by Jeong et al. from Korea,[33] EPLBD without EST was successfully performed in all 38 patients. The mean diameter of the balloon used for large-balloon dilation was 15.5 mm (range 15 to 18 mm). The inflation time was 10 to 60 seconds. Complete duct clearance was achieved in 37 patients (97.4%), irrespective of whether mechanical lithotripsy was used. Complete duct clearance by EPLBD alone (without an additional procedure) occurred in 29 patients (76.3%). In 25 patients (65.8%) the stones were completely removed in the first session by EPLBD alone without using mechanical lithotripsy. A total of 247 patients were reviewed in another study.[59] The mean age of the patients was 71.2 years (76% of patients were ≥65 years). The mean CBD size was 18.1 mm. The mean size of the dilating balloon used was 13.2 mm. The success rate of complete retrieval of stones with the first treatment session was 81.8% (202 of 247); the final success rate after additional treatment sessions was 92.7%.

A retrospective cohort study that compared stone clearance between EPLBD without and with EST showed similar outcomes in overall successful stone removal (96.8% vs 95.7%; $p = 0.738$) and complete stone removal without EML (80.6% vs 73.9%; $p = 0.360$).[65] In a systematic review of 32 EPLBD studies, the initial success rate of EPLBD without EST was significantly lower than that of EPLBD with EST (76.2% vs 84.0%; $p < 0.001$).[64] This was most likely because the opening of the orifice retracted almost immediately to its original size, which is commonly seen with EPBD alone. However, there was no significant difference in the overall success rate between the two groups (97.2% vs 96.5%; $p = 0.432$).[64] Therefore it can be concluded that the overall success rates of EPLBD with and without EST are comparable.

ADVERSE EVENTS OF EPLBD WITHOUT EST

Mild PEP occurred in only one patient (2.6%) after EPLBD without a preceding EST. The serum amylase concentration was increased threefold or more over the normal upper limit without clinical pancreatitis in three patients (7.9%).[60] In another series, pancreatic duct injection was noted in 26.7% (66 of 247). There were three adverse events (1.2%): two cases (0.8%) of mild pancreatitis and one case (0.4%) of mild cholangitis.[59] Possible causes of the low pancreatitis rate include the relatively older patient age in this study (mean age of 71 years)[52,53] and associated progressive decline in pancreatic exocrine function that could protect older patients from pancreatic injury. In addition, the authors tried to selectively cannulate the CBD when performing the ERCP and avoid cannulation of or excessive injection of the pancreatic duct.[59] Although there are still no data comparing EPLBD with and without EST, the incidence (2.6%) of pancreatitis[58] that developed after EPLBD without EST was as low as that of EPLBD with EST in previous studies.[6,24,27,30,46,66,67] Therefore the reason for the lower incidence of PEP in EPLBD with EST compared with EPBD with a small balloon might not reflect EST performed before EPLBD.

Among the ERCP-related adverse events, bleeding theoretically occurs less often if there is no cutting involved before EPLBD.[68] In fact, Baron and Harewood[69] reported that bleeding occurred less frequently with EPBD (EPBD, 0% vs EST, 2.0%; $p = 0.001$) in their meta-analysis of eight prospective randomized trials of EPBD and EST. Performing EST before EPLBD should be avoided in patients with coagulopathy. Although the incidence of postprocedure bleeding ranges from 0% to 9% in previous studies involving EST with EPLBD,[6,24,27,30,46,66,67] minor or major bleeding did not develop after EPLBD without EST in a study by Jeong et al.[33] However, 6 of 247 (2.4%) patients developed intraprocedure bleeding incidents in another study.[59]

Several randomized controlled trials have shown that EPBD might significantly reduce the risk of bleeding compared with EST.[70–72] However, there is not enough evidence supporting the advantages of EPLBD without EST in patients with coagulopathy. Based on the results of a number of EPBD studies, it is suggested that EPLBD without EST may theoretically minimize bleeding. In a well-conducted case-control multicenter study for the analysis of adverse events in 946 patients who underwent EPLBD, underlying liver cirrhosis was found to be an independent predictor of bleeding after EPLBD (OR 8.028, 95% CI 2.022 to 31.883, $p = 0.003$).[42] In a systematic review of 32 EPLBD studies involving 413 patients, no cases of serious bleeding occurred in patients who underwent EPLBD without EST, whereas it was noted in 4 of 2503 patients who underwent EPLBD with EST (nonsignificant).[64] Therefore EPLBD without EST is preferred over EPLBD with EST for removal of large stones in patients with coagulopathy.

The main limitations of two of these studies are the small sample size[58] and retrospective analysis,[58,59] which might have contributed to the underestimation of adverse event rates. In addition, there were many older patients included in these studies and the risk of pancreatitis was possibly underestimated. Therefore there is a possibility that this procedure may cause serious morbidity in younger patients. Study designs may not have been adequate to demonstrate the safety and efficacy of this procedure.

The maximum transverse diameter of the stone induces high resistance at the biliary outlet when the CBD stone is extracted by a basket or retrieval balloon catheter. Often, endoscopists with limited experience with EPLBD tend to undersize the diameter of the balloon catheter in relation to the largest stone. It can be safely applied when the diameter of the balloon matches the size of the stone and the duct.

In conclusion, EPLBD without EST may be simple, effective, and safe in patients with large bile duct stones, similar to previous studies of EPLBD with EST. Therefore EPLBD without EST may be a reasonable alternative for the treatment of large bile duct stones, and sphincterotomy may not be a prerequisite for EPLBD for the treatment of large stones. However, large-scale prospective randomized comparative studies are needed to validate this technique as a useful option and as safe for the removal of large biliary calculi in younger patients.

RECOMMENDATIONS FOR SAFE AND SUCCESSFUL EPLBD

No guidelines or consensus recommendations to avoid adverse effects such as perforation after EPLBD have been developed. Three published papers have proposed recommendations for safe EPLBD and the prevention of fatal adverse events[23,42,64] (Box 18.2).

Park et al.[42] proposed the following guidelines for safe EPLBD: (1) selection of suitable candidates (e.g., EPLBD should be reserved for patients with a dilated CBD but avoided in patients with distal CBD strictures); (2) avoidance of full EST immediately before large-balloon dilation to prevent perforation and bleeding; (3) gradual inflation of the dilating balloon to recognize a narrow distal CBD indicated by a lack of disappearance of the balloon waist; (4) discontinuation of inflation when resistance is encountered in the presence of a persistent balloon waist; (5) not inflating the balloon beyond the maximum upstream size of the dilated CBD; and (6) conversion to alternative stone removal or drainage methods when difficulty in removal of a stone is encountered.

BOX 18.2   Recommendations for Safe EPLBD

- Strict indication
  - Patients with dilated CBD without distal CBD strictures
- Proper methods
  - Avoid full EST immediately before large-balloon dilation to prevent perforation and bleeding.
  - Inflate the balloon gradually to recognize a narrowed distal CBD, indicated by lack of disappearance of the balloon waist (occult stricture).
  - Inflation should be stopped if the balloon waist persists before applying more than 75% of the recommended maximum inflation pressure, and inflate the balloon gradually to recognize occult or undetermined strictures of the distal CBD, shown by persistence of a waist during balloon dilation.
  - Discontinue balloon inflation when resistance is encountered in the presence of a persistent balloon waist.
  - Do not inflate balloon beyond the maximal size of the upstream dilated CBD.
  - If there is a suspicion of strictures, pulling a large inflated retrieval balloon through the site to confirm its existence is recommended.
  - Do not hesitate to convert to alternative stone removal methods such as MLT and EHL when you meet any difficulty in removing stones.

CBD, Common bile duct; *EHL,* electrohydraulic lithotripsy; *EPLBD,* endoscopic papillary large-balloon dilation; *EST,* endoscopic sphincterotomy; *MLT,* mechanical lithotripsy.

Lee et al.[23] also recommended nearly the same for EPLBD in 2012 and recommended that inflation should be stopped if the balloon waist persists before applying more than 75% of the recommended maximum inflation pressure and to inflate the balloon gradually to recognize occult or unexpected strictures of the distal CBD, shown by persistence of a waist during balloon dilation.

Kim et al.[64] also reported recommendations for successful EPLBD that are fundamentally similar to the previous recommendation,[23,42] but added the following details:

1. In patients with obvious distal bile duct stricture, EPLBD should be avoided. If there is a suspicion of stricture, they recommended using the pulling method with a large inflated stone retrieval balloon through the site to confirm its existence.
2. Further balloon inflation must be ceased if the central waist of the balloon does not disappear or the patient indicates severe pain during balloon inflation at any step.

EPBD OF THE NATIVE PAPILLA

After diagnostic ERCP and selective bile duct cannulation, a standard 0.025-inch or 0.035-inch guidewire is inserted into the bile duct. After removing the cannula, a 6-mm to 10-mm balloon catheter is passed over the guidewire (see Fig. 18.3). The balloon is positioned so that two-thirds of it is inside the distal CBD and a third of it is outside the papillary orifice and inflated with diluted contrast (Fig. 18.5). The balloon is expanded slowly with a mixture of contrast medium and saline (1:1), paying close attention to the waist of the balloon. When the waist disappears, the inflation is stopped. Care must be taken to avoid rapid application of excessive pressure. The dilation is maintained for 15 to 30 seconds. When the bile duct is less than 8 mm in diameter, a 6-mm × 2-cm balloon can be used. Other dilating balloons can also be used. The smaller balloons pass readily through a diagnostic channel duodenoscope, whereas the 8-mm balloon requires a biopsy channel of at least 3.2 mm.

INDICATIONS FOR EPBD

In the meta-analysis by Baron and Harewood, the incidence of bleeding was significantly less after EPBD compared with EST.[69] Clinically significant post-EST bleeding occurs in 2% to 5% of EST patients.[12,22] In addition, patients with coagulopathy and those requiring anticoagulation within 3 days of the procedure are at increased risk for bleeding.[12] Thus transient discontinuation of anticoagulation, correction of coagulopathy with fresh frozen plasma, or platelet transfusion is frequently performed to avoid bleeding after EST, though these measures may be inadequate to prevent it. EPBD provides a useful alternative to EST in such cases. No articles have described bleeding after EPBD.[15,17,18,21] In light of this, EPBD should be considered a viable alternative to EST in patients with an underlying coagulopathy or the need for anticoagulation after EST, as such patients have a higher incidence of post-EST bleeding.[12] EPBD may significantly reduce the risk of bleeding compared with EST in patients with advanced cirrhosis and coagulopathy. In these patients, EPBD is recommended over EST for treating small-diameter choledocholithiasis.[73] Another population in which EPBD may be an attractive option is those patients who refuse blood transfusion for religious reasons.

EPBD is a possible alternative to EST for removal of smaller stones, especially in patients with impaired hemostasis. However, large stones may be difficult to remove with EPBD alone. Therefore ideal patients for selecting EPBD over EST (Box 18.3) are those with a limited number of CBD stones (≤3), CBD stones with a maximum diameter of 10 mm, and minimally dilated bile ducts.[21,74–76] It is also important to use extreme caution when EPBD is applied in the following clinical settings: the presence of severe acute cholangitis, a history of previous or ongoing acute pancreatitis, age ≤50 years, and difficult biliary cannulation,[77] especially because of reports describing fatal pancreatitis in younger patients.[71] In must be noted that the early studies of poor outcome of balloon dilation in young patients were before the advent of prophylactic pancreatic duct stents and use of rectally administered nonsteroidal antiinflammatory drugs (NSAIDs) to prevent PEP. In patients who undergo EPBD, especially younger patients, the use of one or both of these preventative measures is recommended.

ADVERSE EVENTS OF EPBD

Early adverse events, defined as those occurring within 24 hours of the procedure, are pancreatitis, bleeding, infection (cholangitis or cholecystitis), and perforation. The meta-analysis of randomized controlled trials by Baron and Harewood showed that the early adverse event rate of EPBD was comparable to EST for removing CBD stones during ERCP.[69] Overall, the early adverse event rates were similar in EPBD and EST (10.5% vs 10.3%, $p = 0.9$). Of note, the bleeding rate was higher in the EST group (2.0% vs 0%, $p = 0.001$), whereas the rates of infection (2.7% for EPBD vs 3.6% for EST, $p = 0.3$) and perforation (0.4% vs 0.4%, $p = 1.0$) were similar. The rate of pancreatitis was higher in the EPBD group (7.4% vs 4.3%, $p = 0.05$) (again, these studies were done before the advent of stents and NSAIDs to prevent PEP). One patient death occurred in each group, yielding a mortality rate of 0.2%.

Hemorrhage is one of the most common and serious adverse events of EST, and the presence of coagulopathy is one of the risk factors for hemorrhage. In the meta-analysis by Baron and Harewood,[69] bleeding was clearly reduced when EPBD was performed compared with EST for the removal of CBD stones, but nearly all comparative studies of EPBD and EST excluded patients with coagulopathy and liver disorders. When bleeding occurs in cirrhotic patients, they may also develop further adverse events such as hepatic failure. Komatsu et al. treated 24 cirrhotic patients with CBD stones using EPBD.[18] Although hemostasis was impaired because of liver dysfunction, no bleeding occurred and all patients responded well to treatment. In particular, no adverse events were seen in four patients with Child-Pugh class C cirrhosis or in six patients with severe coagulopathy. The rate of EST-related hemorrhage was 30% (6 of 20 patients), whereas the rate of EPBD-related hemorrhage was 0% ($p = 0.009$). Regarding the rates of hemorrhage in relation to Child-Pugh class, most ($n = 5$) of the bleeding adverse events occurred in patients with Child-Pugh class C cirrhosis, whereas bleeding occurred in only one patient with Child-Pugh class B cirrhosis.[73] Based on these results, EPBD appears to be the preferred strategy in patients with CBD stones and an underlying coagulopathy and those who require full anticoagulation within 72 hours of stone removal,[78] because these patients are at higher risk for postsphincterotomy bleeding.[12]

Procedure-related pancreatitis needs to be addressed. Five prospective randomized controlled trials of EPBD versus EST have been performed.[17,70,74,75] Of these, the Dutch[12] and UK[74] studies showed similar efficacy and safety between the two methods. Their incidence of pancreatitis was similar in patients undergoing EPBD and EST, in the range of 5% to 7%. In a Japanese study,[70] the rate of pancreatitis was slightly higher with EPBD than with EST; however, there were no reports of severe pancreatitis and all patients recovered with conservative treatment. In addition, Mac Mathuna et al.[15] and Komatsu et al.[18] conducted large-scale studies, but those studies were not randomized controlled trials; the incidence rates of pancreatitis were 5% and 7%, respectively. No severe pancreatitis or fatalities occurred.

The mechanism of post-EPBD hyperamylasemia and pancreatitis is not clear, although it seems to be multifactorial. Balloon compression

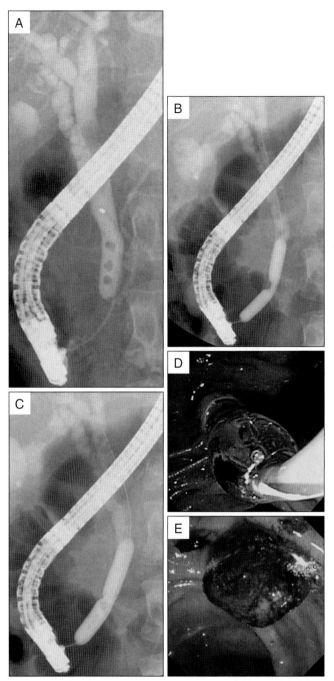

FIG 18.5 Endoscopic balloon dilation in a patient with multiple small CBD stones. **A,** The endoscopic cholangiogram demonstrated multiple stones in the common bile duct. After diagnostic ERCP, a 0.035-inch guidewire was passed through the ERCP catheter into the common bile duct, and the catheter was removed. **B,** A balloon-tipped catheter is inserted into the CBD over the guidewire. Once the balloon is located across the papilla, it is inflated. The biliary sphincter can be seen as a "waist" in the balloon. **C,** The biliary sphincter is considered adequately dilated if the waist has disappeared almost completely. **D,** After cannulation of a guidewire, the balloon catheter is inflated over the guidewire. **E,** After removing the balloon and guidewire, stones are extracted using a retrieval balloon. *CBD,* Common bile duct.

of the papilla or the pancreatic duct orifice may provoke peripapillary edema or SO spasm.[75,79] Bile duct cannulation per se or transpapillary manipulation (stone extraction, nasobiliary drainage, biliary stent placement) may also induce edema or spasm. The peripapillary edema or spasm may in turn obstruct the flow of pancreatic juice and eventually induce pancreatic sedema or pancreatitis associated with hyperamylasemia.[75,79] Contrast medium injection or cannulation of the pancreatic

duct is also likely to have some effect on the pancreas and pancreatic secretions.[80]

SPECIAL SITUATIONS

EST in patients who have undergone Billroth II gastrectomy and in some other postoperative anatomy is more difficult than in patients

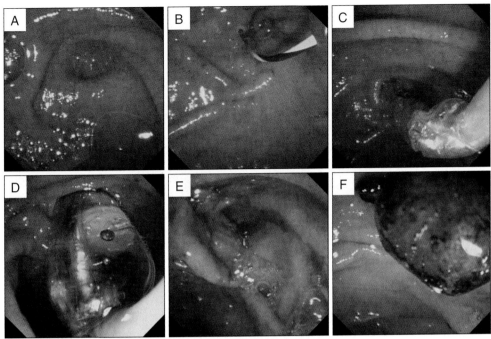

FIG 18.6 Endoscopic images of EPLBD in a patient with a CBD stone and a papilla with an intradiverticular location. **A,** The major papilla is located in the diverticulum. **B,** Small EST is performed. **C** and **D,** After cannulation of a guidewire, the balloon catheter is inflated over the guidewire up to 15 mm. **E** and **F,** After removing the balloon, the stone is evacuated with a basket catheter through the widely opened papilla. *CBD,* Common bile duct; *EPLBD,* endoscopic papillary large-balloon dilation; *EST,* endoscopic sphincterotomy.

BOX 18.3   Ideal Patients for Selecting Endoscopic Papillary Balloon Dilation

- Impaired hemostasis
- Number of stones ≤3
- Size of stones <10 mm
- Minimally dilated common bile duct <12 mm
- No severe acute cholangitis
- No history of previous or ongoing pancreatitis
- Age ≥50 years
- No difficult cannulation

---

with unaltered anatomy because the papilla now has to be approached as an inverted anatomic structure (see Chapter 31). In such a situation, balloon dilation may be preferable to EST.

Jang et al.[81] reported complete CBD stone removal after EPLBD without EST in all Billroth II gastrectomy patients with large or difficult CBD stones without any serious adverse events. However, to date, there are still no randomized controlled trials of EPLBD and EST alone in Billroth II gastrectomy patients. Nonetheless, EPLBD is still regarded as an effective and safe procedure and is commonly used to remove bile duct stones in patients with surgically altered anatomy.

In a retrospective cohort study of EPLBD without a repeat EST and standard balloon and basket extraction techniques in patients with a history of EST and large bile duct stones (>10 mm), the total procedure time was significantly shorter and the frequency of EML use was significantly lower in EPLBD without repeated EST than when performing standard extraction techniques, whereas the rates of

complete stone clearance and procedure-related adverse events were similar in both.[82] Therefore, in patients with previous EST, EPLBD without a repeat EST may be effective and safe for the removal of recurrent stones.

In three retrospective comparison studies in patients with and without periampullary diverticulum (PAD) (Figs. 18.1 and 18.6), there were no significant differences in overall success rates of bile duct stone removal or rates of adverse events after EPLBD with limited EST or EPLBD alone.[83–85] When comparing each subtype of PAD with the controls or between subtypes of PAD in these studies, the rates of total adverse events were comparable,[83,85] whereas the frequency of pancreatitis was significantly higher in PAD type A than in controls (14.3% vs 3.0%, p = 0.047) in one study.[84]

Nevertheless, EPLBD without EST is generally considered to avoid serious adverse events such as perforation and bleeding in patients with PAD. Randomized controlled trials comparing outcomes of patients with and without PAD warrant further investigation, especially based on the type of PAD. A retrospective comparison of patients with and without PAD showed similar stone clearance rates and adverse events in both, after EPLBD with a limited EST.[84] Several studies reported that the presence of a PAD was not associated with a significantly increased rate of adverse events such as pancreatitis, bleeding, or perforation.[42,61,85,86]

There have been six clinical trials of EPLBD in patients with surgically altered anatomy such as that which results from Billroth II surgery (Fig. 18.7)[35,81,87–89] and Roux-en-Y anastomosis.[90] In these, there was complete stone clearance in all patients, with a low incidence of pancreatitis and bleeding. In patients with coagulopathy, EPLBD without EST might be useful but should be undertaken cautiously.[42] Further studies are warranted.

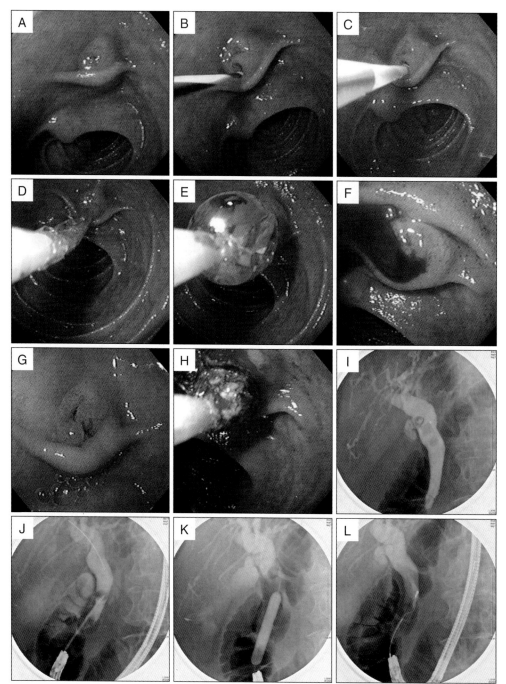

FIG 18.7 Serial endoscopic images **(A–H)** and retrograde cholangiograms **(I–L)** show endoscopic papillary large-balloon dilation of the biliary sphincter in a patient with two bile duct stones and prior Billroth II gastrectomy. **A,** Endoscopy shows an image of the papilla, upside down. **B–E, J,** and **K,** The balloon is advanced over a guidewire and inflated with diluted contrast. **F** and **G,** Transient oozing of blood is observed at the papilla after deflating the balloon, but it does not develop into serious hemorrhage. **I,** Two filling defects are seen on the cholangiogram. **H** and **L,** A stone is removed with a basket catheter.

SUMMARY

Although balloon dilation alone is associated with a higher risk of pancreatitis than sphincterotomy alone for removal of small stones, large-balloon dilation after sphincterotomy does not appear to be associated with a high rate of pancreatitis in patients with large stones. Large-balloon dilation after minimal EST appears to be safe and effective in the setting of bile duct stones that are difficult to extract using EST and conventional techniques. This procedure may reduce the need for EML and shorten procedure time and thus serve as an effective treatment modality for multiple large extrahepatic bile duct stones. Because the use of a larger balloon can tear the sphincter and the bile duct, potentially resulting in bleeding and perforation, a balloon size that is equal to or smaller in diameter than the diameter of the native distal bile duct is recommended. The maximum transverse diameter of the stone and the balloon-stone diameter ratio have a tendency to affect the success or failure of complete removal of stones by large-balloon dilation. One should take into account the size of the native bile duct, the size and burden of stones, the shape and size of the papillary mound, and the presence of the papilla in or adjacent to a diverticulum. In addition, the patient's comorbidities, particularly the presence of coagulopathy or the need for anticoagulation, would seem to favor more emphasis on dilation and less emphasis on sphincterotomy.

Although the types of adverse events and the long-term adverse event rate after EST plus EPLBD are currently unknown, they are unlikely to be much different from those of EST or EPBD alone. EPLBD without EST may be a good alternative for the treatment of large bile duct stones, and sphincterotomy may not necessarily be a prerequisite for EPLBD in the treatment of such calculi. In patients with surgically altered anatomy, PAD, and previous EST, EPLBD without EST may be an effective and safe procedure to remove bile duct stones. However, defining its exact role will require additional clinical experience and investigation.

The complete reference list for this chapter can be found online at www.expertconsult.com.

19

Stone Extraction

Andrew W. Yen and Joseph W. Leung

INTRODUCTION AND SCIENTIFIC BASIS

Biliary stone disease is the most common reason for undertaking therapeutic endoscopic retrograde cholangiopancreatography (ERCP). In Western countries, choledocholithiasis is primarily related to passage of gallstones from the gallbladder into the common bile duct. The clinical presentation of choledocholithiasis varies from no symptoms to biliary colic, jaundice, cholangitis, and/or acute biliary pancreatitis. ERCP plays an important role in managing or preventing biliary complications of biliary stone disease.

After endoscopic sphincterotomy, the majority of stones less than 1 cm in diameter pass spontaneously.[1] Nonetheless, it is current practice to attempt stone extraction and clearance of the bile duct to avoid potential subsequent stone impaction and adverse clinical consequences. Stones are most commonly extracted using a soft, compliant balloon catheter or wire (e.g., Dormia) basket. However, large stones, particularly those greater than 2 cm in diameter, can be difficult to remove and may require some form of stone fragmentation before removal. The most popular method of stone fragmentation is mechanical lithotripsy using large-diameter and robust baskets to break the stone. Other methods include intraductal electrohydraulic or laser lithotripsy and extracorporeal shock wave lithotripsy (ESWL).[2] In rare cases where endoscopic stone extraction fails, surgery or chemical dissolution of the stone may be used.[3-6] When endoscopic extraction fails, temporary biliary stenting provides decompression and is effective in controlling biliary sepsis. Subsequent additional elective endoscopic therapy can be undertaken to attempt stone clearance. Permanent plastic stenting can be used for biliary drainage in selected patients with large nonextractable stones to prevent cholangitis.[7-12] It is worth noting that the advent of large-diameter papillary balloon dilation has not only increased the successful extraction of stones but also reduced the need for mechanical lithotripsy (see Chapter 18).

Diagnostic ERCP is usually performed using undiluted water-soluble contrast, and early filling fluoroscopic images should be carefully analyzed for stones, which are often seen as filling defects with a meniscus sign (Fig. 19.1, *A*, *B*). However, if the bile duct is dilated, diluted contrast should be used to avoid masking small stones by dense contrast in a dilated duct. In patients with suspected intrahepatic stones or stones located proximal to a stricture, an occlusion cholangiogram may also be necessary to visualize the stones (Fig. 19.1, *C*). This may carry a risk of precipitating or exacerbating cholangitis if excess contrast is injected into an obstructed system, causing a rise in intrabiliary pressure.

Although the majority of intraluminal filling defects in the bile duct are caused by stone disease, a filling defect is not pathognomonic for choledocholithiasis. Irregularly shaped or amorphous lesions can be related to other entities such as mucus, as in the case of intraductal papillary neoplasm of the bile duct (IPNB), blood clots, parasites, polypoid malignancies, or other etiologies. An appropriate differential diagnosis should be considered in the clinical context of the patient before attempting extraction of the filling defect.

To achieve successful stone extraction, it is of prime importance to assess the stone size relative to the size of the sphincterotomy and caliber of the distal common bile duct (i.e., the "exit passage"). The sphincterotomy should be of adequate size to allow passage of the stone. One method of gauging sphincterotomy size is to pull a fully bowed sphincterotome across the cut papilla. A generous sphincterotomy should allow easy passage of the bowed sphincterotome. An alternative method to gauge the ease of stone extraction is to pull an inflated stone extraction balloon (about the same size as the stone) through the distal bile duct and sphincterotomy. If the balloon passes easily, stone extraction will likely be simple. If the balloon becomes deformed as it passes through the distal bile duct or excess resistance is felt during balloon passage through the sphincterotomy, it is likely that stone extraction will be difficult and additional therapy—such as balloon dilation of the sphincterotomy and distal bile duct (see Chapter 18)—may be required to facilitate stone extraction. In addition, appropriate accessories should be available to handle any foreseeable complications.

Dilation of a benign bile duct stricture may be necessary to remove stones that occur above a stricture and for intrahepatic stones. Dilation can be achieved using biliary dilation balloons, which are basically low-compliance balloons that can be inflated to a fixed diameter. These balloons are available in sizes ranging from 4 to 10 mm in diameter and can be placed over a guidewire across the stricture. Dilute contrast is used to inflate the balloon to a predetermined pressure as recommended by the manufacturer. The balloon has radiopaque markers that help with the positioning of the stricture at the midpoint of the balloon. The choice of balloon size should be based on the diameter of the normal portion of the bile duct and should not exceed this, in order to avoid unnecessary damage to the bile duct. The balloon is inflated to the recommended pressure, and the persistence or disappearance of the waist on the balloon is noted under fluoroscopy. This will determine the effectiveness of the dilation and ease of subsequent stone extraction through the stricture. If the stricture cannot be dilated adequately, stone fragmentation is necessary before attempting removal. Alternatively, the stricture can be treated (see Chapter 43) without attempting stone removal until it is adequately treated, as the indwelling stents are protected from stone-related clinical adverse events.

Balloon dilation or sphincteroplasty after an initial small sphincterotomy, or in specific cases without a sphincterotomy, has also been more frequently used to facilitate removal of a large stone while avoiding

---

Video for this chapter can be found online at www.expertconsult.com.

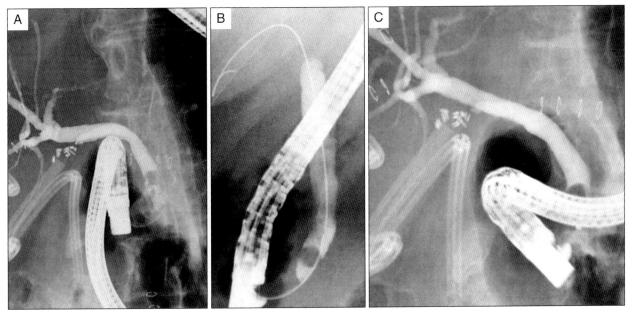

FIG 19.1 A, Cholangiography showing a filling defect that represents an irregular distal bile duct stone. Note that the endoscope is in the long position to expose the stone. **B,** Cholangiography shows a round filling defect consistent with a common bile duct stone. **C,** Occlusion cholangiogram following stone extraction from same patient in **A.** The inflated balloon is seen immediately above the endoscope, which is now in the short position.

the risks of bleeding and perforation from a large sphincterotomy (see Chapter 18).

BILIARY STONE DISEASE AND CONTRAINDICATIONS TO ERCP (SEE CHAPTER 7)

Biliary Stone Disease: Indications and Considerations

1. *Impacted ampullary stone.* Patients presenting with biliary pancreatitis or cholangitis. In general, an impacted ampullary stone precludes easy deep cannulation and a proper sphincterotomy, making stone extraction difficult.
2. *Common bile duct stones.* Patients presenting with abdominal pain or abnormal liver function tests with or without cholangitis.
3. *Intrahepatic duct stones.* Patients are at risk of developing cholangitis.
4. *Failure of standard balloon or basket extraction.* When stones are too large to be removed with standard balloons or wire baskets, large-balloon dilation and/or mechanical lithotripsy is indicated before removal.
5. *Impacted stone-containing basket.* Mechanical lithotripsy can be used to free the basket by fragmenting the stone.
6. *Failed mechanical lithotripsy.* When mechanical lithotripsy fails to remove the stone, particularly large stones that are difficult to capture with the lithotripsy basket or an impacted stone, large-diameter balloon dilation or intraductal (electrohydraulic or laser) lithotripsy is an effective option.
7. *Endoscopic papillary balloon dilation (e.g., sphincteroplasty).* Used as an adjunct for large stones or alternative to endoscopic sphincterotomy (small stones), particularly for anatomy or coagulopathy prohibiting adequate sphincterotomy.

Contraindications

1. Medical conditions that preclude patient undergoing sedated endoscopic procedures.
2. Gastric outlet obstruction that precludes access to the major papilla.

DESCRIPTIONS OF TECHNIQUES

Removal of an Impacted Ampullary Stone

Attempts should be made to disimpact the stone proximally within the bile duct in order to achieve deep cannulation. However, it may be necessary to use a needle knife to cut directly onto the bulging papilla caused by the impacted stone to facilitate deep cannulation (i.e., precut sphincterotomy; see Chapter 15) with subsequent use of a standard sphincterotome and accessories for stone removal. It is possible sometimes to simply extend the cut using the needle knife, eventually delivering the impacted stone.

In cases where a stone is impacted right at the ampullary orifice, as can be seen in patients with acute biliary pancreatitis, a polypectomy snare can be positioned above the impacted stone and closed around the bulging papilla beyond the stone (Fig. 19.2). The wire loop ensnares the bulging papilla and prevents the stone from migrating. With a gentle tug on the closed snare, the impacted stone can be expelled from the orifice.[13] A subsequent sphincterotomy can be performed if residual stones are present in the bile duct. An indwelling biliary stent can be placed to ensure drainage if there is concern about stasis from a swollen papilla to prevent cholangitis.

Balloon Stone Extraction

Extraction balloons are available in various sizes ranging from 8 to 20 mm. The size of the balloon can be adjusted by injecting a varying amount of air into the balloon and regulating the volume with a two-way stopcock (Fig. 19.3, *A*). To size the exit passage before stone extraction and avoid stone impaction, the balloon is inflated to the widest diameter of the common bile duct below the level of the stone and pulled back gently to determine whether there is any resistance to traction removal of the balloon, noting any significant deformity of the balloon. In cases of chronic pancreatitis where the retropancreatic portion of the bile duct may be compressed or fixed, the balloon may deform or become "sausage shaped." This may indicate resistance to stone passage. Triple-lumen balloons allow the catheter to pass over a guidewire and maintain

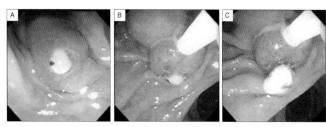

FIG 19.2 **A,** Impacted ampullary stone. **B,** Snare around papilla, above the impacted stone, preventing upward stone migration. **C,** Gentle tugging on the snare expels the stone.

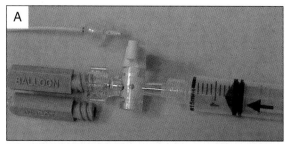

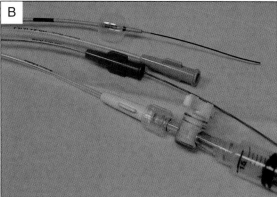

FIG 19.3 **A,** Variable-diameter stone extraction balloon. Balloon (courtesy Boston Scientific, Natick, MA) is inflated to 12 mm in diameter and held in position with two-way stopcock. **B,** Triple-lumen stone extraction balloon (courtesy Cook Endoscopy, Winston-Salem, NC) showing balloon inflated and held in position with two-way stopcock, with a separate lumen for injection of contrast and passage of guidewire.

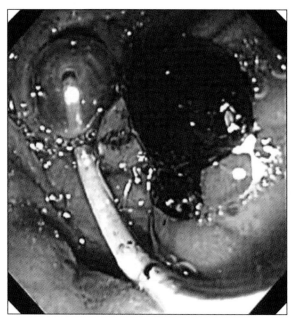

FIG 19.4 Stone extracted with a balloon.

access to the biliary system while allowing injection of contrast (Fig. 19.3, *B*). However, triple-lumen balloon shafts may be stiffer than regular double-lumen balloons.

The tip of the balloon catheter may be gently curved before introduction into the endoscope to facilitate biliary cannulation. Once the catheter is within the bile duct, the balloon is inflated above the stone and pulled back gently until the stone is at the level of the papilla. The scope should be aligned so that the axis of traction is in the same axis as the bile duct to optimize mechanical advantage and avoid ductal damage. The tip of the endoscope is then angled upward against the sphincterotomy. While maintaining gentle traction on the balloon catheter at the level of the biopsy valve, the tip of the scope is deflected downward, expelling the stone from the sphincterotomy (Fig. 19.4). If there is resistance and the stone is not extracted on initial attempt, the tip of the scope is again angled upward with steady traction applied to the catheter, and the "flip down" movement of the scope tip is repeated to remove the stone. It may be necessary to maintain traction on the balloon as the stone is

slowly eased out of the bile duct. If necessary, the scope tip can also be angled downward and rotated to the right to exert more traction force to expel the stone. It is important to remember, however, that an overinflated balloon may give rise to resistance as it is being pulled down, and it may be necessary to deflate the balloon slowly (using the stopcock as a control) to conform to the size of the bile duct and sphincterotomy. If multiple stones are present, the most distal stone should be removed first and then work proximally in the bile duct to avoid stone impaction or rupturing the balloon.

Care should also be taken to avoid overinflating the balloon, as this will stretch the bile duct and cause noticeable pain in the patient who is not under general anesthesia. The balloon should be adjusted in size to fit the diameter of the bile duct. In cases where the balloon goes over a guidewire, excessive scope movement during stone extraction may dislodge the wire. It may be necessary to pull the balloon gently and avoid excess tip deflection of the scope to prevent dislodging the guidewire. An alternative is to insert more guidewire into the bile duct to maintain access before stone extraction. Nonetheless, it should be easy to recannulate the bile duct in the presence of an adequate sphincterotomy even if guidewire access is lost.

Advantages of using a stone extraction balloon include the inflated balloon fully occludes the lumen of the bile duct, facilitating removal of small stones and debris; an occlusion cholangiogram can be performed at the same time to ensure complete clearance of the bile duct; the balloon catheter can be inserted over a guidewire, allowing access to intrahepatic ducts and removal of intrahepatic stones; and finally, it is not possible to impact a balloon catheter in the duct, as can occur with a basket. Drawbacks to using a stone extraction balloon include the possibility of impacting a stone in the distal duct and the possibility of failing to completely clear the bile duct, as balloons can deform around stones in the distal bile duct as they are pulled through the papilla, giving the false impression of duct clearance.

Basket Stone Extraction

Wire baskets are frequently used for stone extraction. A variety of baskets are available in different sizes and configurations, which allow engagement of stones ranging from 5 mm to 3 cm. However, stones larger than

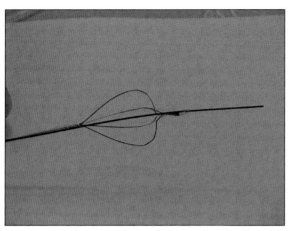

FIG 19.5 Opened wire-guided basket (Olympus America, Lehigh Valley, PA) with the guidewire. Note the much larger gaps between the wires.

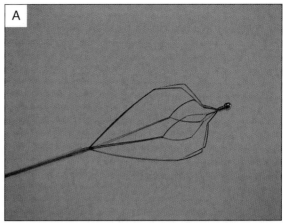

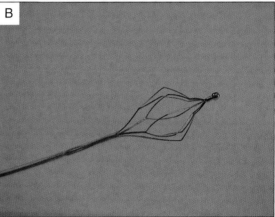

FIG 19.6 **A,** An opened flower basket (Olympus America, Lehigh Valley, PA). Note the smaller mesh size on the upper part of the basket. **B,** Partially closed flower basket showing smaller mesh size, which is better for trapping small stones.

2 cm often cannot be extracted intact and require fragmentation before removal. The four-wire Dormia basket is the most commonly used type (Fig. 19.5). It is hexagonal in shape and made of braided steel or nitinol wires. The stone is engaged between the wires when the basket is closed and removed by continuous traction upon basket withdrawal. Small stones may be difficult to capture with standard baskets that have large gaps between wires. The Olympus flower basket has a modified design, in that the top of the basket is further divided into eight wires, giving more narrow mesh spacing for improved stone engagement when the basket is closed. Small stones are thus more easily trapped than with the regular four-wire basket (Fig. 19.6).

Spiral baskets are also available and may be used to remove relatively small stones (Fig. 19.7). In the spiral configuration, the wires spring closely around the stone as the basket is pushed open. However, spiral baskets are not designed for mechanical lithotripsy. A variety of baskets made for mechanical lithotripsy are designed to engage large stones. The basket wires are much stronger and a spiral metal sheet as support to the basket can be used to mechanically crush the stone. Traction or tension can be applied to the wires either manually or with the help of a special crank handle that is used to tighten the basket wires around the stone and fragment it.

In general, dilute contrast can be injected through the basket to outline the stones in the bile duct. One should avoid injecting an excess volume of contrast to reduce the risk of displacing stones upward into the intrahepatic system. When a single-lumen basket is used, the basket should be opened slightly to allow free flow of dilute contrast. A double-lumen basket allows both injection of contrast through the basket channel and passage of a guidewire through a separate channel. Alternatively, the basket can be advanced over a previously positioned guidewire. This is especially helpful for the removal of intrahepatic stones or stones that may have migrated into the intrahepatic ducts. Traditionally, the guidewire goes through the entire length of the basket catheter. With the short-wire system, only a short length of the basket actually goes over the guidewire and manipulation is done with the wire locked in position. A further modification is the "ropeway" basket, which is a single-lumen system that has a short catheter attached to the tip of the basket, allowing only the tip (instead of the shaft) of the basket to go over the guidewire (Fig. 19.8).

After a stone is visualized on cholangiogram, a closed basket is inserted into the bile duct and advanced proximal to the stone. An alternative approach is to inject contrast using the basket to define the location of the stone(s). After a fresh sphincterotomy or balloon

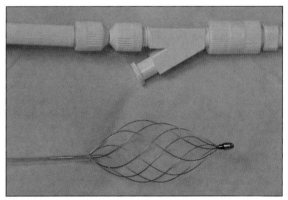

FIG 19.7 Opened helical basket (Cook Endoscopy, Winston-Salem, NC).

sphincteroplasty, it is important that the basket is inserted in the correct axis in the bile duct to avoid dissecting a false plane in the cut tissue and minimize the risk of submucosal trauma and perforation. One way to avoid this potential adverse event is to work with an indwelling guidewire and exchange the basket over the wire. Once in the bile duct, the basket is opened gently above the stone. If necessary, the basket can be opened in the intrahepatic duct and pulled back to engage the stone. Care should be taken to avoid opening the basket below the stone, as the opened basket wires may push the stone proximally up the bile duct or into the intrahepatic system, making removal more difficult.

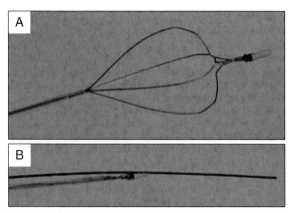

FIG 19.8 A, Olympus ropeway basket showing short segment of catheter attached to tip of opened basket. **B,** Tip of basket going over a guidewire (or over-the-wire technique).

The opened basket is pulled back gently and jiggled alongside the stone to engage it. Once engaged, the basket is closed partially and gently to avoid losing the stone (Fig. 19.9, *A*). The endoscope is then pushed further into the second and third parts of the duodenum to straighten the axis of the basket and the bile duct. Steady traction is applied to the basket catheter at the level of the biopsy valve and the basket containing the stone is withdrawn until it reaches the distal bile duct or the level of the sphincterotomy. With the tip of the scope angled upward close to the sphincterotomy, traction is applied to the basket catheter and at the same time, the tip of the endoscope is angled downward and rotated gently to the right, pulling the stone out of the bile duct (Fig. 19.9, *B*). In most situations, small to medium-sized stones can be removed easily. If the stone does not come out immediately, it is worth repeating the same maneuver while maintaining steady traction on the basket to ease the stone out of the bile duct.

During stone extraction, withdrawing with a fully opened basket (trawling) is less effective, as the loose basket wires tend to cut across the sphincterotomy rather than along the axis of the distal common bile duct. This also tends to pull the stone against the sphincterotomy and results in bruising of the tissue. Closing the basket gently allows the wires to come together, allowing more effective extraction force to be transmitted along the basket catheter for stone removal. However, the basket should not be closed too tightly around the stone to avoid embedding the wires onto the surface of the stone. This is especially important in the case of a large stone, as the basket with the captured stone can become impacted in the distal duct if the stone is too large. When the stone has been tightly engaged in the basket it often cannot be freed from the basket, leading to basket impaction.

One trick to engage small stones/fragments in a dilated bile duct is to open the basket above the stones while aspirating the contrast/bile with a syringe to collapse the bile duct as the basket is withdrawn; this will help trap the stones between the basket wires and improve the success of extraction. For smaller stones that may be difficult to capture, positioning the open basket across the papilla (to open the sphincter) and applying suction in the duodenum may also assist with collapsing the bile duct and facilitating capture of stones in the basket. This maneuver can also be applied in cases of small stones that migrate into the left hepatic duct by positioning the opened basket at the bifurcation and suctioning, which helps to reduce the column of bile and allows the left hepatic duct stones to descend into the common hepatic duct and into the opened basket, which can then be removed.

The advantage that a wire basket offers over an extraction balloon is that it provides more effective traction and therefore is helpful for

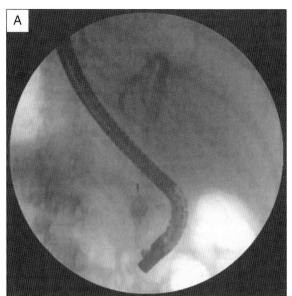

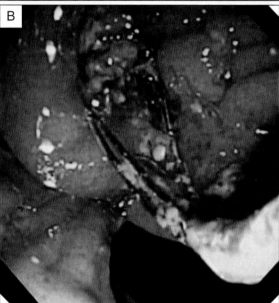

FIG 19.9 A, Stone engaged within a basket. **B,** Stone removed with a wire basket.

removing medium-sized to large stones. However, smaller stones or stone fragments may not be easily engaged by the wires. In addition, intrahepatic stones may be difficult to access because of the smaller caliber of the intrahepatic ducts and the relative lack of flexibility of some baskets, which tend to pass straight (often to the right system), and constraints in opening the basket. In these situations, use of an extraction balloon is preferred.

Recently two randomized trials have compared balloons to baskets for smaller (10 to 11 mm) stones, with mixed results favoring balloons.[13,14]

However, the choice of balloon over basket for smaller-stone removal is often based upon personal preference and geographic variation (east vs west).

Mechanical Lithotripsy

When standard balloon or basket stone extraction fails (Fig. 19.10), fragmentation of the stone within the bile duct may become necessary,

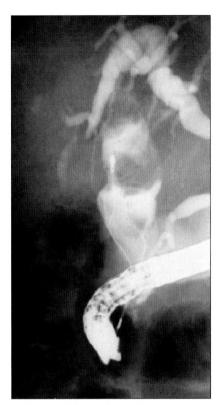

FIG 19.10 Failed basket stone extraction. Three large stones in common bile duct. Basket is too small for the stones.

particularly if the stone is larger than 2 cm or if there is a discrepancy between the stone size and the exit passage (e.g., presence of a distal common bile duct stricture, narrow bile duct, or small sphincterotomy). In some cases, extension of the sphincterotomy is not feasible and may increase the risk of bleeding and perforation. Mechanical lithotripsy is accomplished by capturing a stone within a basket and applying forceful traction to the basket wires around the stone against a metal sheath that is advanced over the basket catheter to crush the stone. In cases of very soft pigment stones (e.g., recurrent or brown pigment stones), however, simply closing a standard Dormia basket tightly around the stone may provide sufficient force to fragment the stone without the use of the metal sheath. However, wire-compatible lithotripsy baskets are preferred in the event that stone entrapment and basket impaction occurs, and a "rescue" non–through the scope (non-TTS) lithotripsy device (which should be available in all endoscopy units) is necessary.

Several lithotriptors are available, which generally fall into two main categories. One requires cutting of the basket handle at the level of the biopsy valve and removal of the endoscope before lithotripsy and is frequently used on an emergency basis ("rescue" lithotripsy) when unexpected stone and basket impaction occurs. The Soehendra lithotriptor (Cook Endoscopy, Winston-Salem, NC) consists of a 14-Fr metal sheath and a self-locking crank handle (Fig. 19.11). The apparatus is compatible with standard extraction baskets or large lithotripsy baskets with stronger wires. It requires cutting of the basket handle to allow removal of the duodenoscope. The plastic sheath around the basket is removed, leaving only the wires exiting the mouth. The metal sheath is then inserted over the basket wires. There are grooves at the tip of

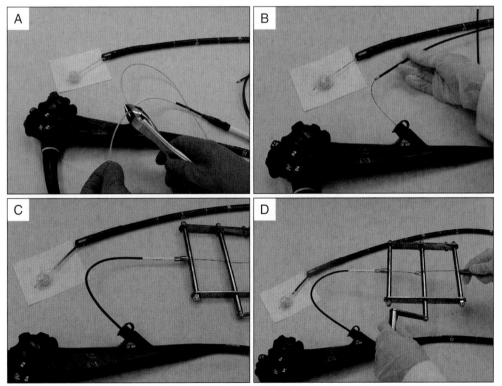

FIG 19.11 For demonstration purposes, an artificial stone is used. **A,** Stone is engaged in the basket. The basket handle is cut and Teflon sheath is then removed. **B,** Metal sheath of the Soehendra lithotripter is inserted over basket wire. **C,** The metal sheath is inserted through the scope channel and advanced to the level of the stone. The cut end of the basket wires is inserted through the shaft of the crank handle. **D,** The basket wires are tied to the shaft of the crank handle and tension is applied as the handle is slowly wound to crush the stone.

the metal sheath. To prevent the bare basket wires from getting stuck in these grooves, a piece of tape may be applied to the end of the metal sheath. This also helps to prevent injury to the posterior pharynx during insertion. It may be helpful to retain the outer basket sheath to facilitate passage of the wires through this 14-Fr metal sheath before removing it. The metal sheath is advanced all the way up to the stone under fluoroscopic visualization. The cut ends of the basket wires are then inserted into the shaft of the crank handle. The metal sheath is attached to the handle by a Luer lock. The wires are then tied to the handle, and the basket is closed tightly around the stone as by winding the crank handle. The basket is closed and drawn into the metal sheath as forceful traction into the metal sheath is applied, crushing the stone against the tip of the metal sheath in the process (Fig. 19.12). It is important to remember that standard baskets are not designed for lithotripsy, and if traction

is applied too quickly the basket wires may break rather than the stone. Winding the crank handle slowly and allowing time for the basket wires to cut through serves to break up the stone and avoids broken basket wires extending toward the mouth (not the basket itself) and stone impaction with the basket.

The latest improvement in design for the Soehendra lithotriptor involves using a smaller 10-Fr sheath, which can be inserted through the scope channel over the basket wires after cutting off the basket handle. In this case it is not necessary to remove the duodenoscope. This TTS setup is used specifically with the Webb basket (Cook Endoscopy) and may not be compatible with other standard baskets. However, unlike other lithotripsy baskets, this basket cannot be reused for repeat stone capture and fragmentation because the handle is cut.

The other types of lithotriptors specifically designed to be used TTS include the BML lithotripsy basket (Olympus, Tokyo, Japan), the Trapezoid basket (Boston Scientific, Marlborough, MA), and the Fusion lithotripsy extraction basket (Cook Endoscopy). These are used in a more elective setting when a large stone, a stone above a stricture, or a difficult stone removal is anticipated.

The BML lithotriptor is a three-layer device consisting of a strong four-wire basket within a Teflon sheath and an overlying metal sheath. The larger lithotripsy basket, or BML-3Q equivalent (BML-201), has a slightly thicker metal sheath and requires a scope with a 4.2-mm working channel. It allows injection of contrast because of the larger diameter. The smaller basket, or BML-4Q equivalent (BML-202, BML-203), passes through a 3.2-mm channel, which makes injection of contrast more difficult. The BML lithotriptor has a reusable version and a disposable version. The reusable system is assembled by inserting the Teflon sheath through the metal sheath, then loading the basket into the Teflon catheter. The wires are soldered together onto a shaft that is connected to the crank handle. Contrast can be injected via the Teflon catheter. The opening and closing of the basket is controlled with the handle. Stone engagement is performed initially with the Teflon catheter and basket. The metal sheath is then advanced over the Teflon catheter up to the level of the stone only when lithotripsy is required (Figs. 19.13 and 19.14).

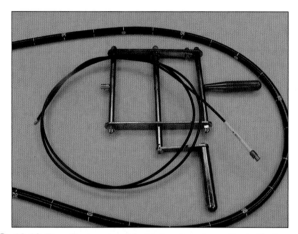

FIG 19.12 The Soehendra lithotripter (courtesy Cook Endoscopy, Winston-Salem, NC) consists of a 10-Fr metal sheath that goes through the instrument channel of the duodenoscope and a self-locking crank handle.

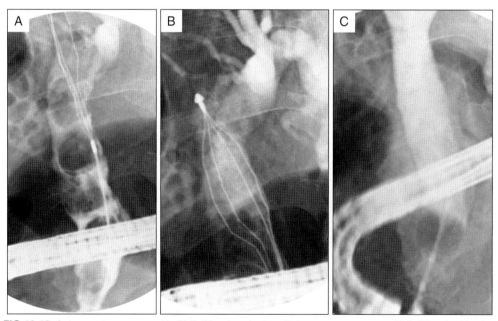

FIG 19.13 A, Large stone engaged in BML lithotripsy basket. **B,** In a separate case, a BML lithotripsy basket is used to engage the stone. **C,** The metal sheath of the lithotripter is advanced over the Teflon sheath, and basket wires tightened around the stone in mid–common bile duct for stone fragmentation.

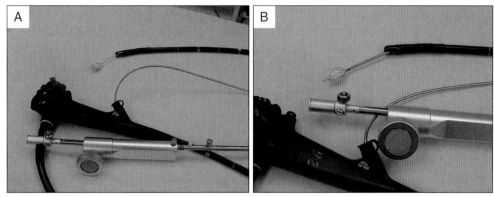

FIG 19.14 A, Through-the-scope BML lithotripter (courtesy Olympus America, Melville, NY) consists of a wire basket within a Teflon catheter, an overlying metal sheath, and the crank handle. **B,** With the stone engaged in the basket, the metal sheath is advanced over the Teflon catheter up to the basket. Basket is closed by turning the wheel and the stone is crushed against the metal sheath.

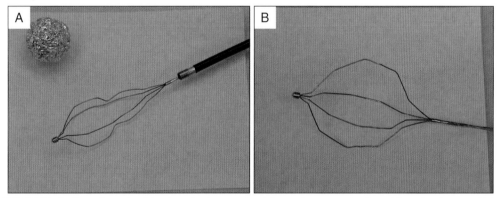

FIG 19.15 A, The wires of a lithotripsy basket can be deformed as a result of crushing a hard stone. **B,** It is necessary to reshape the basket wires to ensure that they open properly for repeat stone engagement.

For the BML basket, although a general shaking and jiggling movement of the basket can be tried to engage the stone, very often a large stone compresses the basket wires, making stone engagement difficult. It may be useful to rotate the basket wires around the stone using rotational movement of the tip of the scope (even better with the help of the metal sheath to transmit a stronger force) to engage the stone. There is a locking mechanism (notches on the metal handle) for the metal sheath to ensure proper engagement of the stone before lithotripsy. It is very important to ensure that the metal sheath is locked in the correct position. This is done by keeping the lithotripsy device straight and avoiding any looping. If the metal sheath is not locked properly (i.e., with a short segment of the Teflon catheter exposed between the stone and the tip of the metal sheath), mechanical lithotripsy will not be effective. If there is recoil or a clicking noise heard when turning the control wheel, lithotripsy is not working, and the position of the metal sheath will need to be adjusted. With the stone properly engaged in the basket and the metal sheath correctly positioned, traction is applied to the wires by turning the control wheel on the handle to crush the stone. The control wheel of the earlier model does not have a built-in self-locking mechanism, and so traction should be applied slowly and continuously to allow time for the wires to cut through the stone. The newer designed crushing handle has a self-locking mechanism that can be used to maintain traction on the basket wires for more controlled stone fragmentation. The reusable system can be taken apart after lithotripsy for cleaning and sterilization. The disposable version comes with the lithotripsy basket, Teflon catheter, and metal

sheath all built into one and is meant for single-use only. If a large and hard stone is crushed, always remove the basket to examine the wires, as they often become deformed as a result of stone breakage (Fig. 19.15). It may be necessary to reshape the basket wires either by hand or with a pair of hemostats to ensure subsequent proper basket opening to trap remaining stone fragments for repeat lithotripsy. In general, mechanical lithotripsy is very effective in breaking large stones. Repeated stone fragmentation may be required in the case of a very large stone because of the larger stone fragments. The reported success rate of mechanical lithotripsy for large stones ranges from 85% to 90%.[16–20]

The Trapezoid basket (Boston Scientific) and, for similar reasons, the Fusion lithotripsy basket (Cook Endoscopy) are both made of nitinol wires and come with a coated and rather flexible metal sheath (Fig. 19.16). The design of these baskets allows them to pass over a guidewire inserted through a separate channel. This is especially handy when used with the short-wire system. The flexibility of the sheath also allows free cannulation with the basket for stone engagement. If stone fragmentation is not necessary, stone extraction can be done in the usual manner because of the flexible sheath. When stone fragmentation is needed, the handle of a rigid balloon insufflator (similar to a caulk gun design) can be fitted to the handle of the basket and traction is then applied to the basket wires to break the stone. This design offers the benefits of allowing selective cannulation over a guidewire and the potential option for stone fragmentation. The baskets come in different sizes to cater to bile duct stones of different diameters.

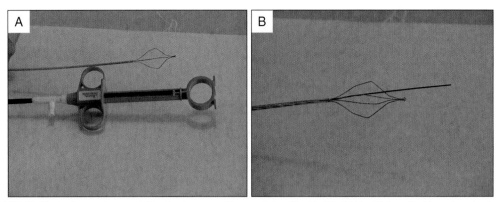

FIG 19.16 A, Opened trapezoid basket (courtesy Boston Scientific, Natick, MA) with handle. Note the plastic-covered metal sheath. The plastic handle can be fitted to a cranking device if lithotripsy is required. **B,** Opened trapezoid basket inserted over a guidewire.

Intraductal Electrohydraulic Lithotripsy

Large-diameter balloon dilation with or without mechanical lithotripsy is so effective and successful that the need for intraductal lithotripsy is reserved for selected cases. Intraductal lithotripsy is available mostly in academic units. Intraductal lithotripsy can be conducted under fluoroscopy using a special balloon that centers the probe in the bile duct, though this is most often performed under direct visual control with peroral cholangioscopy using the "mother and baby" scope system (Olympus) or the SpyGlass (SpyGlass DS) system (Boston Scientific, Natick, MA) (see Chapter 27).

There are two forms of intraductal lithotripsy (IDL): laser lithotripsy and electrohydraulic lithotripsy.[21–25] Each of these types of intraductal lithotripsy is best performed under direct visual control with peroral cholangioscopy.

An older Olympus system consists of a jumbo-sized duodenoscope ("mother" scope) with a 5.5-mm channel and a small fiberoptic cholangioscope ("baby" scope) with an outer diameter of 4.7 mm and a 1.7-mm working channel that has two-way tip deflection. The larger instrument channel allows easier passage of the lithotripsy probe. A newer cholangioscope by Olympus is smaller, with an outer diameter of 3.2 mm and a 1-mm instrument channel, and can be inserted through a therapeutic duodenoscope with a 4.2-mm instrument channel. It is also available in video form. However, because of the small instrument channel, it can accommodate only the small lithotripsy probe or the smaller laser probe.

In recent years, there has been increasing widespread use of a single–operator controlled, single-use peroral system that uses a single-use four-lumen 10-Fr-diameter system that attaches to the duodenoscope head. The SpyScope Legacy (Boston Scientific) access and delivery catheter has four-way steering capability. The initial version had a lumen for insertion of a fiberoptic bundle for direct visualization and a 1.2-mm accessory channel. The remaining two lumens are independent irrigation channels.[26] The second-generation SpyGlass DS, with a 10.5-Fr-diameter access and delivery catheter, has improved digital optics for high-resolution direct imaging and image-guided therapy. The integrated digital sensor eliminates the need for the fragile optical probe used in the first-generation device.[27]

After an adequate sphincterotomy or combined sphincterotomy with balloon sphincteroplasty, the cholangioscope is introduced into the common bile duct. A fluid medium (normal saline, not water) is required to perform electrohydraulic lithotripsy. The electrohydraulic lithotriptor consists of a power generator (e.g., Autolith; Nortech, Elgin, IL) by which the power or energy can be preset based on the size of the probe (3 or 4.5 Fr) used. The tip of the probe has a pair of bipolar electrodes,

which generates a shock wave to fragment the stone when activated in an ionic fluid medium. The frequency of discharge of the shock wave can be preset on the machine and activated by a foot switch either as a single pulse or continuous discharge. Depending on the instrument channel of the cholangioscope, various sizes of probes (1.9, 3, and 4.5 Fr) can be used. Saline irrigation within the bile duct also facilitates examination by cholangioscopy. Care is taken not to overfill the system, in order to minimize the risk of cholangitis. The electrohydraulic lithotripsy probe is placed close to the stone under direct cholangioscopic visualization aided by fluoroscopy. The stone and probe are immersed in saline. The foot switch is activated and stone fragmentation is performed under direct visual control. Stone fragments generated during lithotripsy can obscure the view. Irrigation and suction clears the view. Effective stone fragmentation can be demonstrated under fluoroscopy by injecting contrast into the bile through the cholangioscope duct after the probe is removed or using a Tuohy Borst adapter. Subsequent stone fragment is extracted with a balloon or basket after removal of the cholangioscope, followed by an occlusion cholangiogram to document clearance of the bile duct. Because stone fragments are generated during lithotripsy, it may be helpful to insert the stone extraction basket deep in the bile duct and irrigate the duct with saline flushed through the basket (while applying suction with the scope). This helps to remove the remaining stone fragments from the common duct or at least flushes them toward the distal duct for retrieval. If the jumbo-sized duodenoscope is used for "mother and baby" examination, it may be useful to exchange to a regular therapeutic (4.2-mm channel) duodenoscope for ease of manipulation. In some cases, insertion of a stent or nasobiliary catheter is done to decompress the biliary system, especially if complete stone clearance cannot be assured. This allows stone fragments to settle and avoid the risk of stone impaction and cholangitis. A repeat ERCP is performed at a later time to remove remaining stone fragments for complete duct clearance and stent extraction.

Endoscopic Papillary Balloon Dilation

Papillary balloon dilation can be used to facilitate stone extraction with or without preceding endoscopic sphincterotomy (see Chapter 18). This technique is particularly useful to achieve an adequate opening (i.e., exit passage) to allow retrieval of large stones, in prior failed stone extraction or in difficult anatomy (e.g., diverticulum), or in the presence of patient factors (e.g., coagulopathy) prohibitive of sphincterotomy. Dilation balloons (≤10 mm) available include the Fusion dilation balloon (Cook Endoscopy) and Hurricane balloon (Boston Scientific). Large-balloon dilators (12 to 20 mm) are adapted from CRE balloon pyloric dilators (Cook Endoscopy) or TTS dilators (Boston Scientific). The maximum size of the balloon should preferably not exceed the diameter of the proximal bile duct to avoid perforation, and dilation should be performed slowly and under fluoroscopic guidance to evaluate for disappearance of a waist. The duration of dilation is generally 30 to 60 seconds after disappearance of the waist under fluoroscopy, although a longer duration may be considered, particularly in cases where an endoscopic sphincterotomy was not performed, as this may reduce the risk of pancreatitis (when sphincterotomy is not performed). Large-balloon dilation with endoscopic sphincterotomy has similar outcomes in terms of stone clearance and the advantage of a lower risk of overall adverse events and pancreatitis compared with sphincterotomy alone.[27]

ADVERSE EVENTS AND THEIR MANAGEMENT (SEE CHAPTER 8)

Adverse Events of Extraction Balloons

- Balloon rupture
- Impacted stone

Adverse events may arise when using the balloon. If the balloon is pulled too hard against the stone, rupture of the balloon may occur. If the stone is too large for the sphincterotomy, the air-filled balloon may deform and slip out, leaving the stone impacted at the lower end of the common bile duct or at the level of the papilla. To free an impacted stone, it may be necessary to push it proximally using a stiffer accessory, for example, biopsy forceps. Alternatively, it may be possible to extend the sphincterotomy if a standard sphincterotome can be inserted beyond the stone. Another option is to use a needle knife to cut onto the bulging intraduodenal portion of the distal bile duct and papilla in order to free the stone (Fig. 19.17). If the stone impaction is at the distal duct but not the papilla, a balloon may also be inflated below the impacted stone and contrast injected under pressure to push the stone into the more proximal duct to allow subsequent alternative therapy, including lithotripsy. In the event that the stone is impacted within the bile duct, it is important to ensure drainage of the biliary system by placing a stent or nasobiliary drain to avoid subsequent cholangitis if the stone is not removed. It is therefore preferable to operate the balloon over an indwelling guidewire that maintains biliary access in case of failed stone extraction and to ensure that drainage can be established.

Adverse Events of Extraction Baskets

- Migration of stones into the intrahepatic ducts
- Impaction of stone and basket

During basket stone extraction, the stone(s) may migrate up into the intrahepatic ducts. Capturing a migrated stone within an intrahepatic duct can be challenging. The best method is to avoid using the basket when this occurs. A balloon and guidewire may be used to selectively cannulate the respective segment containing the stone. The balloon is advanced over the guidewire beyond the stone and inflated. The stone is then withdrawn into the common hepatic duct or the common bile duct before further attempts are made to remove the stone, either using the same balloon catheter or exchanging for a basket. Use of a wire-guided basket is also helpful in removing stones from the intrahepatic ducts, although these baskets tend to be rather stiff and manipulation in the intrahepatic ducts can be somewhat difficult.

If stone extraction fails when a basket is used, it may be necessary to free the engaged stone from the basket to avoid basket and stone impaction. This may be achieved by gently advancing the basket and stone up toward and against the bifurcation and opening the basket so that the wires bend back on themselves. In this fashion, the wires are opened and the stone can be dropped from the basket. The basket is then closed slowly above the stone to avoid reengaging it when the basket is pulled back. Once the basket is closed, it can be removed. Further stone extraction may require extension of the sphincterotomy or balloon dilation and/or stone fragmentation using a mechanical lithotriptor.

Another potential complication that may arise is impaction of the basket and stone within the bile duct or at the level of the papilla. This may be because of large stone size, an inadequate sphincterotomy, or inability to enlarge the sphincterotomy. In rare instances, stone and basket impaction has occurred at the level of the head of the pancreas because of a narrowed distal common duct. In these cases, emergent mechanical lithotripsy may be attempted using a Soehendra lithotriptor.

Adverse Events of Mechanical Lithotripsy

- Excess traction on the wires against a very hard stone may lead to breakage of the basket wires.
- Failure can occur if there is stone impaction that prevents proper opening of the large basket around the stone.

The Soehendra lithotriptor may be used as a "rescue" measure in cases of stone and basket impaction. However, the wires of the standard basket are relatively soft and may break in the duodenum, resulting in retained broken basket and stone in the bile duct. Attempts can be made to use a formal TTS lithotripsy basket to engage the broken basket and stone and to fragment the stone and remove the basket. This may

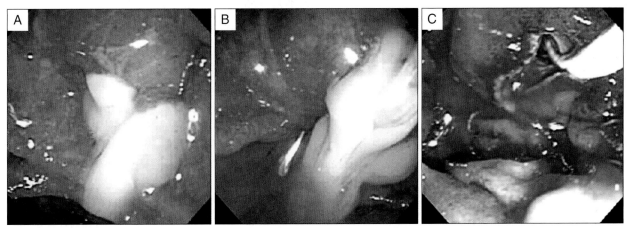

FIG 19.17 Impacted stone. **A,** Note the bulging papilla with pus exiting. **B,** Initial precut was followed by cannulation with sphincterotome. **C,** After extension of sphincterotomy and stone clearance.

also require extension of the sphincterotomy or balloon dilation or use of cholangioscopic lithotripsy to break the stone from inside the basket. If stone/basket engagement is possible, the impacted stone and basket can be successfully removed. As long as adequate drainage can be achieved by insertion of a stent or nasobiliary tube, the situation is not life threatening. In rare cases, surgical exploration may be needed to remove the impacted stone and basket.

The Olympus TTS lithotripsy basket is designed to break at the connection between the basket and the crank handle; alternatively the basket wires are also designed to break at the tip to prevent having a broken basket around an impacted stone in the bile duct. In the unexpected event of the basket breaking at the connection point, Olympus has developed a special metal sheath that resembles the Soehendra rescue lithotriptor. This metal sheath can be inserted over the broken basket after removal of the endoscope. Stone fragmentation can be performed as with the Soehendra lithotriptor. It is not advisable to use the Cook Endoscopy Soehendra lithotriptor handle and adapt it onto a broken Olympus lithotripsy basket, as it is not truly compatible. If that is necessary, it is important to retain the Teflon catheter around the basket wires to offer support for the metal sheath. The design of the metal sheath with the disposable BML system is different, and if tension is applied to the wires without the Teflon catheter, the coils of the metal sheath buckle, thus making lithotripsy ineffective.

TTS mechanical lithotripsy is successful in the majority of cases because these baskets are stronger. Over 80% of large (>2 cm) stones have been fragmented in reported series, giving a common duct clearance rate of over 95%. The main reason for failure is that the stone is too large for the size of the basket, but even then, if part of the stone can be engaged, stone fragmentation can be attempted to reduce the size of the stone, allowing for proper engagement for complete stone fragmentation. Mechanical lithotripsy fails when there is stone impaction or if there is not enough room within the bile duct to open the basket to engage the stone. In this situation, temporary stenting can be attempted to ensure drainage of the biliary system. Subsequent spontaneous stone fragmentation has been observed in 30% of cases, possibly because of the friction between the stone and the stent or because of possible dissolution effects of improved bile flow.

Although relatively uncommon, perforation of the bile duct may occur because of the relative stiffness of the basket when the wires are tightened. In addition, pancreatitis may result from forceful removal of an impacted stone and basket, causing injury to the pancreatic orifice.

Adverse Events of Intraductal Lithotripsy

- Bile duct injury and perforation

Although highly effective, one of the major problems is difficulty with targeting of the shock waves and inadvertent bile duct injury and perforation. The procedure should be performed under direct endoscopic and fluoroscopic guidance by endoscopists with experience in the use of the equipment.

RELATIVE COST

Balloons range in price from $100 to $150 (list price), depending on the manufacturer and whether they are double-lumen or triple-lumen catheters. List prices for baskets range from $150 to $350, depending on the design. Some baskets are disposable, whereas others are reusable. The cost of the startup package for the SpyGlass DS system—which uses a single-use access and delivery catheter that costs around $3000—is about $100,000.

CONCLUSIONS

It is customary to clear the bile duct stones, even when asymptomatic, because of the risk of obstruction, cholangitis, and pancreatitis. Sphincterotomy and sphincteroplasty facilitate access to the biliary system. Basket and balloon catheters are useful for removing the majority of stones up to 1.5 cm in diameter. The use of wire-guided basket or balloon catheters allows proper access to the intrahepatic system to remove intrahepatic stones or migrated stones. Stones above a bile duct stricture require balloon dilation of the stricture before successful removal. The use of mechanical lithotripsy to break up stones facilitates duct clearance of large stones or stones above a stricture. Mechanical lithotripsy is very effective in achieving common duct clearance, and the use of intraductal lithotripsy is limited to about 5% of very difficult ductal stones.

The complete reference list for this chapter can be found online at www.expertconsult.com.

20

Pancreatic Sphincterotomy

Jonathan M. Buscaglia and Anthony N. Kalloo

Since its initial application in 1974, endoscopic biliary sphincterotomy (see Chapter 17) has revolutionized the approach to patients with biliary tract diseases.[1] Biliary sphincterotomy has been used in conjunction with other techniques such as stent placement, balloon and basket extraction of stones, and stricture dilatation, and it has become the standard of care for problems that were once remedied only by surgical procedures. Endoscopic therapy for pancreatic disorders has not advanced quite as rapidly, however. The main reason for this seems to be the long-standing fear of inducing pancreatitis in an organ that frequently expresses its dislike for simple manipulation of the papilla and sphincter alone.[2] Historically, pancreatitis and its associated adverse events have prevented some endoscopists from attempting to apply therapeutic techniques similar to those used in treating biliary tract disorders. In addition, clear-cut indications for endoscopic therapy of the pancreas have been much more difficult to define because of a paucity of well-designed clinical trials justifying its use. Most of the techniques used in previous studies were performed on small numbers of patients and by expert endoscopists. The majority of studies have been retrospective in design without control groups. There is a deficiency of randomized trials that directly compare endoscopic therapy with either surgical or medical therapy.[2]

It is on this background that we begin to discuss endoscopic pancreatic sphincterotomy. This technique is the cornerstone of endoscopic therapy of the pancreas, and it provides initial access to the main pancreatic duct.[3] Once access to the duct is obtained, it may be used as a single therapeutic maneuver (e.g., to treat pancreatic-type sphincter of Oddi dysfunction) or in combination with other endoscopic therapeutic techniques, such as stent placement across a ductal stricture.[4] In chronic pancreatitis, for example, pancreatic sphincterotomy not only decreases pressure within the main pancreatic duct but also may be used to facilitate extraction of calculi and protein plugs.[1]

This chapter focuses on the endoscopic techniques and the equipment used by most experts who regularly perform pancreatic sphincterotomy. The indications and contraindications for this technique, as well as the evidence that supports its basis, are also discussed. The adverse events associated with pancreatic sphincterotomy and their management strategies are outlined. Lastly, we briefly discuss any existing literature associated with the costs and cost savings of pancreatic sphincterotomy.

ENDOSCOPIC PANCREATIC SPHINCTEROTOMY

Preparation

As with all endoscopic procedures, it is imperative to obtain informed consent.[5] This is paramount when discussing with patients and their families the potential risks involved in performing endoscopic retrograde cholangiopancreatography (ERCP) with pancreatic sphincterotomy, as the adverse event rates are higher compared with routine upper

Video for this chapter can be found online at www.expertconsult.com.

endoscopy. Routine blood work, including a complete blood count, and coagulation parameters are verified before the procedure in selected patients (see Chapter 10). Antithrombotic agents are withheld, as appropriate.[5] Antibiotics are administered preprocedurally in an effort to prevent procedure-related infection in the presence of pancreatic pseudocysts and other fluid collections and when incomplete pancreatic drainage is anticipated, as is done for biliary procedures. The data supporting antibiotic prophylaxis before pancreatic sphincterotomy are sparse. Only a few studies have attempted to investigate this issue, and most of them have had small numbers with poorly defined endpoints.[6] Coverage with a second-generation or third-generation cephalosporin appears sufficient. Broader-spectrum antibiotics, such as piperacillin/tazobactam—or vancomycin and gentamicin if there is a penicillin allergy—may be warranted in some instances.

Equipment

Pancreatic sphincterotomy, like biliary sphincterotomy, is performed with a standard side-viewing duodenoscope, the appropriate sphincterotome (papillotome), and an electrosurgical generator.[7] There are a variety of options in terms of commercially available electrosurgical generators (see Chapter 11). Most have both monopolar and bipolar options, and they offer pure cutting, pure coagulation, and blended (cut/coag) current modes.[5] These generators are the same as those used when performing colonoscopic polypectomies. Newer models even allow for cutting options that incrementally splice the sphincter muscle in 1-mm segments, informing the endoscopist with an audible alarm at the end of each segment. This attempts to ensure that the sphincterotomy is performed in a careful, stepwise fashion without producing an unintentional exaggerated cut. However, there are no data that verify the effectiveness of this method.

There is little evidence supporting the use of one current mode over the others when performing biliary sphincterotomy. Some data, however, suggest that pure cutting current may be associated with less post-ERCP pancreatitis compared with blended current.[8] Also, the use of pure cutting current is thought to cause less fibrosis, thus diminishing the risk of papillary stenosis. As a result, some endoscopists advocate using only the pure cutting mode when performing a pancreatic sphincterotomy. It is unclear whether there is an increased risk of bleeding, as some have suggested.

A wide variety of sphincterotomes and guidewires are commercially available for use in pancreatic sphincterotomy. For a more detailed description of endoscopic guidewires and ERCP accessories, refer to Chapter 4. The original Demling-Classen or Erlangen pull-type sphincterotome (bowstring design) is still the most popular choice for performing pancreatic sphincterotomy (Fig. 20.1). There are several variations of this type of sphincterotome based on differences in the length of the exposed cutting wire, the number of additional lumens, and differences in the length of the "nose" of the instrument.[5,7] A shorter nose

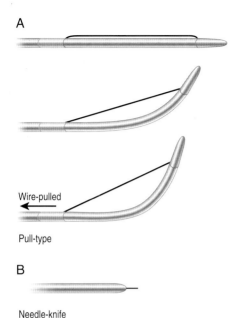

A

Wire-pulled

Pull-type

B

Needle-knife

FIG 20.1 **A** and **B,** Standard sphincterotomes used in pancreatic sphincterotomy. (Reproduced by permission of Division of Gastroenterology and Hepatology, Johns Hopkins Hospital.)

(5 to 8 mm beyond the wire) is sometimes more convenient for cannulation of the major papilla before sphincterotomy. It allows for easier engagement between the sphincterotome tip and the papilla without much interference from the cutting wire. Once the tip is positioned inside the papillary orifice, tension on the wire may be applied to bow the tip into the correct axis and correctly align the instrument for eventual sphincterotomy.[7] Sphincterotomes with longer noses (2 to 5 cm beyond the wire) lose their ability to bow because most of the cutting wire is retained inside the duodenoscope until deep cannulation is attained. The advantage of this type of sphincterotome is the ability to maintain cannulation while the wire is being withdrawn during sphincterotomy. However, now with triple-lumen cannulas and soft-tip and flexible-tip guidewires that cause less injury to the pancreatic duct, a guidewire can be easily left in place within the pancreatic duct in order to maintain cannulation while performing a pancreatic sphincterotomy (wire-guided sphincterotomy). This technique of wire-guided sphincterotomy is now considered the standard of care for both pancreatic and biliary sphincterotomy.

Standard sphincterotomes have a 5-Fr to 7-Fr catheter tip that can accept a 0.035-inch guidewire.[9] Use of a triple-lumen cannula allows for the placement of a preloaded guidewire and simultaneous contrast injection without having to remove the guidewire. When manipulating the papilla and the most proximal portions of the main pancreatic duct before sphincterotomy, many endoscopists prefer an ultratapered catheter tip (5 Fr–4 Fr–3 Fr) for easier cannulation. These sphincterotomes require the use of smaller-caliber guidewires, frequently down to 0.018-inch diameter. Conversely, a special 3-Fr cannula can be passed through the channel of a standard sphincterotome to produce the effect of a tapered-tip catheter.[9]

Endoscopic pancreatic sphincterotomy is performed after deep cannulation of the main pancreatic duct with a guidewire.[10] There are several different types of commercially available guidewires that may be used to perform this technique. Such configurations of guidewires include conventional, nitinol, hydrophilic, and "hybrid." The range in wire diameter is from 0.018 to 0.035 inches.[11] When performing a wire-guided pancreatic sphincterotomy, hydrophilic-coated wires with

soft and floppy tips may be helpful in preventing trauma to the main pancreatic duct and its side branches.[10] As mentioned above, this deep wire-guided technique in pancreatic sphincterotomy has obviated the need for longer-nose sphincterotomes. Maintaining adequate cannulation of the papilla in this manner is less traumatic and more secure.

The Endoscopic Technique

The main principles involved in pancreatic sphincterotomy are similar to biliary sphincterotomy (see Chapter 17). They involve wire-guided cannulation of the duct before cutting and use a slow and stepwise approach that relies on accurate identification of anatomic landmarks. There are essentially two different types of techniques that are used by most expert endoscopists when performing pancreatic sphincterotomy. The first approach, as well as the more popular one, uses a standard pull-type sphincterotome. The second approach uses an endoscopic needle knife to cut the sphincter muscle *after* placement of a pancreatic duct stent. Both techniques have their advantages and disadvantages, and the details surrounding each approach are discussed below. In addition, we will briefly describe the technique of precut or "access" pancreatic sphincterotomy in those instances when the endoscopist is faced with a difficult pancreatic cannulation. Sphincterotomy of the minor papilla is discussed separately in Chapter 21.

As with both biliary and pancreatic sphincterotomy, success starts with accurate cannulation of the correct duct (see Chapter 14). This is, at times, the greatest hurdle for novice therapeutic endoscopists. In general, selective cannulation of the pancreatic duct is easier than that of the biliary duct, assuming that there has not been a previous biliary sphincterotomy. The reason for this is directly related to the anatomic axis of each duct in relation to the wall of the duodenum. Although the main pancreatic duct may be tortuous with multiple side branches, the most proximal portion of the duct courses away from the papilla at a 90-degree angle from the duodenal wall (Fig. 20.2). It then runs more toward the right and straight inside.[12] The most distal part of the common bile duct, on the other hand, assumes more of an acute angle in its relationship with the duodenal wall. It extends in an upward and leftward direction from the papillary orifice. This provides for a more difficult cannulation, depending on how acute the angle of takeoff is from the papilla.

One must remember that a cross-sectional view of the *inner* portion of the ampulla of Vater (the part furthest from the duodenal lumen) is similar to a "double-eyed onion," with each duct running off in its own unique direction.[12] The most proximal portion of the ampulla, however, is a single orifice that leads from the lumen of the duodenum into a common channel. This common channel then merges with the "double-eyed onion." The length of this channel is variable but usually ranges between 1 and 10 mm.[7] Within this channel are several folds of papillary mucosa that may often act as obstacles to selective cannulation with the sphincterotome. Therefore accurate cannulation depends on finding the correct axis with the catheter tip before the guidewire can be pushed all the way out into the main pancreatic duct. Approaching the papillary orifice with the right orientation allows the endoscopist to find the correct axis.

When aiming for the pancreatic duct, the catheter should enter the orifice perpendicular to the duodenal wall. Then, to traverse the correct plane, the catheter tip should be advanced along the *floor* of the orifice to find the pancreatic duct. This is in contrast to biliary cannulation, in which the catheter tip is aimed at the *roof* of the papillary orifice to find the distal common bile duct.[7] The only way to ultimately assure correct cannulation is to (1) gently advance the guidewire into the duct and confirm fluoroscopically the position of the wire in a transverse direction toward and/or across the spine or (2) inject contrast to verify one's position within the duct fluoroscopically. To limit the risk

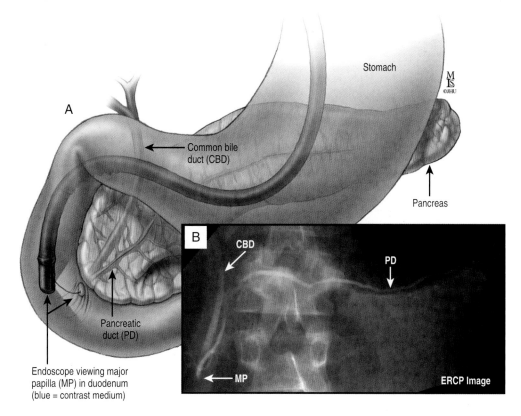

FIG 20.2 A and **B,** Position of the main pancreatic duct and the distal common bile duct in relation to the major papilla. The pancreatic duct runs 90 degrees perpendicular from the duodenal side wall. (Reproduced by permission of Division of Gastroenterology and Hepatology, Johns Hopkins Hospital.)

of pancreatitis, as little contrast as possible should be used in this situation.

The importance of correct ductal axis is paramount. When faced with difficult pancreatic duct cannulation, one may have to lower the catheter tip even further when advancing along the floor of the papillary orifice. This can be achieved by lowering the elevator on the duodenoscope, thus pressing down on the floor.[7] The injection of contrast is done simultaneously in an effort to correctly identify the pancreatic duct.

Pull-Type Sphincterotomy

After successful pancreatic cannulation and advancement of the guidewire into the main pancreatic duct, confirmation of position is usually obtained with a contrast pancreatogram. Assuming that a clear indication for sphincterotomy has been established, this part of the procedure is most often performed with a pull-type sphincterotome (as mentioned above). As with biliary sphincterotomy, the incision should be "hot and slow."[7] It should be directed toward the 1 to 2 o'clock position with the very distal part of the cutting wire.[5,10] In other words, most of the cutting wire should be visible outside the papillary orifice. Note that the direction of the cut is very different from that of a biliary sphincterotomy (Fig. 20.3). When performing biliary sphincterotomy, the cutting direction is in the 11 to 1 o'clock position (preferably the 12 o'clock position). The sphincterotome is slightly bowed while the cutting wire is "walked up" the roof of the papilla in a stepwise fashion.[7] In pancreatic sphincterotomy the same principles apply, but the direction is more toward the right, guiding the cutting wire along the floor of the papillary orifice.

The actual incision should be performed using the pure cutting current with the electrosurgical generator. This prevents further damage to the pancreas and limits the risk of fibrosis and papillary stenosis.[10,13] The length of the cut is generally between 5 and 10 mm. Larger-diameter ducts require longer cuts in order to achieve the largest possible access. Once the sphincterotomy has been completed, a temporary pancreatic stent is usually left in place for a short period in order to facilitate adequate drainage from the duct (assuming that larger stents are not placed for treatment of strictures, leaks, etc.). The edema that ensues after pancreatic sphincterotomy can cause ductal obstruction and acute pancreatitis.[14] Placement of a pancreatic stent after every pancreatic sphincterotomy is nearly universal. However, the stent type chosen and the desired duration of dwell time have been debated.[15]

Early in the era of pancreatic sphincterotomy, many endoscopists advocated *always* performing this procedure in concert with a prior biliary sphincterotomy. Biliary sphincterotomy done immediately before pancreatic sphincterotomy is felt by some to allow for easier identification of clear anatomic landmarks, thus making it safer and more effective. It may provide better exposure of the pancreaticobiliary septum and therefore allow improved access to the desired pancreatic tissue.[16] Also, this approach prevents the rare possibility of biliary adverse events after a primary pancreatic cut.[1] The adverse events include inadvertent damage to the distal bile duct and possible biliary obstruction because of edema adjacent to the biliary duct orifice. Many expert endoscopists recommend a biliary sphincterotomy before a pancreatic sphincterotomy in cases of cholangitis or obstructive jaundice, presence of a common bile duct diameter >12 mm, or an alkaline phosphatase level greater than twice

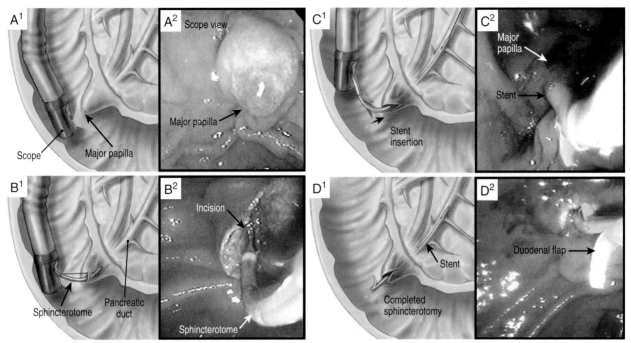

FIG 20.3 **A,** View of the major papilla before pancreatic sphincterotomy. **B,** Sphincterotomy performed with the cutting wire angled toward the 2 o'clock position. **C,** Placement of a pancreatic stent after sphincterotomy. **D,** Completion of the sphincterotomy with the stent in good position. (Reproduced by permission of Division of Gastroenterology and Hepatology, Johns Hopkins Hospital.)

BOX 20.1   The Pull-Type Sphincterotome Technique

- Direction of the incision is along the 1–2 o'clock position.
- Pure cutting current should be used.
- Incision should be "slow and hot."
- Majority of the cutting wire should be outside the papillary orifice.
- Length of the incision is generally between 5 and 10 mm.
- A pancreatic duct stent is inserted after completion.
- May or may not be preceded by a biliary sphincterotomy.

---

normal.[10] It may also be done when it is needed to obtain better access to the main pancreatic duct.[17]

When performing a pancreatic sphincterotomy after a biliary sphincterotomy, the anatomic landmarks are different. Part of the papilla has already been filleted open for this procedure, and so the pancreatic orifice is usually seen at the 5 o'clock position near the right margin of the sphincterotomy.[1] Transient opening of the pancreatic duct will allow for better visualization and more accurate cutting. This may be achieved by gently sucking air into the duodenum with the scope. Once the orifice is correctly identified and cannulated, the sphincterotomy can be carried out in a similar fashion as described above (Box 20.1).

Needle-Knife Sphincterotomy

An alternative method to pancreatic sphincterotomy uses an endoscopic needle knife instead of a standard pull-type sphincterotome (see Fig. 20.1).[16] Cutting with the needle knife is done after placement of a pancreatic duct stent. The tip of the needle knife is placed at the most proximal portion of pancreatic sphincter tissue that is overlying the stent. The stent is used as a guide to direct the cut along the plane of the pancreatic duct, and the needle knife tip is advanced over the top of the stent and down its longitudinal axis (Fig. 20.4). Incision length

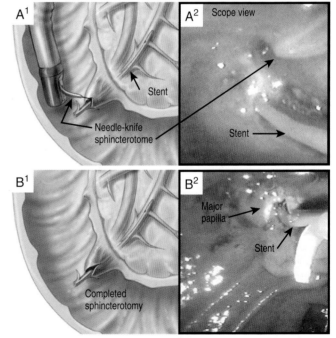

FIG 20.4 **A,** Sphincterotomy performed with a needle-knife sphincterotome. A pancreatic stent is placed before the sphincter tissue is cut. The stent acts as a guide, directing the cut along the plane of the pancreatic duct. Notice that the angle of the cut is in the 2 o'clock position down toward the stent. **B,** Completion of the needle-knife sphincterotomy. (Reproduced by permission of Division of Gastroenterology and Hepatology, Johns Hopkins Hospital.)

BOX 20.2 The Needle-Knife Technique

- A pancreatic duct stent is always inserted beforehand.
- The needle knife is advanced over the top of the stent.
- Pure cutting current should be used.
- Length of incision is between 5 and 10 mm.
- Frequently preceded by a biliary sphincterotomy.

BOX 20.3 Controversies Surrounding Pancreatic Sphincterotomy

- Pull-type sphincterotome technique versus needle-knife technique
- Biliary sphincterotomy before pancreatic sphincterotomy?
- Blended current versus pure cutting current
- Pancreatic stent versus no stent after sphincterotomy
- If stent, what type of stent? How long should the stent stay in place?

TABLE 20.1 Differences in Technique of Pancreatic Sphincterotomy Based on a Survey of 14 Expert Endoscopists

	Always	Often	Sometimes	Never
PTS	3	3	7	1
NK	1	6	5	2
EBS	8	4	1	1
PC	2			
BC	12			
PS	12	2		

Modified from Alsolaiman M, Cotton P, Hawes R, et al. Techniques of pancreatic sphincterotomy: lack of expert consensus. *Gastrointest Endosc.* 2004;59:AB210. With permission.
BC, Blended current; EBS, endoscopic biliary sphincterotomy before pancreatic sphincterotomy; NK, needle-knife technique; PC, pure cutting current; PS, pancreatic stent placement afterward; PTS, pull-type sphincterotome.

is similar to that of sphincterotomy with a pull-type sphincterotome; that is, the length is generally between 5 and 10 mm. Many experts believe that a prior biliary sphincterotomy is especially helpful before using this needle-knife technique.[16] Good exposure of the pancreaticobiliary septum allows for better tissue access and more effective "septotomy."

There are a few limitations to this technique, however. The absolute prerequisite of pancreatic duct stent placement makes it a technique that may not be feasible if a stent cannot be placed. For example, in chronic pancreatitis it may be very difficult to insert a stent without first removing ductal calculi.[10] Furthermore, using the pull-type sphincterotome technique allows a more thorough assessment of sphincterotomy completeness. The endoscopist can reassess the incision and extend the cut, if necessary, with the sphincterotome wire. This is not possible with the needle-knife and stent technique. Lastly, many endoscopists find it simpler and faster to perform the sphincterotomy without having to first place a pancreatic stent (Box 20.2).

Despite the fact that pancreatic sphincterotomy is performed by only two different techniques, survey questionnaires show a lack of expert consensus in terms of the best approach. A previous survey of 14 expert endoscopists in 9 US centers showed that 6 of those 14 gastroenterologists either "always" or "often" used the pull-type sphincterotome technique, whereas 7 of them "always" or "often" used the needle-knife technique.[15] Eight physicians "always" performed a biliary sphincterotomy before pancreatic sphincterotomy, and only 2 of the 14 used pure cutting current during the procedure (Table 20.1). Almost all endoscopists insert a pancreatic stent after sphincterotomy, as it lowers the likelihood of post-ERCP pancreatitis.[14] However, the type of stent used and dwell time are quite variable among those who perform pancreatic sphincterotomy regularly.[15] Questions surrounding these differences among techniques can be answered only with future

randomized trials that examine both the short-term and long-term outcomes of each (Box 20.3).

Precut Pancreatic Sphincterotomy

Precut pancreatic sphincterotomy refers to an endoscopic technique that allows one to gain access to the pancreatic duct without performing prior deep cannulation. It is usually done when access to the duct is impeded (e.g., by an impacted stone).[9,12] Once the pancreatic duct is finally accessed, conventional pancreatic sphincterotomy can then be performed. In general, this technique is not used as often as the precut biliary sphincterotomy because a difficult pancreatic duct cannulation is encountered far less often than a difficult biliary cannulation. The pancreatic precut is done in a manner that is very similar to that of the biliary precut sphincterotomy (see Chapter 15). Most endoscopists will use a freehand needle knife to perform the precut, although there are several options for this technique.[9,18] In the case of a stone that is obstructing the pancreatic orifice, for example, a needle knife can be used to cut the papillary mucosa lying directly over the stone. Once the stone is released and the obstruction is relieved, the pancreatic duct can be cannulated in the usual manner to prepare for a conventional pancreatic sphincterotomy.

INDICATIONS FOR PANCREATIC SPHINCTEROTOMY

Unlike for endoscopic biliary sphincterotomy, scientific evidence to validate the indications for pancreatic sphincterotomy is sparse. There are several reasons for this disparity. First, pancreatic sphincterotomy appears to be mainly performed at specialized referral centers. Physicians performing this procedure usually have years of experience in therapeutic biliary and pancreatic endoscopy. To perform these advanced endoscopic procedures with adequate proficiency, the endoscopist must typically practice in an environment that yields a relatively high volume of ERCP (a workload volume not seen at most centers). This is usually a larger academic or referral center capable of handling all possible adverse events associated with this procedure. Furthermore, it is the relatively high likelihood of adverse events seen with pancreatic sphincterotomy that creates a general uneasiness among endoscopists, contributing to an overall decreased number of physicians performing this technique. As a result, there have been fewer published studies over the years that outline the indications, outcomes, and safety of pancreatic sphincterotomy. It is on this background that we discuss the indications for this technique.

Pancreatic sphincterotomy may be indicated for a variety of diseases and disease-related manifestations that involve the pancreas. In general, it is easiest to think about the indications for pancreatic sphincterotomy in terms of primary therapy and secondary therapy (Box 20.4). In other words, this technique may be performed by itself as the primary treatment modality (e.g., for the treatment of pancreatic sphincter of Oddi dysfunction [SOD]), or it may be used as a secondary treatment modality to facilitate a further intervention (e.g., better access to the main pancreatic

---

BOX 20.4   Indications for Endoscopic Pancreatic Sphincterotomy

EPS as Primary Therapy
- SOD
  - Pancreatic SOD
  - Biliary SOD unresponsive to biliary sphincterotomy
- Chronic pancreatitis with papillary stenosis or stricture
- Pancreas divisum (EPS of the minor papilla)

EPS to Facilitate a Further Intervention
- Chronic pancreatitis with ductal strictures or stones treated with pancreatic stents, lithotripsy, and/or stone removal
- Pancreatic pseudocysts treated with transpapillary drainage
- Resection of an ampullary adenoma
- Pancreatic fistula treated with stent placement
- Pancreatic disease caused by malignancy
  - Primary pancreatic cancer causing strictures, stones, pseudocysts
  - Metastatic disease to the pancreas causing strictures, stones, pseudocysts
- Pancreatoscopy for disease diagnosis, management of stones, and/or preoperative surgical assessment

EPS, Endoscopic pancreatic sphincterotomy; *SOD*, sphincter of Oddi dysfunction.

BOX 20.5   Modified Milwaukee Classification for Pancreatic-Type Sphincter of Oddi Dysfunction

Criteria
a. Pancreatic-type pain
b. Amylase/lipase >1.5–2.0 times normal
c. Pancreatic duct diameter >6 mm in the head or >5 mm in the body

Classification
Type 1 pancreatic-type SOD = (a), (b), and (c)
Type 2 pancreatic-type SOD = (a) plus (b) or (c)
Type 3 pancreatic-type SOD = (a) only*

Adapted from Novack DJ, Al-Kawas F. Endoscopic management of bile duct obstruction and sphincter of Oddi dysfunction. In: Bayless TM, Diehl AM, eds. *Advanced Therapy in Gastroenterology and Liver Disease.* Hamilton, ON: BC Decker; 2005, pp. 766–773, by permission of BC Decker Inc.
SOD, Sphincter of Oddi dysfunction.
*The EPISOD study has questioned SOD as an etiology for pancreaticobiliary-type pain without objective laboratory or imaging abnormalities.

BOX 20.6   Milwaukee Classification of Biliary-Type Sphincter of Oddi Dysfunction

Criteria
a. Biliary-type pain (Rome criteria)
b. Abnormal aspartate aminotransferase (AST) or alkaline phosphatase >2 times normal on two or more occasions
c. Delayed drainage of contrast from the common bile duct on ERCP >45 minutes and a dilated common bile duct >12 mm

Classification
Type 1 biliary-type SOD = (a), (b), and (c)
Type 2 biliary-type SOD = (a) plus (b) or (c)
Type 3 biliary-type SOD = (a) only

Adapted from Novack DJ, Al-Kawas F. Endoscopic management of bile duct obstruction and sphincter of Oddi dysfunction. In: Bayless TM, Diehl AM, eds. *Advanced Therapy in Gastroenterology and Liver Disease.* Hamilton, ON: BC Decker; 2005, pp. 766–773, by permission of BC Decker Inc.
SOD, Sphincter of Oddi dysfunction.

---

duct before dilating a downstream dominant stricture). Overall, there are far more data available regarding the use of pancreatic sphincterotomy in conjunction with an additional intervention (secondary therapy) than regarding using this technique alone (primary therapy).[4] Much of the following discussion concentrates on the indications of pancreatic sphincterotomy as a primary therapy.

Pancreatic Sphincterotomy as Primary Therapy
Pancreas Divisum, Sphincter of Oddi Dysfunction, and Recurrent Acute Pancreatitis

Most of the literature describing pancreatic sphincterotomy as the primary endoscopic therapy of choice is concentrated on the area of pancreas divisum and sphincterotomy of the minor papilla. This topic is covered at length in Chapter 21. Pancreatic sphincterotomy has been shown to provide primary therapeutic benefit in patients with pancreatic-type SOD. A brief review of this disorder is necessary in order to better understand the role of pancreatic sphincterotomy as its main treatment modality.

SOD is a benign obstruction to the flow of bile or pancreatic juice at the level of the pancreaticobiliary junction.[19] It is caused by functional dyskinesia or hypertension of the biliary and/or pancreatic portion of the sphincter. It results in transient noncalculous obstruction, causing abdominal pain or pancreatitis. It can be seen at any age but is most commonly encountered in middle-aged women. SOD should always be suspected in those patients who have had a cholecystectomy and are experiencing biliary-type abdominal pain and/or bouts of otherwise unexplained acute recurrent pancreatitis (see Chapter 52). Presently, the gold standard for making the diagnosis of SOD is biliary or pancreatic sphincter manometry (SOM) (Fig. 20.5). SOM involves passing a pressure-sensing catheter through a duodenoscope into the bile duct or pancreatic duct. Pressures can be measured from both portions of the sphincter (biliary and pancreatic) as the catheter is slowly pulled back and positioned within each of the sphincter zones (see Chapter 16; Fig. 20.6).[19] Elevated pressures may be caused by either sphincter muscle dyskinesia or structural stenosis.

In pancreatic-type SOD, there are essentially three diagnostic criteria: (a) pancreatic-type pain, (b) amylase/lipase >1.5 to 2.0 times normal, and (c) pancreatic duct diameter >6 mm in the head or >5 mm in the body (Box 20.5). Type 1 pancreatic SOD has all three components. Type 2 SOD has pancreatic-type pain plus (b) or (c). Type 3 SOD involves only pancreatic-type pain, although the recent EPISOD study questions the very existence of type 3 SOD.[20] In terms of biliary-type SOD, the criteria are very similar but involve the use of serum liver function tests and delayed drainage of contrast from the biliary tree during ERCP (Box 20.6).

Isolated pancreatic-type SOD may be seen in 15% to 20% of all patients with acute recurrent pancreatitis of unknown etiology.[19] It has been estimated to occur in 25% of all patients undergoing manometry for suspected SOD. The overall clinical response rate of endoscopic sphincterotomy for SOD (biliary and pancreatic) ranges between 55% and 95%. Patients with type 1 pancreatic SOD are most likely to benefit

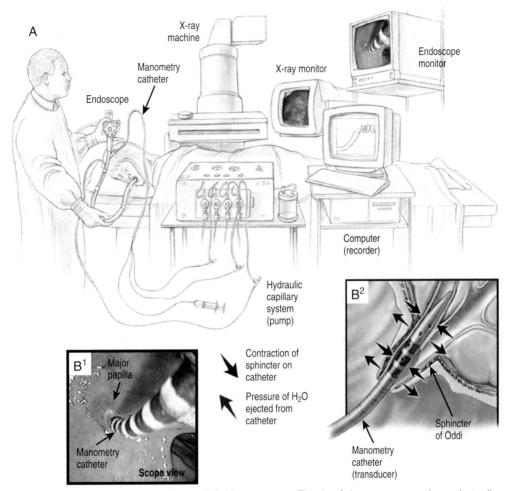

FIG 20.5 A and **B,** Pancreatic sphincter of Oddi manometry. The tip of the pressure-sensing catheter lies within the proximal pancreatic **(B₁)** and bile **(B₂)** ducts. (Reproduced by permission of Division of Gastroenterology and Hepatology, Johns Hopkins Hospital.)

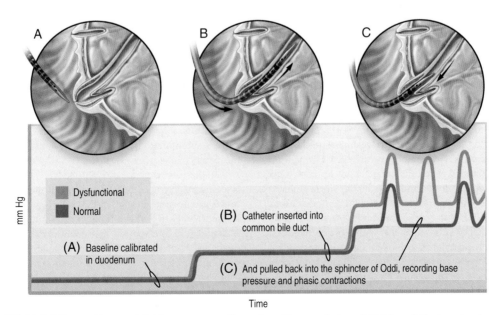

FIG 20.6 Biliary sphincter of Oddi manometry. (Reproduced by permission of Division of Gastroenterology and Hepatology, Johns Hopkins Hospital.)

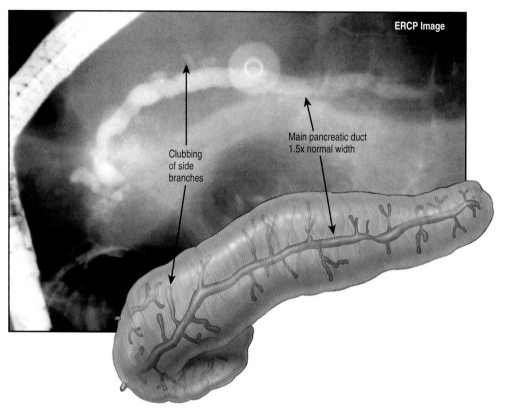

ERCP Image

Clubbing of side branches

Main pancreatic duct 1.5x normal width

FIG 20.7 Changes to the ductal morphology seen in moderate-severity chronic pancreatitis. (Reproduced by permission of Division of Gastroenterology and Hepatology, Johns Hopkins Hospital.)

from a pancreatic sphincterotomy. Several studies have shown that these patients may experience a significant reduction in pain and clinical episodes of pancreatitis. Patients with type 2 pancreatic SOD may also achieve benefit from a pancreatic sphincterotomy, but many experts still prefer to document abnormal pancreatic manometry before undertaking sphincterotomy. More recently, there have been two important clinical studies that have resulted in a change of viewpoint on the topic of sphincterotomy for patients with SOD and/or recurrent acute pancreatitis.

The EPISOD trial, published in 2014 by Cotton et al., was a multicenter, sham-controlled, randomized clinical trial in patients with suspected type 3 SOD.[20] Patients were randomized 2:1 to sphincterotomy ($n = 141$) or sham ($n = 73$), irrespective of manometry findings. Those randomized to sphincterotomy with elevated pancreatic sphincter pressures were randomized again (1:1) to biliary or both biliary and pancreatic sphincterotomies. Interestingly, there was no significant difference in treatment success (improvement in abdominal pain) between those patients who received sphincterotomy versus sham. Furthermore, in those patients with elevated pancreatic sphincter pressures, only 30% in the dual-sphincterotomy group and 20% in the single (biliary)-sphincterotomy group achieved treatment success. The study's overall conclusion was that ERCP with sphincterotomy is not supported for patients with type 3 SOD. In those patients with elevated pancreatic sphincter pressures, there does not appear to be a significant incremental benefit from dual sphincterotomy versus biliary sphincterotomy alone. These particular findings were consistent with an earlier study published in 2012 by Cote et al. in patients with recurrent acute pancreatitis.[21] Among those patients with pancreatic SOD, dual sphincterotomy and biliary sphincterotomy alone both showed similar effects in preventing recurrence of pancreatitis.

Chronic Pancreatitis

A pancreatic sphincterotomy alone is frequently used as the primary treatment modality in moderate to severe chronic pancreatitis (see Chapter 55). The rationale for treating chronic pancreatitis with endoscopic therapy is based on the principle of decreasing pancreatic intraductal pressure. In moderate to severe disease, the development of ductal stones, protein plugs, and ductal strictures may occur. Each of these can cause partial or complete obstruction to the flow of pancreatic juice into the duodenum, resulting in permanent alterations to the duct morphology (Figs. 20.7 and 20.8). Ductal obstruction leads to tissue hypertension and thus to tissue ischemia. Karanja et al. demonstrated a reduction of pancreatic blood flow after ligation of the main pancreatic duct (thereby producing intraductal hypertension) in a feline model of pancreatitis.[22] The reduction of blood flow was partially reversed after relief of the main duct obstruction. It is strongly believed that the symptom of pain in chronic pancreatitis is directly caused by this parenchymal ischemia.[1]

Another consequence of obstruction of the main pancreatic duct is secondary obstruction of the smaller side branch ducts. This ultimately causes parenchymal atrophy. As the tissue begins to atrophy, the pancreas loses its ability to perform both its endocrine and exocrine functions. A therapeutic intervention that could minimize intraductal pressure might help to prevent this dangerous cascade of events, thus diminishing pain and preserving pancreatic function. This is the basis behind sphincterotomy in chronic pancreatitis.

Few studies have specifically examined the role of pancreatic sphincterotomy as the sole endoscopic therapy in chronic pancreatitis. Most studies that have investigated this topic have done so in the context of additional endoscopic interventions; that is, the sphincterotomy is

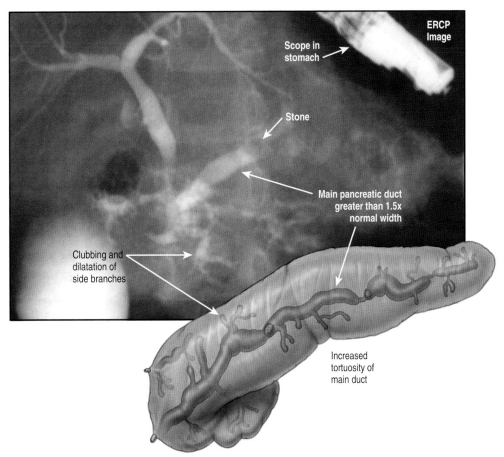

FIG 20.8 Changes to the ductal morphology seen in severe chronic pancreatitis. (Reproduced by permission of Division of Gastroenterology and Hepatology, Johns Hopkins Hospital.)

often performed in conjunction with a further intervention (e.g., stent placement or stricture dilatation). Studies in this area need to be examined closely in order to separate those patients who received a sphincterotomy alone versus those who received a sphincterotomy in concert with an additional endoscopic technique. This is often difficult, especially when the two groups have not been distinguished. Nonetheless, several studies have attempted to evaluate the safety and long-term results of pancreatic sphincterotomy in chronic pancreatitis.

Ell et al. described pancreatic sphincterotomy in 118 patients with chronic pancreatitis.[23] Eighty percent of the patients underwent standard pull-type sphincterotomy, whereas 20% underwent a needle-knife technique. Overall, 98% of the sphincterotomies were successfully performed and the adverse event rate was 4.2% (four cases of moderate pancreatitis, one case of severe bleeding). The results in terms of pain relief were not examined in this study, however.

Okolo et al. retrospectively analyzed 55 patients who had a pancreatic sphincterotomy.[24] Forty patients (73%) underwent the procedure for the treatment of symptomatic chronic pancreatitis. The goal of the study was to assess the long-term efficacy of sphincterotomy, with pain relief being the primary endpoint. After a median follow-up of 16 months, 60% of all patients reported a significant improvement in their pain scores.

Finally, Cahen et al. performed a prospective randomized trial examining both endoscopic and surgical decompression of the main pancreatic duct in patients with chronic pancreatitis.[25] A total of 39 patients underwent randomization, 19 of whom had ERCP with pancreatic sphincterotomy and endoscopic management of their disease.

During the 24 months of follow-up, Izbicki pain scores and physical health summary scores (on the SF-36 questionnaire) were better in the surgical arm compared with the endoscopic arm. At the end of follow-up, 32% of patients in the endoscopic arm had complete or partial pain relief, compared with 75% in the surgical group.

Papillary stenosis appears to be a clear-cut indication for pancreatic sphincterotomy alone in those patients with symptomatic chronic pancreatitis. Without significant ductal abnormalities distal to the papilla that require some additional form of intervention, sphincterotomy can be confidently used as the primary endoscopic therapy of choice in these patients. Similarly, pancreatic sphincterotomy for intraductal papillary mucinous neoplasm (IPMN) involving the proximal main pancreatic duct has also been proposed as potentially efficacious in patients with recurrent pancreatitis, although surgically fit patients may be better treated with pancreatic resection.[4]

Pancreatic Sphincterotomy as Secondary Therapy

Pancreatic sphincterotomy is commonly performed in concert with other endoscopic techniques such as stent placement or balloon dilation of the main duct (see Chapter 55). In this setting, the purpose of the sphincterotomy is to facilitate the primary therapy (e.g., removal of stones from the duct or dilatation of a ductal stricture). There are several diseases and conditions in which pancreatic sphincterotomy is used in this manner (see Box 20.4). The decision to cut the sphincter in these situations is based on sound clinical judgment by the endoscopist and whether it is believed that the risk of a sphincterotomy is outweighed by the potential benefit that may be gained by aiding the primary therapy.

In moderate to severe chronic pancreatitis, ductal strictures and stones are often the norm. Frequently their location within the main duct may be very distal (upstream) to the papilla. Therefore sphincterotomy alone may not be sufficient. Stone removal or stricture dilatation may therefore be the main goal of ERCP for certain patients. Pancreatic sphincterotomy may be needed before the procedure for better access to the duct (precut) or it can be used simply to help reduce intraductal hypertension and allow for easier flow of juice and calculous debris into the duodenum. This also holds true, for example, when treating pancreatic pseudocysts by means of a transpapillary approach. For those pseudocysts that communicate with the main pancreatic duct, a stent is placed within the duct in order to bridge the fistulous connection (see Chapter 56).[26] A pancreatic sphincterotomy in this setting also helps to reduce intraductal pressures and facilitate flow toward the papilla.

Other clinical scenarios for which sphincterotomy has been proposed as secondary therapy include stent placement before surgery for IPMN or surgery on the distal pancreas (e.g., distal pancreatectomy) to prevent postoperative pancreatic duct leak, as well as stent placement for the treatment of pancreatic fistulae (see Chapters 45 and 54).[4] Pancreatic sphincterotomy may also be used in concert with a pancreatic stent after the resection of an ampullary adenoma (see Chapter 25). Here the purpose of the sphincterotomy (and the stent) is to reduce the risk of postprocedural pancreatitis caused by periampullary edema. Finally, sphincterotomy is often indicated for the palliative treatment of strictures, stones, and pseudocysts in malignant obstruction of the pancreas.

ADVERSE EVENTS OF PANCREATIC SPHINCTEROTOMY

Although the first endoscopic pancreatic sphincterotomy was performed almost 35 years ago, the technique has not been used nearly as often as biliary sphincterotomy.[27] The reason for this is partly uncertainty about its precise indications and also concerns over the relatively high likelihood of adverse events.[28] When discussing the adverse events associated with pancreatic sphincterotomy, it must be remembered that studies that have evaluated this topic were generally small in number and had a small number of participants. They were usually performed at expert referral centers only and without control groups.[2] Furthermore, most of the studies report on pancreatic sphincterotomy as it is used to facilitate other endoscopic maneuvers, such as pancreatic stent placement, balloon dilation, and stone removal. Therefore it is often difficult to decipher which maneuver is truly responsible for the adverse event. For example, is the resultant pancreatitis due to the stricture dilation alone or to the sphincterotomy that was first required to access the duct? These issues make interpretation of the literature in this area difficult. It is on this background that we discuss the adverse events associated with pancreatic sphincterotomy.

In general, there are essentially three different types of adverse events associated with pancreatic sphincterotomy: early, late, and stent-related adverse events (Box 20.7).[28] Early adverse events are usually recognized within the first 72 hours after the procedure, but often within the first few hours. They include pancreatitis, severe bleeding, perforation, and pancreatic or biliary sepsis. Late adverse events are encountered at least 3 months after the procedure; this category mainly consists of papillary stenosis and proximal ductal strictures. On the other hand, there are several adverse events that are stent related. The timing of their occurrence is variable. They include pancreatic ductal and parenchymal changes, stone formation, infection, ductal perforation, stent migration, stent occlusion (causing pain and/or pancreatitis), and duodenal erosion.

Within the last 20 years, there have been three studies that have examined the rates of adverse events associated with pancreatic

---

BOX 20.7   Adverse Events of Pancreatic Sphincterotomy

Early Adverse Events (<3 months, typically <72 hours)
- Pancreatitis
- Severe bleeding
- Perforation
- Pancreatic and/or biliary sepsis

Late Adverse Events (>3 months)
- Papillary stenosis
- Proximal pancreatic duct strictures

Stent-Related Adverse Events (Variable Timing)
- Ductal and parenchymal changes
- Stone formation
- Infection
- Ductal perforation
- Stent migration
- Stent occlusion
- Duodenal erosion

TABLE 20.2   Studies Reporting Early Adverse Events of Pancreatic Sphincterotomy

Author	n	Pancreatitis	Total Adverse Events
Kozarek et al.[16]	56	4 (7.1%)	6 (10.7%)
Esber et al.[29]	236	33 (14%)	37 (15.7%)
Parsons et al.[30]	31	1 (3.2%)	1 (3.2%)

Adapted from Sherman S, Lehman GA. Complications of endoscopic pancreatic sphincterotomy. In: Testoni PA, Tittobello A, eds. *Endoscopy in Pancreatic Disease: Diagnosis and Therapy.* Chicago: Mosby-Wolfe; 1997, pp. 167–171, with permission. References 29,30 published in abstract form only.

---

sphincterotomy, and two of these studies were published in abstract form only (Table 20.2).[16,29,30] In a study by Kozarek et al.,[16] 56 patients underwent a pancreatic sphincterotomy. Fifty-four (96%) patients had chronic pancreatitis and two patients had acute recurrent pancreatitis. The indications for the sphincterotomy were as follows: obstructing ductal calculi (26), ductal disruption and leak (13), sphincter stenosis (10), and dominant stricture (8).[16] Forty-seven patients had a pull-type sphincterotomy and 33 of these patients also had a pancreatic stent placed after the sphincterotomy. Nine patients had a needle-knife sphincterotomy over an existing pancreatic stent. Early adverse events occurred in 10.7% of the patients and they included pancreatitis (four patients, or 7.1%) and cholangitis (two patients, or 3.6%). Late adverse events, however, occurred in 30% of the patients: 14% with papillary stenosis and 16% with asymptomatic ductal changes (thought to be stent related).

Esber et al. reported the adverse events of pancreatic sphincterotomy in 236 consecutive patients.[29] A pull-type sphincterotomy was performed in 123 patients, and 87 patients in this group also had a stent placed after the sphincterotomy. Needle-knife sphincterotomy over a pancreatic stent was performed in 113 patients. Seventy-four percent of the patients had a sphincterotomy for the purpose of treating pancreatic-type SOD. Twenty-six percent of the patients had chronic pancreatitis, in which case the procedure was performed to facilitate additional endoscopic maneuvers such as stone removal and stricture biopsy. Overall, post-ERCP pancreatitis occurred in 14% (mild in 76%, moderate in 21%, and severe in 3%). Other various adverse events occurred in only 1.7% of the cases. The rate of pancreatitis was 15.5% in patients with pancreatic-type SOD and 9.7% in patients with chronic pancreatitis. It was suggested that the lower rate of post-ERCP pancreatitis in chronic pancreatitis patients was because of periductal fibrosis and scarring. In other words, the limited amount of nearby healthy pancreatic parenchyma offers some protection against the injury that occurs after a pancreatic sphincterotomy.[17,28]

Parsons et al. evaluated the adverse event rate of performing a stentless pancreatic sphincterotomy.[30] In 31 patients sphincterotomy was done with a pull-type sphincterotome followed by the placement of a nasopancreatic tube. All tubes were removed within 24 hours of placement. Post-ERCP pancreatitis was observed in one patient (3.2%) and no other adverse events (e.g., perforation, bleeding, or sepsis) were seen.

Overall, the rate of pancreatitis after a pancreatic sphincterotomy appears to be approximately 10% to 12%, with a total early adverse event rate (perforation, bleeding, etc.) between 10% and 15%. Pancreatitis occurs more frequently in those patients with pancreatic-type SOD than in those who have the procedure performed for problems associated with chronic pancreatitis. Thorough data concerning the use of pancreatic stents in the prevention of pancreatitis after a pull-type sphincterotomy are somewhat lacking. Sherman et al. showed that a pancreatic stent used with needle-knife sphincterotomy may limit the frequency of postprocedural pancreatitis in SOD patients.[31] The problem, however, is that if the stent is left in place for too long, it may begin to induce unwanted ductal and parenchymal changes itself. Also, patients must undergo an additional procedure to have this endoprosthesis removed if it does not pass spontaneously.

Pancreatitis is the most concerning potential adverse event for those endoscopists who perform pancreatic sphincterotomy. This is mainly because it appears to be the adverse event over which they have the least amount of control and also because its effect may be very severe and sometimes lethal. The decision to place a stent after sphincterotomy is made on a case-by-case basis. Factors weighed in the decision include the perceived risk of early pancreatitis versus the potential for late adverse events and the need for an additional procedure.

THE COST OF PANCREATIC SPHINCTEROTOMY

There is little published information regarding the cost-effectiveness of pancreatic sphincterotomy. We assume that endoscopic therapy for diseases such as chronic pancreatitis and SOD ultimately reduces long-term costs by decreasing the frequency of hospitalizations and the number of required surgical interventions; however, there is truly a lack of data in the current medical literature pertaining to this area of interest. The reason for this may be the enormity and complexity of such a study. To yield useful and effective information, it would need to be conducted over many years and preferably in several different centers. Studies with such difficult endpoints and complex variables are less likely to be initiated by the majority of investigators.

There are some studies, however, that have examined the ability to perform endoscopic pancreatic sphincterotomy safely on an outpatient basis. Presumably, the importance of this idea centers around the reduction of unnecessary overnight observational admissions, thereby reducing the overall costs associated with therapeutic pancreatic endoscopy. Tham et al. reviewed 190 patients undergoing planned outpatient therapeutic ERCP.[32] Five patients had pancreatic sphincterotomy alone and 28 patients had pancreatic stent insertion. Admission was necessary in 31 patients (16%). Five of the 31 patients (3% overall) had unplanned, delayed admission after a median interval of 24 hours after discharge. The other 26 patients (13% overall) were admitted directly from the endoscopy unit because of obvious, discernable postprocedural adverse events. In the 219 consecutive inpatients undergoing ERCP, there was an overall adverse event rate of 13%. The authors claim that "a policy of selective outpatient therapeutic ERCP, with admission reserved for those with established or suspected adverse event, appears to be safe and reduces health care costs."[32] More studies in this area are needed to assess issues of cost and safety in outpatient therapeutic pancreatic endoscopy.

The complete reference list for this chapter can be found online at www.expertconsult.com.

21

Minor Papilla Cannulation and Sphincterotomy

Pier Alberto Testoni and Alberto Mariani

Pancreas divisum (literally "divided pancreas") is a congenital anatomic variant in which the dorsal and ventral pancreatic ducts completely or partially fail to fuse, and drain separately into the medial wall of the duodenum. Thus in most patients with pancreas divisum the vast majority of the pancreatic ductal system drains via the dorsal duct through the minor papilla. This is the most common pancreatic anomaly, occurring in approximately 10% of the general population, though rates vary worldwide from 2.7% to 22%.[1,2] The frequency also varies greatly in different endoscopic retrograde cholangiopancreatography (ERCP) series; a systematic review of endoscopic detection of pancreas divisum found a pooled rate of 2.9%, ranging from 1.5% in Asia to 5.8% in the United States and 6.0% in Europe.[3]

About 15% of pancreas divisum cases are of the incomplete type, in which a small branch of the ventral duct communicates with the dorsal duct. The clinical implications of incomplete and complete pancreas divisum are the same.

Although most patients with pancreas divisum do not suffer pancreatic symptoms throughout their lifetime, about 5% have recurrent mild to severe pancreatic pain, acute pancreatitis (often recurrent), or chronic obstructive pancreatitis. These symptoms or diseases are believed to occur because the minor papilla orifice is so small that intrapancreatic dorsal duct pressure is excessively high during active secretion, resulting in inadequate duct drainage and distension.[4] Persistent or recurrent high intraluminal dorsal duct pressure can cause recurrent bouts of acute pancreatitis, and with time the gland undergoes chronic obstructive changes. Therefore pancreas divisum can be considered a predisposing factor for recurrent and chronic pancreatitis.[5]

Dorsal duct obstruction depends on relative stenosis of the minor papilla rather than the presence of pancreas divisum per se. Lowering the transpapillary pressure gradient across the minor papilla, mainly by ERCP and minor papilla endoscopic sphincterotomy (MiES), appears to be essential when this condition is symptomatic.

Patients with acute recurrent pancreatitis seem to have a significantly better response to MiES than those patients with "pancreatic pain" only and those with chronic pancreatitis.[3] However, because some patients with acute recurrent pancreatitis continue to have attacks after effective dorsal ductal drainage,[6] other nonductal abnormalities such as genetic mutations, alcohol use, and autoimmune pancreatitis[7] may play a pathogenic role. As many as 10% to 20% of patients with pancreas divisum and pancreatitis carry at least one allele of the cystic fibrosis gene product[8] or a higher frequency of SPINK1 gene mutation than healthy controls,[9] suggesting a multifactorial origin of pancreatitis in these cases.

Endoscopic identification, cannulation, and MiES are still challenging, and the decision to perform ERCP in patients with pancreas divisum should not be made lightly in view of the greater potential for adverse events. Although minor papilla cannulation can provide the diagnosis of pancreas divisum, noninvasive imaging techniques such as secretin-enhanced magnetic resonance cholangiopancreatography (S-MRCP), endoscopic ultrasonography (EUS), or thin-slice coronal computed tomography are preferable (see Chapter 34). S-MRCP is the preferred technique, with reported sensitivity, specificity, positive predictive value, and negative predictive value of 73.3%, 96.8%, 82.4%, and 94.8%, respectively.[10] Some radiologists believe that secretin administration during MRCP is essential for diagnosing pancreas divisum, because without hormone stimulation MRCP is nondiagnostic in a substantial proportion of patients. Miss rates of pancreas divisum by MRCP may also be attributable to suboptimal techniques and radiologist inexperience.[11]

This chapter focuses on endoscopic identification and cannulation of minor papilla and on techniques for sphincterotomy and dorsal duct drainage.

INDICATIONS FOR MINOR PAPILLA CANNULATION AND SPHINCTEROTOMY

Box 21.1 lists the indications for minor papilla cannulation and sphincterotomy. The most frequent indications are recurrent pancreatic-type pain with a nondilated pancreatic ductal system, acute recurrent pancreatitis with or without dorsal duct dilation, and obstructive pancreatic-type pain or recurrent pancreatitis in patients with chronic changes of the pancreatic ductal system. In some patients without pancreas divisum, access to the pancreatic duct through the minor papilla and MiES can be useful.[12]

SEDATION, SUPPLEMENTAL DRUGS, AND ERCP ACCESSORIES

Sedation

Endoscopic cannulation and sphincterotomy of the minor papilla is generally a lengthy procedure, requiring appropriate sedation and analgesia. Deep sedation with propofol is therefore preferred, though moderate sedation can be achieved with repeated doses of benzodiazepines (midazolam) and opioids (meperidine, fentanyl) (see Chapter 6).

Antispasmodic Drugs

Antispasmodic agents enhance visualization of the minor papilla and should be readily available for administration. However, these agents should not be administered until the endoscope is passed to the descending duodenum, as gastric distension may occur and make passage through the pylorus difficult. Once the endoscope has been placed in a stable position in front of the minor papilla, in some cases an additional intravenous injection of a smooth muscle inhibitor such as glucagon is required, in 0.25-mg to 0.50-mg increments.

Supplemental Agents

When recognition of the papilla or its orifice is problematic, dyeing techniques or secretin injection can be helpful.

ERCP Accessories

In general, cannulation and papillotomy of the minor papilla can be performed using accessories that are the same as those used for the major papilla (see Chapter 14): a sphincterotome or an ERCP catheter and a soft-tip guidewire (Fig. 21.1, *A*, *B*). If the papillary orifice is very small, a needle-tip catheter (ERCP-1-CRAMER; Cook Medical, Winston-Salem, NC) can be useful. Sometimes a stenotic orifice requires dilation in order to pass standard accessories, which can be done with a tapered 3-Fr to 7-Fr dilator (Soehendra Biliary Dilatation Catheter or Geenen Graduated Dilation Catheter [Cook Medical]; progressive dilation catheter [G-Flex, Nivelles, Belgium]) or a 4-mm balloon-tipped catheter (Titan biliary balloon dilator [Cook Medical]; Eliminator PET biliary balloon dilator [ConMed, Utica, NY]; Hurricane biliary balloon dilator [Boston Scientific, Marlborough, MA]).

The following equipment should be kept in the endoscopy room when attempting minor papilla cannulation and papillotomy:

- **Catheters:** tapered-tip 3-Fr to 5-Fr catheters, some with metal tips (Glo-tip-1-ST or ERCP-1 metal tip or ERCP-1-Huibregtse-Katon, ERCP-1-CRAMER [Cook Medical]; Contour ERCP [Boston Scientific]; PR-V223Q [Olympus])
- **Guidewires:** partially or completely hydrophilic 0.018-inch guidewires (Roadrunner [Cook Medical]; Pathfinder [Boston Scientific]); 0.035-inch guidewires with straight and angled tips (Radifocus [Terumo, Elkton, MD]; METRO or Deltawire or Acrobat [Cook Medical]; Dreamwire or Hydra Jagwire or Jagwire [Boston Scientific])
- **Sphincterotomes:** pull-type short-tip sphincterotome 4-Fr to 5-Fr diameter with a 20-mm to 25-mm cutting wire (Minitome [Cook Medical]) or standard sphincterotome 5.5-Fr to 6-Fr diameter
- **Dilators:** tapered 4-Fr to 7-Fr dilation catheter or 4-mm balloon dilators (as described above)
- **Needle knife:** 4-mm cutting wire with or without a channel for passing a guidewire or for contrast injection (Huibregtse [Cook Medical]; MicroKnife [Boston Scientific])
- **Pancreatic stents:** (a) "prophylactic": 3-Fr to 5-Fr stents, 2 to 5 cm long, flanged or unflanged with or without a duodenal pigtail; (b) "therapeutic": 7 to 10 Fr, 3 to 7 cm long, flanged (Zimmon or Geenen [Cook Medical]; Advanix [Boston Scientific])
- **Nasopancreatic drainage:** 5-Fr diameter (NPDS-5 [Cook Medical]; NPDC-5 [Surgimedic])
- **Cautery unit:** we use an ERBE generator model ICC 200 (ERBE Elektromedizin, Tubingen, Germany) usually set at effect 3, 120 W, and "ENDOCUT" mode.

RECOGNITION OF THE MINOR PAPILLA

The first step of the procedure is to locate the minor papilla. It is usually in the right upper quadrant of the visual field when facing the major papilla, 2 to 3 cm cephalic and anterior to the major papilla, but it may be as close as 1 cm from the major papilla, at the rim of its longitudinal fold (Fig. 21.2). The minor papilla can be very small and difficult to locate or quite prominent and, rarely, located within a diverticulum (Fig. 21.3, *A–C*). High-definition white-light endoscopy and advanced electronic imaging techniques may facilitate the identification of the papilla and its orifice (Fig. 21.4, *A*).

Gentle probing of the duodenal folds may be necessary to identify the minor papilla mound and to make it more prominent, although care must be taken to avoid excessive manipulation-related edema that may make it more difficult to identify the papilla.

The endoscopic appearance of the minor papilla can predict pancreas divisum and underlying pancreatographic findings.[13,14] Bulging of the minor papilla mound and patency of its orifice may differ in patients with normal and abnormal ductography. About 70% of patients with pancreatic dorsal duct abnormalities have substantial bulging and a visible orifice, whereas most cases with a normal pancreatogram have no bulging and/or no visible orifice.[15]

BOX 21.1 Indications for Minor Papilla Cannulation and Sphincterotomy

- Pancreas divisum and acute recurrent pancreatitis
- Obstructive chronic pancreatitis of the dorsal duct (stone removal and/or stricture dilation)
- Santorinicele
- Adenomas of the minor papilla
- Intraductal papillary mucinous neoplasm (IPMN) of the dorsal duct (facilitation of transpapillary mucus drainage)
- Treatment of obstruction in the setting of pancreatic pseudodivisum or acquired dorsal duct syndrome
- Treatment of pancreatic disorders through the minor papilla in nondivisum patients in whom major papilla cannulation fails

---

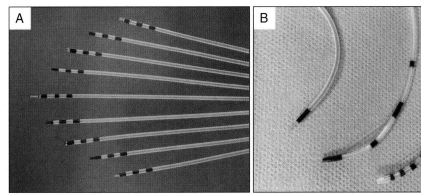

FIG 21.1 A, Various tapered-tip catheters used for minor papilla cannulation; **B,** devices used for papillary sphincterotomy. From left to right: needle-knife, "minitome," and standard sphincterotome.

Supplemental Techniques to Identify the Minor Papilla in Difficult Cases

Despite the endoscopist's experience and advanced imaging, in approximately one-third of cases the papillary orifice is not initially visible. When recognition is problematic, dyeing techniques or secretin injection can be helpful.

Dyeing Solutions

Methylene blue (vital dye) diluted with saline solution (1:10) or, preferably, indigo carmine 0.4% undiluted can be sprayed over the area

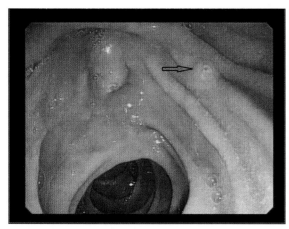

FIG 21.2 Endoscopic view of the minor papilla. It is generally located at the 2 o'clock position *(arrow)*, 1 cm from the major papilla, which is visible at the top of the image.

suspected to contain the minor papilla in order to identify the papillary orifice or the papilla itself, respectively (see Fig. 21.4, *B, C*). Once dye solution has been sprayed, the orifice may appear as a whitish spot emerging on a bluish mucosa or is evidenced by clear juice washing away from the background blue dye.[16,17] In patients with known incomplete pancreas divisum, methylene blue can be diluted 1:10 with contrast medium and injected into the pancreatic ductal system through the major papilla; part of the dyed pancreatic juice flows out through the dorsal duct and minor papilla. With this method it is best to avoid opacifying the entire pancreatic ductal system so as to limit intraductal pressure during contrast-dye injection and thus reduce the risk of post-ERCP pancreatitis (PEP).

Secretin

Secretin, intravenously administered, may facilitate the identification of the minor papilla orifice by stimulating the production of pancreatic juice, which results in a visible flow of juice into the duodenum. Moreover, when pancreatic juice flow is increased, the orifice enlarges, simplifying guidewire or catheter insertion[18] (Fig. 21.5, *A, B*, and Fig. 21.6, *A–C*). Secretin is a 27–amino acid polypeptide that strongly stimulates secretion of water and bicarbonate from pancreatic ductal cells; the enhanced secretion of pancreatic juice may render the minor papilla orifice visible. Secretin stimulates pancreatic juice flow between 1 and 3 minutes after injection with transient ductal dilation, lasting about 15 minutes. However, when the pancreatic ducts are dilated or obstructed, as in severe chronic pancreatitis or dorsal duct stricture, the pancreatic juice flow after secretin may be insufficient to identify the minor papilla orifice. Two synthetic porcine and one synthetic nonporcine secretins are available for widespread clinical application in the United States and Europe, respectively. Secretin is administered intravenously as a

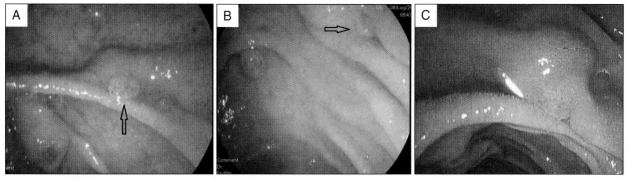

FIG 21.3 Endoscopic appearance of the minor papilla. **A,** Normal *(arrow)*; **B,** flat, not clearly visible *(arrow)*; **C,** prominent.

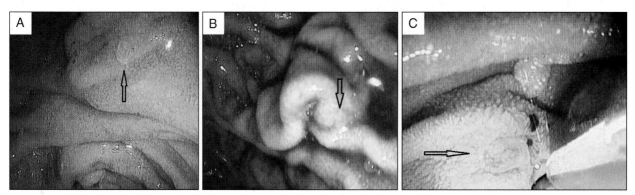

FIG 21.4 Techniques facilitating minor papilla visualization. **A,** High-definition imaging (i-scan) *(arrow)*; **B,** spraying with 0.4% undiluted indigo carmine *(arrow)*; **C,** intravenous secretin injection *(arrow)*.

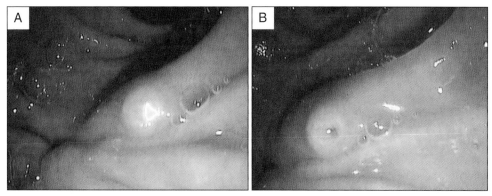

FIG 21.5 A, Minor papilla orifice is not clearly visible before secretin injection; **B,** 2 minutes after secretin injection, the papillary orifice becomes clearly visible.

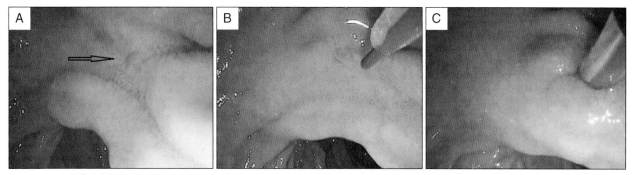

FIG 21.6 A, Flat, nonvisible papilla; **B,** after secretin injection, the orifice can be identified and cannulated by using the guidewire; **C,** deep papillary cannulation with standard sphincterotome.

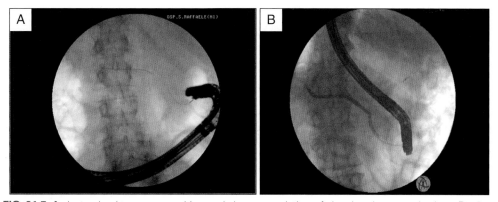

FIG 21.7 A, Long duodenoscope position and deep cannulation of the dorsal pancreatic duct; **B,** short duodenoscope position and opacification of the pancreatic duct. The patient is in the prone position.

bolus dosage of 1 clinical unit per kilogram of body weight. All secretin formulations significantly improve minor papilla cannulation rates and shorten cannulation time.[18,19] A multicenter randomized controlled trial including 29 patients showed significantly higher cannulation rates after secretin injection compared with placebo (81.3% vs 7.7%, $p < 0.01$).[19] However, the use of secretin has some limitations because it is expensive; where it is not readily available, dye spraying is preferred and used before secretin injection.

Intraduodenal hydrochloric acid (HCl) infusion reportedly improves the minor papilla cannulation rate in patients with pancreas divisum during difficult cannulation.[20] Intraduodenal HCl physiologically induces secretin release[21] and is less costly than secretin. However, the available preliminary data need to be confirmed in more patients.

MINOR PAPILLA CANNULATION (VIDEO 21.1)

The patient is generally prone, as for standard ERCP; endoscopists who perform ERCP in the supine position for pancreatic endotherapy prefer the same position for minor papilla cannulation. A standard duodenoscope is used. In some cases a small-caliber, more flexible diagnostic duodenoscope has been reported, because it is believed to be easier to keep the endoscope in a long position along the greater curvature of the stomach, which is nearly uniformly needed to achieve an en face position of the minor papilla (Fig. 21.7, *A, B*). However, our experience does not confirm this and newer therapeutic duodenoscopes are smaller and more flexible than older models. To date, ERCP in pancreas divisum should be done only for therapeutic purposes, and so a standard large-channel duodenoscope is preferable because it allows large-bore stents to be placed, if needed.

The minor papilla can be recognized by carefully withdrawing the endoscope from the position of the major papilla. The long endoscope position makes for easier identification because of the better endoscopic and fluoroscopic views.

Once the minor papilla has been recognized, cannulation is generally best achieved with the endoscope in the long position. However, in this position the endoscope may fall back into the stomach and must be readvanced to maintain the long position.

The papilla can be cannulated by using a 20-mm to 25-mm cutting wire pull-type sphincterotome preloaded with a guidewire (the most commonly used technique), a needle-tip catheter specifically designed for this purpose (ERCP-1-CRAMER), or either a standard-tip or tapered-tip 5-Fr catheters or a 3-Fr catheter. The ERCP-1-CRAMER catheter does not accept a guidewire but dilates the opening of the orifice and facilitates further catheter-assisted and guidewire-assisted deep cannulation. The 5-Fr catheter can be preloaded with a 0.021-inch or 0.035-inch guidewire; 3-Fr catheters can be used only with a 0.018-inch guidewire, which is sometimes too floppy and not easy to manipulate. Catheters without a tapered tip are less helpful.

The guidewire is used to enter the minor papilla orifice directly and should preferably be passed to the midbody of the dorsal duct before touching the papilla with a catheter or sphincterotome. This helps avoid trauma-related edema, which makes subsequent cannulation more difficult. When the orifice is very small or stenotic, the wire will pass into the duct, though the catheter will not. In such cases the wire is left in place and a highly tapered push catheter is passed alongside it, or a precut can be done alongside or over the wire following the path of the wire. In most of these cases, dilation using the push catheter is sufficient. In addition, if one cautiously places the endoscope in the short position, it increases the mechanical advantage to allow a catheter to be passed.

When MiES is planned, it is preferable to begin cannulation using a pull-type sphincterotome preloaded with a guidewire, which is then used to enter the papillary orifice (Fig. 21.8, *A, B*). The sphincterotome also has an advantage when en face orientation to the minor papilla cannot be achieved for initial cannulation: The sphincterotome can "bow" into the correct axis, facilitating cannulation. Once deep cannulation is achieved with the guidewire, if a long position has been maintained it is advisable to withdraw the endoscope into the short position along the lesser curvature of the stomach; this puts it into a more stable position in front of the papilla.

In expert hands and with the appropriate accessories, minor papilla cannulation can be achieved in 90% to 100% of cases.[15] Cannulation may fail for several reasons: the papilla cannot be identified despite a thorough search, papillary distortion is present because of inflammation of either the papilla or the duodenal wall, the papilla is within a diverticulum, duodenal neoplasia is present, or abnormal duodenal anatomy is present.

CANNULATING THE MINOR PAPILLA IN DIFFICULT CASES

EUS is the best complementary technique to identify and cannulate the minor papilla in difficult cases. With ultrasound assistance the main pancreatic duct can be located and punctured transgastrically using a standard fine-needle aspiration needle (see Chapter 33). There are then two ways to achieve transpapillary cannulation. The first involves injecting contrast medium mixed with dilute methylene blue or indigo carmine into the pancreatic duct using a 19-gauge or 22-gauge needle, the latter being less traumatic. The echoendoscope is then withdrawn and exchanged for a standard side-viewing endoscope; the dye can be seen passing out of the minor papilla orifice, which facilitates cannulation. In some cases, secretin stimulation may enhance the bluish pancreatic secretion so as to enhance visualization of the papillary orifice.[22,23]

The other technique is to pass a 0.018-inch to 0.035-inch guidewire under ultrasound guidance through the pancreatic parenchyma into the pancreatic duct and then pass the wire antegrade through the minor papilla into the duodenum. A 19-gauge needle permits the use of a 0.035-inch guidewire and is preferable because when a 22-gauge needle is used it is difficult to pass a 0.018-inch wire through the tip. The echoendoscope is then withdrawn and the duodenoscope is inserted; the wire exiting the minor papilla is captured by a snare or a Dormia basket and retrieved through the working channel of the duodenoscope (Fig. 21.9, *A–F*). With this "rendezvous" technique a standard catheter or a sphincterotome can easily be introduced over the guidewire into the dorsal duct.[24,25]

The echoendoscope-assisted procedure is useful in patients with complete or incomplete pancreas divisum. If an echoendoscope is not available, an internal rendezvous technique can be used in cases of incomplete pancreas divisum. After cannulating the major papilla, a guidewire is passed from the ventral duct to the dorsal duct and then out through the minor papilla (Fig. 21.10). The endoscope is withdrawn to the level of the minor papilla, the wire is grasped and pulled through

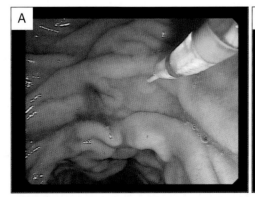
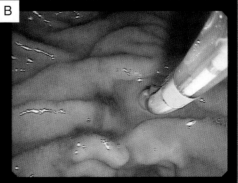

FIG 21.8 Cannulation of the minor papilla. **A,** A 0.035-inch hydrophilic guidewire is gently advanced through the tip of a 5-Fr sphincterotome and directed within the minor papilla orifice; **B,** the minor papilla is cannulated by the sphincterotome preloaded with the guidewire.

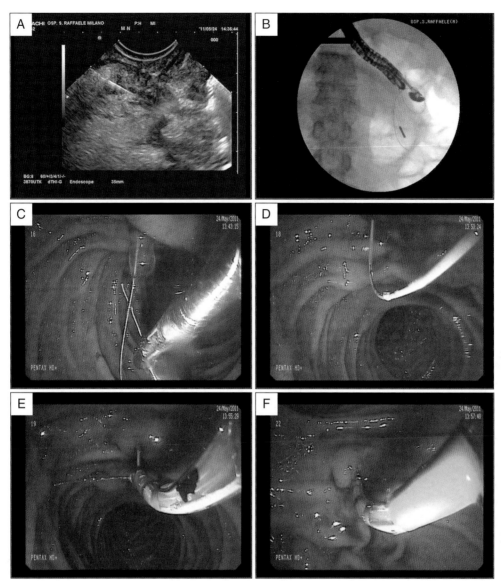

FIG 21.9 EUS-ERCP rendezvous in a patient with failed cannulation of the minor papilla. **A,** Needle puncture by EUS of the main pancreatic duct. **B,** A 0.018-inch guidewire is passed from the pancreatic duct through the minor papilla into the duodenal lumen. **C,** The metallic tip of the guidewire is grasped with a snare. **D,** The body of the guidewire is visible in the duodenal lumen as it is progressively withdrawn through the accessory channel of the duodenoscope. **E,** A sphincterotome is inserted over the guidewire in front of the papilla. **F,** The minor papilla is cannulated with the sphincterotome.

the endoscope, and the minor papilla is cannulated retrogradely over the guidewire. For this maneuver, a more floppy 0.018-inch or 0.021-inch wire is preferable because it easily engages the ductal connection from the ventral and dorsal duct, which may be thin and narrowed.

If these maneuvers fail, precut sphincterotomy of the minor papilla can permit successful cannulation. The technique for precutting the minor papilla is presented in detail later in this chapter.

MINOR PAPILLA SPHINCTEROTOMY

Although some authors report that a true sphincter may be not present and suggest that the term *papillotomy,* rather than *sphincterotomy,* is more appropriate for this endoscopic procedure, manometric studies have identified a sphincter mechanism similar to the major papilla.[26]

Unfortunately, MiES is still a poorly standardized technique because the landmarks for the appropriate extension and depth of the cut are difficult to establish and have never been properly defined, except in patients with a santorinicele, where marked dilation of the dorsal duct close to the papillary orifice causes a well-defined mound protruding into the duodenum (Fig. 21.11).

Techniques for Minor Papilla Sphincterotomy

There are three techniques for sphincterotomy: (1) papillary section using a standard pull-type sphincterotome or "mini" papillotome, generally wire guided; (2) papillary section by a needle-knife cut over a plastic stent placed into the dorsal duct; and (3) papillary section by a wire-assisted needle knife. Sphincteroplasty with balloon dilation has been reported as an alternative to sphincterotomy and shown to be safe and efficient in a small retrospective study.[27]

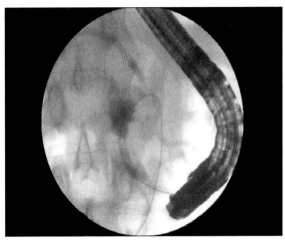

FIG 21.10 Rendezvous technique through the major papilla in case of failed minor papilla cannulation in incomplete pancreas divisum. After cannulating the major papilla, the guidewire is passed from the ventral duct to the dorsal duct and then out through the minor papilla.

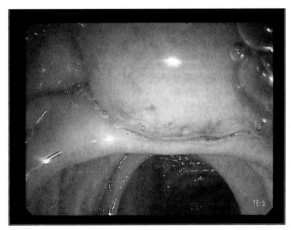

FIG 21.11 Prominent minor papilla in a patient with santorinicele. The marked dilation of the dorsal duct close to the papillary orifice causes a mound protruding into the duodenum.

Sphincterotomy With Pull-Type Sphincterotome

Minor papilla cannulation with the sphincterotome is always done over a guidewire. In general, a 0.018-inch or 0.025-inch guidewire is used for primary cannulation, but a 0.035-inch wire can also be used. If a 0.018-inch wire has been used to cannulate the papilla, once the sphincterotome has been advanced into the dorsal duct this wire may need to be exchanged for a less floppy wire (0.021 to 0.035 inches) for subsequent maneuvers. Once the guidewire has been deeply advanced into the dorsal duct to at least the midbody, the sphincterotome is advanced over the wire through the papillary orifice, with the cutting wire in the 10 to 12 o'clock direction, depending on the long or short duodenoscope position. If the long position is maintained during cannulation, the cutting wire tends to be oriented toward the 10 to 11 o'clock position (Fig. 21.12, *A, B*), whereas if the short position has been achieved, the wire orients more to the 11 to 12 o'clock position (Fig. 21.13, *A, B*).

Any standard wire-guided sphincterotome can be used if the minor papilla orifice has been dilated. A short-tip (2-mm to 3-mm tip extending beyond the cutting wire) 4-Fr-diameter to 5-Fr-diameter sphincterotome with a cutting wire 20 to 25 mm long should be used. A 30-mm cutting wire may be useful for a large minor papilla. Small-diameter sphincterotomes can be inserted without the need for orifice dilation. However, because there is only one channel, the guidewire must be removed to inject contrast and the sphincterotome needs to be inserted deeply over the guidewire before removing the wire and injecting contrast, which is time-consuming. Larger-diameter sphincterotomes allow wire placement and injection of contrast medium at the same time but may require dilation of the papillary orifice to pass into the duct.

Once the wire is in stable position, the sphincterotome is advanced into the dorsal duct. The sphincterotome is positioned with the cutting wire oriented toward 10 to 12 o'clock and inserted 2 to 3 mm into the orifice. The cut is initiated by continuous action on the foot pedal or by repeated taps until the cut is nearly complete, with the cautery unit set with effect 3, 120 W, and ENDOCUT mode on. In general we prefer the step-by-step method, because we have better control of the length and depth of the cut. During the cut, the sphincterotome is bowed to ensure moderate tension on the tissue; this maintains contact with the wire for faster cutting. Pulling back on the bowed sphincterotome further helps to expose the cutting space. The goal is to cut to the upper rim of the minor papilla mound with a depth of at least 3 to 4 mm (Fig. 21.14). In cases with a small minor papilla, the upper rim of the papillary mound may be hard to identify. However, it

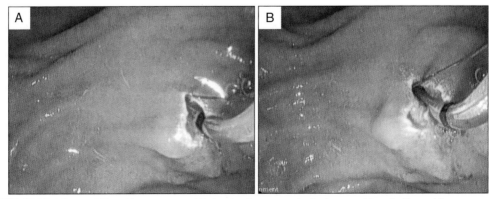

FIG 21.12 Minor papilla sphincterotomy with the duodenoscope in the long position. **A,** The sphincterotome is bowed slightly with the cutting wire oriented toward the 10 to 11 o'clock direction; **B,** papillary section at the end of the sphincterotomy with visible pancreatic dorsal duct lumen.

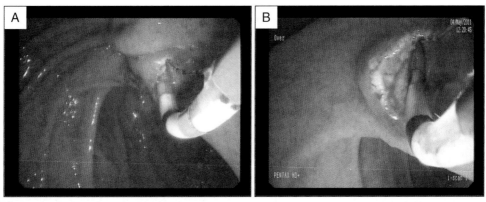

FIG 21.13 Minor papilla sphincterotomy with the duodenoscope in the short position. **A,** The cutting wire is oriented toward the 11 to 12 o'clock direction; **B,** the upper rim of the papillary mound has been cut to a depth of 4 to 5 mm.

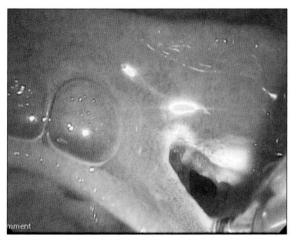

FIG 21.14 Completion of minor papilla sphincterotomy and extended up to the duodenal wall.

becomes more prominent during the sphincterotomy because of heat-induced edema, and so the cephalic margins of the cut become clearer (Fig. 21.15, *A, B*).

Unlike the major papilla, the dorsal duct lumen is visible after the cut only in a minority of cases, generally those with a large papilla or dilated duct (Fig. 21.16, *A, B*).

Cutting requires a fairly dry field, because fluids in contact with the cutting wire divert current away from the target tissue and allow the surrounding tissue to coagulate, rather than cut it. This may make it easier for a stricture to form at the level of the sphincterotomy. It is therefore very important to aspirate fluid from the duodenum during MiES.

If no cutting occurs, it may be because the cutting wire is inserted too deeply in the papilla and in contact with the pancreatic ductal epithelium. This may also cause a thermally induced pancreatic stricture.

Sphincterotomy With Needle Knife Over Pancreatic Stent

Two types of needle-knife sphincterotomes can be used. The one most widely used is a tapered-tip needle knife with a retractable 0.012-inch-diameter, 4-mm-long cutting wire. The small needle permits accurate and rapid cutting and reduces the area of coagulation, limiting the risk of postprocedure strictures. The disadvantage is that it is impossible to cut and inject at the same time. However, during the cut over a stent

there is normally no need to inject contrast medium. A larger-diameter needle knife, with a channel for contrast injection or guidewire insertion, is more difficult to manipulate and the larger needle can reduce the accuracy of the cut and cause more coagulation.

Once the guidewire has been passed through the papilla and advanced proximally to at least the midbody of the dorsal duct, a plastic pancreatic stent, straight or with a pigtail at the duodenal end, is placed over the wire. With a pigtail stent, care must be taken during final delivery to maneuver the pigtail toward the descending duodenum so as to orient the pigtail inferior to the minor papilla and not interfere with needle-knife cutting that takes place superiorly. Placing the stent helps to lift the minor papilla for easier cutting. The needle should be placed into the papillary orifice 1 to 2 mm; the cut is initiated at the orifice and extended cephalad in the 10 to 11 o'clock direction, with repeated 1 to 2 mm cuts deeper into the tissue, until the upper part of the papillary mound is divided. Repeated cuts expose the intramural stent and cutting continues progressively alongside it. Finally, the needle-knife catheter can be advanced with the needle retracted alongside the stent into the dorsal duct. Sphincterotomy with the needle knife is done using pure-cut current (200 W) or ENDOCUT current (200 W cut, 20 W coagulation; tissue effect). An alternative cutting method is to start at the apex of the papillary mound and cut downward onto the stent. This defines the cephalad limit of cutting more precisely, preventing unintentionally cutting more cephalad than required.

Sphincterotomy With Wire-Assisted Needle Knife

Once the guidewire has been deeply advanced into the pancreatic dorsal duct, the needle knife is passed alongside the wire, and cutting is started cephalad in the 10 to 11 o'clock direction by passing the needle knife alongside the wire. The cutting technique is essentially the same as for papillotomy with a needle knife over a pancreatic stent and has comparable efficacy and adverse event rates. However, there are limited comparative data on minor papilla precut techniques.[28]

PULL-TYPE OR NEEDLE-KNIFE SPHINCTEROTOME: PROS AND CONS

The two sphincterotomy techniques are equally effective, with similar rates of adverse events.[29] A pull-type sphincterotome is preferable in cases where it is difficult to keep the endoscope in a stable position in front of the minor papilla, because of an unfavorable angle of approach or difficult control of duodenal motility. In these situations, the pull-type sphincterotome advanced over a deeply placed guidewire helps achieve stability. A pull-type sphincterotome is also more convenient when

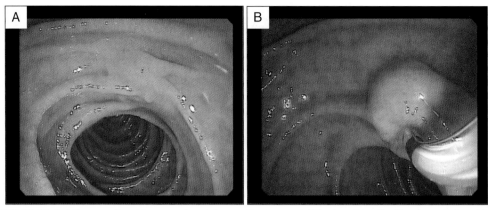

FIG 21.15 A, Minor papilla with upper rim of the papillary mound difficult to identify; **B,** edema induced by papillary manipulation and thermal damage renders the papillary mound prominent and clearly visible.

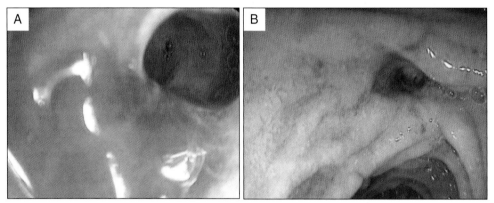

FIG 21.16 Dorsal duct lumen visible at the end of sphincterotomy. **A,** Slightly dilated dorsal duct; **B,** santorinicele.

placement of multiple pancreatic stents is planned. On the other hand, pull sphincterotomy does not permit cutting limited to papillary tissue and the cutting wire can easily come into contact with the prepapillary portion of the dorsal duct, thus extending the thermal effect not only to the papilla but also into the pancreas and leading to stricture formation. The needle knife allows better control of the cut and limits the cautery to the papillary tissue, but difficulties arise when the endoscope is not in a stable position in front of the minor papilla. Although in the past most papillotomies were done using the needle knife over the stent, there appears to be a tendency toward wider use of the pull-type sphincterotome.

PRECUT SPHINCTEROTOMY IN CASE OF FAILED DORSAL DUCT CANNULATION

The technique is essentially the same as for major papilla (see Chapter 15). Precut refers to cutting the papilla with a needle-knife sphincterotome without previous deep cannulation, guidewire passage, or stent placement. However, precut of the minor papilla is more difficult than the major papilla and carries a higher risk of adverse events. This is because of the minor papilla's diminutive size and lack of clearly defined landmarks and because if cannulation fails, protective pancreatic stenting is not possible. Considering these potential risks, we believe that an ultrasound-guided rendezvous technique should be used if available and in a pancreatic duct of sufficient caliber. Otherwise, the need for minor papilla cannulation should be reassessed and the decision to proceed made on a case-by-case basis.

If the minor papillary orifice is visible, the needle knife should be inserted 1 to 2 mm into the papillary tissue at the cephalad rim of the orifice, with the cutting wire extended 1 to 2 mm, and the cut is made in the 10 to 11 o'clock direction, as for needle-knife cutting over a stent. Further short cuts 1 to 2 mm deeper are then made at the base of the first incision, or nearby left or right, until the papillary orifice has been opened completely and pancreatic juice is seen. Cannulation is then attempted with a soft-tip 0.025-inch to 0.035-inch guidewire.

In difficult cases and when the papillary orifice cannot be seen, secretin may be injected to help locate it. Outflow through the papilla is seen as a tiny clear fluid spot against the bluish-stained background mucosa if dye has been sprayed over the papilla surface. If deep guidewire cannulation fails, further short cuts can be made into the base of the original incisions. Once the guidewire is successfully advanced into the pancreatic duct, sphincterotomy is completed with a pull-type sphincterotome or needle-knife cutting alongside the wire or over a pancreatic duct stent.

Precut is more easily performed in patients with santorinicele, a saccular dilation of the distal part of the dorsal duct, beneath the duodenal wall and the papillary mound. Usually the papillary mound is prominent and the duodenal wall is less than 2 mm from the dilation. After contrast injection or secretin stimulation, bulging becomes more evident, and if methylene blue mixed with the contrast medium is injected, a bluish stain can be seen. Because of the thickness of the wall of the santorinicele, an incision that is 2 to 5 mm long and 2 to 3 mm deep with the needle knife is sufficient to enter the ductal lumen. Compared with precutting a normal minor papilla, the needle-knife incision is best made in the most prominent part of the bulge superior to the orifice, similar to precut fistulotomy for biliary access (see Chapter 15). Depending on the size of the santorinicele, the final incision may be up to 8 mm long. Overall, precut of a santorinicele is easier and less risky than normal minor papillae.

POSTPROCEDURAL STENTING OF THE MINOR PAPILLA

Temporary pancreatic stenting or placement of a nasopancreatic drain is essential to prevent PEP. Stent placement may prevent stenosis of the sphincterotomy. Long-term stenting is indicated to treat prepapillary or papillary ductal strictures.

To prevent PEP, stents are placed: polyethylene 3 to 5 Fr, 2 to 5 cm long, unflanged (3 Fr) or flanged, with a pigtail at the duodenal end (Zimmon pancreatic stent [Cook Medical]; Advanix [Boston Scientific]), or 5-Fr straight stents, 3 to 5 cm long (Geenen pancreatic stent [Cook Medical]; Advanix [Boston Scientific]) (Fig. 21.17, A–D). The choice of stent depends on the pancreatic duct diameter, the guidewire used for cannulation (3-Fr stents require a 0.018-inch wire), and endoscopist preference. Although the shortest time for effective postsphincterotomy protection has not yet been defined, 2 to 3 days of drainage seems adequate.

Short 3-Fr and 5-Fr stents tend to migrate spontaneously into the duodenum within a few days, and so stent-related ductal damage is not a concern. A plain abdominal radiograph is obtained 1 week after placement to confirm spontaneous passage; if the stent is still in place (5% to 10% of cases), it must be removed endoscopically.

Very good results have been reported with 3-Fr, 6-cm-long to 8-cm-long Zimmon stents without internal flanges.[30] The small diameter causes less ductal damage, thus avoiding the risk of potentially irreversible chronic pancreatitis ductal changes,[31] including stricture formation.[32,33] These stents have a tendency to migrate out of the duct, though the longer intraductal length serves as a friction anchor to minimize migration. We mainly use a 5-Fr stent (Zimmon [Cook Medical] or Advanix [Boston Scientific]), 2 to 3 cm long, because most of our procedures are done with 0.025-inch or 0.035-inch guidewires; ductal morphologic changes with short-duration stenting have not been observed.

To potentially prevent postsphincterotomy stenosis of the minor papilla, a pancreatic stent with a larger caliber (5 to 7 Fr), flanged or unflanged, can be placed and removed within 1 month (no longer), after a radiograph has excluded the unlikely event of spontaneous passage.

Papillary strictures not manageable by sphincterotomy and prepapillary strictures require large-caliber (10 Fr) plastic stent placement up to 3 months (if the duct is large enough to accommodate), with repeated stent exchange up to 1 year or more until resolution.

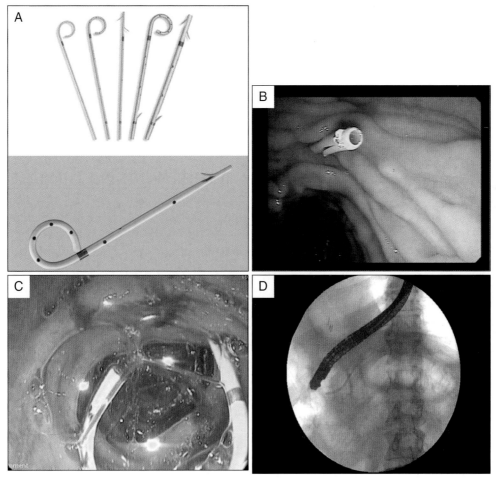

FIG 21.17 A, Different pancreatic plastic stents for prevention of post-ERCP pancreatitis and dorsal duct stenting, with or without pigtail at the duodenal end, and with internal or internal and external flanges. *Above:* Boston Scientific (Advanix). *Below:* Cook Medical (Bloomington, IN). **B,** Plastic pancreatic 5-Fr straight stent. **C,** Plastic 5-Fr stent with pigtail at duodenal end. **D,** Radiograph of a 5-Fr, 5-cm-long plastic straight stent inserted into the dorsal duct. (Courtesy Cook Medical, Bloomington, IN.)

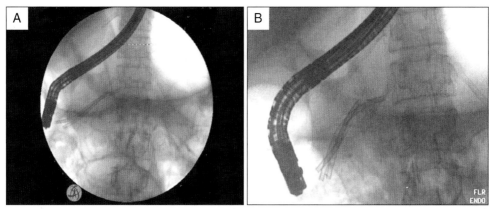

FIG 21.18 Endotherapy of refractory stricture of the prepapillary and distal segment of the dorsal duct. **A,** Two plastic stents have been inserted; **B,** severe stricture treated by placing three plastic stents.

Multiple plastic stents can also be inserted to treat refractory strictures (Fig. 21.18, *A, B*).

REPEAT MINOR PAPILLA SPHINCTEROTOMY

After MiES, stenosis of the minor papilla occurs in approximately 20% of cases. Stenosis may result from the natural healing of the incision or from cautery-induced scar formation. Repeat MiES may be more difficult than the initial sphincterotomy because of the lack of a papillary mound, though it is usually easy to locate the orifice. If there is enough residual tissue between the orifice and the duodenal wall, the cut is extended using a pull-type sphincterotome or needle knife. If no residual tissue is present to allow additional cutting, dilation of the orifice with a 4-mm balloon or a 7-Fr to 9-Fr tapered dilator (Soehendra dilator; Cook Endoscopy) may reveal tissue that can be cut as described above. Similarly, placement of a 3-Fr to 7-Fr stent can also reveal a small amount of residual tissue at the upper rim of the orifice, followed by needle-knife incision over the stent.

Care must be taken to minimize coagulation during repeat MiES to prevent restenosis. In addition, it is advisable to place one 10-Fr, 3-cm-long plastic stent or a smaller and longer plastic stent (depending on the diameter of the duct), to remain in place for 1 to 3 months to prevent restenosis, though the optimal duration of stent placement is unknown.

OUTCOMES OF MINOR PAPILLA SPHINCTEROTOMY

Technical success is defined as complete or partial pancreatic duct drainage obtained at the end of the procedure; clinical success is defined as the disappearance or reduction of episodes of acute pancreatitis, or for patients with pain, a reduction in pain score and narcotic usage and dosage, usually immediately, but especially after long-term follow-up.

In patients with pancreas divisum, the success of MiES depends on the underlying associated clinical presentation and/or underlying pancreatic disease. Clinical presentations include acute recurrent pancreatitis, chronic pancreatitis, or only recurrent pancreatic-type pain. In total, 838 patients with symptomatic pancreas divisum who underwent endotherapy were analyzed in a systematic review of 22 studies.[34] Minor papilla endotherapy provided an overall clinical benefit in 63% of patients: patients with acute recurrent pancreatitis had a response rate ranging from 43% to 100% (median 76%); those with chronic pancreatitis, from 21% to 80% (median 42%); and

those with only abdominal pancreatic-type pain, from 11% to 55% (median 33%).

The results of the main studies of minor papilla endotherapy for pancreas divisum are reported in Table 21.1.[6,35–43] Larger sample sizes, longer follow-up (10 to 20 years), and randomized controlled trials are lacking; there seems to be some reduction in clinical success over time, and multiple procedures are required in about two-thirds of cases. A dilated or irregular dorsal duct does not seem to be related to a better outcome after minor papilla endotherapy compared with a nondilated or regular duct.[42]

Good outcomes of minor papilla sphincterotomy are particularly observed in patients with santorinicele, a cystic dilatation of the terminal end of the dorsal pancreatic duct that is frequently associated with pancreas divisum (Fig. 21.19, *A–D*). In a small study of 15 patients,[44] minor papilla sphincterotomy decreased average pain score and led to complete cessation of narcotic use and a significantly improved quality of life score from 4.5 to 8.4 (on a scale of 1 to 10).

ADVERSE EVENTS (SEE CHAPTER 8)

Minor sphincterotomy can cause immediate, early, or late adverse events similar to those after major papilla sphincterotomy. In the largest published series, 1476 patients with pancreas divisum underwent 2753 ERCPs.[29] Early and immediate adverse events occurred in 7.8% of procedures and included pancreatitis (6.8%), hemorrhage (0.7%), perforation (0.2%), cholecystitis (0.1%), and cardiorespiratory adverse events (0.1%). The frequency and severity of pancreatitis are reported in Table 21.2. MiES was found associated with significantly higher risk of PEP compared with cannulation without MiES (5.9% vs 10.6%) ($p < 0.05$).

In patients with pancreas divisum, multivariate logistic regression indicated that significant predictors of PEP included age <40 years, MiES, female sex, previous PEP, and attempted dorsal duct cannulation, the latter having the highest risk. Underlying severe chronic pancreatitis was protective. The rate of PEP seems to be reduced by placement of a 3-Fr to 5-Fr short pancreatic stent, similar to high-risk patients undergoing ERCP for other indications, or by placement of a 5-Fr to 6-Fr nasopancreatic drain left in situ for 24 to 48 hours. For patients with chronic pancreatitis and a markedly dilated dorsal duct, prophylactic stent placement may not be needed, especially if a large MiES is performed and good drainage is observed. However, prospective studies are needed to specifically assess the benefit of small-caliber prophylactic pancreatic duct stents in patients with pancreas divisum after minor papilla endotherapy.

TABLE 21.1	Clinical Improvement (%) After Minor Papilla Endotherapy for Pancreas Divisum								
				ACUTE RECURRENT PANCREATITIS		PAIN		CHRONIC PANCREATITIS	
Author (Year)	Type of Study	Therapy	Follow-up (mo)	n	%	n	%	n	%
Lans et al. (1992)[35]	RCT	PDS vs none	29*	10	90	0	—	0	—
Coleman et al. (1994)[33]	R	MiES ± PDS	23*	9	78	5	0	20	60
Kozarek et al. (1995)[36]	R	MiES ± PDS	20*	15	73	5	20	19	32
Ertan (2000)[37]	P	PDS	24*	25	76	0	—	0	—
Heyries et al. (2002)[38]	R	MiES ± PDS	39†	24	92	0	—	0	—
Gerke et al. (2004)[39]	R	MiES ± PDS	29†	30	43	9	11	0	—
Attwell et al. (2006)[40]	R	MiES + PDS	60†	69	84‡	32	69‡	83	76‡
Chacko et al. (2008)[41]	R	MiES ± PDS	20†	27	76	8	33	20	42
Borak et al. (2009)[42]	R	MiES	43†	62	71	29	55	22	45
Rustagi and Golioto (2013)[43]	R	MiES ± PDS	ng	18	94	8	50	7	57
Mariani et al. (2014)[6]	P	MiES + PDS	54†	22	74	0	—	0	—
Total				311	77*	86	34*	171	52*

MiES, Minor papilla sphincterotomy; *n,* number of patients; *ng,* not given; *P,* prospective; *PDS,* pancreatic ductal stenting; *R,* retrospective; *RCT,* randomized controlled trial.
*Mean.
†Median.
‡No restenosis.

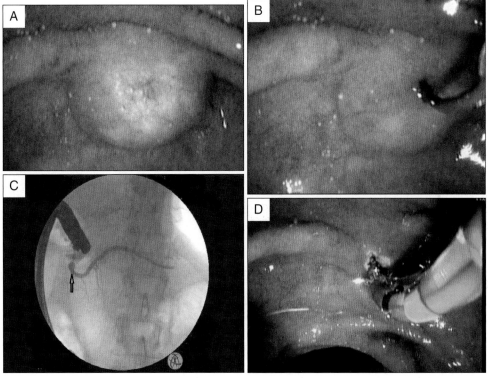

FIG 21.19 A patient with pancreas divisum and santorinicele and acute recurrent pancreatitis. **A,** Endoscopic view of a prominent minor papilla; **B,** minor papilla cannulation by a 0.035-inch guidewire; **C,** radiograph showing complete opacification of the dorsal duct with dilated prepapillary segment; **D,** initial sphincterotomy of the minor papilla using a pull-type sphincterotome.

Among early adverse events, acute bleeding stops spontaneously in most cases or after injection of 0.5 to 2 mL diluted epinephrine (1:10,000) into the bleeding site. Focal bipolar cautery or endoclip placement can be done to treat persistent intraprocedural or clinical postprocedural bleeding. However, application of cautery may increase the risk of postprocedure pancreatitis or induce stenosis at the sphincterotomy site, and clipping may close the papillary orifice because of its small dimension. To prevent the risk of such adverse events, a protective 5-Fr to 7-Fr pancreatic stent should be placed before applying cautery or clips (Fig. 21.20, *A–E*).

Late adverse events include stenosis of the sphincterotomy and ductal changes induced by pancreatic stenting.

TABLE 21.2 **Frequency and Severity of Post-ERCP Pancreatitis After Minor Papilla Sphincterotomy for Pancreas Divisum in the Largest Published Series**

	n	*%*
ERCP	2753	—
PEP	187	6.8
Mild	63	33.7
Moderate	118	63.1
Severe	6	3.2

PEP, Post-ERCP pancreatitis.
From Moffatt DA, Coté GA, Avula H, et al. Risk factors for ERCP-related complications in patients with pancreas divisum: a retrospective study. *Gastrointest Endosc.* 2011;73:963–970.

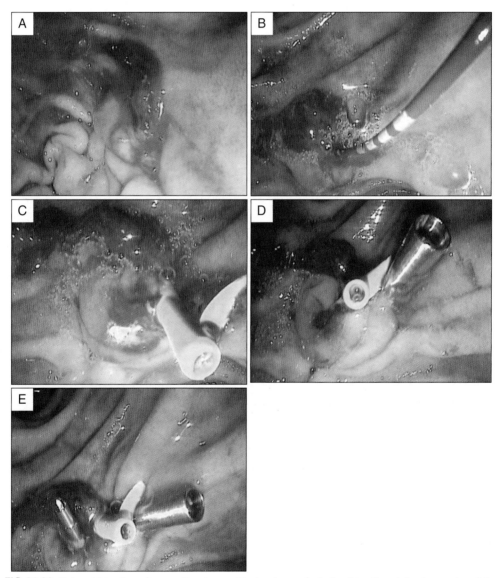

FIG 21.20 Delayed bleeding after papilla minor sphincterotomy. **A,** Active bleeding at the lower rim of the sphincterotomy section; **B,** a guidewire is inserted into the dorsal duct to secure the procedure; **C,** a 5-Fr plastic straight stent is inserted into the dorsal duct over the guidewire; **D,** once the papillary orifice has been protected by the stent, one metallic clip is placed on the bleeding site; **E,** an additional metallic clip is placed to stop bleeding.

The most important late adverse event is papillary restenosis, observed in 11.5% to 19% of patients.[42,45] As previously described, this can be treated by extension of the sphincterotomy or, when there is no residual tissue to cut, by sequential pancreatic stent placement (5 to 10 Fr, depending on ductal diameter). Surgical alternatives include sphincteroplasty or ductal decompression, such as lateral pancreaticojejunostomy, and in some circumstances pancreaticoduodenectomy.[46]

When a pancreatic stent is used not for the prevention of PEP but for therapeutic purposes, especially in patients with a nondilated duct, there is a risk of long-term stent-induced dorsal pancreatic duct changes. These changes are similar to chronic pancreatitis and are observed in 30% to 57% of patients with pancreas divisum who undergo pancreatic stent placement. To reduce this risk, the stent diameter should not be larger than that of the dorsal duct and prolonged stent placement should be avoided.

Prolonged stent placement can also result in pain relapses and/or infection because of stent occlusion and/or proximal migration. Long-term sequelae of pancreatic stenting do not occur when chronic pancreatitis-related ductal changes are present.

The complete reference list for this chapter can be found online at www.expertconsult.com.

22

Plastic Pancreaticobiliary Stents and Nasopancreaticobiliary Tubes: Concepts and Insertion Techniques

Ryan Law and Todd H. Baron

The use of plastic pancreaticobiliary stents for drainage of the bile duct was described more than 3 decades ago.[1] These stents are used for a variety of indications, including malignant and benign conditions, and have proven reliable and safe for decompression of the biliary tree.[2] Palliative insertion of biliary stents relieves distal biliary obstruction as effectively as surgical bypass.[3] Although the use of expandable metal stents has increased and replaced the use of plastic stents for biliary use, plastic stents are preferred for nearly all indications for pancreatic stent placement.

Plastic stents are easy to insert, effective for decompression, and inexpensive to use. Plastic stents are available in a variety of configurations and lengths and are composed of Teflon, polyethylene, or polyurethane (Table 22.1).[2,4] Common configurations are straight, single pigtail, or double pigtail (Fig. 22.1). All plastic stents have limited patency because of occlusion with debris and biofilm (Fig. 22.2)[5] and require periodic replacement when long-term drainage is required. Nearly all stents of the same diameter have similar patency rates. Almost all plastic stents are hollow tubes. Side holes are present in biliary stents to a variable degree but uniformly present in pancreatic duct stents to allow drainage of side branches (Fig. 22.3).

Myriad designs and materials have been proposed and tested to prevent plastic stent occlusion and prolong patency. These include (1) a double-layer design,[6,7] (2) a star-shaped stent with a limited central lumen,[8] and (3) a biliary stent with an antireflux valve (windsock) designed to prevent stent occlusion from food and vegetable material.[9] However, data on such stents have not convincingly demonstrated prolonged patency rates and have not been widely adopted in clinical practice. In addition to alterations in stent design, a recent preclinical study has focused on the development of a hydrophilic coating to deter stent occlusion.[10] Whether this will translate into prolonged patency remains to be seen.

STENT SYSTEMS

A variety of stent systems are available, as discussed in Chapter 4. Stents smaller than 8.5-Fr diameter are usually placed directly over a guidewire using a pusher tube. Stents greater than 8.5-Fr diameter typically include an inner guiding catheter that passes over the guidewire (Fig. 22.4), whereby the stent and pusher tube are passed over the inner guiding catheter (Fig. 22.5). The inner guiding catheter promotes stability and rigidity, which are necessary to allow stent passage across tight strictures.

Endoscope Requirements

Nearly all commercially available duodenoscopes have a therapeutic channel of 4.2 mm that can accommodate stents up to 11.5 Fr in diameter. However, smaller-diameter working channels—such as those in balloon enteroscopes, standard upper endoscopes, and slim (pediatric) colonoscopes—permit placement of only 7-Fr-diameter plastic stents.

Description of Technique: Biliary

Because 10-Fr stents have superior patency to 7-Fr stents, it is recommended that 10-Fr stents be placed whenever possible in patients with malignant disease to limit the number of endoscopic procedures required for palliation.

Distal Biliary Obstruction

The approach to distal biliary strictures is more straightforward than for hilar tumors and will be discussed separately. After successful deep cannulation of the biliary tree, contrast is introduced to clearly elucidate the stricture margins, allowing for selection of the appropriate stent length. The stricture is then traversed with a guidewire. It is important to pass the wire well proximal to the stricture to prevent wire loss and to provide mechanical advantage, although care must be taken to avoid passing the wire too proximally, which can cause ductal perforation. In general, a biliary sphincterotomy is not required for insertion of stents up to 10-Fr diameter[11] and is not protective of post–endoscopic retrograde cholangiopancreatography (ERCP) pancreatitis after stent placement for malignant biliary obstruction.[12] However, one study showed that in patients with bile leaks, placement of 10-Fr stents without sphincterotomy was associated with a higher rate of post-ERCP pancreatitis.[13] A biliary sphincterotomy is required when multiple stents are placed, as is done in the treatment of benign strictures (see Chapter 43).[11]

When placing a single 10-Fr stent, it is rarely necessary to dilate the stricture, especially when placed for a distal stricture, because the mechanical advantage is great enough to overcome resistance. In cases of uncertainty, a 10-Fr dilating catheter (e.g., Soehendra dilator; Cook Endoscopy, Winston-Salem, NC) can be passed through the stricture. If the catheter easily traverses the stricture, balloon dilation is not required. Otherwise, hydrostatic balloon dilation can be performed. When the insertion of multiple stents is planned, stricture dilation is essential. In this setting, more than one guidewire may be placed before insertion of the first stent. Alternatively, a guidewire can be placed after each stent insertion by recannulating the bile duct alongside the stents. A useful tip in placing more than one wire is to pass a large or multilumen catheter over the initial guidewire. This can also be accomplished with a triple-lumen cytology brush sheath by removing the brush and using that lumen for a guidewire. More recently, an "intraductal exchange" can be performed using the Fusion system (Cook Endoscopy) and the short-wire lumen. During each stent placement the wire can be separated

TABLE 22.1 Plastic Biliary and Pancreatic Stents

	Length (cm)	Diameter (Fr)	Shape*	Flap†	Material	Cost: Stent/ System (US$)
Biliary Stents						
Boston Scientific Advanix	5–15	7, 8.5, 10	CB, DB, DP	S	Polyethylene	89/219
Cook Endoscopy‡	1–21	5, 7, 8.5, 10, 11.5§	A, C, DP	S, Q	Various‡	69/145
ConMed Hydroduct	4–15	7, 10, 12§	A, S, C, DP	S	Polyurethane‖	72/146
Hobbs Medical	4–15	7,10	C, DP	S	Soft polymer blend	44/90
Olympus Double Layer & QuickPlace V	3–15	7, 8.5, 10, 12§	CB, DB, S, DP	S, Q	Polyethylene, proprietary¶	78–274/169–365
Pancreatic Stents						
Boston Scientific Advanix	2–18	3, 4, 5, 7, 10	S, SP	S, N	Radiopaque polymer	77–87/170
Cook Endoscopy**	2–22	4, 5, 6, 7, 8.5, 10, 11.5§	S, SP	D	Various**	69/145
Hobbs Medical Freeman Flexi	3–18	3, 4, 5, 7	S, SP	S, N	Soft polymer blend	44–48/50–54

*Shape column: A, angled; C, curved; CB, center bend; DB, duodenal bend; DP, double pigtail; S, straight; SP, single pigtail.
†Flap column: D, 2 internal/external; N, no flaps; Q, 4 internal/external; S, single external/internal.
‡Multiple stent lines available: Cotton-Huibregtse, polyethylene; Cotton-Leung, polyethylene; Cotton-Leung Sof-flex, polyethylene/polyurethane; ST-2 Tannenbaum, Teflon; Solus, polyethylene/polyurethane; Zimmon, polyethylene.
§Stents >10 Fr require a 4.2-mm channel duodenoscope.
‖Covered with hydromer coating.
¶Proprietary stent with perfluoro inner layer, stainless steel middle layer, and polyamide elastomer outer layer.
**Multiple stent lines available: Zimmon, polyethylene; Geenen, polyethylene; Geenen Sof-flex, polyethylene/polyurethane; Johlin Wedge, polyethylene/polyurethane.
From ASGE Technology Assessment Committee, Pfau PR, Pleskow DK, Banerjee S, et al. Pancreatic and biliary stents. *Gastrointest Endosc.* 2013;77:319–327.

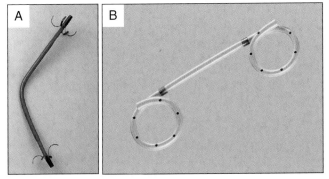

FIG 22.1 Two stents. **A,** Straight 10-Fr biliary stent. **B,** Double-pigtail 10-Fr stent. (**A,** Courtesy Olympus Corporation, Center Valley, PA. **B,** Courtesy Cook Medical, Bloomington, IN.)

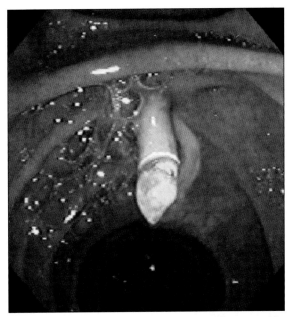

FIG 22.2 Endoscopic photograph of occluded 10-Fr stent exiting the bile duct.

from the delivery system to allow additional stents to be placed sequentially using a single guidewire.

When multiple stents are placed, using a slightly longer initial stent is helpful as the friction created by passage of additional stents during insertion may result in proximal movement. If the first stent is too short, it may migrate into the duct. This is usually of no consequence, assuming that the stent is still across the stricture. The length of the stent chosen is based on the distance from the papilla to the proximal edge of the stricture plus an additional 2 cm. In general, 5-cm-long or 7-cm-long stents are of sufficient length for nearly all biliary strictures resulting from pancreatic cancer. Defining the stricture length can be achieved in several ways. One method is to measure during withdrawal of the initial cannulating catheter. When the catheter tip is at the proximal end of the stricture, the endoscopist holds the catheter just outside the biopsy port. The catheter is withdrawn until it is endoscopically visible in the duodenum just distal to the papilla. The distance from the endoscopist's fingers to the biopsy port is measured and represents the stricture length. Anecdotally, this method seems to overestimate the length of the stricture. Another way is to use the radiograph to measure

the length of the stricture. When the tip of the endoscope is in contact with the papilla, a radiographic image is captured. The distance from the tip of the endoscope to the proximal edge of the stricture is measured. The diameter of the endoscope is used as a comparison measuring point to determine the true stricture length and account for a magnification factor. The following equation is used to solve for the unknown variable X, which is true stricture length (Fig. 22.6):

$$\frac{\text{Actual stricture length}(X)}{\text{Measured stricture length}} = \frac{\text{Actual endoscope diameter}}{\text{Measured endoscope diameter}}$$

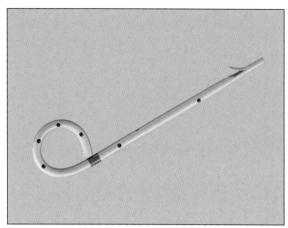

FIG 22.3 Pancreatic duct stent. Note side holes. (Courtesy Cook Medical, Bloomington, IN.)

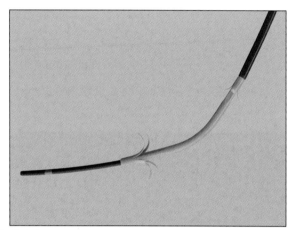

FIG 22.4 Cook Endoscopy stent system showing typical 10-Fr design. Inner guiding catheter, stent (*blue*), and pusher tube are seen. (Courtesy Cook Medical, Bloomington, IN.)

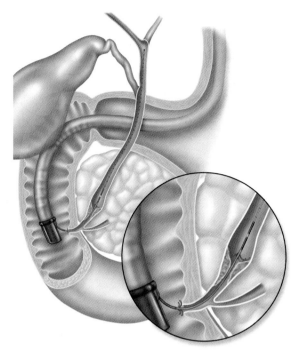

FIG 22.5 Illustration of 10-Fr stent system with stent placed for relief of malignant distal biliary obstruction.

Finally, fluoroscopic markers separated by a known distance are available on some catheters and guidewires and can be used as a reference point to the stricture and papilla. Balloon dilation catheters also have radiopaque markers corresponding to the length of the balloon. Excessively long stents should be avoided. Distal migration tends to occur into the duodenum until the proximal flange or pigtail impacts at the top of the stricture, potentially resulting in the distal end of the stent impacting and perforating the lateral duodenal wall (Fig. 22.7).

Once the stent has been selected, placement is undertaken. If a tapered end is present, this represents the proximal end of the stent. Depending on the type of stent system, either the inner guiding catheter alone or the inner guiding catheter and stent are advanced over the guidewire. It is important that the guidewire and inner guiding catheter do not pass too far proximally into the biliary tree during advancement, as this could cause injury to the intrahepatic ducts or liver capsule. Conversely, excessive traction on the wire or inner guiding catheter may result in wire loss. The stent is then advanced over the guide catheter by advancing the pusher tube. The latter has a larger bore that approximates the diameter of the stent. During advancement down the endoscope channel, the elevator should remain closed. When the stent impacts the elevator, the elevator is opened slightly to allow it to emerge from the endoscope channel. The elevator is closed to direct the stent upward and into the papilla. It is imperative to maintain a short endoscope position with the tip as close as possible to the papilla to maintain maximal mechanical advantage. The stent is ultimately advanced into the bile duct using a series of small movements in which the elevator is sequentially lowered to allow advancement of the stent and then closed to advance the stent in a "ratchet-like" manner. Upward tip deflection and withdrawal of the duodenoscope shaft further shortens the scope and provides forward advancement of the stent. It is important to note that allowing more than a minimal amount of stent to be advanced out of the duodenoscope into the duodenum decreases the mechanical advantage and often prohibits forward advancement because of looping and buckling between the papilla and the endoscope, ultimately risking misdeployment. To facilitate forward movement of the stent, the endoscopy assistant must provide traction on the inner guiding catheter (or guidewire if there is no inner guiding catheter). Once optimal stent position is achieved, the inner guiding catheter and guidewire are removed while the endoscopist maintains forward pressure with the pusher tube against the stent to prevent distal stent dislodgement. If additional contrast is needed to assess drainage or intrahepatic anatomy above the stent, the guidewire can be removed before removing the inner guiding catheter to allow contrast injection (this is possible only when long-wire systems are used). The process is repeated for additional stent placement.

In patients with short, distal bile strictures (e.g., chronic pancreatitis, postsphincterotomy ampullary strictures), three to four 10-Fr, 5-cm-long stents can be mounted on the inner guiding catheter at one time. Once the first stent is placed (Fig. 22.8) the inner guiding catheter and guidewire are withdrawn just enough to release this first stent; the duct is then recannulated alongside the first stent with the second stent, guidewire, and inner guiding catheter. The process is continued until all stents are deployed. Alternatively, the stents can be placed one by one alongside each other (Fig. 22.9).

Stents for Irretrievable Bile Duct Stones

In the absence of a stricture, pigtail stents (see Fig. 22.1, *B*) may be preferable to straight stents when placed into a dilated biliary tree in patients with irretrievable bile duct stones (see Chapter 19) because

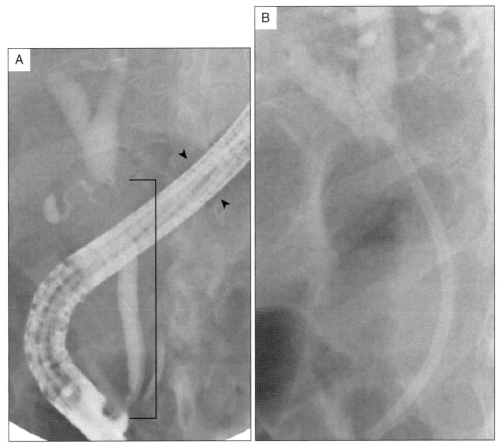

FIG 22.6 Measurement on the radiograph to calculate stent length. **A,** The measurement from the top of the stricture to endoscope tip when positioned at the papilla (*bracket*) compared with the diameter of the endoscope (*arrowheads*) was 7:1. **B,** Because the diameter of the endoscope was 11.5 mm, a 9-cm stent was placed.

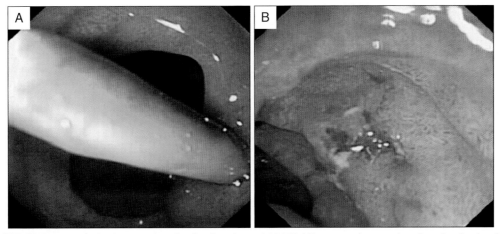

FIG 22.7 Endoscopic photographs of a distally migrated 11.5-Fr biliary stent impacted against the duodenal wall opposite the major papilla. **A,** Before removal; **B,** after removal, a small defect is seen.

they are less likely to migrate distally. Pigtail stents are placed slightly differently from straight stents because the duodenoscope has to be partially withdrawn during final deployment to allow the pigtail to form in the duodenum. The stent should be advanced until the distal portion of the stent just proximal to the distal pigtail is identified endoscopically. The latter is identified by applying an indelible marker before placement (if a visible marker is not already on the stent) at the junction of the straight portion and distal pigtail. The stent is then advanced while simultaneously withdrawing the duodenoscope so that the pigtail is deployed into the duodenum, or by allowing the elevator of the duodenoscope to remain open while advancing the pusher tube and allowing the pigtail to form distally.

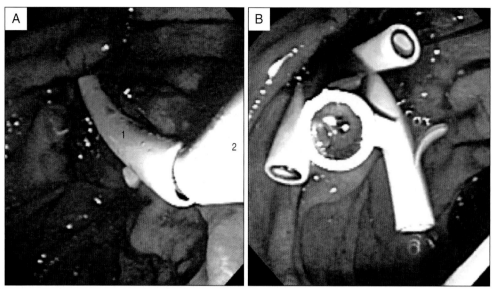

FIG 22.8 Insertion of multiple 10-Fr stents. **A,** The first stent (*1*) is being pushed by the second stent (*2*) because the actual pusher tube is still well above the multiple stents loaded onto the catheter. **B,** Final result of four 10-Fr stents, all placed with one passage of the stent introducer system.

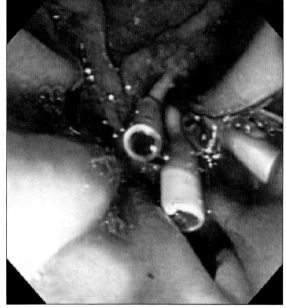

FIG 22.9 Additional stent insertion. Passage of the catheter alongside the initial stents to recannulate and place additional stents.

Hilar Biliary Obstruction

Hilar biliary obstruction differs from distal obstruction in two ways: (1) although a sphincterotomy is not needed for placement of a unilateral stent, limited data suggest that hilar stent placement carries a higher risk of pancreatitis than for distal obstruction, which may be prevented by performing a biliary sphincterotomy, and (2) stricture dilation is frequently required because of loss of mechanical advantage when the resistance of the stricture is away from the tip of the endoscope, and thus both sphincterotomy and stricture dilation are necessary when bilateral stents are placed (Fig. 22.10).

In general, stents used for hilar tumors are at least 12 cm in length, because the distance to the bifurcation from the papilla is approximately 9 cm in most patients. Stents that are of adequate length to cross the stricture may be too short to "anchor" within the intrahepatic system and more prone to migrate distally. Softer, more pliable stents may be less prone to distal migration.[14] If bilateral stent placement is required (see Chapter 40), there are two options for guidewire placement. One option is to place two wires side-by-side, one in each intrahepatic system, before placing either stent (method 1) (see Fig. 22.1). The other option is to place the first stent, recannulate the bile duct alongside it, and pass the guidewire into the opposite intrahepatic system (method 2). There are proponents of both methods, with advantages of method 2 being the lack of friction within the endoscope channel between the first stent (if 10 Fr) and its larger pusher tube and the other guidewire within the endoscope channel. This can be overcome by using a 0.025-inch guidewire as the initial wire. It is important to note that it may not be possible to place bilateral 10-Fr stents during the first session because of either the tightness of the stricture or the diameter of the downstream duct, which is often decompressed and small in patients with hilar obstruction. In that case it may be best to place two 7-Fr or 8.5-Fr stents or one 10-Fr and one 7-Fr stent and then upsize one or both stents at another endoscopic session.

Nasobiliary Tubes

Nasobiliary tubes (NBTs) are essentially extremely long biliary stents that exit the patient's nose after exchange from the mouth. NBTs are placed for many of the same indications as biliary stents, including decompression of the gallbladder. They are not commonly used in the United States because of patient discomfort and risk for dislodgement, as well as difficulty in displacement during the oral-to-nasal transfer. Advantages of NBTs over internal stents are that they allow the practioner to obtain noninvasive cholangiograms and cholecystograms; provide irrigation for hemobilia, mucus, or debris; and remove the tube without the use of endoscopy. They are especially useful for very short-term use in patients with multiple bile duct stones when complete stone clearance is not certain, as a temporizing measure in patients with acute cholecystitis before cholecystectomy[15] (Fig. 22.11), and for delivery of high-dose brachytherapy.[16]

NBTs range in diameter from 5 to 10 Fr and have proximal ends that can be straight or pigtailed. NBT placement begins initially as for

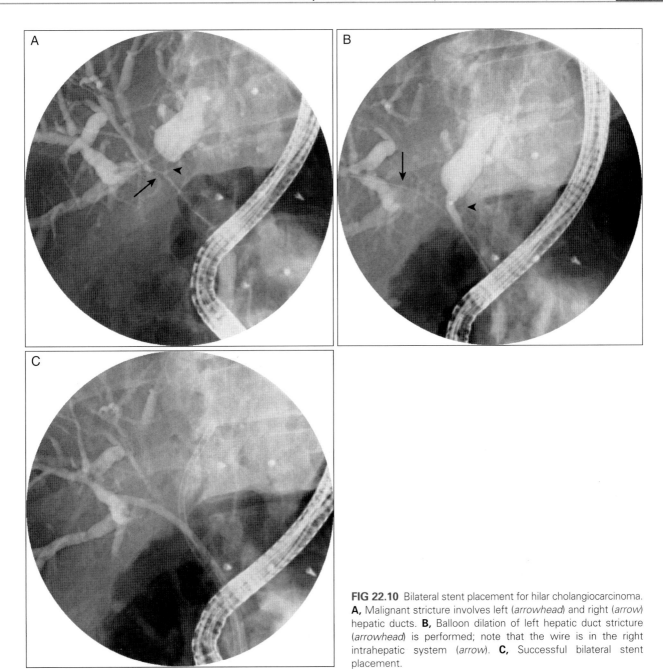

FIG 22.10 Bilateral stent placement for hilar cholangiocarcinoma. **A,** Malignant stricture involves left (*arrowhead*) and right (*arrow*) hepatic ducts. **B,** Balloon dilation of left hepatic duct stricture (*arrowhead*) is performed; note that the wire is in the right intrahepatic system (*arrow*). **C,** Successful bilateral stent placement.

biliary stent placement, although there is no inner guiding catheter for any size. After the drain is in proper position within the biliary tree, the duodenoscope is withdrawn from the patient while simultaneously advancing the NBT. Once the duodenoscope is in the stomach, additional advancement of the NBT allows it to be in a long position along the greater curvature, providing a margin for error so that the tube is not accidentally dislodged during duodenoscope withdrawal or oral-nasal transfer. However, an excessive amount of the NBT should not be placed in the stomach, as loop formation may cause the intraductal portion to be dislodged. After the duodenoscope is removed from the patient, the tube is transferred from the mouth to the nose by the use of a nasal transfer tube included in the NBT kit. This may require passage of the endoscopist's fingers into the patient's mouth, and moderately sedated patients may inadvertently bite down during the process. This can be avoided by using a small-caliber transnasal endoscope to perform the transfer.[17]

Pancreatic Duct Stent Insertion

Pancreatic duct stent placement does not require pancreatic sphincterotomy, especially because these stents are small caliber (3 to 7 Fr). Rarely, 10-Fr stents are placed, and even then pancreatic sphincterotomy for stent placement alone is not absolutely necessary. The diameter of the stent chosen is dependent on the indication (e.g., prevention of post-ERCP pancreatitis, treatment of stricture or leak) and the size of the main pancreatic duct. Small-diameter stents are passed over the guidewire without an inner guiding catheter using only a pusher tube or similar device (e.g., standard catheter, sphincterotome, or balloon catheter). Similar to placement of biliary stents, the site of the pathology is identified, a wire is passed into the tail, and dilation is performed, if necessary. The wire is removed while keeping the pusher tube in position. The pusher tube is then removed, leaving the end of the stent exiting the papilla. One must be careful when placing short and very-small-diameter

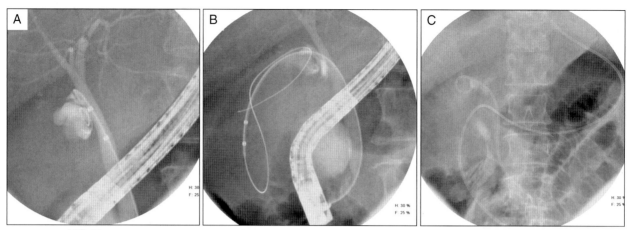

FIG 22.11 Endoscopic placement of nasobiliary tube into the gallbladder. **A,** Occlusion balloon positioned at cystic duct takeoff; note contrast and small amount of guidewire into gallbladder. **B,** Hydrophilic guidewire coiled into gallbladder. **C,** Image after placement of nasobiliary (nasocholecystic) tube and removal of endoscope.

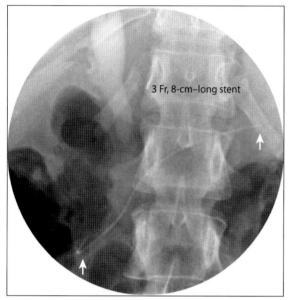

3 Fr, 8-cm–long stent

FIG 22.12 Three-French pancreatic duct stent placed for prevention of post-ERCP pancreatitis. *Arrows* denote ends of stent.

(3 Fr) pancreatic stents, as they can easily be inserted too far into the duct. Some prefer to use single-pigtail stents with the pigtail in the duodenum to avoid inward migration of smaller-diameter stents, as retrieval of these proximally migrated stents can be difficult.[18]

Small-caliber plastic stents (3 to 5 Fr) are commonly used for prevention of post-ERCP pancreatitis in patients who are at high risk (e.g., difficult cannulation, ampullectomy) and/or for the performance of high-risk interventions (e.g., precut biliary sphincterotomy, pancreatic sphincterotomy) (see Chapter 7; Fig. 22.12).[19] These stents are expected to pass spontaneously within a short period to minimize pancreatic duct injury. Available evidence suggests that 5-Fr, 3-cm unflanged pancreatic stents are optimal for prevention of post-ERCP pancreatitis.[20,21]

Nasopancreatic Tubes

Nasopancreatic tubes are rarely placed within the main pancreatic duct. However, the indications for use are similar to pancreatic stents, including transpapillary drainage of pancreatic fluid collections, treatment of leaks and fistulae, and prevention of post-ERCP pancreatitis.[22–27] They also have been used to provide irrigation through the main pancreatic duct after extracorporeal shock wave lithotripsy for treatment of chronic calcific pancreatitis (see Chapter 55) and transmurally for treatment of walled-off pancreatic necrosis (see Chapter 56).

Nasopancreatic tubes, like pancreatic duct stents, have multiple side holes in the distal 10 to 12 cm. The diameter chosen is usually 5 or 7 Fr. Placement is similar to NBTs.

Drainage of Pancreatic Fluid Collections

Double-pigtail stents are placed transgastrically or transduodenally during transmural drainage of pancreatic fluid collections (see Chapters 54 and 56). Transmural placement of double-pigtail stents across the lumen wall into the collection is preferred (Fig. 22.13). Straight stents may be a source of delayed bleeding, as the proximal end within the collection can impact the wall as the cavity collapses. Stents are inserted in similar fashion to biliary stents. It is important to note that the proximal end of some 10-Fr pigtail stents is tapered and does not allow an inner guiding catheter to pass (Zimmon stent; Cook Endoscopy). The tapered portion can be cut to allow an inner guiding catheter to pass through the stent. Alternatively, the inner guiding catheter can be cut shorter such that when the distal end impacts within the proximal tapered portion of the stent, the pusher tube is in contact with the other end of the stent. During deployment of pigtail stents one must be especially careful that an excessive length of stent is not passed into the collection because the entire stent could be inadvertently pushed into the collection.

Indications and Contraindications
Biliary Indications

Malignant biliary obstruction is the most frequent indication for the use of plastic stents. Distal obstruction is most commonly caused by pancreatic adenocarcinoma. Mid to proximal malignant obstruction may be caused by primary cancer of the biliary tree (e.g., gallbladder cancer or cholangiocarcinoma) or from invasion or obstruction of the duct by adjacent malignant metastatic lymph nodes. Plastic stents may be used to relieve obstruction of previously placed metal stents (Fig. 22.14).[28,29] In general, distal bile duct tumors are more effectively palliated with plastic stents than are hilar tumors.

Benign strictures are treated by dilation and placement of multiple plastic stents (Fig. 22.15; see Chapter 43).[30,31] Causes of benign obstruction

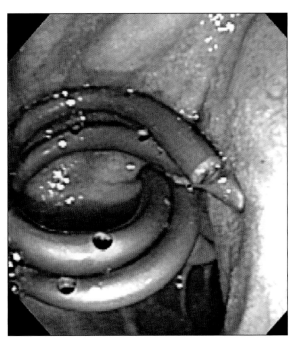

FIG 22.13 Two 10-Fr stents placed transduodenally to drain a pancreatic pseudocyst.

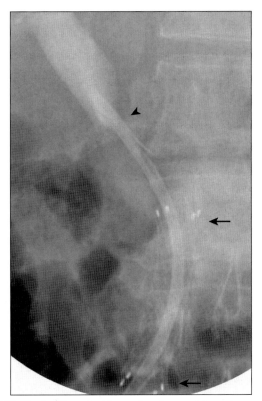

FIG 22.14 Plastic biliary stent (*arrowhead*) passed through an occluded metal biliary stent (*arrows*) that had been placed for palliation of pancreatic carcinoma.

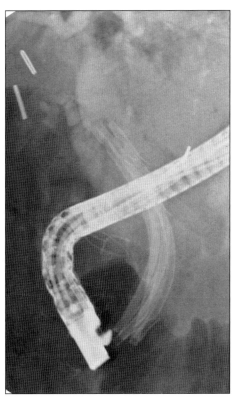

FIG 22.15 Fluoroscopic image after placement of five stents for treatment of benign distal bile duct stricture.

include postsphincterotomy stenosis, chronic pancreatitis, postsurgical injury, ischemia, and anastomotic and nonanastomotic strictures after liver transplantation (see Chapter 44). Biliary leaks and fistulae after biliary surgery, cholecystectomy, and trauma can be treated by short-term stent placement across the papilla with or without sphincterotomy (Fig.

22.16). Stent placement in these scenarios does not need to cross the leak site. The elimination of sphincter pressure promotes flow away from the leak into the duodenum, leading to closure of the leak or fistula. For more complex leaks and major leaks of the common bile duct, it is usually necessary to traverse the leak site.

Pancreatic Indications

Plastic stents are used for relief of pancreatic ductal obstruction caused by chronic pancreatitis. Pancreatic leaks may manifest as pancreatic ascites or pancreatic fluid collections (see Chapters 54 and 56).[32] Occasionally malignant pancreatic ductal obstruction caused by pancreatic cancer will result in pancreatitis or contribute to disabling pain that can be managed with placement of pancreatic stents across the stricture (Fig. 22.17). Temporary stent placement has been proven to prevent post-ERCP pancreatitis in patients at high risk.[33] In the setting of severe acute pancreatitis, pancreatic duct leaks and disruptions can contribute to poor outcome. Pancreatic stent placement may improve the clinical course in a subset of these patients. In patients with traumatic pancreatic duct injury, plastic stents are effective at bridging the injured duct and permitting resolution of the leak (see Chapter 45). Postsurgical pancreatic duct leaks (e.g., due to distal pancreatectomy, inadvertent surgical injury) are effectively treated with pancreatic stents (Fig. 22.18).[34] In patients with chronic calcific pancreatitis, stent placement before extracorporeal shockwave lithotripsy may reduce the cumulative number of shocks necessary for stone fragmentation, ultimately decreasing time to resolution.[35] Finally, a variety of plastic stent configurations have been useful in transpapillary and transmural drainage of pancreatic fluid collections (see Chapter 56).

Adverse Events

When sphincterotomy is performed, adverse events such as hemorrhage (Fig. 22.19) and perforation may occur. Adverse events directly related

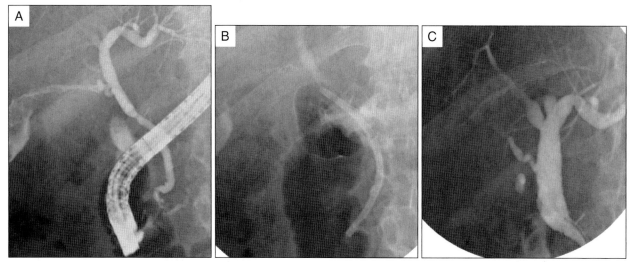

FIG 22.16 Placement of biliary stent for treatment of postcholecystectomy cystic duct leak. **A,** Active leak is seen. **B,** Fluoroscopic image taken immediately after placement of 10-Fr biliary stent. **C,** Follow-up cholangiogram several weeks later showing closure of leak.

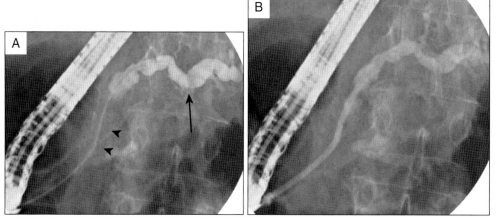

FIG 22.17 Placement of plastic pancreatic stent in a patient with unresectable pancreatic cancer, intractable pain, fever, and hyperamylasemia. **A,** Stricture (*arrowheads*) and dilated main pancreatic duct (*arrow*). **B,** Immediately after placement of stent. Significant improvement in pain was achieved.

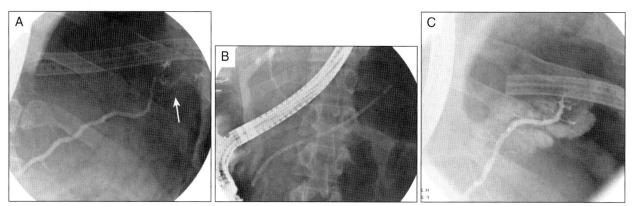

FIG 22.18 Placement of pancreatic stent for treatment of postsplenectomy pancreatic duct leak. **A,** Active leak is seen. **B,** Fluoroscopic image taken immediately after placement of 7-Fr pancreatic stent to tail. **C,** Follow-up pancreatogram several weeks later showing closure of leak.

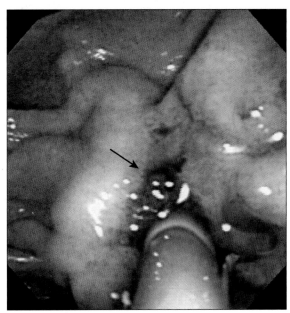

FIG 22.19 Endoscopically visible vessel (*arrow*) identified from post-sphincterotomy bleeding after biliary stent placement. Heater probe therapy was applied and no further bleeding ensued.

to the stent include cholangitis, frequently caused by stent occlusion or migration, and cholecystitis as a result of cystic duct obstruction. Biliary stent occlusion is caused by deposition of bacterial biofilm and/or plant material (see Fig. 22.2) and leads to recurrent biliary obstruction and cholangitis. Stent migration, into or out of the duct, occurs in approximately 5% of cases and may result in recurrent obstruction and cholangitis. Uncommon adverse stent events include perforation of the lateral duodenal wall by the distal end if an excessive amount protrudes into the lumen or if distal stent migration occurs (see Fig. 22.7)[36]; such perforations may be occult and thus recognized only at the time of stent removal or replacement. Rare adverse events as a result of stent

migration completely out of the bile duct include bowel obstruction and perforation.[37]

Removal of inwardly migrated or displaced pancreatic duct stents, particularly those placed for prophylaxis, can be extremely difficult as the duct and stents are small, and the stent may be impacted in a side branch. Additionally, maneuvers to extract the stent may cause the stent to be inadvertently be pushed toward the tail, making extraction more difficult as the duct becomes smaller and the stent wedged into the tail.

Relative Cost

Plastic stents provide rapid relief of biliary obstruction and shorten hospital stay compared with surgical bypass for relief of malignant distal biliary obstruction. Stent placement also may obviate the need for surgery altogether in some patients. Plastic stents cost approximately $100 to $200 and are far less costly than self-expandable metal stents (SEMS), which may exceed $2000, depending on the manufacturer and the presence or absence of a synthetic covering. SEMS have a significantly longer patency than plastic stents, with previous data suggesting that placement of plastic stents is more cost-effective in patients with a distal malignancy who have an anticipated life expectancy of less than 3 to 4 months.[3,38] Recent randomized controlled trial data in patients with malignant biliary obstruction at the level of the extrahepatic bile duct contradict these early data. Plastic stents appear to be the more cost-effective intervention for the index procedure compared with SEMS; however, this cost saving is ultimately offset by higher subsequent costs as a result of hospitalization for premature stent occlusions.[39,40] Moreover, costs were not higher for patients with limited survival who underwent SEMS placement in lieu of plastic stent placement.[40] Similarly, a recent cost-effectiveness analysis revealed that SEMS placement was the dominant strategy, with superior efficacy at significantly less expense.[41] Current Procedural Terminology (CPT) codes and ambulatory payment classifications in the United States for placement and/or removal of plastic biliary stents are available.[2]

The complete reference list for this chapter can be found online at www.expertconsult.com.

23

Biliary Metal Stent Insertion: Indications and Insertion Techniques

Koushik K. Das and Gregory G. Ginsberg

Self-expandable metal stents (SEMS), classified as uncovered (uSEMS), partially covered (pcSEMS), or fully covered (fcSEMS), offer a more durable means to overcome biliary stenosis compared with fixed-diameter plastic stents (PS), which occlude in 30% and 50% of patients within 3 and 6 months, respectively.[1] The outer diameter of PS is limited by the duodenoscope accessory channel diameter to 12 Fr (4 mm). In contrast, SEMS are constrained on a delivery system as small as 6 Fr and expand to up to 10 mm postdeployment.[2] Although SEMS were originally developed to provide durable palliation of malignant biliary obstruction in patients with limited life expectancy, there has been increasing interest in the use of fcSEMS for nonmalignant indications.[3–5] This chapter reviews biliary SEMS, including indications for use, available types, techniques for placement, avoidance and management of adverse events, and relative cost.[2,6]

INDICATIONS

SEMS for Malignant Biliary Stricture

The most common causes of malignant biliary obstruction are pancreatic adenocarcinoma, cholangiocarcinoma, ampullary carcinoma, gallbladder cancer, and extrinsic compression associated with lymphadenopathy caused by lymphoma or metastatic carcinoma. Without therapy, the mean survival for patients presenting with malignant biliary obstruction is <200 days. Because most patients have advanced disease at the time of presentation, operative resection with curative intent is possible in only 10% to 15% of cases.[7] Therefore palliation of mechanical obstruction plays a major role in the management of patients with pancreaticobiliary malignancies (Box 23.1). Options for palliation of malignant biliary obstruction include operative bypass, percutaneous drainage, and endoscopic stent placement. For the vast majority of patients with malignant biliary obstruction, endoscopic stent placement is preferred over operative bypass and percutaneous drainage on the basis of expediency, patient comfort, adverse events, and cost.

SEMS Versus PS

Both PS and uSEMS/pcSEMS can be used for palliation of malignant biliary obstruction. PS, discussed in detail in Chapter 22, are safe and effective, are less expensive than SEMS, and can be removed and replaced if occlusion occurs—usually presenting with a recurrence of jaundice and/or ascending cholangitis. SEMS were designed with a larger internal diameter to extend the duration of patency, thereby reducing the frequency of reintervention. As such, their increased initial cost appears to be offset by a reduction in episodes of cholangitis and the need for elective and emergency interventions. In a meta-analysis of 2436 patients with distal malignant biliary obstruction, SEMS were comparable to PS in technical and therapeutic success rates, mortality, and overall adverse events and were associated with lower rates of obstruction at 4 months.[8] The multicenter US Wallstent study randomized patients to uSEMS or 10-Fr PS for palliation of malignant distal bile duct obstruction.[9] Early stent occlusion as a result of sludge accumulation occurred in ~3% in the PS group compared with 0% in the uSEMS group. During long-term follow-up, uSEMS were associated with one-third the risk of stent occlusion, a significantly reduced adverse event rate (20% vs 31%), and significantly fewer procedures. Numerous subsequent trials,[4,10–14] including a recent multicenter randomized trial from the Netherlands,[15] have similarly confirmed a significantly longer duration of patency, fewer hospital stays, and similar costs after 1 year with SEMS in comparison to PS. In fact, Walter et al. found that even in patients with short survival times (<3 months) the total cost per patient was not significantly different between SEMS and PS.[15]

Covered Versus Uncovered SEMS for Malignant Biliary Obstruction

uSEMS are associated with lower rates of stent migration and can be used anywhere in the bile duct, including the hilum.[16–18] However, tumor ingrowth and lack of removability are limitations of uSEMS. pc/fcSEMS share the same indications as their uncovered counterparts, though they are not advocated for hilar or intrahepatic obstruction because they may block the contralateral intrahepatic system or ipsilateral intrahepatic branches. Similarly, in patients with an intact gallbladder, uSEMS are often preferred when it is anticipated that the stent will cross the cystic duct takeoff; if an fcSEMS is used, it may result in cholecystitis. The anticipated advantage of pc/fcSEMS is the prevention of tissue ingrowth (malignant or hyperplastic) and subsequent stent occlusion while allowing for potential removability (although all but one SEMS are approved by the FDA for only immediate and not delayed removal). However, pc/fcSEMS are considerably more expensive than their uncovered counterparts. Although there are more published data on the use of uncovered stents, there is a substantial body of literature advocating the use of pcSEMS for palliation of malignant biliary obstruction. Studies of pcSEMS have demonstrated very low rates of stent occlusion because of tumor ingrowth.[19,20] However, concerns have been raised about higher rates of stent migration and stent-induced cholecystitis and pancreatitis from cystic duct obstruction and pancreatic duct obstruction, respectively.[13,20–22] Although an earlier meta-analysis of five randomized controlled trials with 781 patients showed that the use of pcSEMS compared with uSEMS was associated with significantly longer stent patency and time to reocclusion,[23] a more recent meta-analysis demonstrated no differences in the number of recurrent biliary obstructions or stent patency after 6 or 12 months.[24] Similarly, a large, single-center retrospective study of 749 patients (171 pcSEMS and 578 uSEMS) demonstrated no difference in recurrent obstruction at 1 year (35% vs 38%), overall or median survival, median time to recurrent biliary obstruction, or rate of adverse events.[25] Of note, however, covered stents may be particularly well suited for

Video for this chapter can be found online at www.expertconsult.com.

recanalization and preservation of occluded indwelling uSEMS. Because many patients with pancreaticobiliary malignancies are experiencing longer, multiyear survival—owing to advances in oncologic therapies such as immunotherapy—enhancing durable endoscopic palliation of biliary obstruction is a welcome challenge.

Preoperative Use of SEMS in Malignant Biliary Disease

When initially introduced into the marketplace, SEMS placement was limited to patients with confirmed, nonoperable, malignant biliary obstruction. However, there has been an evolution in the use of SEMS preoperatively, especially when used for neoadjuvant therapy. Still, in many centers a PS is placed for initial management of suspected but non–biopsy proven malignant biliary obstruction; placement of a SEMS is deferred until occlusion of the initially placed PS, performance status suggesting a greater than 3-month survival, confirmed tissue diagnosis, and/or completed staging to confirm nonoperability. However, recent data suggest a broader application for the up-front use of SEMS. Indeed there are emerging data[26,27] examining the use of fcSEMS in the palliation of malignant biliary obstruction that may support their use up front in patients with a high clinical suspicion of malignant biliary obstruction when a tissue diagnosis is uncertain (because covered SEMS are removable). However, further studies are needed before recommending the routine use of covered SEMS in this setting.

Concerns about the use of routine preoperative placement of PS for biliary decompression for distal biliary obstruction before pancreatectomy have been raised, particularly after a multicenter study demonstrated a significant increase in the complication rate in patients who underwent routine preoperative biliary drainage.[28] It should be noted that successful initial cannulation failure rates in this study were high (25%), as were post–endoscopic retrograde cholangiopancreatography (ERCP)-related adverse events (46%). Furthermore, only PS were used in the study and many patients (26%) developed occlusion-related cholangitis; this may be ameliorated with the up-front use of SEMS. Preoperative biliary drainage may alleviate jaundice and cholestasis-associated adverse events and allow time for delivery of neoadjuvant chemoradiation. Indeed, as multiple therapeutic options for neoadjuvant therapy have evolved for pancreaticobiliary malignancy, meta-analyses have shown that more than one-third of borderline resectable patients can be effectively downstaged to achieve surgical resection.[29,30] Although concerns were raised about SEMS complicating operative resection, this has not been borne out in clinical practice. Several series have detailed the utility of preoperative drainage with SEMS in patients with resectable pancreatic adenocarcinoma. Thus far, these series have consistently reported that preoperative SEMS placement does not impose surgical technical difficulties or influence postoperative course or long-term outcome. Studies have also indicated that for preoperative indications, SEMS require fewer endoscopic interventions than PS.[28,31–33] A Monte Carlo decision analysis that compared several preoperative strategies in patients with resectable distal pancreaticobiliary cancer concluded that placement of short-length uncovered biliary

SEMS provided equal or superior efficacy and reduced overall cost compared with PS placement.[33] Although these published series are neither prospective in nature nor randomized, there is sufficient evidence to support the selective placement of SEMS before anticipated operative resection when considered on an individual basis. Either short-length (4 to 6 cm) uncovered or fully covered SEMS that do not involve the bifurcation are recommended.

SEMS for Benign Biliary Disease

Although SEMS placement has traditionally been used for palliation of malignant bile duct obstruction, a growing body of literature is emerging that supports the use of fully covered (and therefore anticipated as removable) SEMS for management in selected patients with benign biliary conditions (strictures, leaks, fistula, postsphincterotomy bleeding). Benign biliary strictures (BBS) can be caused by postoperative injury, anastomotic (post–liver transplant) chronic pancreatitis (CP), or primary sclerosing cholangitis (see also Chapter 43). Biliary stent placement is frequently required to maintain stricture patency while permitting ductal remodeling. The placement of several large-bore PS side-by-side with periodic elective exchange for up to 1 year or more has been shown to be superior to insertion of only a single 10-Fr PS and is highly effective (80% to 90%) for the treatment of postoperative strictures and moderately effective (50% to 70%) in CP strictures.[34–37] Thus the use of multiple PS is the current recommended approach for the management of the majority of BBS.

The main limitation of PS for BBS is the need to undergo multiple ERCPs for stent exchange, dilation, and upsizing, given the limited duration of PS stent patency. PS predictably promote biofilm accumulation and bile-salt deposition that recruits adherent and aggregated biliary sludge. Once this milieu is established, impedance of flow and lumen occlusion increasingly occurs. The placement of a single fcSEMS instead of multiple PS may be preferable, as the fcSEMS expands to a diameter three times that of 10-Fr PS, resulting in longer duration of patency and more effective dilation. This might reduce the number of endoscopic procedures and offset the initial higher individual stent cost. fcSEMS can be delivered using small deployment systems (8 to 8.5 Fr) that do not require aggressive dilation (if any) at the time of stent placement or biliary sphincterotomy.

Two recent large prospective studies have rigorously examined the use of fcSEMS in BBS. In a prospective multinational study by Devière et al. of 187 patients, a 79.7% (94/118) stricture resolution rate was seen in patients with CP-associated strictures, a 68.3% (28/41) stricture resolution rate in liver transplant anastomotic strictures, and a 72.2% (13/18) stricture resolution rate in postcholecystectomy (post-CCY) strictures.[38] fcSEMS were left in position for 10 to 12 months in CP/post-CCY patients and 4 to 6 months in OLT anastomotic strictures. Migration was noted in <5% and 18.6% of the CP patients at 6 and 12 months, respectively, and 18% and 75% of the liver transplant stricture patients at 3 and 6 months, respectively. Subsequently, an open-label, multicenter, noninferiority clinical trial was completed by Coté et al. of 112 patients with BBS untreated for at least 12 months randomized to either multiple PS with repeat ERCP every 3 months or fcSEMS with repeat ERCP every 6 months.[5] Among liver transplant anastomotic strictures, successful resolution was achieved in 94% (34/36) versus 92% (34/37) with multiple PS versus fcSEMS. Among CP strictures there was 76% (13/17) versus 100% (18/18) successful resolution with PS versus fcSEMS. Importantly, although statistically noninferior in successful resolution at 12 months, the fcSEMS group achieved resolution significantly faster (60% to 80% resolution at 6 months) and required an average of one fewer ERCP. Migration was lower than previously reported and occurred in 25% (14/57) and was more common in post–liver transplant anastomotic stricture patients. In other series,

TABLE 23.1 Common Commercially Available Uncovered SEMS

Model	Manufacturer	Delivery System (Fr)	Material	Length (cm)	Diameter (mm)	Shortening	Recapture Ability
Wallstent RX	Boston Scientific	8.0	Elgiloy	4, 6, 8, 10	8, 10	Yes	Up to 80% full deployment
WallFlex	Boston Scientific	8.0	Platinol	4, 6, 8, 10	8, 10	Yes	Up to 80% full deployment
Zilver 635	Cook Endoscopy	6.0	Nitinol	4, 6, 8	6, 8, 10	No	No
Zilver	Cook Endoscopy	7.0	Nitinol	4, 6, 8	6, 8, 10	No	No
Evolution	Cook Endoscopy	8.5	Nitinol	4, 6, 8, 10	8, 10	Yes	Yes
ALIMAXX-B	Merit Medical Endotek	6.5	Nitinol	4, 6, 8, 10	8, 10	Yes	Yes
X-Suit NIR	Olympus, Inc.	7.5	Nitinol	4, 6, 8, 10	8, 10	Yes	No
Flexxus	ConMed	7.5	Nitinol	4, 6, 8, 10	8, 10	Yes	No
Bonastent Biliary	EndoChoice, Inc.	7.0	Nitinol	5, 6, 7, 8, 9, 10	8, 10	Yes	Up to 76% full deployment
Niti-S S type	Taewoong	8.5	Nitinol	4, 5, 6, 7, 8, 9, 10, 12	8, 10	Yes	No
Niti-S LCD type	Taewoong	8.0	Nitinol	4, 5, 6, 7, 8, 9, 10, 12	6, 8, 10	Yes	No
Niti-S D type	Taewoong	8.0	Nitinol	4, 5, 6, 7, 8, 9, 10, 12	6, 8, 10	Yes	No
Nitinella plus	ELLA-CS	7.0	Nitinol	4, 6, 8, 10	8, 10	Yes	Up to 50% full deployment
BIL-stent	Endo-Flex	8.0	Nitinol	6, 8, 10	10	Yes	No
NIT-BIL-1010	Endo-Technik	8.5	Nitinol	4, 6, 8, 10	10	Yes	Yes
Aixstent Gallengag/ Gallengang BDL-BDH	Leufen Medical	8.5	Nitinol	4, 6, 8, 10, 12	8, 10	Yes	No
Hanarostent	M.I. Tech	8.5	Nitinol	4, 5, 6, 7, 8, 9, 10, 12	8, 10	Yes	Yes
Hanarostent Hilar	M.I. Tech	8.5	Nitinol	8	8	Yes	No
BD Stents Classic or Platinum Line	Micro-Tech	8.0	Nitinol	4, 6, 8, 10	10	Yes	No
EGIS Biliary DC	S and G Biotech	8.0	Nitinol	4, 5, 6, 7, 8, 9, 10, 12	8, 10, 12	Yes	No

fcSEMS migration has been reported in up to 20% to 40% of patients.[39–43] Measures to reduce rates of migration have included placement of a double-pigtail stent through the SEMS and SEMS with anchoring fin designs.[44,45] In light of this exciting research, fcSEMS may be considered in the treatment of BBS. Indeed, one fcSEMS (WallFlex RMV; Boston Scientific, Natick, MA) is approved by the US FDA with an indwell time of up to 12 months for the treatment of BBS from CP.

DESCRIPTION OF TECHNIQUE

Metal biliary SEMS are either woven (braided) or laser-cut to create a hollow, lattice-framework tube with a proscribed radial expansion force. They vary in their degree of postexpansile rigidity and flexibility. Some SEMS are constructed with proximal and distal flares intended to reduce migration. Like large-bore PS, metal biliary stents are deployed on an introducer catheter and advanced over a guidewire through the endoscope accessory channel. Unlike PS, predeployed SEMS are constrained on the introducer catheter by an outer plastic sheath or string release mechanism. The metal component can be composed of nitinol (a combination of nickel and titanium), stainless steel, or platinol (platinum core with nitinol encasement), though nearly all are composed of nitinol. Covered stent coatings may consist of a casing of silicone, polyether polyurethane, polyurethane, polycaprolactone, or expanded polytetra-fluoroethylene fluorinated ethylene propylene (ePTFE). There is insufficient evidence to indicate that any particular stent design, material, or coating provides superior patency.

Currently Available SEMS

There are a variety of commercially available SEMS used for palliation of malignant and benign biliary obstruction in the United States and are detailed in Tables 23.1, 23.2, and 23.3.[2,46] SEMS vary in design, delivery system, configuration, mechanical properties, type of metal, size, and price. Although stents are constantly being introduced into the marketplace, the following are the most commonly available uSEMS: Wallstent (Boston Scientific, Natick, MA) (Fig. 23.1), WallFlex stent (Boston Scientific) (Fig. 23.2), Zilver & Evolution (Zilver, Zilver 635) stents (Cook Endoscopy, Winston-Salem, NC) (Fig. 23.3), ALIMAXX-B stent (Merit Medical Endotek, South Jordan, UT), X-Suit NIR biliary stent (Olympus, Center Valley, PA), Flexxus stent (ConMed, Billerica, MA) (Fig. 23.4), Niti-S S type and Niti-S D type (Taewoong, Seoul, South Korea), T&Y (Taewoong) (Fig. 23.5), and Bonastent Biliary (EndoChoice, Inc., Alpharetta, GA). The Wallstent (Boston Scientific) (Fig. 23.6) and WallFlex (Boston Scientific) (see Fig. 23.2, B) are available in pcSEMS variants. Available fcSEMS include WallFlex (Boston Scientific) (see Fig. 23.2, C), Viabil stent (W.L. Gore, Flagstaff, AZ) (Fig. 23.7), ComVi and Niti-S (Taewoong), and Bonastent Biliary (EndoChoice, Inc.).

Nonmetallic biodegradable and drug-eluting self-expanding stents are currently being investigated for malignant and benign applications. The creation of biodegradable stents may address the limitations of covered SEMS, including removability.[47–50] Several animal trials of biodegradable biliary stents have demonstrated relative safety and efficacy in experimental settings. Such trials include studies of normal canine

TABLE 23.2 Common Commercially Available Partially Covered SEMS

Model	Manufacturer	Material	Length (cm)	Diameter (mm)	Shortening	Recapturability	Shape	Covering
WallFlex	Boston Scientific	Platinol	4, 6, 8, 10	8, 10	Yes	Yes	Two flanges	Permalume
Evolution	Cook Endoscopy	Nitinol	4, 6, 8, 10	8, 10	Yes	Yes	Two flanges	Silicone
SX-ELLA Nitinella Plus	Ella-CS	Nitinol	4, 6, 8, 10	8, 10	Yes	Yes	Two flanges	Silicone
NIT-BIL-1010	Endo-Technik	Nitinol	4, 6, 8, 10	10	Yes	No	Straight	Silicone
Aixstent Gallengang	Leufen Medical	Nitinol	4, 6, 8	8, 10	Yes	No	Two flanges	Polyurethane
Hanarostent BPE	M.I. Tech	Nitinol	8, 10	8, 10	Yes	No	One flange and with flaps	Silicone
BD stents	Micro-Tech	Nitinol	4, 6, 8, 10	10	Yes	No	Two flanges	Silicone
EGIS Biliary DC Stent	S and G Biotech	Nitinol	4, 5, 6, 7, 8, 9, 10, 12	8, 10, 12	Yes	No	Two flanges	PTFE
Niti-S Giobor	Taewoong Medical	Nitinol	8, 10	8, 10	Yes	No	One flange	Silicone

TABLE 23.3 Common Commercially Available Fully Covered SEMS

Model	Manufacturer	Material	Length (cm)	Diameter (mm)	Shortening	Recapturability	Shape	Covering
Allium BIS	Allium Medical	Nitinol	6, 8, 10, 12	8, 10	No	No	Straight with anchoring segment	Polyurethane
WallFlex	Boston Scientific	Platinol	4, 6, 8, 10	8, 10	Yes	Yes	Two flanges	Permalume
Evolution	Cook Endoscopy	Nitinol	4, 6, 8, 10	8, 10	Yes	Yes	Two flanges	Silicone
SX-ELLA Nitinella Plus	Ella-CS	Nitinol	4, 6, 8, 10	8, 10	Yes	Yes	Two flanges	Silicone
Bonastent	Endochoice	Nitinol	4, 5, 6, 8, 10, 12	8, 10	Yes	Yes	Two flanges	Silicone
BIL-stent	Endo-Flex	Nitinol	6, 8	10	Yes	No	Straight	Silicone
Viabil	Gore Medical	Nitinol	4, 6, 8, 10	8, 10	No	No	Straight with anchoring fins	PTFE with/without drainage holes
Aixstent Gallengang	Leufen Medical	Nitinol	4, 6, 8	8, 10	Yes	No	Two flanges	Polyurethane
Hanarostent BCT	M.I. Tech	Nitinol	4, 6, 8, 10	10	Yes	Yes	One flange with flaps and lasso	Silicone
Hanarostent BCS	M.I. Tech	Nitinol	4, 6, 8, 10, 12	10	Yes	No	One flange and with flaps	Silicone
BD stents	Micro-Tech	Nitinol	4, 6, 8, 10	10	Yes	No	Two flanges	Silicone
Niti-S S-type covered	Taewoong Medical	Nitinol	4, 5, 6, 7, 8, 10, 12	6, 8, 10	Yes	No	Two flanges	Silicone
Niti-S Kaffes	Taewoong Medical	Nitinol	4, 5, 6, 7, 8	6, 8, 10	Yes	No	Tapered with long lasso	Silicone
Niti-S Bumpy	Taewoong Medical	Nitinol	4, 5, 6, 7, 8, 10, 12	6, 8, 10	Yes	No	Two flanges	Silicone and PTFE
Niti-S ComVi	Taewoong Medical	Nitinol	4, 5, 6, 7, 8, 10, 12	6, 8, 10	Yes	No	Straight	PTFE

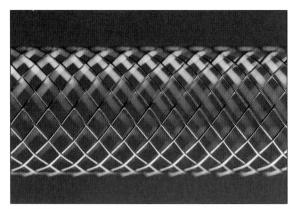

FIG 23.1 Wallstent. (Courtesy Boston Scientific, Natick, MA.)

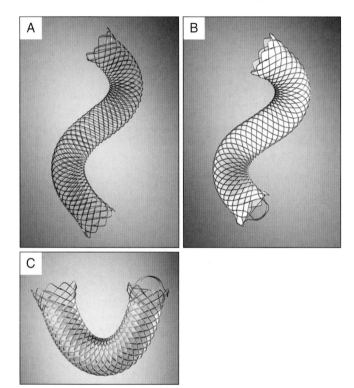

FIG 23.2 WallFlex stents. **A,** Uncovered. **B,** Fully covered. **C,** Partially covered. (Courtesy Boston Scientific, Natick, MA.)

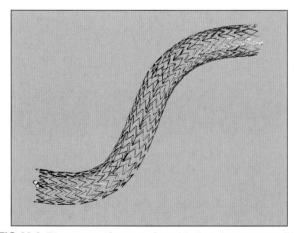

FIG 23.3 Zilver stent. (Courtesy Cook Medical, Bloomington, IN.)

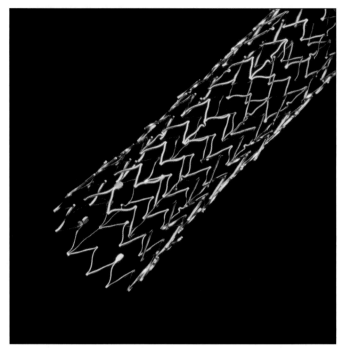

FIG 23.4 Flexxus stent. (Courtesy Merit Medical Endotek, South Jordan, UT.)

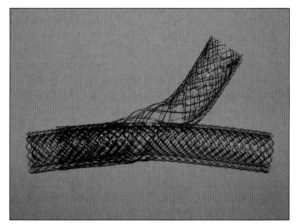

FIG 23.5 Niti-S Y stent. (Courtesy Taewoong, Seoul, South Korea.)

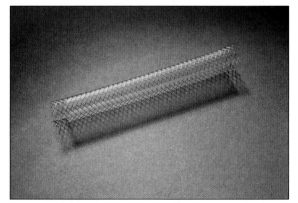

FIG 23.6 Polyurethane covered Wallstent. (Courtesy Boston Scientific, Natick, MA.)

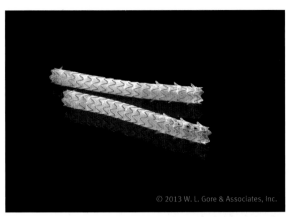

FIG 23.7 Viabil stents: without holes *(top)* and with holes *(bottom)*. (Courtesy W.L. Gore & Associates.)

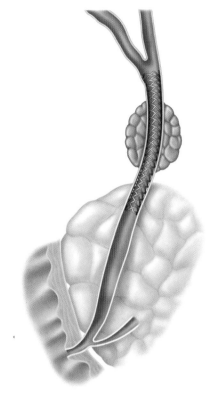

FIG 23.8 Suprapapillary placement of SEMS.

bile ducts, bile duct anastomoses, and cystic ducts after CCY. Thus far, there do not appear to be significant histologic changes to the bile duct after biodegradable stent placement.[51] In a recent multicenter European retrospective analysis of 107 patients with BBS who underwent percutaneous placement of biodegradable stents, they were found to be safe, feasible, and ~70% effective at resolving strictures at 3 years.[50] Drug-eluting stents impregnated with chemotherapeutic agents are being developed. Stents impregnated with 5-fluorouracil, gemcitabine, and paclitaxel have demonstrated local tissue responses in vitro and in vivo.[51] Although the therapeutic potential of these drug-eluting stents is promising, none are currently available at this time for clinical use.

Techniques for SEMS Placement
Guidewire
A guidewire is necessary to traverse biliary strictures, facilitate catheter insertion, and maintain access during device exchange. Larger diameter (0.035 inches) or smaller diameter (0.025-inch wires) with stiff bodies and hydrophilic tips are generally preferred as they enhance device exchange. When placing bilateral stents to palliate hilar strictures in a side-by-side Y configuration, multiple guidewires may be used to maintain access to the specific segments (see Chapter 40).

Stent Size, Positioning, and Sphincterotomy
Although the 10-mm-diameter SEMS is most commonly used, SEMS length selection is based on the length of the stricture, its location, and a desire for suprapapillary or transpapillary placement. Deployed and fully expanded SEMS should extend a minimum of 10 mm beyond the proximal and distal aspects of the stenosis to prevent tumor overgrowth, taking into account device-specific foreshortening. In a suprapapillary position (Fig. 23.8) the sphincter of Oddi remains intact, assuming that sphincterotomy was not performed, potentially reducing reflux of the duodenal contents into the bile duct. Suprapapillary SEMS placement is most commonly performed for strictures at the hilar region or common hepatic duct, in which the SEMS length is insufficient to traverse the ampulla; however, telescoping or layered SEMS placement is possible if the stricture is extensive. A potential disadvantage of suprapapillary SEMS placement is that recannulation of the stent lumen, should it become necessary for management of SEMS occlusion, may prove challenging. Transpapillary SEMS placement with the stent extending 3 to 10 mm into the duodenal lumen allows for easy recannulation and is typically used for common bile duct obstruction (Fig. 23.9). However, excessive transpapillary SEMS overhang into the duodenum should be avoided as it increases the risk for mechanical trauma to the opposite duodenal wall, potentially causing ulceration, bleeding, and even

perforation. A biliary sphincterotomy is not obligatory for SEMS placement in either the suprapapillary or transpapillary position. Routine stricture dilation to facilitate placement is not required as small-diameter delivery systems allow deployment and radial forces permit near-full expansion within 48 hours.

Endoscopic and Fluoroscopic Deployment of SEMS
In addition to the need for quality cholangiography to define the length, localization, and configuration of a biliary obstruction, magnetic resonance cholangiopancreatography (MRCP) or computed tomography may be valuable in the pre-ERCP evaluation of a suspected hilar obstruction in planning unilateral, bilateral, or multisegment drainage (see Chapters 34 and 40).[52] The ports of the stent introducer (depending on the stent) should be lubricated with normal saline to ease advancement over the guidewire and withdrawal of the outer sheath. The tip of the duodenoscope should remain in close proximity to the papilla to prevent accidental loss of guidewire access when the stiff SEMS introducer catheter is being inserted into the ampullary orifice. In a coordinated effort between the endoscopist and the assistant, the guidewire is maintained in a stationary position while the introducer catheter is passed over it. Fluoroscopic markings commonly designate the predeployment and approximate postdeployment proximal and distal ends of the SEMS, and when placed transpapillary, the distal margin of the SEMS is continuously monitored under endoscopic visualization. With the SEMS introducer apparatus in the desired position, the outer restraining sheath or string is incrementally withdrawn by the technician to release the stent. Stents that are delivered by a mechanism of "sheath withdrawal" move away from the endoscope because in actuality the stent is being pushed out of the delivery system and foreshortening of the stent occurs as the SEMS expands. To counter this, during deployment, the endoscopist needs to apply a graded withdrawal of the introducer catheter to achieve precise placement. The proximal end (with respect

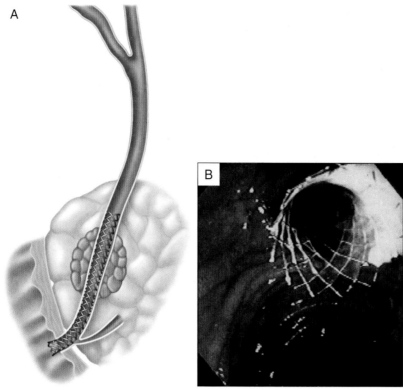

FIG 23.9 **A** and **B,** Transpapillary SEMS placement.

BOX 23.2   Key Points: Technique Summary

- Understand the procedural indication and accessories (available stents, compatible guidewires, etc.).
- Determine appropriate length of stent; obtain high-quality cholangiogram to assist in decision making.
- Maintain a "close" papillary position.
- Use fluoroscopic markings on stent to guide positioning during deployment.
- Adjust for stent foreshortening by withdrawing the stent delivery system during deployment.

---

to the liver) of the stent will gradually open as the outer sheath is withdrawn (Fig. 23.10). The stent position may be adjusted distally by withdrawing the entire apparatus. For more proximal readjustment, it is often necessary to recapture the partially released SEMS, when possible, by advancing the outer sheath. Once the outer sheath is fully deployed, the introducer catheter and guidewire are then removed. When a SEMS is placed across an extremely tight stenosis, complete radial expansion does not occur immediately, which may result in malpositioning of the SEMS during withdrawal of the introducer catheter. To overcome this, the outer sheath may be readvanced as the introducer catheter is withdrawn. This prevents the nose cone of the introducer catheter from engaging with the stent interstices on withdrawal. Postdeployment, although proximal adjustment is not possible, a grasping forceps may be used to reposition the stent distally or remove it altogether, if necessary (Box 23.2).

Hilar Strictures

Cholangiocarcinoma, gallbladder carcinoma, and portal hepatic lymph nodes can lead to obstruction of the bile duct at the level of the hilum of the liver (see also Chapter 40). Palliation of hilar obstruction provides a greater challenge than common bile duct lesions. Although unilateral stenting is effective for the relief of jaundice,[53] bilateral stenting may be required to palliate cholangitis, particularly in patients who have undergone prior instrumentation. It is now generally recommended that both the left and right intrahepatic ducts be drained during the procedure if both sides are opacified during cholangiography (Fig. 23.11). If there is one dominant side identified by MRCP, selective cannulation with a catheter and a guidewire should be attempted, with intentional avoidance of pressure injection of contrast. Bilateral SEMS may be placed alongside one another (side-by-side configuration), or the second SEMS may be deployed through the mesh of the initial SEMS (Fig. 23.12) in Y configuration, though these techniques are considerably more challenging and require higher skill and experience levels.[54] Given these unique circumstances, small introducer SEMS (Zilver 635; Cook; 6-Fr introducer) or SEMS with large interstices to allow the passage of a second stent for Y configuration (Flexxus [ConMed], Niti-S [Taewoong]) should be considered. Two wires are used to maintain access to the right and left biliary systems while placing bilateral stents in a side-by-side fashion. If obstructed intrahepatic ducts remain inadequately drained, adjunctive percutaneous drainage or endoscopic ultrasound (EUS)-guided transmural drainage (see Chapters 32 and 33), in addition to administration of antibiotics, are often required.

Duodenal Obstruction

Up to 10% to 20% of patients with pancreatic and ampullary tumors develop duodenal or gastric outlet obstruction. Enteral stenting is an effective means of palliating malignant gastroduodenal obstruction symptoms.[55–57] Many of these patients have concurrent or imminent bile duct obstruction, and biliary SEMS are recommended before placement of an enteral stent because subsequent access to the bile duct may be lost if the gastroduodenal stent crosses the papilla. Biliary stent

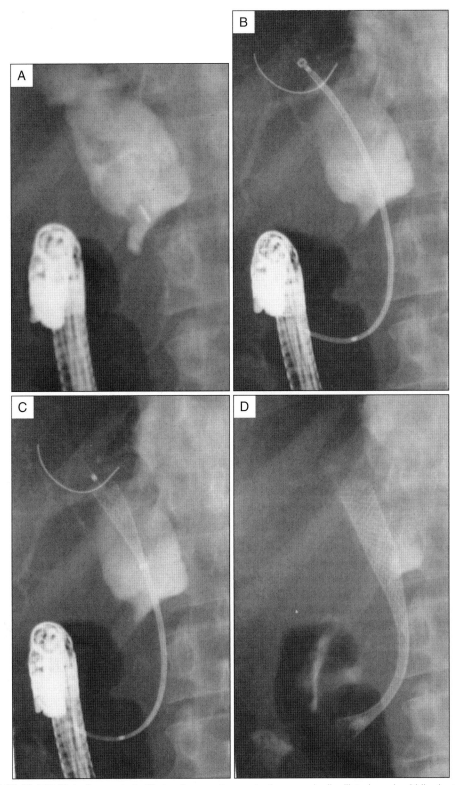

FIG 23.10 SEMS deployment. **A,** Cholangiogram demonstrating a markedly dilated proximal bile duct with a distal stricture. **B,** SEMS introducer advanced over the wire with the proximal end of the stent above the proximal end of the stricture. **C,** Initial withdrawal of the outer sheath. **D,** Full deployment of the SEMS demonstrating fluoroscopic waist of the stricture.

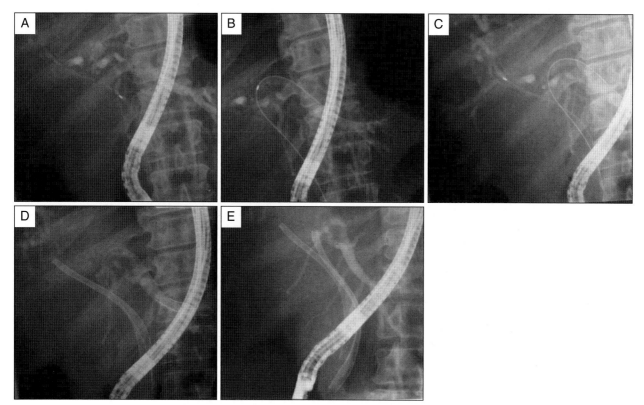

FIG 23.11 Bilateral SEMS placement for treatment of a hilar stricture. **A,** Cholangiography reveals dilated left and right intrahepatic ducts with a hilar stricture. **B,** Wire placed into the left intrahepatic system. **C,** Catheter placed in the right intrahepatic system to facilitate placement of a second wire. **D,** SEMS placed over wire into the right intrahepatic system with a wire in the left intrahepatic system. **E,** Stents placed in both the left and right intrahepatic ducts. The stent in the left intrahepatic duct was placed in a suprapapillary position.

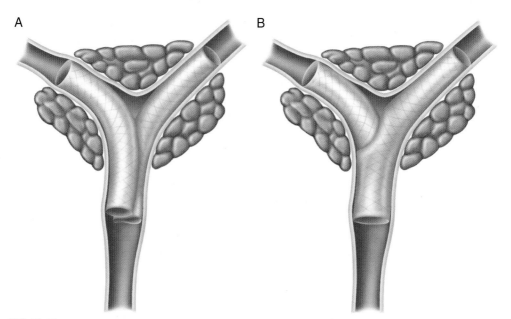

FIG 23.12 Positioning of SEMS in hilar strictures. **A,** Side-by-side stent placement. **B,** One stent through the interstices of another stent, creating a Y formation. (Redrawn from Ahmad NA, Ginsberg GG. Expandable metal stents for malignant biliary obstruction. *Tech Gastrointest Endosc.* 2001;3:93–102, with permission.)

placement may be performed at the same setting (see also Chapter 42).[58] Although feasible in individual cases, it is more difficult to place a biliary stent through the interstices of a previously placed enteral stent. It is our practice, therefore, to dilate the duodenal stricture if necessary to allow ERCP with biliary SEMS placement, followed by enteral stent placement.

ADVERSE EVENTS AND THEIR MANAGEMENT

Adverse events related to SEMS include those associated with ERCP and immediate and delayed SEMS malfunction. Immediate causes of SEMS malfunction include device failure, deployment failure, and malpositioning of the stent. Failure to adequately lubricate the delivery device channels may inhibit withdrawal of the outer sheath. Similarly, excessive articulation of the elevator lever inhibits withdrawal of the outer sheath and may lead to separation of the delivery apparatus at the introducer hub. If the location of the stent is not satisfactory, a second, overlapping stent may be placed at the same setting or the original stent may be removed with a grasping forceps or a snare. For SEMS removal, the stent should be grasped and pulled to the tip of the endoscope and the endoscope should be withdrawn under fluoroscopic guidance. In general, one should avoid withdrawing the stent through the accessory channel of the duodenoscope because the sharp ends can damage the channel and/or the stent may become lodged within the channel if it separates from the grasping device. Removal of uSEMS is best accomplished within 48 hours of insertion, as embedding of the stent within the bile duct wall with or without tissue hyperplasia can occur.

Other early adverse events, defined as occurring within 1 week of stent placement, include cholangitis, hemobilia, and perforation. Ineffective drainage of segments opacified during cholangiography increases the risk of cholangitis. Patients with malignant hilar strictures or coexisting primary sclerosing cholangitis are at greatest risk. Administration of prophylactic antibiotics may be beneficial to prevent or manage cholangitis in selected patients.[59] Persistent cholangitis despite antibiotics requires repeat instrumentation through either a retrograde or antegrade approach. SEMS placement into friable bile duct tumors may induce hemobilia. This bleeding is typically not clinically significant and resolves spontaneously; however, a retained clot may result in biliary obstruction that requires clearance with catheter irrigation or the use of a stone retrieval balloon. A malpositioned SEMS may perforate the bile duct wall or produce ulceration, bleeding, and perforation of the opposite duodenal wall. There are reports of using argon beam plasma coagulation to shorten stents of excessive length within the duodenum that have caused adverse events.[60,61]

The most common late adverse events related to SEMS are stent occlusion and migration. SEMS may become occluded by tumor ingrowth, epithelial hyperplasia, biliary sludge, and refluxed food material. uSEMS have a higher rate of occlusion by tumor ingrowth compared with covered SEMS. Occlusion in either can be managed by insertion of a PS or covered SEMS within the preexisting SEMS or by mechanical clearing of the SEMS, but the approach taken should take into consideration the overall prognosis of the patient. Migration, although rare after uSEMS placement,[16–18] is significantly more common with fcSEMS.[39–43] In addition to migration, cholecystitis occurs in 2.9% to 12% of patients with an intact gallbladder when covered SEMS are placed because of cystic duct obstruction.[20]

RELATIVE COST

For the management of malignant biliary strictures, the cost-effectiveness of SEMS placement compared with PS becomes apparent when multiple PS exchanges are needed, resulting in a higher cost.[10,15] In patients with short expected survival (<3 months) a randomized trial demonstrated that total costs per patient were not significantly different between SEMS and PS,[15] though previous Markov modeling suggested SEMS cost-effectiveness in patients with an anticipated survival of greater than 6 months.[62,63] Given a recent meta-analysis demonstrating no difference in recurrent obstruction, survival, or time to recurrent biliary obstruction between pcSEMS and uSEMS,[24] the additional cost associated with pcSEMS does not seem warranted. As usage of fcSEMS in the management of BBS evolves, initial evidence suggests that longer periods in between repeat ERCPs (i.e., 6-month intervals as opposed to 3-month intervals) lead to cost savings of, on average, one fewer ERCP over a treatment course, thus offsetting the higher up-front costs associated with their placement.[5] As these devices are more widely adopted for this indication, careful evaluation of their ultimate cost-effectiveness needs to be established (Box 23.3).

The complete reference list for this chapter can be found online at www.expertconsult.com.

> ## BOX 23.3   Cost, Adverse Events, and Controversies
>
> - SEMS placement is cost-effective if patient survival is expected to exceed 3 months and in many patients with shorter survival; otherwise, plastic stent may be preferred.
> - Stent migration occurs more often with covered SEMS than uncovered SEMS.
> - Covered SEMS show promise in the treatment of benign biliary disease but their role has yet to be fully established.

24

Pancreaticobiliary Stent Retrieval

Anthony Razzak, Everson Luiz de Almeida Artifon, and Richard A. Kozarek

Pancreaticobiliary stenting is an efficacious and safe method to address biliary manifestations of benign and malignant disease. At present, indications for stent placement include palliative biliary decompression, adjunctive preoperative decompression, treatment of benign biliary and pancreatic strictures, refractory lithiasis, bile leaks, pancreatic ductal disruption, transpapillary gallbladder decompression, prophylaxis of post–endoscopic retrograde cholangiopancreatography (ERCP), pancreatitis (PEP), and treatment of postsphincterotomy-related bleeding.[1–14] The advent of lumen-apposing self-expandable metal stents (LAMS) has broadened the use to include pancreatic fluid collection, and transmural common bile duct and gallbladder drainage.[15–19] Studies to date have demonstrated high technical and clinical success with a favorable safety profile relative to percutaneous and/or surgical interventions.[1,2,20–22]

Removal of pancreaticobiliary prostheses is necessary for most patients with benign disease and for those suffering from stent-related adverse events, including stent occlusion and migration. Plastic stents, with diameters limited by the diameter of the working channel of the duodenoscope, inevitably succumb to multifactorial occlusion with contributions from microbial colonization, precipitation of bile, and biofilm formation.[23] The risk of plastic biliary stent occlusion increases with indwelling time, with a median patency of 4 to 5 months for a 10-Fr stent.[23] Because plastic pancreatic stents tend to be smaller in diameter, most will be occluded within 3 months of placement.[20] Covered self-expandable metal stents (cSEMS) offer the potential advantage of prolonged patency with larger luminal diameters and a design that facilitates retrieval. In published reports of cSEMS for benign biliary strictures, the rates of stent occlusion and migration are estimated to be up to 5% and 10%, respectively.[24] When used indefinitely in the setting of malignant obstruction, recurrent occlusion and migration remain an obstacle, with rates estimated up to 30% and 15%, respectively.[25,26] Data on adverse events from LAMS are limited, but there are reports of migrated and buried stents.[16,21,22,27,28] Ultimately, the timing and technique of removal vary depending on the indication, location, number and type of stents deployed.

The key principles of stent retrieval are:
1. Optimizing patient safety
2. Ensuring complete removal of the foreign body
3. Maintaining intraductal access, when necessary
4. Thoroughly assessing for iatrogenic injury and resolution of the original indication for stent placement.

This chapter will review the indications, timing, and techniques of biliary and pancreatic stent retrieval, as well as introduce the subject of lumen-apposing metal stent removal.

REMOVAL OF BILIARY STENTS

Plastic Biliary Stents (see Chapter 22)

First reported to be used in 1980, endoscopically placed plastic biliary stents (PBS) provided a safe and cost-effective alternative to percutaneous and surgical biliary interventions for relief of malignant biliary obstruction.[29] Removal of PBS is usually performed with ease if performed within months of placement. On the other hand, extraction of PBS is hindered when proximal or distal migration occurs. Risk factors associated with stent migration include the presence of common bile duct dilation, choledocholithiasis, and benign biliary strictures. Proximal strictures and the use of long biliary stents are associated with distal migration, whereas distal strictures and the use of short biliary stents are associated with proximal migration.[30,31] Factors that make proximal migrated stent retrieval more challenging include:

- Migration upstream from a stenotic region
- Migration into the peripheral branches of the intrahepatic biliary system
- Inconsistency between the biliary stent and its axis in patients without biliary dilatation
- Stent impaction into the bile duct wall

Stents are nearly always removable when accessible.[31] Proximally migrated stents are more difficult to retrieve, but the success rate of endoscopic removal ranges from 70% to 100%.[30,31] If endoscopic retrieval is unsuccessful, a second stent can be placed while leaving the first stent in place to facilitate drainage and allow access with subsequent reattempt at retrieval.[32] Distally migrated stents generally pass through the intestine without complication; however, cases of perforation and obstruction requiring surgical intervention and even death have been reported.[31,33]

Self-Expandable Metal Stents

To overcome issues with small-caliber plastic stents, larger-diameter SEMS were designed to provide prolonged patency. At present, SEMS are favored for malignant palliation (see Chapter 39) and cSEMS have an increasing role in the management of benign conditions, including benign strictures, complex bile leaks, biliary perforation, and postsphincterotomy bleeding (see Chapters 8, 43, and 44).[13,14,20,34]

Established and potential risk factors for difficult SEMS extraction include:

- *Type of SEMS.* Data support a favorable retrieval rate for cSEMS at approximately 78% to 99%.[24,35,36] Instances of unsuccessful cSEMS extraction have been attributed to tissue overgrowth and impaction against the bile duct wall. By design, uncovered SEMS (uSEMS) have limited removability because of tissue embedding and ingrowth, and most endoscopists limit their use to palliation. As expected, the reported successful removal rate of uSEMS is poor, ranging between 0% and 38%.[35,36] In a 5-year retrospective review, cSEMS were removed more successfully than uSEMS (24/26 [92.3%] vs 5/13 [38.4%], respectively [$p < 0.05$]).[36]
- *Stent dwell time.* In a study evaluating the efficacy of endoscopic SEMS retrieval, 14/19 patients underwent successful stent extraction. The mean dwell time for those with successfully removed SEMS

was shorter than for those with nonremovable SEMS (94.9 ± 71.5 days vs 166.2 ± 76.2 days, $p = 0.08$),[35] though this was not statistically significant.

- *Stent-specific structural properties.* Familiari et al. hypothesized that an interlaced rather than zigzag mesh design may contribute to more successful stent extraction because of its greater ability to endure longitudinal traction during retrieval. Yet multivariate analysis did not demonstrate a significant correlation (interlaced mesh vs zigzag mesh, $p = 0.258$).[36] Similarly, Ishii et al. correlated differences in the rate of shrinkage and straightening during attempted retrieval with the stent's structural ability to transmit force and ultimately to ease extraction. The authors described that removal of Niti-S Biliary ComVi stents (Taewoong Company, Seoul, South Korea) was slightly more difficult than Wallstents (Boston Scientific, Tokyo, Japan); however, the study was limited by the small number of patients.[35]

Indications and Contraindications

The indication for biliary stent retrieval depends on the nature of disease for which the stent was placed (benign or malignant) and the patient's life expectancy. At present, PBS and cSEMS are used for benign indications, whereas PBS, cSEMS, and uSEMS are used to alleviate malignant obstruction. In benign disease, both PBS and cSEMS must be removed because of the risk of occlusion and cholangitis. The indications to remove PBS and cSEMS are the same and include:

1. *Resolution of underlying biliary disease.* Once the beneficial effect of the stent has been achieved, it should be removed. The timing may vary depending on the nature of the underlying disease. For instance, the outcome after stent placement for chronic pancreatitis-related benign biliary strictures is improved with prolonged stent placement,[20,37] whereas shorter durations of stent placement are necessary for complicated choledocholithiasis and bile leaks.[8,38] Some studies suggest that resolution of disease is the most common indication for stent removal,[39,40] whereas others identify stent-related malfunction (described next), including occlusion, as the leading indication for retrieval.[41]

2. *Stent malfunction.* There are two main causes of biliary stent malfunction. The first is stent occlusion via sludge, debris, duodenal reflux, tissue hyperplasia, or tumor ingrowth and overgrowth. The second is stent migration, either proximally into the biliary tree or distally into the intestine.

   Occlusion of a biliary stent results in obstruction of the biliary tree that can manifest with mixed-type liver injury, jaundice, pruritus, or cholangitis. Sludge formation appears to play a predominant role in the occlusion process. Evaluation of explanted, occluded stents with electron microscopy and biochemical analysis reveals bacteria and/or fungi, microbial byproducts, bilirubin, insoluble dietary residue, proteins, and cholesterol crystals without overt cholesterol or pigment calculi.[23,42] Upon stent insertion, the inner surface is rapidly covered by host proteins that enhance bacterial adherence and subsequent biofilm formation.[23] The biofilm permits bacteria to adhere firmly to the stent, and thus continuous deposition of microbial degradation products and growth of colonies can eventually lead to narrowing of the stent lumen.[43,44] According to Poiseuille's law, as the narrowed lumen slows bile flow, spontaneous and microbial-driven precipitation of bile salts increases bile viscosity and ultimately leads to complete stent occlusion.[23] PBS occlusion with need for reintervention is as high as 40% and appears directly related to stent dwell time.[20] Treatment of PBS occlusion entails retrieval of the occluded stent followed by replacement (if needed), with the number and type of stent(s) dependent on the underlying indication.

With respect to SEMS, hyperplastic tissue and tumor ingrowth are more commonly associated with uSEMS occlusion,[45,46] whereas tumor overgrowth (i.e., occlusion of the stent ends) and sludge formation are associated with occlusion of cSEMS.[46,47] Sludge and refluxed duodenal contents can cause occlusion of both types of SEMS, though the risk may be higher in those with cSEMS.[46,48] Mechanical clearance of the occluded stent with an extraction balloon is one method to address the malfunctioning SEMS and is associated with a high reocclusion rate and short patency.[47] Alternatively, a PBS or SEMS can be placed within an occluded SEMS,[49,50] with supportive data demonstrating prolonged patency relative to mechanical clearance.[47] Data comparing the relative efficacy of PBS versus SEMS for use in stent-in-stent (SIS) SEMS occlusion are limited. In a systematic review of 10 retrospective studies, the risk of reocclusion, patency duration, and overall survival were not significantly different between patients who received PBS versus SEMS for occluded SEMS; however, there was considerable heterogeneity between studies.[51] Because of the lack of significant difference in performance, some have concluded that PBS placement may be the more cost-effective intervention,[52] though data on the subject are limited. Some authors support removal of the occluded stent and deployment of a new SEMS.[35,53,54]

Migration is the other main cause of biliary stent malfunction. Complete external migration usually causes recurrence of symptoms such as abdominal pain, jaundice, or cholangitis, but it may be asymptomatic if the underlying disease process has resolved (i.e., stricture resolution). In those with ongoing or recurrent symptoms, reassessment of the need for repeat stent insertion must be pursued. Externally migrated stents generally pass uneventfully through the intestine, and therefore endoscopic removal is not necessary. Infrequently, migrated stents can cause adverse events that result in the need surgery or even death.[31,33] Stents that migrate distally but remain partially in the common bile duct may embed in the contralateral duodenal wall. In such cases, apart from signs of stent occlusion, mucosal injury, including bleeding and perforation, can occur.[55] Most reported instances of proximal stent migration manifest with clinical symptoms and can be difficult to manage.[31] The reported success rate of removal of proximally migrated stents is favorable and ranges from 70% to 100%.[30–32]

3. *Stent-related adverse events.* Clinical symptoms related to stent insertion can be considered an indication for stent removal. Acute cholecystitis from cystic duct obstruction has been reported as a specific adverse event of cSEMS placement,[56,57] with a variable incidence ranging from 0% to 10%.[13,25,58–61] The risk is believed to be less when cSEMS are placed distal to the cystic duct takeoff and when uSEMS are used. Acute pancreatitis has been associated with large-caliber PBS and SEMS placement, with an incidence ranging from 0% to 9%, though most studies did not control for known contributors to PEP.[62] The predisposing injury is thought to be related to direct or indirect occlusion of the pancreatic orifice. In a recent large retrospective review of 544 patients undergoing stent placement for malignant obstruction, the risk of pancreatitis was significantly higher in those receiving SEMS (7.3%) versus PBS (1.3%) and the frequency did not significantly differ for cSEMS (6.9%) versus uSEMS (7.5%).[62] Most recommend a biliary sphincterotomy before placement of biliary stents because of the potential for reducing PEP, though the data supporting this are conflicting.[63,64] A recent meta-analysis of three randomized controlled trials revealed a reduced incidence of PEP (odds ratio [OR] 0.34, 95% confidence interval [CI] 0.12 to 0.93, $p = 0.04$) but an increased incidence of post–ERCP-related bleeding with biliary sphincterotomy (OR 9.70, 95% CI 1.21 to 77.75, $p = 0.03$).[65] Abdominal pain is rarely reported after placement

of biliary stents.[41,54] In a prospective study evaluating the efficacy of cSEMS in benign biliary strictures, abdominal pain necessitating stent removal was seen in 2/79 patients (2.5%).[39]

Absolute contraindications for stent removal are limited to circumstances when ERCP is also contraindicated. For instance, the development of duodenal stenosis after placement of a biliary stent in patients with benign or malignant biliary occlusion may therefore be considered a contraindication to attempted endoscopic removal. Kahaleh et al. described two patients with duodenal stenosis that precluded initial ERCP and required a period of enteral feeding to allow resolution of duodenal edema before a duodenoscope could successfully traverse the stenosis.[39] Similarly, some retrieval techniques might be contraindicated, including extraction of uSEMS by means of removing individual stent-wire filaments in patients with coagulopathy and extraction of proximally migrated stents in patients with pericholedocal varices or severe portal hypertension. Furthermore, removal of stents should not be attempted in the following situations:

- *Incomplete therapeutic effect and absence of adverse events related to the stent.* The stents should not be removed before the beneficial effect is completed if the patient is asymptomatic and the stent is in good position. An exception to this is scheduled stent exchanges before stent occlusion occurs.
- *Short life expectancy in an asymptomatic patient.* In patients with malignant disease and short life expectancy without symptoms attributable to the biliary stent, there is no need to remove it. It may be reasonable not to try to extract proximally migrated biliary stents in this situation.

Timing of Stent Retrieval

The recommended period that biliary stents should be left in place depends largely on the stent type, stent caliber, and the indication for which the stent is placed. The risk of PBS dysfunction increases with dwell time and is inversely related to the stent's inner diameter. For instance, the median patency of a 10-Fr PBS is estimated at 4 to 5 months, with an occlusion risk that begins to increase progressively after 3 months.[23,66] Early stent occlusion (within 30 days) is rare and, when present, is more likely to be related to stent malposition/migration, blood clots, or mucinous tumor secretions.[66] More commonly, stent occlusion appears to be directly related to the formation of biofilm; however, a meta-analysis of five randomized controlled trials revealed that the use of choleretic agents and/or antibiotics did not significantly prolong stent patency.[67] In addition, previous studies have suggested that stent composition (i.e., polyurethane vs polyethylene) and shape (i.e., straight vs pigtail) do not appear to affect stent occlusion.[66] If prolonged treatment is required, scheduled stent exchanges are recommended to prevent occlusion-related adverse events, with timing intervals typically dictated by local practice.

With regard to the indication for stenting, the treatment of benign biliary strictures requires that the stent remain in place for a prolonged period, typically no less than 1 year.[68] If PBS (single or multiple) are used, stent replacement is usually performed every 3 months until the end of treatment, though one study suggested that for benign disease and multiple stents, occlusion was uncommon at 3 months and the interval to stent exchange could be increased.[69] SEMS are larger in diameter than PBS and therefore can remain in place for longer periods before removal. In a recent multicenter randomized controlled trial comparing cSEMS to multiple PBS in the treatment of benign biliary strictures, cSEMS were not inferior to PBS in achieving stricture resolution and with fewer ERCPs.[70]

Because of the inherent difficulty of uSEMS retrieval, the use of uSEMS should be limited to patients with malignant disease or those with benign indications but a shortened life expectancy. Although long-term follow-up data on the patency of uSEMS are limited,[71] uSEMS appear to maintain function for a median of 20 months (range 4.5 to 60 months) before reintervention, mostly to address occlusion.[40] If a uSEMS is mistakenly placed under an erroneous context (e.g., misdiagnosis) or has migrated, an attempt at retrieval is indicated. In general, uSEMS retrieval becomes more difficult or even impossible if the duration of dwell time exceeds several weeks because of stent embedment and tissue ingrowth.[36,53,72] If removal is unsuccessful, the stents can be mechanically cleaned and additional PBS or SEMS can be placed within the uSEMS; however, this technique will require scheduled maintenance for those with a long life expectancy.

Techniques

Stent removal can be challenging because there are no devices specifically designed for removal other than the Soehendra (Wilson Cook Medical, Winston-Salem, NC) and Carr-Locke (Telemed Systems, Hudson, MA) stent retrievers. The devices most commonly used for stent extraction are polypectomy snares, foreign-body retrieval forceps, and stone extraction baskets. Duodenoscopes with large working channels are recommended if there are multiple stents to remove, there are stents to replace, or bile duct interventions are required. Forward-viewing endoscopes are commonly used when there is a single stent to remove and ERCP is not needed.

For nonmigrated and distally migrated stents, grasping the stent and subsequently removing it through the working channel or simply withdrawing the endoscope while grasping the stent is adequate. Removal of proximally migrated stents is far more difficult and sometimes requires more elaborate devices, intraductal manipulation under fluoroscopic guidance, and, if needed, temporary stenting to ensure ongoing adequate drainage when retrieval is not feasible or is incomplete. During attempted removal, it is important to prioritize patient safety and examination thoroughness with assessment for complete stent retrieval, iatrogenic injury, and resolution of the underlying process that prompted stent placement. Maintaining wire-guided access during the retrieval process can provide safety when intraductal instruments are displaced or biliary orifice visualization becomes impaired from extraction maneuvers.

The choice of retrieval technique is dependent on multiple variables, including the ease of biliary cannulation, presence of biliary duct dilation, type and size of stent requiring retrieval, location of migrated stents, stent impaction, and local expertise. An overview of the more common techniques used for stent retrieval is as follows.

Direct Grasping Technique

The direct grasping technique is a simple technique that involves reaching the second portion of the duodenum with an endoscope and maneuvering a snare to engage the distal intraduodenal end of the stent, which is then tightly grasped and withdrawn from the bile duct. In our experience, comparable to that of other authors,[32,41,73] this is the most commonly used technique (Fig. 24.1). A stone extraction basket or foreign-body forceps (Fig. 24.2) can also be used instead of a polypectomy snare; the basket and the forceps are considered equally efficacious (Video 24.1).[31]

These direct grasping techniques are also used to retrieve distally migrated stents. In a recent multicenter study, 17/30 patients suffered symptomatic distal stent migration. Endoscopic removal was attempted and successful in all 17 patients. Retrieval with a snare was employed in 11 of these patients and with a stone extraction basket in the remaining 6 patients.[31]

Indirect Grasping Technique

The indirect grasping technique uses fluoroscopic imaging to assist in positioning intraductal devices in a manner that facilitates grasping and retrieval. The device must be inserted into the bile duct through the papilla, advanced to the stent, and then maneuvered to grasp and

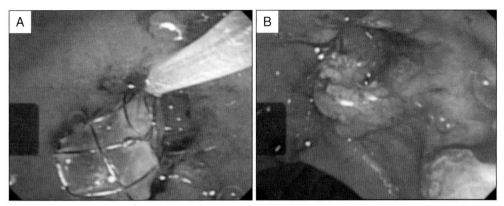

FIG 24.1 Sequence of images demonstrating SEMS removal using direct grasping with a snare. **A,** Snare grasping the distal end of a cSEMS. **B,** Post–stent removal view of the major papilla. *cSEMS,* Covered self-expandable metal stent; *SEMS,* self-expandable metal stent.

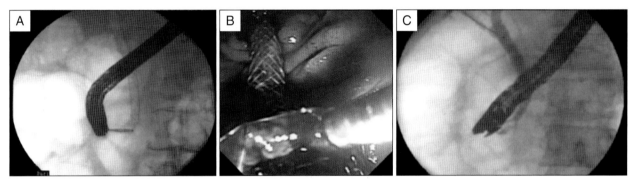

FIG 24.2 Sequence of images demonstrating SEMS removal using direct grasping with forceps. **A** and **B,** Radiographic and endoscopic view of forceps grasping the distal aspect of a cSEMS. **C,** Cholangiogram after stent retrieval. *cSEMS,* Covered self-expandable metal stent; *SEMS,* self-expandable metal stent.

pull it down until the stent exits into the duodenum. This has been successfully used in proximally migrated PBS and SEMS.[30,53] The procedure is most commonly completed by grasping the stent with forceps (Fig. 24.3), although some authors prefer using a snare or stone extraction basket (Fig. 24.4) to retrieve migrated stents.[74]

Lasso Technique

The lasso technique involves inserting a guidewire through the lumen of a stent, and then a partially opened polypectomy snare is passed over the guidewire to grasp the stent. Once the stent is encircled tightly by the snare, it is pulled out over the guidewire, thereby maintaining intraductal access without the need for further cannulation. Special care must be taken in order to remove the stent while keeping the guidewire in place. This technique was originally described by Sherman et al.[75] and required cannulation of the stent with a guidewire. Experiences using variations of the technique by cannulating the duct alongside rather than within the stent lumen have been reported.[76] The main advantage of the lasso technique is that it preserves access to the bile duct, which is especially useful when difficult cannulation is anticipated, including instances of variant anatomy.

The lasso technique does not play a role in the retrieval of distally migrated biliary stents, but it can be applied to proximally migrated stent retrieval. Cannulation of the bile duct must be achieved first to leave a guidewire through or alongside the migrated stent. A polypectomy snare is then threaded over the guidewire and inserted gently into the bile duct, avoiding trauma to the ampulla or bile duct because insertion is performed over the guidewire. Once the snare is at the level of the

distal end of the stent, it is opened and manipulated to hold the stent and retrieve it.

Soehendra Stent Retriever Technique

The Soehendra stent retriever is a single-use, wire-guided metal spiral retrieval device 180 cm in length with a 3-mm to 4-mm screw tip that comes in variable sizes to fit PBS of 5-Fr to 11.5-Fr diameter. The stent retriever size is selected depending on the size of the stent to be removed. It is advanced through the duodenoscope working channel over a guidewire and rotated into the inner lumen of the stent.[77] Exact alignment of the retrieval device with the lumen of the stent is needed to allow the instrument to self-thread into the stent. Once the retriever is securely anchored to the end of the stent, the retriever and stent are withdrawn through the working channel of the duodenoscope. This device has successfully been used to retrieve proximally migrated PBS[31,32]; however, it requires the migrated stent lumen to be cannulated with an appropriately sized guidewire to facilitate adequate alignment.

Dilating Balloon Extraction Technique

Extraction of biliary stents with a dilating balloon can be performed using various techniques. A dilating balloon can be inserted into a cSEMS and inflated to create a retrievable coaxial system. With constant traction applied, the dilating balloon and cSEMS can be pulled through the biliary orifice.[78] To allow the dilating balloon to anchor within the cSEMS with enough integrity to achieve removal, the balloon diameter must be no smaller than the diameter of the cSEMS. For removal of PBS, a 4-mm or 6-mm dilating balloon can be advanced over a guidewire

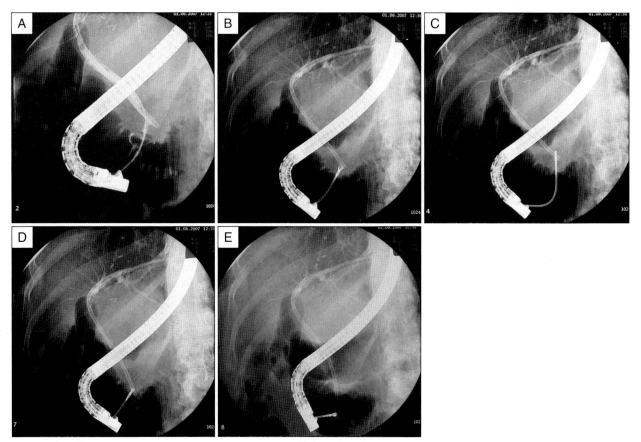

FIG 24.3 Indirect grasping of a proximally migrated PBS with a foreign-body forceps. **A,** The PBS is proximally migrated with the distal end penetrating in the pancreatic head through the bile duct wall. **B,** A foreign-body forceps is gently introduced through the bile duct until it reaches the lower end of the stent. **C,** The stent is grasped and pushed upward to dig it from the bile duct wall. **D,** Once the stent is completely in the bile duct, it is oriented to the ampulla. **E,** The PBS is finally removed from the duct. *PBS,* plastic biliary stent.

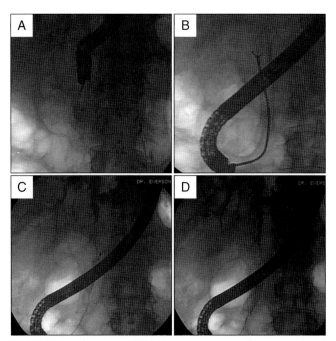

FIG 24.4 Different approaches to the indirect grasping technique removal of proximally migrated SEMS. **A,** Forceps grasping the distal end of the SEMS. **B,** Forceps grasping the proximal end of the SEMS. **C** and **D,** Stone extraction basket grasping the full length of the SEMS. *SEMS,* self-expandable metal stent.

into the stent and inflated. The amount of inflation necessary to provide adequate traction is typically less than that for stricture dilatation. The balloon and stent are subsequently withdrawn with constant traction, whereas the guidewire is kept in place. This method can be used only for PBS with a caliber of at least 10 Fr,[79–81] because balloon catheters are mounted on at least 5-Fr platforms. A variation of this technique is performed for proximally migrated PBS and cSEMS by inserting a dilating balloon over a guidewire alongside the stent. The balloon is then inflated and traction applied until the stent is extracted. The size of balloon required to successfully perform this variation will directly depend on the bile duct caliber.

Stent-in-Stent Technique

Embedment and tissue ingrowth are the main features that limit successful cSEMS and uSEMS removal. In the esophagus, the placement of a fully covered SEMS within an embedded partially covered SEMS is a safe and effective method of achieving successful stent extraction.[82] The radial force imparted on the hyperplastic tissue by the internal stent results in pressure necrosis, thereby freeing up the embedded stent and facilitating removal. The SIS technique has been adapted to and successfully used in the removal of embedded biliary uSEMS and cSEMS (Fig. 24.5). Tan et al. report a case of misdiagnosed pancreatic adenocarcinoma treated with a biliary uSEMS. Six weeks after placement, a cSEMS was placed within the uSEMS and both stents were successfully extracted 2 weeks later.[83] In a series of five cases of embedded cSEMS, Tringali et al. reported successful removal of all five stents within weeks by placing a cSEMS within the embedded stents.[84] Extrapolating from

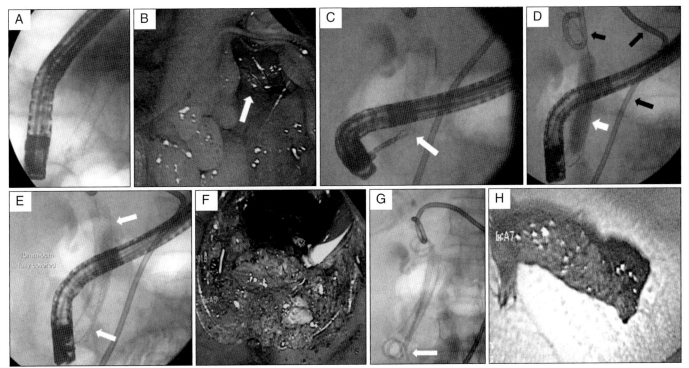

FIG 24.5 Stent-in-stent removal of an embedded biliary cSEMS. **A,** Fluoroscopic view of a cSEMS (10 mm × 4 cm; WallFlex; Boston Scientific) placed for a chronic pancreatitis–related inflammatory stricture. The patient was lost to follow-up and presented 4 years later with ascending cholangitis requiring an emergent PTBD. **B,** Endoscopic view of the major papilla revealing hyperplastic tissue without a clearly identifiable cSEMS. **C** and **D,** Unsuccessful attempts at cSEMS retrieval with rat-tooth forceps and dilating balloon extraction. *Black arrows* highlight the location of the PTBD. **E** and **F,** Fluoroscopic and endoscopic views of a cSEMS (10 mm × 6 cm; WallFlex; Boston Scientific) placed within and completely encompassing the embedded stent. After placement, a significant amount of biliary sludge was noted, which nearly occluded the newly placed stent. **G,** To ensure adequate stent patency, two 7-Fr by 7-cm double-pigtail PBS were placed within the newly placed cSEMS. **H,** Two weeks later the patient returned for stent-in-stent extraction, successfully performed via directly grasping the cSEMS with a rat-tooth forceps. *cSEMS,* Covered self-expandable metal stent; *PBS,* plastic biliary stents; *PTBD,* percutaneous transhepatic biliary drain.

the experience with esophageal SIS extraction, some authors consider that the time between cSEMS placement and removal of both stents should not exceed 18 days.[85] Although promising, further studies evaluating the usefulness of this technique to remove embedded biliary SEMS are warranted.

Trimming of SEMS

SEMS can become partially displaced and impacted in the contralateral duodenal wall, causing occlusion of the SEMS, secondary cholangitis, or duodenal perforation. This situation is challenging, and removal of the stent is difficult. Although not a complete retrieval technique, SEMS trimming with argon plasma coagulation (APC) can be performed to resolve occlusion from a SEMS of excessive length buried against the opposite wall causing bleeding and to minimize the risk of duodenal perforation, or to create a window for biliary access.[35] In a review of eight patients with SEMS migrated into the duodenum, APC trimming was successful in all cases by creating a circumferential amputated stent-stump margin 5 to 15 mm from the papilla. The APC was performed at a power setting of 60 to 80 W and a gas flow rate of 1.5 L/min with a total trimming time ranging from 11 to 16 minutes. The authors noted more efficacious trimming at 80 W relative to 60 W. Gas was suctioned routinely during the procedure to minimize distension. Stent fragments were removed with a retrieval net or forceps. No major adverse events occurred and one patient experienced minor self-limiting

hemorrhage from an esophageal mucosal injury that occurred during stent fragment removal.[35] Of note, in this study there were no differences in trimming time or efficacy with cSEMS versus uSEMS; however, previous studies demonstrated less success with trimming cSEMS and have suggested that the coated membrane predisposes to poor current transmission and heat generation.[86] In addition, although no major adverse events have been reported with APC trimming, a recent case report described the proximal migration of a remnant biliary stent after trimming that required stone extraction basket retrieval.[87] At present, data on SEMS trimming are limited and the indications, techniques, and APC settings are not standardized.

Other Novel Techniques

The first uSEMS removal described entailed a serrated forceps that was used to remove metal filaments one by one.[88] The procedure lasted for 90 minutes and risked damaging the endoscope by removing the sharp wires through the working channel. Apart from the prolonged procedure, it was incomplete, as an abdominal radiograph revealed the presence of remnant metal strands still embedded in the common bile duct. This was hence a laborious, time-consuming technique with a risk of adverse events and endoscope damage and therefore unlikely to become popular.[35,88]

Another technique to remove embedded SEMS is the invagination method. An illustrative case in which it was applied is that of an

85-year-old man with jaundice secondary to pancreatic cancer who was treated with a partially cSEMS. The stent became obstructed within 4 months of placement and initially could not be removed because the proximal uncovered portion was deeply embedded in the bile duct. A biopsy forceps was used to cannulate the stent, grasp the proximal edge, and pull it from the bile duct wall. The proximal edge gradually invaginated into the inner lumen and the stent was finally removed with a snare.[89]

As an alternative to trimming distally impacted SEMS, a closed biopsy forceps may be advanced from the outside of the stent through the mesh and opened within the stent lumen to form an anchor. When the endoscope is withdrawn, the stent can be easily dislodged from the duodenum into the stomach and later removed with a snare. This technique was used in four patients, and although duodenal ulceration was noted, no further adverse events were observed.[90] Ensuring that the SEMS is not deeply impacted within the duodenal wall may reduce the risk of retrieval-related mucosal injury and perforation.

A guidewire-basket "lasso" technique has been described as a means of retrieving a migrated, firmly impacted PBS in the contralateral duodenal wall or in a diverticulum. A guidewire and stone extraction basket are passed side-by-side through the duodenoscope working channel. The basket is passed underneath and the guidewire is manipulated over the impacted PBS. The basket is opened and the guidewire is maneuvered into the basket, which is then closed, thereby creating a lasso around the PBS. With traction, the stent is disimpacted and removed.[91]

A similar looping technique has been described for removal of proximally migrated PBS. A retrieval basket is used to grasp the end of a straight guidewire and both are passed down the duodenoscope working channel. The device is used to cannulate the biliary tree. While still grasping the guidewire end with the basket, additional guidewire is fed into the common bile duct and creates a loop. With manipulation, the loop can be positioned to catch a flap of the biliary stent, tightened, and pulled through the biliary orifice.[92]

A "snare-over-the-scope" technique has been described to retrieve a proximally migrated PBS refractory to balloon extraction. A standard polypectomy snare is taped to the outside of a duodenoscope, oriented along the biopsy channel, and closed around the scope tip. The duodenoscope is advanced to the papilla and a stone extraction balloon is used to cannulate the bile duct and advanced to the migrated stent. The balloon is inflated and pulled through the biliary orifice, dragging the stent alongside. The snare is opened and maneuvered to grasp the stent and extraction balloon shaft. Once tightened, the balloon is deflated and the entire scope is withdrawn.[93]

Additional reports include a "sphincterotome hooking the stent" technique whereby a sphincterotome is passed through a proximally migrated PBS and flexed to form a hook, followed by gentle retraction.[94] Direct cholangioscopy has been used with an ultraslim pediatric endoscope passed into the common bile duct to directly visualize and grasp a proximally migrated PBS with a thin snare.[95]

Adverse Events and Management

Adverse events during or after biliary stent removal are rare, ranging from 0% to 9%.[36,96] The majority of series evaluating the role of biliary stents in different indications report few to no major adverse events. Some reported adverse events include:

- *Bleeding.* In a series of 18 patients with indications for SEMS removal, there was one case of hemobilia after SEMS retrieval that was managed conservatively without the need for blood transfusion.[54] In a series of eight SEMS treated with APC trimming, one patient suffered self-limited bleeding from an injury sustained to the esophageal mucosa during endoscopic stent fragment removal.[35]

- *Biliary leakage.* In a series including 79 patients with benign biliary strictures treated with cSEMS, the development of a bile leak post–cSEMS retrieval was described in one patient and related to a bile duct perforation caused by malpositioning of a dilating balloon used for stent extraction. This was successfully treated with placement of PBS.[39]

- *Acute pancreatitis.* In a review of 37 patients with migrated PBS, one patient developed mild acute pancreatitis during stent retrieval that was managed conservatively.[74] In another review of 44 patients with benign biliary strictures treated with cSEMS, stent retrieval was associated with three cases of PEP, though details on severity and subsequent management were not provided.[96] In addition, it is unclear whether confounding pancreatitis-related contributors were involved or whether standard PEP prophylactic measures were employed.

- *Biliary stricture.* Biliary stenosis can occur from tissue overgrowth at the terminal ends of cSEMS. This is not an adverse event related to stent removal, rather an event related to the stent itself, and can be managed with attempts at retrieval or placement of additional stents.

- *Abdominal pain.* Abdominal pain has been also described following stent removal.[96]

Relative Costs and Choice of Technique

Standardization of endoscopic retrieval of migrated and nonmigrated biliary stents has not been established. Removal is performed according to the imagination, creativity, and skills of the endoscopist, using dedicated and nondedicated devices. Such accessories are readily available in any endoscopy unit and are relatively inexpensive. The costs of endoscopic stent removal should not be considered excessive compared with the available alternatives, which include surgery or percutaneous transhepatic biliary interventions. There are no studies that compare the effectiveness of the various removal techniques. In addition, there are no studies evaluating the cost-effectiveness of such interventions.

Choosing the proper technique is important for successful stent removal and must factor in multiple variables, including available devices, endoscopist experience, type of stent, and location within the bile duct. When managing a nonmigrated stent, the best technique is direct grasping of the intraduodenal end with a snare or forceps. This is a low-cost, simple, and easy technique generally useful for retrieval of PBS, cSEMS, and recently placed uSEMS. If an ERCP is needed after stent removal and difficult cannulation is anticipated, techniques that maintain bile duct access should be chosen, including the lasso technique or its variants, or a dedicated stent retriever. When the distal end of a PBS is impacted against the bile duct wall or the stent is lost within a markedly dilated duct, stent cannulation can be extremely difficult, favoring an indirect grasping technique with forceps or a stone extraction basket. When dealing with an embedded cSEMS or uSEMS, the best choice would probably be the SIS technique, leaving the invagination method as a second option. If the SEMS is partially dislocated and impacted in the contralateral duodenal wall, one could first try to insert a biopsy forceps through the mesh of the stent in order to anchor it and facilitate stent removal. If this is unsuccessful, the guidewire-basket lasso technique could be attempted before considering stent trimming with APC.

Symptomatic distally migrated stents that must be retrieved are best approached with the direct grasping technique. Proximally migrated stents represent a challenge for endoscopic retrieval. In the dilated or nondilated common bile duct with a proximally migrated stent, the indirect grasping technique with forceps is the most commonly used technique, although the dilating balloon extraction technique is useful. The stone extraction balloon or basket technique or the snare technique is especially applicable in patients with choledocholithiasis and a markedly dilated common bile duct. The Soehendra stent retriever is particularly useful when employed over a guidewire in patients with a nondilated common bile duct and a proximally migrated stent.

REMOVAL OF PANCREATIC STENTS

The insertion of pancreatic stents is being performed more frequently because of an increasing number of indications and a better understanding of outcomes. Indications for pancreatic stenting have been described in other chapters, but in summary, stents may be inserted with therapeutic, palliative, or prophylactic intent.[97] Once the intended effect is achieved, nonspontaneously migrated stents must be removed. Successful pancreatic stent insertion and retrieval requires understanding the available techniques, appropriate indications, and potential adverse events.[74] It is strongly advised that an experienced endoscopist perform these procedures to optimize technical and clinical success.[98]

As with the biliary tract, the stents most commonly used in the pancreatic duct are plastic pancreatic stents (PPS)[97]; however, there are increasing data on the use, safety, and efficacy of cSEMS within the pancreatic duct.[99–103] In contrast, there are few indications for uSEMS placement within the pancreas (unresectable malignancy with obstructive complications).

One of the most common indications for pancreatic stent placement is prophylaxis of PEP.[104,105] Typically a small-caliber PPS is placed in high-risk individuals with the intent that spontaneous migration will occur within 4 weeks of placement. This is estimated to occur in 90% of patients.[106,107] At present, more studies have evaluated the use of cSEMS for chronic pancreatitis-related pancreatic stenosis (Video 24.2) than any other pancreas-specific indication. Available reports show comparable results to multiple PPS, though further studies are required to identify the ideal target population and address cost-effectiveness.[100,108]

Indications and Contraindications

Unlike biliary stents, pancreatic stents are nearly always placed for benign indications; therefore the majority need to be removed. An exception to this is stents placed for individuals with shortened life expectancy or for those with evidence of disconnected pancreatic duct syndrome, in whom long-term indwelling transmural plastic stents are safe and appear effective at minimizing recurrence of fluid collection.[109] In addition, stents placed for PEP prophylaxis are intended to migrate spontaneously and only require retrieval in the setting of stent retention.[107]

Besides completion of therapy, the other main indications for pancreatic stent removal are stent-related adverse events:

- *Stent occlusion.* Approximately 50% of pancreatic stents will be occluded by the sixth week after insertion, and nearly all will occlude within 3 months of placement.[20,110] The median time to stent occlusion has been estimated at 35 days, and there are conflicting data on identifiable risk factors to predict occlusion.[111,112] The mechanism of stent occlusion remains unknown, but microscopic evaluation of occluded pancreatic prostheses reveals precipitated pancreatic secretions, calcium carbonate crystals, and bacteria.[113] Although the majority of pancreatic stents become occluded in a short time, some data suggest that only a minority of patients (6%) develop clinical symptoms, including pancreatitis or pain.[110] Stent occlusion can be prevented by means of routine or scheduled stent retrieval and/or exchange. It has been suggested that large-caliber stents may decrease the rate of occlusion. In a study of 23 patients with chronic pancreatitis-related strictures treated with a 10-Fr stent, only 13% of the stents were occluded after 2 months.[114] However, in an evaluation of 47 individuals with chronic pancreatitis treated with PPS,

multivariate analysis identified stent diameter >8.5 Fr as a risk factor for stent occlusion.[111] It was theorized that a larger pancreatic stent may impair a favorable intraductal pressure gradient and result in a slower intrastent pancreatic juice flow that could predispose to precipitation and subsequent occlusion. These conflicting data highlight the importance of using appropriately sized stents driven by stent-specific indications and duct diameter, while ensuring an optimal time frame for stent removal/exchange to minimize the risk of adverse events.

- *Stent migration.* Stent migration may be internal (proximal) or external (distal). The latter does not typically lead to adverse events except those derived from the absence of therapeutic effect or, rarely, stent-related impaction or perforation. Internal migration can carry significant consequences and is typically a serious challenge for the endoscopist. The overall rate of migration is thought to be low and estimated between 4% and 10%.[115] In one of the first published series addressing this issue, an internal migration rate of 5.2% was described, whereas external migration reached 7.5%.[116] Factors associated with internal migration were a previous diagnosis of sphincter of Oddi dysfunction (OR 4.2, 95% CI 1.0 to 16.4) and a stent length greater than 7 cm (OR 3.2, 95% CI 1.01 to 10.0). In a large single-institution retrospective review of 386 PPS, proximal migration occurred in 5 cases (1.5%).[115] In a systematic review comparing cSEMS to multiple PPS for chronic pancreatitis-related strictures, the overall migration rate was 8.2% versus 10.5%, respectively.[100]

  In a retrospective series, 20/26 (77%) proximally migrated PPS could be extracted endoscopically, mostly with a stone extraction balloon or basket. Three of 26 (11%) were left in situ without clinical repercussions and the remaining 3 (11%) required surgical removal.[73] In a more recent series, the endoscopic retrieval rate was similar (18/23 [78%]), with 9 individuals (39%) requiring multiple attempts at retrieval. Most retrieved stents were removed with a stone extraction balloon. Five stents (22%) could not be removed, prompting surgical extraction in four individuals (17%) and observation alone without removal in one patient (5%).[117]

- *Stent-related pancreatic ductal and parenchymal changes.* Chronic pancreatitis-type ductal and parenchymal changes can occur after stent placement. An early report revealed that 36% of individuals treated with PPS developed subsequent pancreatic ductal changes thought related to stent trauma or side branch occlusion.[118] A review of 40 patients treated with PPS revealed that 80% developed new pancreatic duct morphologic changes after PPS retrieval, including duct irregularity, narrowing, and side branch changes. In follow-up, 64% had complete resolution, 32% appeared improved, and 5% remained unchanged.[119] In another study involving 25 patients treated with PPS, 17/25 (68%) developed parenchymal changes when evaluated by endoscopic ultrasonography (EUS) at the time of PPS retrieval. Of these, 16 underwent follow-up pancreatography and 9 patients (56%) were noted to have new ductal changes. Interestingly, 4 individuals underwent long-term follow-up (mean 16 months) using EUS and 2 were found to have focal chronic pancreatitis at the site of prior stent placement.[120] In a recent series including 32 patients treated with pancreatic cSEMS, stent-induced stenosis was seen in 5 patients (15%), of whom 4 patients were treated with a longer length stent for 2 months with complete resolution.[121] Overall, after pancreatic stent retrieval, a majority of stent-induced changes appear to improve; however, a small percentage of individuals are left with the sequelae of pancreatic injury.

Contraindications to pancreatic stent removal are the same as those discussed in the biliary stent removal section.

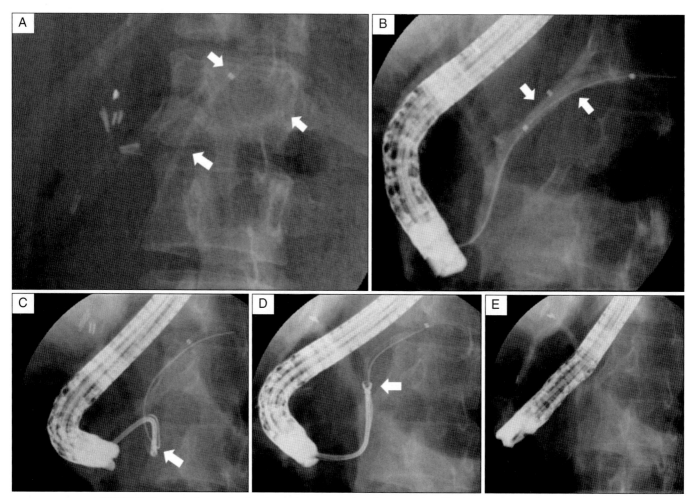

FIG 24.6 Removal of a proximally migrated pancreatic ductal stent assisted by the placement of a guidewire alongside the prosthesis to help direct the retrieval device. **A,** Scout film showing cholecystectomy clips and a proximally migrated, misplaced pigtail stent with the pigtail portion deployed and formed within the pancreas. **B,** A balloon dilator was placed over a guidewire alongside the stent and inflated, but was unsuccessful at stent retrieval. **C–E,** A rat-tooth forceps directed by a guidewire was used to grasp the distal aspect of the stent, reposition it proximally, and then successfully extract the stent from the pancreatic duct.

Timing of Stent Retrieval

Relative to biliary stents, most pancreatic stents are smaller in caliber, and thus stent removal and/or exchange is typically performed earlier. The optimal timing for stent retrieval is based on the number, size, and type of stents used. In addition, the underlying indication for placement can assist in determining the appropriate time interval for removal. For the treatment of chronic pancreatitis–related strictures, a prolonged duration of stent dwell may be required to induce sufficient remodeling.[122] In strictures refractory to a single PPS, multiple larger-caliber PPS can be used, with some reporting dwell times up to 12 months before removal/exchange.[108] An alternative is to place a cSEMS, for which stent retrieval is typically recommended in 3 months.[108]

Regarding assessment for spontaneous prophylactic stent migration, our practice is similar to that reported in the literature.[106] We obtain an abdominal radiograph within 4 weeks of stent placement. If the stent remains in place, it is removed endoscopically.

Techniques

The endoscopic techniques for pancreatic stent extraction are basically the same as those used for biliary stent textraction, with some exceptions. Because of the heightened risk of pancreatitis with manipulation in

patients with normal pancreatic duct caliber and the absence of severe chronic pancreatitis, careful and deliberate atraumatic removal of pancreatic stents is necessary. This minimizes trauma to the pancreatic duct and pancreatic orifice. The presence of chronic pancreatitis allows for more aggressive extraction maneuvers and carries a lower risk of adverse events. Special attention should be paid to establishing intraductal access before the retrieval process if further pancreatic ductal evaluation is needed. This carries heightened importance when performing a minor papilla stent extraction because of the inherent difficulty with minor papilla instrumentation. In addition, a guidewire placed alongside the prosthesis can assist with directing and deflecting retrieval accessories to increase the probability of successful removal (Fig. 24.6).

If a pancreatic ductal stricture is present, it is important to understand the stent location relative to the stricture, as this may dictate which retrieval approach to pursue.[123] Other key principles of stent retrieval include prioritizing patient safety, ensuring complete stent retrieval (Fig. 24.7), and performing a thorough examination to identify iatrogenic injury while assessing for resolution of the disease process that prompted the need for stenting (Fig. 24.8).

Extraction of a correctly placed pancreatic stent is usually accomplished with ease by the same direct grasping techniques described for biliary stents.[117,124] A snare or foreign-body retrieval forceps can be used

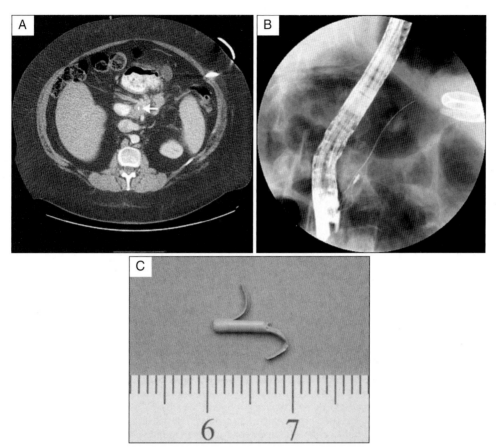

FIG 24.7 Removal of a retained intrapancreatic stent fragment manifesting as a smoldering pancreatic injury. **A,** Computed tomography scan showing a proximally migrated, fragmented tip of a pancreatic duct stent *(arrow)* and a percutaneous drain in a pseudocyst. **B,** ERCP showing retrieval of a proximally migrated, fragmented tip of a pancreatic stent with an over-the-wire basket; a 12-F locking percutaneous pigtail catheter is positioned in a pseudocyst. **C,** Postretrieval fragmented pancreatic duct stent tip. (Reprinted with permission.[117])

to grasp the distal aspect of the stent and extract it from the pancreatic orifice. If stent exchange or follow-up pancreatography is required, stent retrieval with the lasso technique will accomplish stent removal while maintaining pancreatic duct access (Fig. 24.9). With direct grasping techniques, achieving ductal recannulation after removing the stent could be difficult, as the guidewire may enter side branches or follow a false passage and hinder stent replacement. The lasso technique is carried out by cannulating the lumen of the stent with a sphincterotome, as the flexion can facilitate insertion of the guidewire through the stent. This cannulation should be performed with minimal pressure on the stent tip to avoid the potential for advancing the stent more distally (toward the tail), making stent retrieval more difficult (Video 24.3).

Proximally migrated pancreatic stents represent a challenging situation, and the presence of a pancreatic duct stricture, especially distal (upstream) to the migrated stent, can be an additional obstacle to extraction.[123] Many extraction techniques have been proposed, but in the vast majority of reported cases removal is achieved with a stone extraction basket to capture or a stone extraction balloon placed proximal or adjacent to the stent to drag the stent into the duodenum with gentle downward pressure.[73,74,117] In a retrospective review of proximally migrated PPS, 18/23 were endoscopically retrievable, with the most common technique being balloon extraction (8/18 [44%]), followed by indirect grasping (6/18 [33%]), lasso technique (2/18 [11%]), stone extraction basket retrieval (1/18 [5%]), and the use of an interventional radiology loop snare (1/18 [5%]). The majority of these procedures involved

replacing a transpapillary pancreatic stent (15/22 [68%]). Of note, in this series, failure of endoscopic stent extraction was related to the presence of a downstream stenosis.[117]

Because of the difference in size and anatomic shape between the pancreatic and biliary ductal systems, a number of previously mentioned extraction techniques cannot be used for pancreatic stent retrieval. The limited pancreatic duct size prevents maneuvers that require excessive intraductal manipulation, including the formation of loops used to tether or grasp stents. For this reason, other rescue techniques have been reported, including those that use angiographic instruments designed to maneuver in small-caliber spaces.[125]

The lasso technique has proven to be both helpful and easy to perform, allowing the ability to recover proximally migrated stents (Video 24.4). Originally described as a technique to maintain biliary stent position in the setting of malignant obstruction, this technique involves inserting a guidewire through the lumen of the migrated stent[75] or parallel to it.[76] A slightly opened polypectomy snare is then inserted over the guidewire into the pancreatic duct until the distal end of the stent is reached. The snare is then carefully and gently opened and manipulated to seize the stent and remove it by applying soft traction, without closing the snare tightly, which can result in stent fragmentation (Video 24.5).

Direct pancreatoscopy with SpyGlass (Boston Scientific, Marlborough, MA) has been used for difficult PPS retrieval.[126,127] In one case, the SpyGlass system was introduced into the pancreatic duct and advanced to the migrated stent. At that point, the SpyBite forceps (Boston Scientific)

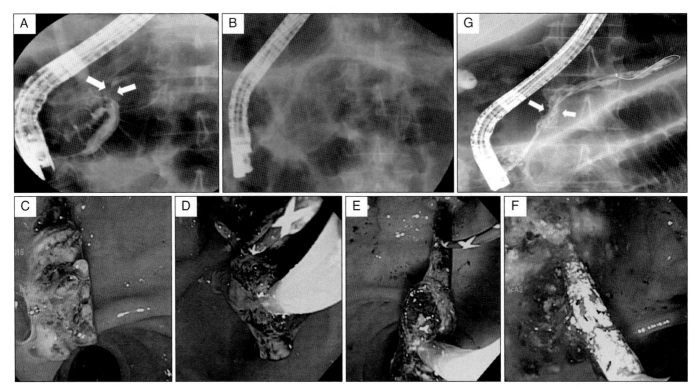

FIG 24.8 Removal of prolonged indwelling pancreatic stents with assessment for stricture resolution. **A** and **B,** Two 7-Fr by 12-cm PBS were placed for a high-grade chronic pancreatitis–related genu stricture *(arrows)* at the site of a prior pancreatitis-related abscess that was drained endoscopically. The patient failed to return for 12 years and presented after a computed tomography abdomen scan revealed two indwelling, ossified pancreatic stents with extensive peristent calcifications. **C,** Endoscopic view of the indwelling stents. **D** and **E,** Guidewire access was obtained alongside the stents and each was individually removed by directly grasping the distal stent tip with a snare. **F,** Representative balloon extraction with removal of multiple soft pancreatic stones and debris. **G,** Pancreatogram revealing resolution of the previous high-grade genu stricture *(arrow highlighting prior site of stricture).* In the setting of chronic pancreatitis and the patient's poor medical compliance, no further stenting was pursued.

was used to capture and remove the stent.[127] In another case the SpyGlass was used to visualize the distal end of the stent and cannulate its lumen with a guidewire. Afterward the SpyGlass system was removed and the stent was retrieved with a Soehendra stent retriever.[126] It is important to note that the current iteration of the SpyScope has a 10-Fr distal tip and efforts should be made to ensure that the pancreatic duct diameter is sufficient.

Other novel techniques to address pancreatic stent retrieval have been described. To remove a proximally migrated 10-Fr PPS, a guidewire was placed through the stent lumen and a 7-Fr PPS was advanced into the 10-Fr PPS. The 7-Fr/10-Fr system was directly grasped and successfully retrieved.[128] For those with postsurgical anatomy not amendable to pancreatic duct cannulation, an EUS rendezvous can be used to access the main pancreatic duct and facilitate stent extraction (Fig. 24.10). In a single-center retrospective review, EUS permitted successful extraction of two retained postsurgical pancreatic stents using a 19-gauge needle and a guidewire to dislodge and advance the stents into the jejunum.[129]

Adverse Events and Management

Procedural adverse events in the previously cited series reached 13%, including pancreatic duct disruption with subsequent leakage (1/23 [4.3%]), stent fragmentation (1/23 [4.3%]), and PEP (1/23 [4.3%]).[117] Moffatt et al. described PEP occurring in 3% of patients in a large series of retained prophylactic pancreatic stents.[124] A retrospective review of 36 cases of proximally migrated PPS retrieval included 5 PEP (13.9%), 1 infection (2.8%), and 1 hemorrhage (2.8%).[130]

Relative Costs and Choice of Technique

A standard protocol for endoscopic retrieval of pancreatic stents has not been established. Like the approach for bile stent extraction, pancreatic stent removal is commonly performed using accessories found in most endoscopy units, and so the procedure should not be considered costly.

Definitive extraction of nonmigrated stents should be performed with direct grasping techniques. If pancreatic duct access is needed, the lasso technique will facilitate stent retrieval while maintaining a guidewire within the pancreatic duct.

For proximally migrated PPS, Price et al. reported success in the majority of cases with a stone extraction balloon and indirect grasping technique.[117] If possible, cannulation of the stent facilitates removal, although this is not easy to accomplish, especially for proximally migrated stents. Difficult cases with downstream stenoses require a series of ductal balloon dilations before retrieval. If the aforementioned techniques fail, multiple case reports of stent retrieval with direct pancreatoscopy exist, but caution must be used to ensure that the pancreatic duct caliber can accommodate the 10-Fr device.

REMOVAL OF LUMEN-APPOSING METAL STENTS

The introduction of LAMS has broadened the indication for gastrointestinal tract stenting to include transmural drainage of the common bile duct and gallbladder, while providing an additional accessory to

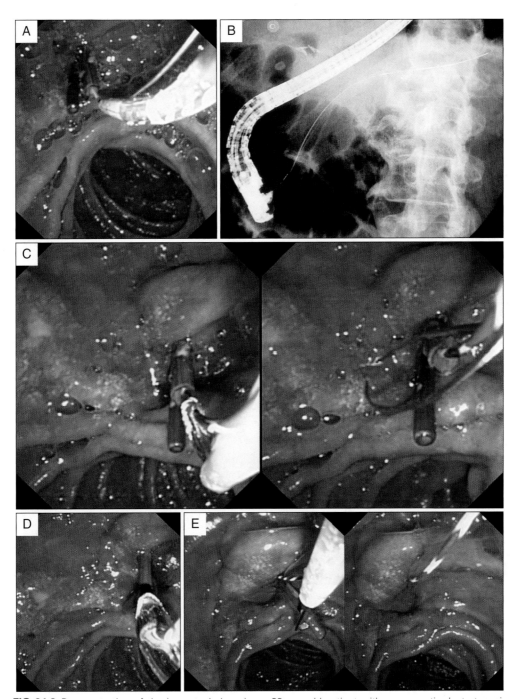

FIG 24.9 Demonstration of the lasso technique in an 83-year-old patient with a pancreatic duct stenosis treated with two PPS (5 and 7 Fr). Six weeks later, stent exchange is scheduled. **A,** The 7-Fr PPS lumen is cannulated with a sphincterotome. **B,** The guidewire is passed through the stent lumen into the pancreatic tail. **C,** A polypectomy snare is threaded over the guidewire and advanced to grasp the stent. **D,** The stent is seized with the snare and extracted over the guidewire, which remains in place in the pancreatic duct. **E,** The second stent is extracted by directly grasping with the snare along the guidewire. *PPS,* Plastic pancreatic stents.

address symptomatic pancreatic fluid collection. Inherent in its design is a dumbbell shape with dual antimigration flanges to facilitate the apposition of two opposing lumens. The preliminary data on efficacy are promising,[15,19,22,131,132] and additional indications for LAMS placement have included benign enteric strictures[133] and creation of gastroenteric anastomoses.[134]

Indications, Contraindications, and Timing of Stent Retrieval

At present there is little to no standardized approach to the use of LAMS for pancreatic and biliary drainage, and therefore no universal protocol exists to dictate the practice of removal.

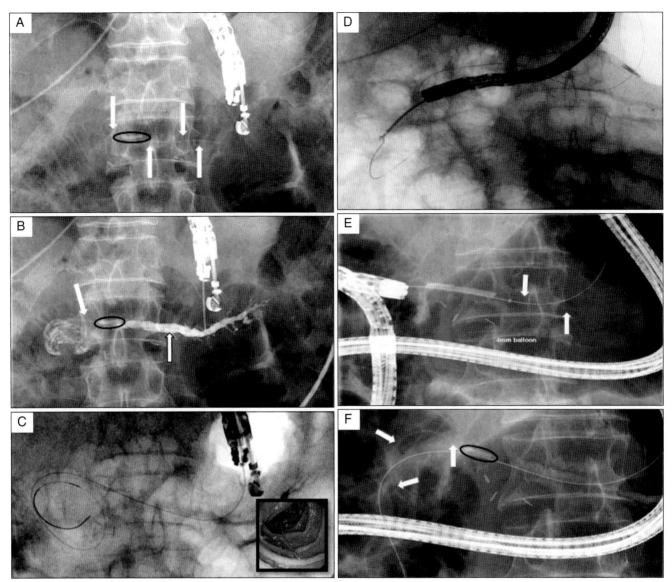

FIG 24.10 EUS rendezvous–assisted removal of proximally migrated postsurgical pancreatic stent not amenable to enteroscopic retrieval because of inability to visualize the pancreaticojejunal anastomosis. **A,** Scout film (*arrows* highlight the location of the retained pancreatic stent and a *black oval* encircles a surgical clip). **B,** EUS pancreatography. **C,** Placement of a guidewire through the pancreatic duct into the jejunum (*arrows* highlight the location of the stent). **D,** Guidewire grasped by a rat-tooth forceps. **E** and **F,** A dilating balloon is used to extract the stent. *EUS,* endoscopic ultrasonography.

For pancreatic fluid collection drainage, LAMS retrieval should be performed once the pancreatic fluid collection has been adequately treated, with timing dependent on clinical context and local practice.

For biliary drainage (i.e., choledochoduodenostomy and cholecystoduodenostomy), LAMS are used for palliation and limited life expectancy; therefore retrieval is limited to specific patient circumstances.

Techniques

The basis of LAMS retrieval is direct grasping, either with a rat-tooth forceps or a snare placed around the antimigration flange. The use of an endoscope with a large working channel is favored, either a therapeutic endoscope or a duodenoscope. Once grasped, the LAMS is secured and will collapse while being removed through the working channel. If the stent is unable to be pulled through the endoscope channel, the entire scope is withdrawn.

In instances of buried stents, it is of utmost importance to attempt to identify a migration tract. Anecdotally, we have achieved success at maintaining a tract via the use of a short double-pigtail stent placed through the LAMS (Fig. 24.11); however, this is not a universally accepted intervention and must be tailored to the individual endoscopist's preference. If identified, a cannula or dilating balloon can be used to inject contrast and confirm communication with the buried stent. The tract can be dilated, and success with direct grasping and an inside-out stent retrieval method via a rat-tooth forceps has been reported.[135]

There are little data available on the risk of external stent migration or the success of passing a luminally migrated LAMS through the digestive tract. Intestinal obstruction requiring exploratory laparotomy for successful stent extraction has been reported.[27]

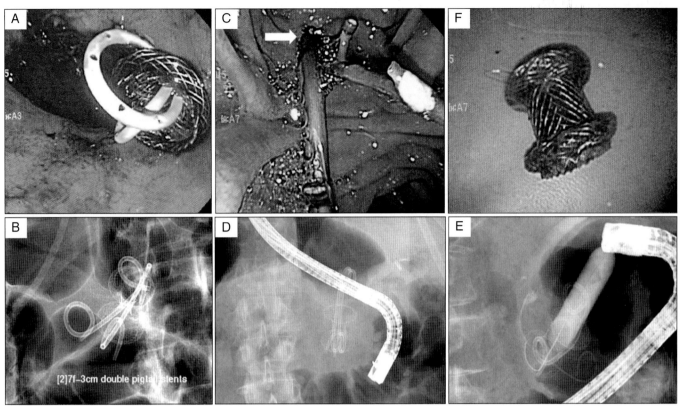

FIG 24.11 Retrieval of a buried lumen-apposing metal stent (LAMS) used to create a cystogastrostomy in a patient with chronic pancreatitis and symptomatic pseudocyst. **A** and **B,** Fluoroscopic and endoscopic views of a newly placed LAMS cystogastrostomy with two 7-Fr by 3-cm double-pigtail stents within the stent. **C** and **D,** Endoscopic and fluoroscopic view of the buried LAMS on follow-up endoscopy. *Arrows* highlight the site of the buried bumper. Note that the presence of the double-pigtail stents ensured patency of the migration tract to facilitate retrieval. The tract was cannulated, and once the position was confirmed fluoroscopically, the tract was balloon dilated **(E)** and the stent was successfully retrieved with a rat-tooth forceps. **F,** Endoscopic view of the extracted stent.

SUMMARY

Endoscopic removal of biliary and pancreatic stents can be challenging, with success dependent on many factors, including access to appropriate accessories, experience with certain therapeutic procedures, multidisciplinary decisions, and, finally, respect for the professional, institutional, and anatomic limitations. The introduction of LAMS for pancreaticobiliary drainage is promising, but additional studies with longitudinal and outcomes data are needed to standardize an approach to retrieval.

The complete reference list for this chapter can be found online at www.expertconsult.com.

25

Papillectomy and Ampullectomy

Shayan Irani and Richard A. Kozarek

Ampullary neoplasms (see Chapter 38) are rare, with an annual incidence of 3000 in the United States and a reported prevalence of 0.04% to 0.12% in autopsy series.[1,2] Endoscopically the papilla can appear enlarged and abnormal because of various tumors (benign or malignant) and other etiologies such as papillitis, gastric foveolar metaplasia, or pancreatic acinar hyperplasia (Fig. 25.1). Ampullary tumors can be classified based on their layer of origin: those that arise from the epithelium (e.g., adenomas, adenocarcinomas, lymphomas) and those that arise from the subepithelium (e.g., neuroendocrine tumors, lipomas, leiomyomas, gastrointestinal stromal tumors, lymphangiomas, fibromas, hamartomas). Ampullary adenomas are by far the most common of these. Although uncommon in the general population (representing <10% of all periampullary tumors),[3] they are increased twofold to threefold in genetic polyposis syndromes, especially familial adenomatous polyposis (FAP) and its variants.[4] Between 40% and 100% of FAP patients will also develop duodenal adenomas, which are frequently numerous with a similar malignant potential. Ampullary adenomas can arise from the surface or the inner epithelium of the ampulla.[5]

Historically, ampullary adenomas presented late, with a high incidence of underlying malignancy.[1,2] Endoscopic management in the early years consisted mainly of palliation of obstructive jaundice with biliary sphincterotomy and stent placement. Patients often become symptomatic when the lesions are large enough to cause obstruction, presenting with cholestasis, cholangitis, pancreatitis, nonspecific abdominal pain, and, less commonly, bleeding.[6,7] With increased awareness among endoscopists and the increasing use of cross-sectional imaging (computed tomography [CT] and magnetic resonance imaging [MRI]), these lesions are being recognized at earlier stages with a lower incidence of underlying malignancy. Asymptomatic lesions are being recognized more commonly in patients undergoing endoscopy for unrelated reasons such as gastroesophageal reflux disease (GERD), surveillance of Barrett esophagus, and dyspepsia or, alternatively, in patients undergoing surveillance for FAP.[8,9]

TREATMENT OPTIONS

Once diagnosed with a biopsy-proven ampullary adenoma, patients have four options: close endoscopic surveillance with biliary stent placement (for cholestasis) or without biliary stent placement endoscopic papillectomy, surgical ampullectomy/local resection, or pancreaticoduodenectomy (Whipple operation). There are no clinical trials comparing one approach to another. The decision regarding treatment choice is influenced by various factors, including patient preference, associated comorbidities that may affect fitness for surgery, local endoscopic and surgical expertise, characteristics of the lesion, and whether sporadic or in the setting of FAP. For patients with large lesions (greater than 4 to 5 cm), presence of high-grade dysplasia or carcinoma in situ, or obvious nodal disease on cross-sectional imaging or endoscopic ultrasonography (EUS),

pancreaticoduodenectomy should be considered.[10–12] However, small series have demonstrated the ability to completely resect focal, low-grade, early-stage T1 ampullary adenocarcinoma via endoscopic papillectomy.[13–15]

Although associated with the highest cure rates and lowest recurrence rates, pancreaticoduodenectomy carries a morbidity rate of 25% to 63%, with mortality ranging from 0% to 13% (higher rates are reported in patients with malignant disease).[16–18] Surgical local resection is associated with lower morbidity (14% to 27%) and mortality (0% to 4%), but recurrence rates vary from 0% to 32% (mean, 18% to 20%), thus necessitating continued postoperative endoscopic surveillance.[19–22] In a retrospective review of 38 patients, surgical ampullectomy was associated with lower operative time (169 minutes vs 268 minutes), estimated blood loss (192 mL vs 727 mL), mean hospital stay (10 days vs 25 days), and overall morbidity (29% vs 78%) compared with pancreaticoduodenectomy.[23] As colonoscopic polypectomy has become routine for even large colonic polyps, and with the acceptable morbidity, mortality, and recurrence rates of surgical local resection for papillary adenomas, endoscopic papillectomy emerged as an acceptable alternative to surgery.

Endoscopic papillectomy was first described by Suzuki et al. in 1983,[24] and the first large case series was reported by Binmoeller et al. in 1993.[10] Over the last 2 decades, many more studies have been published showing high success rates, low morbidity, and minimal mortality. Endoscopic papillectomy has therefore gained increasing acceptance as the treatment of choice for the vast majority of patients with ampullary adenomas.

CONSIDERATIONS IN FAP

In patients with FAP, ampullary adenomas develop in 80% in their lifetime, with up to a 5% risk of developing malignancy.[25] The management of ampullary adenomas in the setting of FAP is further complicated because complete excision does not eliminate the risk of recurrence or new upper gastrointestinal tract cancers. Fortunately, the risk of histologic progression of upper gastrointestinal tract adenomas in patients with FAP appears to be low.[25,26] In one of the largest studies on surveillance of duodenal and ampullary adenomas in 114 patients with FAP, duodenal polyps progressed in size in 26%, number in 32%, and histology in 11% of patients. Morphology and histology of the papilla progressed in 14% and 11% of patients, respectively, with only one patient developing a periampullary cancer over a mean follow-up of 51 months.[25] This has prompted some experts to propose surveillance endoscopy with biopsies only, rather than excision, for FAP patients with ampullary adenomas in the absence of rapid growth or high-grade dysplasia on endoscopic biopsy. The obvious benefit of this approach is avoidance of the risks associated with excision of these lesions. The limitation of surveillance with biopsies alone is the potential to miss occult foci of high-grade dysplasia or carcinoma. In a study of 33 patients with ampullary adenomas (not necessarily FAP) in whom endoscopic biopsies

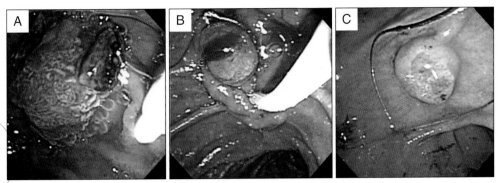

FIG 25.1 Enlarged prominent papilla that could be mistaken for an ampullary adenoma because of papillitis (**A**), gastric foveolar metaplasia (**B**), and pancreatic acinar hyperplasia (**C**).

BOX 25.1   Summary of the Technique

- Staging of ampullary adenomas with cross-sectional imaging (computed tomography or magnetic resonance imaging) is not routine, although in the setting of significant weight loss and dilated ducts should be done to evaluate for the presence of nodal and metastatic disease.[8]
- Endoscopic ultrasonography is very helpful in defining lesion size, depth of invasion, ductal involvement, and anatomy but is not routine, especially in small lesions and in the absence of jaundice, history of acute pancreatitis, or dilation of the pancreatic or bile ducts.
- Endoscopic retrograde cholangiopancreatography before papillectomy is indicated in all patients to assess whether intraductal involvement is present and to identify pancreatic duct anatomy for conditions such as pancreas divisum.
- A duodenoscope is used to perform the papillectomy in a similar manner to colonoscopic snare polypectomy, usually using blended current.
- Thermal ablation may be used in select cases as adjunctive therapy.
- Prophylactic pancreatic sphincterotomy and stent placement should be attempted in all patients.
- Routine biliary sphincterotomy is recommended, although biliary stent placement is not routine in the presence of good biliary drainage.
- Surveillance is critical after complete resection because of known local recurrences.

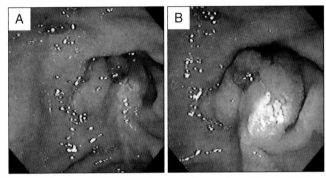

FIG 25.2 A, Ampullary adenoma obscured by a periampullary diverticulum. **B,** Better appreciated after eversion of the surrounding mucosa.

were obtained, carcinoma was found at final surgical pathology in 5/10 patients with high-grade dysplasia and in 3/19 patients with low-grade dysplasia.[27] Because of these competing issues, the management of ampullary adenomas in FAP patients is determined on a case-by-case basis, taking into consideration all of the aforementioned factors in addition to the patient's wishes and risk tolerance.

TECHNIQUE (BOX 25.1)

The role of endoscopic papillectomy was reviewed in a guideline statement published by the American Society for Gastrointestinal Endoscopy in 2006.[28]

Initial Endoscopic Assessment
Conventional Endoscopy

Visualization of the ampulla is possible with a conventional forward-viewing endoscope but is best performed with a duodenoscope. A large periampullary diverticulum can hinder visualization (Fig. 25.2). Ampullary adenomas can have varied appearances, ranging from appearing normal in the setting of FAP, to a slight enlargement, to flat laterally spreading, to granular or polypoid, with or without ulceration

(Fig. 25.3). The use of endoscopic tools such as narrow band imaging (NBI), flexible spectral imaging color enhancement (FICE), or magnification endoscopy may help further characterize lesions in certain cases.[29] Although some endoscopic features alone should raise the suspicion of an associated underlying malignancy (large, friable, ulcerated, indurated lesions), endoscopic biopsies are needed to confirm the pathology. Endoscopic biopsies, however, can be suboptimal at detecting underlying malignant foci. The reported rates of malignancy in ampullary adenomas are approximately 20% to 30%.[9,16,30] Detection rates for cancer present within adenomas based on biopsy alone range from a dismal 40% to 89%.[19–20,31–35] These arguments may suggest favoring a radical surgical approach in all patients; however, this is mostly based on data obtained from surgical series. Nowadays, many ampullary lesions are diagnosed at routine endoscopy, with a much higher percentage being detected at earlier stages. In the more recent and larger endoscopic series (over 100 patients in each), incidental or asymptomatic presentation of ampullary adenomatous lesions was seen in 25% to 33%.[2,9,36] Rates of malignancy in papillectomy specimens ranged from 6% to 8%.[2,9,36] In addition, there are clinical, endoscopic, and imaging features that should give the clinician pause before considering endoscopic papillectomy, even if biopsies alone do not reveal cancer—specifically, clinical features such as significant weight loss and jaundice and endoscopic features such as large (>4 cm), friable, ulcerated, fixed lesions and evidence of dilated ducts, especially with intraductal extension, as seen on EUS, MRCP, or during cholangiography at the time of removal. In our series of 102 patients who underwent papillectomy, 8 (7%) were found to have invasive cancer. Of these eight patients, two were referred by surgeons because of significant comorbidities precluding pancreaticoduodenectomy. Thus only 6 of 102 (5%) patients who appeared endoscopically resectable and who underwent papillectomy had invasive cancer on final pathology.[9] Therefore, although it is true that biopsy alone has a

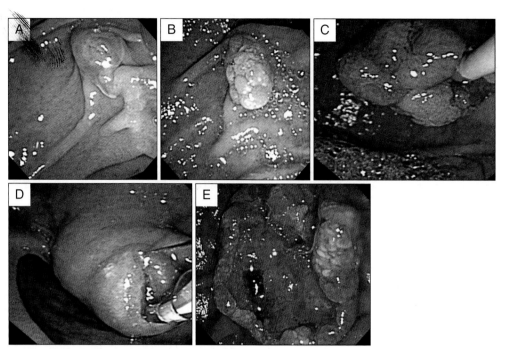

FIG 25.3 Endoscopic appearance of various ampullary adenomas. **A,** Normal-appearing papilla harboring microadenomas in familial adenomatous polyposis. **B,** Flat ampullary adenoma. **C,** Granular and polypoid adenoma. **D,** Purely intraductal adenoma. **E,** Depressed ampullary adenocarcinoma.

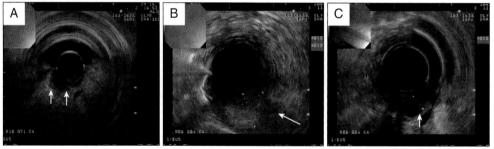

FIG 25.4 Endoscopic ultrasonography examination of ampullary lesions. **A,** Lesion limited to the submucosa with an intact muscularis propria (*arrows*). **B,** Lesion (*arrow*) invading through the muscularis propria precluding papillectomy. **C,** Intraductal extension into the bile duct (*arrow*) precluding papillectomy.

definable miss rate in diagnosing invasive cancer, only a minority of patients with invasive cancer seem to have endoscopically resectable lesions. Most authors propose that EUS in selected patients could help decrease this unnecessary papillectomy rate even further, with many centers performing EUS routinely for all ampullary adenomas.[37,38] More recently, in a study of 56 ampullary tumors, histology and immunohistochemical characteristics helped further with selecting the appropriate surgical or endoscopic approach. They demonstrated that periampullary tumors, intestinal histology, and high CK20-positive rate can be regarded as good indications for endoscopic papillectomy. On the other hand, tumors that are either pancreatobiliary or intestinal type without CDX2 expression have a higher chance of intraductal involvement and may be better suited for a surgical approach.[39]

Endoscopic Ultrasonography and Intraductal Endoscopic Ultrasonography

Some authors recommend performing EUS in all patients with ampullary adenomas, whereas others recommend EUS only for selected cases.[9,37,38,40]

As mentioned above, clinical features of weight loss and jaundice, cross-sectional imaging features of dilated ducts, and endoscopic appearance (friable, ulcerated, indurated, and in our practice lesions >2 cm) should prompt performance of EUS before papillectomy. EUS is very useful in evaluating tumor size, depth of invasion of the duodenal wall, and involvement of the biliary or pancreatic ducts and periampullary lymph nodes (Fig. 25.4).[28,38,41–43] The T-staging accuracy of EUS is very good (83% to 90%) and superior to CT and MRI.[38,44–47] N-staging accuracy in some studies is reported to be better than CT (84% vs 68%),[43] whereas in others it is reported to be comparable to CT and MRI (68% vs 59% vs 77%).[48] Prior sphincterotomy and the presence of a biliary or pancreatic stent, however, can decrease EUS T-stage accuracy.

The optimal management of patients with intramucosal cancer (pT1) remains debatable. In these patients, lymphatic or vascular invasion and lymph node metastases do not occur.[49,50] Local resection can be justified if biliary or pancreatic duct infiltration can be confidently excluded. The evaluation of tumor invasion of the sphincter of Oddi remains challenging. Intraductal endoscopic ultrasonography (IDUS) can be performed in a transpapillary or percutaneous fashion. IDUS has excellent resolution because of the use of high-frequency ultrasound (20 to 30 MHz) compared with standard EUS (at most usually 7.5 to 10 MHz). There are three studies comparing EUS with IDUS in ampullary cancer. Itoh et al.[38] reported the diagnostic accuracy of IDUS and EUS in 32 patients with ampullary cancer who underwent surgical resection. The TNM staging accuracy of IDUS was comparable to EUS (88% vs 90%) but the depiction of the sphincter of Oddi and detailed staging were better with IDUS. Menzel et al.[51] reported the results of a prospective study on 27 patients with ampullary neoplasm (adenoma in 12, adenocarcinoma in 15) who underwent surgical management. They concluded that IDUS was significantly superior to EUS with regard to tumor visualization and staging (staging accuracy 93% vs 62%). Ito et al.[41] performed EUS and transpapillary IDUS in 40 patients (adenocarcinoma in 33, adenoma in 7). IDUS had a slightly better T-stage accuracy (78% vs 62%) but was no better at detecting ductal involvement (90% vs 88%). Because of the paucity of data and similar performance of IDUS and EUS, IDUS cannot be routinely recommended at this time. However, as probe technology improves it may become more commonly used to differentiate more subtle, early invasive cancers of the ampulla, thus precluding unnecessary papillectomies.

Endoscopic Retrograde Cholangiopancreatography

Although EUS is generally performed before resection to improve staging accuracy, endoscopic retrograde cholangiopancreatography (ERCP) is performed at the time of papillectomy to exclude intraductal tumor involvement and to perform pancreaticobiliary sphincterotomy and stent placement. If EUS is unavailable or if the findings at EUS are equivocal, performance of ERCP is critical before resection (Fig. 25.5). Surgical referral should be considered if there is evidence of intraductal involvement, especially if there is extension >1 cm into the biliary or pancreatic duct. Cholangiopancreatography outlines the ductal anatomy to help access the pancreatic and bile ducts after papillectomy. In addition, the presence of pancreas divisum can obviate the need for pancreatic duct stent placement.

Endoscopic Papillectomy

Endoscopic resection is limited to the mucosa and submucosa of the duodenal wall and the tissue around the biliary and pancreatic duct orifices located at the major duodenal papilla.[52] Endoscopic papillectomy makes it difficult to remove tumor tissue invading the common bile duct or pancreatic duct. In clinical practice, the terms *endoscopic papillectomy* and *endoscopic ampullectomy* are used interchangeably. However, ampullectomy consists of circumferential resection of the ampulla of Vater, with separate reinsertion of the bile duct and pancreatic duct into the duodenal wall. This cannot be achieved using translumenal endoscopic therapy and necessitates a surgical duodenotomy and resection of pancreatic tissue in the area of anatomic attachment of the ampulla to the duodenal wall.[53] Therefore the term *endoscopic papillectomy* is more appropriate than *endoscopic ampullectomy*.

The goal of endoscopic resection is to achieve complete excision of the ampullary neoplasm. There are currently many different techniques to perform a papillectomy, with no consensus on one method and a lack of large comparative studies.[54] In deciding how best to remove an ampullary adenoma, the endoscopist must clearly define the margins of the lesion (which may sometimes be difficult in very flat, spreading lesions or when associated with a periampullary diverticulum). In general, papillectomy is accomplished in a manner similar to colonoscopic snare polypectomy using a duodenoscope. Although there are no data to support administration of antibiotics before endoscopic papillectomy, the procedure is similar to an ERCP and other submucosal resections. We routinely give antibiotics before papillectomy and in cases of concern for injury to the duodenal muscularis propria, and we continue for 2 to 3 days after resection.

Snare Excision

Papillectomy is typically performed with a standard monopolar diathermic snare used for colonoscopic polypectomy. In most studies neither the size of the snare nor the direction of snaring is mentioned.[6,10,11,55,56] Polypectomy snares of various diameters ranging from 11 to 27 mm are used depending on the size of the lesion.[12,36,57,58] Some authors prefer softer, more flexible snares (e.g., 2.5-cm AcuSnare; Cook Medical, Winston-Salem, NC) and some prefer stiffer, more rigid snares (e.g., 2-cm oval snare with spiral wires, SnareMaster; Olympus America, Center Valley, PA).[59,60] The softer, more flexible snares allow easier manipulation over the elevator. A stiffer snare can be more easily positioned parallel to the plane of dissection and perpendicular to the catheter for a uniform excision to the level of the muscularis propria (Fig. 25.6). We prefer a softer snare for pedunculated or bulkier lesions and a stiffer snare for flatter, laterally spreading lesions. The lesion, together with the papilla, is grasped and excised using a blended current to decrease the risk of bleeding. Two studies advocated snaring the tumor from the cephalad to the caudal side (snare apex placed at the superior margin of the lesion), citing that ensnaring the entire papilla

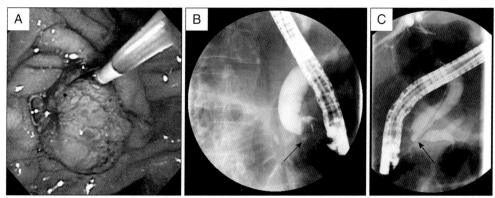

FIG 25.5 Endoscopic retrograde cholangiopancreatography examination of ampullary adenomas. **A,** Visualization and performance of ductography. **B,** Intraductal extension into bile duct (*arrow*) beyond the ampulla precluding papillectomy. **C,** Intraductal extension into the pancreatic duct (*arrow*) beyond the ampulla precluding papillectomy.

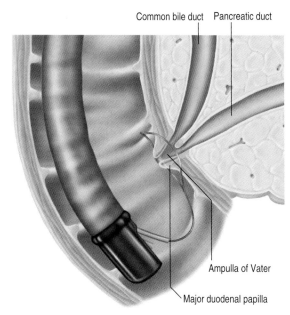

Common bile duct   Pancreatic duct

Ampulla of Vater

Major duodenal papilla

FIG 25.6 Schematic drawing demonstrating the exact plane of resection during endoscopic papillectomy.

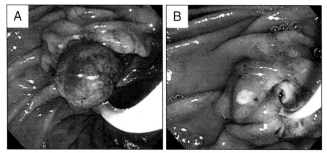

FIG 25.7 En bloc endoscopic papillectomy. **A,** Lesion is snared from cephalad to caudal side. **B,** Appearance of the same lesion after papillectomy.

was easier, although secure snaring is feasible from either direction (Video 25.1).[58,61]

Electrosurgical Currents: Cutting Versus Coagulation

There is no established consensus or guidelines regarding power output or the mode of electrosurgical current for endoscopic papillectomy, and in most studies these settings are not specified.[62] When specified, monopolar current was used in all studies[63–65] and the power output ranged from 25 to 150 W, with effect of two or three.[11,12,36,64] The mode of the current also varied, with some authors using blended electrosurgical current and others using pure cutting current (usually 40 to 50 J).[6,36,64,65] The rationale for the use of pure cutting current is to avoid edema caused by the coagulation mode.[2,10,44,63] In the absence of any randomized trials it is difficult to compare various power outputs and modes of current. In our practice, we use a monopolar blended current at a setting of 25 W.

En Bloc Versus Piecemeal Resection

En bloc resection of the lesion should be attempted whenever possible, with only one study demonstrating a decreased incidence of tumor recurrence when en bloc rather than piecemeal papillectomy is performed (Fig. 25.7).[66] Based on general principles of oncologic surgery, en bloc

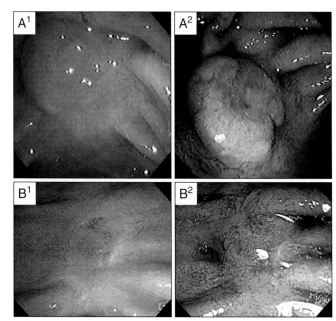

FIG 25.8 Vital dye staining. **A1,** Ampullary adenoma with indistinct borders. **A2,** Same lesion with well-defined borders after methylene blue staining. **B1,** A small recurrent adenoma after prior papillectomy is better visualized with (**B2**) indigo carmine staining.

resection is preferred because of a higher likelihood of complete tumor excision and better histologic analysis of the resection margins.[63,67,68] En bloc resection can be technically more difficult and may incur a higher risk of bleeding and perforation, especially in the presence of one or more of the following: large tumor size, limited endoscopic accessibility, and laterally spreading lesions. In these cases, piecemeal resection may be undertaken, frequently with adjuvant ablative therapy, if needed. Also, piecemeal excision may require several sessions to achieve complete removal of the lesion.[11] Vital dye staining with indigo carmine or methylene blue or use of narrow band imaging may help to delineate the tumor margins before resection (Fig. 25.8). In our center, when feasible, en bloc resection is performed; when this is not feasible, piecemeal resection is undertaken.[9,10,12,36,53,61,69]

Role of Submucosal Injection

The use of submucosal injection with solutions such as normal saline or dilute epinephrine remains somewhat controversial. Extrapolating from the practice of submucosal injection before mucosectomy, there is a theoretical benefit that this reduces the risk of perforation and bleeding. The inability to "lift" the lesion after submucosal injection has been used by some to predict the presence of invasive cancer and preclude attempting endoscopic papillectomy.[58]

If submucosal injection is performed, a sclerotherapy needle is used and the number of injections and total volume of solution vary with the size of the lesion.[11] Methylene blue can be added to the solution to improve tumor visualization, especially the margins.[67] However, ampullary tumors differ from mucosal neoplasms in other locations within the gastrointestinal tract because the biliary and pancreatic ducts are embedded and traverse the submucosa to emerge at the mucosal surface. A submucosal injection will fail to raise the lesion at the site of ductal insertion, making complete resection down to the sphincteric muscle difficult and potentially hindering subsequent access to the pancreatic and biliary ducts.[70] Furthermore, submucosal injections may increase the risk of postprocedure pancreatitis. In the majority of series, submucosal injections have not been used. This does not appear to make complete resection difficult or increase the rate of adverse events.[6,10,49,55,69] In our practice we do not perform submucosal injections unless dealing with laterally spreading lesions, and in these cases, submucosal injections close to the papilla are avoided.

Infrequently Performed Novel Techniques

Some novel but infrequently performed techniques to facilitate endoscopic papillectomy have been proposed. A few authors have reported successful resection of ampullary adenomas with intraductal extension using a balloon catheter linked to a snare, with the inflated balloon in the common bile duct providing traction toward the duodenal lumen.[63,71] Soma et al.[72] similarly reported a double-snare retracting technique to provide retraction before resection in 12 patients with ampullary lesions with good outcomes. To maintain pancreatic duct access after papillectomy, Kim et al.[71,73] inserted a guidewire into the pancreatic duct before papillectomy in 72 patients with ampullary adenomas. A snare was passed over the wire, and immediately after papillectomy a pancreatic duct stent was placed. Complete resection was achieved in 90% and pancreatitis occurred in 8%, with a recurrence of 8% reported over a mean follow-up of 24 months. In a multicenter, prospective, randomized study, 22 patients underwent wire-guided papillectomy (WP) and 23 patients underwent conventional papillectomy (CP). Although a significant difference was noted in pancreatic duct stent placement (100% WP vs 65% CP), no difference was noted in resection rates or pancreatitis rates.[54] More studies are needed to confirm the feasibility and safety of these inventive methods.

Specimen Retrieval and Preparation

The retrieval of all resected specimens for submission to histopathology is essential for detection of small malignant foci. Specimens should be retrieved immediately after resection with a net, snare, basket, or suction cap (Fig. 25.9). Intravenous glucagon administered just before papillectomy may help prevent the downstream loss of tissue because of peristalsis. Some authors have suggested pinning the specimen on polystyrene plates for orientation before submission.[62] The size, gross appearance, histology, microscopic depth, and involvement of the margins and ducts should be reported in detail.[62]

Preresection Sphincterotomy

The rationale for preresection pancreatic sphincterotomy is to allow easier access to the pancreatic duct after papillectomy. In one series of

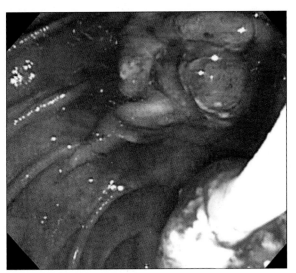

FIG 25.9 Specimen retrieval with a snare after en bloc papillectomy.

41 patients, preresection sphincterotomy and pancreatic duct stent placement were performed to reduce papillectomy-related adverse events and permit more aggressive treatment.[11] After pancreatic sphincterotomy, a 5-Fr, 5-cm long pancreatic duct stent was placed. Subsequent endoscopy was performed 1 month later and further thermal ablation was performed to treat residual adenomatous tissue with the stent still in place to protect against thermal injury.[11] The rationale proposed by those who favor performing preresection biliary sphincterotomy is that it allows a more complete excision by facilitating access to tissues in the biliary orifice and also increases the diagnostic accuracy before resection.[11,74] Despite these advantages, there are significant potential disadvantages, including increased risk of postsphincterotomy bleeding in ampullary adenomas.[75] However, postsphincterotomy bleeding occurred in only 1 of 41 patients who underwent preresection biliary sphincterotomy.[11] Other potential risks of preresection sphincterotomy include perforation or penetration of the duodenal wall, which may theoretically lead to tumor seeding if the lesion harbors malignancy.[75] However, no perforations occurred in the previously mentioned study, nor are there reports of tumor seeding in the literature. Probably the most important reason to consider avoiding a preresection sphincterotomy is the thermal and mechanical injury that affects precise histopathologic staging and the potential to miss foci of malignancy. Lastly, the presence of a stent in the pancreatic or bile duct may limit the ability to perform en bloc resection. At our institution, neither preresection sphincterotomy nor preresection stent placement is performed.

Postpapillectomy Sphincterotomy

After papillectomy, separate biliary and pancreatic duct orifices can usually be readily identified (Fig. 25.10). Mixing methylene blue with contrast during pancreatography before papillectomy or administering secretin after resection may facilitate identification of the ductal orifice when difficulty is encountered.[76] The role of prophylactic sphincterotomy to reduce the risk of adverse events such as cholangitis, pancreatitis, and papillary stenosis remains controversial. Sphincterotomy allows exposure of the distal biliary and pancreatic ducts, thereby occasionally allowing the detection of intraductal involvement that might have been missed on preresection ductography.[2] This benefit has to be weighed against the risks of bleeding and perforation. We perform postresection biliary and pancreatic sphincterotomies in patients with any suspicion for residual duct involvement, unless there is a concern for a risk of perforation.

Postpapillectomy Stents: Pancreatic and Biliary

Pancreatic duct stent placement has been shown to reduce the incidence of post-ERCP pancreatitis (PEP) when ERCP is performed in patients at high risk for this adverse event.[77–79] While there is only one, small randomized trial demonstrating the benefit of pancreatic duct stents after papillectomy,[80] there seems to be consensus that stents reduce the risk of postpapillectomy pancreatitis and perhaps papillary stenosis as well. Pancreatic stents of various diameters, lengths, and shapes have been used.[2,9,11,12,36,55,56,69] Some authors, however, advocate pancreatic stent placement only if delayed drainage of contrast is noted after papillectomy.[6,10,58,59] With selective placement of pancreatic stents, Norton et al.[64] found that PEP developed in 2/10 patients (20%) with pancreatic stent placement and 2/18 patients (11%) without a stent, but this difference was not statistically significant ($p > 0.5$), likely because of small sample sizes. The function of the minor duodenal papilla may affect the development of postpapillectomy pancreatitis.[52] In one study, a patent duct of Santorini identified at ERCP was protective of PEP and obviated the need for pancreatic duct stent placement after papillectomy.[63] In a larger study using 5-Fr to 7-Fr pancreatic stents, Catalano et al.[36] found a reduced rate of acute pancreatitis and papillary stenosis

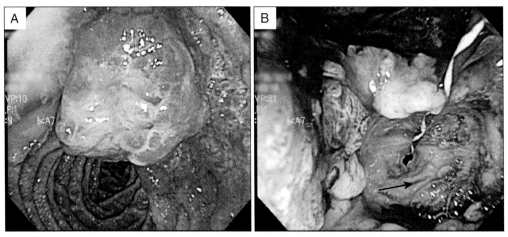

FIG 25.10 A, A large indurated ampullary adenoma with concern for malignancy (nonsurgical candidate). **B,** Postpapillectomy, separate entrances to bile duct (with a guidewire in it) and pancreatic duct *(arrow)* are easily seen.

in patients in whom a stent was placed (17% vs 3% for pancreatitis and 8% vs 3% for stenosis). However, no randomization was done and the total number of patients with adverse events of pancreatitis (5 of 103) and papillary stenosis (3 of 103) was small. Similarly, in a study by Cheng et al.[12] 4/41 patients (10%) developed pancreatitis when a single 3-Fr to 5-Fr stent was placed compared with 1/4 patients (25%) without stents. This difference was also not statistically significant (p = 0.33). Zadorova et al.[55] observed that postpapillectomy pancreatitis occurred in 0% and 20% of patients with and without a pancreatic stent, respectively. The only prospective randomized controlled trial of prophylactic pancreatic stent placement after endoscopic papillectomy was reported by Harewood et al.[70] Pancreatic stents (5 Fr) were placed immediately after papillectomy without performance of a pancreatic sphincterotomy. Pancreatitis developed in 3/19 patients (16%) in the nonstent group versus 0/10 patients in the stented group (p = 0.02). The study was terminated early because of the institutional review board's concerns about the risk of pancreatitis in the unstented group. An important point to note is that the number of patients enrolled was smaller than the intended 25 patients in each arm. Hence a single episode of pancreatitis in the stented group would have resulted in a nonsignificant p value.[81] Further larger-scale prospective studies are needed to prove conclusively that prophylactic pancreatic stent placement decreases adverse events after endoscopic papillectomy. Nonetheless, current data from difficult or complex ERCP and the bulk of the evidence support empiric pancreatic stent placement. As such, it is our practice to routinely place pancreatic stents in all patients undergoing papillectomy who do not have pancreas divisum (unless the adenoma arises from the minor papilla) (Fig. 25.11). The optimal duration of pancreatic stenting is unknown, but probably ranges from 2 to 7 days.[10,36,64] Because the main purpose of pancreatic stent placement is the prevention of postpapillectomy pancreatitis while minimizing stent-induced ductal change,[82] most endoscopists prefer to place a small-caliber stent (3-Fr stent without flaps) for the shortest duration possible.[9,12,84] An abdominal radiograph is obtained 2 to 4 weeks later to confirm spontaneous stent migration. A retained stent is removed endoscopically without the need for ductography.

In contrast to pancreatitis, cholangitis after endoscopic papillectomy is rare, resulting from the same pathogenesis as postpapillectomy pancreatitis.[9,36,64] Most authors do not routinely recommend biliary stent placement, although there have been occasional reports using plastic biliary stents (7 to 10 Fr) after endoscopic papillectomy.[9–11,56,58]

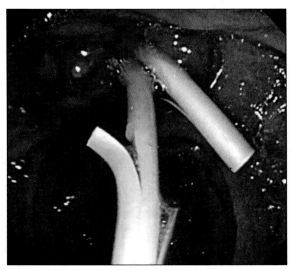

FIG 25.11 Bile duct stent placed in addition to routine placement of pancreatic duct stent because of poor drainage of contrast from biliary tree after endoscopic papillectomy.

If there is any doubt about the adequacy of contrast drainage after biliary sphincterotomy or if any adjunctive thermal therapy is performed, we place a 10-Fr biliary stent to reduce the risk of cholangitis and to prevent subsequent stenosis. After resection of large laterally spreading lesions, fully covered self-expandable metal stents (SEMS) may be better than plastic stents for a few theoretical reasons. SEMS may provide closure in the event of a microperforation. Radial expansion may provide tamponade, mitigating delayed bleeding to some degree (Fig. 25.12). Finally, a 10-mm stent results in distal duct dilation, facilitating direct endoscopic assessment of the biliary orifice at the time of subsequent surveillance.[83] Using SEMS in selected cases seems logical, and it is our practice to use them in the above setting. However, this has not been subjected to systematic study.

Adjunctive Therapy and Thermal Ablation

Although thermal ablation was initially used as a primary therapy with acceptable success,[65] it is now almost universally applied only as an adjunctive treatment. When used alone, thermal ablation precludes

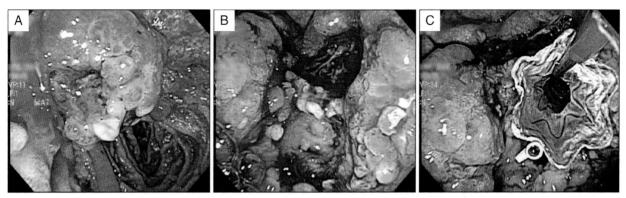

FIG 25.12 A, A large indurated ampullary adenoma with concern for malignancy (nonsurgical candidate). **B,** Postpapillectomy, given concern for depth of injury and some ongoing bleeding. **C,** A fully covered self-expandable metal stent is placed in the bile duct.

histopathologic evaluation and risks incomplete treatment. If residual tissue is identified that is not amenable to further snare resection or removal with biopsy forceps after papillectomy, adjunctive thermal ablation can be used.[12,64] In addition, thermal ablation can be used for hemostasis, palliation in patients with inoperable neoplasms, or intraductal extension in nonsurgical patients. Modalities to achieve adjunctive ablation include argon plasma coagulation (APC),[27,55,59,64,85] monopolar and bipolar coagulation,[11,59,64,85] photodynamic therapy (PDT),[86] neodymium:yttrium aluminum garnet (Nd:YAG) laser,[59,85,86] and most recently intraductal radiofrequency ablation (RFA).[87,88] A preliminary report using RFA to treat intraductal extension of adenoma (>1 cm) from three centers, including ours, found complete elimination of adenoma in 10/13 patients over a median follow-up of 16 months. Mild pancreatitis was noted in one patient, pancreatic stricture in one patient, and biliary stricture in three patients (all managed endoscopically).[89] The selection of adjuvant therapy depends on availability and the preference of individual endoscopists. Nd:YAG laser may cause deep tissue injury and is considered inferior to other modalities.[67] Adjunctive thermal ablation has not been consistently used or evaluated in most studies and there has been only one retrospective study evaluating its efficacy. The overall success rates were similar between patients who had thermal ablation and those who did not (81% vs 78%). However, there was a nonstatistically significant lower recurrence rate in patients treated with thermal ablation.[36]

We use a 7-Fr APC probe for visible residual adenomatous tissue after snare excision at a power of 40 to 60 W and a flow rate of 0.8 to 1 L/min, and have used RFA at a setting of 10 W for 90 seconds in inoperable patients with intraductal extension. We also routinely place pancreatic and biliary stents before or after any thermal ablation, especially if therapy is applied close to the papilla, to protect the pancreatic and biliary epithelia and reduce the risk of stenosis.

Postpapillectomy Surveillance

Surveillance duodenoscopy and ERCP apply predominantly to ampullary adenomas, but the same principle can be used to monitor for recurrences of rare nonadenomatous lesions. Final histopathology and sporadic adenomas versus adenomas associated with FAP are the two main determinants of follow-up care. In a study by Heidecke et al.[30] the impact of the grade of dysplasia on prognosis was assessed. There was an increased risk of postoperative recurrence and development of invasive carcinoma in adenomas with high-grade dysplasia, whereas no recurrences were observed in the low-grade dysplasia group.[30] If final histopathology reveals high-grade dysplasia (previously known as carcinoma in situ), additional surgery should be considered.[30] However, in patients who are poor surgical candidates or who refuse surgery, close follow-up with periodic ERCP and biopsy may be sufficient.[67]

Duodenoscopy should be performed with multiple biopsies from the papillectomy site, even in the absence of macroscopic recurrence. We recommend performing ductography at least during the first one to two follow-ups, especially if there was evidence of intraductal involvement at final histopathology. There have been rare reports of late intraductal lesions that developed in the absence of a local recurrence at the ampulla.[9] There are no standard guidelines regarding appropriate postpapillectomy surveillance intervals, but some authors have provided recommendations. In general, small (<3 cm) adenomas with clean resection margins are reevaluated at 3 months. Once there is a biopsy-proven lack of residual adenoma, follow-up endoscopy is undertaken at 6-month to 12-month intervals for at least 2 years and then as clinically needed.[9–12,36] In patients with FAP, a similar protocol is followed, and after 2 years without recurrence further surveillance is performed based on the duodenal polyp burden, but no more than every 1 to 2 years.[9,36,59] For large (>3 cm) adenomas excised piecemeal and for lesions with positive resection margins, repeat papillectomy with possible thermal ablation and ductography should be performed every 2 to 3 months until biopsy-proven eradication is established.[9–11,36] Subsequently, follow-up duodenoscopy with biopsies and ERCP should be performed every 6 months for a minimum of 2 years. Surgery should be strongly considered for intraductal tumor extension found on subsequent follow-up.

INDICATIONS AND CONTRAINDICATIONS (BOX 25.2)

Careful patient selection in centers with substantial experience with pancreaticobiliary disease is a prerequisite for successful endoscopic papillectomy. Indications for endoscopic papillectomy are the collection of features that can predict complete removal of adenomas while minimizing procedure-related morbidity. These are not yet fully established and at this time are individualized based on the patient's preference, general health, lesion characteristics, association with FAP, and local expertise. Patient selection criteria have varied among studies, but in general the following features have been considered important:

1. Biopsies showing no evidence of malignancy (usually at least 6 biopsies).[10]
2. Maximum size for endoscopic resectability. Binmoeller et al.[10] suggested 4 cm and Cheng et al.[12] suggested 4.5 cm. Desilets et al.[11] and

BOX 25.2   Indications and Contraindications

- In general, endoscopic papillectomy is indicated in patients with benign ampullary lesions without evidence of intraductal involvement.
- Endoscopic papillectomy may be considered in patients with high-grade dysplasia or intramucosal cancer, intraductal involvement, or early invasive cancer (pT1) who are not surgical candidates or who refuse surgery.
- Endoscopic papillectomy should be performed by appropriately trained and experienced endoscopists because of the potential for serious adverse events.
- Contraindications to papillectomy include metastases, invasive cancer, and advanced intraductal involvement. Patients unwilling to undergo postpapillectomy surveillance should be advised against undergoing the procedure.
- With improving techniques and increasing experience, indications for endoscopic papillectomy may be expanded or modified.

BOX 25.3   Adverse Events

- Adverse events occur commonly (average 22%) but are usually mild, and most are managed nonoperatively. They include acute pancreatitis, bleeding, cholangitis, perforation, and stenosis of the pancreaticobiliary orifices.
- Death as a result of endoscopic papillectomy is very rare but may be underreported.

BOX 25.4   Controversies

- Given the lack of randomized controlled studies comparing endoscopic papillectomy to local surgical resection and pancreaticoduodenectomy, the optimal treatment for ampullary adenomas is based on multiple factors, including local expertise. Some of this controversy stems from the limited ability of biopsies alone to detect foci of malignancy in ampullary adenomas.
- Some authors propose using endoscopic ultrasonography for staging all ampullary adenomas, whereas others use it more selectively. There are no available studies that compare outcomes of one approach to another. The role of intraductal endoscopic ultrasonography remains unclear at this time.
- Several opinions and controversies exist on the technique of papillectomy, including the use of submucosal injection, thermal ablation, sphincterotomy, and prophylactic biliary stent placement.
- The optimal strategy for postpapillectomy surveillance is unknown.

Irani et al.[9] suggest half the duodenal circumference. In some studies a maximum size for resectability has not been mentioned.[36,56]

3. Endoscopic characteristics of the lesion suggesting benignity. Most authors have been consistent and include lesions with well-defined margins that are not friable, ulcerated, or indurated and are soft on probing as features indicative of noninvasive lesions.[2,9–12,36]

4. Intraductal involvement on EUS or ERCP. Some authors found any ductal involvement a contraindication for endoscopic papillectomy,[10] whereas others have allowed some intraductal extension up to 1 cm.[2,9,58] Minimal intraductal extension does not seem to be an absolute contraindication for endoscopic papillectomy because the tumor can be exposed and resected completely after sphincterotomy or with a balloon sweep. A potential option for treatment of intraductal extension >1 cm may be intraductal biliary RFA.[87,88,89]

The three absolute contraindications for endoscopic papillectomy at this time are obvious metastases, invasive cancer beyond the mucosa, and intraductal extension that cannot be fully exposed with a sphincterotomy or with balloon/double snare extraction techniques (usually ≥1 cm into the duct). Relative contraindications include tumor size greater than 4 to 5 cm, early/T1 cancers, poor patient compliance with follow-up, and lack of expertise with pancreaticobiliary endoscopy. It is worth noting that these inclusion and exclusion criteria may be modified as endoscopic techniques and novel diagnostic modalities improve. Papillary adenomas up to 7 cm in diameter[55] and lesions with intraductal growth up to 1 cm[2,9,58] have been successfully managed endoscopically. Although previous studies suggest that up to 50% of T1 ampullary cancers may have lymph node involvement at the time of pancreaticoduodenectomy, a handful of such cases have also been successfully treated endoscopically.[90–97] In the largest series to date on 15 patients with T1 ampullary cancers, Petrone et al.[93] reported a success rate of 57% at a mean follow-up of 34 months. No tumor-related deaths were seen in patients when cancer infiltration depth was <4 mm.

ADVERSE EVENTS AND THEIR MANAGEMENT (BOXES 25.3 AND 25.4)

Overall adverse events based on some of the larger endoscopic papillectomy series (Table 25.1) average approximately 22% (range 10% to 58%) and can be classified as early (pancreatitis, bleeding, perforation, cholangitis) and late (papillary stenosis).[36,66,98,99] Procedure-related mortality is very low, averaging 0.03% (range 0% to 7%). The most commonly reported adverse events are postpapillectomy bleeding (10%) and mild to moderate pancreatitis (10%). Perforation,[35,41] cholangitis,[9,58,61] and papillary stenosis[37,41] are much less common. Most pancreatitis is mild to moderate and is managed conservatively. In the two reported deaths caused by severe necrotizing pancreatitis, attempted pancreatic stent placement failed in both.[58,98] In a prospective study of 25 FAP patients who underwent endoscopic papillectomy with adjunctive thermal ablation, 15% developed pancreatitis despite stent placement.[100] Patients with FAP and those with adenocarcinoma may have higher adverse event rates.[9] Immediate bleeding can be controlled with endoscopic epinephrine injection, electrocautery, or clip placement. Delayed bleeding may require blood transfusion. Embolization is rarely required.[9] Applying clips through a duodenoscope is technically challenging owing to the angulation at the end of the working channel. It is important to keep the elevator down when opening the clip (thus opening the clip blindly), lift the elevator to bring the opened clip into view for proper positioning, and then bring the elevator down again when deploying the clip (again blindly).

Duodenal perforations have been reported in 14 patients.[9,12,56,64] All but one patient (successful surgical repair)[9] improved with conservative management alone consisting of bowel rest, biliary and pancreatic stent placement, and administration of antibiotics for 5 to 10 days. Two authors described clip closure of perforations (Fig. 25.13).[9,64] Cholangitis is rare after papillectomy and easily managed with antibiotics and ERCP with extension of sphincterotomy and/or biliary stent placement.[9,58,61] Stenosis of the pancreatic and biliary orifices is a late adverse event that may occur weeks to years after papillectomy.[9,64–66,98] In one study it occurred more frequently when short-term pancreatic duct stents were not placed (15.4% vs 1.1%).[36] Treatment is endoscopic sphincterotomy and balloon dilation with or without stent placement. There was one patient in the above series who required surgical sphincteroplasty because of failed endoscopic cannulation.[9,12,36,64]

TABLE 25.1   Adverse Events Related to Endoscopic Papillectomy as Reported in Larger Published Series

Reference	N	Bleeding, n (%)	Pancreatitis, n (%)	Perforation, n (%)	Cholangitis, n (%)	Papillary Stricture, n (%)	Overall Morbidity, n (%)	Mortality, n (%)
Binmoeller et al.[10]	25	2 (8)	3 (12)	0	0	0	5 (20)	0
Fukushima et al.[104]	31	4 (13)	4 (13)	0	0	0	8 (26)	0
Norton et al.[64]	26	0	4 (15)	1 (4)	0	2 (8)	7 (27)	0
Bohnacker et al.[2]	106	18 (21)	11 (13)	0	0	0	29 (34)	0
Catalano et al.[36]	103	2 (2)	5 (5)	0	0	3 (3)	10 (10)	0
Cheng et al.[12]	55	4 (7)	5 (9)	1 (2)	0	2 (4)	12 (22)	0
Kahaleh et al.[58]	56	2 (4)	4 (7)	0	1 (2)	0	7 (13)	1 (2) (pancreatitis)
Hirooka et al.[61]	60	8 (13)	6 (10)	0	2 (3)	0	16 (26)	0
Han et al.[62]	33	6 (18)	0	1 (3)	1 (3)	3 (9)	11 (33)	0
Irani et al.[9]	102	5 (5)	10 (10)	2 (2)	1 (1)	3 (3)	21 (21)	0
Ridtitid et al.[66]	151	23 (13)	7 (4)	3 (2)	0	3 (2)	41 (22)	1 (0.5) (myocardial infarction)
Napoleon et al.[98]	79 (110 procedures)	11 (10)	22 (20)	4 (4)	5 (5)	2 (2)	39 (35)	1 (1) (pancreatitis)
Ismail et al.[99]	61	6 (10)	4 (7)	2 (3)	0	0	12 (19)	0
TOTAL	888	91 (10)	85 (10)	14 (1.5)	10 (1)	18 (2)	218 (25)	3 (0.3)

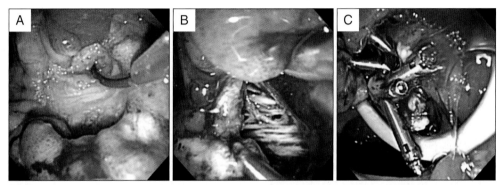

FIG 25.13 Endoscopic closure of postpapillectomy perforation. **A,** Deep defect identified after papillectomy with wire access into bile duct. **B,** Obvious separation of circular fibers of the muscularis propria. **C,** Multiple clips were placed to approximate the perforation after stent placement.

SUCCESS

Complete tumor eradication rates based on some of the larger published series average more than 80% (range 46% to 92%) (Table 25.2; Fig. 25.14). Because of the lack of consensus on the definition of "success" after endoscopic papillectomy, it is difficult to compare outcomes among studies. Conventionally, success may be defined as complete resection of the adenoma with endoscopic papillectomy. However, success can be defined as complete eradication despite the need for additional thermal ablation for positive margins or treatment of residual tissue, regardless of the number of sessions required. There are several factors that affect the success rate. Catalano et al.[36] found the following factors to be associated with successful outcome: age >48 years, male gender, size of lesion <2.4 cm, and sporadic lesions compared with adenomas associated with FAP (86% vs 67%). Bohnacker et al.[2] found comparable recurrence rates between patients with and without intraductal extension (14% vs 15%); however, the long-term success rate was significantly higher in the group without intraductal involvement (83% vs 46%, p < 0.001). We[9] found that lesions <2 cm and absence of dilated ducts were associated with successful outcomes. Kahaleh et al.[58] failed to identify any factors (age, size, EUS stage, or "lifting sign") to be predictive of successful endoscopic resection. More recently, Ridtitid et al.[66] found that jaundice, intraductal extension at ERCP, adenocarcinoma on final histology, and failure to perform en bloc resection were associated with a high failure rate. There is also a lack of consensus on the definitions of "recurrence" and "residual tissue," with some authors choosing not to differentiate the two. Some authors consider adenomatous tissue found on biopsy 3 months after papillectomy a recurrence, whereas others consider this residual tissue. Recurrent or residual ampullary adenoma after endoscopic papillectomy averages around 12% (range 0% to 33%). Most recurrences are usually benign and can be treated by further endoscopic therapy,[2,9,12,36,55,64] though some intraductal recurrences require surgical management.[2,9,69]

RELATIVE COST SAVINGS

Although direct cost and outcome comparisons between surgical and endoscopic resection of ampullary adenomas are lacking, indirect comparisons can be made (Table 25.3). The mean duration of hospital stay after surgical local resection ranges from 11 to 13 days and 15 to

TABLE 25.2 **Outcomes of Endoscopic Papillectomy for Ampullary Adenomas as Reported in Larger Published Series**

Reference	N	FAP	Endoscopic Success (%)	Incomplete Resection	Recurrence (%)	Malignant Foci (%)	Need for Surgery (%)	Mean Follow-Up (Months)	Mean Number of Procedures
Binmoeller et al.[10]	25	NA	23 of 25 (92)	2	6 of 23 (26)	0	3 (12)	37	1.1
Bohnacker et al.[2]	93	6	74 of 93 (73)	13	15 of 93 (17)	9 (10)	8 (9)	43	1.5
Catalano et al.[36]	103	31	83 of 103 (81)	20	10 of 103 (10)	6 (6)	16 (16)	36	1.8
Cheng et al.[12]	55	14	39 of 55 (71)	0	9 of 27 (33)	7 (13)	4 (7)	30	1.3
Hirooka et al.[61]	60	NA	49 of 60 (82)	11	1 of 60 (2)	NA	2 (3)	60	NA
Han et al.[62]	33	NA	20 of 33 (61)	13	2 of 29 (6)	3 (9)	2 (7)	8	NA
Irani et al.[9]	102	17	86 of 102 (84)	14	14 of 102 (8)	8 (8)	16 (16)	35	1.4
Ridtitid et al.[66]	151	29	91 of 107 (85)	44 of 151	16 of 107 (15)	12 (8)	44 of 151 (29)	23	NA
Napoleon et al.[98]	79 (110 procedures)	21	64 of 79 (81)	6	6 of 79 (8)	13 (16)	14 (18)	36	NA
Ismail et al.[99]	61	16	46 of 61 (75)	5	5 of 51 (10)	10 (16)	15 (25)	14	NA
TOTAL	888	134 of 770 (17)	575 of 718 (80)	128 (14)	84 of 677 (12)	68 (8)	124 (14)	32	

FAP, Familial adenomatous polyposis; *NA,* not applicable.

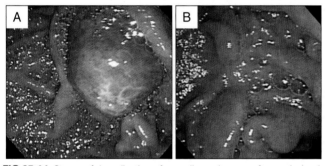

FIG 25.14 Successful eradication of ampullary adenoma after endoscopic papillectomy. **A,** A 2-cm ampullary adenoma. **B,** The same lesion 3 months after endoscopic papillectomy showing no residual tumor.

TABLE 25.3 **Comparison of Outcomes Between Endoscopic Papillectomy, Surgical Local Resection (LR), and Pancreaticoduodenectomy (PD) for Adenomas of the Ampulla of Vater**

	Endoscopic Papillectomy	Surgical LR	PD
Recurrence rate	70 of 573 (16%)	15 of 117 (26%)	0 of 31 (0%)
Morbidity	144 of 651 (22%)	22 of 80 (29%)	8 of 31 (26%)
Mortality	2 of 651 (0.03%)	3 of 117 (0.03%)	4 of 31 (13%)
Duration of hospital stay	0–2 days	1–3 weeks	2–4 weeks
Need for endoscopic surveillance	Yes	Yes	No
Need for laparotomy	No	Yes	Yes

23 days after pancreaticoduodenectomy.[17,19] By comparison, endoscopic papillectomy is usually performed as an outpatient procedure using moderate sedation, with an observation period of 2 to 24 hours. As mentioned previously, the rates of morbidity and mortality after endoscopic papillectomy are significantly lower than those after surgical alternatives, with recurrence rates similar to or better than surgical local resection. Complete eradication after endoscopic papillectomy is achieved in >80% of patients, with the mean number of procedures to achieve eradication <2 (range of 1.2 to 2.7 procedures per patient), which still translates to substantial savings compared with surgery. Finally, in patients with FAP, where recurrence rates are high even after surgical local resection,[47] patients require lifelong surveillance for duodenal polyps.

SUBEPITHELIAL LESIONS

Subepithelial tumors arising from the major or minor duodenal papilla are extraordinarily rare. These are similar to the subepithelial tumors found in other locations in the gastrointestinal tract and include neuroendocrine tumors (carcinoids), lipomas, leiomyomas, gastrointestinal stromal tumors, lymphangiomas, fibromas, and hamartomas (Fig. 25.15). Of these, the most frequent are neuroendocrine tumors, accounting for 0.3% of all gastrointestinal carcinoids.[101] Neuroendocrine tumors of the ampulla of Vater are very rarely hormonally active.[102] Cholestasis is the presenting symptom in 55% of patients[103]; endoscopic biopsies are often not diagnostic, and EUS is the primary modality used for locoregional staging.[48,105] Cross-sectional imaging and somatostatin receptor scintigraphy can be useful. Pancreaticoduodenectomy has been recommended by some authors for all ampullary neuroendocrine tumors regardless of size, given that metastases have been discovered in some patients with small lesions.[102,103,106,107] However, given the significant morbidity and mortality associated with

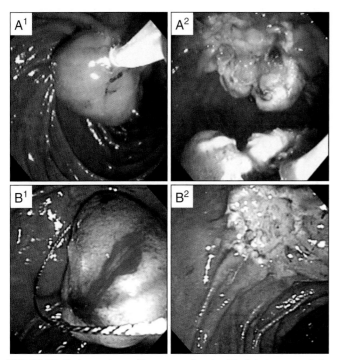

FIG 25.15 Endoscopic papillectomy of subepithelial tumors of the ampulla. **A1,** Endoscopic resection of a 2.5-cm ampullary neuroendocrine tumor in a patient who refused pancreaticoduodenectomy. **A2,** Papillectomy site after en bloc resection of the same lesion. **B1,** Endoscopic removal of a bleeding ampullary gangliocytic paraganglioma. **B2,** Papillectomy site after en bloc resection of the same lesion. Neither lesion has recurred in more than 3 years of follow-up.

pancreaticoduodenectomy[108] and data that demonstrate long-term disease-free survival and safety of surgical local resection,[109,110] endoscopic excision has been proposed as a preferred method in patients with medical comorbidities, advanced age, or tumor size <1 cm,[109-111] as tumors larger than 1 cm have a greater propensity to metastasize.[112-114] Follow-up endoscopy is recommended 2 to 3 months later to ensure complete resection in these patients. We follow a similar surveillance protocol as for adenomatous lesions and, depending on the grade of the tumor, consider surveillance beyond 2 years as well. CT or MRI should be considered to rule out development of adenopathy 1 to 2 years postresection.

There are rare case reports[115-116] of ampullary Peutz-Jeghers hamartomas treated with local surgical resection and two reports of successful endoscopic papillectomy.[117,118] Because of their premalignant potential, follow-up endoscopic surveillance is recommended and should be individualized according to the tumor histology, resection margins, and patient comorbidities.

Gangliocytic paragangliomas of the ampulla of Vater are very rare tumors and occur in middle-aged men, often presenting with gastrointestinal bleeding and abdominal pain.[119,120-123] Although thought to be benign, metastatic lymphadenopathy, bile duct infiltration, and the need for radiation therapy have been reported.[119,124] There are several case reports and a case series of successful endoscopic resection of these lesions.[117,123,125-129]

Adverse events after the endoscopic resection of subepithelial ampullary lesions are unknown, although they should be similar to those occurring after endoscopic papillectomy for ampullary adenomas.

SUMMARY

Although endoscopic resection of potentially curable ampullary lesions is increasingly being performed, significant discretion in patient selection should be exercised. Clinicians should be cognizant of the possibility of false-negative results on the endoscopic biopsy specimens and the risk of procedural and postprocedural adverse events. Surgery is recommended for treatment of operative patients who have lesions that harbor invasive cancer. Finally, long-term follow-up is essential in all patients with endoscopically resected benign tumors to exclude residual disease, recurrence, and progression to cancer.

The complete reference list for this chapter can be found online at www.experconsult.com.

26

Pancreatoscopy

Tadashi Kodama and Tatsuya Koshitani

Peroral pancreatoscopy, in which a small-caliber fiberscope ("baby scope") is inserted into the pancreatic duct from the papilla through the working channel of a duodenoscope ("mother scope"), was first described by Japanese investigators Takagi and Takegoshi[1] in 1974. Although the idea was very attractive and several investigators studied its feasibility, pancreatoscopy was not widely adopted because of poor visibility and instrument fragility, as well as the relatively large diameter of the instrument compared with the pancreatic duct. The description of intraductal papillary mucinous neoplasm (IPMN) by another group of Japanese investigators, Ohashi et al.,[2] made an impact on pancreatoscopy in the early 1980s. This tumor was characterized by mucin secretion with a patulous papilla and a dilated pancreatic duct and was a good indication for pancreatoscopy. Since then, pancreatoscopy has been reassessed as a useful modality for the diagnosis of IPMN showing characteristic endoscopic findings.

Two types of fiberoptic pancreatoscopes were mainly used in previous studies. One is a thin fiberscope (diameter 3.1 to 3.7 mm) that has two-way tip deflection and a working channel. Biopsies can be taken under direct vision, but pancreatic sphincterotomy is usually needed for endoscope insertion because of its large diameter. To insert the scope into a nondilated pancreatic duct, an ultrathin pancreatoscope (diameter 0.75 to 0.8 mm) was also developed by decreasing the number of optical fibers. This scope can be inserted via a standard endoscopic retrograde cholangiopancreatography (ERCP) cannula without the need for sphincterotomy; however, neither tip deflection nor a working channel is present. Cytology sampling and injection of saline were performed through the outer cannula. These fiberscopes suffered the same problem of poor visibility, contingent on the number of optical bundles.

Several recent developments have rekindled interest in pancreatoscopy. The first is the emergence of video (electronic) pancreatoscopes, first made by our group with the development of a miniature charge-coupled device (CCD) video chip in 1999.[3] Video pancreatoscopes provide drastically improved resolution of images of the pancreatic duct compared with those obtained using fiberoptic pancreatoscopes (Fig. 26.1). This development has led to pancreatoscopy with adjunct imaging techniques such as narrow-band imaging (NBI). The second is the development of the SpyGlass Direct Visualization System. This single-operator cholangio-pancreatoscopy system was first applied to the biliary tree in 2006.[4] The external diameter (10.5 Fr) of the current miniscope is greater than that of most normal pancreatic ducts and may limit pancreatic applications. However, SpyGlass pancreatoscopy has been applied in the investigation of the dilated pancreatic duct (see Chapter 37) with IPMN and in endo-therapy for pancreatic stones in selected patients with chronic pancreatitis (see Chapter 55).

EQUIPMENT AND TECHNIQUE

Video Pancreatoscope

At present, Olympus Medical Systems Co. (Tokyo, Japan) offers two types of video pancreatoscopes in Japanese markets. The first type (CHF-BP260) is a thin scope with a 2.6-mm outer diameter and a 0.5-mm working channel. The second type (CHF-B260) is a larger scope with a 3.4-mm outer diameter and a 1.2-mm working channel that permits use of a 0.035-inch guidewire, a 3-Fr biopsy forceps, and an electrohydraulic or laser lithotripsy probe (Fig. 26.2). These scopes use a field sequential imaging system and can be passed through the 4.2-mm working channel of a therapeutic duodenoscope. In the United States these video pancreatoscopes are not commercially available, and only the use of a prototype digital pancreatoscope (CHF-Y0002B; Olympus) is reported.[5] The specifications of available fiberoptic and video pancreatoscopes are compared in Table 26.1. All baby scopes require a dedicated light source and image processor. Both video pancreatoscopes (CHF-BP260, B260) can be used with a processor (CV-260SL/CV-290; Olympus) for NBI examinations. The baby scope image is projected onto a separate video monitor (Fig. 26.3).

Two-Operator "Mother–Baby" Method

Peroral pancreatoscopy is performed during ERCP, usually with the patient in the prone position. Using a two-operator method, one endoscopist operates the mother duodenoscope and the other operates the baby scope (Fig. 26.4). The duodenoscope is positioned at the ampulla and the baby scope is inserted through the working channel of the duodenoscope. A prior pancreatic sphincterotomy or balloon sphincteroplasty is typically needed when inserting a relatively large pancreatoscope. Intubation with the baby scope is performed by the endoscopist who operates the duodenoscope. Given that the baby scope is fragile at the bending part of its tip, care is taken to advance the baby scope with the elevator of the duodenoscope when maximally opened. For baby scopes equipped with a 1.2-mm working channel, inserting the baby scope over a guidewire reduces the need for elevator use and minimizes the risk of scope damage. Alternatively, for baby scopes with a 0.5-mm working channel, the scope must be inserted directly into the pancreatic duct.

Once in the pancreatic duct, the baby scope can be advanced deeply under both direct endoscopic and fluoroscopic guidance. The torturous pancreas head is the most difficult part to pass. The baby scope is mainly steered by the endoscopist handling the duodenoscope, while repositioning the duodenoscope relative to the papilla. The endoscopist handling the baby scope can fine-tune the view using tip deflection. Water irrigation is usually needed to optimize visualization. Protein plugs in the

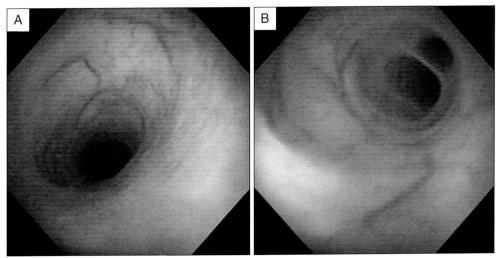

FIG 26.1 Video pancreatoscopic images of the pancreatic duct in a normal subject. Fine capillary vessels are clearly visualized on the surface of the pancreatic duct. (**A,** From Kodama T, Sato H, Horii Y, et al. Pancreatoscopy for the next generation: development of the peroral electronic pancreatoscope system. *Gastrointest Endosc.* 1999;49:366–371. **B,** From Kodama T, Koshitani T, Sato H, et al. Electronic pancreatoscopy for the diagnosis of pancreatic diseases. *Am J Gastroenterol.* 2002;97:617–622.)

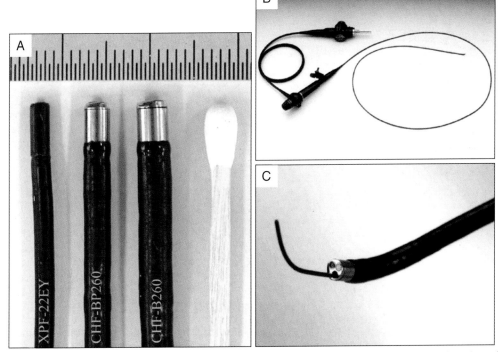

FIG 26.2 **A,** Comparison of the outer diameters of various types of video pancreatoscopes. **B,** Overview of the 3.4-mm video pancreatoscope (CHF-B260; Olympus, Tokyo, Japan). **C,** Distal tip of the same model (note the accessory channel).

pancreatic duct may impair visualization and need to be irrigated with sterile saline solution. Intravenous secretin (100 units) has been used to stimulate pancreatic juice flow in an effort to improve visualization of the pancreatic duct.[6] To facilitate insertion of accessories such as biopsy forceps or a lithotripsy probe, the elevator of the duodenoscope needs to be relaxed and the angulation of both the duodenoscope and the baby scope reduced.

Single-Operator Cholangiopancreatoscopy

The SpyGlass Direct Visualization System (Boston Scientific, Marlborough, MA), although only recently developed, has been applied for pancreatoscopy. The first-generation system had a 10-Fr disposable four-lumen catheter (SpyScope, now called Spy Legacy) containing a 0.9-mm channel for the SpyGlass fiberoptic probe, a 1.2-mm instrumentation channel, and two dedicated 0.6-mm irrigation channels. The current

TABLE 26.1   Specifications of Available Fiberoptic and Video Pancreatoscopes and Single-Operator Cholagiopancreatoscopy Systems

	Imaging System	Tip Diameter (mm)	Working Channel (mm)	Tip Deflection (Degrees)	Field of View (Degrees)
CHF-BP30 (Olympus)	Fiberoptic	3.1	1.2	2-way, 160/130	90
FCP-9P (Pentax)	Fiberoptic	3.0	1.2	2-way, 90/90	90
CHF-BP260* (Olympus)	Video (field sequential)	2.6	0.5	2-way, 70/70	90
CHF-B260* (Olympus)	Video (field sequential)	3.4	1.2	2-way, 70/70	90
SpyGlass DS (Boston Scientific)	Video	3.4	1.2/0.6/0.6	4-way, 30/30/30/30	70

*Not commercially available in the United States.

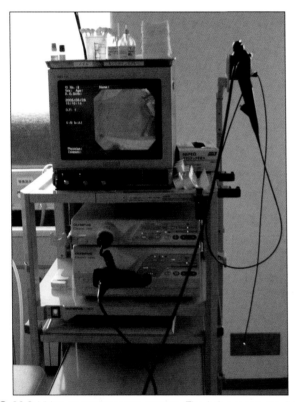

FIG 26.3 Video pancreatoscopy system. The baby scope requires a dedicated light source, image processor, and separate video monitor.

system has two light-emitting diode lights on the catheter tip and a single complementary metal-oxide semiconductor chip for imaging that provides improved resolution (×4) and a 60% wider field of view than the first-generation system.[7] The SpyScope catheter has four-way tip deflection (each more than 30 degrees), is strapped to the duodenoscope just below the operating channel, and is operated by a single endoscopist (see Table 26.1) (Fig. 26.5).

The SpyScope is inserted through the 4.2-mm working channel of a therapeutic duodenoscope. In most cases, a small pancreatic sphincterotomy is required to insert the scope into the pancreatic duct. The SpyScope is usually inserted over the guidewire under combined fluoroscopic and visual guidance. The clarity of the luminal visual field improves significantly with water irrigation via two dedicated irrigation channels connected to the irrigation pump. Intermittent sterile saline irrigation at the minimal setting is recommended for pancreatic use. Biopsy specimens can be obtained using the 3-Fr SpyBite forceps under direct visualization. The 1.2-mm working channel of the SpyScope also allows insertion of an electrohydraulic or laser lithotripsy probe for stone fragmentation under direct vision.

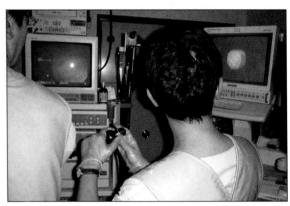

FIG 26.4 Two-operator method. A second endoscopist operates the baby scope.

Other Techniques

Direct peroral pancreatoscopy has been recently described for investigation of the markedly dilated pancreatic duct in patients with IPMN.

Ultraslim gastroscopes (diameter 4.9 or 5.0 mm) are used, employing two different techniques. In the first technique an overtube for balloon enteroscopy can be used to prevent loop formation in the stomach during insertion of the ultraslim gastroscope (GIF-N260; Olympus) over a guidewire positioned in the main pancreatic duct. The overtube is punctured at 70 cm from the distal tip to allow passage of the ultraslim gastroscope.[8] In the second technique a 5-Fr anchoring balloon catheter is inflated in the main pancreatic duct and an ultraslim gastroscope (GIF-XP260N; Olympus) advanced directly through the major papilla into the pancreatic duct assisted by the intraductal balloon catheter. NBI and forceps biopsy can be performed.[9]

DIAGNOSTIC INDICATIONS

Intraductal Papillary Mucinous Neoplasm

IPMN is a premalignant or malignant tumor of the pancreas that is characterized by mucin secretion.[2] The tumor spreads along the pancreatic duct, replacing the normal epithelium, and includes a broad spectrum of histopathologic disorders such as hyperplasia, adenoma, and adenocarcinoma.[10] IPMNs are usually classified into three types: main duct, branch duct, and mixed type, according to the site and extent of involvement. IPMN is the best indication for pancreatoscopy because of the patulous papilla and dilated pancreatic duct (Fig. 26.6).[11,12] In patients with IPMN and equivocal radiographic findings, pancreatoscopy may provide valuable information for the differential diagnosis of amorphous filling defects in the main pancreatic duct and may allow a definite diagnosis to be obtained based on the characteristic appearance of papillary tumors. Biopsies can be taken from abnormal-appearing

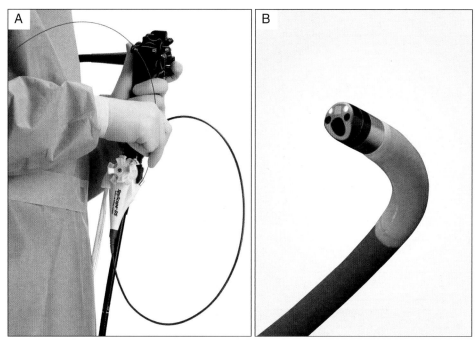

FIG 26.5 Single-operator cholangiopancreatoscopy system. **A,** The SpyScope strapped to the duodenoscope just below the operating channel is operated by a single endoscopist. **B,** Distal tip of the SpyScope (note an instrumentation channel and two dedicated irrigation channels).

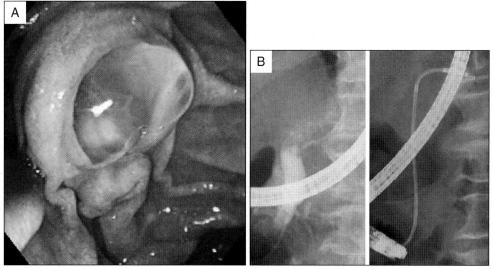

FIG 26.6 Observation of main duct–type intraductal papillary mucinous neoplasm. **A,** A patulous ampullary orifice with mucus secretion. **B,** A dilated main pancreatic duct with filling defects on ERCP. A pancreatoscope was easily inserted into the pancreatic duct.

mucosal lesions under direct visualization when a larger pancreatoscope with a working channel is used. Pancreatoscopy may provide valuable information in assessing the location and extent of IPMN in order to select the best surgical procedure (Fig. 26.7 and Video 26.1; Fig. 26.8 and Video 26.2).

Current data suggest that fiberoptic pancreatoscopy and video pancreatoscopy successfully identify ductal lesions in 67% to 83% of patients with IPMN.[13–16] This diagnostic rate is comparable to that of endoscopic ultrasonography (EUS) and ERCP and is significantly better than that of transabdominal ultrasonography (US) and computed tomography (CT), but less than that of intraductal ultrasonography (IDUS). In a series[13] of 31 patients with surgically resected IPMN, detection rates were compared among various imaging techniques. The detection rates for papillary tumorous lesions of ≥3 mm in maximum height (adenocarcinoma) were 29% with transabdominal US, 21% with CT, 86% with EUS, 100% with IDUS, and 83% with pancreatoscopy.

Differentiating malignant from benign IPMN with pancreatoscopy may be challenging. In a series[15] of 60 patients with surgically resected IPMN, findings of pancreatoscopy and IDUS were compared with histopathology of resected specimens. Fish-egg–like protrusions with vascular images, villous protrusions, and vegetative protrusions were

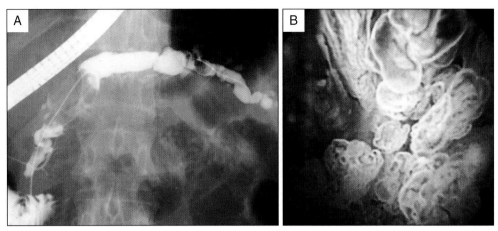

FIG 26.7 A case of main duct–type intraductal papillary mucinous neoplasm (adenocarcinoma). **A,** Endoscopic retrograde pancreatography. The main pancreatic duct was dilated, with an amorphous filling defect at the pancreas head. **B,** Video pancreatoscopic image. Villous tumors with dilation of capillary vessels were observed corresponding to the filling defect.

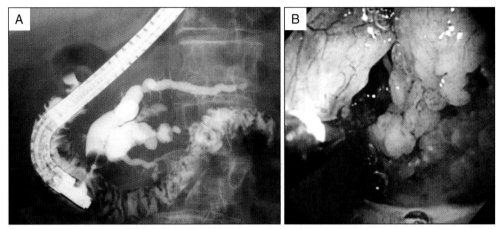

FIG 26.8 Branch duct–type intraductal papillary mucinous neoplasm (adenoma). **A,** Endoscopic retrograde pancreatography. The main pancreatic duct was dilated with a cystic dilation of the branch duct at the pancreas head. **B,** Video pancreatoscopic image. Papillary tumors were clearly visualized inside the branch duct and tumor biopsy was undertaken under direct vision.

considered to be malignant on pancreatoscopy. With these criteria, the sensitivity, specificity, and accuracy of pancreatoscopy in differentiating malignant from benign IPMN were 65%, 88%, and 75%, respectively. When the pancreatoscopic findings were combined with IDUS findings of diagnosing lesions protruding ≥4 mm to be malignant, the sensitivity, specificity, and accuracy improved to 91%, 82%, and 88%, respectively.

Introducing enhanced digital imaging, such as addition of NBI, to the miniscope is an encouraging area of investigation. Video pancreatoscopy combined with NBI provided high-contrast imaging of the pancreatic duct and the fine surface structure of IPMN. Furthermore, it provided excellent visualization of vascular patterns and tumor vessels that are harbingers of malignancy.[17,18]

In a prospective study[19] of 44 patients with suspected IPMN investigated by single-operator pancreatoscopy, the targeted region of the pancreatic duct was reached in 41 patients. Of 17 patients with a final diagnosis of main duct IPMN and 9 patients with branch duct IPMN, 76% and 78% were correctly identified by pancreatoscopy, respectively. Single-operator pancreatoscopy was found to have provided additional diagnostic information in the vast majority of the cases and to affect clinical decision making in 76%.

Diffuse or multifocal lesions have been described in 7% to 54% of IPMN cases.[20] Appropriate surgical treatment of such pancreatic lesions can be challenging in the face of preoperative imaging limitations. Several investigators[20,21] reported that intraoperative pancreatoscopy was effective for determining the resection line of the pancreas during surgery for IPMN.

Indeterminate Pancreatic Duct Strictures (Benign or Malignant)

EUS has a high diagnostic yield in identifying pancreatic masses that may not be detected by noninvasive imaging. The addition of fine-needle aspiration (FNA) capability further enhances diagnostic accuracy for pancreatic cancer, with a sensitivity ranging from 80% to 95%.[22,23] The role of pancreatoscopy in cancer diagnosis has yet to be defined. However, pancreatoscopy might help to characterize indeterminate main pancreatic duct strictures in highly selected cases with inconclusive findings from EUS-guided FNA (Fig. 26.9).

In a series[24] of 52 patients (8 with pancreatic cancer, 19 with chronic pancreatitis, and 25 normal cases), 42 (81%) were observed successfully with the ultrathin pancreatoscope (0.8 mm). Pancreatoscopic findings in the seven malignant strictures were friability and erythema (100%),

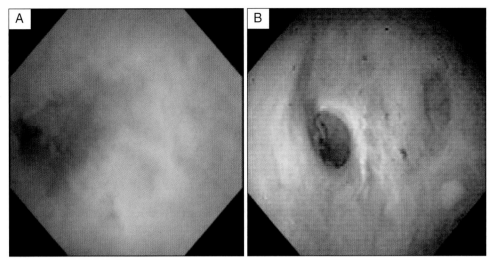

FIG 26.9 Video pancreatoscopic images of ductal stenosis. **A,** Ductal stenosis caused by pancreatic cancer. Friable mucosa with erythema and erosive changes were observed around the stenosis. **B,** Ductal stenosis caused by chronic pancreatitis. The lumen was narrowed by scar formation. (From Kodama T, Koshitani T, Sato H, et al. Electronic pancreatoscopy for the diagnosis of pancreatic diseases. *Am J Gastroenterol.* 2002;97:617–622.)

nodularity (71%), and erosive changes (57%). Strictures with scarred appearance were observed in 12/15 (80%) of cases with chronic pancreatitis.

In another series[16] of patients, 35 with pancreatic cancer and 20 with benign ductal stenosis, 22 (63%) and 16 (80%) were adequately seen with the ultrathin pancreatoscope. Tumor vessels and papillary tumors were observed when pancreatic cancer was small (<2 cm). Stenosis without significant mucosal changes was observed in 62% of cases with benign ductal stenosis. Coarse mucosa and friability were observed more frequently in association with pancreatic cancer than benign ductal stenosis.

Sampling

Tissue sampling during pancreatoscopy is technically difficult because of the limited maneuverability of the biopsy forceps in the pancreatic duct. Cytopathologic examination of pancreatic juice collected during pancreatoscopy may be more useful, particularly in patients with IPMN.

In a series[25] of 103 surgically resected IPMN patients, the usefulness of peroral pancreatoscopy for pancreatic juice cytology was assessed. The sensitivity of pancreatic juice cytology for IPMN was 62.2% when pancreatic juice was collected from suspicious lesions by pancreatoscopy and was 38.2% when it was collected using a catheter. The cytologic yield was higher in patients with IPMN than in those with pancreatic carcinoma (25.4%).

In another series[26] of 17 patients with possible IPMN with main pancreatic duct dilation, the targeted biopsy during single-operator pancreatoscopy had 25% sensitivity and 100% specificity for detecting malignancy. However, SpyGlass pancreatoscopy with irrigation cytology had 100% sensitivity and 100% specificity for detecting malignancy. These results indicate that irrigation cytology seems to be better than targeted biopsy during pancreatoscopy for the detection of malignant IPMN.

THERAPEUTIC INDICATIONS

Intraductal Lithotripsy in Patients With Chronic Pancreatitis

Extracorporeal shockwave lithotripsy (ESWL) is a well-established modality for removing main pancreatic duct stones (see Chapter 55); however, it requires special equipment and expertise. Conventional endoscopic removal by ERCP is less invasive than surgery but unlikely to be successful for stones >10 mm in diameter, a downstream stricture, or stone impaction.[27] Pancreatoscopy allows intraductal lithotripsy of pancreatic stones under the safety of direct vision.[28,29]

In a study[30] that included 28 patients, SpyGlass pancreatoscopy-guided laser lithotripsy was performed and 9 of the 28 patients (32%) had prior ESWL sessions. A median of 2 stones sized 15 mm was identified in the head (32%), neck (11%), body (32%), tail (4%), or multiple sites (21%). Technical success was achieved in 22 of 28 patients (79%), with complete stone clearance and clinical improvement noted in 25 of 28 patients (89%) at a median of 13 months of follow-up.

ADVERSE EVENTS AND MANAGEMENT

Possible adverse events of peroral pancreatoscopy, with or without pancreatic sphincterotomy, include bleeding, perforation, and pancreatitis. Acute pancreatitis may be induced by mechanical trauma of the pancreatoscope passage or excessive intraductal irrigation, which is required for improved visualization.

The reported frequency of pancreatoscopy-related pancreatitis in the largest series ranged from 10% to 12%.[31] The least amount of irrigant volume possible must be used and the flow rate of water irrigation should be reduced. Particular care is needed for inspection in those patients with nondilated main pancreatic ducts who might be at high risk for postprocedural pancreatitis.[19] To avoid possible infection, intravenous administration of prophylactic antibiotics is also recommended after the procedure.

RELATIVE COST

There are no published data on cost comparisons between pancreatoscopy and alternative techniques; there are no cost-effectiveness studies for pancreatoscopy either. However, pancreatoscopy can be expensive because it requires a second light source and a suitable processor for a baby scope. In addition, the reusable baby scope involves significant maintenance costs because of its fragility.

CONCLUSIONS

Pancreatoscopy plays an important role in both the diagnosis and treatment of pancreatic disorders, especially those that cannot be readily differentiated by noninvasive imaging techniques and conventional tissue sampling. Single-operator cholangiopancreatoscopy has simplified direct visualization of the bile and pancreatic ducts and largely replaced traditional mother–baby systems. Although SpyGlass is the dominant technology in today's market, CCD chip pancreatoscopes still have an advantage in their optics that enables high-resolution digital images. The addition of imaging enhancement such as NBI further improves diagnostic accuracy. Pancreatoscopy could be improved further by including one or more imaging enhancements in a smaller catheter.

REFERENCES

1. Takagi K, Takegoshi T. Endoscopic diagnosis of pancreatic cancer [in Japanese]. *Stom Intes.* 1974;9:1533–1541.
2. Ohashi K, Murakami Y, Maruyama M. Four cases of a mucous secreting pancreatic cancer [in Japanese]. *Prog Dig Endosc.* 1982;20:348–351.
3. Kodama T, Sato H, Horii Y, et al. Pancreatoscopy for the next generation: development of the peroral electronic pancreatoscope system. *Gastrointest Endosc.* 1999;49:366–371.
4. Chen YK, Pleskow DKL. Results from the first human use clinical series utilizing a new peroral cholangiopancreatoscopy system (SpyGlass Direct Visualization System). *Gastrointest Endosc.* 2006;63:AB88.
5. Parsi MA, Jang S, Sanaka M, et al. Diagnostic and therapeutic cholangiopancreatoscopy: performance of a new digital cholangioscope. *Gastrointest Endosc.* 2014;79:936–942.
6. Kodama T, Koshitani T, Sato H, et al. Electronic pancreatoscopy for the diagnosis of pancreatic diseases. *Am J Gastroenterol.* 2002;97:617–622.
7. Navaneethan U, Hasan MK, Kommaraju K, et al. Digital, single-operator cholangiopancreatoscopy in the diagnosis and management of pancreatobiliary disorders: a multicenter clinical experience (with video). *Gastrointest Endosc.* 2016;84:649–655.
8. Prachayakul V, Aswakul P, Kachintorn U. Overtube-assisted direct peroral pancreatoscopy using an ultraslim gastroscope in a patient suspected of having an intraductal papillary mucinous neoplasm. *Endoscopy.* 2011;43:E279–E280.
9. Cheon YK, Moon JH, Choi HJ, et al. Direct peroral pancreatoscopy with an ultraslim endoscope for the evaluation of intraductal papillary mucinous neoplasms. *Endoscopy.* 2011;43:E390–E391.
10. Yamada M, Kozuka S, Yamao K, et al. Mucin-producing tumor of the pancreas. *Cancer.* 1991;68:159–168.
11. Koshitani T, Kodama T. The role of endoscopy for the diagnosis of intraductal papillary mucinous tumor of the pancreas. *Tech Gastrointest Endosc.* 2005;7:200–210.
12. Ringold DA, Shah RJ. Peroral pancreatoscopy in the diagnosis and management of intraductal papillary mucinous neoplasia and indeterminate pancreatic duct pathology. *Gastrointest Endosc Clin N Am.* 2009;19:601–613.
13. Mukai H, Yasuda K, Nakajima M. Differential diagnosis of mucin-producing tumors of the pancreas by intraductal ultrasonography and peroral pancreatoscopy. *Endoscopy.* 1998;30:A99–A102.
14. Yamaguchi T, Hara T, Tsuyuguchi T, et al. Peroral pancreatoscopy in the diagnosis of mucin-producing tumors of the pancreas. *Gastrointest Endosc.* 2000;52:67–73.
15. Hara T, Yamaguchi T, Ishihara T, et al. Diagnosis and patient management of intraductal papillary-mucinous tumor of the pancreas by using peroral pancreatoscopy and intraductal ultrasonography. *Gastroenterology.* 2002;122:34–43.
16. Yamao K, Ohashi K, Nakamura T, et al. Efficacy of peroral pancreatoscopy in the diagnosis of pancreatic diseases. *Gastrointest Endosc.* 2003;57:205–209.
17. Itoi T, Neuhaus H, Chen YK. Diagnostic value of image-enhanced video cholangiopancreatoscopy. *Gastrointest Endosc Clin N Am.* 2009;19:557–566.
18. Miura T, Igarashi Y, Okano N, et al. Endoscopic diagnosis of intraductal papillary-mucinous neoplasm of the pancreas by means of peroral pancreatoscopy using a small-diameter videoscope and narrow-band imaging. *Dig Endosc.* 2010;22:119–123.
19. Arnelo U, Siiki A, Swahn F, et al. Single-operator pancreatoscopy is helpful in the evaluation of suspected intraductal papillary mucinous neoplasms (IPMN). *Pancreatology.* 2014;14:510–514.
20. Navez J, Hubert C, Gigot JF, et al. Impact of intraoperative pancreatoscopy with intraductal biopsies on surgical management of intraductal papillary mucinous neoplasm of the pancreas. *J Am Coll Surg.* 2015;221:982–987.
21. Pucci MJ, Johnson CM, Punja VP, et al. Intraoperative pancreatoscopy: a valuable tool for pancreatic surgeons? *J Gastrointest Surg.* 2014;18:1100–1107.
22. Afify AM, al-Khafaji BM, Kim B, et al. Endoscopic ultrasound-guided fine needle aspiration of the pancreas: diagnostic utility and accuracy. *Acta Cytol.* 2003;47:341–348.
23. Eloubeidi MA, Jhala D, Chhieng DC, et al. Yield of endoscopic ultrasound-guided fine-needle aspiration biopsy in patients with suspected pancreatic carcinoma. *Cancer.* 2003;99:285–292.
24. Tajiri H, Kobayashi M, Niwa H, et al. Clinical application of an ultra-thin pancreatoscope using a sequential video converter. *Gastrointest Endosc.* 1993;39:371–374.
25. Yamaguchi T, Shirai Y, Ishihara T, et al. Pancreatic juice cytology in the diagnosis of intraductal papillary mucinous neoplasm of the pancreas. *Cancer.* 2005;104:2830–2836.
26. Nagayoshi Y, Aso T, Ohtsuka T, et al. Peroral pancreatoscopy using the SpyGlass system for the assessment of intraductal papillary mucinous neoplasm of the pancreas. *J Hepatobiliary Pancreat Sci.* 2014;21:410–417.
27. Sherman S, Lehman G, Hawes R, et al. Pancreatic ductal stones: frequency of successful endoscopic removal and improvement in symptoms. *Gastrointest Endosc.* 1991;37:511–517.
28. Nguyen NQ, Binmoeller KF, Shah JN. Cholangioscopy and pancreatoscopy (with videos). *Gastrointest Endosc.* 2009;70:1200–1210.
29. Shah RJ. Innovations in intraductal endoscopy. *Gastrointest Endosc Clin N Am.* 2015;25:779–792.
30. Attwell AR, Patel S, Kahaleh M, et al. ERCP with per-oral pancreatoscopy-guided laser lithotripsy for calcific chronic pancreatitis: a multicenter U.S. experience. *Gastrointest Endosc.* 2015;82:311–318.
31. Tringali A, Lemmers A, Meves V, et al. Intraductal biliopancreatic imaging: European Society of Gastrointestinal Endoscopy (ESGE) technology review. *Endoscopy.* 2015;47:739–753.

27

Cholangioscopy

Raj J. Shah and Takao Itoi

Historically, cholangioscopy was performed with a fiberoptic mother (large-caliber duodenoscope) and daughter (cholangioscope) system requiring two endoscopists, two light sources, and two video monitors, if the endoscopy unit was fortunate enough to have two video cameras to interface with the respective endoscopes.[1] The development of a video mother endoscope made the endoscopy suite a bit less cluttered, although even after video daughter endoscopes were markedly improved and variably marketed, equipment expense, fragility, and maintenance costs limited their use. It took the introduction of disposable daughter endoscopes, initially fiberoptic and currently digital, to change endoscopic retrograde cholangiopancreatography (ERCP) from a procedure in which virtually all diagnostic and therapeutic procedures were facilitated by fluoroscopy to one in which the endoscopist can look directly into the pancreaticobiliary tree both to improve diagnosis and to facilitate therapy. In recognition of this technological dichotomy, the authors have tried, Solomon-like, to split this chapter into two parts. We will leave it to the individuals performing cholangioscopy to decide whether they adopt one, both, or neither of these technologies and instead rely on interventional radiologists to provide access to the biliary tree through a transhepatic percutaneous biliary drain (PTBD) using the subsequent track as the cholangioscope entry port.

SINGLE-OPERATOR CHOLANGIOSCOPY

Introduction

The advantages of single-operator cholangioscopy using the catheter-based fiberoptic SpyGlass system (FSOC; SpyGlass Direct Visualization System; Boston Scientific, Marlborough, MA) include the ability of a single endoscopist to perform cholangiopancreatoscopy and the use of a disposable 4-lumen 10-Fr catheter, reusable optical fiber, and four-way tip deflection (up–down and left–right) that is passed through the working channel (4.2 mm) of a standard therapeutic duodenoscope.[2] The device is approved by the Food and Drug Administration (FDA) for both biliary and pancreatic applications. In February 2015, a fully disposable digital single-operator cholangioscope (DSOC) was introduced in the United States.[3]

In an ex vivo study with FSOC, Chen compared four-quadrant access, simulated biopsy, irrigation flow rates, and optical resolution between FSOC and an endoscope-based system (CHF BP-30; Olympus Medical Systems, Tokyo, Japan).[4] The author reported that the ability to access four quadrants for visualization and biopsy with FSOC was better than with the two-way tip deflection of the endoscope-based system (odds ratio 1.7 to 2.94, $p < 0.001$). A preliminary ex vivo study that included five investigators compared optical quality and maneuverability between DSOC and FSOC.[5] A biliary tract model contained fixed and variable color targets. Runs (passes of the scope) were randomized, and DSOC outperformed FSOC by a higher percentage of visualized targets (96% vs 66%), successful targeting per run, and faster run times (all comparisons $p < 0.01$). Further, subjective parameters of image quality and ease of use were superior ($p < 0.001$).

Equipment

FSOC has a control section that houses three ports: irrigation that feeds into two 0.6-mm channels, a 0.77-mm optical probe, and a 1.2-mm accessory channel that permits passage of guidewires, intraductal lithotripsy fibers, and miniature biopsy forceps.[4] The control section is secured with a Silastic belt just below the working channel of the duodenoscope. The disposable 3.4-mm insertion tube has four steering wires embedded in its length. The 6000-pixel optical probe is a collection of light fibers that surround optical fiber bundles and is incorporated into a polyimide sheath, providing approximately a 70-degree field of view. The connector section entails a camera processor with 1/4-inch charge-coupled device (CCD) chip, a light source, an optical coupler that interfaces the optical probe with the light source and video camera head, a medical-grade isolation transformer, and a travel cart with a three-joint arm for extension. An irrigation pump with foot pedal and monitor are available through separate vendors.[6] The DSOC has a complementary metal-oxide semiconductor (CMOS) chip for higher resolution, magnification, and field of view (120 degrees). It has a thin copper cable for digital transmission and lacks a separate fiber optic probe that may contribute to improved catheter tip articulation. A separate suction connection with the working channel seems to permit improved irrigation capability. The processor is portable for simplified setup.[5]

Technique

For FSOC, the optical probe is preloaded into the access/therapeutic catheter and advanced to within a few millimeters of the catheter's bending portion to reduce the potential for damage during passage across the duodenoscope's elevator and ductal strictures. The DSOC system has the optical bundle incorporated into the catheter. Advancement through the duodenoscope's working channel is similar to the endoscope-based cholangioscope. Once the duct is entered with the access catheter, the optical probe is advanced gently beyond the catheter's tip for intraductal inspection. If resistance is encountered, the control section knobs should be unlocked and fluoroscopy may be used to determine whether the catheter's tip is straight. The endoscopist has control of the four-way steering dials and may periodically lock the dials to stabilize scope position at a target during tissue acquisition or intraductal lithotripsy. Irrigation is performed through two dedicated channels facilitated by a foot pedal. Irrigation rates should be kept as low as possible to reduce the risk of cholangitis.[7]

Clinical Use and Efficacy
Intraductal Lithotripsy

Electrohydraulic lithotripsy (EHL) or laser lithotripsy (LL) can be used to treat both bile duct and pancreatic duct stones (Fig. 27.1, *A–E,* and Fig. 27.2, *A–E*). Cholangioscopic or pancreatoscopic visualization during intraductal lithotripsy helps to avoid duct injury. The 1.9-Fr nitinol EHL fiber contains two coaxially insulated electrodes ending at an open

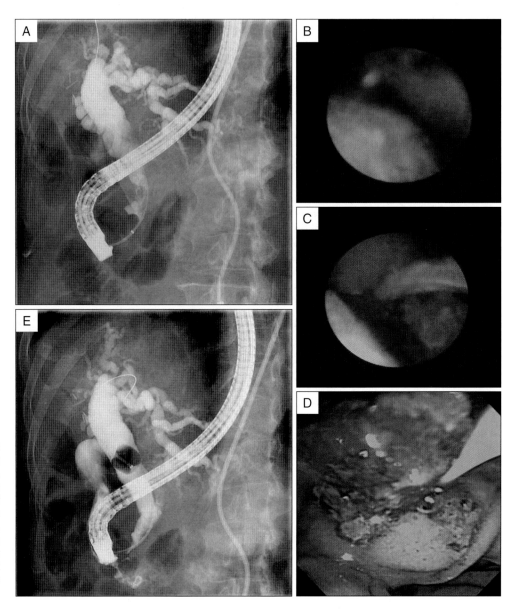

FIG 27.1 A, Fluoroscopic view of a lateral wall of bile duct filling defect consistent with impacted stones. **B,** FSOC view of two large common bile duct stones. **C,** FSOC view of common bile duct stone fragments after electrohydraulic lithotripsy. **D,** Duodenal view of removed stone fragments. **E,** Balloon occlusion cholangiogram after common bile duct stone clearance. *FSOC,* Fiberoptic single-operator cholangioscope.

tip. Water or saline immersion is necessary and, as an advantage over endoscope-based cholangioscopes, the dedicated channels for irrigation provide a sufficient medium. During immersion, sparks are generated that produce high-amplitude hydraulic pressure waves for stone fragmentation.[8] A generator produces a series of high-voltage electrical impulses at a frequency of 1 to 20 per second, with settings ranging from a power of 50 to 100. The tip of the EHL fiber should protrude no more than 2 to 3 mm from the scope and be positioned en face with the stone while the generator's foot pedal is depressed to deliver energy.[9]

During LL, a laser beam is transmitted via a flexible quartz fiber through the working channel of the cholangiopancreatoscope. LL requires more precise localization of the stone, and though fragmentation is enhanced by direct contact, it can lead to a "drilling" effect. The application of repetitive pulses of laser energy to the stone leads to the formation of a gaseous collection of ions and free electrons of high kinetic energy. This plasma rapidly expands as it absorbs the laser energy and then collapses, inducing a spherical mechanical shockwave between the laser fiber and the stone, leading to stone fragmentation.[10]

Clearance of Difficult Biliary Stone Clearance Using FSOC

A multicenter US experience using FSOC with LL included 69 patients, 89% of whom had extrahepatic or cystic duct stones and the remainder had intrahepatic stones.[11] All patients had a minimum of one prior failed attempt at ERCP for stone extraction and required a mean of 1.2 LL sessions to achieve an impressive 97% complete clearance rate with a 4% adverse event rate. In a large, single-center FSOC series from India, holmium LL was used in 60 patients with previously failed attempts of mechanical lithotripsy (44%) or other factors such as Mirizzi's syndrome or stone impaction that precluded attempts at basket capture or large-balloon sphincter dilation.[12] The mean stone size was 23 mm (range 15 to 40 mm) and 100% complete clearance was reported after a mean of 1.2 LL sessions. Interestingly, 24 potentially eligible patients were excluded because of portal hypertension or extensive stone burden occupying most of the bile duct and mostly referred to surgery without attempt at FSOC. In a small but significant series of 13 patients with cystic duct stones (four with Mirizzi's syndrome type 1), FSOC was used to achieve complete clearance of the cystic duct and bile duct in 10/13 (77%) patients during a total of 17 FSOC sessions.[13]

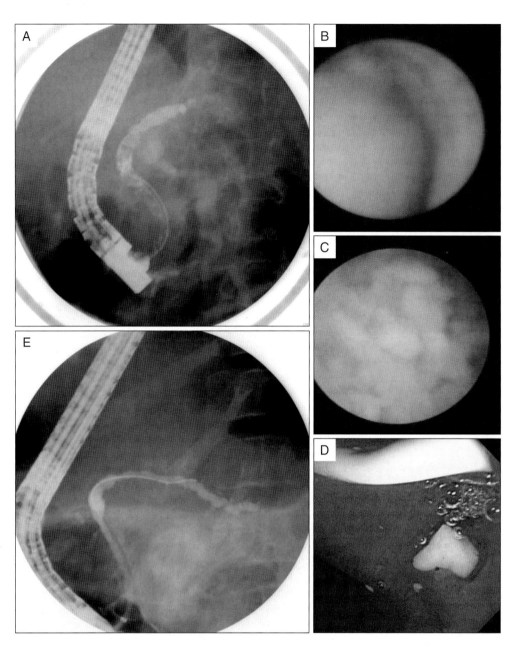

FIG 27.2 A, Pancreatogram with stones in the head and genu. **B,** FSOC view of impacted pancreatic duct stone in head. **C,** FSOC view of pancreatic duct stone fragments after electrohydraulic lithotripsy. **D,** Duodenal view of pancreatic stone fragment after endoscopic removal. **E,** Pancreatogram revealing clearance of stones from head and genu. *FSOC,* Fiberoptic single-operator cholangioscope.

In a multicenter international prospective registry study using FSOC, 66 of 297 total cases were for the treatment of difficult biliary stones and included EHL (*n* = 50) and LL (*n* = 16).[14] The median stone size was 19 mm and the duration of index intraductal lithotripsy was 38 minutes. Ductal clearance was achieved in 100%: 47/66 (71%) at index study single-operator cholangioscopy (SOC) and the remaining 29% after an average of one to two ERCPs. Overall, in the appropriately identified patient, the treatment of difficult biliary stones remains an indispensable indication for single-operator cholangioscopy-guided intraductal lithotripsy.

Pancreatic Stone Therapy Using FSOC

A potential advantage of peroral pancreatoscopy (POP) over extracorporeal shock wave lithotripsy (ESWL) as a primary modality in the approach to patients with main pancreatic duct (MPD) stones is the ability to fragment and remove stones during the same procedure. In a single-center study of 46 patients undergoing either endoscope or FSOC pancreatoscopy

with EHL or LL for MPD stones, 14 underwent FSOC.[15] Overall, complete or partial stone clearance was achieved in 91%, with complete clearance in 70%; complete or partial clearance was similar between those undergoing FSOC and those undergoing endoscope-based pancreatoscopy (*p* = 0.294), although the disposable system with four-way tip deflection seems particularly advantageous for treating pancreatic duct stones (personal observation). Mild POP-related adverse events occurred in 3/25 (12%) procedures in the FSOC group. Overall clinical success at a median follow-up of 15 months was 74% and similar between endoscope-based and FSOC groups (*p* = 0.149).

From a multicenter LL working group, 28 patients were retrospectively identified who underwent FSOC for MPD stones.[16] Before index FSOC with LL, 32% had undergone adjunctive ESWL and 25% had failed or incomplete stone fragmentation with FSOC ± EHL. Median stone size was 15 mm (4 to 32 mm) and located in the head or neck (*n* = 12 [42%]) or body/tail (*n* = 10 [36%]), or multiple sites (*n* = 6 [21%]). Overall, there was 90% per protocol technical success with complete

(22/28 [79%]) and partial (3/28 [11%]) clearance associated with clinical success in 89% of patients at a median 13-month follow-up based on a 50% reduction in pain, narcotic usage, or hospitalizations. Of note, a 29% rate of mild postprocedural adverse events occurred.

FSOC Evaluation of Indeterminate Biliary Strictures

Although comparative series of endoscope-based cholangioscopes and FSOC have not been performed, cohort series of FSOC have shown encouraging findings in patients with indeterminate pancreaticobiliary pathology (Fig. 27.3, A–F). It is likely that the ability to navigate and sample different quadrants of a stricture may be enhanced with four-way tip deflection and a compressible catheter tip.[4] Lesions suggestive of malignancy have been based primarily on studies using the endoscope-based cholangioscopes and include (1) exophytic lesions, (2) ulceration, (3) papillary mucosal projections, and (4) dilated tortuous vessels.[2,17,18]

For FSOC, interobserver agreement of video clips to distinguish malignant from benign lesions revealed only slight to fair agreement and may be only modestly improved with the DSOC system. Accuracy by the investigators to distinguish benign from malignant was 70% (20% higher than with FSOC) and there was moderate interobserver agreement specifically for papillary projections.[18-20]

Intraductal biopsy with the FSOC technique can be performed using two methods previously described for the endoscope-based cholangioscope.[17] Cholangioscopy-directed biopsy is performed by passing a miniature cholangioscope biopsy forceps with a span of 4.1 mm (SpyBite; Boston Scientific) through the 1.2-mm working channel of the FSOC.[3] Cholangioscopy-assisted biopsy is performed by localizing the target biopsy site using cholangioscopic visualization. For example, for distal biliary strictures in which passage of the miniature forceps may be technically difficult, obtain fluoroscopic spot films of the cholangioscope

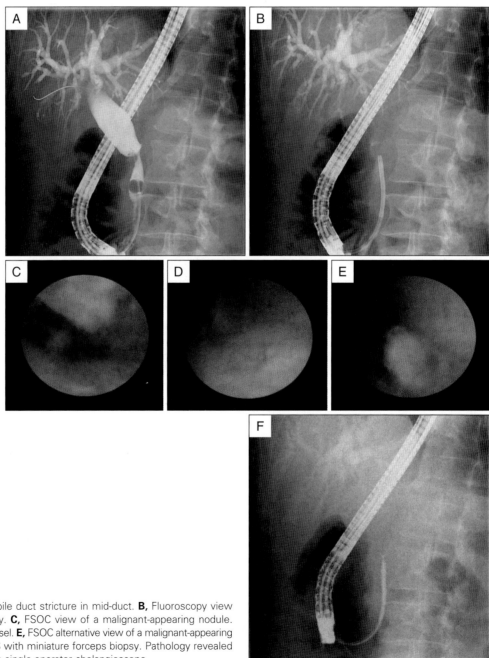

FIG 27.3 **A,** Cholangiogram of main bile duct stricture in mid-duct. **B,** Fluoroscopy view of FSOC position at level of pathology. **C,** FSOC view of a malignant-appearing nodule. **D,** FSOC view of a suspected tumor vessel. **E,** FSOC alternative view of a malignant-appearing nodule. **F,** Fluoroscopic view of SOC-S with miniature forceps biopsy. Pathology revealed high-grade dysplasia. *FSOC,* Fiberoptic single-operator cholangioscope.

tip positioned at the target lesion. After removing the cholangioscope, a conventional biliary biopsy forceps is then passed through the working channel of the duodenoscope to obtain tissue samples under fluoroscopic guidance.[17]

Clinical feasibility studies reveal adequate histologic specimens for the miniature forceps in 95% to 97% of samples when the target lesion is reached.[2,17] In a prospective small series, 26 patients with indeterminate biliary strictures underwent, per protocol, single-operator cholangioscopy using catheter-based SpyGlass system (FSOC)–directed biopsy followed by brush cytology and fluoroscopy-guided biopsy.[21] Most patients (85%) had previous nondiagnostic tissue sampling and 46% were hilar strictures. Sensitivity, specificity, and accuracy of cytology (6%, 100%, 39%), standard forceps biopsy (29%, 100%, 54%), and miniature-forceps biopsy (77%, 100%, 85%) were reported, with significant differences noted when comparing the miniature-forceps biopsy with the other methods for sensitivity and accuracy ($p < 0.0001$ and $p = 0.0215$ for cytology and standard forceps biopsy, respectively). Whether brush cytology and conventional biopsy were performed by referencing a spot film of the cholangioscope at the target area is unknown. Further, there is not a satisfactory explanation provided as to the extremely low sensitivity of brush cytology in this series.

In a study from India, data from a 9-month prospective enrollment period were reported in which approximately 10% of patients ($n = 36$) with indeterminate biliary strictures underwent FSOC for further characterization.[22] Overall, adequate histology was obtained in 82%. A high proportion of hilar strictures (21/36 [58%]) may partially explain the lower rates of adequate histology from the miniature forceps because of limited access. The accuracy of the visual impression of SOC-S using the malignancy criteria described above was 89% (95% sensitivity and 79% specificity) and for histology using the miniature forceps was 82% (82% sensitivity and specificity). Benign appearance was suggested by smooth surface mucosa without definite neovascularization and homogenous granular mucosa.

The largest multicenter trial on cholangioscopy included 15 centers from Europe and the United States in which FSOC was prospectively used for indeterminate pancreaticobiliary pathology and difficult stone disease.[14] Chen and coinvestigators evaluated 226 patients with indeterminate biliary pathology who underwent diagnostic SOC-S; 140 had directed miniature forceps biopsy (median of 4 bites, 20% hilar, and histologic adequacy of 88%). Complete ERCP, FSOC, and biopsy data were available for a subset of 95 patients. The sensitivities and specificities of cholangiographic impression, FSOC visualization, and FSOC-directed tissue biopsies for detecting malignancy were 51% and 54%, 78% and 82%, and 49% and 98%, respectively. In a meta-analysis of FSOC, eight studies that evaluated operating characteristics of visual impression and use of directed SpyBite sampling were reported.[23] The authors noted the sensitivity and specificity of the FSOC visual impression to be 90% and 87%, respectively (area under the curve [AUC] 0.94). The use of SpyBite sampling had a 69% sensitivity and 98% specificity in detection of neoplasia (AUC 0.93).

With the introduction of DSOC, the hope is that improved optics will enhance the ability to detect and exclude neoplasia (Figs. 27.4 and 27.5). The first preliminary US multicenter clinical series using DSOC was by Shah et al. and included 121 patients: 85 for stricture and ductal dilatation evaluation and 36 with difficult stones.[24] The patients with stones (29 biliary, 7 pancreatic) achieved 100% clearance using intraductal lithotripsy techniques. Eight patients underwent DSOC to assess the extent of cholangiocarcinoma (CCA), and two were found to have unsuspected, multifocal intrahepatic CCA. Of the 77 with indeterminate stricture/dilatation, 40% had confirmed neoplasia, of which 81% were positive by SpyBite sampling. Overall, the use of DSOC in the detection of neoplasia in the indeterminate cohort was found to carry sensitivity,

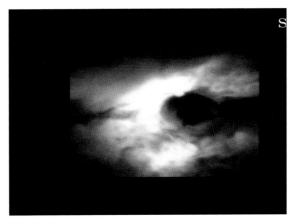

FIG 27.4 Digital single-operator cholangioscope view of an infiltrative stricture with tumor vessels.

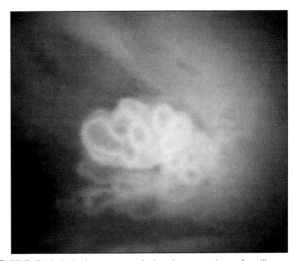

FIG 27.5 Digital single-operator cholangioscope view of a villous mass of a biliary intraductal papillary mucinous neoplasm.

specificity, PPV, and NPV of 97%, 96%, 94%, and 98%, respectively (all confidence intervals [CIs] ranged from 0.87 to 1.0). An additional smaller series included 105 patients, 73 of whom had the examination for diagnostic purposes.[25] There was a relatively low (27%) prevalence of neoplasia, and diagnostic SOC without biopsy was noted in a high proportion of examinations (40%). Indications and findings included PSC, posttransplant stricture, benign strictures from stones, and normal examinations, which are low-yield indications for the use of cholangiopancreatoscopy. Overall, the authors found the sensitivity and specificity of DSOC clinical and visual impression for diagnosis of malignancy to be 90% and 96%, respectively, and those of DSOC-guided biopsies to be 85% and 100%, respectively. An on-site pathologist performed immediate wet-prep evaluation of the specimens, which may have helped to improve the diagnostic yield of sampling.

Because tissue sampling remains the key to further triaging and managing of patients with suspected neoplasia, perhaps the optimal use of SOC may be in the identification of suspicious lesions, followed by directed tissue sampling by either cholangioscopy-directed or cholangioscopy-assisted methods, in conjunction with brush cytology, to provide the highest probability of obtaining tissue confirmation of suspected lesions. If tissue sampling is nondiagnostic but the visual impression is concerning for neoplasia, then a close surveillance interval and sampling are recommended. Although a fully disposable DSOC is now available and simpler to use, given the lack of pass-through code and limited reimbursement, it is wise to be more selective in the use of this costly technology. A good clinical impression and cholangiography technique may help to avoid the need for some cholangioscopy use described in published series. Lastly, with the anticipated introduction of competing disposable digital cholangioscopes, retail costs for the technology may decrease.

Reimbursement and Limitations

As of 2009, a current procedural terminology add-on code with ERCP exists for cholangiopancreatoscopy.

Despite the described advances, there remains a limited ability of the 10-Fr-diameter catheter to traverse tight strictures without preinspection dilation, which, when performed, may alter visual interpretation. Although four-quadrant inspection of mucosa may be achieved with four-way tip deflection and the application of torque on the duodenoscope, circumferential views and the ability to advance accessories through the working channel may be difficult, depending on duodenoscope angulations, downstream duct strictures, small duct diameter, and intraductal debris. Aspirating debris and fluid through a Y-adapter fixed to the working channel while simultaneously irrigating through the flushing port can improve the latter.[6] Circumferential visualization may also be difficult in the presence of markedly dilated ducts. During inspection of strictures, stent-associated changes may alter the mucosal appearance to include papillary mucosal projections, making visual diagnosis of malignancy very difficult.[26]

If resistance is encountered during accessory passage, advancing the cholangioscope to the upstream duct or increasing the loop of the cholangioscope within the duodenum may allow passage of the device beyond the point of angulations. The EHL and LL fibers are fragile and sometimes require preloading through a straight cholangioscope to facilitate introduction.[9,27] During intraductal lithotripsy, there can be recoil of the fiber into the working channel because of transmitted energy, contact with fragmented stones, or a deflected scope tip. As blood and stone debris may reduce visualization, careful and frequent confirmation that the tip of the fiber is in the appropriate position by endoscopic and fluoroscopic visualization is necessary to reduce duct injury or optical fiber damage. If passage of the biopsy forceps is unsuccessful, cholangioscopy-assisted fluoroscopy-guided biopsy can be performed.[17]

Although the optical probe in the FSOC is reprocessed, use may be limited to 10 cases, beyond which image quality may diminish because of broken fiber bundles. In the presence of a lithotripsy fiber or biopsy forceps within the working channel, the dedicated irrigation channel provides higher flow rates compared with reusable cholangioscopes.[4] The access catheter lacks a conventional suction button, and intermittent manual aspiration using a syringe attached to a Y-port adapter and/or intermittent duodenoscope suctioning is required to reduce intraductal pressure and gastroduodenal fluid reflux.[6] For DSOC, a suction apparatus connected to the working channel provides improved irrigation ability (i.e., the ability to flush and aspirate) to improve visualization.[3]

Adverse Events

Although not specific to FSOC, a single-center series of ERCP alone compared with ERCP and cholangiopancreatoscopy found that cholangiopancreatoscopy may be associated with a significantly higher rate of procedure-related adverse events than ERCP alone.[7] This increased risk was observed in overall adverse events (7.0% vs 2.9%), consensus adverse events (pancreatitis, perforation, cholangitis, or bleeding; 4.2% vs 2.2%), and specifically with postprocedural cholangitis (1.0% vs 0.2%). Studies specific to FSOC reveal adverse event rates ranging from 5% to 13% and include mostly cholangitis and pancreatitis.[12,13,22,24]

Prophylactic IV antibiotics are therefore recommended when performing intraductal cholangioscopy.

Summary

Single-operator cholangioscopy using SpyGlass has been demonstrated to be an established modality in the treatment of difficult biliary stones. When used in the evaluation of indeterminate biliary strictures by endoscopists experienced in recognizing intraductal pathology, it increases the diagnostic yield of tissue sampling. Results remain limited and mostly preliminary in its use for pancreatic duct stones and in the evaluation of pancreatic neoplasia. The digital imaging system provides a simplified setup and improved optical resolution.

VIDEOCHOLANGIOSCOPY USING THE MOTHER–BABY SYSTEM

A videocholangioscope can provide outstanding quality digital images compared with conventional fiberoptic cholangioscopy.[28–36] Two videocholangioscopes have been used in the mother-baby cholangioscopy system (Table 27.1). At present, however, their use is limited to a few countries. Recently, newly designed digital cholangioscopy (SpyGlass DS, Boston Scientific), which is available as a single-operator system, has been developed.[37,38] (See details in the previous section.)

Description of the Technique

The therapeutic duodenoscope that is used as the mother scope has a 4.2-mm working channel that helps prevent kinking of the baby videocholangioscope. Endoscopic sphincterotomy is needed to facilitate scope passage across the papilla. Two videocholangioscopes (CHF-B260/B160 and CHF-BP260, with outer diameters of 3.4 and 2.6 mm and working channel diameters of 1.2 and 0.5 mm, respectively; B260 and BP260 [Olympus Medical Systems, Tokyo, Japan] and B160 [Olympus America Inc., Center Valley, PA]) are available (Fig. 27.6). They are advanced through the 4.2-mm working channel of therapeutic duodenoscopes into the bile duct with or without a 0.035-inch/0.025-inch guidewire. Both have two-way tip angulation. The wire-guided insertion technique is used with the CHF-B260 but not with the CHF-BP260 because of the diameter of the working channel. Saline irrigation and CO_2 insufflation are used during cholangioscopy because of reports of air embolism.[34,35] Endoscopic observation is usually performed using white-light imaging. Observation using narrow-band imaging (NBI) is available with the NBI system (CV-260SL, CVL-260SL,

TABLE 27.1 Mother–Baby Videocholangioscopy		
	CHF-BP260*	CHF-B260/B160*
Angle of view, degrees	90	90
Observed depth, mm	3 to 20	3 to 20
Outer diameter, mm		
Distal end	2.6	3.4
Insertion end	2.9	3.5
Bending section, degrees		
Up/down	70/70	70/70
Right/left	NA	NA
Working length, mm	2000	2000
Working channel diameter, mm	0.5	1.2
Image-enhanced endoscopy	NBI	NBI

NA, Not available; *NBI*, narrow-band imaging.
Olympus Medical Systems, Tokyo, Japan.

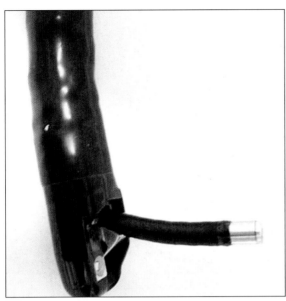

FIG 27.6 Videocholangioscopy using the mother–baby system.

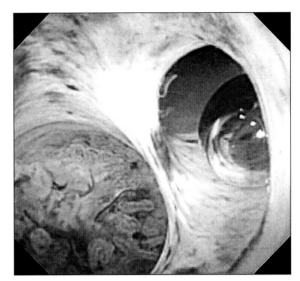

FIG 27.7 Papillary lesions in the intrahepatic bile duct.

TABLE 27.2   Summary of Diagnostic Ability of Mother–Baby-Type Videocholangioscopy

Author (Year)	n	Study	Sensitivity (%)	Specificity (%)	PPV (%)	NPV (%)	Accuracy (%)
Itoi (2010)[33]	144	R	99	96	99	99	98
Nishikawa (2013)[40]	33	P	100	92	96	96	97
Osanai (2013)[39]	87	P	94	92	NA	NA	93

NA, Not applicable; *NPV*, negative predictive value; *P*, prospective study; *PPV*, positive predictive value; *R*, retrospective study.
All data including visual impression + biopsy.

CVL-290SL/CV-180, CLV-180, CLV-S190, light source; Olympus Medical Systems).

Technique: Diagnostic and Therapeutic

Videocholangioscopy provides better-quality digital images and offers enhanced mucosal detail compared with conventional fiberoptic cholangioscopes (Fig. 27.7 and Video 27.1). Thus it can delineate fine mucosal structures like shallow pseudodiverticula, papillary or granular lesions, and fine vessel patterns, leading to differentiation between benign and malignant lesions to include the indeterminate filling defects and biliary strictures as noted on cholangiography. A recent retrospective study[33] and prospective studies[39,40] of the ability of videocholangioscopy to differentiate between indeterminate filling defects and biliary strictures revealed that videocholangioscopy provided high diagnostic ability (accuracy, 93% to 98%; sensitivity, 94% to 100%; specificity, 92% to 96%; positive predictive value, 96% to 99%; negative predictive value, 96% to 100%) (Table 27.2). However, videocholangioscopy cannot always differentiate benign from malignant lesions. For instance, in cases of IgG4-related cholangitis, cholangioscopic images are often similar to those visualized in cholangiocarcinoma, for example, presence of thick and tortuous vessels.[41] Thus cholangioscopic imaging alone is limited and biopsy appears to be mandatory in such cases.

Mucinous-producing neoplasms in the bile duct can produce a large amount of mucin, resulting in misdiagnosis of tumor location when only cholangiography is employed. Videocholangioscopy is very useful for accurate localization of the primary site of the tumor.[36] Detailed observations make it possible to not only detect abnormal findings but also accurately target biopsy sites by direct inspection (Fig. 27.8).

Bile duct neoplasms, in particular papillary growth type or mucinous-producing neoplasms, often show a longitudinal tumor spreading from the primary bile duct lesions. Detailed visualization of enlarged images obtained by videocholangioscopy permits detection of tiny abnormalities, regardless of benign or malignant nature.[32,36] Furthermore, videocholangioscopy biopsy using a directed 3-Fr biopsy forceps further improves diagnostic capability.[33] When a biliary stricture is too tight to allow passage by a videocholangioscope, balloon dilation or temporary 10-Fr plastic stent placement can increase the luminal diameter to allow for subsequent cholangioscopy.

Image-enhanced videocholangioscopy using NBI clearly displays fine biliary mucosal structures and capillary vessels (Fig. 27.9, *A*, *B*; Video 27.2) and helps to distinguish benign from malignant lesions.[31,39,41,42] Primary sclerosing cholangitis increases the lifetime risk of cholangiocarcinoma. A recent study suggested that cholangioscopy allowed visualization of tumor margins in CCA compared with traditional fluoroscopy-based ERCP.[43]

Although therapeutic videocholangioscopy is limited because of its small working channel, 1.9-Fr to 3-Fr EHL and LL using holmium YAG and FREDDY have been performed under direct videocholangioscopic visualization (Fig. 27.10 and Video 27.3).

Adverse Events and Limitations

Videocholangioscopy can cause procedure-related adverse events such as cholangitis and pancreatitis. There are several limitations of the mother–baby videocholangioscopy system because of endoscope fragility, expense of repair, and need for two skilled endoscopists. On NBI cholangioscopy, bile resembles blood, which can lead to poor images, and it is time-consuming to clean the bile duct without a dedicated irrigation channel.[31]

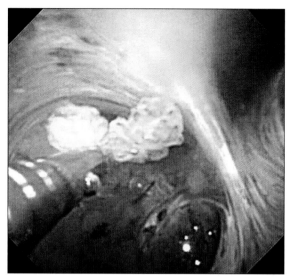

FIG 27.8 Biopsy under direct inspection.

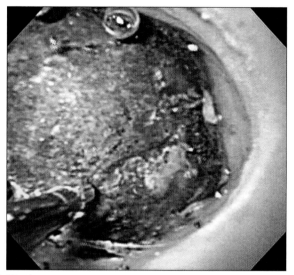

FIG 27.10 Baby cholangioscopy–assisted intraductal electrohydraulic lithotripsy for large bile duct stone.

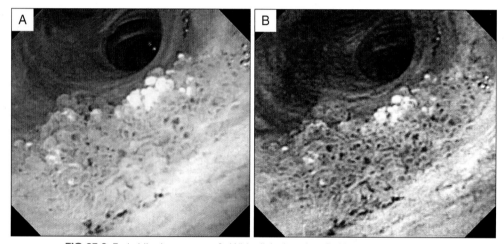

FIG 27.9 Early bile duct cancer. **A,** White-light imaging. **B,** Narrow-band imaging.

VIDEOCHOLANGIOSCOPY BY THE DIRECT INSERTION SYSTEM

Direct peroral fiberoptic cholangioscopy is performed by the direct insertion technique was first described by Urakami et al. 3 decades ago using a standard upper gastrointestinal (GI) endoscope.[44] However, this method has not become common because of the technical difficulty of passing a large-diameter endoscope into the biliary tree. In 2006 the first case series using ultraslim upper GI videoendoscopes was reported by Larghi and Waxman.[45] Since then, diagnostic and therapeutic direct peroral videocholangioscopy (DPVCS) have become increasingly performed.[46–54]

Description of the Technique

DPVCS is usually performed using conventional ultraslim upper GI endoscopes (Table 27.3). However, because they have a 5-mm to 6-mm outer diameter, endoscopic sphincterotomy is mandatory. On occasion, papillary balloon dilation is added to facilitate endoscope passage across the papilla. These instruments have four-way tip angulation and a 2-mm working channel.

At present, five approaches for direct bile duct access have been reported: (1) free-hand insertion without any assisting devices, (2) wire-guided insertion, (3) balloon overtube–assisted insertion, (4) occluded duodenal balloon–assisted insertion, and (5) intraductal anchoring balloon–assisted insertion[55] (Fig. 27.11). In general, free-hand scope insertion is usually difficult when using a conventional ultraslim upper GI videoendoscope, and therefore either wire-guided insertion or intraductal anchoring balloon-assisted insertion is most frequently used. Early studies showed that the success rate of intraductal balloon catheter–assisted insertion was higher (20/21 [95.2%]) than that of wire-guided insertion (5/11 [45.5%]) or balloon overtube–assisted insertion (10/12 [83.3%]).[46,47]

For wire-guided insertion, initially a 0.035-inch or stiff-type 0.025-inch guidewire is inserted into the bile duct through a standard duodenoscope, which is then removed, leaving the guidewire in place. An ultraslim endoscope is then advanced into the bile duct using an over-the-wire technique. It is relatively easy to advance the tip of the endoscope into the lower bile duct in either an angulated or straight position. A combination of pushing and pulling techniques is needed for scope insertion up to the hilum. When we use the 5-Fr anchoring balloon for scope insertion into the bile duct, the anchoring balloon is advanced into the right or left intrahepatic bile duct and inflated as an anchor. A 0.018-inch or 0.025-inch guidewire is used for placing the 5-Fr anchoring balloon. Then, an ultraslim endoscope is advanced to the hilum or intrahepatic bile ducts using the pushing and pulling techniques in combination

TABLE 27.3   Direct Peroral Videocholangioscopy

	OLYMPUS MEDICAL SYSTEMS			Fujinon EG-530NW/530N2	Pentax EG-1690K
	GIF-XP160	GIF-XP180N	GIF-XP260N		
Angle of view, degrees	120	120	120	140	120
Observed depth, mm	3 to 100	3 to 100	3 to 100	4 to 100	4 to 100
Outer diameter, mm					
Distal end	5.9	5.5	5.0	5.9	5.4
Insertion end	5.9	5.5	5.5	5.9	5.3
Bending section, degrees					
Up/down	180/90	210/90	210/90	210/90	210/120
Right/left	100/100	100/100	100/100	100/100	120/120
Working length, mm	1030	1100	1030	1100	1100
Working channel diameter, mm	2	2	2	2	2
Image-enhanced endoscopy	NBI	NBI	NBI	FICE	i-SCAN

FICE, Flexible spectral imaging color enhancement; *NBI,* narrow-band imaging.

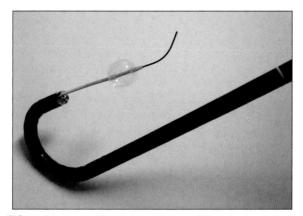

FIG 27.11 Direct videocholangioscopy with anchoring balloon.

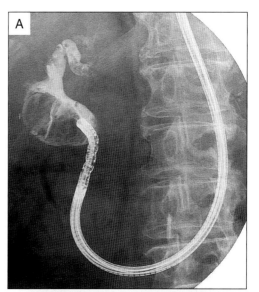

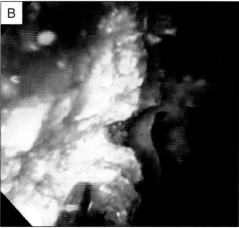

FIG 27.12 Direct videocholangioscopy–assisted electrohydraulic lithotripsy for large bile duct stone. **A,** Radiographic finding. **B,** Endoscopic imaging.

with the anchoring balloon. At this time, the shape of endoscope shows an α-loop or U-loop scope position. Saline irrigation and CO_2 insufflation are used to facilitate endoscopic visualization in the bile duct.

Recently a prototype dedicated DPVCS with a multibending tip has been developed.[56] It has two bending sections: the proximal section can be deflected in a single plane (90° up or 90° down), and the distal section can also be deflected in a single plane (160° up or 100° down). The endoscope is forward-viewing, with a working length of 133 cm, a field of view of 90°, and an outer diameter of the distal end and the insertion tube of 5.2 and 7.0 mm, respectively. The ratios of the distal bending section and the distal plus proximal bending section compared with the GIF-XP180N (Olympus Medical Systems) are 0.6 and 2.2, respectively. The endoscope has two accessory channels of 2.2 and 0.85 mm diameter. It also has suction and insufflation capabilities. The latest generation of dedicated DPVCS has shown an extremely high success rate (97%) using only the free-hand technique.[54] For successful free-hand insertion of the dedicated DPVCS, the tip of cholangioscope is inserted into the distal bile duct using up-angle and torque of the cholangioscope shaft. The manipulation is similar to that of a colonoscope inserted into the terminal ileum, or "blinded" terminal ileum insertion. Once the tip of the cholangioscope is inserted into the bile duct, it is easily advanced to the hilum using scope angulation and by direct advancement. In contrast to a conventional ultraslim upper GI endoscope, the dedicated DPVCS is stable in the bile duct during scope manipulation.

Technique: Diagnostic and Therapeutic

After reaching the bile duct segment of interest, DPVCS enables several diagnostic and therapeutic procedures, including visualization alone,

biopsy for diagnosis, electrohydraulic or LL (Fig. 27.12, *A* and *B*) tumor ablation using argon plasma coagulation, and photodynamic therapy or passage of guidewires to facilitate biliary stenting using plastic or metallic stents through the 2-mm working channel. However, 2-mm accessories are not commonly available (Fig. 27.13).

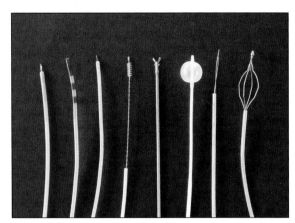

FIG 27.13 5-Fr Accessories for direct cholangioscopy.

TABLE 27.4		**Summary of Insertion Success Rate of Direct Peroral Cholangioscopy**		
Author (Year)	**n**	**Endoscope**	**Assistant Devices**	**Insertion Success (%)**
Larghi (2007)[45]	15	UGI	GW	78
Choi (2009)[46]	12	UGI	Balloon overtube	83
Moon (2009)[47]	11	UGI	GW	46
Tsou (2010)[48]	21	UGI	AB	95
	14	UGI	Balloon overtube	93
Pohl (2011)[49]	25	UGI	AB	72
Mori (2012)[50]	40	UGI	Duodenal balloon	93
Farnik (2014)[51]	40	UGI	AB	98
Itoi (2014)[52]	7	DDPVCS	Free-hand	0
	34	DDPVCS	GW and/or AB	94
Weigt (2015)[53]	42	UGI	AB	90
Beyna (2016)[54]	67	UGI	AB	88
	74	DDPVCS	Free-hand w/wo AB	90

AB, Anchoring balloon; *DDPVCS,* dedicated diagnostic and therapeutic direct peroral videocholangioscopy; *GW,* guidewire; *UGI,* upper gastrointestinal endoscopy.

Based on the high success rate of scope insertion (Table 27.4) and the durability of DPVCS, as well as cost benefit (no need for two light sources or two skilled endoscopists), DPVCS appears to be the first choice for cholangioscopy when ducts are dilated and the target lesion is in the proximal bile duct.

Image-enhanced endoscopy, enabling delineation of fine mucosal structures and vessels, is possible using various processor systems as follows: (1) NBI (Olympus Medical Systems), (2) flexible spectral imaging color enhancement (FICE; Fujifilm, Tokyo, Japan), and (3) i-Scan (Pentax, Tokyo, Japan).

Adverse Events and Limitations

DPVCS also causes procedure-related adverse events. The most serious adverse event is cardiac or cerebral air embolism if the procedure is performed using air insufflation rather than saline irrigation or CO_2 insufflation.[57] Ultraslim endoscopes do not always match the size of the bile duct or papilla as frequently as the smaller-diameter dedicated cholangioscopes. Care should be taken, because this size mismatch may cause unexpected serious adverse events, including bleeding, pancreatitis, and perforation of the duodenum at the site of sphincterotomy.

Acknowledgment

We are indebted to Professor Edward Barroga, Department of International Medical Communications of Tokyo Medical University, for his editorial review of the English manuscript.

The complete reference list for this chapter can be found online at www.expertconsult.com.

28

Endomicroscopy in the Pancreaticobiliary Tree

Anthony J. Choi and Michel Kahaleh

The concept of confocal microscopy was first patented in 1957.[1] Since then, this technology has been used with much success in the laboratory, and more recently this has translated into use in various clinical settings, first described in the field of gastroenterology in 2004 for diagnosing colorectal lesions.[2]

Confocal laser endomicroscopy (CLE) combines the principles of confocal laser microscopy with the endoscope to allow high-resolution images of the gastrointestinal (GI) tract mucosa in real time. In essence, a low-power laser is shot through a pinhole and lens onto the tissue of interest at a certain depth.[3] Only the light reflected back through the same lens and pinhole is detected by the collection system, which is on the same plane as the laser—thus the term "confocal." Any scattered or unfocused reflected light is excluded from detection, leading to great spatial resolution at the plane of interest. Combined with a flexible endoscope, in vivo "optical biopsies"[4] of the GI mucosa at the cellular level are made possible.

CONFOCAL LASER ENDOMICROSCOPY

Although two confocal microscopy imaging systems exist, fluorescence and reflectance, the former is used primarily during GI endoscopy. With fluorescence, intravenous and topical contrast agents are used to highlight different structures. Intravenous fluorescein courses along the vasculature to highlight the extracellular matrix and lamina propria of the surface epithelium, allowing the differentiation of normal and abnormal structures.[5] Topical agents such as acriflavine and cresyl violet achieve nuclear staining but are less popular in the West.[6] In the reflectance type, no contrast agent is required, but it provides limited architectural analysis.

Intravenous fluorescein is the most commonly used contrast agent for CLE, with the most common dose being 2.5 to 5 mL of 10% sodium fluorescein.[7] Becker et al. reported an optimal window ranging from 0 to 8 minutes after injection for viewing the time-dependent CLE imaging, with interpretable images lasting up to 30 minutes.[8] Topical contrast involves removing the mucin layer with *N*-acetylcysteine or acetic acid, flushing with water, and using a spraying catheter to apply the agent. However, this nuclear staining has raised concerns for DNA damage and is not currently FDA-approved.[9,10]

Two endoscopic modalities exist. Probe-based CLE (pCLE) uses a separate probe requiring an accessory channel, needle, or catheter, whereas endoscope-based CLE (eCLE) uses endoscopes with already-integrated CLE systems. Specifically, the pCLE system comprises a fiberoptic bundle with an integrated distal lens that is connected to a laser-scanning unit.[3] Depending on the manufacturer, the required diameter of the accessory channel (0.9 to 2.8 mm), reusability of the probe (10 to 20 examinations), depth of imaging (40 to 70 μm), and resolution (1 to 3.5 μm) differ. The eCLE is too large for pancreaticobiliary imaging and is no longer commercially available, so with the focus of this chapter in mind, any mention of CLE going forward will refer to pCLE.

TECHNIQUE

A miniprobe is inserted into the common bile duct through an endoscopic retrograde cholangiopancreatography (ERCP) catheter or accessory channel of a cholangioscope. With the aid of its radiopaque tip, the probe's position is identified fluoroscopically. The probe is placed in direct contact with the mucosa of the biliary duct, as perpendicular as possible to improve image quality. Once in place, any movement or tissue disruption should be carefully avoided as both may cause visual artifacts. After the injection of intravenous contrast, the fluorescent signal returning from the tissue is converted into an image using a detector, and processed and displayed via a software–hardware system,[10] and is then interpreted and/or saved. Based on visualization, a targeted biopsy can be obtained at this time by removing the probe and passing a biopsy forceps through the endoscope channel (Video 28.1).

DIAGNOSTIC AND SAFETY DATA

Despite advances in imaging and sampling methods in the biliary system, sensitivities for confirming malignancy remain low in the biliary tree, with a meta-analysis showing that sensitivities for endoscopic brush cytology, intraductal biopsy, and both combined were 45%, 48.1%, and 59.4%, respectively.[11] With CLE, however, the diagnostic sensitivity of biliary pathology is improved by interpreting images according to published diagnostic criteria (Table 28.1).

The Miami classification was created and validated[12] to differentiate healthy bile duct mucosa (Fig. 28.1) from that involved with malignant biliary strictures. It consists of four criteria: (1) epithelial structures, (2) thick dark bands (>40 μm), (3) thick white bands (>20 μm), and (4) dark clumps, and the presence of three criteria is highly suggestive of malignancy (Fig. 28.2). Because of false-positive interpretation in the setting of inflammation, the criteria were further refined for inflammatory strictures, called the Paris Classification,[13] which also consist of four criteria: (1) vascular congestion, (2) granular pattern with scales, (3) increased interglandular space, and (4) thickened reticular structures (Fig. 28.3). In a study of 60 cases, the Paris Classification was introduced to aid interpretation of CLE images and further improved overall accuracy to 82% and increased specificity to 83%.[13] As diagnostic criteria continue to be refined, advances will continue to minimize delays in diagnoses and the need for repeat procedures for definitive diagnosis.

TABLE 28.1 Observations and Studies in the Biliary Duct

Study	Purpose	Study Details	Results	Adverse Events
Loeser et al. (2011)[14]	Evaluate utility of CLE in indeterminate biliary strictures	14 patients Prospective 1 center	Normal reticular pattern without loss of mucosal structures or irregular-appearing epithelium is a good predictor of benign biliary stricture.	Not reported
Meining et al. (2011)[12]	Develop and validate classification of CLE images in pancreaticobiliary system	102 patients Prospective 1 center	Diagnosis of malignancy using Miami classification: SN 97% SP 33% PPV 80% NPV 80%	Not reported
Chennat et al. (2011)[15]	Assess utility of CLE in management of bile duct lesions	4 patients Retrospective 1 center	CLE is a promising diagnostic tool for biliary neoplasia.	Not reported
Talreja et al. (2012)[16]	Assess interobserver agreement of CLE of indeterminate biliary strictures	25 lesions Prospective 5 centers	Interobserver agreement for final diagnosis was $K = 0.195$.	Not reported
Heif et al. (2013)[17]	Evaluate CLE in PSC patients	15 patients Retrospective 1 center	Diagnosis of PSC with CLE: SN 100% SP 61.1% PPV 22.2% NPV 100%	No complications
Bakhru et al. (2013)[18]	Assess interobserver agreement of CLE of ampullary lesions	12 lesions Prospective 5 centers	Overall interobserver agreement was $K = 0.02$ for final diagnosis.	Not reported
Caillol et al. (2013)[13]	Assess impact of CLE in management of bile duct strictures	61 patients Prospective Single center	Diagnosis of bile duct stenotic lesions with CLE: SN 83% SP 77% PPV 62% NPV 91% AC 79% Diagnosis with CLE + endobiliary and EUS biopsy: SN 100% SP 69% PPV 60% NPV 100% AC 79%	Not reported
Peter et al. (2014)[19]	Compare CLE interpretation between endoscopists and GI pathologists for various GI lesions	66 patients Prospective Single center	Agreement between endoscopists and pathologist was $K = 0.19$ (95% CI: −0.26 to 0.63) for pancreaticobiliary lesions.	Not reported
Slivka et al. (2015)[20]	Validate CLE for indeterminate biliary strictures	36 patients Prospective 6 centers	Diagnosis with ERCP and CLE using Paris criteria: SN 89% SP 71% PPV 84% NPV 78% AC 82%	Not reported
Karia and Kahaleh (2016)[21]	Compare findings of inflammatory strictures in PSC and non-PSC	35 patients Retrospective 1 center	In patients with inflammatory strictures, components of Paris Classification are present in higher frequency in non-PSC patients.	Not reported
Yang et al. (2016)[22]	Compare diagnostic accuracy of CLE and cholangioscopic biopsy for indeterminate biliary strictures	195 patients Retrospective 1 center	Sensitivity and diagnostic accuracy are similar between CLE + cytology and cholangioscopic biopsy.	Not reported

AC, Accuracy; *CLE,* confocal laser endocmicroscopy; *EUS,* endoscopic ultrasonography; *GI,* gastrointestinal; *NPV,* negative predictive value; *PPV,* positive predictive value; *PSC,* primary sclerosing cholangitis; *SN,* sensitivity; *SP,* specificity.

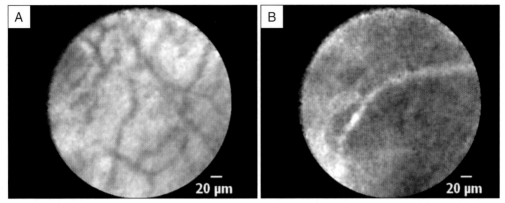

FIG 28.1 Probe-based confocal laser endomicroscopy (pCLE) findings in a healthy bile duct. **A,** Reticular network of thin dark branching bands (<20 μm) with light-gray background. **B,** Vessels <20 μm.

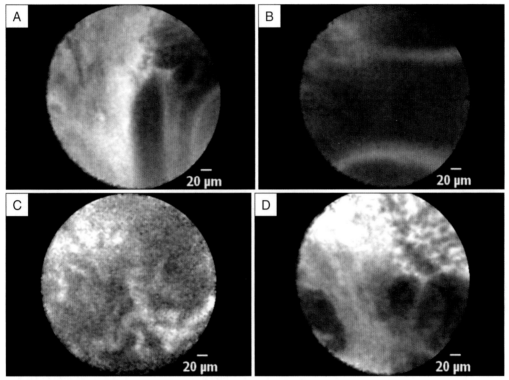

FIG 28.2 The Miami Classification for malignant pancreaticobiliary strictures. **A,** Epithelial structures. **B,** Thick dark bands (>40 μm). **C,** Thick white bands >20 μm. **D,** Dark clumps.

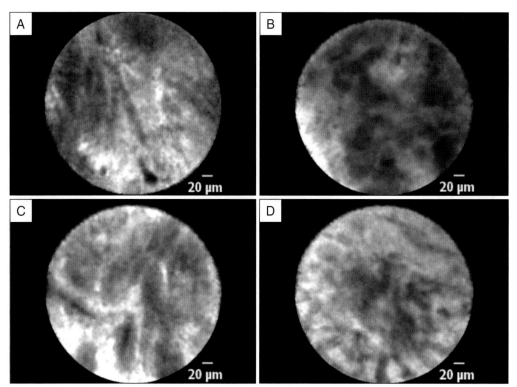

FIG 28.3 The Paris Classification for inflammatory strictures. **A,** Vascular congestion. **B,** Dark granular pattern with scales. **C,** Increased interglandular space. **D,** Thickened reticular structures.

OPTICAL COHERENCE TOMOGRAPHY

Optical coherence tomography (OCT) provides wide-field, cross-sectional imaging at the microscopic level. First-generation OCT technology has been previously shown to increase sensitivity in diagnosing malignant biliary and pancreatic duct strictures.[23,24] A newer device using OCT imaging is now available, allowing for in vivo cross-sectional imaging of the ductal wall (Fig. 28.4). Future studies are required to validate its significance and utility.

CONCLUSION

CLE has been shown in multiple studies to be safe and effective at providing useful diagnostic information at the time of ERCP. pCLE in particular has been shown to have higher performance characteristics in the evaluation of indeterminate pancreaticobiliary strictures than brushing and intraductal biopsy, possibly reducing the need for repeat procedures and decreasing cost. However, further studies on its cost-effectiveness are needed to improve its acceptance and widespread distribution.

The complete reference list for this chapter can be found online at www.expertconsult.com.

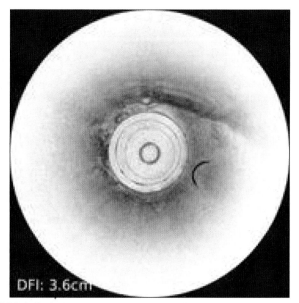

FIG 28.4 Optical coherence tomography of the distal bile duct showing loss of integrity of the biliary wall between 5 and 10 o'clock, compatible with malignancy.

29

ERCP in Children

Victor L. Fox

Endoscopic retrograde cholangiopancreatography (ERCP) was introduced into pediatric medicine in the late 1970s and is now routinely used for the diagnosis and treatment of biliary tract and pancreatic diseases in children throughout the world. With the advent of high-quality magnetic resonance cholangiopancreatography (MRCP) and endoscopic ultrasonography (EUS) (see Chapter 33), ERCP in children is now predominantly used for anticipated therapeutic interventions. This parallels practice in adult medicine. Recent pediatric reports have focused on technical success, safety, and therapeutic efficacy.[1–10] Data from hospitalized children in the United States show a trend of both increasing volume of ERCP and increasing percentage of therapeutic application.[11] Although technical expertise continues to remain concentrated literally in the hands of adult-medicine endoscopists, pediatric specialists should collaborate closely on patient selection and preprocedural and postprocedural management.[12] In high-volume tertiary pediatric referral centers, ERCP is increasingly performed by expert pediatric endoscopists working independently.[13]

This chapter highlights unique aspects of pediatric ERCP, distinguished by differences in childhood behavior, physiology, anatomy, and disease spectrum compared with adults.

DESCRIPTION OF TECHNIQUE

Patient and Family Preparation

Preparation for high-risk procedures in children involves preparing both the child and the parents or guardians. This process may resemble preparation for adults who are elderly or disabled and dependent on the assistance of family for medical decision making. The current and past medical history must be carefully reviewed to include prior anesthesia and operative history, current medications, and allergies to medications, contrast agents, and latex. Problems that may have followed a prior similar procedure should be reviewed to identify opportunities for improvement or risk reduction. Additional vulnerabilities that are unique or more common in children include behavioral issues such as exaggerated fears, emotional lability, oppositional behavior, occult metabolic or hematologic conditions, undiscovered congenital abnormalities, and thermal instability in young infants. A detailed family history assumes greater importance for young children undergoing their first procedure, because anesthetic risk attributable to hereditary conditions such as malignant hyperthermia or other metabolic disorders may be revealed.

Infants are unusually sensitive to seemingly minor hemorrhage because of their small total circulating blood volume. Supportive blood products should be held in reserve for procedures in which significant bleeding may develop. Infants are also more vulnerable to compromised ventilation when excessive insufflation restricts movement of the diaphragm or an endoscope compresses the relatively soft trachea.

Older children and adolescents may join their parents in the process of obtaining informed consent for a procedure. The parents must understand the potential risks, benefits, and alternatives and be offered additional consultation with a surgeon or interventional radiologist when appropriate. Families are most reassured by a team management approach.

Procedure Environment

The procedure environment must have equipment and staff available to support complex therapeutic procedures and adverse events that might arise. Busy adult endoscopy units have highly experienced staff who can anticipate and efficiently assist with the technical aspects of ERCP. Pediatric units and their staff are disadvantaged by the relative infrequency of this procedure. Periodic review of basic principles, hands-on simulation, and consistent staff participation can build and reinforce skills and improve teamwork in a pediatric unit. Ideally, recovery unit nurses with pediatric experience should be available to recognize emerging problems and expedite supportive care. Although ERCP can be performed safely on an ambulatory or outpatient basis, overnight hospital admission for observation of children is advisable because the signs and symptoms of adverse events can evolve many hours after the procedure and may not be reliably reported or recognized early by a child. Immediate access to subspecialty consultation by pediatric anesthesiologists, gastroenterologists, surgeons, and radiologists is essential when providing safe and effective care.

Endoscopist

Who should perform pediatric ERCP relates to issues of skill, knowledge, and environment. High-volume ERCP and advanced endoscopic skills reside within adult medicine centers of excellence supported by experienced assistants with abundant accessories, ensuring the likelihood of technical success. However, technical success alone may not be sufficient for optimal care of children. Pediatricians have important clinical knowledge about when and how to use ERCP in a particular child or situation, but they may be excluded from important decision making once a child is transferred to an adult medicine facility. Endoscopists who have an adult practice are reluctant to perform ERCP in a pediatric facility where properly trained assistants and an adequate inventory of accessories may be lacking. Adult and pediatric endoscopists must consider these factors and the availability of alternative therapy before embarking on ERCP in pediatric patients.

Pediatric endoscopists who seek training in ERCP require either supplemental training with adult patients or a very long training period with pediatric patients to achieve experience with several hundred procedures, a number shown to correlate with achieving technical success in adult patients.[14] The volume and complexity of cases required to achieve a comparable level of initial competence and, importantly, to maintain competence in pediatric ERCP are unknown. A special interest group (SIG) of pediatric endoscopists performing ERCP in tertiary care centers around the world was recently formed under the sponsorship of the North American Society for Pediatric Gastroenterology, Hepatology, and Nutrition (NASPGHAN). Members of this SIG are collaborating on a prospective multicenter database that will soon provide information about technical success and clinical outcomes when ERCP is performed by pediatric endoscopists.[15]

Sedation

Most pediatric gastroenterologists prefer general anesthesia or deep sedation for technically challenging procedures in children. This is similar to a trend toward more frequent use of deep sedation and anesthesia in adults undergoing particularly uncomfortable or lengthy endoscopic procedures. Although ERCP in older children and adolescents may be performed successfully with intravenous moderate sedation, general anesthesia with endotracheal intubation affords safer airway management with assured analgesia and hypnosis during a potentially lengthy or difficult procedure. Once the airway has been secured, either prone or supine positioning can be safely used; when the prone position is selected, adequate use of padding and bolsters allows for sufficient chest excursion and reduced abdominal compression.

Fluoroscopy (see Chapter 3)

Children are more vulnerable than adults to radiation injury during fluoroscopy.[16] They are more sensitive to the effects of radiation, have a longer life expectancy than adults during which the long-term adverse events from exposure (stochastic effects) such as cancer may evolve, and may receive unnecessary high-dose radiation exposure if equipment is not adjusted for a smaller body. Therefore the assistance of a radiation technologist with pediatric experience for equipment support and the availability of a radiologist with pediatric training for consultation are critically important for safe and effective fluoroscopy during ERCP. The desire for high-resolution imaging must be balanced against the risk of greater radiation exposure to the child.

Fluoroscopy for pediatric ERCP may be performed using a fixed table in a dedicated fluoroscopy suite or a portable C-arm in a separate procedure room. The advantages of the C-arm device are portability, lower cost, and easier oblique imaging. Modern digital devices provide excellent image quality. The x-ray equipment should be adjusted to accommodate the smaller body of a young child and reduce the radiation dose rate. Shielding of reproductive organs is important and should be performed for all patients. Good fluoroscopic technique by the examiner can minimize radiation exposure to the child and to personnel (see also Chapter 3). The following rules or principles will help advance this goal: (1) position the child so that the beam takes the shortest distance through the body—that is, avoid unnecessary oblique projection; (2) position the image intensifier or receptor above the patient; (3) minimize the distance of the intensifier and maximize the distance of the x-ray tube to the child's body; (4) use the least magnification necessary and use field collimators to focus on areas of interest; (5) avoid the use of a grid; (6) minimize beam-on time and use the slowest pulse rates that produce acceptable imaging for a given task; and (7) use the "last image hold" feature when capturing images to avoid additional exposure. Either low-osmolar nonionic or high-osmolar water-soluble contrast media in the range of 150 to 300 mg/mL may be used.

Supplemental Medications

Drug dosing for children is based on units per kilogram body weight ranging up to maximum adult doses. In addition to limited use for endocarditis prophylaxis, antibiotics are recommended for high-grade biliary or pancreatic duct obstruction, biliary or pancreatic duct disruption, and pancreatic fluid collections (see also Chapter 10). Ampicillin/sulbactam (100 to 200 mg/kg/day intravenous [IV] divided every 6 hours, maximum 4 g sulbactam per day), a broad-spectrum cephalosporin such as cefazolin (50 to 100 mg/kg/day IV divided every 8 hours, maximum 6 g/day), or a fluoroquinolone such as ciprofloxacin (20 to 30 mg/kg/day IV divided every 12 hours, maximum 800 mg/day) is usually adequate. Intravenous glucagon can be used to briefly reduce duodenal contractions during cannulation. A dose of 0.25 to 0.5 mg IV is appropriate for most ages and can be repeated. Intravenous secretin 0.2 mcg/kg may be used to facilitate successful cannulation of the minor papilla (see Chapter 21). The efficacy of rectal indomethacin for prevention of post-ERCP pancreatitis in children has not been studied. However, given the low risk of single-dose administration and the potential benefit extrapolated from adult data (see Chapter 8), rectal indomethacin should be considered for use in children. This author uses the dose of rectal indomethacin, 2 mg/kg (maximum 100 mg), for all children undergoing ERCP unless performed during an episode of acute pancreatitis. This can be achieved by cutting 50 mg rectal suppositories and using 2 mL of a 5 mg/mL liquid oral suspension for rectal administration in children under 10 kg.

Endoscopic Equipment

Although there are no duodenoscopes specifically designed for use in children, patients of all ages and sizes, including full-term neonates, can undergo diagnostic and therapeutic ERCP using duodenoscopes that are commercially available. Standard diagnostic duodenoscopes with insertion tube diameters in the range of 11 to 12 mm can be used effectively in children older than 2 years and with difficulty between 1 and 2 years of age. These endoscopes generally have operating channels that will accommodate catheters and stents up to 7 to 8 Fr, which is adequate for most interventions. Whereas "therapeutic" duodenoscopes containing operating channels in excess of 4 mm are needed to place 10-Fr stents, such large endoprostheses are rarely needed in young children. These larger endoscopes are easily used in most adolescents.

Neonates and infants require a small-diameter instrument in the range of 7 to 8 mm that will pass easily through the pylorus and allow effective positioning of the tip adjacent to the major papilla. Currently, there is only one commercially available duodenoscope suitable for use in small infants, the PJF-160 (Olympus America, Inc., Lehigh Valley, PA). This endoscope has a working length of 1240 mm, a maximum distal tip diameter of 7.5 mm, an operating channel diameter of 2.0 mm, an elevator, and a noninsulated metal tip. The length is poorly suited for use in small infants (Fig. 29.1). Basic diagnostic and therapeutic maneuvers are possible with this endoscope, although the repertoire of available accessories that will fit through the small operating channel is limited. Catheter tips that taper to a diameter of 3 to 4 Fr are helpful in order to selectively cannulate biliary and pancreatic ducts in infants. However, deep selective cannulation into normal ducts is not always

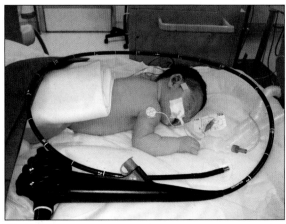

FIG 29.1 Olympus PJF-160 duodenoscope and young infant.

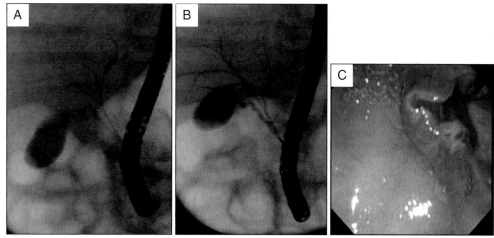

FIG 29.2 Cholestasis in a 2-month-old infant caused by biliary sludge. **A,** Guidewire advanced into left hepatic duct. **B,** Deep cannulation of main bile duct. **C,** Sphincterotomy performed, followed by irrigation of ducts to clear sludge.

possible in young infants because of their narrow caliber. An ultratapered (3.5 Fr) cannula, a retrieval balloon catheter, and a wire basket catheter that will fit the 2.0-mm channel of the PJF-160 duodenoscope are available from Olympus. Other highly tapered cannulas such as the precurved Glo-Tip (GT-5-4-3) (Cook Endoscopy, Winston-Salem, NC) may be used. A tapered-tip sphincterotome catheter with a short cutting wire such as the UTS-15 (Cook Endoscopy) can be advanced with some resistance through the operating channel of the PJF-160 endoscope. Olympus does not endorse the use of this endoscope for sphincterotomy because of the potential risk of thermal injury from electrical current conducted through the metal tip. Nonetheless, this author and others have used this instrument for sphincterotomy without incident.

Equipment for irrigation and hemostasis must be readily available when performing therapeutic ERCP. The 2.0-mm operating channel of the PJF-160 endoscope is too narrow for hemostatic clip devices and bipolar cautery probes, but small-diameter (1.8 mm) sclerotherapy catheters (Boston Scientific Corp., Marlborough, MA) and small-diameter (1.5 mm) argon plasma coagulation catheters (Erbe USA, Inc., Marietta, GA) can be used for injection and cautery hemostasis, respectively.

CO_2 insufflation substituted for air insufflation may reduce the risk of abdominal distension in infants and air embolism. Although air embolism is rarely reported in pediatric endoscopy, CO_2 embolism may be better tolerated based on animal studies.[17–19] This author uses CO_2 insufflation for all ERCPs.

Technique

The techniques for ERCP in children are the same as those for adult patients and are discussed in detail in other chapters. The procedure can be conducted with a child either prone or supine on the examining table. Prone positioning is most comfortable for the endoscopist and preferred by this author. The basic endoscopic maneuvers are technically challenging in young children, because the equipment has not been optimally designed for smaller-scale anatomy. In young children and infants, the endoscope tip is forced close to the papilla. This limits the length of the catheter that can be advanced into view while attempting cannulation. Although precurved cannulas are available, selective biliary cannulation is most easily achieved using a tapered-tip, pull-type sphincterotome with a short cutting wire. Tightening the cutting wire increases the angulation of the catheter tip within a short working distance to the papilla. Also, by starting the procedure with a sphincterotome, the endoscopist can proceed directly with therapy when

indicated. Wire-guided access, using a soft-tipped, hydrophilic, narrow-gauge wire, may be preferred over contrast-guided cannulation to avoid repeated unintentional injection of the pancreatic duct when biliary access is sought.[20] A guidewire also secures selective duct cannulation during sphincterotomy. Stiff catheters such as those used for stricture dilation or stone retrieval are also more likely to require wire-guided entry. In young infants a soft-wire retrieval basket will enter the duct more easily if partially opened because the basket wires are more flexible when extended out from the stiffer plastic sheath. Alternatively, placing the endoscope in the long position may achieve a more favorable position in front of the major papilla, similar to the position generally used to cannulate the minor papilla. However, tip control is compromised with the endoscope in the long position. Sphincterotomy, stone extraction, and temporary stent placement have all been successfully performed in very young infants using small-diameter endoscopes (Fig. 29.2).

Although the PJF-160 duodenoscope with a 2.0-mm operating channel will accept accessory catheters of 5-Fr diameter, the catheters tend to bind in the channel when the endoscope tip is angulated. In addition, air and fluid cannot be evacuated when a catheter is in the channel. It is also difficult to maintain a stable tip position when using a small-diameter endoscope in an infant, because much of the long flexible insertion tube remains unanchored outside of the child. Assistance is sometimes needed to maintain torque stability on the insertion tube.

The endoscopist must be careful to avoid excessive distension of the bowel with gas, which can impede movement of the diaphragm and acutely compromise ventilation in an infant. Also, the soft tissues of an infant are fragile. Repeated impaction of catheters or wire guides against the papilla in a young infant can render the structure unrecognizable because of traumatic edema. A false tract can easily be created using surprisingly little force while advancing a catheter or wire into the ampulla of Vater or into the minor papilla.

INDICATIONS AND CONTRAINDICATIONS (BOX 29.1)

Diagnostic and Therapeutic Indications

Although the necessity of diagnostic ERCP has been diminished by advances in MRCP, subtle diagnostic findings are still best resolved with direct contrast injection. This is particularly true for young children who cannot cooperate with breath-holding sequences required for magnetic resonance imaging (MRI) and for conditions that may require fine spatial resolution such as early sclerosing cholangitis, bile duct paucity syndromes, biliary atresia (BA), anomalous pancreaticobiliary junction (APBJ), and pancreas divisum. The principal roles for ERCP in children are to relieve obstruction, improve drainage, and divert leakage from the bile ducts and the pancreas.

Biliary Indications
Neonatal Cholestasis

Neonatal cholestasis is the only biliary condition unique to pediatrics in which purely diagnostic cholangiography has a role. The most common causes of neonatal cholestasis are idiopathic neonatal hepatitis and prolonged administration of total parenteral nutrition, both frequently encountered in neonates compromised by premature birth, congenital abnormalities requiring surgical intervention, or other acute illnesses of the newborn. These conditions are characterized by hepatocellular and canalicular dysfunction rather than bile duct obstruction. However, they can sometimes be difficult to distinguish from ductal obstruction because of inspissated bile (seen with cystic fibrosis or idiopathic causes), bile duct paucity (e.g., Alagille syndrome), or obliteration of the duct caused by BA. Of these conditions, the correct diagnosis most urgently needed is for BA, because surgical intervention by portoenterostomy (Kasai procedure) substantially reduces long-term morbidity and mortality if undertaken during the early weeks and months of life.[21] If left untreated, BA leads to liver failure and organ transplantation or death by 1 to 2 years of age.

The role of ERCP in the diagnosis of BA remains controversial because of variations in clinical practice; interpretation of liver histology; access to high-quality diagnostic ultrasonography, MRI, and scintigraphy imaging; and availability of highly skilled biliary endoscopists. Most pediatric gastroenterologists, hepatologists, and surgeons continue to rely on a combination of clinical presentation, serum chemistry profile, ultrasonography, biliary scintigraphy, and liver histology rather than ERCP to identify infants in need of surgical exploration with intraoperative cholangiography and possible portoenterostomy. However, published series of ERCP in infants with unexplained cholestasis consistently report high positive and negative predictive values exceeding 90% with only rare minor adverse events.[22–26] Appropriate equipment and technical proficiency are required by endoscopists who use ERCP for this indication, because cannulation of the ampulla in a neonate is quite difficult. The endoscopic findings suggestive of BA include absence of visible bile within the duodenum, partial filling of the bile duct with abnormal termination, and failure to fill the bile duct despite filling of the pancreatic duct[27] (Figs. 29.3 to 29.5). Complete filling of the bile duct, including hepatic branches, excludes the diagnosis of BA (Fig. 29.6). ERCP is most helpful when the diagnosis of BA is unlikely but cannot be definitely excluded without cholangiography. In this situation, an unnecessary exploratory laparotomy can be avoided by demonstrating a patent bile duct.

Cholelithiasis and Choledocholithiasis

Choledocholithiasis, usually associated with cholelithiasis, is the predominant indication for ERCP in children. Black pigment bilirubinate material is commonly found in infants and in children with underlying hemolytic conditions such as sickle cell disease or spherocytosis, or in a child with a history of multiple blood transfusions (Fig. 29.7). Light-colored cholesterol stones are more typical in adolescent patients. Stringer and colleagues reported a detailed analysis of the chemical composition of gallstones in a series of 20 children ranging in age from 0.3 to 13.9 years.[28] Ten had black pigment stones, two had cholesterol stones, one had brown pigment stones, and seven (35%) had calcium carbonate stones, a form uniquely found in children.

Asymptomatic neonatal cholelithiasis may resolve spontaneously, and even symptomatic choledocholithiasis can clear without the need for aggressive intervention.[29,30] Therefore a brief period of supportive care with dietary fasting, IV fluids, and antibiotics can be justified to avoid unnecessary invasive therapy. Otherwise, symptomatic small stones and impacted sludge can be definitively treated endoscopically without resorting to surgical intervention or more challenging percutaneous transhepatic techniques. Sphincterotomy with removal of stone or sludge material can be performed successfully with appropriate equipment even in very young infants,[31–34] (Fig. 29.8). Osanai and colleagues reported a small series of five children ranging in age from 7 to 13 years who underwent successful papillary balloon dilation for removal of bile duct stones.[35] Three of five patients developed hyperamylasemia, but no clinical pancreatitis or other severe adverse events were reported.

Some pediatric surgeons advocate a total laparoscopic approach at the time of cholecystectomy for primary therapy of choledocholithiasis, reserving intraoperative or postoperative ERCP for intraductal calculi that cannot be cleared laparoscopically.[36] However, there are no data to support routine cholecystectomy in young children or infants without an underlying condition that predisposes to stone formation. Small gallstones and sludge may pass spontaneously after endoscopic sphincterotomy alone.[34]

Choledochal Anomalies (see also Chapter 35)

Choledochal anomalies include cystic malformations of the bile duct and anomalous junctions between the bile duct and pancreatic duct.[26,37,38] Choledochal cyst (CDC) (described in more detail in Chapter 35) is a descriptive term used when there is segmental rounded or fusiform distension of the bile duct. An anatomic classification scheme proposed by Todani and associates subcategorizes the condition into types I through V depending on the shape and location[39] (Figs. 29.9 to 29.11). When APBJ accompanies a cystic deformity of the bile duct, stenosis at the junction is often present and surgery is appropriate treatment for definitive decompression and to reduce the long-term risk of biliary cancer. ERCP may be useful in complicated choledochal cysts to relieve obstruction before surgery.[40]

Soares and colleagues used a large multi-institutional database, including 394 patients (135 children), to analyze differences in clinical presentation and clinical outcomes between children and adults.[41] Children were less likely to present with pain and more likely to present with jaundice. Predominant morphologic categories were type I in children and type IV in adults. Concurrent biliary malignancy was found in only 2 (1.5%) children (embryonal rhabdomyosarcoma) compared with 8

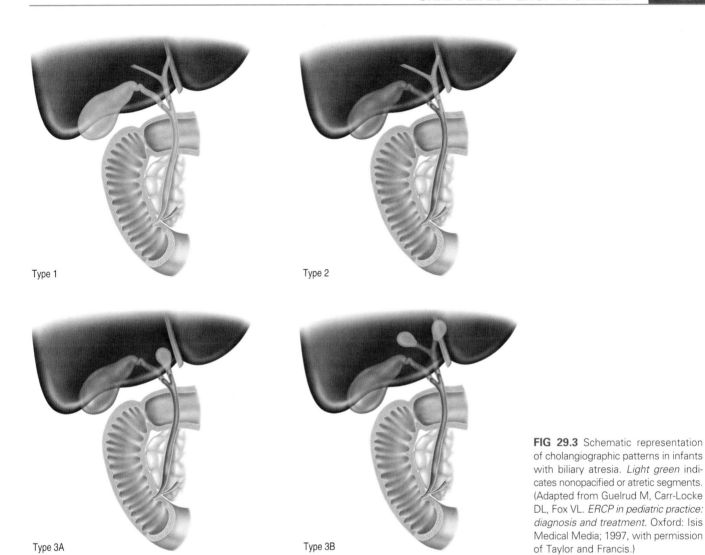

Type 1

Type 2

Type 3A

Type 3B

FIG 29.3 Schematic representation of cholangiographic patterns in infants with biliary atresia. *Light green* indicates nonopacified or atretic segments. (Adapted from Guelrud M, Carr-Locke DL, Fox VL. *ERCP in pediatric practice: diagnosis and treatment.* Oxford: Isis Medical Media; 1997, with permission of Taylor and Francis.)

FIG 29.4 Two-month-old infant with severe cholestasis, nonexcreting hepatobiliary iminodiacetic acid (HIDA) scan, valve and peripheral pulmonic stenosis, and liver biopsy equivocal for biliary atresia. **A,** Successful cannulation of major papilla but no contrast filling of bile duct was noted on subsequent cholangiography (not shown). **B,** Small amount of bile emerged from papilla, suggesting patency. Hereditary bile duct paucity (Alagille's syndrome) subsequently confirmed with novel mutation in the *JAG1* gene.

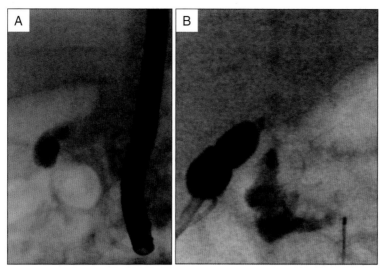

FIG 29.5 Seven-week-old infant with acholic stool, cholestasis, and normal gallbladder on ultrasonography examination; alpha 1 antitrypsin deficiency with ZZ phenotype; and liver biopsy equivocal for biliary atresia. **A,** Contrast entered gallbladder but failed to enter hepatic ducts. **B,** Intraoperative cholangiogram confirmed type 2 pattern of atresia with absent filling of the hepatic ducts. Contrast fills the gallbladder and flows into the duodenum.

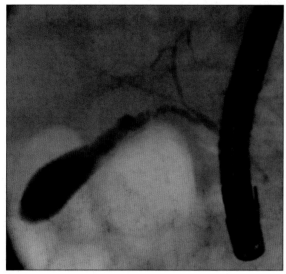

FIG 29.6 Ten-week-old infant with cholestasis, nonexcreting hepatobiliary iminodiacetic acid (HIDA) scan, contracted gallbladder on ultrasonography examination, and equivocally abnormal liver biopsy. Complete filling of hepatic ducts excluded biliary atresia.

(3.1%) adults (adenocarcinoma). A major indication for early surgical resection of the bile duct is prevention of biliary cancer. Urushihara and colleagues reported long-term outcomes in 120 patients operated at a mean age of 4 years.[42] No biliary malignancies were found after a mean postresection interval of 16.6 years (range 3 to 34 years).

APBJ may also be found incidentally without associated cystic changes in the bile duct or may be seen in association with recurrent acute pancreatitis (see Chapter 52).[43,44] Endoscopic sphincterotomy may relieve symptoms or assist the preoperative management of this problem.[45]

Distal common bile duct obstruction in infants from choledocholithiasis can cause fusiform distension mimicking type I choledochal cyst (Fig. 29.12). ERCP is therefore important in this situation to clarify the diagnosis and relieve the obstruction, avoiding unnecessary surgery.

Biliary Strictures and Leaks

Most pediatric biliary strictures are caused by benign acquired conditions. Primary sclerosing cholangitis (PSC) is the most common inflammatory etiology (see Chapter 48). In children, PSC is predominantly associated with chronic inflammatory bowel disease, especially ulcerative colitis.[46] It is also the most common hepatic complication of primary immunodeficiency disorders.[47] The diagnosis of PSC is established on the basis of a suggestive history, compatible laboratory findings, and most importantly by cholangiography and liver histology. The condition in children is further subclassified as large-duct PSC and small-duct PSC (defined as typical histology with normal cholangiogram), where the latter may be an earlier or milder form. Overlapping features with autoimmune hepatitis occur in approximately 30% of patients with both large-duct and small-duct disease.[46] Rossi and colleagues compared MR cholangiography with endoscopic cholangiography in a small series of children with PSC.[48] The diagnostic accuracy was comparable, but endoscopic cholangiography produced better image quality and superior resolution of peripheral hepatic duct branches, especially in younger children. A pattern of diffusely irregular intrahepatic ducts with alternating thin and thick caliber is essentially pathognomonic for large-duct PSC. Because the bile duct epithelium is diffusely inflamed extending to the papilla, an early feature is dilation of the common bile duct caused by mild or intermittent functional papillary stenosis. A characteristic observation during ERCP is underfilling of the intrahepatic ducts during simple contrast injection despite deep cannulation to the level of the common hepatic duct (Fig. 29.13). Pressurized injection through a retrieval balloon catheter positioned above the cystic duct takeoff using occlusion technique is required to fill the intrahepatic branches. Dominant strictures are uncommon in children but may be amenable to endoscopic dilation when indicated by pain, jaundice, or recurrent bacterial cholangitis. Secondary biliary malignancy is quite rare in childhood but must be considered when there is a dominant stricture or significant rise in CA19-9 antigen level. Deneau and colleagues reported cholangiocarcinoma in 8 of 781 (1%) children with a diagnosis ranging in age from 15 to 18 years.[46] Brush cytology and intraductal biopsy may be performed as in adult patients with suspected malignancy.

Biliary complications occur in 10% to 35% of pediatric liver transplant recipients (see also Chapter 44).[49] Laurence and colleagues reported 22

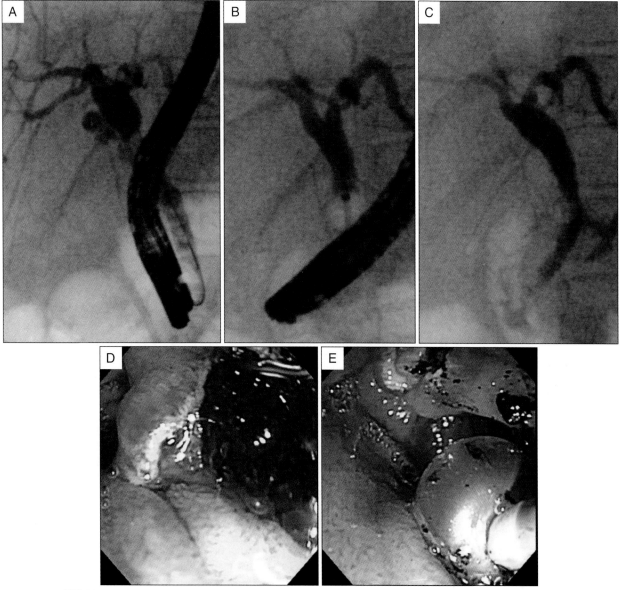

FIG 29.7 Bilirubinate stones in an 8-year-old boy with hemoglobin SS disease. **A,** Multiple stones and sludge stacked within a dilated common bile duct and in the cystic duct. **B** and **C,** Clearing debris from common bile duct using balloon catheter. **D** and **E,** Endoscopic appearance of black pigment stones and sludge material.

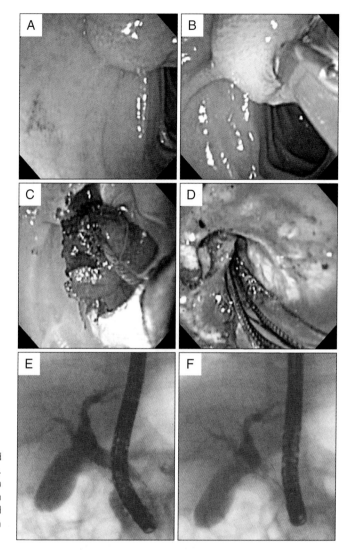

FIG 29.8 A 4-month-old, 4.8-kg infant presenting with acholic stool and jaundice 6 weeks after surgery for complex congenital heart disease. **A,** Endoscopic views of a darkened bulging papilla. **B,** Cannulation with sphincterotome. **C** and **D,** Removal of impacted soft pigment stone with retrieval basket after sphincterotomy. **E** and **F,** Cholangiogram shows dilated intrahepatic and extrahepatic ducts, small filling defects within common bile duct, and retrieval basket open within common bile duct.

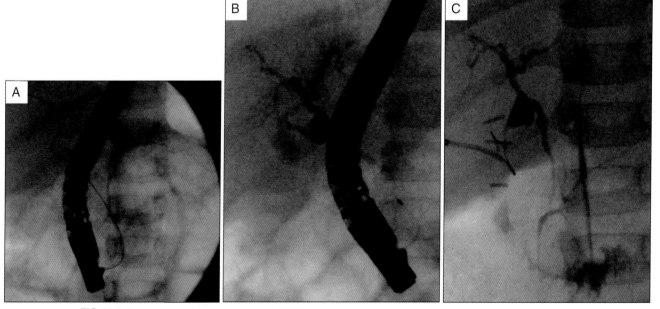

FIG 29.9 Saccular type I choledochal cyst (CDC) in 4-year-old girl presenting with recurrent abdominal pain and elevated amylase and lipase levels. **A,** Deep cannulation over wire guide in bile duct shows unexpected selective filling of pancreatic duct. **B,** Selective cholangiogram using a cannula with a highly tapered tip (3.5 Fr) that could cross the stenosis at the pancreaticobiliary junction. **C,** Intraoperative cholangiogram confirming type I CDC and anomalous pancreaticobiliary junction.

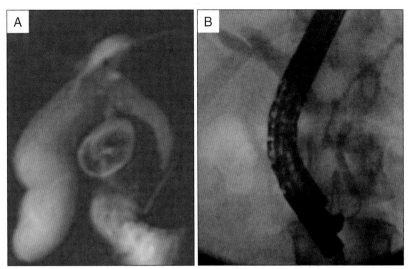

FIG 29.10 Fusiform type I choledochal cyst in adolescent female patient presenting with intermittent episodes of abdominal pain because of either acute pancreatitis or acute cholestasis and elevated transaminase levels. **A,** Magnetic resonance cholangiopancreatography showing fusiform dilation of common bile duct proximal to stenosis at junction with pancreatic duct. **B,** Injection of contrast into common channel simultaneously fills pancreatic duct and bile duct.

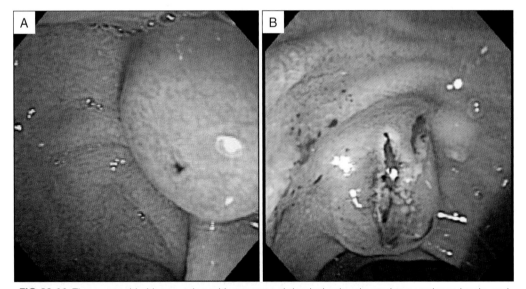

FIG 29.11 Three-year-old girl presenting with recurrent abdominal pain, elevated transaminase levels, and dilated common bile duct on abdominal ultrasonography examination. **A,** Bulging papilla with stenotic orifice, suggesting type III choledochal cyst. **B,** Sphincterotomy begun with needle-knife incision and completed with pull-type sphincterotome. Symptoms and findings remained resolved 5 years later.

(12.7%) biliary strictures and 12 (7%) leaks in a single-center cohort of 173 pediatric recipients.[50] Anderson and colleagues reported strictures in 15 of 66 (23%) transplant cases, of which 12 (71%) were successfully treated nonoperatively, primarily by percutaneous approach.[49] Valentino and colleagues reported biliary complications in 23 of 99 (23%) cases, including 14 (14%) strictures and 9 (9%) leaks, of which more than half (13) required surgical revision of the anastomosis.[51] BA is the most frequent indication for liver transplantation in childhood, and biliary drainage must be established by Roux-en-Y choledochojejunostomy. Gaining access for endoscopic treatment in such altered anatomy (see Chapter 31) is technically challenging in adult patients and even more difficult or impossible in a small child. Therefore treatment often requires a percutaneous transhepatic approach by an interventional radiologist

or direct surgical revision. For other types of liver disease, children will either undergo whole-organ or split-organ graft transplantation with duct-to-duct anastomosis. Anastomotic strictures and leaks after duct-to-duct anastomosis are managed the same as in adult patients, using dilation and stent therapy[52,53] (Fig. 29.14).

Biliary leaks occur in children after partial hepatectomy, cholecystectomy, and blunt abdominal trauma. ERCP can be used to confirm the source and treat the leak by transpapillary stent placement (Fig. 29.15).[54–56] Spontaneous perforation of the bile duct occurs in infants and young children. In a review of 60 cases over 20 years, the median age at presentation was 4 months and 24 (40%) showed a leak at the junction of the common bile duct and cystic duct.[57] ERCP with stent placement may eliminate the need for surgery in some cases.[57–59]

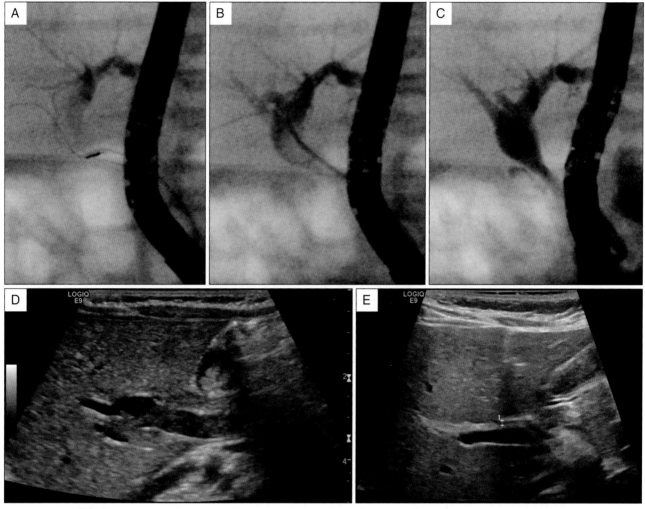

FIG 29.12 Obstruction caused by impacted biliary sludge mimicking fusiform type I choledochal cyst in 16-day-old neonate. **A,** Wire-guided deep cannulation of bile duct with sphincterotome. **B,** Balloon catheter extraction of sludge. **C,** After sludge removal, saccular dilation of proximal bile duct and absence of anomalous pancreaticobiliary junction. **D** and **E,** Abdominal ultrasonography images showing dilated bile duct filled with sludge before endoscopy and complete resolution (1.3 mm common bile duct) 4 months later after sphincterotomy and sludge removal.

FIG 29.13 Adolescent male patient presented with mild jaundice, elevated inflammatory markers, abnormal liver chemistry profile, dilated common bile duct on abdominal ultrasonography examination, poorly defined hepatic ducts on magnetic resonance cholangiopancreatography, and liver biopsy with overlapping features of autoimmune hepatitis and sclerosing cholangitis. **A,** Injection of contrast after deep cannulation of the bile duct shows filling of the common bile duct and gallbladder but little filling of the hepatic ducts. **B,** Injection of contrast using occlusion balloon technique demonstrates characteristic pattern of diffuse peripheral bile duct strictures found in primary sclerosing cholangitis.

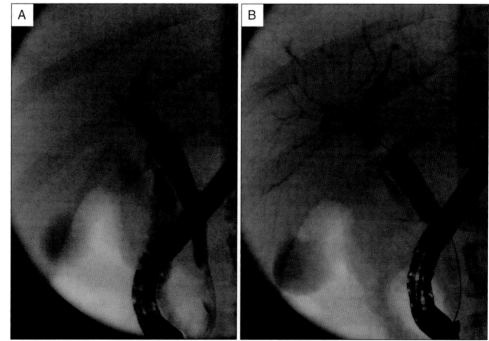

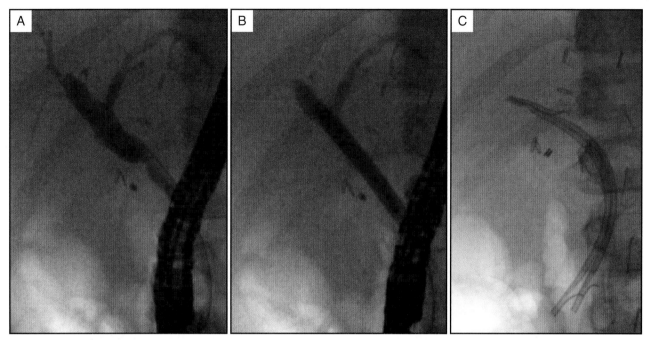

FIG 29.14 Anastomotic stricture after liver transplantation with duct-to-duct anastomosis in a 9-year-old boy. **A** and **B,** Deep cannulation of bile duct followed by balloon catheter dilation. **C,** Two side-by-side stents placed after dilation.

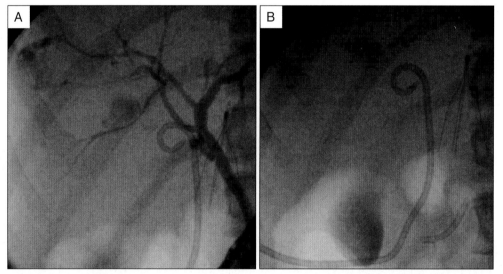

FIG 29.15 Grade IV liver laceration in a 15-year-old male patient caused by blunt abdominal trauma. Note inferior vena cava filter and percutaneous drainage catheter. **A,** Bile leak demonstrated by extravasation of contrast from multiple branches of the right hepatic duct. **B,** Placement of short 10-Fr transpapillary stent resolved the leak.

Idiopathic strictures found at the junction of the main left and right hepatic ducts have been rarely reported in children and are presumed to be congenital in origin[60] (Fig. 29.16). These have been successfully managed both surgically and endoscopically.

Malignant biliary obstruction in children is rarely caused by bile duct epithelium–derived tumors. Rather, most obstructing lesions are solid tumors of the abdomen, causing extrinsic compression. Neuroblastoma is the most frequent solid tumor of childhood and has been implicated as the cause of biliary obstruction in rare case reports.[61] Percutaneous or endoscopic drainage can provide temporary relief of obstruction while awaiting definitive therapy.[62,63]

The "double duct sign" or coexistent narrowing of both the distal bile duct and the head segment of the pancreatic duct is considered ominous in adults, suggesting a pancreatic malignancy. However, children presenting with abdominal pain or jaundice and this finding are much more likely to have a benign self-limited inflammatory process than a primary pancreatic malignancy (Fig. 29.17). Primary pancreatic tumors are extremely rare in childhood. Only 18 cases were found in a 90-year retrospective review at a major tertiary referral hospital.[64] Imaging by MRI, computed tomography (CT), or EUS should be performed to exclude a tumor or mass lesion within the pancreatic head. There may be localized or diffuse pancreatic swelling. When in doubt, EUS-guided or CT-guided needle biopsy of the pancreas can be obtained to exclude tumor. Early reports of this condition applied the term "idiopathic fibrosing pancreatitis" based on pancreatic biopsy or resection specimens that revealed a lymphoplasmacytic infiltrate, fibrosis, and edema of the

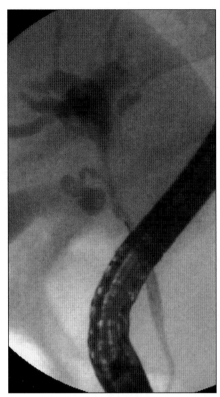

FIG 29.16 Presumed congenital stricture of the common hepatic duct presenting with advanced cirrhosis and portal hypertension in a 10-year-old girl.

parenchyma.[65] Early published cases were managed by partial pancreatectomy and biliary diversion. However, endoscopic dilation of the stenosis and placement of a temporary stent relieves the obstruction while awaiting resolution of the pancreatic swelling.[66] These findings are now increasingly recognized as a form of autoimmune pancreatitis in children, and treatment with corticosteroids may be substituted or used as adjunctive therapy to suppress the inflammatory activity.[67] Although long-term follow-up of this condition has not been reported, short-term outcomes have included exocrine and endocrine insufficiency in 16% and 11%, respectively, of small numbers of patients, but relapsing biliary obstruction has not been described.[67] Therefore, conservative nonsurgical management should be pursued.

Unusual Biliary Infections

Human immunodeficiency virus (HIV)–associated cholangiopathy has been described in children.[68] As in adults, the biliary abnormalities include irregularities of contour and caliber of the intrahepatic and extrahepatic ducts and papillary stenosis. The changes may result from concomitant infection with opportunistic organisms such as cytomegalovirus and *Cryptosporidium parvum*. Ascariasis infestation may be the most prevalent biliary infection worldwide, although concentrated within tropical climates.[69] Among 214 children hospitalized in northern India for management of hepatobiliary and pancreatic ascariasis, 20 (9%) underwent endoscopic intervention and 7 (4%) underwent surgical intervention.[70]

Sphincter of Oddi Dysmotility (see Chapters 16 and 47)

Sphincter of Oddi dysmotility is sometimes considered in children with unexplained abdominal pain that may be accompanied by a dilated

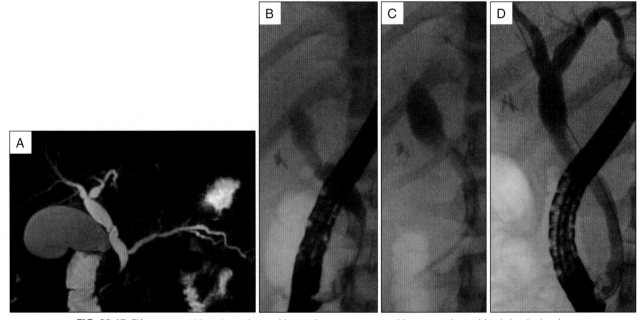

FIG 29.17 Fifteen-year-old male patient with autoimmune pancreatitis presenting with abdominal pain, jaundice, and mildly elevated amylase and lipase levels. Cholecystectomy was initially performed for suspected gallstone pancreatitis. **A,** Magnetic resonance cholangiopancreatography shows tapered narrowing of distal bile duct and narrowed pancreatic duct in head portion with upstream dilation. **B,** Endoscopic cholangiogram shows extrinsic compression of distal bile duct. **C,** Biliary obstruction relieved by endoscopic dilation and placement of temporary stent. **D,** Biliary stenosis resolved after 3 months.

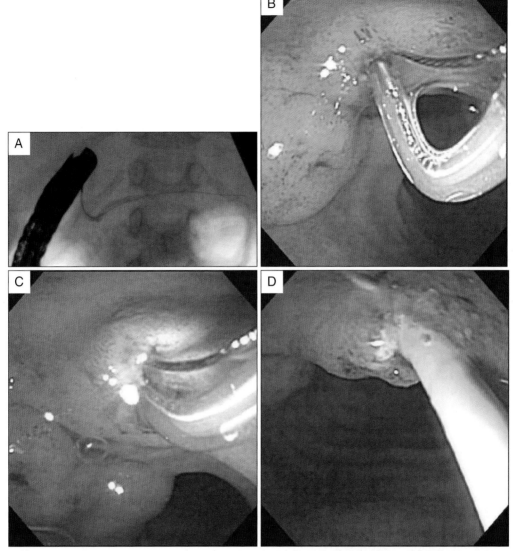

FIG 29.18 Pancreas divisum in a 3-year-old girl presenting with recurrent acute pancreatitis. **A,** Wire-guided cannulation of minor papilla and injection of contrast into dominant dorsal pancreatic duct. **B–D,** Endoscopic cannulation of minor papilla with tapered-tip sphincterotome, followed by sphincterotomy and stent placement.

common bile duct on ultrasonography or delayed gallbladder emptying during scintigraphy. Although no normal manometric values have been established for children, some experts apply adult normal data and perform interventions such as biliary sphincterotomy when basal pressure exceeds 40 mm Hg. Improvement after sphincterotomy has been reported in small numbers of patients, but no controlled outcome data exist for children.[71–73] Moreover, sphincter of Oddi dysfunction cannot be diagnosed in the setting of an intact gallbladder.[74]

Pancreatic Indications
Acute Pancreatitis
Biliary pancreatitis is a major cause of acute pancreatitis in children, accounting for 10% to 30% of cases.[75,76] ERCP with sphincterotomy and stone or sludge removal will improve drainage and reduce the risk of cholangitis or recurrent obstruction without necessarily changing the course of pancreatitis. For children with residual gallbladder stones or an underlying condition that is predisposing to stone or sludge formation, operative cholecystectomy is recommended without delay.[77]

Developmental anomalies involving the pancreas have been reported in association with acute pancreatitis, especially with recurring acute episodes.[78,79] These include pancreas divisum, APBJ, and enteric duplications. Endoscopic papillotomy of the minor papilla in children with pancreas divisum may improve drainage and reduce the frequency or severity of pain attacks (Fig. 29.18). However, recurring acute pancreatitis in children with pancreas divisum and coexistent mutations in *SPINK1* and *CFTR* genes may represent emerging chronic pancreatitis (Fig. 29.19). ERCP is superior to MRCP for imaging the pancreatic duct and APBJ[80] (Fig. 29.20). Whereas APBJ is usually accompanied by a choledochal cyst that requires surgery, patients with isolated APBJ may be treated with endoscopic sphincterotomy alone to prevent recurrent pancreatitis (Fig. 29.21). Cholecystectomy has been recommended in such patients to prevent the long-term risk of adult-onset gallbladder cancer, especially in high-risk ethnic groups.[81,82]

Endoscopic pancreatography can most accurately document communication of the pancreatic duct with enteric duplication cysts, preoperatively guiding surgical intervention[83,84] (Fig. 29.22).

Englum and colleagues analyzed pediatric pancreas trauma data from the American College of Surgeons–sponsored National Trauma Data Bank during the years 2007 to 2011.[85] ERCP was performed in 19 of 674 (2.8%) cases of blunt pancreatic injury and 14 of these 19 cases were managed nonoperatively. Early ERCP can assess duct integrity and provide internal drainage by placement of a transpapillary stent when appropriate and technically feasible. Endoscopic therapy is not indicated for contained intraparenchymal leaks, which usually heal spontaneously (Fig. 29.23). Indications for surgery remain controversial among pediatric surgeons[86–88] (Fig. 29.24).

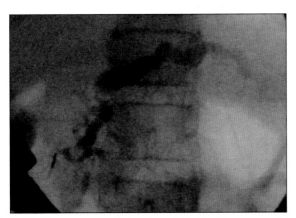

FIG 29.19 Chronic pancreatitis in a 6-year-old girl with pancreas divisum, a dilated irregular pancreatic duct with stone, and single-allele mutations in *SPINK1* and *CFTR* genes.

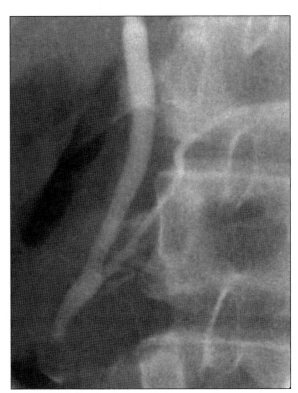

FIG 29.21 Anomalous pancreaticobiliary junction with long common channel treated with sphincterotomy in a 14-year-old girl presenting with recurrent acute pancreatitis.

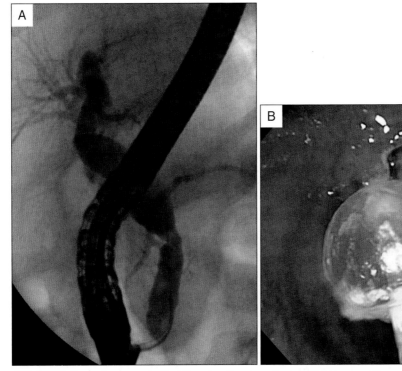

FIG 29.20 Anomalous pancreaticobiliary junction in a 3-year-old girl presenting with acute pancreatitis. **A,** Contrast injection after wire-guided deep cannulation of presumed bile duct revealed a dilated common channel with multiple filling defects, fusiform dilation of the proximal common bile duct, and simultaneous filling of the main and accessory pancreatic ducts via a T-shaped connection not revealed by prior magnetic resonance cholangiopancreatography. **B,** Soft white pancreatic-type stones were removed with retrieval balloon after sphincterotomy.

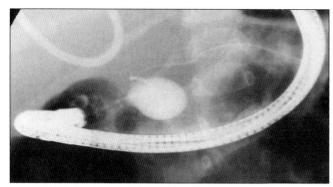

FIG 29.22 Eighteen-month-old infant presented with recurrent acute pancreatitis and persistent pancreatic cyst. Pancreatogram revealed a cyst in continuity with the main pancreatic duct. Enteric duplication cyst was confirmed by histology after surgical excision.

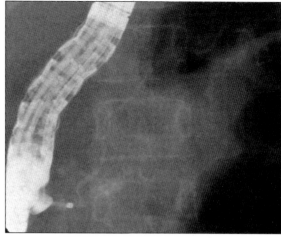

FIG 29.23 Pancreatogram shows faint intraparenchymal extravasation of contrast in the pancreatic head in a 9-year-old girl after a lap belt injury that occurred during an automobile accident.

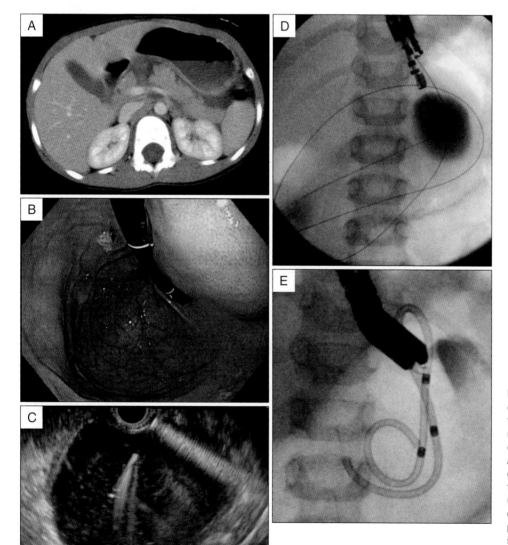

FIG 29.24 Seven-year-old boy with pancreatic injury caused by blunt abdominal trauma. The patient was successfully managed nonoperatively, with subsequent endoscopic drainage of a large pseudocyst. **A,** Computed tomography scan showing complete transection of pancreas at junction of head and main body of pancreas (grade IV laceration). **B,** Endoscopic view of extrinsic compression of stomach by pseudocyst. **C** and **D,** Endoscopic ultrasonography–guided transgastric needle puncture and placement of guidewire into pseudocyst. **E,** Placement of two double-pigtail transgastric stents using a duodenoscope.

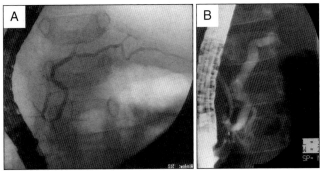

FIG 29.25 Repeat pancreatogram 6 years later shows progressive dilation of the main duct in a child with chronic pancreatitis.

In tropical countries, parasites, primarily *Ascaris lumbricoides,* are the predominant cause of acute pancreatitis in children living in endemic areas (see Chapter 49).[70,89] Endoscopy is indicated to remove obstructing worms that fail to pass after drug therapy.

SOD has also been reported as a cause of recurrent pancreatitis in children that improves after endoscopic pancreatic sphincterotomy.[71,73,90] As with biliary manometry, basal pressures considered normal for adults have been used for normal baseline values in children.

Chronic Pancreatitis (see Chapter 55)

Chronic pancreatitis in children features the same anatomic changes seen in adult, patients, including early progressive dilation and tortuosity of the main duct, followed by strictures and intraductal stones, ectatic side branches, and parenchymal atrophy and calcifications (Fig. 29.25). These abnormalities are easily seen with noninvasive imaging using transabdominal ultrasonography, MR, and CT techniques. The principal role of ERCP is to relieve duct obstruction and improve drainage by performing sphincterotomy, stricture dilation, stone extraction, and temporary stent placement (Figs. 29.26 and 29.27). Several published pediatric series suggest that pain and frequency of acute attacks can be reduced by therapeutic ERCP, in some cases supplemented by extracorporeal shock wave lithotripsy to fragment large stones.[91–93] Surgical drainage operations and total pancreatectomy with islet cell autotransplantation are alternatives to repeat endoscopic procedures in children with disabling pain.[94–98]

Pancreatic Fluid Collections

Pancreatic fluid collections (PFCs), pseudocysts, and walled-off necrosis are managed in children as they are in adults (see Chapter 56). Pseudocysts in children occur most often after blunt abdominal trauma, resulting in disruption or a leak from the main pancreatic duct (see Fig. 29.24). Acute pancreatitis progressing to necrosis is fortunately uncommon in children. Although drugs, especially L-asparaginase and valproate, are often implicated, necrotizing pancreatitis can result from a variety of insults, including idiopathic or metabolic disorders, trauma, and gallstones[99] (Figs. 29.28 and 29.29).

Fluid collections that cause persistent clinical symptoms because of compression of adjacent structures may be drained endoscopically using a transpapillary, transmural, or combination approach, as discussed in Chapter 56. An EUS-guided approach is preferred for transmural drainage. An EUS scope can be used alone or in combination with a duodenoscope for cystogastrostomy with stent placement (see Figs. 29.24 and 29.28). Experience in children with endoscopic and EUS-guided drainage of PFCs using both plastic and metal stents is limited to case reports and small series.[100–106]

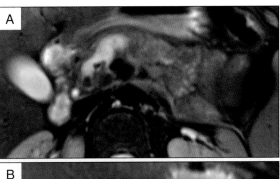

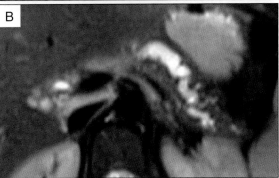

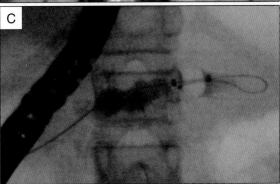

FIG 29.26 Ten-year-old girl presenting with abdominal pain and chronic pancreatitis associated with homozygous N34S *SPINK1* mutation and single-allele *CFTR* mutation. **A** and **B,** Magnetic resonance cholangiopancreatography shows dilated tortuous main pancreatic duct and ectatic side branches along with stones in the head portion of the main duct. **C,** Retrieval balloon catheter is used to sweep out stones and protein plugs from the main duct.

ADVERSE EVENTS

Statistically equivalent high rates of technical success and low rates of adverse events were found in one retrospective case-controlled study of 116 children and 116 adults matched for procedure complexity.[107] Post-ERCP pancreatitis (PEP) is the most common adverse event in children. Rates in early series ranged from 3% to 17%, with higher rates associated with therapeutic procedures.[12] Giefer and colleagues reported rates of 7.7% and 1.1% for PEP and bleeding, respectively, in a recent series of 425 ERCPs (81% therapeutic) in 276 children.[10] The highest rates of PEP in children were reported by Cheng and colleagues in patients who underwent sphincterotomy for SOD: 30% with biliary sphincterotomy alone, 25% with biliary sphincterotomy followed by placement of a temporary pancreatic duct stent, and 20% with pancreatic sphincterotomy followed by placement of a pancreatic duct stent.[71] Other adverse events, such as perforation and infection, occur rarely in pediatric ERCP series. A single case of air embolism during ERCP in a child has been reported.[18] The incidence of delayed adverse events

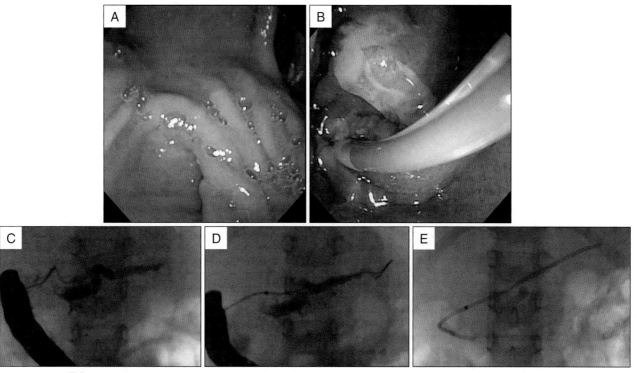

FIG 29.27 Three-year-old girl presenting with acute pancreatitis and magnetic resonance cholangiopancreatography showing a dilated pancreatic duct with suspected obstructing duct stone, and a history of repaired duodenal atresia. Genetic testing detected three heterozygous variants in *CFTR*. **A** and **B,** Endoscopic view of distorted anatomy after duodenoduodenostomy, and purulent drainage from ampulla during cannulation. **C,** Stone obstructing the ventral duct. **D** and **E,** Wire-guided access and stenting across the dorsal duct.

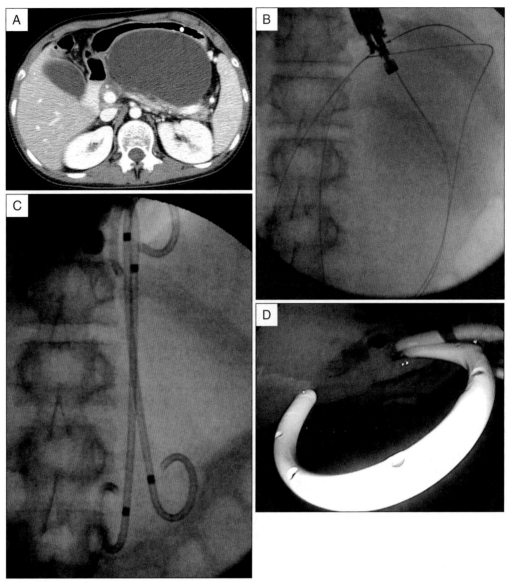

FIG 29.28 L-asparaginase-induced walled-off necrosis in a 15-year-old boy undergoing treatment for leukemia. **A,** Computed tomography scan showing large fluid-filled cyst compressing stomach. **B,** Endoscopic ultrasonography–guided wire coiled within large cyst cavity. **C** and **D,** Fluoroscopic and endoscopic views of two double-pigtail stents placed across cystogastrostomy.

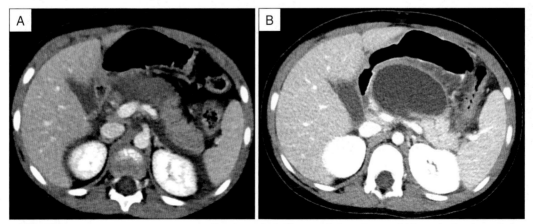

FIG 29.29 Blunt abdominal trauma resulting in walled-off necrosis in a 7-year-old boy. **A,** Focal area of ischemia seen during early contrast-enhanced computed tomography scan. **B,** Cystic fluid collection compressing stomach.

resulting from early childhood sphincterotomy is unknown although this has recently been addressed in a large retrospective Korean series and in an accompanying editorial.[108] Adverse events of sedation or anesthesia must also be considered as part of the total risk to children undergoing ERCP.

RELATIVE COSTS

There are no published data comparing the cost of ERCP with alternative diagnostic and therapeutic approaches such as percutaneous transhepatic cholangiography and direct surgical exploration. Anesthesia contributes a large fraction of the total cost of each approach. Surgical fees likely exceed those of either endoscopy or interventional radiology. The expense of maintaining costly specialized endoscopes and a reasonable inventory of accessories can be prohibitive for many pediatric facilities. Sharing equipment and accessories with a busy adult medicine service is most cost-effective.

The complete reference list for this chapter can be found online at www.expertconsult.com.

30

ERCP in Pregnancy

Thiruvengadam Muniraj and Priya A. Jamidar

Pancreaticobiliary diseases such as choledocholithiasis and gallstone pancreatitis during pregnancy are challenging to manage because of increased risk to both the mother and fetus. Physiologic alterations during pregnancy, such as weight gain and hormonal changes, increase the risk of cholelithiasis. Elevated estrogen levels are believed to enhance biliary saturation, increasing bile lithogenicity, whereas a rise in progesterone causes smooth muscle relaxation and bile stasis, reducing gallbladder motility, thereby promoting gallstone formation.[1–4] The incidence of gallstones in the general population is approximately 10%, with gallstones and biliary sludge reported in up to 12% and 30% of pregnant patients, respectively.[1,5] Most pregnant women with gallstones are asymptomatic, and stone and sludge may spontaneously resolve during the postpartum period. Symptomatic choledocholithiasis during pregnancy is much less frequent and has been reported to occur in 1 in 1200 deliveries.[6] Common bile duct (CBD) stones (Fig. 30.1) may lead to such complications as pancreatitis and cholangitis and generally require therapeutic intervention. Biliary stone disease is the most common cause of pancreatitis during pregnancy.[7]

Older literature suggests that open cholecystectomy with CBD exploration during pregnancy poses significant risks to the fetus.[8] Although newer reports suggest that laparoscopic cholecystectomy in pregnancy is safer, the presence of choledocholithiasis still necessitates endoscopic retrograde cholangiopancreatography (ERCP) or, rarely, CBD exploration.[9] Although ERCP during pregnancy has become increasingly used, it was not always accepted as an appropriate therapeutic modality. Concerns about potential teratogenic effects of fluoroscopy and adverse events that could potentially harm both the mother and fetus (e.g., pancreatitis) were raised. It was not until 1990 that Baillie and colleagues at Duke University Medical Center reported the first experience of ERCP during pregnancy. Five pregnant women underwent ERCP with sphincterotomy without adverse events to the mother or fetus.[10] Since then, several case reports and case series of ERCP during pregnancy have been reported.[11–22] ERCP is now considered a safe and effective procedure during pregnancy.

INDICATION

It is essential to have a strong indication before performing an ERCP during pregnancy. ERCP in pregnancy is most commonly performed for management of choledocholithiasis. Strong suspicion for the presence of a CBD stone is necessary before considering ERCP. For asymptomatic and minimally symptomatic patients, it may be reasonable to manage expectantly, understanding that there remains a risk for development of cholangitis and gallstone pancreatitis if stones are left untreated. There is no place for diagnostic ERCP, given the advancements in diagnostic imaging. ERCP has also been performed during pregnancy for cholangitis, biliary pancreatitis, and bile duct injury.[12,23] There have been a few reports of performing ERCP in pregnant patients for management of

choledochal cysts, parasitic infestation of the biliary tree, and pancreatic adenocarcinoma.[24–26] Unusual situations such as these warrant careful evaluation on a case-by-case basis with a thorough assessment of the risks and benefits before pursuing ERCP. Serious obstetric complications such as placental abruption, eclampsia, rupture of membranes, and imminent delivery are contraindications to endoscopy. Rapid pregnancy testing before endoscopy is now commonplace and should be considered the standard of care before ERCP in women of childbearing age. Box 30.1 lists the indications for ERCP in pregnancy.

DIAGNOSTIC IMAGING MODALITIES

Advances in diagnostic imaging have enabled endoscopists to often confirm a diagnosis before proceeding with ERCP, yielding the highest probability of therapeutic intervention. This is especially important in the pregnant patient, as these imaging modalities can often prevent unnecessary ERCP procedures.

Transabdominal ultrasonography is commonly used because of its safety profile and low cost. It is a sensitive method of detecting gallstones but has a low sensitivity for detecting CBD stones.[27] It should still be used as an initial test, as a dilated CBD in the appropriate clinical setting (e.g., cholangitis) is often sufficient evidence to pursue ERCP. It is important to keep in mind that the symptoms of biliary disease (e.g., nausea, vomiting, abdominal pain) can often be encountered as a part of normal pregnancy, potentially obscuring the clinical picture.

Computed tomography scan is not recommended in the pregnant patient because of radiation exposure and poor sensitivity for choledocholithiasis.[28] Magnetic resonance cholangiopancreatography (MRCP) is an excellent imaging tool for detection of CBD stones, with a reported sensitivity of 92%.[29] There are no known deleterious effects of magnetic fields on the fetus. Magnetic resonance imaging is indicated in pregnancy with diagnostic-therapeutic urgency when the information needed cannot be obtained by other nonionizing imaging.[30] It should be kept in mind that paramagnetic contrast agents (gadolinium) cross the placenta. Although there are no reports of harmful effects on the fetus, the molecule theoretically remains in the fetoplacental system, and for this reason these agents are generally not recommended for use in the pregnant patient.[31] Fortunately, MRCP does not require paramagnetic contrast to image the biliary and pancreatic ductal systems, although imaging of other structures is limited without contrast. It should be noted that MRCP is less sensitive for detection of smaller stones (<6 mm).[32]

Endoscopic ultrasonography (EUS) has emerged as a highly sensitive and specific test for choledocholithiasis (Fig. 30.2) and can reduce the need for intervention in cases with low or moderate probability.[33,34] Only a few cases of EUS in pregnancy have been reported.[11] The risk of diagnostic EUS during pregnancy is believed to be minimal. It is reasonable to consider EUS immediately before ERCP in indeterminate cases of biliary obstruction if MRCP is not available, is contraindicated,

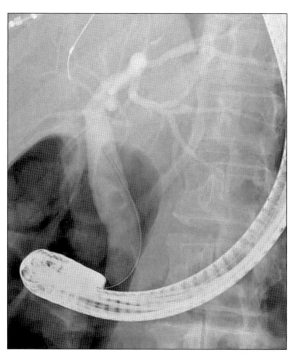

FIG 30.1 Cholangiogram demonstrating a mid–common bile duct stone.

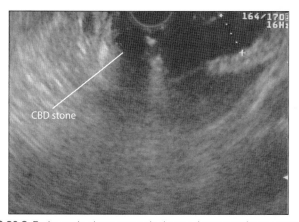

FIG 30.2 Endoscopic ultrasonography image demonstrating a common bile duct stone.

BOX 30.1   Indications for ERCP During Pregnancy

- Choledocholithiasis
- Cholangitis
- Biliary pancreatitis
- Biliary or pancreatic ductal injury

Adapted from ASGE Guidelines.[43]

---

or is nondiagnostic in the setting of high clinical suspicion for CBD stones.[21]

TIMING

The optimal time to perform ERCP is during the second trimester, although it has been performed safely throughout gestation. ERCP during the first trimester should be avoided if possible because of fetal exposure to ionizing radiation during the period of organogenesis and the risk of spontaneous abortion. In the general population, 15% to 20% of clinical pregnancies end in spontaneous abortion, with most of these occurring during the first trimester.[35] This may represent a confounding factor if miscarriage occurs after an ERCP performed in the first trimester. ERCP during the third trimester may be complicated by distortion of anatomy by the gravid uterus and the risk of preterm labor and therefore should be preferably delayed beyond 36 weeks or ideally after delivery. In the presence of an urgent indication, ERCP should be performed regardless of the stage of pregnancy. It is advisable to have an obstetrician involved in the care of these patients. In some centers, fetal monitoring is performed preprocedurally and postprocedurally and, in some cases, intraprocedurally.

Surgery for gallbladder disease during pregnancy is controversial. Some surgeons favor early surgical management, whereas others prefer to wait until after delivery.[9] If possible, surgery should be avoided in the first trimester during the period of organogenesis. Laparoscopy in the third trimester may be problematic because of the enlarged uterus, which can obscure surgical anatomy and limit access to the gallbladder fossa. The second trimester and early third trimester provide the best window should surgery be necessary.[5] Recent reports suggest that laparoscopic cholecystectomy can be performed safely throughout gestation.[9]

RADIATION EXPOSURE DURING ERCP (SEE CHAPTER 3)

Exposing the fetus to ionizing radiation is of major concern when performing ERCP during pregnancy. Exposure to radiation from fluoroscopy can occur in multiple ways. Primary exposure results from the x-ray source emitting a focused beam of radiation toward the patient. Secondary or "scatter" radiation occurs when x-ray photons strike an object (e.g., the patient) and then deviate from a straight trajectory. This type of radiation can affect the fetus by "scattering" within the mother's body. Anyone present in the fluoroscopy suite will be exposed to secondary scatter radiation. Another form of exposure, called "leakage," can occur when radiation escapes from the protective shielding of the source.

The risks of radiation to the fetus include abnormalities in growth and development, malformations, and increased risk of future cancer. Deterministic effects on growth and development have a threshold of approximately 100 mGy and are at greatest risk of occurring between the 2nd and 15th weeks of gestation.[36] According to the American College of Obstetricians and Gynecologists, "exposure to less than 5 rad [50 mGy] has not been associated with an increase in fetal anomalies or pregnancy loss."[37] The risk of developing cancer from radiation, although small, is a stochastic effect and has no threshold level.[36] (For gamma radiation: 100 rem = 100 rad = 1 gray = 1 sievert). Multiple studies have estimated levels of radiation exposure to the fetus and have reported an average exposure between 10 and 310 mrad.[13,38] The largest study, by Kahaleh et al.,[20] examined radiation exposure in 15 pregnant women undergoing ERCP. Techniques were used to minimize fluoroscopy time, and exposure levels were monitored by thermoluminescent dosimeters. The mean estimated fetal exposure level was 40 mrad (range 1 to 180 mrad), which is well within the accepted teratogenic threshold. Samara et al.[39] studied potential conceptus radiation doses using simulated mathematical models in 24 nonpregnant patients undergoing ERCP. These models took into account not only the effect of the primary radiation beam on the fetus but also internal "scatter" radiation. The authors found that radiation exposure to the fetus may occasionally exceed 10 mGy. Although most pregnant patients are probably exposed to much lower levels, this finding underscores the importance of minimizing radiation exposure to pregnant women.

STRATEGIES TO MINIMIZE RADIATION RISK TO THE FETUS

A variety of techniques can be used to reduce radiation exposure to pregnant women and fetuses (Box 30.2). The most effective method to reduce radiation is to minimize the fluoroscopy time and limit overall radiation dose. Short "taps" of fluoroscopy can be used. A sphincterotome should be used for the procedure to avoid unnecessary catheter exchanges. Aspiration of bile through the sphincterotome channel confirms biliary cannulation. "Hard copy" images should be avoided as they expose the patient to higher levels of radiation. Instead, brief snapshots of the "last-minute hold" feature should be used to review and document the study. Low-dose-rate pulsed fluoroscopy should be used with tight collimation in the area of interest to reduce the amount of scatter radiation. The x-ray tube should be kept as far from the patient as possible, whereas the image receptor should be kept as close as possible. Magnification can amplify radiation levels and its use should be avoided.[40] Lead shielding can also be used to protect the fetus. It is important to place the lead apron beneath the patient, where the x-ray beam originates (Fig. 30.3). Lead shielding may reduce levels of primary radiation to the fetus but will not affect scatter radiation within the mother. Some have found the effect of lead shielding to be negligible.[39] Nonetheless, it is still recommended as a simple method of decreasing radiation

---

BOX 30.2   Techniques to Reduce Radiation Exposure

- Use sphincterotome for cannulation to aspirate bile and also avoid catheter exchanges.
- Use short "taps" of fluoroscopy.
- Avoid "hard copy" images.
- Use "last-image hold" feature to review images.
- Avoid use of magnification.
- Use low-dose-rate pulsed fluoroscopy.
- Collimate x-ray beam to smallest possible field.
- Place patient far from radiation source and close to image receptor.
- Use lead shielding.
- Use novel lead-free radiation protection drape.
- Use bile aspiration technique.
- Consider use of choledochoscopy or endoscopic ultrasonography to confirm clearance of common bile duct.

---

exposure without adding any additional risk. A dosimeter may be attached over the gravid abdomen to estimate levels of exposure to the fetus, although this is not performed in our practice.[20]

A recent randomized double-blind sham-controlled trial showed 90% reduction in radiation exposure for endoscopists by hanging a novel drape made of bismuth and antimony around the image intensifier, thereby preventing scatter radiation (Fig. 30.4).[41] This lead-free drape could potentially also be used to minimize the radiation to the mother and fetus, although the majority of fetal radiation occurs as a result of scatter radiation within the mother's body.[39] Consultation with a radiation physicist may be helpful in planning an ERCP in a pregnant patient. In recent years, novel techniques have evolved for performing ERCP without fluoroscopy. This approach will be covered later in this chapter.

POSITIONING, SEDATION, AND MEDICATIONS

Early in pregnancy, the patient may be placed in the standard prone position. Selecting the optimal position plays an important role in minimizing radiation. However, the gravid abdomen may make this position difficult during the second and third trimesters. In this case a left lateral position or a semiprone oblique position can be used (see Fig. 30.3). A pelvic wedge may be helpful in maintaining this position. During the third trimester, the supine position should be avoided as the gravid uterus can compress the inferior vena cava or aorta, resulting in decreased perfusion to the mother and fetus, known as "supine hypotensive syndrome."[42] When sphincterotomy is performed (Fig. 30.5), the grounding pad should be placed such that the uterus does not lie between the sphincterotome and the pad; this will avoid conduction of electrical current through the amniotic fluid.[43] Maternal-fetal monitoring is preferred during the procedure and fetal heart tones should be confirmed before and after the procedure.

In general, moderate sedation in nonpregnant patients is achieved with a combination of intravenous benzodiazepines, such as diazepam or midazolam, and opioids, such as fentanyl or meperidine. During pregnancy, the choice of medication may need to be altered, as certain medications may pose additional risk to the fetus. For example, diazepam and midazolam are considered category D drugs. Diazepam in particular has been associated with cleft palate malformation.[44] Both of these drugs should generally be avoided in pregnancy. If use of a benzodiazepine is absolutely necessary, midazolam is preferred over diazepam. Meperidine is a category C drug (category D if used for a prolonged period at term), as is fentanyl. These analgesic drugs can probably be used safely during pregnancy. The reversal agents naloxone and flumazenil are classified

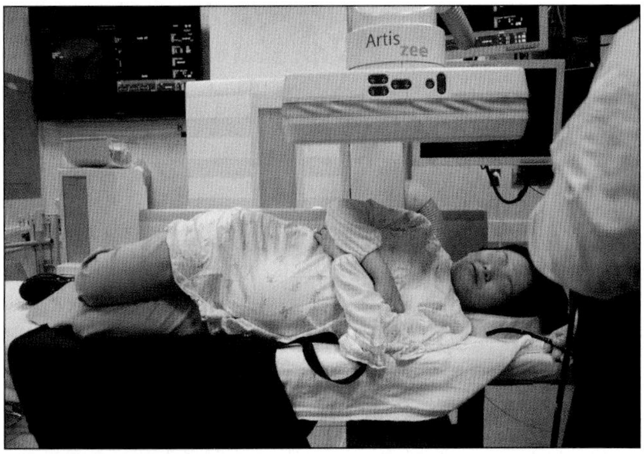

FIG 30.3 Pregnant patient lying in the left lateral position with a lead apron placed underneath the lower abdomen.

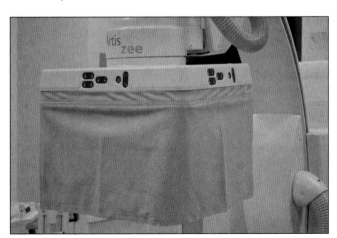

FIG 30.4 Radiation-attenuating drape hanging over the image intensifier.

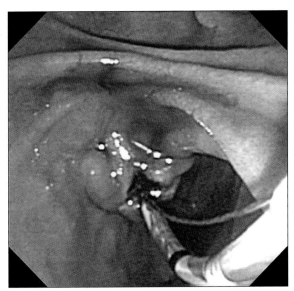

FIG 30.5 Duodenal papilla postsphincterotomy.

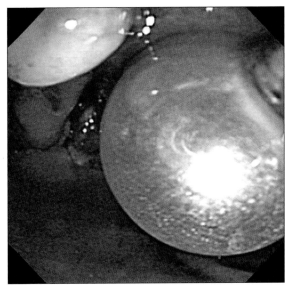

FIG 30.6 Extraction of a common bile duct stone using a balloon catheter.

TABLE 30.1 Sedative Medications for ERCP During Pregnancy

Drug	Pregnancy Safety Category	Evidence From Literature
Propofol	B	Low risk in animal studies. Inadequate data in first trimester.
Meperidine	C (D with prolonged use at term)	Toxic metabolites may accumulate with large doses, limiting use during pregnancy to 50–75 mg
Fentanyl	C	May be used during pregnancy at low doses (<125 mcg). Some risk may exist with use in third trimester.
Diazepam	D	Early studies demonstrated possible association with cleft palate. Use discouraged, especially during first trimester.
Midazolam	D	Little human data exist. Avoid during first trimester because of same mechanism of action as diazepam.

as categories B and C, respectively. These agents should be used only if absolutely necessary for a medication overdose. If moderate sedation is being used, consultation with a pharmacologist before the procedure may be helpful.[45]

Propofol is now being increasingly used to achieve moderate to deep sedation during ERCP. Being a category B drug, propofol is an attractive alternative to conscious sedation in pregnancy. However, propofol can rapidly cause respiratory depression and should be used in the pregnant patient only with the support of an anesthesiologist.[45] General anesthesia with intubation should also be considered to protect the airway. Hormonal changes during pregnancy can decrease lower esophageal sphincter tone, which can cause gastroesophageal reflux and increase the risk of aspiration.[46] Table 30.1 summarizes the safety data of sedative medications that may be used for ERCP during pregnancy.

The indications for antibiotics are the same in pregnant and non-pregnant patients. Antibiotics should be used in cases of biliary obstruction and cholangitis. Most penicillin derivatives (e.g., amoxicillin, ampicillin, cephalosporins) are category B drugs and considered safe during pregnancy. Clindamycin or erythromycin can be used safely in penicillin-allergic patients.[43]

TECHNIQUES

In 1990, the first case series of ERCP during pregnancy was reported.[47] Four women underwent sphincterotomy for visualized CBD stones, and the first empiric sphincterotomy was performed on a patient with cholelithiasis and a normal cholangiogram. Since that time, there have been significant developments in ERCP techniques used in pregnant patients. Binmoeller and Katon[48] reported the first use of a needle knife to remove an impacted CBD stone. This was also the first reported ERCP without the use of fluoroscopy in a pregnant patient. Axelrad and colleagues[38] were the first to describe a case of prophylactic CBD stenting during pregnancy. The patient had recurrent pain weeks after an ERCP with sphincterotomy and balloon extraction of CBD stones. A repeat ERCP demonstrated gallstones and a normal cholangiogram. A CBD stent was placed to prevent further episodes. Jamidar et al.[17] reported the first minor sphincterotomy in a pregnant patient with pancreas divisum. It was unknown at the time of the procedure that the patient was pregnant. Both the mother and baby did well, but this underscores the importance of pregnancy testing before performing ERCP.

Several techniques have been described to minimize the use of fluoroscopy during ERCP. Initial cannulation should be performed with a sphincterotome to avoid unnecessary catheter exchanges. ERCP can be performed without fluoroscopy by using a wire-guided cannulation technique. Uomo and colleagues[49] first described the "bile aspiration" technique in 1994 after performing ERCP in two pregnant patients without the use of fluoroscopy. Once the catheter is inserted into the duct, aspiration of bile is used to confirm selective cannulation of the CBD. If clear fluid is seen, cannulation is reattempted. If bile is seen, biliary sphincterotomy is performed, followed by balloon extraction of stones without fluoroscopy (Fig. 30.6).

The advent of these techniques has enabled some endoscopists to successfully perform ERCP without fluoroscopy. This approach avoids radiation exposure to the fetus; however, it may be difficult to exclude residual stones or debris in the duct without fluoroscopic imaging. Furthermore, the bile aspiration technique does not help differentiate between cannulation of the cystic duct and the common hepatic duct. Consequently, some have performed nonradiation ERCP by using alternative imaging. One group described their successful use of transabdominal ultrasonography during ERCP to confirm CBD cannulation.[50] This method did not confirm clearance of the duct once stones had been removed. Shelton and colleagues[12] reported a case series of 21 pregnant women who had ERCP without fluoroscopy. Of these 21 patients, 5 had peroral choledochoscopy using an optical probe (SpyGlass; Boston Scientific, Marlborough, MA). In one patient, choledochoscopy revealed cannulation of the cystic duct. The other four patients were free of residual stones. No complications of choledochoscopy occurred in these patients. If cholangioscopy is not available, another option is to perform diagnostic EUS after balloon extraction is performed to confirm clearance of the duct. Although this technique has not been formally studied, it would probably add minimal risk, though the resultant air within the biliary tree may obscure residual stones.[21]

Long and complicated procedures, such as removal of large or multiple CBD stones, may be problematic during pregnancy, as they pose an additional risk of adverse events and prolonged fluoroscopy time. Balloon dilation of the sphincter should be avoided because of an increased risk of pancreatitis with this technique.[51] However, if undertaken, placement of a temporary pancreatic duct stent is recommended. Recently balloon dilation *after* sphincterotomy has become a popular technique for removing large CBD stones, although its use has not yet been reported in the pregnant patient. Alternatively, biliary stents can be placed for decompression with the intent to repeat the procedure postpartum and to avoid excessive fluoroscopy. This alternative needs to be weighed against the risk of potential stent occlusion and cholangitis. A two-stage approach has been described in all cases, whereby pregnant patients are initially treated with sphincterotomy and stent placement, with definitive ERCP and stone clearance performed after delivery.[52] However, as stent placement would require subsequent procedures, which may occur during the course of the pregnancy, the risks and benefits of

repeat ERCP with potential radiation must be considered before deciding on the optimal management strategy. It may also be reasonable to consider prophylactic pancreatic duct stenting in complex procedures to reduce the risk of severe post-ERCP pancreatitis (PEP; see Chapter 8).

Although sphincterotomy is clearly warranted in cases of choledocholithiasis or cholangitis, the management of biliary pancreatitis with a normal cholangiogram is controversial. Endoscopic sphincterotomy may provide protection against recurrent pancreatitis, which has led some to advocate empiric sphincterotomy in the absence of CBD stones on cholangiogram.[53] One must be cautious in this approach, with careful consideration of the risks and benefits, as sphincterotomy may increase the likelihood of adverse events from ERCP. Again, placement of a biliary stent is an alternative to empiric sphincterotomy.

OUTCOMES AFTER ERCP DURING PREGNANCY

To date, more than 1000 ERCP procedures in pregnant women have been reported. Table 30.2 summarizes the outcomes of the larger studies (>10 patients), including the recent retrospective matched-cohort study on 907 pregnant patients who underwent ERCP compared with matched nonpregnant female patients.[22]

Studies with fewer than 10 patients and abstracts have been excluded from analysis. These studies include a total of 200 patients who underwent 217 procedures. ERCP was performed 62 times in the first trimester (29%), 75 times in the second trimester (35%), and 79 times in the third trimester (36%). PEP occurred after 19 procedures (9%). No cases of severe pancreatitis were reported. Two cases of postsphincterotomy hemorrhage occurred (1%), which were controlled by epinephrine injection and endoclip placement. Fetal outcomes included eight preterm deliveries (4%), one spontaneous abortion (0.5%), and two cases of preeclampsia (1%). One neonatal death has been reported, but there was no clear causal relationship to the ERCP procedure. No maternal deaths were reported.

TABLE 30.2	**Outcomes of Large Studies on ERCP in Pregnancy**				
Author	No. of Patients (No. of Procedures)	Trimester Procedure Performed	Maternal Complications	Fetal Outcomes	Interesting Notes
Inamdar et al.[22]	907 (907)	NA	PEP (*n* = 108)	PTD (*n* = 17)	Largest database study to date Showed pregnancy as independent risk factor for PEP
Tang et al.[15]	65 (68)	1st (*n* = 17) 2nd (*n* = 20) 3rd (*n* = 31)	PEP (*n* = 11)	PTD (*n* = 5) EAB (*n* = 1) LBW (*n* = 4)	
Bani Hani et al.[55]	10 (10)	1st (*n* = 2) 2nd (*n* = 5) 3rd (*n* = 3)	PEP (*n* = 1)	No adverse outcomes	
Daas et al.[56]	10 (17)	1st (*n* = 5) 2nd (*n* = 3) 3rd (*n* = 5)	None	EAB (*n* = 1)	
Shelton et al.[12]	21 (21)	1st (*n* = 8) 2nd (*n* = 6) 3rd (*n* = 7)	PEP (*n* = 1) Residual CBD stones (*n* = 1)	IUGR + PTD (*n* = 1)	All without fluoro (5 with SpyGlass)
Sharma and Maharshi[52]	11 (11)	1st (*n* = 2) 2nd (*n* = 6) 3rd (*n* = 3)	None	No adverse outcomes	All with biliary stenting and ERCP postpartum
Gupta et al.[57]	18 (18)	1st (*n* = 4) 2nd (*n* = 6) 3rd (*n* = 8)	PEP (*n* = 1) Bleed (*n* = 1)	PTD (*n* = 1)	US used in some cases to confirm CBD

TABLE 30.2   Outcomes of Large Studies on ERCP in Pregnancy—cont'd

Author	No. of Patients (No. of Procedures)	Trimester Procedure Performed	Maternal Complications	Fetal Outcomes	Interesting Notes
Kahaleh et al.[20]	17 (17)	1st ($n = 4$) 2nd ($n = 9$) 3rd ($n = 4$)	PEP ($n = 1$) Bleed ($n = 1$)	Preeclampsia ($n = 2$)	Estimated fetal radiation exposure
Tham et al.[13]	15 (15)	1st ($n = 1$) 2nd ($n = 5$) 3rd ($n = 9$)	PEP ($n = 1$)	PTD ($n = 1$)	
Farca et al.[58]	10 (11)	1st ($n = 3$) 2nd ($n = 5$) 3rd ($n = 2$)	Proximal stent migration, both removed ($n = 2$)	No adverse outcomes	Only stent placed; no sphincterotomy or stone extraction
Jamidar et al.[17]	23 (29)	1st ($n = 15$) 2nd ($n = 8$) 3rd ($n = 6$)	PEP ($n = 3$); all in same patient after 3 procedures	SAB ($n = 1$) EAB ($n = 2$) Neonatal death ($n = 1$)	Largest multicenter study

CBD, Common bile duct; *EAB*, elective abortion; *IUGR*, intrauterine growth retardation; *LBW*, low birth weight; *PEP*, post-ERCP pancreatitis; *PTD*, preterm delivery; *SAB*, spontaneous abortion; *US*, ultrasonography.
Only studies with $n > 10$ patients are included in the table.

In a retrospective matched-cohort study that used a national hospital database, Inamdar et al.[22] compared outcomes of ERCP among 907 pregnant women with those of 2721 nonpregnant women. ERCP-associated adverse events of perforation, infection, and bleeding were similar and infrequent in both groups; however, PEP occurred in 12% of pregnant women and 5% of controls ($p < 0.001$), with an adjusted odds ratio of 2.8 (95% confidence interval, 2.1 to 3.8) for pregnant versus nonpregnant ERCP patients. Rectal indomethacin is commonly used in nonpregnant patients to decrease the risk of PEP, but it is a class C drug for use in pregnancy and a recent study showed increased risk of spontaneous abortion with indomethacin compared with other nonsteroidal antiinflammatory drugs in pregnancy.[54] Therefore it is not uncommon to see restricted use of rectal indomethacin in pregnant patients, putting them at higher risk for PEP.

CONCLUSIONS

ERCP is now considered the standard of care for treatment of choledocholithiasis during pregnancy. Because of its inherent risks, it should be used only if therapy is planned. In patients with a low or intermediate probability of having CBD stones, alternative imaging modalities such as MRCP and EUS should be considered before ERCP. This approach can prevent unnecessary ERCP procedures. Only the most experienced endoscopists should perform ERCP on pregnant women and all efforts should be undertaken to curtail radiation exposure. Newer techniques to minimize or even eliminate the use of fluoroscopy should be used whenever possible. In complex cases, temporary biliary stent placement with planned elective repeat ERCP postpartum for definitive treatment should be considered, rather than subjecting the patient to a long and potentially risky procedure. Prophylactic pancreatic duct stents should be used when the risk of PEP is felt to be high. ERCP can be performed safely and effectively during pregnancy when done judiciously with the support of an experienced multidisciplinary team.

The complete reference list for this chapter can be found online at www.expertconsult.com.

31

ERCP in Surgically Altered Anatomy

Simon K. Lo

Endoscopic retrograde cholangiopancreatography (ERCP) is generally considered the technically most difficult procedure in gastrointestinal (GI) endoscopy because of the complex maneuvers necessary to gain ductal access and perform therapies within the bile duct or pancreas. Altering the upper GI tract or pancreaticobiliary anatomy invariably adds to procedure complexity and technical challenges. Thorough understanding of surgically altered anatomy is essential to ensure technical success and minimize procedure-related adverse events. In virtually all these cases, careful preprocedure planning is mandatory (Box 31.1). This chapter provides a basic review of the anatomic considerations and some practical tips on overcoming some of the challenges.

SURGERY THAT MAY AFFECT THE PERFORMANCE OR INTERPRETATION OF ERCP

The combination of thorough understanding of altered anatomy, use of a specific endoscope, and application of a special skill set may be needed to reach the pancreatic and biliary systems. Some operations simply remove or bypass a portion of the bile duct or pancreas but do not create any hardship when performing ERCP. Conversely, there are extreme surgical consequences that would not allow endoscopic access of the biliary tract regardless of experience, equipment, and skill. We will explain most of these operations and attempt to bring to light relevant points pertaining to the performance of ERCP.

ESOPHAGEAL RESECTION

Mostly done for esophageal neoplasm or premalignant conditions, esophageal resection results in a high esophageal anastomotic stricture in up to 22% of cases.[1] In addition, a small diverticulum or misaligned lumen may form proximal to the anastomosis. When passing a duodenoscope, care must be taken to avoid forceful advancement through a diverticulum or anastomosis. If resistance is encountered, the duodenoscope should be withdrawn and an end-viewing upper endoscope inserted to inspect the esophageal reconstruction. Esophageal resection also results in the stomach being brought up into the chest and turned into a tubular sack with a midgastric diaphragmatic pinch, which may frustrate the endoscopist because of trouble visualizing the distal stomach. Once the duodenoscope has passed the pylorus, the major papilla is easily identified by a slight clockwise rotation, but keeping the scope in a stable position is difficult because of the straightened upper GI tract. Sometimes a long scope position may offer a better and more secure view of the major papilla for cannulation.

GASTRIC RESECTION

There are many forms of gastric resection, which range from a simple Billroth I with very little loss of gastric volume to total gastrectomy.

Video for this chapter can be found online at www.expertconsult.com.

Thus the impact of gastric resection on ERCP can be either minimal or profound.

Billroth I

In a Billroth I surgery, only the antrum and pylorus are removed and the stomach is attached to the duodenum along its greater curvature (Fig. 31.1). Endoscope passage into the duodenum is typically easier than usual because of the loss of the pylorus, but the papilla is actually harder to find. As expected, both the major and minor papillae are more proximally located than usual. In the short-scope position, the papilla is seen after an exaggerated rotation of the endoscope. Additionally, anchoring the endoscope is difficult without the antrum and pylorus, and achieving a stable scope position for cannulation may be quite difficult. Occasionally, working in the long-scope position may be more desirable because the papillary orifice is better visualized and the scope is more stably situated. Because it is difficult to cannulate the bile duct in a sharply retrograde fashion, using a sphincterotome and guidewire in combination may overcome the intrinsic issues in Billroth I cannulation.

Billroth II

Before proton pump inhibitors were introduced, peptic ulcer surgery was common. Currently, most Billroth II procedures are done for resection of distal gastric cancers and involve antrectomy and creation of a gastrojejunostomy. The result is an end (stomach)-to-side (jejunum) anastomosis with two jejunal lumens (Fig. 31.2, *A, B*) immediately beyond the gastric staple line. The afferent limb travels proximally and ends as a duodenal stump proximal to the major and minor papillae, whereas the efferent limb restores intestinal continuity with the rest of the GI tract. The major papilla is typically located within a few centimeters of the duodenal stump, and its orifice is pointing down at the endoscope.

There are several considerations when performing ERCP in a Billroth II stomach, the first of which is the choice of endoscope. It was initially believed that an end-viewing endoscope was preferred because of the ease in navigating the convoluted small bowel and cannulating the biliary orifice. Many experienced biliary endoscopists have since switched to duodenoscopes to take advantage of the large channel, instrument elevator, and unique side-viewing design to inspect the papilla. Selection of endoscopes may be simply a matter of personal preference, as a Korean prospective, randomized study demonstrated no difference between side-viewing and end-viewing endoscopes in cannulation success and sphincterotomy.[2] In fact, end-viewing endoscopes were safer to use. Regardless of which endoscope is used, it is difficult to perform ERCP in a Billroth II gastrectomy. In a study involving 185 Billroth II ERCP procedures, the failure rate was as high as 34%.[3]

There is no definite way to correctly identify the afferent lumen in a Billroth II gastrectomy, even though there is the common impression

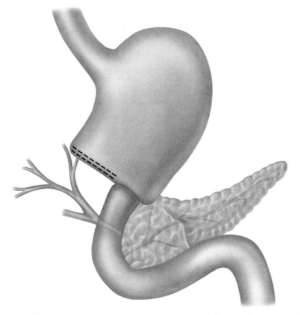

FIG 31.1 Billroth I gastrectomy. Antrectomy is followed by connection of the stomach to the duodenum in end-to-end fashion. The lesser curvature side of the cut end of the stomach is closed to allow creation of the gastroduodenostomy.

that it arises from the more awkwardly located orifice. The afferent limb can be attached to the stomach along either the lesser (antiperistaltic) (Fig. 31.2, A) or greater (isoperistaltic) curvature (Fig. 31.2, B). Scope passage with an end-viewing device is intuitive, and the major challenge is in visualizing and cannulating the papilla. Because the instrument channel of most endoscopes is located at the 5 to 7 o'clock position, it is best to situate the papilla at the bottom of the endoscopic view. Unfortunately, typically a sharp angle is encountered between the transverse and descending duodenum that makes visualizing the papillary orifice difficult. A soft transparent cap at the tip of the end-viewing endoscope may help stabilize the papilla during cannulation.

Scope passage with a side-viewing duodenoscope can be very difficult or even impossible and begins with attempting to gain entry into the afferent lumen. Endoscope passage is even more difficult if the afferent limb is sutured to the lesser curvature after it has exited the gastrojejunostomy, as this form of operation creates a fixed and significantly angulated point of entry[4] (Fig. 31.3, A, B). The technique of entering the gastrojejunostomy orifice is the same as for the pylorus. When the lumen can be visualized only in the retroflexed (maximally up-angulated) position, attempting to glide the scope gently toward it rarely works. Suctioning excess gastric air may make gliding a little easier. A technique of entering the lumen by rotating the endoscope 180 degrees at the orifice and pointing the tip of the scope downward until the small bowel lumen is clearly in sight can be used. This can theoretically be done with the endoscope facing the opening rather than "backing in." However, the endoscope is blinded by mucosa and visual inspection during the maneuvering is more difficult. Hand-compressing the midabdomen or extending a polypectomy snare into the intended lumen has been reported to assist in intubation of a difficult gastrojejunostomy orifice.[5] Passage of the duodenoscope alongside or over a stiff guidewire that has been placed into the afferent limb with an end-viewing endoscope may occasionally be helpful. Even in tertiary biliary centers, the rate of failure to enter the afferent limb is as high as 10%.[3]

Once the side-viewing duodenoscope has securely entered the afferent jejunal lumen, passage forward is safe and effective by constantly orientating the intestinal channel in the 6 o'clock position (Fig. 31.4, A). This would simulate the view of driving a car in a long tunnel. It is common to see two lumens when a duodenoscope is partially retroflexed, and it creates confusion regarding where to advance the endoscope. A good rule of thumb is to orientate the two lumens along the vertical midline, and the lower lumen is the one that the endoscope should enter (Fig. 31.4, B). Natural intestinal redundancy and tortuosity rarely allow unimpeded forward advancements. Rather, successful passage requires a combination of gentle rotation, dial redirection, and alternating withdrawal and advancement. The forward blinded-gliding technique, commonly applied in colonoscopy passage, should not be practiced because of the risk of perforation. For the same reason, care must be taken to minimize sudden or forceful manipulations. One series reported a 5% perforation rate when advancing duodenoscopes through the afferent limb.[3] In another study, jejunal perforation occurred in 18%.[2] Using an older, more flexible duodenoscope may reduce the chance of traumatizing the intestinal wall. Minimizing air insufflation helps keep the lumen straight and the bowel wall soft and pliable. Abdominal compression or rotation of the patient is occasionally effective in advancing around seemingly improbable turns. With experience and special care, an acceptable risk of perforation can be achieved.[6]

After passing some distance, it is wise to take a fluoroscopic picture to confirm that the endoscope is passing through the transverse duodenum (Fig. 31.5). If the tip of the endoscope is seen in the pelvis, it is likely to be in the efferent limb and should be withdrawn to search for the other intestinal orifice. Some afferent limbs seem to be longer and more tortuous than others. This impression is indeed correct, as

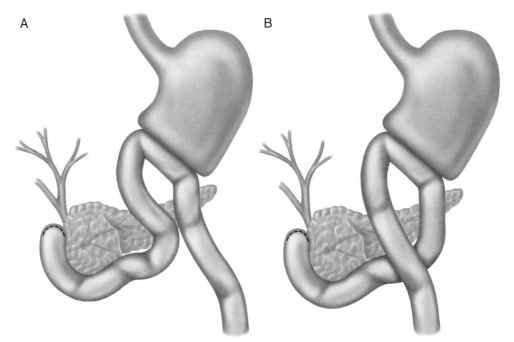

FIG 31.2 A, Billroth II gastrectomy with an antiperistaltic gastrojejunostomy anastomosis. In this case the afferent limb is accessed through the stomal orifice located near the lesser curvature. **B,** Billroth II gastrectomy with an isoperistaltic anastomosis, where the afferent limb is attached to the greater curvature.

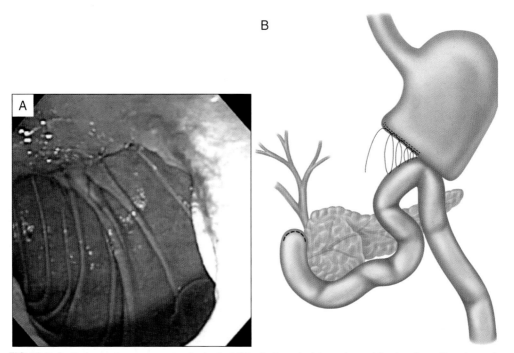

FIG 31.3 A, Endoscopic appearance of a typical Billroth II gastrojejunostomy. Viewing from the stomach, the two jejunal limbs are located at the extreme right and left of this image. **B,** Billroth II gastrectomy with the greater curvature side of the stomach attached to the jejunum in an end-to-side fashion. The lesser curvature side of the stomach is closed surgically. Some surgeons choose to suture the jejunum onto this area to protect the suture line. If the afferent limb is tagged down in this manner, endoscope entry into this limb may be quite difficult.

the afferent loop may be created in antecolic fashion over the transverse colon (Fig. 31.6, *A, B*). Correct endoscopic intubation of the afferent loop is readily confirmed if fluoroscopy shows that the scope has quickly crossed the midline into the right upper abdomen.

On the way to the proximal duodenum, an anastomosis that connects the afferent to the efferent limb may be encountered, which is indicative of a Braun procedure, a modification of the Billroth II operation. This is performed to reduce bile reflux into the stomach or to lessen the chance of duodenal obstruction (Fig. 31.7) and is recognized because of the finding of three exiting lumens. It should not influence the endoscopic passage if the scope does not cross the anastomotic stable line. On some occasions the duodenal stump, which appears as a blind sac with a distinctly flat mucosa and possibly surgical staples, is reached without identifying the major papilla. The minor and then major papilla should be readily identified upon gradual withdrawal of the endoscope (Fig. 31.8, *A–C*).

The major papilla is almost always found near the 12 o'clock position of the duodenum when a duodenoscope is used (Fig. 31.8, *C*). If the intestinal lumen is kept in view ahead of the endoscope, the bile duct should be straight or slightly to the right ahead of the papillary orifice (Fig. 31.9, *A* and Fig. 31.10). To keep the cannulating catheter or guidewire tangential to the duodenal wall for biliary access, the papilla should not be approached up close (Fig. 31.8, *C*). Rather, the scope should be pulled back slightly with its elevator partially lowered for catheter passage. Conversely, the pancreatic duct is easier to cannulate by advancing the endoscope close to the papilla and keeping the elevator in a lifted position (Fig. 31.8, *B*). Some endoscopists prefer to use straight-tip catheters for biliary cannulation,[5] whereas others like to use straight guidewires. However, perhaps the most effective way to enter the bile duct is to use a catheter bent into an S-shape, with its tip pointing downward (Fig. 31.9, *B*). A cap-assisted approach has been described to improve

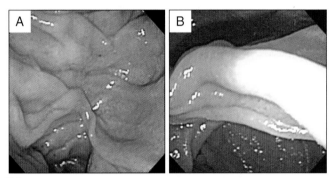

FIG 31.4 **A,** The typical view of the jejunal lumen when a side-viewing duodenoscope is being advanced. Note that the upper half of the lumen should always be kept in the 6 o'clock position. **B,** A similar duodenoscopic view of the distal lumen in the 6 o'clock position. Note that the upper lumen always represents a retroflexed view. An attempt to pass the scope toward the 12 o'clock direction would cause either perforation or the scope to fold backward.

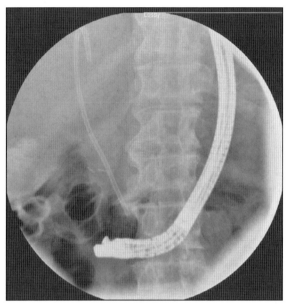

FIG 31.5 Fluoroscopy shows that the duodenoscope is facing the right direction and crossing the transverse duodenum.

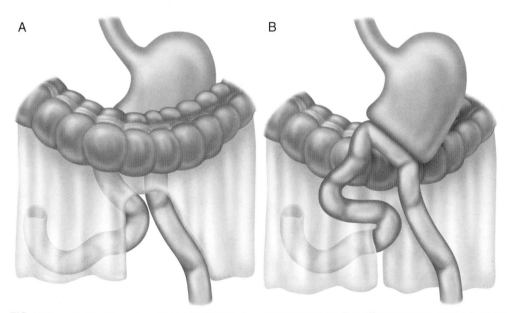

FIG 31.6 **A,** Retrocolic construction of a Billroth II gastrojejunostomy. The afferent limb is relatively short in this case. **B,** Antecolic Billroth II gastrojejunostomy. The afferent limb is significantly longer than that in **(A)**.

cannulation of a Billroth II papilla when an end-viewing endoscope is used[7] (Fig. 31.11). On some occasions when pancreas divisum is suspected, the minor papilla should be correctly identified for cannulation. As a rule, it is located slightly farther away from (cephalad to) and to the left of the superiorly located major papilla (Fig. 31.8, A and Fig. 31.10).

Biliary sphincterotomy is accomplished using either a wire-guided Billroth II sphincterotome or a needle knife to cut over an indwelling biliary stent. A Billroth II sphincterotome is designed in an opposite fashion to a conventional traction sphincterotome, with its cutting wire loosened to form a half loop over a straight sphincterotome catheter. With the wire protruding, the sphincterotome is pushed forward to cut the papillary hood along the 6 o'clock position of the superiorly located papilla. Sphincterotomy done in this manner is slightly less well controlled than in the normal setting because of the pushing motion and suboptimal visualization of the proximal papillary mound. A modified sphincterotome that forces its tip into an S-shape when the cutting wire tightens may also be used to perform sphincterotomy in this setting.[8] However, many endoscopists choose needle-knife cutting over a biliary stent because it avoids injury to the pancreatic sphincter and allows controlled tissue cutting.[4,9] Balloon sphincter dilation, commonly done with an 8-mm balloon, is technically easy to perform and can be done

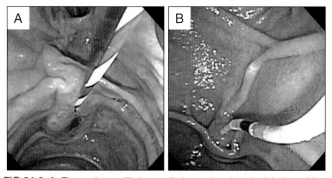

FIG 31.9 A, The major papilla is usually located at the 12 o'clock position. Here the guidewire points in the direction of the bile duct. **B,** This S-shaped biliary cannula is best used for intubating the bile duct.

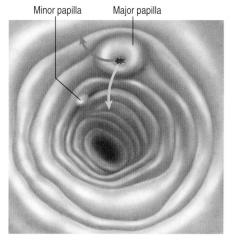

FIG 31.10 A schematic illustration of the relationship between the major and minor papillae and the directions of the bile duct (*yellow arrow*) and pancreatic duct (*blue arrow*).

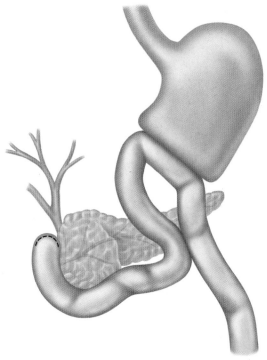

FIG 31.7 A Braun modification of a Billroth II operation. Here the afferent and efferent limbs are connected via a side-to-side anastomosis.

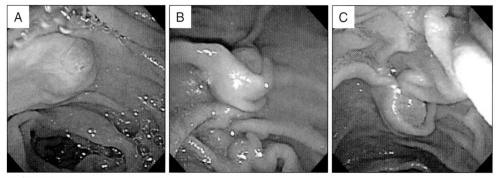

FIG 31.8 A, The minor papilla, which is quite prominent in this case, is located more cephalad to and to the left side of the major papilla. Further into the afferent lumen is the duodenal stump. **B,** As the scope is withdrawn from the duodenal stump, the major papilla is seen up close and perpendicular to the duodenoscope. This position favors cannulation of the pancreatic duct. **C,** The duodenoscope is withdrawn further, and farther away from the major papilla. This position favors cannulation of the bile duct.

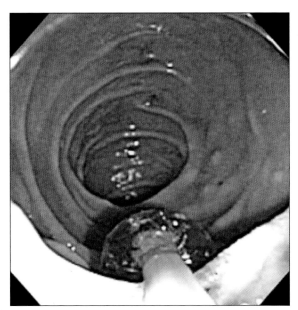

FIG 31.11 A balloon dilator is being used to perform sphincteroplasty using an end-viewing endoscope. Note that a short soft cap has been fitted to the tip of the endoscope. This cap is believed to improve the ability to cannulate the papilla.

as a solo therapy or in combination with a limited sphincterotomy. A randomized study showed that balloon sphincter dilation was just as effective as sphincterotomy at facilitating stone extraction, with fewer adverse events, in the Billroth II setting.[9] Additionally, pancreatitis was not encountered.

Roux-en-Y Gastrectomy

Aimed to reduce reflux of pancreatic and biliary fluids into the stomach after a partial gastrectomy, Roux-en-Y gastrectomy creates a gastric outlet that appears similar to that of a Billroth II surgery. However, one end of this end-to-side anastomosis is a short blind stump (Fig. 31.12). The other lumen, the Roux limb, extends around 40 cm before a jejunojejunostomy anastomosis is encountered. At this point two or three lumens (Fig. 31.13, A, B) will be identified, depending on whether the two jejunal limbs are connected end-to-side (Fig. 31.13, C) or side-to-side (Fig. 31.13, D). If done side-to-side, one of the three outlets will be a short blind stump. If the afferent limb is correctly entered, the endoscope will pass sequentially up the proximal jejunum, ligament of Treitz, transverse duodenum, and finally the descending duodenum. This long path makes it nearly impossible for a 125-cm-long duodenoscope to reach the major papilla. Many longer-length endoscopes have been used to perform ERCP in this setting, including pediatric and adult colonoscopes and push enteroscopes.[10] A special oblique-viewing endoscope, which is no longer available commercially, was reported to be useful for this purpose.[11] Double-balloon enteroscopes, which can routinely reach the ileum per-os, were introduced to the United States in 2004 (Fig. 31.14, A–D). Their use in performing diagnostic and therapeutic ERCP in patients with Roux-Y hepaticojejunostomy was soon reported.[12] Until now, all forms of deep enteroscopes, including single and enteroscopes used through a spiral overtube, are routinely employed for a variety of pancreatic and biliary conditions in this postoperative setting.

The challenge of performing ERCP in a Roux-en-Y gastrectomy patient lies not just in traveling a great length and recognizing the proper intestinal lumen but also in selectively cannulating the bile duct and pancreatic duct. It is common to pass the endoscope past the anastomosis into the efferent jejunal limb without recognizing the

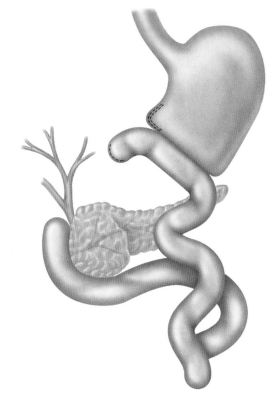

FIG 31.12 A typical Roux-en-Y gastrojejunostomy.

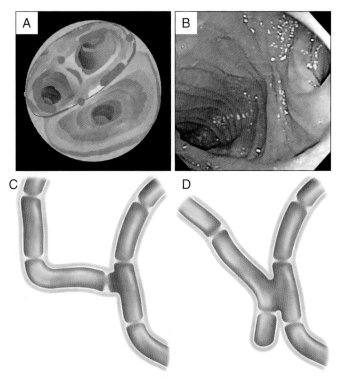

FIG 31.13 A, A schematic illustration of three lumens at the point of a jejunojejunostomy anastomosis. The single distal lumen on the same side of the anastomosis should be the efferent limb. One of the two lumens on the other side of the anastomosis is a blind stump, whereas the other is the afferent limb. **B,** Endoscopic picture of the two lumens seen beyond an anastomosis. One of these two orifices should lead to the afferent limb. **C,** Illustration of an end-to-side jejunojejunostomy anastomosis. **D,** Illustration of a side-to-side jejunojejunostomy anastomosis.

jejunojejunostomy. A clue to the vicinity of the anastomosis is the presence of bilious fluid. Once bile is seen, endoscope advancement should be slowed to identify the intestinal bifurcation. The afferent limb is always found across the circular rim of anastomosis and is typically entered via the straighter of the two orifices. All end-viewing endoscopes have an inherent difficulty in visualizing the major papilla because of its location along the sharply turned, interior aspect of the duodenal C-loop. Even when identified, cannulation is extraordinarily difficult because of the awkward orientation and unstable endoscope positioning (Fig. 31.15, *A–B*). In the hands of ERCP experts, the success rate is a mere 67%.[13] Yamamoto and colleagues reported the success of performing diagnostic and therapeutic ERCP with a double-balloon enteroscope in five patients.[12] Interestingly, the authors fitted a small plastic cap on the tip of the enteroscope to enable cannulation. The added advantage of a plastic cap was also reported by another endoscopy group using the single-balloon enteroscope.[14] Given the difficulty and frequent failure of performing ERCP in this postoperative anatomy, it is best to refer these types of cases to a tertiary biliary center or choose an alternative method such as a percutaneous transhepatic or endoscopic

ultrasonography (EUS)–guided approach. Performing ERCP with the intent to evaluate and treat a pancreatic condition is particularly problematic, as a transhepatic procedure cannot intubate the pancreatic duct. We prefer to use a long-length (320 cm) 5-Fr diagnostic ERCP catheter preloaded with a hydrophilic guidewire to perform cannulation when a double-balloon or single-balloon enteroscope is employed. Contrast can be injected with this setup if a Y-adapter is used. To circumvent the technical challenge in performing ERCP with an ultralong endoscope, some endoscopists advocate an intraoperative transjejunal method. This surgery-assisted procedure creates an enterotomy at 20 cm distal to the ligament of Treitz to allow a gas-sterilized duodenoscope to advance up the afferent limb.[15]

Total Gastrectomy

Usually performed for gastric cancer or postoperative complications, total gastrectomy leads to an end-to-side esophagojejunostomy. One lumen of the esophagojejunostomy is a blind end, whereas the other is the jejunal Roux limb (Fig. 31.16). A short distance distal is a side-to-side or end-to-side jejunojejunostomy to receive pancreatic and biliary contents. Similar to Roux-en-Y gastrectomy, the peroral endoscope must enter the proximal jejunum before arriving at the duodenum. Unlike in Roux-en-Y partial gastrectomy, a duodenoscope can actually reach the major papilla because of its straighter and shorter upper GI route. Once the major papilla is identified with the duodenoscope, the approach to ERCP cannulation and therapy is as for Billroth II anatomy. When a duodenoscope cannot negotiate the jejunojejunostomy or is too short to reach the descending duodenum, a long end-viewing endoscope must be used. Again, the challenge lies in cannulating and treating disease processes without the benefits of an elevator and side-viewing capability. The same techniques used for a Roux-en-Y gastrectomy apply to this situation.

UPPER GI BYPASS SURGERY WITHOUT RESECTION

Loop Gastrojejunostomy

The indications for gastrojejunostomy without resection of any part of the stomach include an obstructing pancreatic head mass, benign chronic duodenal obstruction, and unresectable duodenal malignancy with stricture. Gastrojejunostomy may occasionally be done in combination with surgical closure of the pylorus to prevent food from entering a perforated duodenum (pylorus exclusion). When inspecting the stomach during ERCP, this loop gastrojejunostomy is usually located along the

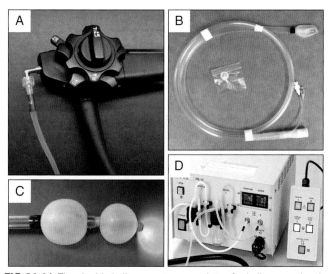

FIG 31.14 The double-balloon system consists of a balloon on the tip of a thin endoscope **(A)** and a balloon on an overtube **(B)**. **C,** Both balloons are inflated. **D,** Balloon inflation device that controls air insufflation, deflation, pressure reading, and an alarm with a yellow light indicating excessive pressure.

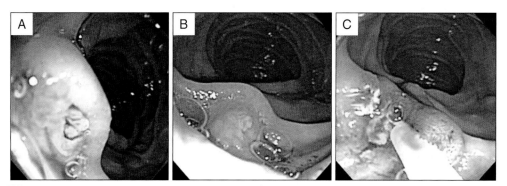

FIG 31.15 A, The major papilla seen with an end-viewing endoscope. Note the very tangential view with an awkward position for cannulation. **B,** After rotating the end-viewing endoscope, the major papilla appears to be optimally positioned for cannulation. The papilla is still tangentially located and it is difficult to maintain this view for long. **C,** A catheter has been successfully inserted into the bile duct with this end-viewing endoscope.

dependent portion of the stomach. However, it may be slightly toward the anterior or posterior wall along the greater curvature (Fig. 31.17, A, B). Although most anastomoses for bypass of obstructive diseases are expected to be large, some of these gastrojejunostomy openings appear to be quite small. Immediately through the rim of an anastomosis two jejunal orifices will be found, and either opening can be the one

that leads to the afferent limb. When it is the more distal orifice, an antiperistaltic connection has been performed and the afferent limb is relatively short. This distance becomes longer if the surgery is done in the antecolic fashion because the intestine has to drape over the transverse colon. This limb may become even longer if the gastrojejunostomy is created in an isoperistaltic manner. On some occasions a second anastomosis is noted beyond the gastrojejunostomy. It may be a Braun procedure (Fig. 31.17, B), done to add further bypass of contents between the afferent and efferent limbs to reduce alkaline biliary reflux into the stomach or to provide a safety net to minimize the chance of an afferent limb obstruction. If the endoscope passes through a Braun anastomosis, it has a 50% chance of returning to the stomach via the other limb of the gastrojejunostomy. When a Braun procedure is suspected, it is best to stay on the same intestinal limb without advancing through the second anastomosis. If the loop gastrojejunostomy is combined with suture closure of the pylorus as a short-term fix for duodenal perforation, the pylorus may reopen within a few months. It is best to first examine whether the pyloroduodenal stricture is patent before going through one of the gastrojejunostomy lumens.

Because the major papilla is intact in this setting, a duodenoscope is preferred for ease of inspection and cannulation unless it is proven to be of inadequate length. In practice, reaching the descending duodenum is often not the key issue. Instead, inspection and cannulation are a bigger challenge, because most of these cases have a highly stenotic duodenum as the reason for creating the loop gastrojejunostomy. Fortunately, duodenal obstruction from pancreatic head cancer is often located proximal to the major papilla, leaving sufficient room to carry out an ERCP. In the event of inadequate spacing, balloon dilation of the duodenal stricture can be performed, but the resultant mucosal trauma and hemorrhage may add more obstacles to the procedure. A transhepatic approach to biliary drainage, either percutaneously or using EUS guidance, is frequently necessary in this situation. Alternatively, a rendezvous procedure, in which a transhepatic catheter or guidewire is passed across the biliary sphincter, via percutaneous transhepatic or EUS guidance can be done for endoscopic access. There are occasions when the bypass surgery is done for gastroparesis and performing an ERCP in the usual antegrade fashion is preferred. In this situation, the

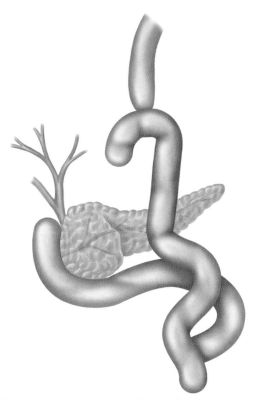

FIG 31.16 A total gastrectomy with a Roux-en-Y esophagojejunostomy. In spite of the significant distance, a side-viewing duodenoscope is usually long enough to reach the papilla.

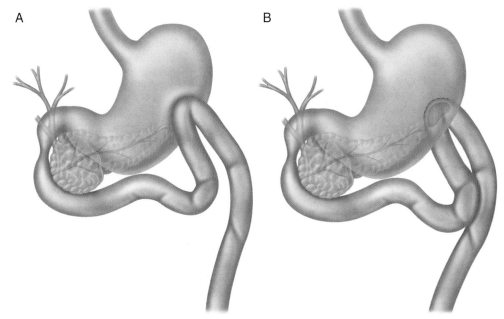

FIG 31.17 A, Gastric bypass via loop gastrojejunostomy with an anteriorly located gastrojejunostomy. B, Gastric bypass with a posteriorly located gastrojejunostomy. Note a Braun procedure that connects the afferent and efferent jejunal limbs.

duodenoscope has to be rotated slightly to glide along the anterior gastric wall to reach the pylorus and avoid inadvertently passing into the gastrojejunostomy.

Duodenal Bypass

Duodenal perforations are occasionally treated by a duodenojejunostomy. Even though this form of operation is uncommon, identification of two or more intestinal lumens beyond the pylorus or at the descending duodenum may create confusion for the endoscopist. If there is no associated duodenal narrowing, the procedure is straightforward and the key is to carefully inspect each lumen until the major papilla is found. If a mildly to moderately stenotic duodenal lumen is found, gentle balloon dilation may be attempted to ease passage of the endoscope. Alternatively, a pediatric ERCP scope with a 7.5-mm outer diameter and 2.0-mm instrument channel can be used. However, the small working channel allows only limited therapeutic possibilities such as sphincterotomy, stone extraction, and placement of a 5-Fr stent. On very rare occasions, duodenoduodenostomy (Fig. 31.18, A, B) is done on a newborn to bypass a congenital duodenal stricture or annular pancreas. Depending

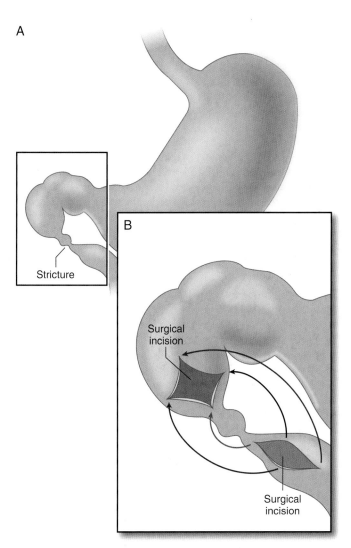

A

B

Stricture

Surgical incision

Surgical incision

FIG 31.18 A, Graphic illustration of congenital duodenal stricture or stenosis caused by annular pancreas. **B,** Duodenoduodenostomy is constructed by creating surgical incisions above and below the stricture and then suturing these incision edges together.

on the level of the stricture relative to the major papilla when this patient reaches adulthood, the endoscopist may find the papilla recessed above or below the stricture as if it was located inside a deep-seated diverticulum. The techniques and challenges of cannulating the ampullary orifice are very similar to those with the usually identified duodenal diverticulum.

BARIATRIC SURGERY

There are many forms of bariatric surgery to induce weight loss. Roux-en-Y gastric bypass (RYGB), once the dominant operation, is now performed approximately 32% of the time.[16] Vertical sleeve gastrectomy is currently the most often performed surgery (54%), whereas adjustable gastric band (<5%) is now rarely performed.[16] In the United States nearly 40% of all weight-reduction operations were performed in the South, whereas only 13% were done in the West in recent years. As the American obesity epidemic continues, the rates of weight-reduction operations will probably continue to rise. Because gallstone disease and abdominal pain are common issues in patients with rapid weight loss or extensive abdominal surgery, biliary and pancreatic evaluations are commonly requested for these bariatric patients. At the same time, ERCP in RYGB patients is the most difficult to perform because of the need to pass through an extremely long intestine to get to the proximal duodenum. Variations of techniques and surgeons' preferences add further challenges to this already-difficult ERCP population.

Malabsorptive Jejunoileal Bypass

This form of weight-reduction surgery is mentioned primarily for historical purposes. It is neither practiced today nor does it affect the performance of ERCP. Rarely, a consultation for ERCP may be requested for a patient with a prior jejunoileal bypass surgery because of jaundice. In this case the cause of jaundice is more likely hepatic failure rather than biliary tract disease. This operation, popular before 1980, may consist of transecting and connecting a large jejunoileal segment to the distal colon. Alternatively, the proximal jejunum is transected and connected to the distal ileum in an end-to-side manner, excluding a long jejunum and ileum from contact with intestinal nutrients (Fig. 31.19). The result of this form of operation is a very short functioning small bowel that causes weight loss by malabsorption and maldigestion. Chronic diarrhea, stone disease, and fatal liver dysfunction are reasons that all patients who underwent this surgery should have the bypass reversed.[17] Theoretically, if such a patient needs an ERCP, it can be done in the normal manner, although one of the editors of this book has done an ERCP successfully retrograde through the colon using a balloon-assisted enteroscope.

Biliopancreatic Diversion and Duodenal Switch

These are two other forms of malabsorptive operations that are still practiced today. Their metabolic complications are reportedly seen less often seen than in those associated with jejunoileal bypass. Both operations require resection of most of the stomach and connection of either the duodenum or the stomach remnant to the ileum (250 cm proximal to the ileocecal valve) (Fig. 31.20, A, B). The excluded section of duodenum–jejunum–ileum is then anastomosed to the distal ileum approximately 100 cm proximal to the ileocecal valve. Peroral ERCP is not possible, whether it is biliopancreatic bypass or duodenal switch, because the intact major papilla can be reached only by passing through most of the small intestine.

Restrictive Surgery

Until recently, there were two forms of this operation aimed at restricting gastric food passage by creating a mere 15 mL proximal gastric pouch

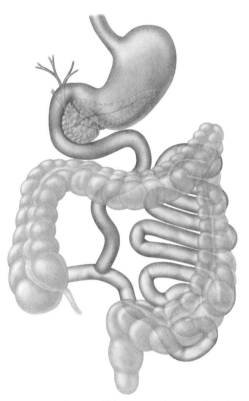

with a small outlet roughly 1 cm in diameter. Vertical band gastroplasty, popular in 1980s, consists of cutting off the fundus with staples and limiting the pouch outlet with a 5-cm circumferential Marlex band[17] (Fig. 31.21, *A*). The vertical band gastroplasty is easily recognized endoscopically because of the tiny gastric pouch that leads to a small firm outlet that barely allows passage of an upper endoscope. The outlet channel is typically 1 to 2 cm in length. If a restrictive gastroplasty is suspected, it is best to start the procedure with a standard upper endoscope to assess the degree of narrowing at the outlet. If difficulty passing a duodenoscope is anticipated, dilating the ring outlet with a 13.5-mm or 15-mm balloon before the procedure can be safely done. Once the duodenoscope has reached the distal stomach, no special ERCP techniques are needed, even though there are some subtle restrictions in straightening the endoscope and how the major papilla is approached. In patients who have regained weight after a vertical band gastroplasty, the stomach may appear normal because of spontaneous breakdown of the gastroplasty partition or fistula formation between the two gastric compartments.

A more modern alternative is the laparoscopic adjustable gastric banding procedure, whereby a silicone band is placed and wraps around the gastric cardia (Fig. 31.21, *B*). The band can be tightened by inserting a needle into a reservoir embedded in the abdominal wall. The gastric band is not typically recognized and no resistance during endoscope passage is encountered unless the patient complains of associated obstructive symptoms.

Vertical sleeve gastrectomy or gastric sleeve resection is the latest restrictive and most popular bariatric operation. Previously a component of the duodenal switch procedure, it is now a stand-alone surgery

FIG 31.19 Jejunoileal bypass. This surgery does not interfere with the performance of ERCP.

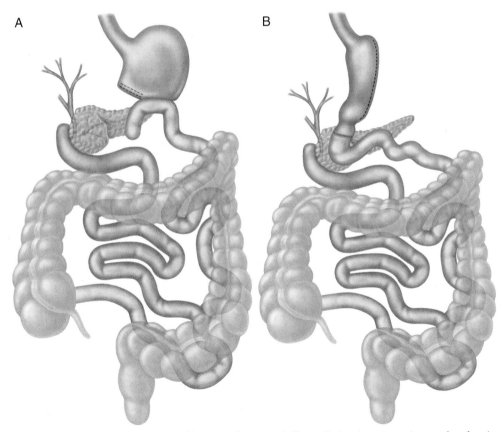

FIG 31.20 A, Biliopancreatic diversion. The long efferent and afferent limbs prevent any chance of performing ERCP in this case. **B,** Duodenal switch procedure. Very similar to the biliopancreatic diversion surgery, it is not possible to perform ERCP in this situation.

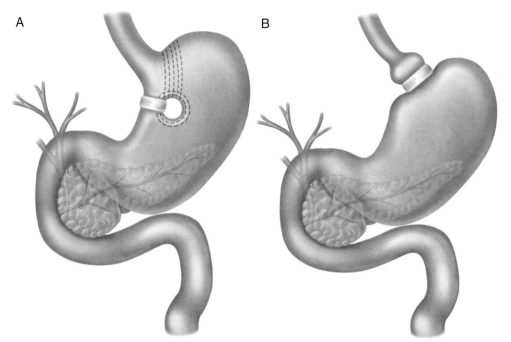

A

B

FIG 31.21 A, Vertical banded gastroplasty, with a small aperture that allows food passage. This channel may have to be dilated in order to pass a duodenoscope through. **B,** Laparoscopic adjustable gastric banding. The degree of constriction in the proximal stomach is adjustable externally.

performed by removing the greater curvature portion of the stomach and converting it into a tubular organ. It should pose no major technical challenge to performing ERCP.

Roux-en-Y Gastric Bypass

The Roux-en-Y gastric bypass surgical procedure works by restricting food intake with a small (<50 mL) gastric pouch and by creating maldigestion because of late contact between ingested food and pancreatic and biliary fluids in the jejunum. This is the most difficult form of Roux-en-Y surgical anatomy on which to perform ERCP. To reach the papilla, the endoscope must travel through 40 cm of the esophagus, a tiny gastric pouch, and a 75-cm to 150-cm Roux limb, followed by a variable-length afferent limb (Fig. 31.22). After arriving at the descending duodenum, the tip of the endoscope has to be flexible enough to visualize the major papilla but sufficiently stable to perform cannulation. Even a 250-cm-long push enteroscope is usually too short because of looping and stretching of the intestine. Working with long accessories to perform ERCP in this setting poses additional technical challenges that even elite endoscopists consider overwhelming.

There are several ways of performing ERCP in this very difficult situation (Box 31.2). The simplest approach, though most likely to fail, is to use the longest endoscope available and cannulate the papilla with extra long accessories. Attempting the procedure with a pediatric colonoscope or duodenoscope is rarely effective and is frustrating in maneuvering through the jejunojejunostomy, and the length is exhausted long before reaching the descending duodenum. A more logical alternative is to use a balloon enteroscope, which is thinner, more flexible, and able to travel over long segments of the intestine. We presented our initial experience of using double-balloon enteroscopy and modified accessories to perform ERCP on 40 patients with RYGB and an intact papilla at an annual society meeting.[18] The procedure involved passage of a double-balloon enteroscope through the small gastric pouch and the jejunal Roux limb. After reaching the jejunojejunostomy, the afferent limb was identified and entered. We typically advanced the endoscope

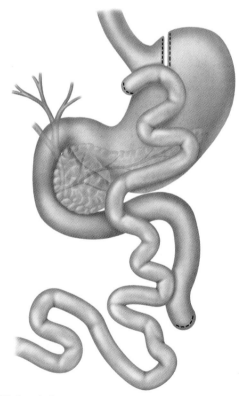

FIG 31.22 Gastric bypass surgery for weight reduction by combining restrictive and malabsorptive principles. This increasingly common operation creates one of the most challenging surgically altered anatomies for performing ERCP.

into the stomach to allow anchoring, followed by shortening the endoscope and advancing the overtube into the general area of the ligament of Treitz. After straightening, the endoscope was gradually withdrawn to the descending duodenum, where the minor papilla was readily visualized. We would then withdraw further to find the major papilla and orientate it at the 6 to 7 o'clock position, although the 12 o'clock position was occasionally used. A commercially available 320-cm sphincterotome or ERCP cannula was then used to approach the papilla. Because it was often not possible to cannulate the bile duct directly with a catheter, we typically preloaded the device with a 450-cm-long hydrophilic guidewire and a side-arm adapter and prefilled the catheter with contrast. If engaging the papillary orifice was not immediately successful, we would use the guidewire to probe gently until the bile duct was accessed. Fluoroscopy was important to determine whether the guidewire was coursing properly in the biliary direction. If the papilla could not be cannulated despite numerous attempts, we would modify the long sphincterotome into a needle knife and perform precut biliary sphincterotomy to access the bile duct. Even if the bile duct was entered smoothly with a guidewire, cutting the papilla still required the needle knife that had been inserted over the guidewire, because the long sphincterotome does not orient in proper cutting position. It is important to recognize that instrument exchange could not be performed over the conventional 450-cm or 480-cm guidewire, though it is possible to perform a hydraulic exchange with a totally hydrophilic wire (e.g., Terumo). Since our initial experience, a 600-cm, 0.035-inch guidewire has become available (Metro; Cook Endoscopy, Winston-Salem, NC). Balloon dilation was typically done to ensure an adequate papillary opening without risking perforation or bleeding. With this technique, our initial success rate of performing therapeutic ERCP on those 40 RYGB patients was 90%. Since then, we have done more than 200 such procedures and our rate of technical success is close to 95%. Interestingly, there have been multiple reports and presentations[19] suggesting that enteroscope-assisted ERCP in RYGB patients is only moderately successful at around 50%, and the reason for the discrepancy relative to our experience is unclear.

In theory, the enteroscopy-assisted technique can be used with the single-balloon or spiral enteroscope. Because the spiral overtubes have limited availability, they are no longer an option for most centers, though the possibility of a newly designed commercial version exists. The single-balloon device may have difficulty negotiating the jejunojejunostomy and tends to have insecure footing, and technical success may be less than that of double-balloon enteroscopy.

If biliary cannulation is not possible despite successful endoscope advancement to the major papilla, then there are several alternatives. One method is to create a percutaneous endoscopic gastrostomy (PEG) by utilizing the Russell PEG placement technique once the enteroscope has entered into the excluded stomach. One group has even described immediate ERCP by placing a large-diameter self-expandable metal stent through this percutaneous tract.[20] Otherwise, after the large-bore gastric fistula has matured, a duodenoscope can be inserted through it to perform ERCP. A similar and less technically challenging alternative is to have a surgical gastrostomy tube placed for the performance of ERCP after the tract has matured.[21] An EUS-assisted transgastric method to distend the excluded stomach to provide a target for PEG insertion has also been described.[22] It is also possible to perform either an open surgical or laparoscopic gastrostomy to allow intraoperative duodenoscope insertion and ERCP.[23] All these transgastric ERCP approaches have a common problem, which is the restriction from passing a duodenoscope at the epigastrium. Performing ERCP through a short route, in a sharply angulated position, with the patient lying supine, and working with suboptimal fluoroscopic images are many challenges to overcome. Alternatively, a transjejunal retrograde operative approach for duodenoscope advancement at 20 cm below the ligament of Treitz may be attempted.[14] Likewise, a rendezvous procedure with the insertion of a percutaneous transhepatic guidewire into the duodenum or jejunum may help enteroscopic advancement as well as gain access into the bile duct.

Recently an EUS-guided transgastric-transhepatic approach to directly dilate the biliary sphincter in an antegrade manner and allow biliary therapy has been successfully performed in a limited number of patients.[24] If biliary access is achieved and a guidewire can be passed into the duodenum but dilation of the transhepatic tract is not performed, then the transampullary wire can be advanced down the jejunum to allow the performance of an "internal rendezvous" procedure using a single-balloon endoscope-passed retrograde. Finally, not all biliary diseases require endoscopic manipulations and a solely percutaneous transhepatic approach may be sufficient. It is still unclear which endoscopic or combined procedure should be attempted in this difficult setting. Clearly the best option is one that would take advantage of the endoscopist's skill, local endoscopic resources, and surgical and interventional radiology expertise. Regardless of the options, these procedures are intrinsically difficult and best done in a tertiary care environment. EUS approaches to biliary drainage are discussed in Chapters 32 and 33.

PANCREATIC RESECTION

Conventional Whipple Procedure

The most recognized name in abdominal surgery is Whipple, who developed the pancreaticoduodenectomy, done for resection of the pancreatic head. Although the concept of resection is simple, the multiple anastomoses in this operation create a great deal of confusion. Because the bile duct, pancreatic duct, and duodenum are interrupted, at least three separate connections are made to reestablish pancreatic, biliary, and intestinal continuity. When an endoscope is passed into the midstomach, two small bowel orifices should be seen in the conventional Whipple procedure (Fig. 31.23, A). One gastrojejunostomy ascends the afferent limb and joins the bile duct and eventually the pancreatic duct. The other gastrojejunal anastomosis leads to the efferent limb and remainder of the GI tract. Because the usual challenge of cannulating an intact papilla is absent, ERCP can be readily performed with either an end-viewing or side-viewing endoscope. Indeed, we routinely start

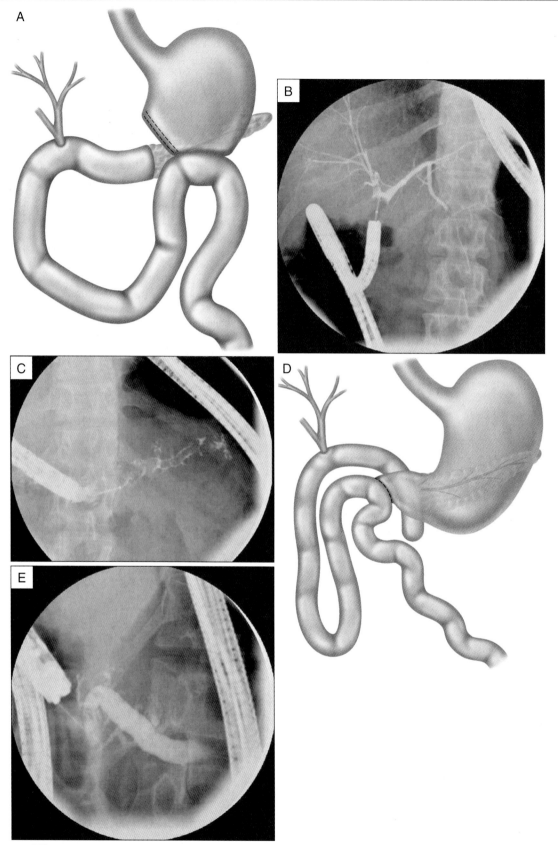

FIG 31.23 A, Conventional Whipple procedure. Note that the pancreatic duct is found at the upper end of the afferent limb. **B,** A cholangiogram obtained through a hepaticojejunostomy anastomosis with a pediatric colonoscope. **C,** A pancreaticogram showing a markedly dilated pancreatic duct after Whipple procedure. **D,** Pylorus-preserving Whipple procedure with an intact stomach and a very short duodenal bulb before the lumen splits into the afferent and efferent limbs. Note that in this case the pancreaticojejunostomy is fashioned on the side of the proximal afferent limb before the intestinal lumen ends. **E,** A corresponding radiograph showing the relationship between the endoscope and a tortuous and markedly dilated pancreatic duct due to stenosis of the pancreaticojejunostomy. The afferent jejunum ends a few centimeters straight away from the tip of the endoscope.

this procedure with a diagnostic or therapeutic upper endoscope to take advantage of the easy maneuverability. In spite of the short length, an upper endoscope can reach the hepaticojejunostomy in more than two-thirds of cases. However, reaching the pancreatic anastomosis is significantly more challenging with a short-length scope. Abdominal compression and aggressive gastric decompression are effective means to aid in endoscope advancement. If a diagnostic upper endoscope is too short, then a pediatric colonoscope or duodenoscope should be able to reach the bilioenteric or pancreaticoenteric anastomosis (Fig. 31.23, *B*). Fluoroscopy may occasionally be of benefit to confirm if the endoscope is within the afferent limb and to assist in reducing loops.

In our experience, approximately 90% of afferent gastrojejunostomy lumens in both classic and pylorus-sparing operations are located at or around the 10 o'clock position. Correctly inserting the endoscope into the afferent limb saves time and avoids the frustration of passing into a lumen without knowing if it is the wrong limb or an excessively long one. Fluoroscopy usually helps to locate the biliary anastomosis, as it always arises from the most cephalad portion of the bowel gas in the right upper quadrant. Pneumobilia seen on fluoroscopy represents a patent hepaticojejunostomy. Endoscopically, a normal bile duct anastomosis is readily identified as a round orifice with bile exiting. The opening is frequently located eccentrically or retracted behind an intestinal fold and is typically seen on the left side. Determining whether a hepaticojejunostomy is mildly or moderately narrowed by endoscopic visualization is subjective. In the presence of a severe stenosis, the opening can appear as a pinhole or be covered by a film of whitish scar tissue and pneumobilia is distinctively absent on fluoroscopy. The pancreaticojejunostomy is notoriously difficult to identify or cannulate, which is the main cause of diagnostic or therapeutic failure.[25] Whereas the pancreaticojejunal anastomosis may be seen at the very proximal end of the afferent limb (Fig. 31.23, *A, C*), the pancreatic anastomosis is most commonly found at 5 to 10 cm beyond the biliary orifice in an end-to-side fashion (Fig. 31.23, *D, E*). A clue that the endoscope is in the vicinity of the pancreaticojejunostomy is the presence of a large amount of flat tissue, most commonly located at between the 6 and 9 o'clock positions. In addition, when the endoscope is seen facing medially directly toward the spine on fluoroscopy, the pancreatic orifice is in the vicinity.

Pylorus-Preserving Whipple Procedure

Aimed to minimize delayed gastric emptying and other surgery-related morbidity, a pylorus-preserving Whipple procedure is different from the conventional Whipple procedure with a completely intact stomach and a tiny cuff of proximal duodenal bulb (Fig. 31.23, *D*). However, the theoretical advantage of keeping the antrum and pylorus has not been proven.[26] When performing an ERCP, the stomach and pylorus appear normal. Immediately beyond the pylorus are two duodenoje-junostomy orifices, with the left upper lumen likely to be leading to the biliary and pancreatic anastomoses. As opposed to conventional Whipple surgery, this anatomy makes it harder to reach the bilioenteric anastomosis because of the longer distance to travel and the sharper angle it takes to turn deeply into the afferent limb. As such, it is often necessary to start the procedure with a duodenoscope or pediatric colonoscope.

Pancreaticogastrostomy

A pancreaticoduodenectomy can be further modified to have the main duct of the body and tail of the pancreas implanted into the posterior wall of the stomach[27] (Fig. 31.24). In this case the bilioenteric anastomosis is found along the afferent limb in the usual manner. However, the pancreatic orifice is no longer near the end of the proximal jejunal

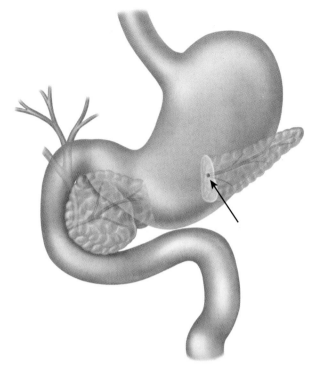

FIG 31.24 Pancreaticogastrostomy. The *arrow* points to the pancreatic duct that is directly anastomosed to the posterior wall of the stomach. Endoscopic pancreatography is possible if this gastric anastomosis is identified.

stump. Rather, it is located along the posterior gastric body and seen as a small opening. Finding the anastomosis among the gastric rugal folds can be difficult, but parenteral injection of secretin and spraying a color dye on the gastric mucosa should help with identification. In spite of the gastric location of this anastomosis, it may be easier to identify and approach the pancreatic duct with a duodenoscope than with the end-viewing upper endoscope.

Other Pancreatic Resective Surgery (see also Chapter 45)

Resection of the tail of the pancreas does not alter any gastric, duodenal, or pancreaticobiliary anatomy. Pancreatogram shows a shortened duct. Likewise, midpancreatic resection for a benign condition may result in a normal anatomy in the head of the pancreas and a short distal pancreatic duct that drains proximally into a loop of jejunum. Studying the pancreaticojejunostomy in this setting is difficult. When the tail of the pancreas is anastomosed to the posterior wall of the stomach, accessing the pancreatic duct is much easier.[28]

PANCREATIC DUCT DRAINAGE PROCEDURES

Puestow Procedure

The Puestow procedure is a longitudinal pancreaticojejunostomy procedure that is used to decompress a dilated, obstructed pancreatic duct for relief of pain from chronic pancreatitis. The procedure involves opening the pancreatic duct from the head to the tail of the pancreas and creating a side-to-side anastomosis between the open edges of the pancreatic duct and jejunum.[29] There is obviously no anatomic alteration in the upper GI tract and ERCP is done in the usual manner. Pancreatography shows a short Wirsung duct followed by immediate spillage of contrast outside of the duct with opacification of the jejunum. Although determining whether there is a stricture between the Wirsung duct and the jejunum is relatively easy, there is no certainty whether the duct beyond that point is fully decompressed.

Frey Procedure

This procedure combines removal of tissue within the head of the pancreas and the Puestow (longitudinal pancreaticojejunostomy) procedure while preserving the duodenum and the bile duct.[30] As in the Puestow procedure, injection of contrast should identify a Wirsung duct that drains into the small bowel. Despite resection of a large portion of the head of the pancreas, pancreatic duct continuity is maintained and there is no altered GI anatomy.

Duval Procedure

One of the original pancreatic duct drainage procedures, this surgery involves resection of the tail of the pancreas and the spleen and creation of an end-to-end pancreaticojejunostomy. The principal function of this surgery is to allow backward drainage of an obstructed pancreatic duct into the jejunum. However, this operation has a high incidence of treatment failure and is now rarely performed. A pancreatogram should reflect a slightly shortened pancreatic duct that connects to an intestinal lumen.

BILIARY SURGERY

Choledochoduodenostomy

Choledochoduodenostomy is a simple form of surgery that provides midextrahepatic bile duct drainage for benign conditions such as distal bile duct stricture or recurrent choledocholithiasis. It is usually done in a side-to-side fashion between the proximal duodenum and the midextrahepatic bile duct, without ductal or duodenal transection (Fig. 31.25, A). However, an end-to-side anastomosis may be created occasionally by ligating off the distal bile duct. The side-to-side anastomosis may be complicated by recurrent fever, abdominal pain, liver abscess, pancreatitis, or cholangitis. Bile duct impaction caused by trapped debris distal to a side-to-side choledochoduodenostomy is referred to as sump syndrome (Fig. 31.25, B, C, F). Interestingly, symptoms of sump syndrome occur 5 to 6 years postoperatively.[31] Inspection of biliary complaints in this situation should aim at studying the bile duct via the major papilla. However, the biliary sphincter may be so stenotic as to not allow access through the duodenum. Therefore contrast injection or guidewire passage antegrade via the anastomosis may be required to assess drainage at the level of the papilla and to pass a wire antegrade across the papilla to allow internal rendezvous. Identification of the choledochoduodenal anastomosis, which is normally about 0.5 to 1 cm in diameter, is difficult because it is located in the medial aspect of the proximal descending duodenum (Fig. 31.25, D). Nonetheless, careful inspection and gentle rotation of the duodenoscope should reveal this opening. A biliary sphincterotomy may provide relief from sump syndrome for up to several years.[31] Jaundice and recurrent cholangitis may also occur because of stenosis of the choledochoduodenostomy; balloon dilation and stenting through the strictured anastomosis are necessary in this situation. Direct choledochoscopy through the choledochoduodenostomy can be done with an ultrathin upper endoscope and is sometimes required to inspect the distal and proximal bile duct segments and to perform electrohydraulic lithotripsy. In an end-to-side choledochoduodenostomy, the common hepatic and intrahepatic ducts can be accessed only through the duodenal anastomosis. Because the proximal end of the common bile duct is a blind stump, food debris cannot enter from the duodenum and sump syndrome does not occur; however, contamination of the common hepatic and intrahepatic ducts may still occur and lead to cholangitis and liver abscesses. ERCP can be performed with either

a duodenoscope or a thin upper endoscope in these patients. If the endoscopist is unaware of the surgical bile duct transection, he/she might mistake the proximal end of the common bile duct for a high-grade stricture. Excessive probing of the stump must be avoided to prevent perforation.

Roux-en-Y Hepaticojejunostomy

The hepatic duct is surgically connected to the jejunum for biliary anastomosis during liver transplantation and to treat a variety of conditions, including recurrent biliary stones, benign distal biliary strictures, cholangiocarcinoma, choledochal cyst, and iatrogenic bile duct injury. When done for extensive intrahepatic stone disease and benign biliary stasis, disease recurrence is common and further endoscopic access is desirable. In that case, continuity of the biliary tract may be maintained and the biliojejunal anastomosis is constructed in a side-to-side manner (Fig. 31.26, A). The clue to this surgery is continuous spillage of contrast into what appears to be the duodenal bulb through the common hepatic duct, even though the "spilled" contrast cannot be captured with endoscope suctioning. In this case, quality cholangiograms can be obtained only by injecting contrast superior to the hepaticojejunostomy or occluding the common hepatic duct with a stone-retrieval balloon.

Most of the time, a hepaticojejunostomy is created in conjunction with transection of the mid–bile duct. In this situation a cholangiogram via the major papilla shows termination at the proximal common bile duct (Fig. 31.26, B). If this is known in advance, performing a standard ERCP via the major papilla to study the biliary tract is unnecessary and raises the risk of an otherwise negligible chance of pancreatitis. Sometimes the surgically ligated stump is misinterpreted as a tight biliary stricture, and ductal perforation may result from aggressive probing with catheters and wires.

Studying the biliary system proximal to the transected bile duct in a Roux-en-Y hepaticojejunostomy is difficult. It requires a long endoscope that can travel through the entire duodenum, ligament of Treitz, proximal jejunum, jejunojejunostomy, and the afferent limb. A pediatric colonoscope is the ideal endoscope for this purpose, although a commercially made push enteroscope, therapeutic colonoscope, or balloon enteroscope may also be used. Because there is no major papilla involved, accessing the bile duct is relatively straightforward once the proximal afferent limb is reached, assuming that the hepaticojejunal anastomosis is visualized and patent. Identifying the hepaticojejunostomy or choledochojejunostomy requires experience. The biliary anastomosis is frequently hidden behind a sharp turn or a recessed fold. En face viewing is often difficult because it may only be partially visible near the edge of an endoscopic image, but fluoroscopy may guide endoscope passage and biliary catheterization with an air cholangiogram. Cannulation may be possible with the use of a guidewire. An immediate bifurcation may be noted if the anastomosis is created in the proximal hepatic duct. On rare occasions, two or three separate orifices may be identified if the bilioenteric anastomosis is created very proximally in the liver. Even more rarely, two separate biliary implantations in the jejunum may be found several centimeters apart. When the anastomosis is severely stenosed, a seemingly complete closure by a film of whitish scar tissue may be observed. It is essential to look for a fully opacified intrahepatic cholangiogram. If a part of the intrahepatic distribution is missing, then a ductal stricture or an occluded separate orifice should be suspected.

Cholecystojejunostomy

This operation was once commonly employed to bypass an obstructed bile duct by an unresectable pancreatic head cancer. This form of surgery is an unreliable means to decompress the bile duct because of the potential for tumor extension to involve the cystic duct. The surgery is a very

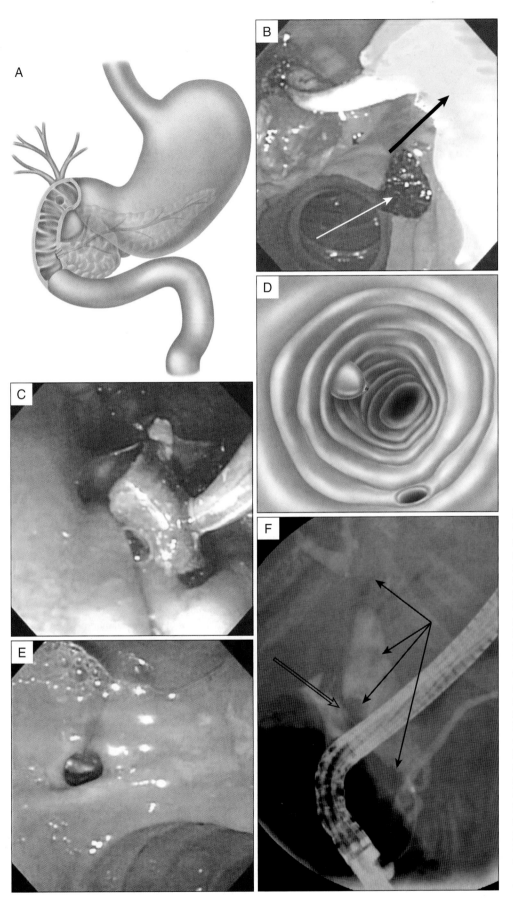

FIG 31.25 A, A choledochojejunostomy without interruption of the bile duct. The bile duct can be accessed either through the major papilla or the choledochoduodenostomy. **B,** A pigmented stone (*thin arrow*) and a large piece of fresh vegetable (*large arrow*) were swept into the duodenum after a sphincterotomy. **C,** More foreign body–like biliary debris was extracted from the bile duct of the same patient. This material appears to have been in the bile duct for a long duration. **D,** A schematic illustration of the usual relationship between the choledochoduodenostomy and the major papilla. Finding the anastomosis can be quite difficult because of its usual location in the posterior wall of the proximal descending duodenum. **E,** A biliary stent was visualized through a choledochoduodenostomy as expected. **F,** A cholangiogram typically seen in sump syndrome. The *open arrow* points toward the choledochoduodenostomy, where biliary contrast escapes laterally into the duodenum. *Thin arrows* show filling defects throughout the dilated bile duct.

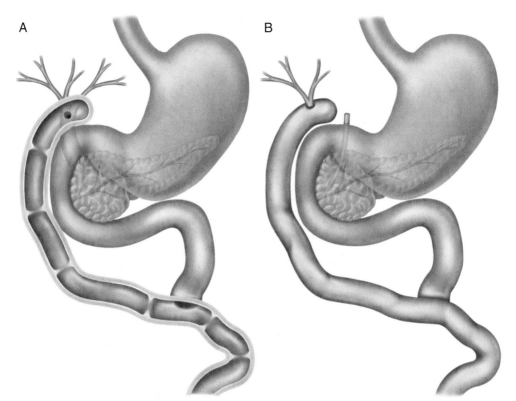

FIG 31.26 A, Roux-en-Y hepaticojejunostomy without transection of the bile duct. ERCP is done in the usual fashion and contrast is seen flowing outside of the bile duct via the biliary bypass into the jejunum. **B,** Roux-en-Y hepaticojejunostomy without biliary continuity. In this case the only possible way to study the bile duct is by passing a long endoscope through the proximal jejunum and up the afferent jejunal limb. Injection of the major papilla to evaluate the bile duct should be avoided to prevent causing pancreatitis.

simple one, whereby the distended gallbladder is opened and anastomosed to a jejunal limb (Fig. 31.27). Today, this operation is mostly reserved for the intraoperative finding of an unresectable and obstructing cancer that is too large to allow access to the proximal bile duct to create a hepaticojejunostomy. This surgery does not alter the upper GI anatomy and poses no additional difficulty for standard ERCP. In fact, the result of this surgery is not readily recognized unless the bile duct is overfilled with contrast.

Liver Transplantation (see Chapter 44)

The bile duct anastomosis in liver transplantation is usually a duct-to-duct connection or choledochocholedochostomy. There is no special anatomic challenge to the performance of ERCP in this situation. When the transplantation is done for primary sclerosing cholangitis or other conditions in which the distal bile duct conduit cannot be used, then a Roux-en-Y choledochojejunostomy or hepaticojejunostomy is constructed (Fig. 31.26, B). Living donor liver transplantation cases also often use Roux-en-Y hepaticojejunostomy because of difficulty in matching the native main bile duct with the donor right hepatic duct. As previously mentioned, a long endoscope is mandatory when performing ERCP in these Roux-en-Y cases.

Hepaticocutaneous Jejunostomy

This form of biliary surgery is rarely encountered in the United States but is occasionally done in Southeast Asia, where recurrent pyogenic cholangitis is prevalent. The persistent nature of pyogenic cholangitis mandates access to the bile duct for periodic clearance of intrahepatic biliary stones.[32] This is essentially a Roux-en-Y hepaticojejunostomy

with an extension of the afferent limb to the abdominal wall as a permanent stoma or a concealed "port" within the subcutaneous tissue. Via this stoma a choledochoscope, bronchoscope, or pediatric upper endoscope can be inserted into the intrahepatic ducts for stricture dilation and stone extraction. This cutaneous stoma provides a highly convenient means of biliary access without having to perform numerous difficult ERCPs and peroral choledochoscopies. It theoretically reduces the risk of post-ERCP cholangitis, cumulative radiation exposure, and repeated prolonged sedation.

ENDOSCOPIC TECHNIQUES COMMONLY EMPLOYED FOR ERCP IN SURGICALLY ALTERED ANATOMY

External Rendezvous Procedure

There is no single rendezvous technique uniformly adopted by gastroenterologists for endoscopic biliary access using a percutaneous transhepatic biliary guidewire or catheter. Most of these procedures are done in two steps and possibly in two locations within a medical center.[33] An interventional radiologist first inserts a needle into a dilated peripheral intrahepatic duct, most often through the right lobe of the liver. A guidewire between 250 and 450 cm in length is then passed through the needle into the bile duct and eventually into the duodenum, or jejunum if there is a biliojejunal anastomosis. The external end of the guidewire is then secured onto the abdominal wall with heavy dressing. Some radiologists prefer to slide a thin-caliber biliary catheter over the guidewire to protect the liver and biliary tissue from slicing injuries

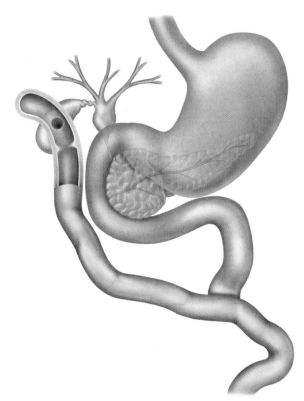

FIG 31.27 Schematic drawing of a partially exposed proximal afferent jejunum to illustrate biliary decompression through a patent cystic duct. This form of surgery does not interfere with the performance of ERCP and may not even be recognized if only a small amount of contrast is injected above an obstructed distal bile duct.

from a thin, tightly wound wire.[32] The patient is then transferred to an endoscopic suite where ERCP is performed, unless the two procedures are performed in the same suite. If endoscope passage is met with technical difficulty, such as in the case of a long afferent limb in a Whipple procedure, the guidewire can be floated down the intestinal lumen under fluoroscopy guidance until it is seen endoscopically. The guidewire is grasped with a snare and pulled into the endoscope channel until it can be secured externally. With slight traction on the guidewire, the endoscope may be advanced along the lumen. However, the assumption that an externally placed wire may readily pull an endoscope up the afferent tract is inaccurate. In fact, excessive tension on a tightly drawn wire can injure the intestine or liver tissue and must be avoided. A previously inserted "external-internal" transhepatic drainage catheter can also be used as the conduit for this type of rendezvous procedure.

For the most part, a rendezvous procedure is done to gain biliary access in the setting of a difficult papilla (e.g., intradiverticular) or tight biliary stricture. The free end of the wire is snared and pulled into the endoscope channel until it can be secured externally. During guidewire manipulation, the external end must be secured with a clamp to prevent it from being drawn into the liver or small intestine. Once the guidewire has been withdrawn through the instrument channel, a sphincterotome, balloon dilator, or biliary stent is readily passed over the guidewire into the bile duct to complete the ERCP. Alternatively, a needle-knife sphincterotomy can be done over a transhepatic-transpapillary guidewire or catheter to create space in the papilla for subsequent biliary cannulation. Yet another way to complete a rendezvous procedure is to slide a catheter directly onto the free end of the guidewire that is barely exposed

through the papilla to perform a sphincterotomy, stricture dilation, or stenting. Finally, a two-step procedure that combines transhepatic placement of an 8-Fr external-to-duodenal biliary catheter with a subsequent ERCP session to cannulate the bile duct alongside the biliary drain has been described.[34] Rendezvous procedures are best done with monitored anesthesia (MAC) or general anesthesia because of potential injuries that may result from the patient waking up during light sedation with a long wire traversing the various organs.

Internal rendezvous and other EUS-guided procedures have been discussed elsewhere (see Chapters 32 and 33). These approaches take advantage of the transmural needle access capability of EUS. By inserting a needle into the pancreatic or bile duct, a diagnostic cholangiogram or pancreatogram is readily obtained. Guidewire passage through a 22-gauge or 19-gauge FNA needle provides luminal access whereby subsequent dilation, stenting, or advancement of the wire beyond the papilla or biliary enteric anastomosis can be performed. Rapid growth in this area will likely become a key component of therapeutic pancreaticobiliary procedures. However, in their current form, EUS-access ERCPs are technically challenging, are associated with significant adverse events,[35] and should be done in established tertiary care centers.

Selection of an Anastomotic Limb to Enter

It is often confusing when the endoscope reaches an anastomosis with more than one exiting lumen. Correctly identifying the afferent limb among several orifices is a difficult but important task, as incorrect selection may lead to tremendous energy and time wasted. If an alternative lumen is chosen, it becomes a stressful situation to decide between withdrawing the scope to start over versus continuing on the same path with the hope that the endoscope is in the correct lumen. There is no quick solution other than examining the anatomy carefully and systematically. A thorough understanding of small-bowel surgeries may minimize frustration with these kinds of procedures. Recognizing which lumen has been examined is also crucial to prevent entering the same lumen over and over. Some endoscopists use India ink to mark the examined lumen, whereas others take superficial biopsies or leave cautery marks to help recognition. However, placing permanent tattoo marks is not advisable in this setting, as it may cause confusion in subsequent procedures. In the event of endoscope withdrawal because of the concern of being in the wrong intestinal limb, a more practical method of leaving a trail is to insert a long guidewire into the lumen as the endoscope is being withdrawn.

In a loop gastric bypass, there are two gastrojejunostomy openings, where one lumen leads back to the duodenum and the other down the efferent limb. In total gastrectomy, the esophagus bifurcates into a short blind jejunal limb and a long Roux lumen. At the end of the Roux limb is a jejunojejunostomy, which further branches into the afferent pancreaticobiliary and efferent jejunoileal lumens. In all jejunojejunostomies, whether they are done for RYGB or hepaticojejunostomy, the afferent limb is typically found beyond the circumferential surgical staple line. It is important to know that there are either two or three lumens at any given jejunojejunostomy anastomosis, depending on whether they are the result of a side-to-side (three lumens) or end-to-side (two lumens) reconstruction (Fig. 31.13, A–D). It is equally important to know that the afferent limb is usually not a direct extension of the Roux limb. Therefore it is crucial to observe where the suture line is and pass the endoscope across it. Once this is done, the decision is to enter one of the two small bowel exits. Contrary to common belief, the afferent lumen is typically the orifice that is easy to visualize and is usually close to the staple line. In our experience performing more than 500 Roux-en-Y cases, we can correctly "guess" the afferent limb in over 95% using this concept as our guide. An exception is when a Braun procedure is found, and it should be suspected whenever a second anastomosis in a series is noted. In Whipple surgery, whether it is the conventional operation or pylorus-preserving procedure, the afferent lumen is commonly found at the 10 o'clock position. Because many of these procedures must be repeated in the future, it is important to construct a roadmap by carefully documenting how the afferent limb and papilla or bilioenteric anastomosis are found.

Navigation Through the Small Intestine

Passing an endoscope through the small intestine is like navigating the lumen of a tortuous colon, and simple endoscope shaft advancement does not advance the tip of the endoscope. Whether working with a side-viewing or end-viewing endoscope, gentle rotation and intermittent shortening are essential maneuvers. Handling a side-viewing duodenoscope requires extra care to avoid perforation at fixed corners. When a duodenoscope is used, the scope should constantly be adjusted so that the top half of the intestinal lumen is situated at the 6 o'clock position before it can be advanced forward. Sudden rotation and forceful pulling should be avoided to prevent trauma to the intestine. Minimizing air insufflation is equally important, as it reduces bowel tortuosity and allows pliability with less chance of injury to the intestinal wall. When repeated passages result in the same paradoxical movements, hand compressions of the various regions of the abdomen may have positive effects, like the maneuvers used in passing a colonoscope. Rotating the patient may straighten an angulated segment of the intestine and allow further passage. On rare occasions, fluoroscopic examination may visualize a redundant gastric or jejunal loop that can be gently straightened before making further advancement. Some highly angulated intestine behaves like a blind pouch and the downstream lumen may be identified only by probing with a hydrophilic wire or infusing contrast into the intestinal lumen. Finally, it is important to be willing to stop a procedure if repeated attempts fail to lead to any forward progress.

With the increasing applications of double-balloon enteroscopy, single-balloon enteroscopy, and even spiral enteroscopy to perform ERCP, today's biliary interventionists should be familiar with these procedures. Virtually all tertiary biliary centers should have someone with expertise in one of the deep enteroscopies. Because it can be time-consuming to perform both enteroscopy and ERCP, care must be taken to avoid excessive intestinal distention. A highly effective way is to equip the endoscopy system with carbon dioxide, which, unlike room air, rapidly diffuses across the small intestine mucosa and is readily exhaled through the lungs. Indeed, carbon dioxide has been found to induce less postprocedure abdominal discomfort after ERCP and balloon enteroscopy.[36–38]

ERCP ACCESSORIES

Billroth II gastrectomy may be the most common surgically altered anatomy encountered when performing an ERCP. All commercially available ERCP accessories can be used; however, they may have to be modified in order to gain access to the tangentially and upside-down-oriented bile duct (Fig. 31.28, *A*). Sphincterotomes are also specially made to accommodate the distorted anatomy (Fig. 31.28, *B*). The techniques for using these catheters and sphincterotomes are intuitive but can be difficult during the first few uses. Despite the concern for inducing acute pancreatitis,[39] balloon sphincter dilation is an important therapeutic option if the endoscopist is unfamiliar with sphincterotomy performance in this setting. In fact, a small study showed no disadvantage in employing balloon dilation for biliary stone removal in Billroth II cases.[9] When a colonoscope is used, most standard diagnostic and therapeutic ERCP accessories are sufficiently long. However, a few instruments, such as many biliary balloon dilators and some sphincterotomes, are too short to go through the colonoscope channel. Each

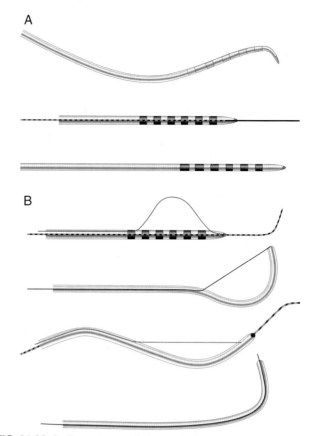

FIG 31.28 A, Three types of diagnostic instruments are commonly used for cannulating the Billroth II bile duct. A tapered ERCP catheter bent into an S-shape is probably the most useful instrument. Some endoscopists prefer to use a catheter with a straight hydrophilic wire. Other endoscopists find it helpful to start with a straight, uncurved cannula. **B,** Sphincter-cutting accessories include a push-type sphincterotome with a protruding loop when the cutting wire is loosened, a sphincterotome with the cutting wire at the very tip, an S-shape sphincterotome, and the needle knife.

endoscopy unit should consult with its accessories manufacturers to compile a complete set of supplies for this purpose.

It is far more challenging to find the right accessories to use through a balloon enteroscope, which is 200 cm in length. Most ERCP accessories, except colonic dilators and retrieval balloons, are of insufficient length for these enteroscopes. Some accessories manufacturers have made available 320-cm-long diagnostic catheters and sphincterotomes. A 600-cm guidewire makes it possible to exchange instruments without having to shorten these devices during exchange over standard 450-cm wires. Because it is difficult to perform ERCP in a Roux-en-Y anatomy, every effort must be made to reduce the need for future procedures. Therefore nasobiliary drainage catheters are more likely to be used in this setting than in patients with a normal upper GI anatomy. Biliary metal stenting is difficult to place using a deep enteroscope. After placement of a stiff guidewire across the stricture, the enteroscope is removed while leaving the enteroscope overtube in place. The stenting device can then be advanced over the guidewire for stent release under fluoroscopic guidance.

CONCLUSIONS

Performing ERCP in surgically altered anatomy is a uniquely challenging experience. Preprocedure planning, stocking of appropriate accessories, and knowledge of surgical procedures are as important as good endoscopic skills in achieving technical success. ERCP in Billroth II predisposes to a high risk of perforation and should be done only by those with a record of acceptable safety. Accessing the bile duct through the afferent limb of a Roux-en-Y anatomy, once considered an improbability, is increasingly accomplished by expert endoscopists. However, the bar of technical difficulty has been raised by the recent rise in volume of bariatric operations. Other than an occasional case of favorably short Roux and afferent limbs, bariatric gastric bypass makes ERCP far too challenging a procedure to perform in the community setting in the absence of laparoscopic assistance. Balloon enteroscopy–assisted ERCP has been reported to be highly successful in a few centers, but most endoscopists would prefer to perform ERCP in conjunction with laparoscopy in these patients. EUS-guided biliary access and therapy will likely become an essential component of ERCP interventions in the setting of altered GI anatomy in the future.

The complete reference list for this chapter can be found online at www.expertconsult.com.

32

Endoscopic Ultrasonography–Guided Biliary Drainage

Manuel Perez-Miranda

Endoscopic ultrasonography (EUS) has gradually replaced many percutaneous image-guided interventions, such as tissue sampling of pancreatic tumors. Similarly, EUS-guided biliary therapeutics mirror percutaneous intervention on the biliary tract. Three anatomic structures can be targeted for biliary drainage under EUS guidance: the bile duct, the gallbladder, and the gastrointestinal (GI) tract, giving rise to three distinct procedures, EUS-guided biliary drainage (EUS-BD), EUS-guided gallbladder drainage (EUS-GBD), and EUS-guided enteroanastomosis (EUS-EA). Endosonography-guided cholangiopancreatography (ESCP) involves EUS-guided needle access and contrast injection under fluoroscopy into the target duct, much like endoscopic retrograde cholangiopancreatography (ERCP) with cannulation of the papilla.[1] ESCP was introduced in 1996 and is the parent procedure of the three variant techniques of EUS-BD: rendezvous, antegrade, and transmural interventions. Some authors consider EUS-guided rendezvous (EUS-RV) to be separate from EUS-BD, as drainage is accomplished by ERCP rather than by ESCP. The use of the term "ESCP" to define procedural boundaries between EUS-guided "ductal" access and other forms of EUS-BD has been proposed. This is in keeping with the ERCP paradigm, where one name designates a range of diagnostic and therapeutic interventions.[2] This proposal has not been widely accepted. Nonetheless, in this chapter "EUS-BD" will be used to encompass all three variant EUS-guided bile duct access and drainage techniques described above, namely, rendezvous, antegrade, and transmural drainage. The other two EUS-guided interventions for biliary drainage not primarily involving the bile duct, EUS-GBD and EUS-EA, are discussed in Chapters 33 and 42.

As indicated above, EUS-BD, EUS-GBD, and EUS-EA are alternative endoscopic approaches to percutaneous access, reserved for cases in which the initially preferred/attempted endoscopic therapeutic approach fails or is not feasible. For EUS-BD and EUS-EA the failed preferred therapeutic approach is ERCP, although the specific percutaneous approach that is replaced differs for each procedure. EUS-BD is commonly used after failed ERCP as an alternative to percutaneous transhepatic biliary drainage (PTBD), especially for palliation of malignant biliary obstruction. In expert hands, EUS-BD has been shown to be equally efficacious but with fewer adverse events.[3] EUS-EA has only been preliminarily evaluated for malignant or benign biliary obstruction in patients who have one of three types of surgically altered anatomy: Roux-en-Y gastric bypass[4] (RYGB), Roux-en-Y hepaticojejunostomy, or afferent loop syndrome.[5] Because of patient heterogeneity and limited evidence, there is no single best option for EUS-EA, as different approaches are possible after failed retrograde endoscopic therapy. These range from percutaneous transgastric or transjejunal biliary interventions[6] to revisional surgery,[7] including combined endoscopic-surgical approaches, such as intraoperative transgastric ERCP in RYGB patients.

Cholecystectomy is the standard treatment for symptomatic gallbladder disease, but percutaneous transhepatic gallbladder drainage (PTGBD) is often used in poor surgical patients.[8] EUS-GBD can replace PTGBD as a temporizing measure before cholecystectomy with equal efficacy and fewer adverse events[9] but only when small-caliber plastic drains are used. In short, EUS-GBD can be viewed as an internal PTGBD, much as EUS-BD can be considered an internal form of PTBD from within the GI tract and EUS-EA a transluminal adaptation of previously reported percutaneous transenteric biliary interventions.

Endoscopists performing these complex EUS-BD interventions require proficiency in both ERCP and linear EUS. Until recently, diverging training and practice pathways for ERCP and EUS resulted in EUS-BD putting expert therapeutic endoscopists and master endosonographers outside of their respective comfort zones.[10] A steep learning curve partially explains the slow dissemination of EUS-BD and the lingering skepticism about EUS-guided interventions, a pattern seen with laparoscopic cholecystectomy during the early 1990s, and with ERCP itself during the early 1980s. Critics of EUS-BD often cite lack of evidence, lack of procedural standardization, lack of dedicated devices, lack of trained operators, and lack of "true" indications—assuming that state-of-the-art ERCP, current percutaneous approaches, and surgery adequately address all possible clinical scenarios in which EUS-BD is being considered. The degree to which some of these five criticisms rightly apply varies greatly across EUS-BD proper, EUS-GBD, and EUS-EA (Box 32.1). Even if progress in EUS-BD has been slow, it has been steady, consistent, and exponential. Milestones along two decades of EUS-BD can be summarized in 5-year intervals. In 1996, diagnostic ESCP was introduced.[1] In 2001, EUS-BD (i.e., therapeutic ESCP) was first described as choledochoduodenostomy[11] (CDS). By 2006, hepaticogastrostomy (HGS), rendezvous, and antegrade stenting had all been reported within a couple of dozen EUS-BD cases originating from just five centers in Europe and the United States.[12] In 2011, the cumulative number of reported cases reached more than 200, after the active development of EUS-BD in Asia since 2006. In 2016, with over 2000 cases reported worldwide, including several level I evidence studies, EUS-BD had definitely become an established salvage procedure after failed ERCP.[13] On the other hand, a decade after the original description,[14] with only 200 cases reported and several unanswered questions, EUS-GBD is still an evolving procedure requiring further evaluation.[9,15] Finally, EUS-EA remains truly experimental, with approximately two dozen published cases.

DESCRIPTION OF TECHNIQUE

The three EUS-guided procedures mentioned above are performed in the ERCP room by experienced therapeutic endoscopists assisted by fully trained personnel under fluoroscopy and optimal sedation (often general anesthesia or endoscopist-directed propofol sedation). Standard therapeutic oblique-viewing linear echoendoscopes are typically used. Forward-viewing linear echoendoscopes can also be used, but they lack

BOX 32.1 Indications for Endoscopic Ultrasonography–Guided Biliary Drainage Interventions

- Established indications:
  - EUS-RV for failed cannulation after precut
  - EUS-BD for palliation of MBO not amenable to ERCP
  - tEUS-GBD in severe cholecystitis (small plastic stents only)
- Possible indications:
  - Antegrade EUS-BD for BBO in altered anatomy
  - pEUS-GBD in nonsurgical relapsing cholecystitis
  - pEUS-GBD for palliation of MBO not amenable to EUS-BD
  - EUS-EA for afferent loop syndrome
- Controversial indications:
  - EUS-RV for failed cannulation as alternative to precut
  - EUS-BD in potentially resectable MBO after failed ERCP
  - EUS-BD for palliation of MBO instead of ERCP
  - Transmural EUS-BD for BBO
  - EUS-GBD with LAMS or SEMS in potentially operable patients
  - EUS-EA for biliary access in Roux-en-Y anatomy

BBO, Benign biliary obstruction; *EUS-BD,* endoscopic ultrasonography–guided biliary drainage; *EUS-EA,* EUS-guided enteroanastomosis; *EUS-RV,* EUS-guided rendezvous; *LAMS,* lumen-apposing metal stent; *MBO,* malignant biliary obstruction; *pEUS-GBD,* permanent EUS-GBD; *SEMS,* self-expandable metal stent; *tEUS-GBD,* temporizing EUS-guided gallbladder drainage.

an elevator and the limited available literature does not show distinct advantages over oblique-viewing linear echoendoscopes. Carbon dioxide insufflation prevents air leakage during transmural puncture and should routinely be used over standard air insufflation. EUS-BD, EUS-GBD, and EUS-EA largely involve standard steps and devices common to all EUS-guided drainage interventions, of which pseudocyst drainage is the paradigm procedure. As opposed to the characteristically large, adherent pseudocysts, EUS-BD interventions target smaller, usually mobile anatomic structures. We will first discuss the steps common to EUS-BD, EUS-GBD, and EUS-EA and then focus on specific techniques for performing EUS-BD proper.

Steps and Devices Common to Different EUS-BD Procedures

All EUS-guided drainage procedures replicate the Seldinger technique through an echoendoscope using very similar devices, regardless of the target organ. The original percutaneous Seldinger technique allows safe access into a hollow organ by advancing a blunt dilating catheter over a guidewire introduced into the target organ through a sharp needle. The following sequential five steps common to EUS-BD, EUS-GBD, and EUS-EA are taken.

Target Identification Under EUS

This relatively simple step should not be overlooked. Before the initial puncture, the endoscopist must carefully explore different access sites within the GI tract so as to choose the optimal approach based on shorter distance to the target, absence of interposed vessels, endoscope stability and least degree of angulation of the echoendoscope, and overall ergonomics. Changes in endoscope position throughout the subsequent steps may compromise procedure success, so time used to assess for the best possible access site is time well spent. As will be discussed below, fluoroscopic landmarks during EUS imaging of the target are also critical for EUS-BD (Fig. 32.1).

Needle Access Into the Target Organ

Standard EUS needles of 19G caliber are most often used, because they reliably allow passage of 0.025-inch and 0.035-inch guidewires. The stiffness of different commercially available 19G needles varies. When the endoscope is in the long position (i.e., within the duodenum), the more flexible 19G needles offer an advantage over stiffer ones. Blunt-tipped 19G needles have also been specifically designed for EUS-BD to prevent wire shearing but have not come into general use. For nondilated targets such as the bile duct or a collapsed small bowel, particularly if there is hard, fibrotic tissue interposed or if the target is very mobile, 22G needles may be used. Some 22G needles allow 0.021-inch guidewires, which is the minimum size required for adequate stiffness to pass accessories. Some 22G needles allow only 0.018-inch guidewires, which are usually too floppy for transmural intervention. For targets requiring 22G needle access, another alternative is the graded injection technique.[16] Two punctures are sequentially made, the initial one with a 22G needle, through which saline and/or contrast is injected to distend the target. Next, the 22G needle is rapidly removed and replaced with a 19G needle, which is then thrust into the distended target. Even when needle access is not a limiting step for EUS-BD, difficulties may be encountered occasionally when trying to puncture ducts across fibrotic tissue. Tenting may occur, with the needle pushing the target away instead of entering it. A quick needle thrust beyond the intended target is often required, and then access is gained by slowly pulling the needle back toward the echoendoscope. Reverse tenting may also occur during needle withdrawal, with the opposite wall of the target catching on the needle. Confirmation of needle access is readily obtained by EUS alone for larger targets. For nondistended small bowel or intrahepatic ducts, aspiration of fluid through the needle and visual confirmation that the aspirated fluid is not blood is useful before proceeding to injection of contrast (Fig. 32.2). If the aspirate is bloody, the needle must be removed into the GI lumen and flushed with saline to prevent clogging. Some authors remove the stylet from the needle before the puncture to allow either priming with contrast or preloading with a guidewire in order to decrease procedure time. However, leaving the stylet in place during puncture may optimize needle performance. Furthermore, a preloaded guidewire prevents fluid aspiration and contrast injection through the needle to confirm entry and fluoroscopic mapping.

Historically, "free-hand" EUS-guided access to the bile duct using needle knives or other cautery-tipped devices was used, but this has been abandoned. More recently, lumen-apposing metal stents (LAMS) with a cautery-enabled delivery system have been successfully used for EUS-guided drainage of pancreatic fluid collections (PFCs; see Chapter 56). The free-hand access technique of cautery-tipped LAMS may simplify drainage of PFCs; however, over-the-wire insertion appears to be safer than free-hand insertion of LAMS into the gallbladder or the bile duct. The guidewire protects the contralateral wall from cautery injury during LAMS insertion and helps maintain access in the unlikely (but possible) event of delivery catheter malfunction. These potential difficulties during free-hand access are not an issue when drainage of large, adherent PFC is undertaken but may have serious consequences during biliary or small bowel access. Therefore needles remain the time-honored, standard devices for access under EUS guidance. Low-risk, low-difficulty targets may allow this standard to be changed. But for other types of targets, the challenges for needle access described above may escalate when trying free-hand access with larger-diameter devices, especially when used by less-experienced operators.

Before puncture is attempted, it must be borne in mind that, compared with EUS-guided PFC drainage or cannulation of the papilla during ERCP, the chances for repeat needle access into the bile duct and—to a lesser extent—into the gallbladder are limited. Once an obstructed

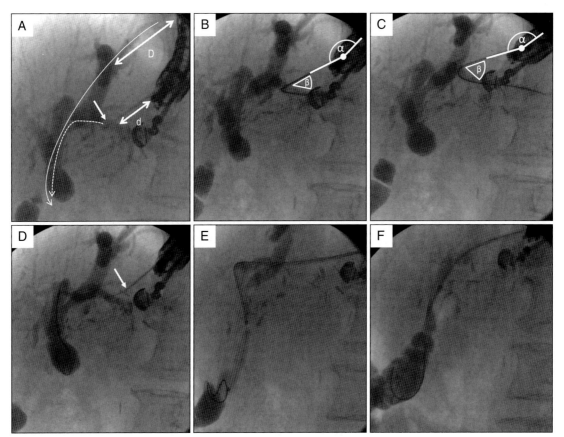

FIG 32.1 Fluoroscopic landmarks and guidewire management during intrahepatic endoscopic ultrasonography–guided biliary drainage (EUS-BD). EUS-guided antegrade biliary balloon dilation in a patient with benign hepaticojejunostomy (HJ) stricture. **A,** Segment II intrahepatic duct (B2) offers a straighter trajectory (*solid line arrow*) for antegrade EUS-BD than segment III (B3, *dotted line arrow*). However, longer distance to dilated B2 branches (*D*) precluded sonographic visualization in this case. Distance to dilated B3 was shorter (*d*), allowing needle (*short arrow*) access. **B,** Despite adequate needle orientation on fluoroscopy toward the hilum, the guidewire initially passed toward the periphery. **C,** Careful elevator and scope reorientation (α) allowed alteration of the angle of needle entry into the duct (β). **D,** The needle was then withdrawn into the liver parenchyma (*arrow*) to prevent shearing of the guidewire during withdrawal before redirecting it toward the hilum and common bile duct (CBD). **E,** A flexible over-the-wire catheter was required for antegrade passage of the guidewire from the CBD across the HJ anastomosis into the jejunum. **F,** Insufficient guidewire coiling into the afferent jejunal limb was overcome by using a flexible catheter, resulting in larger coils to improve support for antegrade interventions.

biliary system is punctured, it rapidly decompresses, making subsequent attempts at puncture more challenging (see Fig. 32.2). Contrast and (unintended) air injection further compromise the success of repeated puncture attempts by blurring the ultrasonographic view. Therefore the intended goal is to obtain a successful puncture at the first attempt, both to minimize trauma and the attendant risk of leakage and to maximize the chances of success. This is the reason why the seemingly mundane step number one above is of critical importance.

Contrast Injection and Guidewire Insertion

Contrast delineation under fluoroscopy of the target structure is critical for bile duct drainage and small-bowel anastomosis procedures and very useful but not mandatory for EUS-GBD. Successful cholangiography or enterography eventually serves to confirm access and provide additional guidance throughout the procedure. Even if the gallbladder can be readily imaged and EUS-GBD performed under EUS alone, fluoroscopy is helpful to monitor guidewire looping inside the gallbladder (Fig. 32.3) and to check for contrast leakage, whether iatrogenic from instrumentation or spontaneous from underlying cholecystitis.

Guidewire insertion into the gallbladder or into the GI tract after needle access is straightforward. Standard 0.025-inch or 0.035-inch guidewires are typically used. A more detailed consideration of the type of guidewire is required for EUS-BD, where guidewire manipulation is more demanding (see Fig. 32.1). For the gallbladder and the GI tract, guidewire looping is aimed for providing stability throughout the next step of tract dilation, and it is usually easily achieved. Stiff guidewires may push away mobile targets such as the gallbladder or the small bowel. To prevent this, EUS monitoring of the target is maintained during guidewire insertion. The specifics of guidewire insertion and manipulation during EUS-BD will be discussed below.

Puncture Tract Dilation

Dilation is routinely required before transmural stent placement into any target but is often not necessary before transpapillary bile duct drainage (see "Transpapillary Drainage" section). Over-the-wire needle exchange for a flexible catheter, the defining step of the Seldinger technique, is also the limiting step of transmural EUS-BD.[17] Similar to pseudocyst drainage, two types of over-the-wire dilating methods can

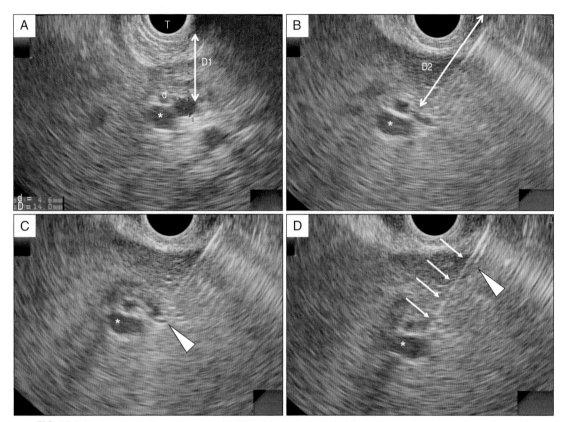

FIG 32.2 Endoscopic ultrasonography (EUS)–guided intrahepatic bile duct needle access. Transducer (*T*) below the cardia readily images the left liver lobe. **A,** Perpendicular distance of 14.0 mm (*D1*) measured between the transducer and a 4.6-mm diameter (*d*) left intrahepatic duct branch next to a vessel (*). **B,** The bile duct collapses when pressed by the relatively thick 19G needle before the actual puncture. Note that ultrasonographic identification of the needle tip is subtle and that the actual distance of the oblique needle path (*D2*) is longer than *D1*. **C,** Despite the seemingly intraductal location of the needle (*arrowhead*), bile aspiration is required to confirm access before contrast injection for cholangiography. If inadvertent parenchymal injection occurs, the ultrasonographic window is instantly lost. **D,** The needle is withdrawn from the duct (*arrowhead*). After fluoroscopic confirmation of intraductal placement, the guidewire must be kept under ultrasonographic view (*arrows*) throughout the steps of dilation and stent insertion. Note the relative difficulty of ultrasonographic identification of the bile duct in **B**, **C**, and **D** compared with **A** (despite larger zoom size in **B**, **C**, and **D**), in contrast to the unchanged appearance of the vessel (*). This is caused by needle pressure (**A**), puncture (**B**), and postpuncture decompression (**C**) and is the reason why more than one attempt at needle access is often not possible during intrahepatic EUS-guided biliary drainage.

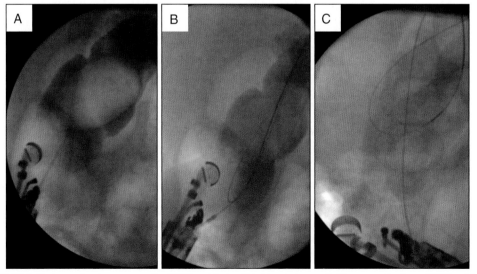

FIG 32.3 Endoscopic ultrasonography (EUS)–guided gallbladder drainage. **A,** Fluoroscopic view of EUS-guided gallbladder puncture after 19G needle access and contrast injection. **B,** Puncture tract dilation with a 6-Fr cystotome passed over a guidewire coiled inside the gallbladder. **C,** Lumen-apposing metal stent (LAMS) deployed across the puncture tract being balloon dilated up to 15-mm nominal diameter.

be used, cautery or noncautery. Cautery methods include needle knife, cystotome, and cautery-enabled LAMS delivery catheters. Noncautery methods include tapered-tip ERCP cannulae, stepped axial dilating ERCP catheters, balloon dilators, and a novel dedicated tapered metal tip stent delivery catheter.[18] Most endoscopists tend to avoid cautery dilation when possible. This is the purpose of the graded dilation technique originally described for EUS-guided drainage of PFCs. It consists of sequential over-the-wire dilation with devices of increasing diameter: cannula, axial dilator, and balloon catheter.[19] The classic graded dilation technique therefore requires four over-the-wire exchanges to achieve transmural stent placement, taking a median procedure time of 75 minutes during the learning curve of PFC drainage and decreasing to 25 minutes after 25 procedures. For successful graded dilation, the ultrasound plane must be maintained to allow axial transmission of the pushing force. The ultrasound plane is confirmed by sonographic monitoring of the guidewire throughout dilation (see Fig. 32.2), which requires that the echoendoscope stays in the same position and with the same orientation as it did when the needle first punctured the target. A simplified graded dilation technique with just three exchanges (cannula, axial dilator, and stent delivery catheter) was used successfully for bile duct drainage in 75% of HGS and 20% of CDS in one study, with a median procedure time of 18 minutes[20] (decreased from 26 minutes during the learning phase). In this study, needle-knife electrocautery was used to salvage failed graded dilation, resulting in 96% overall procedure success. However, needle-knife use was also found to be the single risk factor for postprocedure adverse events.[20] A thin-caliber (6-Fr) cystotome (not available in the United States) has the advantage over a needle knife in providing coaxial cautery. Thin-caliber cystotomes

appear to be safer over-the-wire dilating devices than needle knives for EUS-BD.[21] Anecdotal experience suggests that dilation with cystotomes larger than 6 Fr is associated with serious bile leakage during EUS-BD, although apparently not during EUS-GBD.[22] Prolonged unsuccessful noncautery attempts at dilation may incur a greater risk of leakage and loss of access than coaxial thin-caliber cautery (cystotome) while carefully maintaining the ultrasound plane. Ineffective attempts at noncautery dilation increase the number of exchanges, procedure time, and eventually the chances of technical failure. The dilemma between noncautery and cautery dilation during difficult tract dilation is similar to the choice faced during difficult ERCP cannulation between changing to a precut approach or persisting with standard catheters and wires. Our standard approach is to use the 6-Fr cystotome over the wire with a short burst of cautery while applying firm traction on the wire for both EUS-GBD and extrahepatic EUS-BD.[23] For intrahepatic EUS-BD the chances of successful mechanical dilation and the risk of cautery-induced bleeding are higher, and so we initially try noncautery passage of the 6-Fr cystotome unless the tactile feedback from the preceding needle puncture suggests that the liver parenchyma is firm (Fig. 32.4). If the initial noncautery attempt fails, the same device is used for cautery access. Before metal stent delivery catheter insertion (typically 8 to 10 Fr in diameter), we routinely perform 4-mm biliary balloon dilation, maintaining the dilation for 1 minute, to allow subsequent smooth stent insertion. After balloon deflation, continuous suction is applied until the stent enters the target across the transmural tract. This minimizes potential leakage of bile between the bile duct and the GI lumen, which can occur during the time after balloon dilation/deflation/exchange and stent placement.

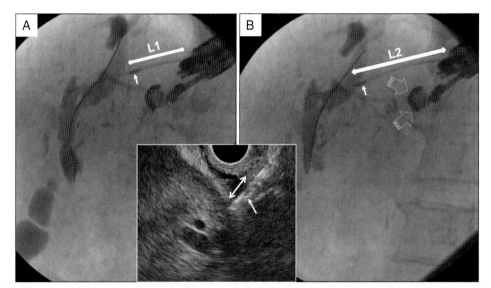

FIG 32.4 Over-the-wire dilation of intrahepatic puncture tract during endoscopic ultrasonography–guided biliary drainage (EUS-BD). Same procedure as in Figs. 32.1 and 32.2. When the 6-Fr cystotome (*small arrow* in **A** and **B**) is advanced over the wire for graded dilation, there is a failure to enter the bile duct accompanied by pushback of the echoendoscope tip (*block arrows* in **B**). This is manifested by the fluoroscopic and ultrasonographic triad of (1) increased length of cystotome catheter between the working channel and the contour of the bile duct on cholangiography (from *L1* to *L2*); (2) changed position of the echoendoscope tip—seen here relative to the stitches in the background; and (3) tenting away of the liver surface (*double arrow* in *inset*), with the cystotome tip (*single arrow* in *inset*) already beyond the gastric wall. These imaging findings correlate with the tactile feedback of resistance, as opposed to the yield that is felt during successful tract dilation. Failure to enter the bile duct with graded dilation in this case was attributable to fibrotic liver parenchyma secondary to long-standing biliary obstruction caused by a benign anastomotic stricture. It was overcome by a short burst of cautery applied to the cystotome. Perhaps a more tapered noncautery device, such as a 4-Fr cannula, might have also succeeded at graded dilation, but at the expense of requiring an additional over-the-wire exchange.

There are two final points concerning guidewire management. First, keeping the echoendoscope in position during dilation not only helps with axial transmission of the pushing force but also prevents looping of the guidewire within or outside the GI tract. If looping of the guidewire occurs at any time during EUS-BD, access is almost invariably lost, and a repeat puncture is required to salvage the procedure. Second, the endoscopist has to coordinate during the final dilating movement into the target with the assistant holding the guidewire and often with a second assistant stabilizing the echoendoscope. The endoscopist signals the exact moment when the final thrust into the target is made so that the first assistant applies traction to the guidewire and the second assistant gently pushes the echoendoscope forward to prevent rebound of the dilating device against the wall.

Cautery and noncautery one-step stent delivery catheters allow over-the-wire dilation and transmural stent insertion with just one exchange and will be discussed later. These novel devices appear to ease transmural stent insertion. However, adherence to the technical principles outlined above is still required, just as guidewires or precuts are not substitutes for lack of proper technique during cannulation at ERCP.

Transmural Stent Placement

Straight or pigtail plastic stents, standard tubular biliary self-expandable metal stents (SEMS), LAMS, and different combinations of the above have been used variably for EUS-BD and EUS-GBD. The stent type chosen is closely related to the target and the indication for the procedure (see "Transmural Drainage" section). There is a trend to avoid transmural plastic stents in favor of covered SEMS or LAMS to minimize the risk of adverse events.[13,20] When temporary transmural stenting is sought, a nasobiliary drain is sometimes used. Examples of this use include temporizing EUS-GBD before elective cholecystectomy[9] and preventing bile leakage after antegrade stone removal in patients with Roux-en-Y gastrectomy.[24] As a more convenient alternative to nasobiliary drains, temporary placement of single-pigtail plastic stents has also been used to prevent leakage after antegrade stone removal in altered anatomy patients.[25]

Specific Considerations for EUS-BD (Therapeutic ESCP)

Compared with other anatomic structures targeted for biliary drainage under EUS, the bile duct has two distinctive features: a variety of potential access sites, and the option of a transpapillary route as an alternative to transmural drainage. Commonly used access sites for EUS-BD are the left intrahepatic duct from the cardia or lesser gastric curvature (see Fig. 32.1) and the common bile duct (CBD) from the duodenum or distal gastric antrum (Fig. 32.5). Access to the right intrahepatic duct from the duodenum or distal gastric antrum is also possible but is technically more challenging and infrequently used.[26] Individual approaches to EUSBD result from the combination of these two possible sites of access to the bile duct (intrahepatic and extrahepatic) with the three possible drainage techniques (transmural, retrograde transpapillary or rendezvous, and antegrade transpapillary) (Fig. 32.6). In practice, however, some of these theoretically possible access/drainage combinations are much more commonly used than others. In a recent review including nearly 800 patients, CDS represented around 40%, extrahepatic RV 25%, HGS 20%, intrahepatic RV 10%, and antegrade (mostly intrahepatic) around 5% of the total published EUS-BD cases.[27] When examining access site and drainage technique, instead of the tandem combination, the breakdown is 65% extrahepatic versus 35% intrahepatic access, and 60% transmural versus 40% transpapillary drainage.

Choice of Approach

Access site is largely dictated by patient anatomic factors (Fig. 32.7), such as level of obstruction (hilar vs distal) and upper GI tract anatomy

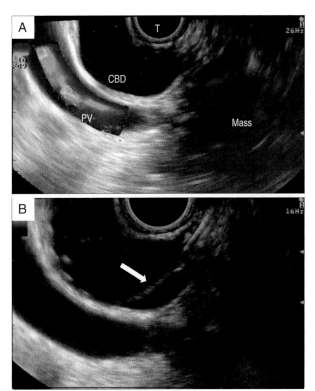

FIG 32.5 Endoscopic ultrasonography (EUS)–guided extrahepatic bile duct needle access. Transducer (*T*) in the duodenal bulb provides a longitudinal ultrasonographic view of a dilated common bile duct (*CBD*) above a pancreatic mass. **A,** Portal vein (*PV*) adjacent to the CBD readily identified by color Doppler. **B,** A 0.035-inch guidewire (*arrow*) through 19G needle, entering into the *CBD*. Keeping the guidewire in ultrasonographic view is required for adequate transmission of axial force during over-the-wire advancement of any flexible devices (e.g., catheters to achieve antegrade guidewire passage during rendezvous, dilator passage before choledochoduodenostomy). Extrahepatic bile duct needle puncture and guidewire insertion are steps common to both choledochoduodenostomy (CDS) and rendezvous (RV). However, CDS requires a long echoendoscope position with the tip oriented upward, whereas RV is best achieved in the short position pointing downward.

(native vs surgically altered). Drainage route is primarily determined by the underlying diagnosis (malignant vs benign) and secondarily by operator preference. Hilar obstruction and surgically altered anatomy require intrahepatic access. In benign disease, transmural drainage is characteristically avoided, whereas transpapillary (rendezvous or antegrade) drainage is preferred.[28] Malignant distal biliary obstruction with native upper GI anatomy represents a patient subset for whom intrahepatic or extrahepatic access can be chosen based on operator preference alone. For successful intrahepatic access a peripheral duct of at least 4 to 5 mm diameter within a maximum distance of 20 mm to the transducer should be targeted (see Fig. 32.2). Smaller intrahepatic ducts may require a compromise in needle size, which in turn has consequences for guidewire selection. In a recent study, intrahepatic ducts of 5 mm or greater in diameter could be accessed with 19G needles in 75% of cases but only in 20% of smaller-sized ducts.[25] In contrast to PTBD, "blind" access is not possible during EUS-BD, and so if dilated ducts are not identified by EUS, intrahepatic access cannot be attempted. The CBD is readily apparent next to the duodenal wall, particularly in the setting of malignant distal biliary obstruction (see Fig. 32.5). Even if the intrahepatic bile duct is a smaller target than the CBD, some authors favor intrahepatic access initially, leaving extrahepatic access

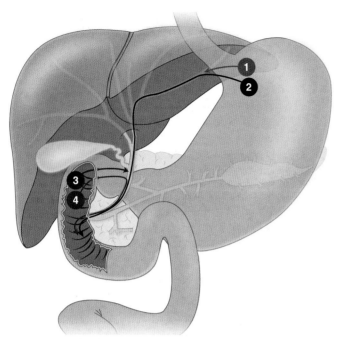

FIG 32.6 Endoscopic ultrasonography–guided biliary drainage (EUS-BD) access sites and drainage routes. The two dominant EUS-BD access sites: left intrahepatic (*1, 2*) and extrahepatic (*3, 4*). After ductal access, drainage can be accomplished transmurally over an intraductally placed guidewire (*1, 3*) via hepaticogastrostomy (*1*) or choledochoduodenostomy (*3*). Alternatively, transpapillary guidewire placement (*2, 4*) allows either retrograde access via rendezvous endoscopic retrograde cholangiopan-creatography (ERCP) or antegrade stent placement (*2, 4*). Rendezvous requires an accessible papilla and is preferentially performed after extrahepatic access for benign disease. Antegrade transpapillary EUS-BD is well suited to complex postoperative anatomy, which dictates intrahepatic access, and is performed for either benign stricture dilation or malignant stricture stenting. Two access sites combined with three drainage techniques give rise to the six variant EUS-BD approaches. Of these six, choledochoduodenostomy and extrahepatic rendezvous are the two most common, representing two-thirds of the total number of cases reported. (Adapted from Perez-Miranda M, de la Serna C, Diez-Redondo P, et al. Endosonography-guided cholangio-pancreatography as a salvage drainage procedure for obstructed biliary and pancreatic ducts. *World J Gastrointest Endosc.* 2010;2:212–222; with permission from Baishideng.)

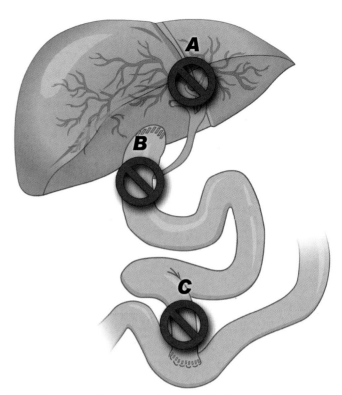

FIG 32.7 Anatomic factors associated with failed endoscopic retrograde cholangiopancreatography (ERCP) determining an endoscopic ultraso-nography–guided biliary drainage (EUS-BD) approach. Extrahepatic access is suitable for distal biliary obstruction in patients with native antroduodenal anatomy despite the presence of ascites or nondilated intrahepatic ducts (*B*). Any prior surgery involving distal gastrectomy with gastrojejunostomy (*C*) precludes EUS imaging of the common bile duct (CBD), dictating the need for intrahepatic access. Similarly, a hilar stricture causing intrahepatic duct dilation (*A*) requires intrahepatic access. Only a minority of patients with biliary obstruction and failed ERCP lack all three anatomic factors that determine access site. In this small patient subset of EUS-BD candidates, access site is left to the operator's preference. (Reprinted from Perez-Miranda M, de la Serna C, Diez-Redondo P, et al. Endo-sonography-guided cholangio-pancreatography as a salvage drainage procedure for obstructed biliary and pancreatic ducts. *World J Gastrointest Endosc.* 2010;2:212–222; with permission from Baishideng.)

for cases without intrahepatic dilation.[29,30] Overall, there appear to be no differences in outcomes between intrahepatic and extrahepatic access.[13] Transpapillary drainage is *a priori* less invasive but also more technically demanding than transmural drainage. Most proposed EUS-BD algorithms recommend transpapillary drainage initially and leave transmural approaches for salvage of failed transpapillary drainage or predefined unfavorable cases for transpapillary drainage[27,28,30] (e.g., malignant stricture of the second duodenum). Despite these recommendations, it is unclear whether transpapillary drainage has any advantage over transmural drainage in patients with unresectable malignant biliary obstruction. Furthermore, different approaches are not mutually exclusive and are increasingly being used complementarily. Examples of combined EUS-BD approaches include failed rendezvous or antegrade EUS-BD salvaged by EUS-CDS or EUS-HGS (a commonly used cross-over strategy[28,29]), antegrade and transmural stenting in the same patient (either simultaneously[31] [Fig. 32.8] or sequentially[32,33]), and simultaneous bilateral transmural stenting.

Transpapillary Drainage

The limiting step for antegrade and rendezvous techniques is transpapil-lary guidewire passage.[17] Specific steps are required for each individual technique after this common step of antegrade transpapillary guidewire passage: antegrade EUS-BD requires tract dilation, similar to transmural EUS-BD, whereas RV requires retrograde biliary access. Once the needle is inside the bile duct, there is very limited opportunity for guidewire manipulation, because pulling the guidewire back may result in wire shearing. To increase the chances of successful antegrade guidewire passage, the optimal access site and needle orientation should be sought with the help of fluoroscopy before puncture (see Fig. 32.1). Overall the success rate of rendezvous is 81%, but it is only 65% for intrahepatic RV versus 87% for extrahepatic RV.[27] Therefore, if RV is intended and extrahepatic access is available, it should preferably be chosen over intrahepatic access. Furthermore, after extrahepatic access, the chances for successful guidewire passage are higher if the puncture is made from the second duodenal portion, closer to the papilla, with the echoendoscope in the short position and pointing downward, as opposed to from the bulb in the long position. However, this optimal short

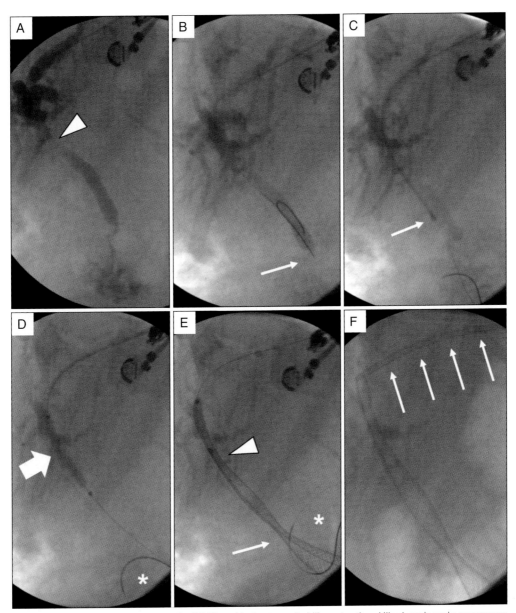

FIG 32.8 Endoscopic ultrasonography (EUS)–guided antegrade biliary stenting. Hilar lymph node recurrence in a patient with Roux-en-Y subtotal gastrectomy for gastric cancer. **A,** Dilated segment II intrahepatic duct (B2) needle access allows antegrade guidewire passage directly through the needle across the hilar stricture (*arrowhead*). **B,** However, the guidewire coils at the papilla (*arrow*); **C,** requiring manipulation with a 6-Fr cystotome (*arrow*) for antegrade passage into the jejunum. **D,** In addition to cystotome dilation of the puncture tract, 4-mm balloon dilation (*block arrow*) facilitates insertion of the stent delivery catheter across the hilar stricture, located at a straight angle from the intrahepatic access site. Jejunal guidewire coils indicated by asterisk (*). **E,** After stent deployment, subtle upper waist (*arrowhead*) denotes hilar stricture location, whereas lower waist (*arrow*) denotes location of the papilla. **F,** Additional hepaticogastrostomy with a 7-Fr straight plastic stent (*arrows*) both to minimize risk of postprocedure leakage and to facilitate future revision should antegrade stent dysfunction occur.

echoendoscope position for extrahepatic RV is only possible in 50% of cases[34] (Fig. 32.9) and may be less stable. Patients with altered anatomy require intrahepatic access to obtain transpapillary drainage, typically with the antegrade technique. Intrahepatic RV has also been occasionally reported with enteroscopes as crossover salvage of failed antegrade EUS-BD. Failed antegrade EUS-BD may result from failure to dilate the puncture track before stent insertion or from failed antegrade stone removal.[27,29] After intrahepatic access, the chances of successful antegrade transpapillary guidewire passage appear higher if segment II of the liver

is accessed instead of segment III, as segment II offers a straighter trajectory toward the papilla[28] (see Fig. 32.1). In addition to careful needle orientation and selection of the exact entry point, a range of hydrophilic angled or straight-tipped guidewires should be available. An assistant experienced in guidewire torque and manipulation is critical for successful guidewire passage. Regardless of access site, needle orientation, guidewire performance, and assistant expertise, there is an occasional need to advance steering cannulas or catheters by the Seldinger technique into the bile duct to effectively direct the guidewire across the papilla[28,35]

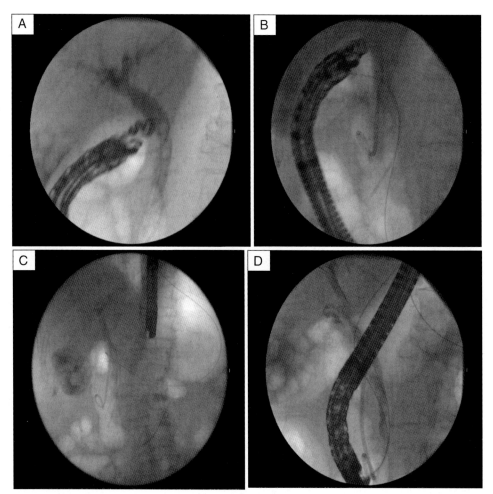

FIG 32.9 Potential difficulties during endoscopic ultrasonography–guided rendezvous (EUS-RV). Nondilated common bile duct (CBD) with distal stones after failed endoscopic retrograde cholangiopancreatography (ERCP) in a patient with a juxtadiverticular papilla, despite precut over a pancreatic stent. **A,** Guidewire courses up toward the right intrahepatic duct. A more caudad initial puncture and/or short scope position may have resulted in a downward course but could not be obtained in this case. **B,** To avoid a second puncture into a nondilated, contrast-filled CBD or prolonged manipulation of the guidewire to redirect it antegrade, the proximally coursing guidewire was used to place a 7-Fr plastic pigtail for salvage temporizing choledochoduodenostomy (CDS). Wireless RV with methylene-blue cholangiography might have been chosen as a less-invasive salvage strategy but was not considered in this case. After drainage was ensured, parallel cannulation alongside the pigtail with a sphincterotome allowed antegrade guidewire passage across the papilla. **C,** Duodenoscope being advanced into the stomach after echoendoscope removal. Here, insufficient guidewire coiling in the duodenum and intragastric looping severely risked guidewire dislodgment from the bile duct. **D,** Eventually successful cannulation was achieved with parallel RV. Thus three procedures were sequentially performed in one session: failed ERCP with precut and prophylactic pancreatic stenting, EUS-guided biliary drainage (EUS-BD) with temporary CDS and parallel antegrade guidewire passage, and successful rendezvous ERCP with sphincterotomy and stone removal. The pancreatic stent and temporary CDS pigtail stent were removed electively at follow-up endoscopy 1 month later.

(see Fig. 32.8). These flexible catheters are often useful to help form several loops of guidewire in the small bowel distal to the papilla (see Figs. 32.1 and 32.8), a very convenient step to enhance stability before antegrade interventions and to minimize the risk of guidewire dislodgment during endoscope exchange during RV (see next paragraph).

Retrograde biliary access after transpapillary guidewire placement during RV is most commonly achieved by over-the-wire removal of the echoendoscope and insertion of a duodenoscope or enteroscope (in altered anatomy cases) alongside the guidewire. The process of endoscope exchange requires fluoroscopic monitoring of the guidewire and delicate coordination between the endoscopist and the assistant.

During echoendoscope removal, the guidewire is carefully advanced by the endoscopist while the assistant is ready to hold the guidewire at the patient's mouth, whereas during duodenoscope advancement, traction is applied on the guidewire by the assistant. Careful precautions are aimed at preventing looping inside the stomach, which can easily result in guidewire dislodgment from the bile duct (see Fig. 32.9). The final step of the so-called "classic" RV involves guidewire retrieval, typically by grasping and withdrawing it through the duodenoscope working channel using a polypectomy snare or a forceps device. While the guidewire is being withdrawn into the endoscope, the assistant must advance the guidewire from its proximal end in coordination with the endoscopist. Friction is progressively met during the process of guidewire retrieval into the endoscope working channel. This increasing friction may result in the guidewire slipping from the grasp of the snare or forceps, usually when it is nearing the end of the working channel. If the guidewire slips out of grasp, the duodenoscope has to be removed, leaving the wire exiting the mouth. The guidewire is then further withdrawn and the endoscope back-loaded over it down to the papilla. Duodenoscope back-loading requires attention to avoid forming a knot in the stomach by crisscrossing the proximal (i.e., antegrade entry to the bile duct) and distal (i.e., end pulled into the endoscope channel) ends of the guidewire. As an alternative to classic RV there is parallel RV, by which cannulation alongside the guidewire exiting through the papilla is attempted with a sphincterotome loaded with a second guidewire (see Fig. 32.9). Parallel RV is convenient, as it avoids the cumbersome step of guidewire retrieval described above. If parallel RV is unsuccessful, classic RV can be tried. The ultimate simplification of RV is "wireless" RV, by which contrast injected into the duct after EUS-guided needle access facilitates subsequent ERCP. Wireless RV can be used either primarily or as salvage of failed antegrade guidewire passage across the papilla during classic RV. Contrast is typically mixed with methylene blue, and a sufficient volume (5 to 15 mL, depending on duct size) is injected to distend the duct. If contrast is seen flowing across the papilla during EUS-guided cholangiography, ERCP with standard cannulation is successful in 90% of cases, despite prior failed retrograde cannulation or RV guidewire passage across the papilla.[36]

Transmural Drainage

As mentioned above, transmural drainage is the most commonly used form of EUS-BD in practice,[27] even if transpapillary approaches are favored in theory.[27,28,30] Despite having a higher success rate than transpapillary EUS-BD, transmural EUS-BD is more invasive. In addition to the techniques discussed earlier for needle access and puncture tract dilation, stent factors are also relevant to the safety and efficacy of transmural EUS-BD. Acute postprocedure leakage and late stent dysfunction are the two main concerns. Both CDS and HGS are associated with a higher incidence of adverse events when plastic stents are used compared with covered SEMS.[13] Covered SEMS allow more effective sealing of the transmural tract and provide longer patency than plastic stents. On the other hand, transmural placement of SEMS can be relatively challenging, largely because of difficulties during stent deployment. Transmural biliary SEMS may result in more severe leakage than plastic stents in the event that foreshortening beyond the GI tract wall into the peritoneal cavity occurs. Technical points relevant to access site for CDS and HGS have already been discussed above. We will now focus on stent issues specific to CDS and HGS.

EUS-guided choledochoduodenostomy. EUS-guided CDS involves stent placement across the duodenal wall into the extrahepatic bile duct with the echoendoscope in the long position, usually with the tip directed up toward the hepatic hilum (see Fig. 32.4). Guidewire insertion into the intrahepatic bile duct is helpful to provide stability for dilation and stent insertion. During early experiences with EUS-BD, straight plastic stents of 7-Fr to 10-Fr diameter were used for CDS, but the use of plastic stents has now largely been replaced by covered (usually partially) biliary SEMS. When covered SEMS are used for CDS, the biliary end of the stent must not cross the confluence of the right and left hepatic ducts, which would result in contralateral branch blockage and cholangitis. Even if the CBD is seen under EUS closely adjacent to the duodenal wall before puncture, some separation invariably occurs during transmural EUS-BD. For this reason, SEMS of 60-mm length are typically required to safely bridge that ensuing gap. More recently, a dedicated biliary LAMS of only 8-mm length has been introduced for CDS, with or without a cautery-tipped delivery system (Axios; Boston Scientific,

Marlborough, MA). In a multicenter evaluation of this novel LAMS for CDS, a high technical success rate of 95% with a mean procedure time of 22 minutes was found. However, major adverse events occurred in 7% and late stent dysfunction caused by sump syndrome or stent migration occurred in an additional 10% of patients.[37] The delivery catheter of this dedicated LAMS has unique features compared with delivery catheters of standard SEMS that allow operator-controlled independent release of the distal (bile duct) and proximal (GI tract) flanges. Although these features are intended to simplify stent placement, they have some disadvantages: increased stiffness and limited depth of insertion of the delivery catheter, retrograde foreshortening of the LAMS during distal flange deployment, and much higher cost of the device. It remains to be seen if the purported benefits of this promising new biliary LAMS outweigh its disadvantages to allow justification of its use over standard SEMS for CDS. However, its unique design allows CDS with a metal stent in situations where standard covered SEMS cannot be used, such as when the guidewire initially courses distally toward the papilla[38] or when the extrahepatic access site is close to the hepatic confluence (Fig. 32.10).

EUS-guided hepaticogastrostomy. EUS-guided HGS involves stent placement across the gastric wall, usually with the echoendoscope in the proximal stomach with the tip pointing rightward toward the hepatic hilum (see Fig. 32.1). Plastic stents were used for HGS during the early years but have gradually been abandoned in favor of SEMS. Migration before a mature fistula forms between the bile duct and the stomach is the overwhelming concern with SEMS for HGS.[39] This early migration is often caused by SEMS foreshortening. To prevent SEMS foreshortening into the peritoneal cavity after HGS, different strategies have been used. Initial placement of an uncovered SEMS deeply into the intrahepatic duct followed by placement of a second, overlapping covered SEMS more proximally into the stomach is one option.[32] Another strategy is antegrade stenting combined with HGS.[31] Both strategies require sequential placement of two separate SEMS. An alternative to these relatively inefficient strategies includes one single hybrid SEMS with distal (biliary) uncovered and proximal (gastric) covered ends. One such hybrid HGS-specific SEMS mounted on a 7-Fr introducer with a tapered dilating tip allows one-step insertion without any cautery. This novel SEMS has been tested in a randomized trial against standard 8-Fr fully covered SEMS with antimigration flaps. Despite impressive success rates close to 100% in both study arms, the one-step delivery hybrid SEMS outperformed the conventional fully covered SEMS in procedure time (10 vs 15 minutes) and early adverse event rate[18] (6% vs 30%). Until such dedicated SEMS become widely available, alternative means against foreshortening can be used, such as forced expansion of standard covered SEMS immediately upon deployment by means of balloon dilation, and coaxial double-pigtail insertion (Fig. 32.11). One non-foreshortening fully covered SEMS is available in the United States (Viabil; W.L. Gore, Flagstaff, AZ), which has been successfully used for HGS. Endoclip attachment of the SEMS to the gastric wall is another low-cost, low-tech option sometimes used empirically against migration after HGS. Finally, a dedicated tapered 8-Fr single-pigtail plastic stent for HGS has also been developed and tested with promising results in a pilot study.[25]

INDICATIONS AND CONTRAINDICATIONS

Contraindications to EUS-BD interventions are similar to those of ERCP, that is, any situation preventing therapeutic upper GI endoscopy, such as active perforation, hemodynamic instability, or uncorrectable coagulopathy. Certain anatomic factors, such as lack of intrahepatic dilatation, massive ascites, and collapsed gallbladder, may represent relative contraindications. In other words, anatomic factors precluding

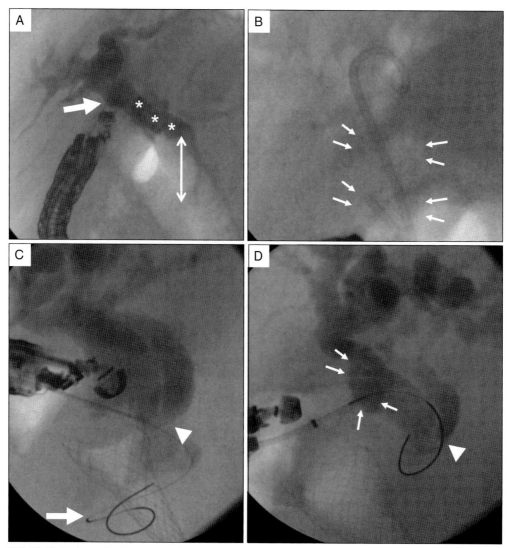

FIG 32.10 Endoscopic ultrasonography–guided choledochoduodenostomy (EUS-CDS) with lumen-apposing metal stent (LAMS). **A** and **B,** Lymph node metastasis from lung cancer resulted in a long, narrow distal biliary stricture (*double arrow*) and secondarily distended cystic duct above (*asterisks*), so that the common hepatic duct near the confluence (*short arrow*) was the best EUS-guided biliary access site. Note minimal intrahepatic dilation. Barely visible biliary LAMS (flanges denoted by *thin arrows*) deployed across puncture tract with coaxial plastic double-pigtail stent. **C** and **D,** Pancreatic cancer with distal biliary stricture involving cystic take-off (*arrowhead*) and duodenal stricture with metal duodenal stent across the papilla. Extrahepatic bile duct punctured at upper margin of biliary stricture with guidewire coursing distally across the papilla into false tracks (*short arrow*), precluding transpapillary drainage. Deployed biliary LAMS (distal flange denoted by *thin arrows*) allows choledochoduodenostomy (CDS) despite downward guidewire course. During CDS, LAMS distinctly prevents stent-induced cystic duct blockage, in contrast to what happens with SEMS.

target identification can preclude the feasibility of EUS-BD and EUS-GBD. Finally, as with all invasive procedures requiring proficient operators, lack of proper indication and of adequate individual or institutional expertise may also be viewed as contraindications.

There are three levels of indications for EUS-BD interventions: established, possible, and controversial. Established indications have been tested in large numbers of patients from different centers, with comparable results among them, and through results of randomized trials. Established indications include RV for failed ERCP cannulation using standard and advanced methods such as precut,[34,40] any form of EUS-BD for the palliation of unresectable malignant biliary obstruction, either when ERCP fails or in cases that are highly demanding and unlikely to succeed, such as in Roux-en-Y anatomy.[27,28] Lastly, temporary

gallbladder drainage using nasobiliary drains is not yet widely used but has been proven to be as effective as PTGBD at relieving acute cholecystitis preoperatively.[9]

Regarding possible indications, antegrade EUS-BD seems reasonable in patients with stones or benign anastomotic strictures and altered anatomy but is more challenging than rendezvous or standard transmural EUS-BD, and its relative merits compared with enteroscopy-assisted EUS-BD are not yet well studied.[24,28] Similarly, there is mounting evidence regarding the safety and efficacy of permanent EUS-GBD using either SEMS or LAMS in nonoperable candidates,[22,23] but its role relative to other endoscopic (e.g., transcystic gallbladder stenting) or percutaneous (e.g., PTGBD) approaches remains to be elucidated. The very long-term outcomes of EUS-GBD with metal stents and the reproducibility of

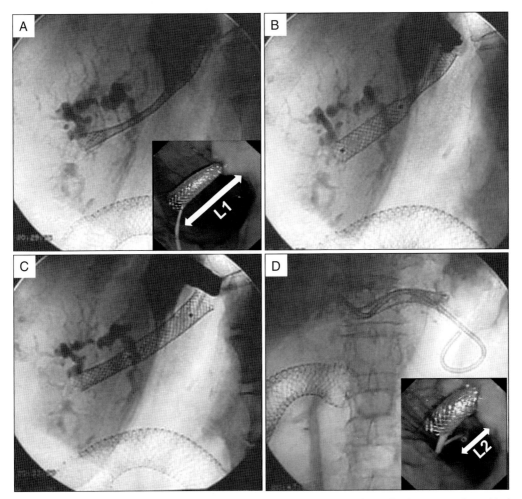

FIG 32.11 Self-expandable metal stents (SEMS) anchoring strategies at endoscopic ultrasonography–guided hepaticogastrostomy (EUS-HGS). **A,** Partially covered biliary SEMS immediately upon deployment with long intragastric segment 20-mm deep inside the stomach (*L1* on *inset*). **B,** Fluoroscopic monitoring of balloon expansion of the distal (intrahepatic) end of the SEMS. **C,** The waist from the transmural segment disappears after a second balloon dilation toward the proximal end of the SEMS. **D,** A double-pigtail stent placed across the SEMS provides further anchoring to prevent migration and potentially mitigates the risk of dysfunction caused by ingrowth and/or angulation at the distal (biliary) end. Note that the intragastric segment is significantly shorter (*L2* on *inset*) after complete SEMS expansion. Balloon dilation to achieve forced SEMS expansion results in SEMS foreshortening in a controlled, predictable manner.

the procedure in different practice settings need further evaluation. Particularly challenging clinical problems for which there are no satisfactory alternatives have also been addressed in a few cases by EUS-guided drainage, such as malignant biliary obstruction after failed ERCP and failed EUS-BD successfully salvaged by EUS-GBD.[41] Equally challenging to manage is biliary obstruction secondary to afferent loop syndrome. The handful of cases reported all show very promising results.[5]

EUS-BD interventions have also been used for controversial indications. The first group includes using EUS-BD as an alternative rather than after failed ERCP, for instance, for palliation of malignant biliary obstruction or for difficult biliary access as an alternative to precut sphincterotomy.[40] Transmural drainage other than for cholecystitis using nasobiliary drains in any patient who may later undergo cholecystectomy has also been reported but is controversial. Also technically feasible but debatable is the use of transmural EUS-BD for benign disease, such as stones or strictures, and transmural stents across the GI tract wall to facilitate conventional ERCP. These procedures have evolved from approaches where EUS puncture of the excluded distal antrum was

done to facilitate percutaneous access for ERCP as an alternative to laparoscopic-assisted transgastric ERCP in RYGB patients.[42] A recent pilot study showed the feasibility of a temporary gastrogastric anastomosis using LAMS,[43] at the expense of stent migration in 69%. Anecdotal reports also point toward using this strategy with patients with benign[44] or malignant Roux-en-Y hepaticojejunostomy strictures.[45] Breaching the integrity of the GI tract in this context deserves proper evaluation before it can be recommended.

PROCEDURAL OUTCOMES AND ADVERSE EVENTS

Procedural outcomes of EUS-BD and EUS-GBD are summarized in Tables 32.1 and 32.2. Morbidity from EUS-BD is an important consideration. Adverse events arise from two sources: breach of the integrity of the duct and GI walls inherent to all approaches, and trauma to the papilla. Breach of transluminal integrity is minimal in cases where only ductal needle puncture is performed (e.g., during rendezvous) and maximal where transmural drainage is performed (e.g., CDS, HGS). It

TABLE 32.1 **Outcomes of Endoscopic Ultrasonography–Guided Biliary Drainage**

	N	Technical Success (%)	AEs (%)	Failures and AEs (%)
Overall	764	87	16	29
Rendezvous	267	81	11	30
Antegrade	39	77	5	28
CDS	300	94	19	25
HGS	158	87	27	39

AE, Adverse events; *CDS,* choledochoduodenostomy; *HGS,* hepaticogastrostomy.
Adapted from Iwashita T, Doi S, Yasuda I. Endoscopic ultrasound-guided biliary drainage: a review. *Clin J Gastroenterol.* 2014;7:94–102.

TABLE 32.2 **Outcomes of Endoscopic Ultrasonography–Guided Gallbladder Drainage**

	N	Technical Success (%)	Clinical Success (%)	Adverse Events (%)
Overall	196	96	93	12
Plastic*	52	100	100	18
SEMS	73	99	94	12
LAMS	71	92	90	10

LAMS, Lumen-apposing metal stent; *SEMS,* self-expandable metal stent.
*Plastic includes pigtail stents and nasobiliary drainage catheters.
Adapted from Anderloni A, Buda A, Vieceli F, et al. Endoscopic ultrasound-guided transmural stenting for gallbladder drainage in high-risk patients with acute cholecystitis: a systematic review and pooled analysis. *Surg Endosc.* 2016;30:5200–5208.

may lead to intraperitoneal or retroperitoneal bile leakage ranging in severity from mild, self-limiting abdominal pain accompanied by elevation in white blood cell count (a clinical scenario often labeled as "pneumoperitoneum") to biloma (sometimes requiring drainage) or bile peritonitis (with free fluid on cross-sectional imaging). Postprocedure pancreatitis may be a consequence of prior failed ERCP or antegrade transpapillary instrumentation (e.g., balloon dilation or metal stent insertion) during transpapillary EUS-BD. Similarly, bleeding may arise from prior precut or from endoscopic sphincterotomy (in cases where the rendezvous approach is used), but severe bleeding most commonly arises from transmural instrumentation (e.g., repeat transhepatic punctures during difficult intrahepatic access) or, more typically, from cautery tract dilation. As stated earlier, use of a needle knife has been identified as the single most significant predictor of complications during EUS-BD.[20]

There are several confounding factors to establish the true incidence of EUS-BD adverse events, which is estimated at 23% overall in a systematic review.[13] More than half of all adverse events are accounted for by bleeding, bile leakage, pneumoperitoneum, and stent migration. Therefore, even if severe adverse events such as biloma, peritonitis, and perforation are possible, they are also uncommon. Most adverse events can be managed conservatively, and although death is rare, it is a possible outcome.

There are two important risk factors for adverse events: level of experience and technique. In a multicenter study pooling data from the first procedures of 20 endoscopists, technical success was lower than 70%. Failures were accounted for by the ERCP-related steps of EUS-BD, namely, guidewire manipulation, tract dilation, and stent insertion. Adverse events were within range. However, there were five deaths resulting from peritonitis, perforation, and bleeding.[17] Another author reported outcomes of an initial 80 cases over a 10-year period. Overall success was 84% and complications 31%. However, highly significant differences in success and adverse events rates were found between the first and last 40 cases.[46] These findings indicate that the learning curve for EUS-BD is long and steep, with a sharp impact on procedural outcomes.

The complete reference list for this chapter can be found online at www.expertconsult.com.

33

Endoscopic Ultrasound and EUS-Guided Endotherapy

S. Ian Gan

OVERVIEW

Endoscopic ultrasonography (EUS) was first introduced in the 1980s and has since become a cornerstone of endoscopic diagnosis of pancreaticobiliary disease, tissue acquisition via fine-needle aspiration (FNA), and staging of gastrointestinal malignancy. As experience with directed needle access into adjacent organ systems increased, endoscopists were able to expand the utility of EUS to therapeutic interventions. This evolution includes EUS-guided drainage of pancreatic fluid collections, abscesses, cholangiography, biliary drainage, pancreatic duct access, gallbladder drainage, directed cancer therapies, celiac nerve block and neurolysis, cyst ablation, and, most recently, enteroenteral anastomosis. In this chapter, the role of EUS-directed intervention in pancreaticobiliary disease will be reviewed in detail, and the indications, the mechanics, the outcomes, and the adverse events will be examined.

ENDOSCOPIC ULTRASONOGRAPHY

EUS combines luminally based endoscopic video capabilities with an ultrasound probe. Echoendoscope designs include catheter-based miniprobes and radial array echoendoscopes that provide a 360-degree sonographic view. For therapeutic purposes, curvilinear (or "linear") scopes with a 100-degree to 120-degree view allow for sonographically directed advancement of needles, stents, and devices. Both forward and oblique endoscopic viewing linear scopes exist, and device channels range from 2.8 to 4.2 mm in diameter. All current models of EUS scopes have Doppler capability for vascular imaging.

EUS imaging provides detailed and rich diagnostic information in pancreaticobiliary disease. Imaging quality is dependent on the echo-endoscope itself, the ultrasound processor, and ultimately the end-user's ability. The entire pancreas, including the pancreatic parenchyma, pancreatic duct, and uncinate processs, can be seen. The bile duct is easily visible and accessible, as is the left lobe of the liver, the gallbladder, and lymph nodes in the porta hepatis, the celiac region, and the gastrohepatic ligament. As such, in the hands of experienced endosonographers, EUS is highly sensitive and useful in the diagnosis of chronic pancreatitis, pancreatic malignancy, choledocholithiasis, cholangiocarcinoma, and pancreatic cysts.

EUS-guided endotherapy is widening in its reach in the pancreaticobiliary system and now includes a number of indications:

1. Celiac nerve block and celiac neurolysis
2. Drainage of pancreatic fluid collections (pseudocysts and walled-off necrosis [WON]) (Chapter 56)
3. Pancreatic duct access and drainage
4. Biliary drainage (see Chapter 32)
5. Gallbladder drainage
6. EUS-guided ablation and cancer therapy

CELIAC NERVE BLOCK AND NEUROLYSIS

Both pancreatic cancer and chronic pancreatitis can cause debilitating pain. Narcotic medications are frequently necessary for pain control, but as pain becomes increasingly intractable and as dosage increases, medication side effects such as nausea, constipation, and drowsiness may result. Celiac plexus neurolysis (CPN) with ethanol injection for pancreatic cancer patients and celiac plexus block (CPB) with steroids for chronic pancreatitis patients can both be useful adjuncts in the palliation of chronic pain. The celiac plexus surrounds the celiac artery trunk, and several ganglia lie interconnected in the region, transmitting pain signals from the pancreas to the splanchnic nerves and then to the central nervous system. In the case of pancreatic cancer, it is believed that the pain is caused by perineural invasion of the pancreatic nerves.[1] Neurolysis with ethanol, or less commonly with phenol, aims to destroy the ganglia and neural pathways, resulting in neuronal degeneration and fibrosis, but histopathologic evidence suggests only axonal and fascicular damage by chemical injection, allowing for the persistence of neuronal tissue and only short-term benefit. Direct ganglionic injection may increase neuronal damage and thus provides a more effective and durable response. In the case of chronic pancreatitis, CPB with triamcinolone and bupivacaine theoretically treats the perineural inflammation associated with chronic pancreatitis, although bupivacaine alone has been shown to be equivalent to a mixture of the two.

CPN and CPB can be performed percutaneously under radiologic guidance, surgically, or under EUS guidance. Percutaneous posterior approaches are effective, but rarely (<1%) spinal cord trauma or ischemia can occur and result in neurologic complications such as lower limb weakness, paresthesias, and paraplegia. Thus anterior approaches using EUS-guided CPN are more attractive. Regional anatomy and landmarks are generally easily visualized with linear echoendoscopes, and fine-needle injection can be performed precisely and safely.

All patients with pancreatic cancer or chronic pancreatitis and chronic abdominal pain are potential candidates for CPB/CPN. It is generally suggested that the technique be reserved for patients with pain severe enough to require narcotics, and particularly if there is evidence of adverse effects from chronic opioid use.

Technique

The celiac plexus is located around the trunk of the celiac artery. Ganglia are variably visible sonographically, and detection rates vary greatly, from 73% to 89%.[2,3] (Fig. 33.1). If a central approach is taken, the needle is advanced just superior and anterior to the celiac artery take-off. If a bilateral approach is taken, the scope is rotated clockwise and counterclockwise to either side of the celiac axis until the artery is no longer visible, and the needle is advanced into the space adjacent to the trunk. Different needles can be used, generally 22-gauge or 19-gauge FNA needles, or specially designed fenestrated 20-gauge needles (Cook

Medical, Winston-Salem, NC). If ganglia are targeted, sonographers should look for hypoechoic oblong structures measuring between 0.5 and 4.5 cm with central hyperechoic foci or bands.[4] Mixtures vary, but 5 to 10 mL of 2.5% bupivacaine mixed with 15 to 20 mL of absolute ethanol is injected centrally or divided and injected bilaterally or into visualized ganglia. In CPB, ethanol is included as part of the injectant, but most sonographers use a mixture of 5 mL of diluted triamcinolone (40 to 80 mg) and 10 to 20 mL of bupivacaine, injected centrally in the celiac region above the trunk.

Efficacy

Overall efficacy of CPN for pain reduction in inoperable pancreatic cancer is estimated at 80% in meta-analysis.[5] In a meta-analysis, EUS-CPN has been shown to reduce pain compared with opioids at 4 and 8 weeks and to reduce opioid consumption.[6,7] Central injection has been shown to be as effective as bilateral injection. If ganglia are identified, direct ganglia injection has been shown to be more effective than standard CPN,[8] with an almost 30% absolute improvement in partial and complete response rates.

Alcohol-based CPN for chronic pancreatitis has been shown to provide relief in 59.4% of patients.[9] CPB for chronic pancreatitis has been shown in meta-analysis to provide significant relief of pain in 51.4% of patients and is more effective compared with percutaneous CPB.[10] No difference has been found in randomized controlled trials of central versus bilateral injection[11] or in a randomized controlled trial of bupivacaine alone versus bupivacaine and triamcinolone. Duration of response is estimated at 10 weeks (range 1 to 54 weeks) after the initial procedure, and repeated CPB appears safe and effective if there is response to the initial CPB.[12]

Adverse Events

The most common adverse events from CPB/CPN are transient hypotension (1%), diarrhea (4% to 15%), and transient increase in pain (9%). Infections are also reported, including retroperitoneal abscess, and some sonographers recommend administration of prophylactic antibiotics. Despite improved safety compared with percutaneous approaches, anterior spinal cord infarction with paralysis has been reported.[13] There are also rare reports of lethal complications such as necrosis and perforation of the stomach and aorta.[14]

DRAINAGE OF PANCREATIC FLUID COLLECTIONS

EUS-guided drainage of pancreatic fluid collections (EGDPFC) is now a well-established procedure. The nomenclature for pancreatic fluid collections has evolved and it is important to recognize the differences between subtypes, as successful drainage and avoidance of adverse events (AEs) is partly dependent on recognition of subtypes and how to best manage them (see Chapter 56).[15] Acute fluid collections form shortly after the onset of pancreatitis, within the first 4 weeks. They are homogeneous and without debris or encapsulation. Most will not become infected and will resorb without intervention. Pseudocysts are often the result of a maturing acute fluid collection. They do not have necrotic material and are normally round, with a thick wall, and usually do not become infected (Fig. 33.2, *A*). If large, they may be symptomatic and require drainage. If a significant amount of necrosis is present, resulting computed tomography (CT) findings are defined as acute necrotic collections, with nonenhancing areas of variable attenuation. Over time, generally 4 weeks after onset, these mature and develop a wall, referred

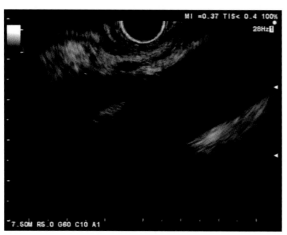

FIG 33.1 Celiac axis viewed with linear echoendoscope, with visible celiac ganglion *(white arrow)*.

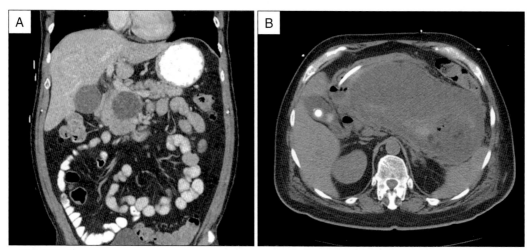

FIG 33.2 Pancreatic fluid collections vary in etiology, appearance, composition, and behavior. **A,** An example of a pseudocyst within the uncinate process. Note round, thick-walled appearance. **B,** Typical walled-off necrosis 4 weeks after onset of severe acute pancreatitis. Note heterogeneous enhancement with small pocket of air and start of rind formation around the fluid collection.

to as WON, which can cause unremitting pain, gastric or duodenal obstruction, or infection (Fig. 33.2, *B*).

Treatment of pancreatic fluid collections should be reserved for organized collections (pseudocysts and WON) that are causing symptoms or complications. Acute fluid collections are rarely infected and should generally not require drainage, and attempting drainage of unorganized fluid or necrosis will often lead to worse outcomes. Recent efforts have been targeted at endoscopic management of WON, and EUS has become a cornerstone of therapy, as it has been shown to be clearly superior to conventional "blind" endoscopic drainage, with lower cost and shorter hospital stay compared with surgical cystgastrostomy.[16] Several variations of care now exist, there are no clear standard approaches, none can be generalized, and the approach taken is often more dependent on local practice and expertise. Transgastric or transduodenal stenting can be performed with plastic stents, covered self-expanding metal stents (SEMS), or lumen-apposing stents (LAMS). Some have advocated for the use of nasocystic drains for repeated flushing, whereas others have had remarkable success with dual-modality drainage, in which a percutaneous drain is placed in addition to transgastric stents and gradually upsized to allow for drainage of liquefying necrotic tissue.[18] More recently, endoscopic necrosectomy has been performed in centers worldwide, to debride the necrotic cavity after access through dilated transluminal tracts or through preexisting metal stents (Fig. 33.3).

Technique

An appropriate site for necrogastromy or duodenostomy is identified sonographically. Ideally, the distance from the transducer to the inside of the collection should be <10 mm, without evidence of intervening blood vessels and with adherence of the area of WON, usually foretold by obliteration of the wall layers of the gastric or duodenal wall and no intervening fat planes. A 19-gauge FNA needle or blunt-tipped access needle is introduced into the cavity, and entry can be confirmed with contrast injection. A 0.035-inch or 0.025-inch guidewire is then coiled in the pseudocyst or WON cavity under fluoroscopic guidance. The tract is dilated with a graduated dilator (4 to 6 Fr) and/or balloon catheter (6 to 10 mm diameter). Once adequately dilated, stents can be placed, either two double-pigtail plastic stents, a SEMS device, or a non–cautery-tipped LAMS device. Pseudocysts can be treated with plastic or metal stents. It should be emphasized that WON cannot be effectively treated with plastic stents alone and only in conjunction with irrigation using nasocystic tubes or percutaneous drains.[18] In the author's experience, plastic stents may be advantageous in the setting of disconnected duct syndrome, where they can remain in place indefinitely to allow egress of pancreatic juice from the disconnected tail, preventing formation of another fluid collection after stent removal. In the absence of percutaneous drains, metal stents (SEMS, LAMS) must be used with or without endoscopic necrosectomy. Techniques of endoscopic necrosectomy are discussed in more detail in Chapter 56, but include lavage, sometimes with hydrogen peroxide, baskets, snares, and retrieval nets.

Efficacy

Over 55 studies of EGDPFC were collated in a systematic review including more than 2100 patients, with mean technical and clinical success rates of 97% and 90%, respectively, but it should be clear that WON and pseudocysts were not subdivided.[10] Time to complete drainage is unclear

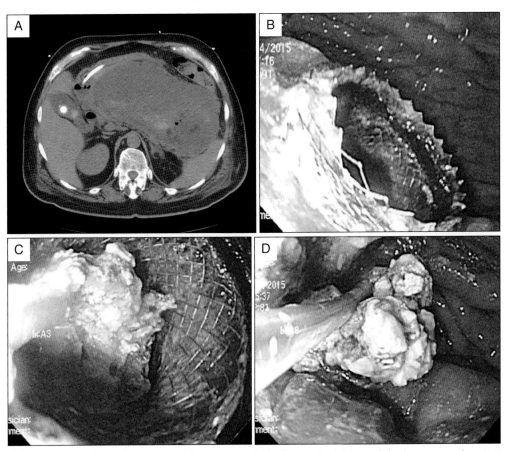

FIG 33.3 Necrosectomy in a 46-year-old man with walled-off necrosis. A 15-mm Axios lumen-apposing stent was placed transgastrically into the necroma **(A)** and the necroma was entered **(B)**. The majority of necrosectomy was performed using a snare **(C** and **D)**.

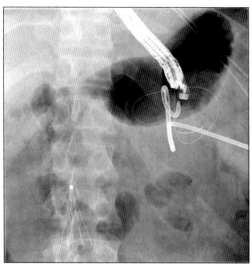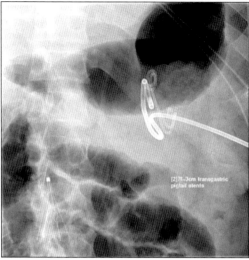

FIG 33.4 Fluoroscopic images of dual-modality drainage; percutaneous drain has already been placed. Endoscopic ultrasonography was used to place two transgastric 7-Fr 3-cm double-pigtail stents.

from the literature. For pseudocysts, direct comparisons of plastic stents, SEMS, and LAMS have not shown superiority of one stent type. Meta-analysis of almost 700 patients has not shown significant differences in treatment success rates, AE rates, and recurrence rates for pseudocysts. A large recent study found a statistically significant higher rate of complete resolution with SEMS (98%) than with plastic stents (89%) and lower rates of AEs (16% vs 31%). Initial reports of LAMS for pseudocyst drainage show high rates of technical (89% to 95%) and clinical (93% to 100%) success.[19-21] Successful treatment of WON with transgastric stents alone has not been shown to be effective, with reported success of 63.2%.[22] Ross et al. demonstrated 100% technical and clinical success of WON with dual-modality drainage (percutaneous drain and transgastric stents) in 103 patients, without need for surgical necrosectomy or procedure-related mortality (Fig. 33.4).[18] Nasocystic drains have been shown to reduce stent occlusion rates[23] and can be used in conjunction with transgastric stenting. A recent multicenter retrospective series of 124 patients who underwent LAMS placement for WON reported 100% technical success and 86.3% clinical success within 3 months. Necrosectomy was performed in 78 patients and the median number of debridement interventions was 2.[24] Hydrogen peroxide can also be used to aid in necrosectomy and may reduce AEs, procedure time, and number of necrosectomy sessions.

Adverse Events

In Fabbri's systematic review, the mean overall AE rate was 17% for EGDPFC.[10] AEs included hemorrhage (3.2%), superinfection (2.4%), stent migration (2.4%), perforation (1.2%), and pneumoperitoneum (0.8%). There were five procedure-related deaths (0.2%). The AE rate after necrosectomy is estimated at 22%.[25] The most common AE is bleeding (11%), followed by perforations and pneumoperitoneum (3%) and air embolism (0.4%). It is for this reason that CO_2 insufflation is suggested during necrosectomy.

PANCREATIC DUCT ACCESS AND DRAINAGE

When standard attempts at transpapillary access to the pancreatic duct by ERCP fail, EUS-guided pancreatic duct access (EUSPDA) is an increasingly commonly used option. Failure to gain wire access to the pancreatic duct can occur for a variety of reasons, including difficult cannulation, divisum anatomy and a small or nonvisible

minor duct orifice, duct tortuosity, strictures, failure to locate or cannulate a pancreaticojejunostomy, and disconnected pancreatic duct syndrome.

Technique

The pancreatic duct is located with a linear echoendoscope, and access is achieved most commonly with a 19-gauge needle, most often within the body of the pancreatic duct. Contrast injection will confirm ductal access and outline the pancreatic duct. The author generally uses a 19-gauge blunt-tipped access needle (19A EchoTip; Cook Medical), as there is less risk of wire shearing with the blunt-tipped needle. Nineteen-gauge needles allow the passage of both 0.035-inch and 0.025-inch guidewires. If the gland is particularly fibrotic, a 22-gauge needle may be necessary to puncture the gland, requiring the use of a 0.018-inch guidewire, which may not have the stiffness required for maneuvering through tight strictures. In rendezvous procedures, the guidewire is advanced antegrade into the downstream bowel, and the echoendoscope is removed and replaced with a side-viewing scope (in native anatomy) or a forward-viewing scope (in cases of surgically altered anatomy, like pancreaticojejunostomy). The guidewire is grasped with a snare or forceps and pulled through the endoscope, allowing for retrograde therapeutic maneuvers like dilation and stenting (Fig. 33.5). In direct pancreaticogastrostomy, the tract is created after wire access using dilation catheters, balloon catheters, needle knife, and cystotomes. Plastic stents are then placed after the tract has been successfully dilated.

Efficacy of EUSPDA is variable in the literature. Technical success is quoted between 50% and 100% and overall success rate is 78%.[10] AE rates range between 7% and 55% and are higher in cases of anterograde transluminal stent placement as opposed to rendezvous techniques. AEs include pancreatitis, pancreatic duct leak, bleeding, and perforation.

BILIARY DRAINAGE

Conventional biliary drainage with ERCP is safe and highly effective, but biliary cannulation is not always successful, even in the most experienced hands. Reasons for failure include inability to reach the papilla because of duodenal obstruction, inability to find the papilla, and altered anatomy. EUS-guided biliary drainage (EGBD) is an increasingly used alternative in these situations. Variations of the procedure

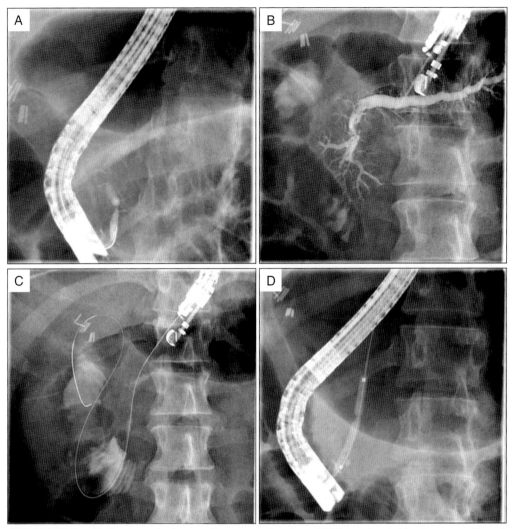

FIG 33.5 EUS-guided pancreatic duct rendezvous: during three ERCPs performed by three experienced endoscopists, guidewire passage beyond a seemingly mild stricture failed in a 28-year-old woman with recurrent acute pancreatitis **(A)**. EUS-guided rendezvous was performed. Nineteen-gauge needle was advanced into the pancreatic duct in the body **(B)** and a 0.025 angled guidewire was passed anterograde beyond the stricture into the duodenum **(C)**. Balloon dilation was performed retrograde after rendezvous with a duodenoscope **(D)**, followed by pancreatic duct stenting. *EUS,* Endoscopic ultrasonography.

include EUS-guided choledochoduodenostomy (EGCD), EUS-guided hepaticogastrostomy (EGHG), and EUS-guided biliary rendezvous (EGBRV). All such procedures should be undertaken with caution, as serious AEs can occur. It is suggested that only highly experienced endosonographers attempt these procedures, and training and mentoring may be necessary.

The decision to use these techniques also depends heavily on local expertise, as percutaneous transhepatic biliary drainage (PTBD) by skilled interventional radiologists has a very high success rate, 100% in some series,[26] although with higher AE and reintervention rates. If local expertise favors endoscopic intervention or if expertise is equivalent, EGBD may be preferable for patients, as percutaneous drainage does not reduce quality of life. A single-center retrospective study showed similar technical success rates (91.6% PTBD vs 93.3% EGBD) but higher rates of reintervention (4.9% vs 1.3%), pain (4.1% vs 1.9%), and late AEs (53.8% vs 6.6%) with PTBD. EGBRV generally has a lower success rate than PTBD and EGBD. Systematic reviews and a recent multicenter trial show a success rate of 74% to 80%.[27,28] Experts therefore suggest

that EGBRV should be reserved for patients with benign disease and normal anatomy in whom normal biliary cannulation fails.[29]

Two approaches to luminal drainage of the biliary tree are EGCD and EGHG. In cases in which there is no access to the duodenal bulb, only EGHG is possible. When both procedures are possible, studies comparing the two techniques show similar success rates, between 85% and 93%,[30] but some studies show EGHG to have significantly higher AE rates than EGCD (30.5% vs 9.3%; 19% vs 13%)[30,31] and greater 1-year stent patency.[30] No difference in survival times was reported. Recent reports of use of LAMS for EGCD have been promising,

Technique

For EGCD, the bile duct is identified from the duodenal bulb and punctured with a 19-gauge needle. Contrast can be injected to obtain cholangiography. Access with a 0.035-inch guidewire is obtained and the tract is dilated using a graduated dilator, balloon, needle knife, or coaxial cystotome, depending on availability. Stents can be placed in the proximal common bile duct if the EUS scope is in a long position

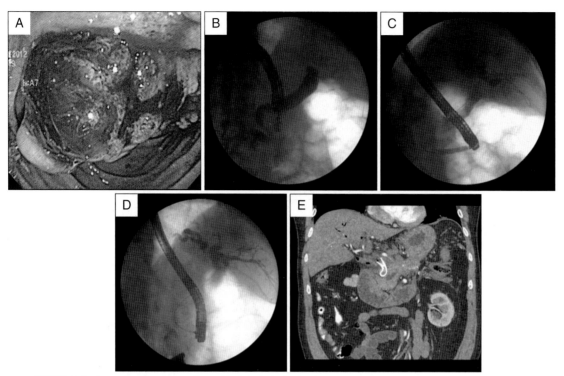

FIG 33.6 Endoscopic ultrasonography–guided choledochoduodenostomy in a 54-year-old man with metastatic ampullary adenocarcinoma. ERCP was not possible, as the biliary orifice was not evident despite innumerable attempts at cannulation because of the size and distortion of the mass **(A)**. Common bile duct access was gained with the linear echoendoscope in a short position and a 19-gauge needle. A 0.035 guidewire was advanced into the duct **(B)**, and the echoendoscope was exchanged for a duodenoscope (with a 4.2-mm therapeutic device channel). The tract was dilated with a 4-mm dilating balloon **(D)**, and a 10-mm × 6-cm stent was placed across the choledochoduodenostomy **(E)**.

facing superiorly, or into the distal common bile duct if in a short position and facing toward the ampulla (Fig. 33.6). Either plastic or metal stents can be placed, but most prefer fully or partially covered SEMS, which have longer patency rates and fewer AEs.[29] For EGHG, the left biliary tree is accessed from the stomach, with ultimate placement of a long covered SEMS.

Adverse Events

AEs from EGBD occur in approximately 29% of cases (3% to 77%) and include bile peritonitis, perforation, pneumoperitoneum, hemorrhage, and stent migration.[10] As transhepatic stents can occlude biliary segmental branches, focal cholangitis can occur. Long-term AEs include stent-induced hyperplasia, particularly if stent size and duct size are mismatched.

GALLBLADDER DRAINAGE

Acute cholecystitis often occurs in patients with multiple comorbidities and contraindications to surgery. Nonsurgical means of gallbladder drainage are often required as temporizing or definitive treatment. Before the advent of recent developments in EUS, decompression of the gallbladder required percutaneous radiologic drainage procedures or cystic duct stents or drainage tubes, placed during ERCP. Percutaneous drainage is successful in 90% of patients[32]; however, it often causes significant discomfort but remains necessary in patients too sick to undergo surgery or endoscopy. Other risks include bile leak, dislodgment, fistula, pneumothorax, and infection.[33] Endoscopically placed transpapillary cystic duct stents or nasocholecystic drains are also effective means of

gallbladder decompression, with an 80% to 90% success rate,[34] but success can be limited by access into and through the cystic duct because of an angulated or narrow take-off, tortuosity of the duct, or by the spiral valves.

EUS-guided cholecystoduodenostomy or gastrostomy (EGCG) has proven to be an effective means of gallbladder drainage in cases where surgery and transpapillary stenting are not possible. Initially, plastic stents were used but have since been superseded by self-expandable metal stents (SEMS) and lumen-apposing metal stents (LAMS). Plastic stent placement can be associated with bile leakage and bile peritonitis, and covered SEMS were thought to have the advantage of creating a seal between the gallbladder and the bowel/gastric lumen. LAMS have taken this one step further, with a dumbbell configuration of flanges and a 10-mm or 15-mm lumen diameter.

Technique

Using a therapeutic linear echoendoscope, the gallbladder is located and apposed to the gastrointestinal lumen, normally from the duodenal bulb or the gastric antrum. A 19-gauge FNA needle or a 19-gauge blunt-tipped "access" needle is introduced into the gallbladder and a 0.035-inch or 0.025-inch guidewire is advanced under fluoroscopic guidance into the gallbladder lumen. The tract is dilated enough to allow passage of the stent (usually 4-mm biliary balloon dilator to allow a 7-Fr or 10-Fr plastic stent, or a metal stent introducer) and the stent is deployed thereafter. The Axios (Boston-Scientific, Natick, MA) LAMS is deployed in a stepwise fashion, with the distal end deploying first under fluoroscopic and sonographic guidance and the proximal flange deploying after with direct endoscopic visualization (Fig. 33.7). The

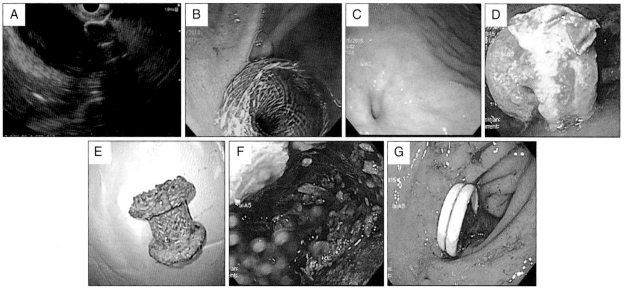

FIG 33.7 EUS-guided gallbladder stent placement. **A,** EUS image of deployment of the internal flange of lumen-apposing stent within the gallbladder. **B,** Endoscopic view of fully deployed 15-mm Axios lumen-apposing cholecystogastrostomy stent. **C,** Endoscopic appearance of the previously placed stent 6 months later, now migrated internally and almost granulated over. **D** and **E,** Stent appearance after tract dilation and retrieval. **F,** Tract appearance after stent retrieval. **G,** Two double-pigtail stents were left in place across the cholecystogastrostomy tract instead of placing a second lumen-apposing stent. *EUS,* Endoscopic ultrasonography.

AXIOS-EC "Hot Axios" device (Boston-Scientific) avoids the need for needle and guidewire advancement, as it has a diathermic ring and cut-wire that allows direct access into adjacent organs with electrocautery.

Efficacy

A systematic review of 22 cases reported that the technical and clinical success was 100% and 100% for plastic stents, respectively, and 98.6% and 94.6% for SEMS, respectively. Clinical success rate was significantly higher for partially covered SEMS than fully covered SEMS (98% vs 78%).[35] Technical and clinical success rates for LAMS ECGC were reported to be 91% and 90.1%, respectively. Long-term follow-up was studied by Walter et al. of 30 patients from a multicenter prospective trial.[36] Technical success (placement of stent) and clinical success (resolution of symptoms and decrease in parameters of infection) were reported to be 90% (27 patients) and 96% (26 of 27 patients), respectively. Two patients developed recurrent cholecystitis because of stent occlusion, and 50% of patients had LAMS removed after a mean duration of 91 days. In the other 15 patients, 5 (33%) died before removal, and 10 could not be removed because of other causes, including 2 with significant tissue overgrowth, but also because of "poor clinical condition of the patient," patient refusal, and ongoing cholelithiasis.

Adverse Events

AEs of plastic stents had a pooled frequency rate of 18.2% and included pneumoperitoneum, bile leaks, and bile peritonitis. Late stent migration occurred in 1 patient (out of 22).[35] The pooled AE rate in SEMS was 12.3%, and AEs more commonly occurred with covered SEMS than with partially covered SEMS. These included pneumoperitoneum, duodenal perforation, stent migration, and stent occlusion. LAMS

EGDG had an AE frequency of 9.9%. In the Walter study, there was 7% stent-related/procedure-related mortality and an overall stent-related severe AE rate of 13% (aspiration, infection, hemorrhage, and jaundice).

EUS-GUIDED ABLATION AND CANCER THERAPY

EUS-guided therapy also includes fine-needle injection and delivery of antitumor therapy. Successful pancreatic cyst ablation with ethanol with and without paclitaxel has been performed with clinical success rates between 33% and 79%.[37–39] AEs included acute pancreatitis, pain, and fever. Neuroendocrine tumors have also been treated with ethanol ablation in case series and case reports, as have hepatic metastasis, adrenal metastasis, and gastrointestinal stromal tumors lesions.[10] Direct antitumor therapy with injection of adenovirus vectors (ONYX-015; TNFerade), cryothermal therapy, and brachytherapy have been reported.[40–43] The safety and efficacy of these treatments, although feasible, are not yet clear from the limited literature.

CONCLUSIONS

The range and capacity of EUS for endotherapy in the gastrointestinal tract continue to expand. As such, EUS has evolved into an important tool in the management and therapy of pancreaticobiliary disease, providing access to structures often not within the reach of conventional endoscopes. Further research and innovation will continue to consolidate its role and expand its indications for benign and malignant disease.

The complete reference list for this chapter can be found online at www.experconsult.com.

34

Pancreaticobiliary Disorders: What Are the Roles of CT, MRCP, and EUS Relative to ERCP?

Andres Gelrud and Ajaypal Singh

Endoscopic retrograde cholangiopancreatography (ERCP) was first described in 1968 (see Chapter 1).[1] Despite being technically challenging because of the limited range of available endoscopes and accessories at that time, it became an important modality for diagnostic evaluation of the pancreaticobiliary system in Japan and Europe.[2–4] The therapeutic role of ERCP was recognized and developed after the introduction of sphincterotomy in 1972 by Classen and Demling from Germany[5] and Kawai et al. from Japan.[6] The therapeutic utility of ERCP expanded from removal of bile duct stones to relief of malignant hepatobiliary obstruction after the development of bile duct and pancreatic stents in the 1980s.[7] Despite initial concerns about its utility and safety, ERCP was subsequently accepted in the United States. The use of ERCP in the United States reached a peak in the mid-1990s. Along with the development of formal ERCP training, the introduction of laparoscopic cholecystectomy in 1989 may have also contributed to the increased use of ERCP in the early 1990s.[8,9]

Since the initial development of ERCP, imaging of the pancreaticobiliary tract has undergone a remarkable transition with the development of high-resolution computed tomography (CT), endoscopic ultrasonography (EUS), and magnetic resonance imaging with cholangiopancreatography (MRI/MRCP). With the availability of these less invasive, safer imaging modalities, the role of ERCP has now transitioned mainly to a therapeutic tool, especially because of the recognition of the high risk of potential adverse effects associated with diagnostic ERCP (see Chapter 8). High-quality prospective studies have also led to the recognition of conditions where ERCP is now not the best management option.

In a study published in 2007 using the National Inpatient Sample (NIS) database, Jamal et al. showed that the use of ERCP in the United States increased from 1988 to 1996, but from 1996 to 2002 showed a steady decline.[10] The age-adjusted ERCP rate declined approximately 20% from 1996 to 2002. The study also concluded that the declining trend was mainly attributable to a decrease in the use of diagnostic ERCP, as the utilization of therapeutic ERCP continued to increase during the study period. The trend of declining ERCP use was also noted in the outpatient ambulatory centers from the Stage Ambulatory Surgery Database (SASD) during the same period. It is our assumption that the use of ERCP has continued to decline since then, and with the recent EPISOD trial showing no benefit of ERCP in patients with suspected type III sphincter of Oddi dysfunction (SOD) (see Chapter 47), this trend will likely continue.[11] In the pediatric population, the

use of therapeutic ERCP increased from 2000 to 2009 but diagnostic ERCP use showed a significant decrease.[12]

The reason for the declining role of ERCP is twofold. First, the high and, in most cases, unacceptable risk of adverse events, and second, the availability of alternate noninvasive and less risky imaging modalities.[13] The adverse events associated with ERCP and how to minimize these have already been discussed in Chapter 8 and will not be discussed here in detail. We summarize here the literature comparing ERCP with EUS, MRI, and CT imaging for various diagnostic purposes in the major pancreaticobiliary diseases. The therapeutic role of ERCP in obtaining biliary and pancreatic duct drainage and treatment of choledocholithiasis is well established and will not be reviewed here. Cost of care is an important consideration in current-day medicine and should play a role in deciding the choice of diagnostic evaluation. Along with the increased risk of adverse events, studies have shown that ERCP is less cost-effective than less invasive modalities such as EUS and MRCP for evaluation of the biliary tree in patients with suspected biliary disease, especially in a population with low disease prevalence.[14] There are multiple studies comparing the cost and diagnostic yield of MRI/MRCP versus EUS for diagnosing biliary diseases.[15,16] However, in patient populations with a high prevalence of pancreaticobiliary disease, where the probability of performing therapeutics is greater than 50%, ERCP is more cost-effective than EUS and MRCP.[17] Such patients include those with indeterminate biliary strictures, obstructive jaundice, and high likelihood of choledocholithiasis based on clinical criteria.

ROLE OF NONINVASIVE IMAGING AND EUS COMPARED WITH ERCP IN BENIGN HEPATOBILIARY DISEASES

Stone Disease

Choledocholithiasis is the most common indication for ERCP. Because laparoscopic cholecystectomy is commonly not associated with bile duct exploration, ERCP is the preferred and first-line therapeutic modality for the management of bile duct stones. Given the risk of adverse events, there is not a diagnostic role for ERCP in all patients in whom bile duct stones are expected. Among those with symptomatic cholelithiasis and suspected choledocholithiasis, it is important to select patients carefully for ERCP.

Even though CT imaging is sensitive for detecting the presence and level of bile duct dilation, the sensitivity of CT imaging for choledocholithiasis is relatively low (around 75%) and CT imaging should ideally not be used in patients with suspected choledocholithiasis.[18,19] MRI/MRCP (Fig. 34.1) has a sensitivity >90% for the diagnosis of choledocholithiasis but is lower for stones <6 mm in diameter, where the sensitivity is approximately 75%; it is also decreased in the presence of dilated bile ducts.[20–24] Both EUS and MRI/MRCP have very high sensitivity and specificity for diagnosing bile duct stones, with EUS (Fig. 34.2) being slightly superior to MRI/MRCP especially for small distal bile duct stones.[25–27] The American Society for Gastrointestinal Endoscopy (ASGE) practice guidelines categorize symptomatic cholelithiasis patients with

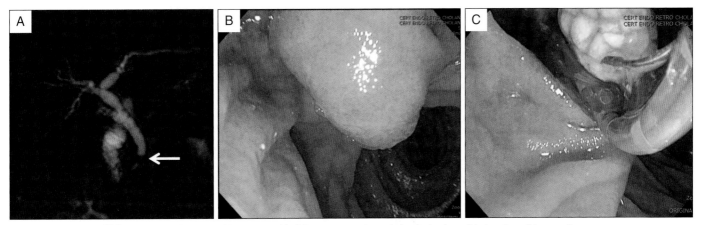

FIG 34.1 Thirty-five-year-old woman with right-upper-quadrant abdominal pain, mild elevation of transaminases, and total bilirubin of 2.1 mg/dL. Abdominal ultrasonography revealed "prominent bile duct" and was unable to visualize the distal duct because of air in small bowel. **A,** Magnetic resonance cholangiopancreatography (MRCP) revealed a small obstructing stone in the distal common bile duct (*arrow*). **B,** Endoscopic retrograde cholangiopancreatography (ERCP) image with bulge in major papilla (suggestive of impacted stone). **C,** Biliary sphincterotomy with stone extraction.

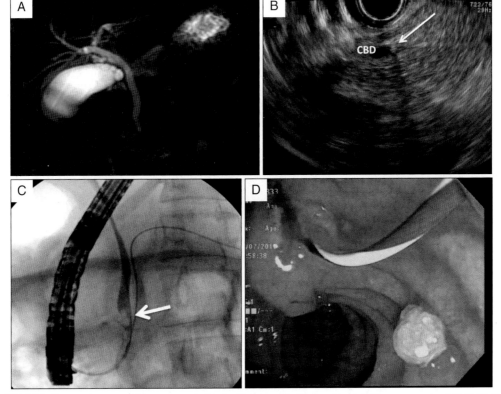

FIG 34.2 Twenty-four-year-old woman admitted with 1 month of intermittent right-upper-quadrant abdominal pain, now with mild elevation of transaminases and normal bilirubin. **A,** Magnetic resonance cholangiopancreatography (MRCP) images revealed a normal biliary system. Pain persisted and endoscopic ultrasonography (EUS) **(B)** was performed with visualization of small stone in distal common bile duct (*white arrow*) with distal shadow (*red arrow*). **C,** Endoscopic retrograde cholangiopancreatography (ERCP) with filling defect in distal common bile duct (arrow). **D,** Small-stone extraction.

suspected choledocholithiasis into three groups based on the likelihood of the presence of common bile duct stones.[28] This categorization uses clinical presentation, laboratory, and transabdominal ultrasonographic findings. Patients with high likelihood of choledocholithiasis (defined as >50% probability) should undergo preoperative ERCP, whereas those with low likelihood (<30%) should undergo cholecystectomy directly. Those

patients with medium likelihood (30% to 50%) should undergo either preoperative MRI or EUS or intraoperative cholangiography (Fig. 34.3) to confirm the presence of choledocholithiasis before undergoing ERCP.

Chronic Pancreatitis
Role in Diagnosis

The major manifestations of chronic pancreatitis (CP) that require endoscopic diagnosis or management include pain, presence of a biliary stricture (Fig. 34.4), pancreatic duct stricture, and treatment of pancreatic fluid collections (see Chapter 55). There is little role for endoscopic therapy in the management of exocrine pancreatic insufficiency, and the role of endoscopy in pain management is also not clearly defined,[29-31] except when ductal obstruction is present. ERCP should not be the first-line modality to diagnose CP because of lack of visualization of parenchyma and also because of the risk of acute pancreatitis associated with pancreatography. The sensitivity to diagnose mild-severity or moderate-severity chronic pancreatitis is also low for ERCP. All of the other imaging modalities (EUS, CT, and MRI/MRCP) allow evaluation of the parenchyma and the ductal anatomy and hence are preferred for diagnosis of chronic pancreatitis (Fig. 34.5). They also allow for visualization of any mass lesions in the pancreas, as risk of pancreatic cancer is increased in the setting of CP. However, all imaging modalities have poor sensitivity in detecting pancreatic cancer in the setting of chronic pancreatitis.

Pain Management

The pathogenesis of pain in chronic pancreatitis is complex and still not fully understood. Pancreatic duct strictures can lead to upstream duct dilation and increased intraductal pressure and is believed to be one of

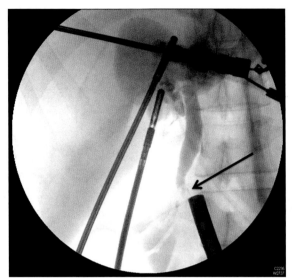

FIG 34.3 Forty-eight-year-old man underwent laparoscopic cholecystectomy for the treatment of symptomatic cholelithiasis. Intraoperative cholangiogram revealed a small distal common bile duct stone (*arrow*).

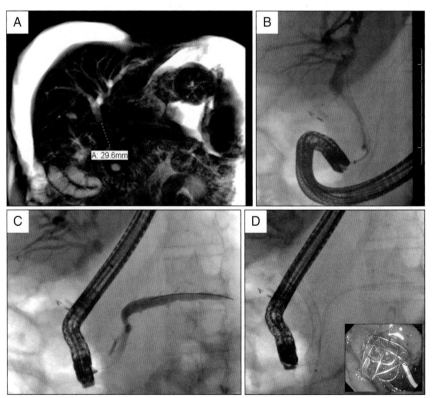

FIG 34.4 Fifty-two-year-old patient with chronic calcific pancreatitis was admitted with jaundice. **A,** Magnetic resonance cholangiopancreatography (MRCP) with stricture in the intrapancreatic portion of the distal common bile duct and intrahepatic ductal dilation. **B,** Endoscopic retrograde cholangiopancreatography (ERCP) with cholangiogram showing "mirror" image of MRCP. **C,** ERCP showing dilated pancreatic duct of chronic pancreatitis. **D,** Fluoroscopic and endoscopic view after placement of metal biliary and plastic pancreatic stents.

the many processes contributing to pain. Although endoscopic drainage with dilation and stent placement is still being used for pain control in many patients, randomized studies have shown that outcomes are much better with surgical drainage in these patients compared with endoscopic drainage.[32–34] Before surgical drainage, a road map of the pancreatic ductal and parenchymal anatomy may be indicated and cross-sectional imaging

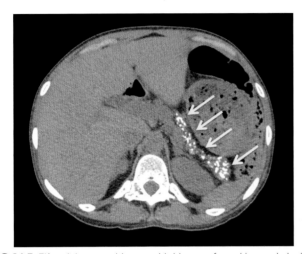

FIG 34.5 Fifty-eight-year-old man with history of smoking and alcohol-induced chronic calcific pancreatitis. Abdominal computed tomography scan shows innumerable parenchymal pancreatic stones (*yellow arrows*).

either with CT or MRI/MRCP is very important. There are currently no randomized trials comparing the two modalities and the approach is usually surgeon dependent. One important role of MRI/MRCP is to evaluate for ductal leak and to identify ductal communications with a pseudocyst (discussed later). EUS-guided celiac plexus block is an alternative to ERCP-guided pancreatic therapy for pain control, especially in CP patients with disabling pain and absence of ductal obstruction/dilatation. However, the data for celiac plexus block in CP are not as robust as the data for pain control in patients with pancreatic cancer.[35] Fifty-five percent to 70% patients experience temporary improvement in abdominal pain, but long-term data are not promising and depend on the underlying etiology of the chronic pancreatitis. The efficacy is further limited in patients with prior pancreatic surgery and those younger than 45 years. The published data have suggested better pain relief with EUS-guided celiac plexus block compared with CT-guided percutaneous block.[36–38] Celiac plexus neurolysis with absolute alcohol should be used with caution, if at all, in patients with benign disease because of the potential for severe adverse events.

Symptomatic Pancreatic and Peripancreatic Fluid Collections

Symptomatic pancreatic and peripancreatic fluid collections in the setting of chronic pancreatitis are usually related to pancreatic duct leaks with underlying downstream obstruction. The management approach to pancreatic pseudocysts in the setting of acute pancreatitis and chronic pancreatitis is slightly different, but most of the recent literature regarding endoscopic management of these collections does not differentiate between the two forms of pancreatitis. EUS-guided transmural drainage of pseudocysts (Fig. 34.6) has emerged as the

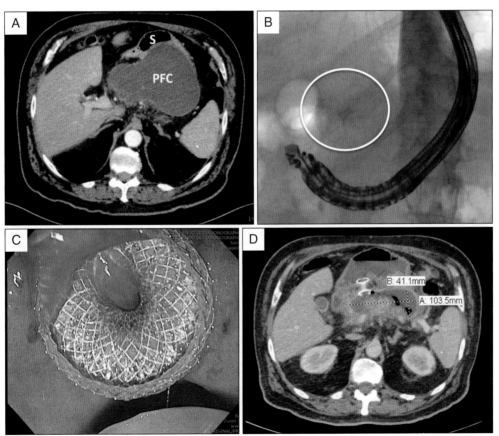

FIG 34.6 Thirty-four-year-old man after 5 weeks of an episode of pancreatitis with early satiety and abdominal pain. **A,** Abdominal computed tomography (CT) with pancreatic fluid collection (*PFC*) compressing the stomach (*S*). **B** and **C,** Endoscopic ultrasonography–guided drainage using a lumen-apposing metal stent (*ellipse*). **D,** Abdominal CT with resolving PFC.

first-line therapy and has nearly completely replaced transpapillary drainage. Some published studies suggested that ERCP with pancreatic duct stenting might be helpful in management of pancreatic fluid collections, particularly in the setting of pancreatic duct disruption or with a duct leak communicating with the fluid collection[39–42] (Fig. 34.7). This is technically difficult in many instances, and a recent multicenter study involving tertiary care centers with high expertise in advanced endoscopy showed that it was successful in only 17 of 47 patients in whom a leak was identified.[43]

SUSPECTED PANCREATICOBILIARY MALIGNANCY

The role of ERCP in malignant obstructive jaundice is therapeutic, with a major focus on preoperative and palliative drainage with biliary stenting. The diagnostic roles of ERCP, EUS, and cross-sectional imaging for pancreaticobiliary malignancies depend on the presence of a discrete

mass on imaging or presentation with a biliary stricture and jaundice without a mass.

In patients who have a pancreatic mass and biliary obstruction, EUS has been shown to have the highest sensitivity for detecting pancreatic tumors (Fig. 34.8), especially those <2 cm.[16,44–46] High-resolution CT scanning with pancreas protocol consisting of arterial, venous, and delayed phase imaging has a high sensitivity for detection of a mass lesion but can miss smaller lesions. EUS provides the additional ability to obtain tissue for histologic diagnosis. The role of ERCP in these situations is usually palliative drainage, but it can be used for diagnostic purposes in patients with inconclusive EUS-guided sampling. ERCP assumes a more diagnostic role in patients with cholangiocarcinoma who present with jaundice (Fig. 34.9) in the absence of a discrete mass. Whereas CT imaging is usually sufficient to proceed with tissue sampling and drainage in patients with pancreatic head cancer and jaundice, in patients with cholangiocarcinoma, especially of the hilar type, noninvasive

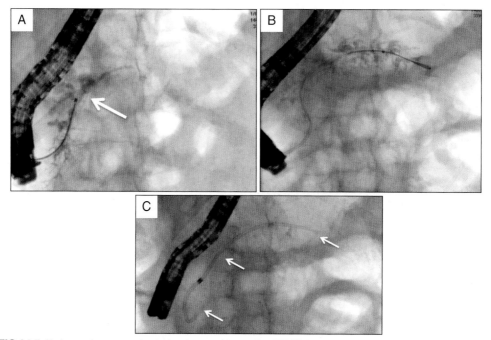

FIG 34.7 Endoscopic retrograde cholangiopancreatography (ERCP) pancreatogram revealed pancreatic duct disruption **(A)** able to bypass the leak site **(B)** with pancreatic duct stent placement **(C)**.

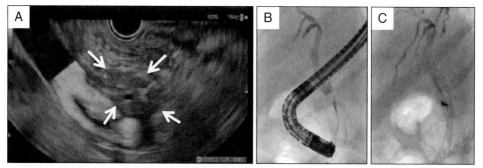

FIG 34.8 Sixty-two-year-old man admitted with painless jaundice and abdominal computed tomography with 1.8 cm × 1.5 cm lesion in the head of the pancreas (HOP). **A,** Endoscopic ultrasonography with small lesion in HOP (*arrows*); fine-needle aspiration revealed pancreatic adenocarcinoma. **B** and **C,** Endoscopic retrograde cholangiopancreatography (ERCP) with obstructed distal bile duct and metal stent placement.

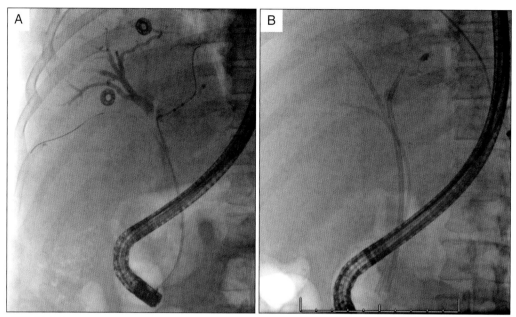

FIG 34.9 Seventy-two-year-old patient with painless jaundice and weight loss (see Fig. 34.10 for MRCP image). **A,** Cholangiogram with hilar malignant-appearing stricture involving the intrahepatic ducts. **B,** Placement of three plastic stents in the opacified intrahepatic ducts.

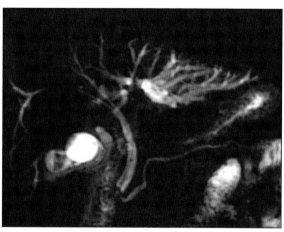

FIG 34.10 Patient from Fig. 34.9. Magnetic resonance cholangiopancreatography with hilar malignant-appearing stricture with intrahepatic duct dilation.

cholangiography using MRCP (Fig. 34.10) is of great help in providing a road map of the biliary tract before attempting ERCP (see Chapter 40). MRCP has similar sensitivity and specificity to ERCP for assessing the level and morphology of biliary strictures.[47,48] A meta-analysis of 67 studies that included 4711 patients with biliary obstruction showed sensitivity and specificity of 88% and 95%, respectively, for diagnosing malignancy.[21] Use of diffusion-weighted imaging can further improve the diagnostic yield of MRI for indeterminate biliary strictures. In patients with biliary strictures without an obvious mass, a pancreas protocol CT might be sufficient if the level of obstruction is in the distal bile duct, but if the stricture is proximal, MRI/MRCP should be favored.

Along with delineating the stricture extent and allowing biliary drainage, ERCP also allows for tissue sampling using either brush cytology or intraductal biopsies. The specificity of diagnosing malignancy with ERCP sampling of bile duct strictures approaches 95%, but the sensitivity is low for brush cytology (23% to 56%) and biopsy (33% to 65%).[49–53] Obtaining both biliary brushings and intraductal biopsies during ERCP can increase the diagnostic yield to 60% to 70%.[54–56]

The role of EUS in biliary obstruction without a definite mass is not as well established as its role in fine-needle sampling of pancreatic masses. Initially reported in 2000, EUS has been used for evaluation of biliary strictures, and multiple studies have shown sensitivity ranging from 40% to 90% for EUS fine-needle aspiration (FNA) of biliary strictures.[57–62] Even though no studies have shown needle track seeding after FNA of biliary strictures, it has been reported with FNA of pancreatic masses and hence is a theoretical concern.[63–65] Some centers that offer liver transplant for cholangiocarcinoma consider prior FNA a contraindication to transplantation, even though a recent study showed no increase in mortality or adverse outcomes after EUS-FNA of cholangiocarcinoma.[66–68] Thus ERCP should still be the primary modality of tissue acquisition in these patients, if needed. Intraductal sonography and cholangioscopy are other available options for evaluation of the biliary tract, and both of these require ERCP to access the bile duct.

CONCLUSIONS

There has been a decrease in the use of ERCP. This is because of a combination of two factors. First, there are many diseases for which ERCP is not the right choice, as in patients with the now-debunked diagnosis of SOD type III. Second, with the development of CT, EUS, and MRI/MRCP, safer alternatives for diagnosis and are now available. This is true for many medical technologies during their development, when enthusiasm leads to widespread use followed by realization and quantification of the risks and benefits of all applications. ERCP as a technology appears to have passed through this stage and has matured enough to realize its true potential. Although some experts have raised concerns that the decrease in use and resultant low volumes might lead to poorly trained endoscopists, especially a lack of exposure to technically challenging cases, ERCP could be replaced by other modalities such as EUS-guided transmural drainage procedures that might someday be the primary method for palliation of malignant distal biliary obstruction. It is also important to note that EUS is currently going through the same stages of excitement and widening of therapeutic applications, similar to ERCP in the 1980s and early 1990s.

Appropriate trials will determine the respective roles for each of these modalities.

The complete reference list for this chapter can be found online at www.expertconsult.com.

35

Pancreas Divisum, Biliary Cysts, and Other Congenital Anomalies

Mark Topazian

Anomalies of the biliary and pancreatic ducts are commonly encountered during endoscopic retrograde cholangiopancreatography (ERCP) and are important to both surgeons and gastroenterologists. This chapter reviews the diagnosis, clinical relevance, and therapy of these variants.

AMPULLARY ANOMALIES

Ectopic Major Papilla

The major papilla, which is typically located in the mid-duodenum or distal second duodenum, is occasionally located in the third duodenum.[1] Ectopic distal location of the ampulla is associated with anomalous pancreaticobiliary junction (APBJ), congenital biliary dilatation, and biliary cysts.[2] The distal displacement of the papilla may correspond to the length of an abnormally long common channel[3] and may reflect failure of the ducts to migrate normally into the duodenum during embryologic development. Rarely the major papilla may be located in the duodenal bulb.[4] Double papilla of Vater has been described.[5] When the papilla is in an anomalous location, the oblique intramural course of the bile duct is often absent,[6] leaving less room for endoscopic biliary sphincterotomy.

Anomalous Pancreaticobiliary Junction

The bile duct and pancreatic duct typically form a common channel of 1 to 6 mm in the papilla of Vater.[7] Less commonly a long common channel is present (Fig. 35.1), which may be termed the anomalous pancreaticobiliary junction (APBJ). Synonyms include anomalous union of pancreaticobiliary duct,[8] anomalous arrangement of the pancreaticobiliary duct, or anomalous pancreaticobiliary union.[9] APBJ may be subdivided into pancreaticobiliary malunion (PBM), in which the junction of the bile duct and pancreatic duct lies outside of the duodenal wall, with free communication between the ducts when the ampullary sphincter is contracting,[10] and high confluence of pancreaticobiliary ducts (HCPBD), in which contractions of the duodenal wall or sphincter interrupt communication between the ducts.[11] APBJ can also be subclassified according to the presence or absence of pancreas divisum, a dilated common channel, and an acute angle between the bile duct and pancreatic duct.[12] These findings may influence treatment strategy in symptomatic patients, particularly those with biliary cysts. APBJ promotes reflux of pancreatic juice into the biliary system, and a bile amylase concentration of >8000 IU/L may be considered diagnostic of an anomalous ductal junction.[13]

APBJ appears to be a risk factor for the development of malignancy in a biliary cyst, as discussed in the next section. Patients with APBJ and no biliary cyst have an increased risk of biliary cancer and develop gallbladder cancer at an earlier age (Fig. 35.2).[14,15] The risk of gallbladder cancer in patients with HCPBD may be somewhat lower than the risk seen with PBM.[11] Either way, the finding of an isolated APBJ should

prompt consideration of prophylactic cholecystectomy and perhaps longitudinal surveillance of the bile duct. Unexplained thickening of the gallbladder wall identified on transabdominal ultrasonography has been associated with underlying APBJ.[16]

BILIARY ANOMALIES

Variations of Bile Duct Anatomy

Couinaud[17] described the liver as being composed of four sectors, defined by the three hepatic veins.[18] The four sectors can be further subdivided into eight segments, which are drained by segmental bile ducts (Fig. 35.3). Ducts from segments II, III, and IV form the left hepatic duct, and ducts from segments V, VI, VII, and VIII form the right hepatic duct. The right and left hepatic ducts then form the biliary confluence. The caudate lobe (segment I) is typically drained by several short, small ducts into both the right and left hepatic ducts, and the caudate branches are generally not well seen during ERCP.

The right hepatic duct drains into the biliary confluence and is typically formed by a right anterior sectoral duct (draining segments V and VIII) and a right posterior sectoral duct (draining segments VI and VII). On cholangiography the right anterior duct arises superiorly and often takes a relatively straight course to the confluence. The right posterior duct has a more horizontal course, arising laterally or inferiorly and appearing to cross over the right anterior duct before inserting into the confluence medially (Fig. 35.4; see also Figs. 35.6 and 35.7).[18] Moving away from the confluence along the left hepatic duct, the first visualized branches generally drain segment IV, which may be drained by one to three segmental ducts. Moving farther to the left, the left main duct is formed by the confluence of the segment II and III ducts (see Fig. 35.4).[18]

Variants of confluence anatomy are common, and the normal confluence anatomy described above is seen in only 57% of persons. The commonest variations involve the right anterior and posterior ducts and are shown in Fig. 35.5. These include low drainage of one of the right sectoral ducts into the common duct (seen in 20%) (Fig. 35.6), a "triple confluence" in which the two right sectoral ducts drain separately into the confluence (12%), and drainage of a right sectoral duct into the left duct (6%). In about 2% a right sectoral duct drains into the cystic duct, as shown in Fig. 35.7. These variants of right duct anatomy may increase the risk of a bile duct injury during cholecystectomy. They are also important to the endoscopist when managing hilar malignant obstruction and evaluating postoperative biliary strictures and leaks. When a right sectoral duct draining into the cystic duct is divided and clipped during laparoscopic cholecystectomy, resulting in a Bismuth V ductal injury (see Chapter 44), cholangiographic diagnosis is difficult and requires a high degree of suspicion to recognize that a right sectoral duct is not visualized.

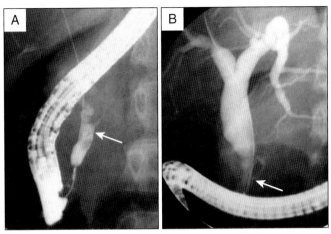

FIG 35.1 Anomalous pancreaticobiliary junction (APBJ) (*arrows*) and pancreas divisum in a 14-year-old with recurrent pancreatitis. **A,** A long, dilated common channel is present, which contains a stone. **B,** The common bile duct is dilated, suggestive of a type I choledochal cyst.

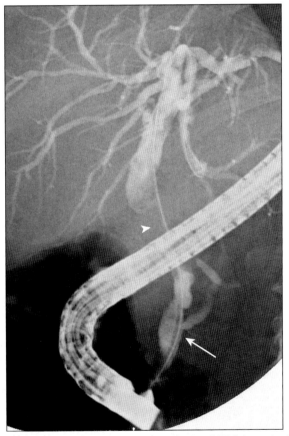

FIG 35.2 Anomalous pancreaticobiliary junction (APBJ) (*arrow*) with a bile duct stricture (*arrowhead*) caused by gallbladder cancer in a 32-year-old with obstructive jaundice. APBJ is a risk factor for development of gallbladder cancer. Note the absence of a bile duct cyst.

Variants of segmental duct anatomy also commonly occur (particularly segments IV, V, VI, and VIII) and are shown in Fig. 35.8. Ectopic drainage of the gallbladder and cystic duct may occur and is discussed elsewhere.[18] The cystic duct may drain into the ampulla separately from the common bile duct.[19]

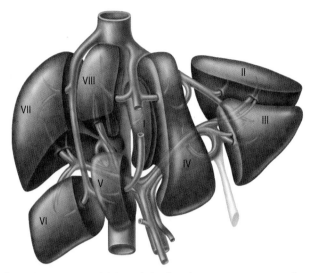

FIG 35.3 Functional division of the liver into segments, according to Couinaud's nomenclature. (From Blumgart LH, Fong Y, eds. *Surgery of the Liver and Biliary Tract.* Philadelphia: Saunders; 2002. Reproduced with permission.)

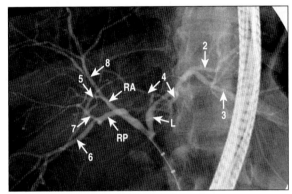

FIG 35.4 Normal intrahepatic ductal anatomy. Note that the right anterior duct has a relatively vertical and medial course and the right posterior duct has a more horizontal and lateral course. See also Figs. 41.6 and 41.7. *L,* Left duct; *RA,* right anterior duct; *RP,* right posterior duct; numbers indicate drained hepatic segments.

Biliary Cysts

Biliary cysts, also called choledochal cysts, are cystic dilatations of the biliary tree. One widely adopted classification of biliary cysts was described by Alonso-Lej et al.[20] and modified by Todani et al.[21] and is shown in Fig. 35.9. Type I cysts, which are commonest, are dilatations of the common bile duct, often in association with an APBJ. They can be subdivided into types 1a, 1b, 1c, and 1d based on the presence or absence of an APBJ, fusiform or segmental ductal dilation, and involvement of the cystic duct, as shown in Figs. 35.1, 35.9, and 35.10. Type II cysts are diverticula of the common duct. Type III cysts involve the major papilla and may also be termed "choledochoceles"; they are often lined by duodenal rather than biliary mucosa. Type III cysts may be further subdivided into type IIIA (in which the bile duct and pancreatic duct enter the cyst proximally, and the cyst drains through a separate distal opening into the duodenum) (Fig. 35.11) and type IIIB (a diverticulum of the intraampullary common channel). Type IV cysts are multiple cysts located in both the intrahepatic and extrahepatic

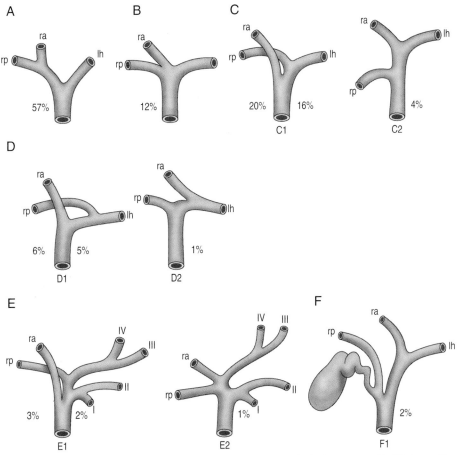

FIG 35.5 Common variations of biliary confluence anatomy. **A,** Typical anatomy. **B,** Triple confluence. **C,** Ectopic drainage of a right sectoral duct into the common hepatic duct. **D,** Ectopic drainage of a right sectoral duct into the left hepatic duct. **E,** Absence of a confluence. **F,** Ectopic drainage of the right posterior sectoral duct into the cystic duct. *lh,* Left hepatic duct; *ra,* right anterior; *rp,* right posterior. (From Blumgart LH, Fong Y, eds. *Surgery of the Liver and Biliary Tract.* Philadelphia: Saunders; 2002. Reproduced with permission.)

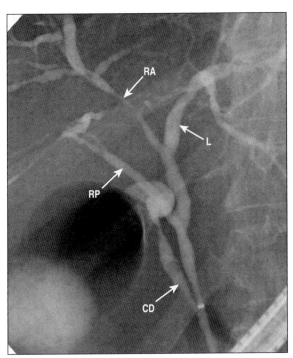

FIG 35.6 Ectopic drainage of the right posterior duct into the common hepatic duct. *CD,* Cystic duct; *L,* left duct; *RA,* right anterior duct; *RP,* right posterior duct.

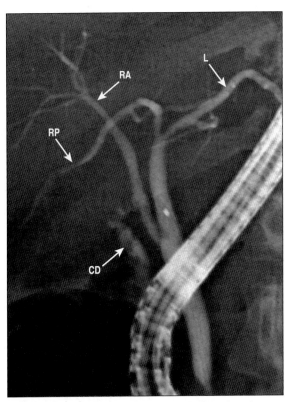

FIG 35.7 Ectopic drainage of the right anterior duct into the common hepatic duct. The cystic duct drains into the right anterior duct. *CD,* Cystic duct; *L,* left duct; *RA,* right anterior duct; *RP,* right posterior duct.

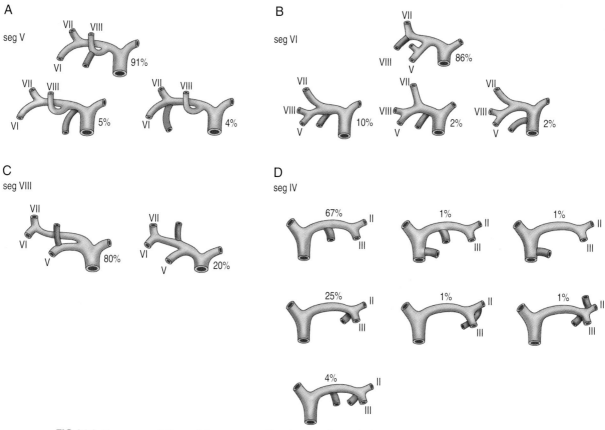

FIG 35.8 Common variations of the segmental intrahepatic ducts. **A,** Segment V. **B,** Segment VI. **C,** Segment VIII. **D,** Segment IV. (From Blumgart LH, Fong Y, eds. *Surgery of the Liver and Biliary Tract.* Philadelphia: Saunders; 2002. Reproduced with permission.)

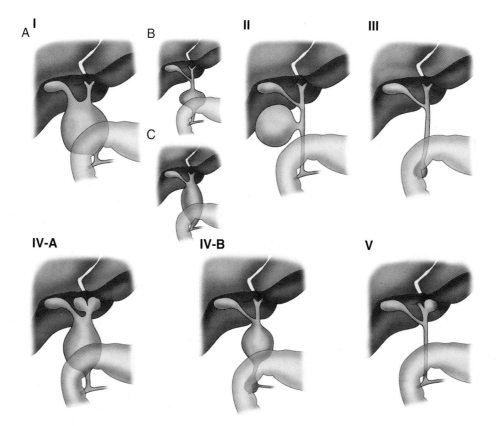

FIG 35.9 Classification of biliary cysts. (From Todani T, Watanabe Y, Toki A, et al. Classification of congenital biliary cystic disease: special reference to type Ic and IVA cysts with primary ductal stricture. *J Hepatobiliary Pancreat Surg.* 2003;10:340–344. Reproduced with permission.)

ducts (IVA) (Fig. 35.12) or in the extrahepatic biliary tree (IVB). Type I cysts with associated dilation of central intrahepatic ducts can be distinguished from type IVA (combined intrahepatic and extrahepatic cysts) by the presence of a distinct change in ductal caliber at the distal end of a true intrahepatic cyst.[21] Type V cysts, also called Caroli's disease, are segmental cystic dilatations of the intrahepatic ducts (Fig. 35.13). Type VI cysts are isolated cystic dilatations of the cystic duct and have recently been described.

Periampullary choledochal diverticula are small diverticular outpouchings of the distal bile duct at the superior edge of the biliary sphincter. These lesions are most often incidental, are not associated with APBJ, and may be associated with sphincter of Oddi dysfunction. These small diverticula should probably be distinguished from type II biliary cysts and have not been associated with biliary malignancy.[22]

Various mechanisms probably lead to formation of biliary cysts, as reviewed elsewhere.[23] Biliary cysts are often congenital but may be

acquired, and an APBJ may predispose to formation of a type 1 cyst after cholecystectomy.[24] In many patients with extrahepatic cysts an APBJ is present, with bile amylase levels > 8000 IU/L,[11] and chronic reflux of pancreatic juice into the bile duct may lead to ductal dilatation, biliary mucosal inflammation, and metaplasia. Sequelae may include pancreatitis, ductal stones, biliary dysplasia, and cholangiocarcinoma. The risk of cholangiocarcinoma increases with age and is low (0.4%) in patients younger than 18 years but is 5% to 14% in young adults[25,26] and 50% in older adults[27] presenting with symptomatic complications of their cysts; the prevalence of cancer in asymptomatic cysts is lower but is certainly increased compared with the general population. The risk of cholangiocarcinoma may also be somewhat lower in biliary cyst patients without an APBJ.[9,13] The possibility of cholangiocarcinoma should always be considered in an adult patient with a newly diagnosed biliary cyst.

Diagnosis of a biliary cyst requires a high degree of clinical suspicion, particularly for type I cysts, which may have a similar cholangiographic appearance to a chronically obstructed bile duct. The absence of biochemical, imaging, or endoscopic evidence of obstruction is a key diagnostic finding, although patients with biliary cysts may become symptomatic only when an obstruction (because of stone or malignancy) occurs. Subtle distal bile duct obstruction may be difficult to fully exclude, and chronic narcotic or ketamine use can cause fusiform dilatation of the bile duct mimicking a type 1c biliary cyst,[28] presumably by inducing sphincter of Oddi spasm or a subtle stricture. An APBJ, when present, is an important clue to diagnosis of an extrahepatic biliary cyst.

Biliary atresia is an important differential diagnosis in neonates with cystic dilation of the bile ducts. Biliary atresia generally requires surgery within 60 days of birth to prevent irreversible cirrhosis and liver failure, whereas biliary cysts can be safely observed through infancy and childhood. Neonates with biliary atresia have persistent jaundice, higher blood bilirubin and bile acid levels, and less impressive ductal dilatation than those with biliary cysts.[29] The differential diagnosis of biliary cysts also includes biliary mucinous cystic neoplasms (cystadenoma and cystadenocarcinoma), which typically present as solitary intrahepatic cystic lesions communicating with the bile ducts.

When a cholangiocarcinoma develops in a type 1 biliary cyst, the bile duct is typically dilated both proximal and distal to the malignant stricture; the malignancy may be missed during ERCP unless the extrahepatic duct, biliary confluence, and central intrahepatic ducts are all visualized. It may be difficult to fill the entire dilated duct with contrast, and guidewire cannulation of the intrahepatic ducts can facilitate passage of a catheter above the biliary cyst and visualization of the cyst's proximal extent. Diagnosis of early, nonobstructing cholangio-carcinoma in a dilated segment of bile duct is difficult because the

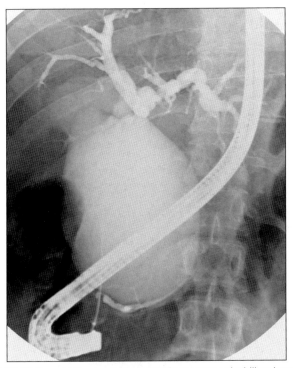

FIG 35.10 Type I biliary cyst. An anomalous pancreaticobiliary junction was also present.

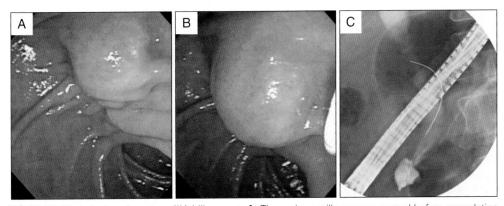

FIG 35.11 Choledochocele or type IIIA biliary cyst. **A,** The major papilla appears normal before cannulation. **B,** The intramural duct balloons outward after cholangiography. **C,** Cholangiography demonstrates a cystic dilation of the intraampullary common channel.

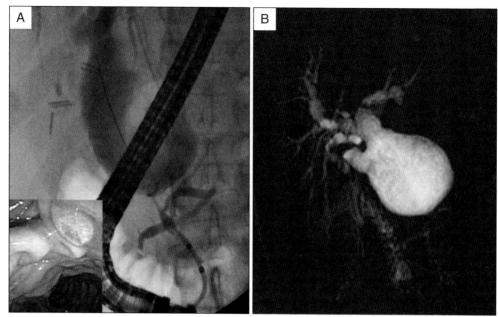

FIG 35.12 Type IVA biliary cysts. **A,** Anomalous pancreaticobiliary junction with a cyst of the common bile duct. Bile drains to the duodenum via the minor papilla (*inset*). **B,** Magnetic resonance cholangiopancreatography (MRCP) demonstrates both intrahepatic and extrahepatic cystic dilations of the bile ducts. (Images courtesy Dr. Naoki Takahashi.)

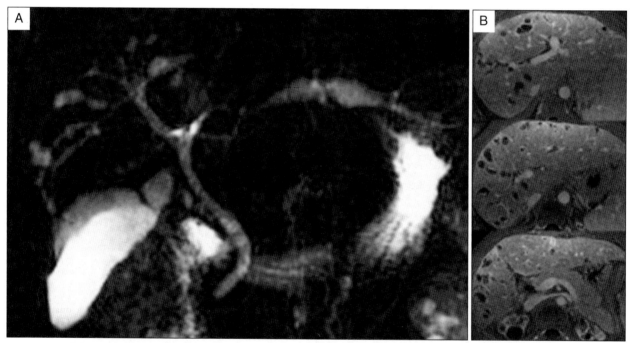

FIG 35.13 Type V biliary cysts (Caroli disease). Magnetic resonance cholangiopancreatography (MRCP; **A**) and cross-sectional magnetic resonance imaging (MRI; **B**) demonstrate segmental cystic dilations of the intrahepatic bile ducts. (Images courtesy Dr. Naoki Takahashi.)

lesion may be obscured in the large column of contrast required to obtain full cholangiography. Endoscopic ultrasonography (EUS) and intraductal ultrasonography (IDUS) are probably more sensitive than cholangiography for detection of early cholangiocarcinoma in this setting.

Types I, II, and IV biliary cysts are best treated with surgical resection, which manages local complications of the disease and decreases the risk of subsequent malignancy. Surgical drainage procedures such as cystenterostomy are associated with a higher rate of subsequent benign complications such as recurrent biliary stones, strictures, and cholangitis, as well as a persistently high cancer risk.[30,31] Efforts should be made to resect the entire intrapancreatic portion of type 1 cysts, to the pancreaticobiliary junction if necessary, because retained cyst remnants may develop stones or malignancy. Preoperative placement of a pancreatic duct stent may help the surgeon to determine the distal extent of resection of a type I cyst. Type IV cysts may require partial hepatectomy. Laparoscopic resection of types I and IV cysts appears to be safe and effective.[32] Although resection of a biliary cyst decreases the risk of cancer, cholangiocarcinoma may occur decades after complete cyst excision.[33]

Exceptions to the general principle of surgical resection include type III cysts or choledochoceles, which can be treated with endoscopic sphincterotomy[34] (type IIIA) or endoscopic resection[35] (type IIIB). Cancer is uncommon in choledochoceles but does occur,[34] and endoscopic biopsy of the cyst lining (to assess for dysplasia) should be considered at the time of endoscopic treatment and again 1 year later.

Although most type 1 cysts are best treated by surgical resection, endoscopic treatment may also be required, particularly in patients with stones in a long common ductal channel. IDUS is probably the most sensitive imaging test currently available to identify small tumors in unresected biliary cysts, but the accuracy of IDUS screening is unknown.

Patients with type V cysts (Caroli's disease) typically present with pain and cholangitis because of intrahepatic stones and sludge. The management of type V cysts varies based on the distribution of cysts, stones, and strictures within the liver. Hepatic resection is often performed, sometimes in combination with endoscopic or percutaneous treatment of disease in segments of the liver that are not resected. Liver transplantation may be required.[36]

PANCREATIC ANOMALIES

Pancreas Divisum

Embryology and Terminology

The embryologic development of the pancreatic ductal system is shown in Fig. 35.14. The pancreas develops from dorsal and ventral pancreatic buds that appear in the dorsal mesentery during the fifth week of embryologic development. The dorsal bud is larger and eventually forms the pancreatic tail, body, neck, and portions of head, including the uncinate process. The ventral bud arises together with the bile duct and eventually forms part of the periampullary pancreatic head. Growth and rotation of the duodenum bring the ventral bud around the posterior aspect of the duodenum toward the dorsal bud. The two buds fuse, as shown in Fig. 35.14. Typically the ducts within the buds also fuse, and the main pancreatic duct drains both the dorsal and ventral pancreas into the duodenum via the major papilla. In pancreas divisum the ducts do not fuse or fuse incompletely, and the dorsal pancreatic duct drains the bulk of pancreatic exocrine secretions into the duodenum via the minor papilla.

Pancreas divisum can be subdivided into cases in which there is no communication between the ventral and dorsal pancreas (complete pancreas divisum; Fig. 35.15) and cases in which the dorsal duct drains to the minor papilla and also communicates with the ventral pancreatic duct (incomplete pancreas divisum; Fig. 35.16). Patients with complete divisum usually have a small ventral pancreatic duct communicating with the major papilla, but this cannot always be demonstrated. Incomplete pancreas divisum is best used to describe cases in which a narrow connecting duct joins the ventral and dorsal pancreas, and the bulk of pancreatic exocrine secretion drains through the minor papilla (dominant dorsal duct drainage) (see Fig. 35.16).

Diagnosis

Diagnosis of pancreas divisum can typically be made by computed tomography (CT), magnetic resonance imaging (MRI), or EUS, although this may require review of diagnostic images with attention to the possibility of divisum. Pancreatography in complete divisum demonstrates a diminutive, arborizing ventral pancreatic duct in divisum,

which does not cross the midline (see Fig. 35.15). The pancreatic uncinate process is part of the dorsal pancreas, and the uncinate branch does not fill with major papilla injections in divisum, another clue to diagnosis.[37] When divisum is diagnosed on the basis of a ventral pancreatogram alone, the possibility of pseudodivisum (in which an obstruction of the main pancreatic duct in the head simulates divisum) should be considered (Fig. 35.17). Pseudodivisum typically causes an eccentric, rapidly tapering, or abrupt terminus of the ventral pancreatic duct, whereas in true divisum the ventral duct arborizes. In some clinical situations, cannulation of the minor papilla to confirm the diagnosis of divisum may be necessary to exclude pseudodivisum. With advances in imaging and EUS, pseudodivisum is rarely an enigma.

Association with Pancreatitis (see also Chapter 52)

Pancreas divisum probably contributes to the pathogenesis of pancreatic disease, but only in a small minority of persons with this anatomic variant. Pancreas divisum is common, with a prevalence of 5% to 10% at autopsy,[38,39] and a population-based MRI study found no association between divisum and either chronic pancreatitis or pancreatic exocrine insufficiency.[40] Because less than 0.1% of the population is admitted to hospital yearly with pancreatitis of any cause,[41] divisum must be asymptomatic in the great majority of affected persons. An early study found pancreas divisum in 25% of patients with idiopathic pancreatitis presenting for ERCP,[42] but in subsequent larger studies divisum was not seen more commonly in ERCP patients with a history of acute, chronic, or idiopathic pancreatitis compared with those with no history of pancreatic disease.[43] Referral bias may explain the high incidence of divisum seen at some centers. In one community-based study, the population incidence of divisum as determined by MRI was 2.6%, whereas 35% of consecutive patients with unexplained pancreatitis undergoing MRI had divisum.[44] Divisum was associated with idiopathic chronic and acute recurrent pancreatitis in that study but not lone bouts of acute pancreatitis. In many pancreatitis patients, divisum may be an incidental finding rather than a cause of disease.

Factors that may link divisum directly to pancreatitis include obstruction to outflow at the minor papilla and the presence of underlying genetic abnormalities associated with pancreatitis. A stenotic minor papilla orifice or spasm of the minor papilla sphincter[45] might result in divisum-related pancreatitis because of relative obstruction of dorsal duct drainage. Several lines of evidence lend some support to this hypothesis. In a surgical series, minor papilla sphincteroplasty was of most benefit in divisum patients whose minor papilla was stenotic by intraoperative assessment with lacrimal probes.[46] In a small randomized, prospective study, endoscopic stenting of the minor papilla resulted in significantly better outcomes than sham therapy in patients with pancreas divisum and at least two attacks of unexplained acute pancreatitis.[47] The occasional finding of a santorinicele, or a dilated terminus of the dorsal pancreatic duct in the duodenal wall, may also be taken as evidence of pancreatic outflow obstruction in some patients with pancreas divisum. Secretin-stimulated MRI in patients with santorinicele demonstrates larger pancreatic duct diameters and delayed drainage into the duodenum compared with divisum patients without a santorinicele.[48] Manometry of the minor papilla and dorsal pancreatic duct has shown increased dorsal duct pressures, although normal control data are not available.[45] In one small series, botulinum toxin injections into the minor papilla predicted subsequent response to minor papilla sphincterotomy, presumably by decreasing sphincter or duodenal wall contractions.[49]

The obstruction theory has led to widespread adoption of endoscopic therapy for idiopathic pancreatitis associated with pancreas divisum (see Chapters 14 and 21). In addition to the randomized controlled

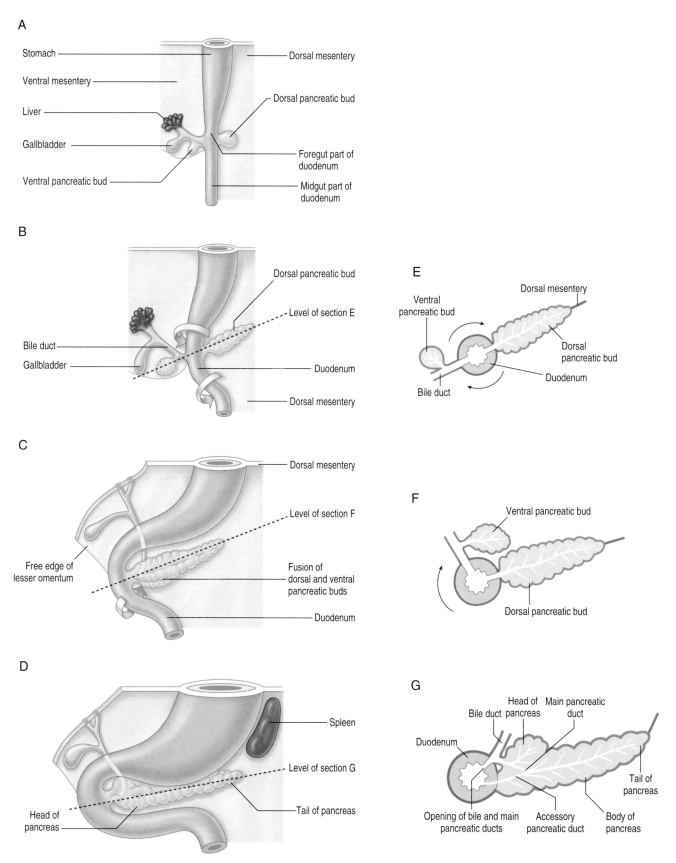

FIG 35.14 Embryologic development of the pancreas and pancreatic ductal system. (From Moore KL, Persaud TVN. *The developing human: clinically oriented embryology.* 7th ed. Philadelphia: Saunders; 2003. Reproduced with permission.)

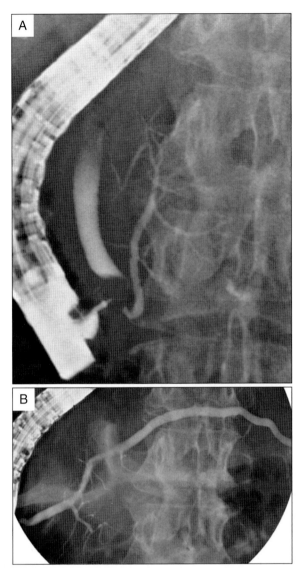

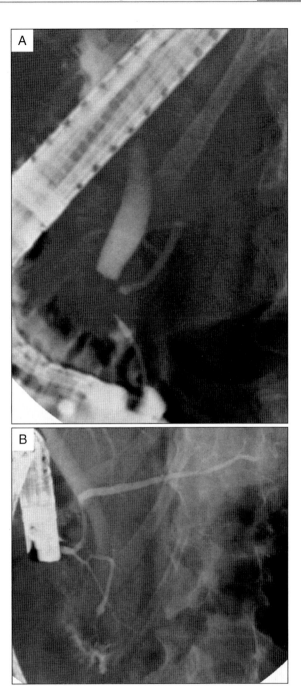

FIG 35.15 Complete pancreas divisum. **A,** Cannulation of the major papilla demonstrates an arborizing ventral pancreatic duct that does not cross the midline or give rise to an uncinate branch. **B,** Cannulation of the minor papilla demonstrates a dominant dorsal pancreatic duct, with no communication to the ventral pancreas. The uncinate branch arises from the dorsal pancreatic duct.

FIG 35.16 Incomplete pancreas divisum. **A,** Cannulation of the major papilla demonstrates a small ventral pancreatic duct without filling of the dorsal duct. **B,** Cannulation of the minor papilla demonstrates a dominant dorsal pancreatic duct with communication to the ventral pancreatic duct and major papilla. The uncinate branch arises from the dorsal pancreatic duct.

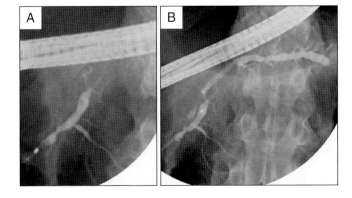

FIG 35.17 Pseudodivisum. **A,** Cannulation of the major papilla demonstrates an arborizing ventral pancreatic duct, suggestive of pancreas divisum, but with some filling of an irregular duct superiorly. **B,** With deep cannulation of the ventral pancreatic duct and further injection, a stricture of the main pancreatic duct is demonstrated. Biopsies showed adenocarcinoma.

series described above, uncontrolled surgical and endoscopic reports indicate that about 70% of persons with divisum and idiopathic recurrent acute pancreatitis will improve after sphincterotomy or stenting of the minor papilla. These relatively good outcomes are reported in patients with recurrent acute pancreatitis who have no evidence of chronic pancreatitis; patients with chronic pancreatitis and divisum are less likely to respond, and patients with chronic upper abdominal pain and no history of pancreatitis will improve only about 30% of the time.[50] A randomized trial of minor papilla sphincterotomy versus sham therapy in divisum patients with pain alone, reported in abstract form, did not show a significant benefit to endoscopic treatment.[51]

Difficulties with the obstruction theory persist. Those patients who respond best to endoscopic therapy do not have pancreatographic evidence of chronic ductal obstruction. Endoscopists have not developed a reliable method of assessing the minor papilla for stenosis or spasm at the time of ERCP: normal values for minor papilla manometry are not known, and delayed drainage has not been studied as a predictor of outcome after endoscopic treatment. More recent series report poorer response to endoscopic treatment than previously seen, with immediate improvement in the majority but later recurrence in most patients.[52-54] Finally, minor papilla cannulation and sphincterotomy carry increased risk of adverse events compared with ERCP performed at the major papilla.[55]

These difficulties have led investigators to look for other factors responsible for pancreatitis in divisum patients. An early study found cystic fibrosis transmembrane receptor (CFTR) gene mutations significantly more often in divisum patients with pancreatitis (22%) than in divisum patients without pancreatitis (0%).[56] The true prevalence of these mutations in persons with divisum and pancreatitis is probably higher, because about 1000 CFTR mutations have been described and the authors tested for 13 common mutations. CFTR function, assayed by nasal transepithelial potential difference testing, is intermediate between normal controls and classic cystic fibrosis in patients with divisum and pancreatitis, a result that parallels findings in other adult-onset, single-organ diseases linked to partial loss of CFTR function.[57] Divisum was found in 7% of patients with idiopathic pancreatitis and wild-type CFTR and PRSS1 (cationic trypsinogen) genes but was present in up to 47% of those with idiopathic pancreatitis and mutated alleles[58]; in another recent study, polymorphisms of the monocyte chemoattractant protein 1 gene (MCP-1) were common in patients with divisum and idiopathic pancreatitis.[59] The evidence increasingly suggests that underlying genetic variations may contribute to the development of pancreatitis in persons with pancreas divisum. In the case of CFTR, diminished function may result in more viscous pancreatic secretions, potentially contributing to ductal obstruction. There are currently no large series assessing whether genetic testing identifies divisum patients likely to benefit from endoscopic intervention. In one small study of 12 divisum patients, only 2 with diminished CFTR function improved after endoscopic or surgical therapy.[57]

A noninvasive test that identified obstruction to pancreatic duct outflow and predicted response to minor papilla therapy would be useful. Secretin-stimulated ultrasonography or MRI has been used for this purpose. After secretin administration, changes in pancreatic duct diameter are measured using either transabdominal ultrasonography, MRI, or EUS. Transient dilation of the pancreatic duct occurs after secretin administration in normal subjects, but ductal dilation of more than 1 mm persisting for at least 10 minutes after secretin administration may indicate ductal obstruction. In some series this technique has been a strong predictor of clinical response to minor papilla therapy in pancreas divisum.[46,60] Other investigators, however, have not reproduced these findings.[61] In one study, abnormal secretin ultrasonography results were seen after episodes of acute pancreatitis due to a variety of causes.[62]

The major concern with secretin-stimulated imaging is the potential for false-positive results; false-negative results are likely to be seen only in patients with chronic pancreatitis and exocrine insufficiency. Secretin MRI has theoretical advantages over secretin ultrasonography, because the entire pancreatic duct is visualized, and the timing and volume of pancreatic juice secretion into the duodenum can be estimated.[63,64] Currently the value of secretin MRI for predicting response to endoscopic therapy in pancreas divisum is unclear.

In summary, endoscopic minor papilla therapy probably helps a minority of patients with recurrent acute pancreatitis and pancreas divisum, but its role is limited, and optimal patient selection requires further clarification. A practical approach to divisum patients based on current evidence is to discourage endoscopic therapy in patients with pain alone or one episode of pancreatitis and to consider endoscopic therapy in those who have had at least two episodes of otherwise unexplained acute pancreatitis, recognizing that even these patients face a substantial chance of persistent or recurrent disease after endoscopic treatment. The possibility of genetic predisposition to pancreatitis should be discussed with divisum patients. Before endoscopic treatment, both secretin-stimulated MRI and genetic testing may be considered, although more data are needed regarding the predictive value of these tests. If testing is performed for CFTR mutations, it should include uncommon mutations associated with adult-onset, single-organ disease. If the patient is having frequent episodes of pancreatitis, botulinum toxin injection of the minor papilla may be considered as a therapeutic trial, based on limited data. Patients considering minor papilla sphincterotomy or stenting should be told about the variable outcomes reported with these interventions, the chance of recurrent symptoms, and the possibility of adverse events and postsphincterotomy stenosis.

Incomplete Pancreas Divisum

As discussed earlier, incomplete pancreas divisum is characterized by communicating ventral and dorsal pancreatic ducts, with a patent minor papilla and dominant dorsal pancreatic duct drainage. Despite having two routes of pancreatic drainage, some patients with incomplete divisum may nevertheless have symptoms related to pancreatic outflow obstruction, perhaps because of stenosis of both the major and minor papilla, or due to an underlying genetic predisposition to pancreatitis.

As with complete pancreas divisum, incomplete divisum is a common anatomic variant, and most persons with incomplete divisum are asymptomatic. It seems likely that incomplete divisum occasionally causes or contributes to disease, as in the reported case of an adult with acute relapsing pancreatitis, incomplete divisum, and a carcinoid tumor of the minor papilla causing partial obstruction.[65] However, the caveats discussed above regarding pancreas divisum are germane to incomplete divisum as well. There is no randomized controlled trial of endoscopic therapy for incomplete divisum, and convincing evidence of benefit from endoscopic treatment is lacking. Two series of endoscopic treatment for incomplete divisum report short-term improvement in 50% to 60% of patients, though without long-term follow-up.[66,67] Therapy was most successful in patients with recurrent acute pancreatitis. The decision to direct endoscopic treatment at the minor papilla, major papilla, or both is affected by the degree of dominant dorsal duct drainage.

Annular Pancreas

Annulus is the Latin word for ring, and an annular pancreas is a ringed pancreas partially or completely encircling the duodenum. As shown in Fig. 35.18, the likely embryologic basis of annular pancreas is encirclement of the duodenum by the ventral pancreas during duodenal rotation

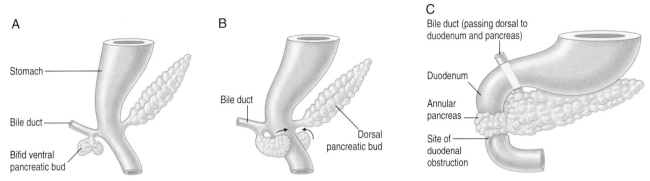

FIG 35.18 Embryologic basis of annular pancreas. (From Moore KL, Persaud TVN. *The Developing Human: Clinically Oriented Embryology.* 7th ed. Philadelphia: Saunders; 2003. Reproduced with permission.)

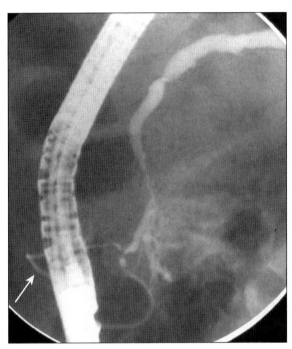

FIG 35.19 Annular pancreas. The ventral pancreatic duct encircles the second duodenum *(arrow)*. This patient also has a stricture of the main pancreatic duct, caused by pancreatic adenocarcinoma.

in the fifth to eighth week of fetal development. The encircling ring of pancreas typically involves the second duodenum or the apex of the duodenal bulb. The commonest clinical presentation of annular pancreas is duodenal obstruction, most often diagnosed in infancy but occasionally presenting later in life. Cases of annular pancreas associated with pancreatitis and pancreatic cancer have been reported, but it is unclear if annular pancreas predisposes to these diseases.

Annular pancreas in adults is typically diagnosed by CT. EUS is also useful for diagnosis, showing a ring of ventral pancreatic tissue encircling the duodenum proximal to the papilla. At pancreatography a ventral pancreatic duct is seen encircling the duodenum, as shown in Fig. 35.19.

The complete reference list for this chapter can be found online at www.expertconsult.com.

36

Dilated Bile Duct and Pneumobilia

Koushik K. Das and Michael L. Kochman

DILATED BILE DUCT

Defining Dilated Bile Ducts

There is no consensus definition for what constitutes a dilated bile duct. Rather, it is important to understand that the definition is contextual and depends on the site of measurement, the imaging modality used, and the clinical scenario. Even with parameters such as these, definitions can vary widely based on individual patient characteristics and imaging study characteristics. Dilation may be present in isolated intrahepatic ducts, diffusely in the intrahepatic ducts, in the extrahepatic duct, or combinations thereof. If dilation is secondary to obstruction in the distal duct, diffuse dilation of intrahepatic and extrahepatic bile ducts will usually be seen. If obstruction is at a more proximal site, focal intrahepatic dilation will usually be observed. Normal intrahepatic ducts as small as 1 to 2 mm are seen as scattered and nonconfluent biliary branches on abdominal computed tomography (CT) or ultrasonography, and become confluent and more easily imaged as they move centrally, with diameters exceeding 2 mm (Fig. 36.1).[1,2] Abnormally dilated intrahepatic ducts are present when duct diameter exceeds 40% of the diameter of the adjacent intrahepatic portal vein and when the ducts appear as parallel tubes coursing together.[1] An increase in diameter of the extrahepatic bile ducts, in particular the common hepatic duct (CHD) or common bile duct (CBD), is most often what is referred to as biliary dilation. The normal size of the duct varies at different levels, varies from person to person, and may even vary in estimation based on time of day, respiration, or patient positioning.[1-6]

The imaging modality used to evaluate the biliary system can influence the reported duct diameter.[2] Transabdominal ultrasonography (TUS) measures the internal diameter of the duct (Fig. 36.2).[3,7] Measurements of the CHD are typically obtained at the level of the hepatic artery in the porta hepatis, anterior to the main or right portal vein; measurements of the CBD are obtained more proximal to this site.[1,8] Using TUS, most studies have placed the upper limit of normal for the diameter of the CBD at 6 to 8 mm and that of the CHD at 6 mm.[1,8-10] However, a study using ultrasonography to measure CBD diameters in asymptomatic patients recorded normal values up to 8 to 10 mm.[9] This may reflect variation among operators obtaining the measurements and among interpreters of these imaging modalities. By CT, values of 8 to 10 mm are more commonly accepted as normal for the CBD (Fig. 36.3).[1,3] This difference is in part attributable to measurements performed at different locations along the duct. Unlike ultrasonography, CT can more easily image the midportion to distal portion of the CBD, which are often larger in diameter.[11] It also more readily identifies the fat around the duct, and measurements by CT generally include the duct wall. Evaluation of the biliary system with cholangiography, by either endoscopic retrograde cholangiopancreatography (ERCP) or percutaneous transhepatic cholangiography (PTC), may also yield results different from those with other imaging techniques. A study of 135 patients who underwent imaging of the extrahepatic bile ducts with ultrasonography and ERCP or PTC demonstrated normal duct size of up to 4 mm by ultrasonography compared with 10.4 and 10.6 mm by ERCP and PTC, respectively.[12] This was likely a result of radiographic magnification of the cholangiogram and may also reflect distension from contrast injection.

Patient characteristics can affect measurement of duct size. Some studies have shown that CBD diameters increase in older individuals,[9,13] prompting authors to suggest adding 0.4 mm to the upper limit of normal for duct size for each decade of life or 1 mm per decade of life after age 60 years.[14,15] However, results from a large TUS study of 1018 asymptomatic adults showed a slight trend toward an increase in duct size with age but not as large as previously reported, with a mean diameter of 3.6 mm at age 60 and 4 mm at age 85.[16] In this study, 99% of patients had a CBD diameter less than 7 mm. Since Oddi first predicted the phenomenon of ductal dilation after cholecystectomy in 1887,[17] some studies have found no dilation,[18,19] whereas others have found a slight trend.[20-23] In a study of 234 patients undergoing cholecystectomy, the CBD increased 1 to 2 mm after surgery from a mean of 5.9 mm before cholecystectomy to 6.1 mm at an average of 393 days after cholecystectomy.[21] Although most patients have minimal, if any, dilation after cholecystectomy, there are those who clearly manifest profound asymptomatic ductal dilation.

Given all possible circumstances that may affect the measurement of the extrahepatic biliary system, it is difficult to define an absolute measurement that will by itself yield satisfactory predictive values for pathologic dilation of the bile duct. Instead, duct diameter should be interpreted in the context of potential causes of obstructive or nonobstructive biliary dilation so that any pertinent findings from the clinical presentation or biochemical tests may be considered in the decision to pursue further diagnostic evaluation (Fig. 36.4).

Etiology

Dilated bile ducts may be secondary to obstructive lesions (neoplastic or benign; Table 36.1) or to nonobstructive lesions.[1,2,24-26] Benign etiologies of bile duct dilation include choledocholithiasis and, uncommonly in the United States, infections such as parasitic diseases. In one study, endoscopic ultrasonography (EUS) was used in the evaluation of a dilated biliary tree in 90 patients with a nondiagnostic TUS, and the study found that 40 patients had choledocholithiasis, 13 malignancy, 8 benign stricture, 2 choledochal cysts, and 1 ascariasis, and in 24 there was no evidence of an obstructing lesion.[27] Other studies have confirmed common causes of biliary obstruction leading to ductal dilation, in order of decreasing prevalence: choledocholithiasis, pancreatic cancer, ampullary carcinoma, and cholangiocarcinoma.[2,16,28]

Clinical Evaluation

A thorough history should be obtained, including history of malignancy and the presence or absence of symptoms such as abdominal pain,

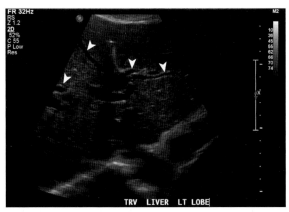

FIG 36.1 Transabdominal ultrasonography examination demonstrating intrahepatic ductal dilation (*arrowheads*).

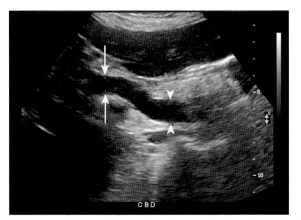

FIG 36.2 Transabdominal ultrasonography examination demonstrating a dilated common bile duct (*arrowheads*) and dilated common hepatic duct (*arrows*).

fever, weight loss, jaundice, pruritus, acholic stools, dark urine, or steatorrhea. The physical examination may be limited in its utility, but special attention should be paid to the presence of abdominal tenderness or mass, hepatomegaly, jaundice, or lymphadenopathy. A positive history or physical examination may serve to lower the threshold for further diagnostic evaluation in those patients with an equivocal duct size on initial imaging.

Biochemical Evaluation

Integral to the biochemical evaluation of obstruction are serum bilirubin and liver-associated enzymes (LAEs) (alkaline phosphatase [AP], alanine

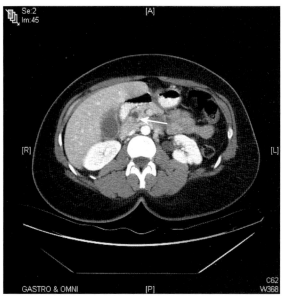

FIG 36.3 Abdominal computed tomography demonstrating a dilated common bile duct (*arrow*) in a patient with choledocholithiasis.

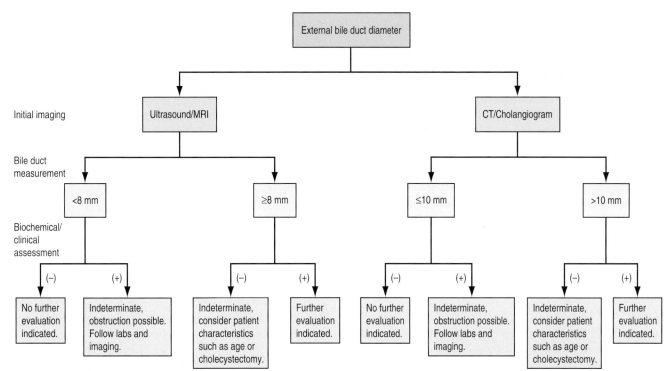

FIG 36.4 Algorithm for assessment of the common bile duct for obstruction. *CT,* Computed tomography; *MRI,* magnetic resonance imaging.

TABLE 36.1   Common Causes of Biliary Obstruction

Intrahepatic	Porta Hepatis	Suprapancreatic	Intrapancreatic
Primary sclerosing cholangitis (PSC)	Cholangiocarcinoma	Pancreatic carcinoma	Pancreatic carcinoma
Space-occupying liver lesion	PSC	Cholangiocarcinoma	Pancreatitis
	Gallbladder carcinoma	Metastatic disease	Choledocholithiasis
	Hepatocellular carcinoma	Direct extension and nodal metastases of gastric/colon/gallbladder carcinoma	Ampullary stenosis/carcinoma
	Malignant lymph nodes		Duodenal carcinoma
	Liver metastases	Carcinoma	Cholangiocarcinoma
	Nodal metastases	Pancreatitis	PSC
		PSC	

aminotransferase [ALT], and aspartate aminotransferase [AST]). The principal markers of cholestasis are elevated bilirubin and AP.[29–31] The total bilirubin present in the serum represents a balance between input from production and output from hepatobiliary clearance. In obstructive jaundice the serum bilirubin is principally conjugated (water soluble). Transient elevations of AST/ALT within 1 to 2 days with levels into the thousands may occur in acute CBD obstruction, from trauma, or more typically in the presence of choledocholithiasis with subsequent rapidly declining levels.[29–31] Aminotransferase levels may also rise from other subacute or chronic obstructions but typically remain less than 500 IU/dL. Hepatobiliary AP is present on the apical membrane of the hepatocyte and in the luminal bile duct epithelium. Increases in AP result from increased synthesis and release into the serum. As a result, levels may not rise until 1 to 2 days after biliary obstruction occurs. In addition, the enzyme has a half-life of 1 week and may therefore remain elevated for several days after the resolution of biliary obstruction. Levels of AP up to three times normal are relatively nonspecific and occur in a variety of liver diseases. However, higher elevations are more specific for biliary obstruction (intrahepatic or extrahepatic) and infiltrating liver diseases. As AP can be produced in sources outside the liver, it may be necessary in certain instances to use other biochemical tests such as the AP isoenzymes, gamma-glutamyl transpeptidase, or 5′-nucleotidase to confirm a hepatobiliary etiology of an elevated AP.

In general, there is an increased likelihood of choledocholithiasis with abnormalities in bilirubin, AP, and transaminase levels. It would be unusual for a lesion to cause biliary obstruction and dilation without any clinical or biochemical abnormality. However, this is not universal, and there have been case reports of patients with normal LAEs in the presence of dilated ducts and choledocholithiasis.[32] In the era of laparoscopic cholecystectomy, models of clinical features in addition to biochemical values have been developed to predict choledocholithiasis before surgery.[29,33–35] More recently, the American Society for Gastrointestinal Endoscopy has adopted guidelines for the evaluation of suspected choledocholithiasis, grouping presenting factors as being very strong (CBD stone on abdominal ultrasonography, clinical ascending cholangitis, bilirubin >4 mg/dL), strong (dilated CBD on abdominal ultrasonography >6 mm, bilirubin 1.8 to 4 mg/dL), and moderate (abnormal liver biochemical tests, age older than 55 years, clinical gallstone pancreatitis[36]).[37] The presence of very strong predictors or strong predictors should trigger further evaluation with ERCP.

Imaging

Imaging of the biliary tract continues to evolve with the enhancement of noninvasive techniques for cross-sectional evaluation and with biliary reconstruction techniques. Each technique has strengths and limitations in the common goal of confirming the presence of an obstruction and defining its location, extent, and etiology.

Transabdominal Ultrasonography

Transabdominal ultrasonography (TUS) is often the first-line imaging technique in the evaluation of the bile duct, gallbladder, and liver, as it is widely available, is noninvasive, is inexpensive, and can be performed rapidly. It does, however, require experience in technique and interpretation and may be limited (particularly in the distal bile duct) because of interference from gas within the surrounding bowel or body habitus. TUS is highly sensitive and specific for both cholelithiasis (up to 99%) and biliary ductal dilation (more than 90%).[8,38–41] However, the ability of ultrasonography to define the site and cause of biliary obstruction is less reliable. Estimates of sensitivity of ultrasonography for determining the level of obstruction range from 27% to 95% and the etiology of the obstruction from 23% to 81%.[40,42–45] Because of overlying bowel gas, the distal CBD is well visualized only in 40% to 50% of patients.[8] Clearly the ease of use, widespread availability, and few contraindications place TUS early in the algorithm for evaluation of the biliary tract, but further studies are often needed, as it is often inconclusive because it does not provide adequate information in the setting of suspected neoplasms.

Computed Tomography

Multidetector CT can obtain images at thin 1.25-mm to 2.5-mm intervals to create excellent axial images and reproductions of the biliary tree.[1,11,46,47] Although unenhanced scans can highlight the presence of calcification, intravenous (IV) contrast agents are necessary to provide vascular landmarks and organ opacification to maximize visualization of the bile ducts.[46] CT cholangiography, used extensively in Asia and Europe, employs the administration of IV contrast material to highlight the biliary tree. However, biliary obstruction limits contrast excretion into the bile ducts and there is a higher incidence of adverse reactions to contrast agents.[48] In a study evaluating the presence of biliary obstruction, defined as extrahepatic bile duct diameter >8 mm, the sensitivity and specificity of CT for diagnosing dilated ducts were 96% and 91%, respectively.[46] CT is also accurate at defining the level of obstruction in 88% to 97% of cases and the cause of obstruction in 70% to 95% of cases.[45,46,49,50] However, there are several limitations to CT, including the need for IV contrast for enhanced images, which may lead to adverse reactions, including potential nephrotoxicity. It also lacks sensitivity for a common cause of obstruction, choledocholithiasis, as 20% to 25% of biliary stones are isoattenuating with bile, making them difficult to detect on CT.[1,46] Sensitivity of CT for choledocholithiasis ranges from 70% to 94%, depending on the use of indirect signs of obstruction that typically coincide with choledocholithiasis.[1,51,52]

Magnetic Resonance Imaging

Since it was first introduced in 1991, magnetic resonance cholangiopancreatography (MRCP) has gained popularity as a noninvasive

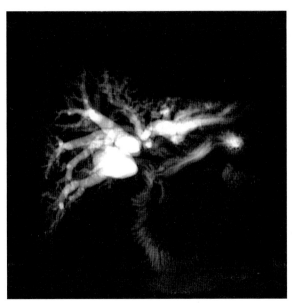

FIG 36.5 Magnetic resonance cholangiopancreatography image demonstrating markedly dilated bile ducts proximal to a Klatskin-type bile duct tumor.

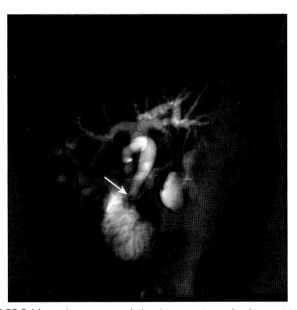

FIG 36.6 Magnetic resonance cholangiopancreatography demonstrating choledocholithiasis (arrow).

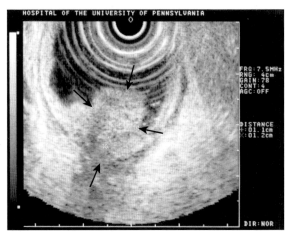

FIG 36.7 Radial endoscopic ultrasonography demonstrating ampullary adenoma (arrows).

modality for imaging of the biliary system. The static or slow-moving fluid within the pancreatic and biliary system produces a different signal compared with solid tissue.[24,25] Images can be obtained without use of IV contrast and are routinely performed in the axial and coronal planes (Figs. 36.5 and 36.6). MRCP has high accuracy in detecting the level and cause of biliary obstruction. It has been shown to have a sensitivity of 91% to 97% and specificity of up to 99% for the diagnosis of biliary obstruction.[28,53–55] Unlike TUS and CT, which can be limited in their ability to correctly identify the level and etiology of an obstructed biliary system, MRCP can more accurately define these parameters, similar to the use of direct cholangiography. The level of obstruction can be determined by MRCP in 87% to 98% of cases.[28,53,55–57] A large

meta-analysis confirmed a sensitivity and specificity of MRCP of 92% and 97%, respectively, for cholelithiasis and 88% and 95%, respectively, for malignancy.[53] However, the reported accuracy in discerning a benign from a malignant obstruction has varied from 30% to 98% across studies, with a mean accuracy of 88% reported in a meta-analysis. Adding conventional T1-weighted and T2-weighted images to MRCP allows for the evaluation of extraductal soft tissue, increasing the diagnostic accuracy by demonstrating tumor extension, lymph nodes, or metastatic disease.[57,58] In one study this increased the sensitivity, specificity, and accuracy 17% to 20% for differentiation of benign and malignant causes of biliary obstruction.[59]

The major advantages of MRCP over other imaging techniques are the avoidance of invasive procedures, IV contrast, and ionizing radiation and the ability to visualize the biliary system above and below an obstruction. However, it is unnecessary in cases where there is a high pretest probability of a need for intervention (e.g., cholangitis in the setting of suspected choledocholithiasis).[37] Technical and interpretive difficulties can simulate or miss pathologic conditions of the biliary system. Static images demonstrating a contraction of the sphincter of Oddi can simulate a stenosis, for example.[60] Other drawbacks include its high cost; the extended time to perform an examination, leading to patient intolerance; and contraindications such as implanted metallic objects.

Endoscopic Ultrasonography

Endoscopic ultrasonography (EUS) allows for diagnostic evaluation of the pancreaticobiliary system with high-resolution images obtained from a transgastric or transduodenal position.[61–63] Unlike TUS, EUS allows for superior visualization of the extrahepatic biliary tree without the interference of bowel gas as the CBD passes posterior to the duodenal bulb. Additionally, EUS offers accurate and systematic visualization of the wall of the duodenum, including the papillary region (Fig. 36.7). In the setting of choledocholithiasis, EUS has consistently demonstrated sensitivities >90% and specificities up to 100%.[63–68] EUS may be particularly useful for detecting microlithiasis (stones <3 mm), though such small stones would be less likely to lead to biliary obstruction and dilation (Fig. 36.8).[68,69] The close proximity of the stomach and duodenum to the pancreas allows for sensitive evaluation of pancreatic lesions such as neoplasms and cysts, which may lead to biliary obstruction. EUS has demonstrated greater sensitivity than other imaging modalities in the detection of pancreatic carcinoma, especially small lesions, with sensitivities and accuracies ≥90% (Fig. 36.9).[70–73]

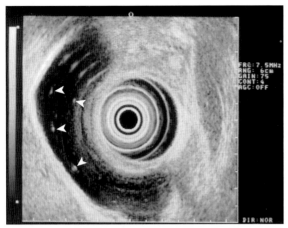

FIG 36.8 Radial endoscopic ultrasonography demonstrating microlithiasis (*arrowheads*).

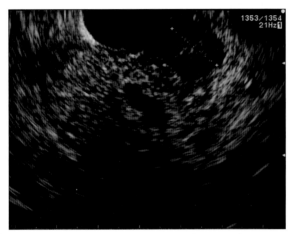

FIG 36.9 Radial endoscopic ultrasonography demonstrating a pancreatic head carcinoma.

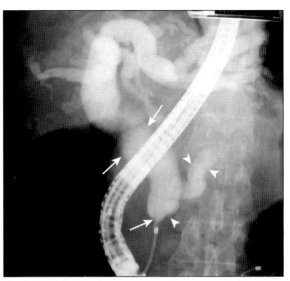

FIG 36.10 Endoscopic retrograde cholangiopancreatography demonstrating a "double-duct" sign in pancreatic carcinoma with proximal biliary dilation (*arrows*) and dilated pancreatic duct (*arrowheads*).

common location for cholangiocarcinoma, with ERCP and MRCP demonstrated both to be very effective at detecting the presence of obstruction, with a sensitivity of 100%.[75,76] However, MRCP was superior in its ability to image the biliary tree cephalad to the obstruction and to characterize the intraductal extension. ERCP and EUS remain the best means of diagnosing ampullary cancers because of direct visualization and the ability to biopsy.[39,62,76]

Biliary Scintigraphy

Scintigraphy employs the administration of IV radioisotopes to evaluate the biliary system. The radioisotopes are taken up by the hepatocytes and excreted into the bile with concentration in the gallbladder. The sensitivity and specificity for biliary obstruction in patients with jaundice are 97% and 89%, respectively, based on the duration until the appearance of radiotracer in the duodenum.[77] This test may help elucidate whether obstruction is present in the setting of a dilated bile duct, but little, if any, information is gained regarding the etiology of obstruction.

Approach to the Dilated Duct

The heterogeneity of techniques in defining an upper limit of normal for duct size makes it difficult to assign a value representing pathologic dilation. In general, a CBD with diameter >7 mm on ultrasonography or >10 mm on CT should be considered abnormal, because diameters less than these are rarely seen in the presence of biliary obstruction. However, these are not absolute diameters, and based on the anatomic information from the initial imaging study and the clinical and biochemical assessment of the patient, one must estimate the clinical probability that an underlying obstructive lesion is present and will require further evaluation (Fig. 36.11). The subsequent approach must be individualized based on the clinical scenario, with consideration of the possible underlying etiology. In clinically stable patients, the algorithm should start with noninvasive testing. However, patients presenting with obstruction and signs and symptoms of cholangitis (fever, right-upper-quadrant abdominal pain, jaundice) may require diagnostic and therapeutic intervention acutely; ERCP would be an appropriate initial procedure. Patients without an emergent indication for biliary drainage will likely benefit from cross-sectional imaging with either CT or magnetic

The limitations of EUS for the evaluation of biliary dilation include poor visualization of obstructive lesions located more proximally in the biliary system, such as in the hilum or in the right hepatic duct. Poor visualization of the distal CBD also occurs when the pancreas is markedly calcified, during an episode of acute pancreatitis, when there is altered anatomy such as from previous gastric surgery, and when there is air within the biliary tract from prior iatrogenic interventions. Adverse events from diagnostic EUS are uncommon and similar to upper endoscopy, with a major adverse event rate of approximately 0.5%.[74]

Cholangiography

Cholangiography performed via ERCP, percutaneously (PTC) or intraoperatively (IOC), remains the gold standard for assessment of the bile duct. Each route affords an anatomic view of the bile ducts and a functional assessment of biliary drainage. PTC should be employed only for patients who warrant therapeutic biliary intervention but are not candidates for ERCP, those with inaccessible papillae, or after failed endoscopic biliary access. With recent advances in MRCP, purely diagnostic indications for ERCP have been significantly reduced given the invasive nature and increased risk of adverse events of the latter (see Chapters 7 and 8). In some scenarios, such as the diagnosis of pancreatic cancer, ERCP has an inferior sensitivity to MRCP (70% vs 84%) (Fig. 36.10).[57] Evaluation of perihilar biliary obstruction, the most resonance imaging (MRI)/MRCP (depending on contraindications to IV contrast with CT, intolerance of MRI, and metal objects precluding MRI). Availability of testing, cost, patient characteristics, and probability of the underlying etiology must be considered when choosing between these tests. Based on the findings from subsequent imaging, more invasive procedures such as EUS or ERCP may be needed to obtain tissue for definitive diagnosis (Fig. 36.12).

PNEUMOBILIA

Defining and Imaging Pneumobilia

Pneumobilia is defined as the presence of air in the biliary system, indicating a possible communication between the biliary system and the gastrointestinal tract. This is generally represented by the collection of isolated bubbles of air ranging from 2 to 5 mm within the biliary system and most commonly clustered in a central location toward the liver hilum (Fig. 36.13).[78] Pneumobilia may appear on plain supine abdominal radiography with an air bubble accumulation in the left intrahepatic duct and the CBD, creating the shape of a saber.[78–80] However, it is more commonly identified incidentally on ultrasonography or CT. Ultrasonography will identify pneumobilia as multiple highly reflective areas in the liver, often with prominent shadowing

behind. In fact, a study comparing 25 patients with pneumobilia with concurrent ultrasound and CT imaging demonstrated that CT better characterized this finding.[81] On ultrasonography, pneumobilia may be seen in conjunction with emphysematous cholecystitis, leading to the "effervescent gallbladder" sign, though this finding is not pathognomonic.[82] On CT scan, pneumobilia is generally seen as a branching pattern of air. Additionally, reflux of oral contrast material in the biliary duct may be seen and can support the diagnosis of pneumobilia. CT can also suggest an etiology to the presence of the pneumobilia. For example, it may identify biliary stents or the presence of dilated bile ducts; it may suggest the possible diagnosis of cholangitis with inflammatory stranding of the bile duct or the presence of cholecystitis; or it may confirm postsurgical anatomy or anastomoses. In addition to CT, MRI/MRCP, especially with the combination of both T1-weighted and T2-weighted images, is highly sensitive and specific for intrahepatic pneumobilia.[83] Once identified on imaging, pneumobilia must be differentiated from portal venous air, as the two entities may have similar appearance on ultrasonography and may require CT scan with contrast to differentiate. Portal venous air tends to appear more confluent, may extend to the liver capsule, and may have a more branching pattern than pneumobilia. The use of IV contrast can assist in localizing the identified air bubbles.[81] Ultimately, a complete analysis of history and physical

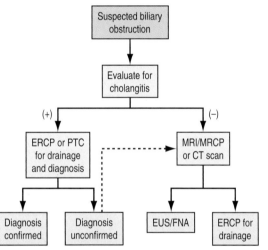

FIG 36.11 Algorithm for the evaluation of an obstructed bile duct. *CT*, Computed tomography; *ERCP*, endoscopic retrograde cholangiopancreatography; *EUS*, endoscopic ultrasonography; *FNA*, fine-needle aspiration; *MRCP*, magnetic resonance cholangiopancreatography; *MRI*, magnetic resonance imaging; *PTC*, percutaneous transhepatic cholangiography.

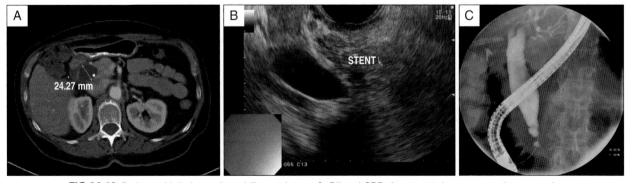

FIG 36.12 Patient with indeterminate biliary stricture. **A,** Dilated CBD documented on computed tomography scan. **B,** Dilated CBD documented on radial endoscopic ultrasonography. **C,** Dilated CBD documented on endoscopic retrograde cholangiopancreatography. *CBD,* Common bile duct.

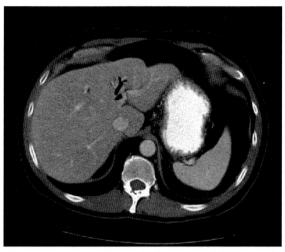

FIG 36.13 Computed tomography scan demonstrating pneumobilia in a patient after endoscopic retrograde cholangiopancreatography.

TABLE 36.2	**Etiology of Pneumobilia**		
Surgical Pneumobilia	**Sphincter of Oddi Incompetence**	**Biliary-Enteric Fistula**	**Infection**
Choledochoduodenostomy	Post-ERCP sphincterotomy	Passage of stone	Cholecystitis
Choledochojejunostomy	Passage of stone	Malignancy	Liver abscess
Pancreaticoduodenectomy	Endoscopy	Liver abscess	Ascariasis
	Blunt trauma	Peptic ulcer disease	
	Ascariasis		

ERCP, Endoscopic retrograde cholangiopancreatography.

findings must be completed to determine the clinical significance of this finding.

Etiology

The etiology of pneumobilia is generally attributable to one of four possible causes: surgical manipulation of the biliary system, incompetence of the sphincter of Oddi, benign or malignant fistulas, or infection (Table 36.2). Surgically created anastomoses between the biliary system and the small intestine can result in free communication of air between the biliary system and the gastrointestinal lumen. Most commonly, pneumobilia is seen secondary to choledochoduodenostomy, choledochojejunostomy, or pancreaticoduodenectomy (Whipple procedure) and is without clinical significance.[78] Pneumobilia secondary to incompetence of the sphincter of Oddi is expected after ERCP with biliary sphincterotomy and is a clinically insignificant entity. Prior biliary sphincterotomy is the most common etiology of pneumobilia. Sphincter of Oddi incompetence can also result after passage of stones through the ampulla of Vater. Additionally, several case reports have documented pneumobilia after upper endoscopy or double-balloon enteroscopy, in which it is hypothesized that the high pressure of air in the bowel lumen overcame the pressure of the sphincter of Oddi, resulting in transient pneumobilia.[84] Pneumobilia has also been rarely reported after blunt abdominal trauma, possibly because of a similar mechanism.[85] Pneumobilia secondary to iatrogenic or noniatrogenic sphincter of Oddi incompetence is generally benign and requires no further evaluation. Pneumobilia may also occur in response to spontaneous biliary-enteric fistulas. Fistulas between the biliary system and the intestine most commonly form as a consequence of cholelithiasis

with resultant necrosis and inflammation. However, malignancy and, rarely, peptic ulcer disease can result in fistulas between the biliary tract and the enteric system.[86–89] Although cholecystoduodenal fistula represents the majority (70%) of these fistulas, cholecystocolic fistula, cholecystogastric fistula, or choledochoduodenal fistula may occur.[78,89,90] Biliary-enteric fistula can result in the rare adverse event of gallstone ileus. Additionally, gastric outlet obstruction secondary to stone impaction in the duodenal bulb after the passage of a stone through a cholecystogastric or cholecystoduodenal fistula may occur, known as Bouveret syndrome.[91,92] These entities are diagnosed by a combination of clinical symptoms, radiographic imaging, and endoscopic evaluation. The final etiology for pneumobilia is secondary to infection. This can include the subcategories of gas-producing infection, such as those seen in association with emphysematous cholecystitis or cholangitis, liver abscess (e.g., caused by Klebsiella infection), and parasitic infections such as ascariasis, which can lead to obstruction of the sphincter of Oddi and pneumobilia.[78,93]

Clinical Evaluation

The clinical history and physical examination may be useful in identifying the etiology of pneumobilia and determining the urgency with which treatment (if any) is needed. A history of prior surgical intervention or ERCP with biliary sphincterotomy or stent placement obviates further evaluation or clinical intervention. However, the absence of this history raises the concern for infection or fistula. On physical examination, the presence of signs or symptoms of infection is important to recognize. Right-upper-quadrant abdominal pain or a positive Murphy sign narrows the differential diagnosis.

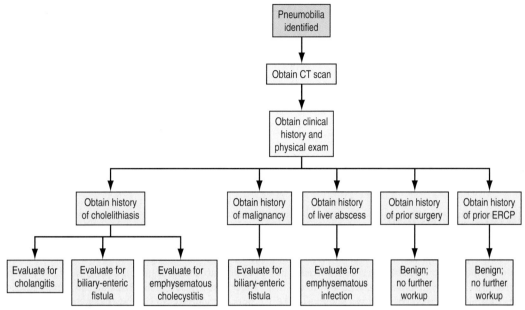

FIG 36.14 Algorithm for the evaluation of pneumobilia. *CT,* Computed tomography; *ERCP,* endoscopic retrograde cholangiopancreatography.

Approach to the Patient With Pneumobilia

The initial step in the evaluation of pneumobilia is to obtain a CT scan to further characterize the finding of air in the liver. Review of the CT scan is essential to confirm the presence of air in the biliary tree compared with the portal vein. Subsequently, a thorough history should be gathered to determine whether the patient has had any endoscopic or surgical procedure within his or her lifetime that may explain the findings. This will remove the most common causes of pneumobilia, including incompetence of the sphincter of Oddi through sphincterotomy or stone passage and postsurgical anatomy. If these are not present, the patient should be evaluated for biliary-enteric fistula or biliary infection such as cholangitis or emphysematous cholecystitis. Symptoms may be similar in these two entities and evaluation of underlying cholelithiasis or malignancy must be considered (Fig. 36.14).

The complete reference list for this chapter can be found online at www.expertconsult.com.

37

The Dilated Pancreatic Duct

Douglas G. Adler and Michelle A. Anderson

BACKGROUND AND DEFINITIONS

The pancreas arises in utero from the fusion of the ventral and dorsal pancreatic buds. The dorsal pancreatic bud gives rise to the pancreatic body and tail, and the ventral pancreatic bud gives rise to the pancreatic head and uncinate process. The main pancreatic duct (also known as the duct of Wirsung) forms when the dorsal and ventral pancreatic buds fuse at the genu (or neck), with the primary location for pancreatic drainage into the duodenum being the major papilla, also referred to as the ampulla of Vater. A remnant of the dorsal pancreatic bud that is in continuity with the minor papilla contains the duct of Santorini. In patients with pancreas divisum, occurring in approximately 7% to 10% of the population, the major route of pancreatic drainage is through the duct of Santorini and the minor papilla rather than the major papilla.

The average dimension of the pancreatic duct varies from patient to patient and with respect to its location within the pancreas. In general, the main pancreatic duct diameter is approximately 3 to 4 mm in the head, 2 to 3 mm in the body, and 1 to 2 mm in the tail. Pancreatic duct dilation would then refer to a ductal dimension that exceeds the accepted upper limit of normal at each anatomic section. Causes for dilation of the pancreatic duct can broadly be divided into those associated with benign conditions and those associated with malignant or premalignant conditions (Box 37.1). In some patients the pancreatic duct can dilate physiologically with age in the absence of a disease state.

When a duct is distended relative to the downstream duct, it can be considered dilated even if it falls within the normal range. In other words, the pancreatic duct should taper as one moves from head to body to tail. When this pattern is not seen, underlying pathology may be present. This frequently occurs in the setting of a focal stricture or obstructing mass lesion. In contrast, it is normal to have a focal narrowing at the genu without upstream dilation, as this represents the location of fusion between the dorsal and ventral pancreatic ducts.

Several clinical and autopsy studies have suggested that the pancreatic duct likely dilates with age in the absence of underlying pancreatic pathology. In one autopsy study of 112 patients without known pancreatic disease, 18 (16%) had pancreatic duct diameters greater than 4 mm. This becomes important when a physician is asked to evaluate a patient with an asymptomatic dilated pancreatic duct—a very common reason for consultation.[1] Hastier and colleagues compared pancreatograms obtained at endoscopic retrograde cholangiopancreatography (ERCP) from 105 subjects older than 70 years with those obtained from a control group of patients younger than 50 years.[2] Subjects with pancreatic pathology were excluded from both cohorts. These authors found that the mean main pancreatic duct diameter in the head of the pancreas was 2 mm wider (5.3 mm compared with 3.3 mm, $p < 0.05$) in the older cohort and that 20% of the subjects in the elderly group had pancreatic duct diameters that were more than two standard deviations above normal. In a prospective endoscopic ultrasonography (EUS) study of age-related changes in the pancreas, patients older than 60 years had wider pancreatic ducts in the head of the pancreas [median diameter in mm (interquartile range) = 2.9 (2.2 to 3.5)] than patients younger than 40 years [2.0 (1.6 to 2.2)].[3] Similarly, duct diameters in the pancreatic body were greater in patients older than 60 years, at 1.8 (1.3 to 2.1), compared with 1.5 (1.2 to 2.0) in patients younger than 40 years, whereas duct diameters in the tail of the pancreas did not differ significantly between these two groups.

EVALUATION

Clinical

A patient with a dilated pancreatic duct may present with abdominal pain, acute or chronic pancreatitis, exocrine insufficiency, or a pancreatic duct leak, or may be completely asymptomatic. Often the dilated pancreatic duct is detected as an incidental finding on a cross-sectional imaging study that was ordered to investigate a completely different problem, such as a computed tomography (CT) scan to evaluate for nephrolithiasis.

The most important aspect is the clinical setting (patient characteristics, symptoms, associated imaging features) in which the abnormality is found, and thus a detailed history is imperative. Abdominal pain associated with pancreatic ductal dilation is thought to result from increased pressure within the duct, as well as the related parenchymal hypertension and localized ischemia and inflammation. If a dilated duct is found in the setting of concomitant weight loss, a double-duct sign (biliary duct dilation in concert with pancreatic duct dilation), presence of pancreatic atrophy found on imaging studies, and other "red flag" symptoms such as new-onset or worsening diabetes mellitus or depression, the chance of malignancy being present is substantial (Fig. 37.1). Alternatively, if the patient has significant pain with pancreatic calcifications on imaging tests, then a diagnosis of chronic pancreatitis with associated pancreatic duct distension with or without a downstream stricture is more likely. In this case a history of recurrent bouts of acute pancreatitis is reassuring, although patients with chronic pancreatitis can harbor malignancy.

If the patient is truly asymptomatic, it may influence the decision regarding further treatment or investigation. This is particularly true if the patient is of an advanced age or has multiple and/or significant comorbidities, wherein a potential endoscopic procedure or surgical resection may not affect the natural history of the disease or improve the length or quality of life. In contrast, because one-third of patients with isolated pancreatic duct dilation without chronic pancreatitis are diagnosed with an underlying pancreatic malignancy, it is generally prudent to obtain further diagnostic information in the majority of patients.[4]

BOX 37.1   Differential Diagnosis of the Dilated Pancreatic Duct

Benign
- Chronic pancreatitis (with and without pancreatic stones or strictures)
- Ampullary stenosis
- Iatrogenic (e.g., stent-induced stricture, stricture of surgical anastomosis)
- Pancreas divisum
- Obstructing cystic lesions (e.g., serous cystadenoma, pseudocyst)
- Pancreatic necrosis leading to disconnected pancreatic duct
- Age associated
- Idiopathic
- Cystic fibrosis

Malignant or Premalignant
- Pancreatic adenocarcinoma
  - Ampullary adenoma or adenocarcinoma
  - Intraductal pancreatic mucinous neoplasm
  - Mucinous cystadenoma or cystadenocarcinoma with obstruction of main pancreatic duct

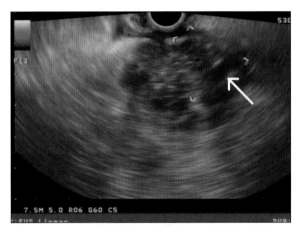

FIG 37.1 A 7.5-MHz endoscopic ultrasonography image of a pancreatic body mass detected in a patient with a dilated pancreatic duct found as an incidental finding on a noncontrast computed tomography scan to rule out nephrolithiasis. The mass is well seen as a hypoechoic solid lesion, and the pancreatic duct (*arrow*) is dilated and obstructed by the mass itself.

Laboratory Evaluation

Laboratory values can help to identify signs of pancreatic inflammation and exocrine insufficiency with associated fat malabsorption and steatorrhea. The presence of elevated serum tumor markers may raise the suspicion for malignant lesions, though their relative specificity and sensitivity can vary depending on cutoff values and comorbid conditions.

Serum Amylase and Lipase

These values can be elevated in the setting of pancreatitis, pancreatic cystic lesions, and pancreatic neoplasms. Amylase and lipase levels may also be increased in the absence of pancreatic disease in the setting of renal insufficiency, intestinal injury, or gastrointestinal ischemia. Some healthy individuals will manifest elevated serum amylase and lipase levels in the absence of any pancreatic parenchymal or ductal disease.[5] Nevertheless, a serum lipase greater than three times the upper limit of the normal level is a reliable diagnostic criterion for acute pancreatitis in the appropriate clinical setting. In patients with chronic pancreatitis,

normal levels of amylase and lipase do not exclude a flare of acute pancreatitis. Persistent but mild elevations can be seen in chronic pancreatitis.

Fecal Fat

Elevated levels of fecal fat imply an element of fat malabsorption, typically from exocrine pancreatic insufficiency. This can be tested in a qualitative manner as a one-time stool test. A timed quantitative 72-hour cumulative collection can be used as a screening or confirmatory test in the setting of a high-fat diet (often 100 g/day). The upper level of normal is a measurement greater than 7 g of fat per 24-hour period.

Fecal Elastase-1 and Chymotrypsin

The fecal elastase-1 test is used to measure the concentration of elastase-3B enzyme in the stool, a zymogen that is secreted by the pancreas. Levels of less than 200 µg/g of stool suggest exocrine pancreatic insufficiency.

Serum CA 19-9

CA 19-9 has limited utility as a screening test and is commonly employed as a surveillance test for disease recurrence in those patients in whom levels are high before treatment. Serum CA 19-9 lacks specificity for the diagnosis of pancreatic cancer and can be elevated in a variety of nonpancreatic cancers, including colon cancer, hepatoma, and gastric cancer, as well as in noncancerous disease states, including acute and chronic pancreatitis, choledocholithiasis with or without cholangitis and cirrhosis of the liver, and biliary obstruction of any cause.[5,6] The presence of hyperbilirubinemia is particularly confounding in the interpretation of elevated serum CA 19-9 levels. In one retrospective study, serum CA 19-9 was elevated in 41% (25/61) of subjects ultimately found to have obstructive jaundice from benign causes.[7] The same study showed that normalization of or a significant drop in CA 19-9 levels (to <90 U/mL) after biliary drainage was highly suggestive of a benign etiology. It is possible that alternative assays for CA 19-9 may improve specificity in the future,[8] but at present this marker should be considered adjunctive information in the particular setting where pancreatic ductal dilation is identified, as a markedly high level (>1000 U/mL) would argue for a malignant etiology. For a detailed discussion of the utility and limitations of CA 19-9 in the evaluation of patients with suspected pancreatic cancer, the reader is referred to either of two comprehensive reviews on the topic.[9,10]

Fluid Carcinoembryonic Antigen

Fine-needle aspiration (FNA) with measurement of fluid carcinoembryonic antigen (CEA) level has been used to help guide the diagnosis of cystic pancreatic lesions (including mucinous cystic neoplasms and intraductal papillary mucinous neoplasms [IPMN]) by providing information that is complementary to clinical and imaging data. As CEA is secreted in high levels from mucinous cystic lesions as opposed to serous cystadenomas, it is thought that higher levels of CEA suggest a higher likelihood of mucinous neoplasm. Studies have shown that fluid CEA levels greater than 192 ng/mL are highly sensitive and specific for mucinous cystic lesions but cannot definitively differentiate between benign and malignant lesions.[11] The diagnosis of IPMN in a patient with an isolated dilated pancreatic duct is typically made using imaging results in combination with clinical history, although the use of fluid CEA level obtained via EUS-FNA and endoscopic retrograde pancreatography (ERP) has been described.[12–14]

Imaging and Endoscopy

Radiologic studies are widely used to assess and follow patients with a dilated pancreatic duct. A pancreatic protocol CT scan includes fine (1

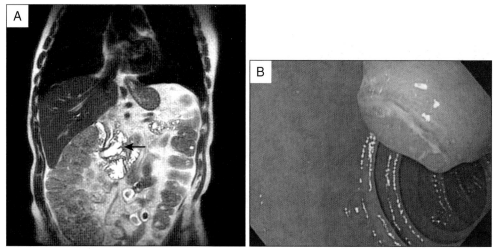

FIG 37.2 A, A 74-year-old man underwent magnetic resonance imaging for evaluation of hematuria. Image shows a dilated main pancreatic duct (*arrow*). **B,** Endoscopic image from the same patient that shows a patulous pancreatic orifice with thick mucin being extruded. Endoscopic ultrasonography confirmed the diagnosis of intraductal papillary mucinous neoplasm and showed a 12-mm pancreatic duct filled with mucin and evidence of papillary projections. (Images courtesy Richard S. Kwon, MD.)

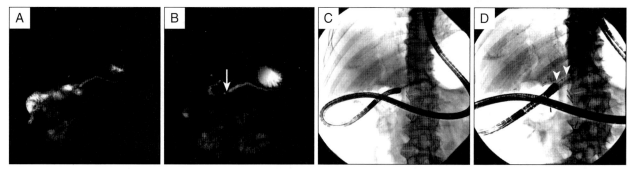

FIG 37.3 MRCP (**A** and **B**) and ERCP (**C** and **D**) images of a 71-year-old man after pancreaticoduodenectomy for main duct intraductal papillary mucinous neoplasm. MRCP images 1 minute (**A**) and 10 minutes (**B**) after secretin infusion. Note the dilation of the main pancreatic duct and side branches with evidence of a stricture (*arrow*) near the anastomosis. ERCP images demonstrating an anastomotic stricture (**C**) that was treated successfully with balloon dilation (**D**). (MRCP images courtesy Hero Hussain, MD.) *ERCP,* Endoscopic retrograde cholangiopancreatography; *MRCP,* magnetic resonance cholangiopancreatography.

to 3 mm) cuts through the pancreas, with timed arterial contrast injection to provide higher-resolution imaging of the pancreas. Even when traditional abdominal CT identifies a dilated pancreatic duct, a pancreatic protocol CT can provide a significant amount of information about the nature of the dilation. Similarly, direct endoscopic visualization of the pancreatic orifice may reveal a patulous opening with mucin being visible or extruded. This finding is pathognomonic for main duct IPMN (Fig. 37.2).

Magnetic resonance cholangiopancreatography (MRCP) is another noninvasive imaging study that provides a great deal of information with regard to pancreaticobiliary anatomy and has effectively supplanted ERCP in the evaluation of pancreatic ductal dilation. MRCP has been proven to be as sensitive as ERCP for the diagnosis of pancreatic cancer and more accurate at providing a measurement of the diameter of the main pancreatic duct in patients with chronic pancreatitis.[15,16] MRCP with secretin stimulation (MRCP-S) can be used to induce some degree of ductal dilation of the main pancreatic duct, sometimes enhancing imaging features. Measures of the difference in the absolute diameter of the duct preinjection and postinjection can be used as an indirect indicator of sphincter function and pancreatic outflow (Fig. 37.3).[17] If

significant dilation is noted, this suggests the presence of a stricture or stenosis, which may warrant further diagnostic evaluation and/or therapy.

EUS provides diagnostic information through the assessment of the pancreatic parenchyma, identification of strictures and associated masses, and evaluation of adjacent vasculature and lymph nodes. EUS has become the mainstay for evaluation of the pancreatic duct and the surrounding pancreatic parenchyma at most centers. EUS-guided pancreatic duct aspiration can provide fluid for cytology and/or testing of tumor biomarkers, although this procedure is rarely performed given the risk of pancreatic duct leak at the puncture site. In one small study, 12 patients with isolated dilation of the pancreatic duct underwent EUS evaluation with FNA.[18] Among these patients, nine had no associated mass and FNA of the pancreatic duct with aspiration of pancreatic fluid resulted in a diagnostic yield of 100%.

The role of ERCP as a diagnostic tool for the evaluation of patients with pancreatic duct dilation without a clear cause is limited. ERCP in this setting exposes patients to the risk of pancreatitis when other less invasive but equally effective tests such as EUS and MRCP can often look for masses, stones, or strictures with much less risk. A relatively new area in which endoscopy is being used in patients with a dilated

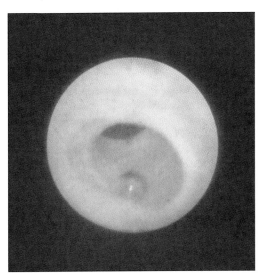

FIG 37.4 Image obtained at pancreatoscopy in a patient with a dilated main pancreatic duct. Absence of mucin helped to exclude the diagnosis of intraductal papillary mucinous neoplasm.

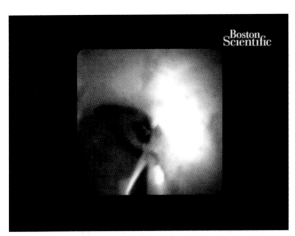

FIG 37.5 Digital pancreatoscopy image of a dilated pancreatic duct in a child with a 6-mm pancreatic duct detected via magnetic resonance cholangiopancreatography during evaluation for pain.

pancreatic duct is direct pancreatoscopy (see Chapter 26). For patients with suspected cystic pancreatic neoplasms, pancreatoscopy can be used to differentiate main-duct from side-branch IPMN, define the extent of duct involvement, and provide tissue samples for a histopathologic diagnosis (Fig. 37.4).[19] Pancreatoscopy is also widely used in patients with dilated pancreatic ducts in the setting of chronic pancreatitis to evaluate for stones, strictures, or malignancy (see Chapter 26) (Fig. 37.5).

TREATMENT

In general, treatment of patients with a dilated pancreatic duct should be focused on excluding malignancy and treating and obstructing pancreatic duct strictures or stones. Other objectives of therapy include improvement in exocrine insufficiency and resolution of pancreatic duct leaks. A dilated pancreatic duct in an asymptomatic patient does not typically warrant endoscopic or surgical intervention. Furthermore, in patients with a dilated pancreatic duct due to an obstructing pancreatic mass, decompression of the pancreatic duct itself is usually not undertaken.

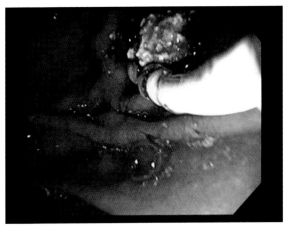

FIG 37.6 A 1-cm obstructing pancreatic duct stone removed via ERCP in a patient who was initially referred for surgical treatment after failed prior outside ERCP. The patient was pain-free after stone removal and was able to avoid surgery. *ERCP*, Endoscopic retrograde cholangiopancreatography.

Endoscopic Therapy

Endoscopic therapy of the dilated pancreatic duct is based on the concept that the ductal dilation results from increased intraductal pressure. Because of this, treatments are directed toward relief of the obstructive element and restoration of the normal flow of pancreatic juice to the duodenum. Similarly, nonobstructive dilations, as can be seen in patients with an atrophic pancreas, often do not require endoscopy.

Decompressive endoscopic therapies available to treat a dilated and obstructed pancreatic duct include pancreatic sphincterotomy (major and minor), pancreatic duct stone removal (often with extracorporeal shockwave lithotripsy [ESWL] or electrohydraulic lithotripsy [EHL]), pancreatic duct stricture dilation, pancreatic stent placement, pseudocyst drainage, and endoscopic necrosectomy (see Chapters 54, 55, and 56). Surgery has been shown to produce more significant and durable reduction in pain in patients with chronic pancreatitis than endoscopic therapy in one often-cited study, but as a rule endoscopic therapy is usually attempted before considering surgery given its risks and invasiveness.[20] Most endoscopic therapies for chronic pancreatitis and/or a dilated, obstructed pancreatic duct have lower morbidity and mortality, making endoscopic treatment more attractive for poor surgical candidates (Fig. 37.6). Endoscopic therapies do not preclude surgical intervention if treatment fails. Technical success is assessed by resolution of the targeted lesion and normalization of the pancreatic duct diameter on repeat imaging, whereas clinical success is measured by improvement of patient symptoms.

In patients with chronic pancreatitis the most common indication for endoscopic therapy for a dilated pancreatic duct is treatment of pancreatic stones, strictures, or both, as the two conditions often arise simultaneously; that is, a stricture predisposes the patient to stone formation, and stones can produce inflammation that leads to strictures. The effectiveness of endoscopic therapy is variable and reflects the myriad of approaches used by endoscopists and the complexity of pain in this population.[21,22]

A trial of endoscopic therapy is usually undertaken if definite pathology such as stones and strictures can be treated, particularly if there is upstream pancreatic ductal dilation (Fig. 37.7). Most pancreatic endotherapy is initiated by guidewire access to the pancreatic duct and followed by pancreatic sphincterotomy (Figs. 37.8 and 37.9). These two fundamental maneuvers pave the way for other interventions to be carried out in the pancreatic duct.

For treatment of pancreatic strictures, dilation may be achieved with graduated dilation catheters, balloon dilators, or Soehendra-type screw stent extractors, which can be used to core through very tight strictures (Fig. 37.10). A general rule is to select dilating devices that are the same or only slightly broader in diameter than the downstream duct to avoid perforation and/or duct disruption. After the dilation, a plastic stent is placed across the pancreatic duct stricture over a guidewire (Fig. 37.11). Pancreatic stents are constructed using more compliant material than that utilized for standard plastic biliary stents. In addition, pancreatic stents commonly have multiple side holes to allow drainage of side branches of the pancreatic duct. The use of covered, removable metal biliary stents in patients with pancreatic duct strictures has been explored to a limited extent. The concept behind this notion is that these stents, with their larger diameters and radial forces, may be more

effective and durable at treating refractory pancreatic duct strictures. It is unclear whether covered metal stents are more effective than one or more plastic stents, but it is reasonable to use metal stents to treat pancreatic duct strictures in selected patients for intervals of 3 to 4 months.[23–25]

Similar to the endoscopic approach to treating chronic pancreatitis–associated biliary strictures, some have advocated the placement of multiple plastic stents in the pancreatic duct to treat pancreatic duct strictures.[26] Adverse events of pancreatic duct stenting include migration of the stent upstream into the proximal duct or out of the duct into the intestinal lumen; iatrogenic stricture formation from localized trauma because of the stent; acute injury to the pancreatic duct, including duct disruption; stent-induced mucosal ulcers; and stone formation upstream from the stent. Premature stent occlusion may result in acute pancreatitis and, rarely, pancreatic sepsis. Endoscopic pancreatic therapy in a patient with a cyst or pseudocyst carries a small (1% to 2%) risk of infection, and the administration of preprocedural antibiotics is recommended.

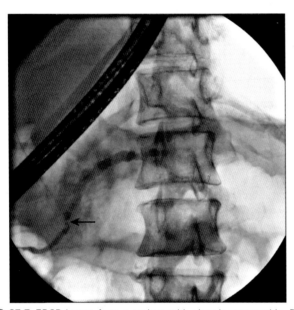

FIG 37.7 ERCP image from a patient with chronic pancreatitis. Pancreatogram reveals a stricture (*arrow*) in the head of the pancreas with upstream dilation of the pancreatic duct.

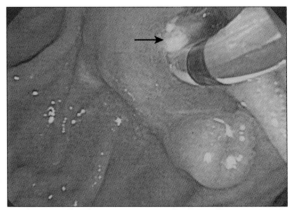

FIG 37.8 ERCP image from the same patient shown in Fig. 37.7. A pancreatic sphincterotomy was performed to facilitate passage of accessories to treat the stricture. A small stone (*arrow*) is seen exiting the pancreatic duct immediately after pancreatic sphincterotomy. The image also shows extension of a previously performed biliary sphincterotomy.

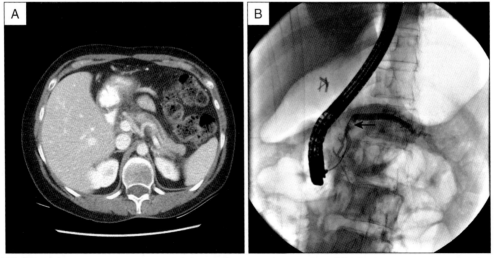

FIG 37.9 Images from a 64-year-old woman with recurrent pancreatitis. **A,** Computed tomography image showing dilation of the pancreatic duct in the body and tail with a transition point near the genu. **B,** ERCP image showing a stone (*arrow*) in the neck of the pancreas with upstream dilation of the pancreatic duct. The patient was treated with pancreatic sphincterotomy and stone extraction.

Oral antibiotics for 3 to 7 days after endoscopic therapy is reasonable in patients who have contrast remaining within the pancreas at the completion of the procedure.

Patients with chronic pancreatitis and pancreatic duct stones frequently have downstream strictures that contribute to stone formation and must be addressed before stone extraction can be performed (Fig. 37.12). This is particularly true in the patient with multiple strictures where complete ductal clearance is difficult to accomplish, and associated with lower rates of technical success and clinical improvement.[27] Other factors associated with greater difficulty and lower rates of successful clearance include the presence of multiple stones, large or impacted stones, and stones in the tail of the pancreas. In select centers, ESWL is used in conjunction with ERCP-directed therapy to achieve stone clearance. In the setting of chronic pancreatitis and a dilated pancreatic duct without underlying stones or strictures, the benefits of endoscopic therapy are likely to be limited to EUS-guided celiac plexus block/

neurolysis. For a more detailed discussion of endoscopic therapy in the patient with chronic pancreatitis, the reader is directed to Chapter 54.

Occasionally, ERCP is used in the treatment of ampullary stenosis associated with acute recurrent or chronic pancreatitis. In this setting, the goal of therapy is to enlarge the pancreatic orifice, allowing a lower resistance to the outflow of pancreatic secretions. This is typically accomplished by performing a pancreatic sphincterotomy. True ampullary stenosis is a rare finding, and the definition of ampullary stenosis is often very subjective. True ampullary stenosis may develop after a prior endoscopic sphincterotomy that has undergone stenosis.[28]

A prophylactic pancreatic duct stent is usually placed to reduce the risk of post-ERCP pancreatitis. For a detailed discussion of pancreatic sphincterotomy, including technique, devices, and potential adverse events, please see Chapter 20.

The clinical implications of pancreas divisum remain controversial, although new data suggest that in patients with an underlying genetic mutation, pancreas divisum may predispose to pancreatitis.[29] Endoscopic therapy of acute recurrent pancreatitis commonly involves minor papilla sphincterotomy with placement of a prophylactic pancreatic stent. Because of the high rate of ERCP-related adverse events in this population, endoscopic therapy of the minor papilla should be performed by experienced endoscopists.

The role of endoscopy in the patient with a dilated pancreatic duct caused by an obstructing cystic neoplasm is mainly diagnostic and most commonly involves the use of EUS with or without FNA. Although prospective studies examining the role of EUS in the treatment of cystic neoplasms show promise, this work is still considered experimental and is directed at cyst ablation rather than correction of pancreatic duct dilation.[30]

Conversely, ampullectomy for ampullary adenoma will typically result in resolution of pancreatic duct dilation, particularly if the duct has not been dilated for a prolonged period. This procedure is being performed with increasing frequency at centers offering advanced therapeutic endoscopy and has acceptably low adverse event rates when performed by experienced endoscopists.[31] For further discussion of ampullectomy, please see Chapter 25.

Surgical Therapy

Surgical intervention for the patient with a dilated pancreatic duct is undertaken with one of two goals: resection of an obstructing lesion (whether benign or malignant) or decompression of the duct with the intention of reducing pain. In the former, the most common scenario

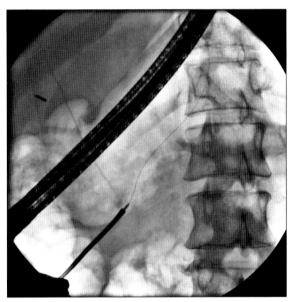

FIG 37.10 ERCP image from a patient with a tight stricture of the pancreatic duct. After attempts to treat the stricture with rigid and balloon dilators failed, a Soehendra stent extractor was used successfully to core through the stricture.

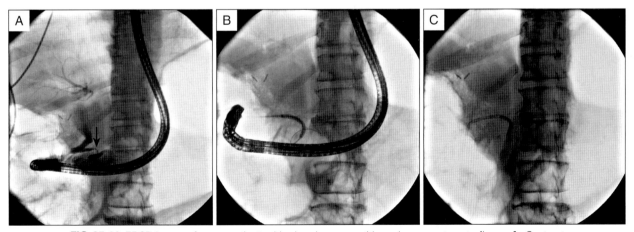

FIG 37.11 ERCP images from a patient with chronic pancreatitis and recurrent acute flares. **A,** Contrast injection revealed a stricture (arrow) in the head of the pancreas with upstream dilation of a tortuous duct. The stricture was treated with balloon dilation **(B)** followed by placement of a pancreatic stent **(C)**.

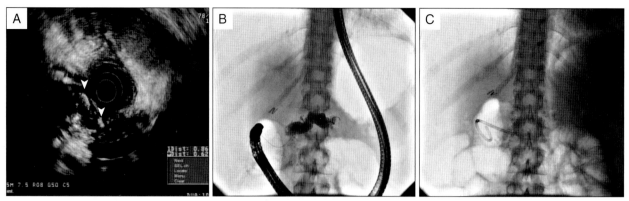

FIG 37.12 **A,** Endoscopic ultrasonography image showing pancreatic duct stones (*arrowheads*) in a 54-year-old woman with chronic pancreatitis and increased pain. **B,** ERCP demonstrates a dilated pancreatic duct with multiple filling defects consistent with stones and a stricture in the head of the pancreas. **C,** The patient was treated using a combination of pancreatic sphincterotomy, stricture dilation, and lithotripsy. A temporary pancreatic stent was placed at the conclusion of the procedure.

is that of a patient with a solid or cystic mass and upstream pancreatic ductal dilation. In the case of a neoplastic pancreatic head mass, pancreaticoduodenectomy (Whipple procedure) is usually performed when possible. Less frequently, a mass in the body is resected using an extended distal pancreatectomy or a midpancreatic resection. In the situation of a malignant lesion, the goal is primarily removal of the tumor, with little concern for treatment of the underlying pancreatic duct distention.

There are a number of surgical approaches that have been developed for resection of an inflammatory lesion in the head of the pancreas in the patient with chronic pancreatitis, a dilated pancreatic duct, and chronic pain. These include the Frey procedure and the Beger procedure. Both of these involve a partial resection or coring out of the head of the pancreas and decompression of the remaining pancreas via lateral pancreaticojejunostomy. In the patient with chronic pancreatitis, a dilated pancreatic duct, and diffuse involvement of the gland without a predominant head mass, the Puestow procedure or lateral pancreaticojejunostomy is the operation of choice. In this surgery, the pancreas is "filleted" longitudinally along the main pancreatic duct and then anastomosed to a loop of jejunum, which is similarly incised longitudinally. Partial or complete relief of pain after surgical drainage ranges from 65% to 85%, although sustained relief in long-term follow-up is significantly less (30% to 50%).[20]

CONCLUSIONS

The differential diagnosis in the patient with a dilated pancreatic duct is diverse and runs the gamut from benign, asymptomatic, coincidental findings to harbingers of underlying malignancy. The successful evaluation of such patients rests on a critical assessment of patient history and a careful evaluation of laboratory and imaging test results. Given the complexity of these cases and the potential consequences of therapy, dedicated training and experience in pancreatic endotherapy are recommended. As the medical community moves toward less invasive approaches, endoscopic therapy, including EUS and ERCP, will continue to play a central role in the evaluation and treatment of the patient with a dilated pancreatic duct.

The complete reference list for this chapter can be found online at www.expertconsult.com.

38

Ampullary Neoplasia

Paul Fockens and Ian D. Norton

Malignant tumors of the ampulla of Vater are uncommon. Fewer than 1 in 50,000 people older than 40 years are diagnosed with ampullary malignancy each year.[1] Much more common is a heterogeneous group of malignancies occurring in the *peri*ampullary region, including tumors of the adjacent part of the pancreatic head, the distal common bile duct, adjacent duodenal mucosa, and the ampulla of Vater. Before surgical resection the exact origin of a periampullary tumor is often not clear. However, the tissue of origin has important prognostic implications, with tumors arising from the pancreas carrying a worse prognosis (Fig. 38.1).[2] Conversely, tumors in this region often present relatively early because of biliary and/or pancreatic obstruction and therefore have a better prognosis than pancreaticobiliary malignancy. An autopsy series from the Mayo Clinic reported 25 periampullary lesions out of 4000 consecutive autopsies (0.6%), and at most only 20% of these lesions were symptomatic.[3]

The most common benign tumor of the ampulla of Vater is an adenoma. An adenoma-carcinoma sequence analogous to what occurs in the colon exists, and therefore all adenomas should be considered for resection. Many adenomas will be suitable for endoscopic resection (see Chapter 25). However, adenomas extending well into the ductal system or lesions with malignant transformation usually require pancreaticoduodenectomy (Whipple procedure). This chapter discusses lesions arising from the ampulla.

SYMPTOMS AND SIGNS

Fortunately, patients with ampullary lesions often develop symptoms and signs relatively early in the course of the disease. This is the result of the lesion arising from the junction of the pancreatic and bile ducts, thus impeding flow of bile and/or pancreatic secretions. Jaundice is the presenting symptom in the majority of patients. Unlike patients with pancreatic head malignancy, jaundice may initially be intermittent. Biliary obstruction may also be associated with signs and symptoms of cholangitis. In addition, nonspecific symptoms such as weight loss, abdominal discomfort, nausea, and vomiting may be seen. Obstructive jaundice, anemia caused by blood loss, and a palpable gallbladder* make up the classic triad of ampullary cancer, though this is seen in a small minority of patients.

Benign ampullary lesions present less often with jaundice, reflecting their small size. Vague abdominal pain may occur. Bile duct calculi

---

*Courvoisier sign, often misquoted, indicates that jaundice in the setting of a palpable gallbladder is not likely to be caused by gallstones (in which case gallbladder fibrosis will prevent obstructive dilation). The sign is often misquoted to state that painless jaundice in the presence of a palpable gallbladder is caused by malignant biliary obstruction, usually a pancreatic malignancy.

related to bile stasis may cause obstructive symptoms. Increasingly, patients with benign ampullary adenomata are diagnosed while asymptomatic, usually in one of three contexts:

1. Surveillance for duodenal/ampullary lesions in patients with familial adenomatous polyposis (FAP) syndrome
2. Incidental lesions discovered at upper endoscopy
3. Investigation of biliary dilation where imaging was performed for an unrelated indication (see Chapter 36)

In an endoscopic series of 55 ampullary adenomas, 45% were asymptomatic, 16% had abdominal pain, 15% had jaundice, 9% had pancreatitis, and 15% had miscellaneous symptoms.[4]

Presentation with acute gastrointestinal bleeding is uncommon but has been described with ampullary adenomas, carcinomas, metastatic malignancy, and mesenchymal tumors. In all cases they result from necrosis and ulceration of the overlying mucosa.[5]

There are no specific laboratory findings associated with ampullary tumors. Biliary obstruction results in elevation of alkaline phosphatase, gamma-glutamyl transpeptidase, and eventually bilirubin. Transaminases may also be elevated, especially in the setting of acute obstruction or cholangitis. Tumor markers have little role but may be useful for prognostic purposes. Serum CA 19-9 and carcinoembryonic antigen (CEA) levels have sensitivities for ampullary adenocarcinoma of 78% and 33%, respectively. The specificity of both markers is low.[6]

DIAGNOSTIC WORKUP AND EVALUATION

Endoscopy

For complete endoscopic assessment of the ampulla, the examination *must* be done with a duodenoscope. Examination with an end-viewing endoscope will cause a significant proportion of abnormalities to be missed. Two recent studies have demonstrated that duodenoscopy with a forward-viewing endoscope missed 50% of gross lesions visible with the side-viewing endoscope.[7,8] Endoscopy usually allows diagnosis of ampullary tumors and provides information regarding degree of lateral spread. A wide variation exists in the appearance of the ampulla, which often appears quite villiform. Endoscopy permits biopsy of the ampulla, although in one study endoscopic biopsy failed to diagnose deeper malignancy in 7 of 23 cases.[9] Furthermore, care should be taken to avoid direct biopsy of the papillary orifice, as even cold biopsy has been associated with acute necrotizing pancreatitis. Biopsies from the interior of a biliary sphincterotomy may diagnose ampullary pathology more accurately.

Macroscopically, ampullary masses conform to one of four well-recognized variations (Figs. 38.2 and 38.3):

- *Macroscopically normal papilla:* Suspicion of an ampullary lesion is usually attributable to pancreatic and biliary ductal dilation down to the level of the duodenal wall on cross-sectional imaging. Completely intraampullary neoplasms may become apparent only when a sphincterotomy is performed but may also be well visualized with endoscopic ultrasonography (EUS). In a series of 52 cases of adenomas or carcinomas, Ponchon and co-workers noted an ampulla appearing endoscopically normal in 37%.[10] In these cases an underlying tumor became evident only after biliary sphincterotomy.

- *Intramural protrusion:* A bulge underneath a normal-appearing papilla ("prominent infundibulum"). The differential diagnosis of this appearance also includes type III choledochal cyst and impacted biliary or pancreatic duct stones.
- *Exposed protrusion:* Neoplastic-appearing tissue extending out from the papilla.
- *Ulcerating tumor:* This situation is suspicious for malignancy (Fig. 38.4, *A*). Another feature suggestive of malignancy is failure of the lesion to lift when a submucosal injection is performed (sometimes included in the technique of endoscopic ampullectomy; see Chapter

25).[11] Other features suggesting malignancy include friability and induration. A recent study suggested that narrow band imaging (NBI) may be useful in differentiation of inflammatory lesions from neoplastic ampullary lesions.[12]

Sporadic lesions are solitary, whereas those associated with FAP syndrome are usually accompanied by other duodenal polyps. These may have a varied appearance, ranging from discrete villous lesions to thickened plaques of tissue to myriad tiny dots scattered over the mucosa ("miliary" appearance).

Endoscopic Retrograde Cholangiopancreatography

The introduction of magnetic resonance cholangiopancreatography (MRCP) and EUS has lessened the diagnostic role for endoscopic retrograde cholangiopancreatography (ERCP). Nonetheless, ERCP continues to play an important therapeutic role in establishing biliary

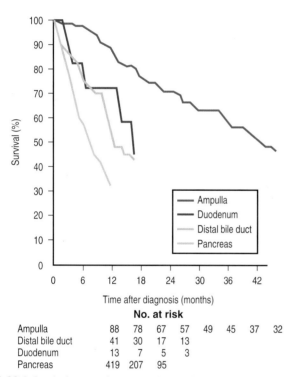

FIG 38.1 Survival curves for 561 patients with periampullary tumors, stratified by site of origin. (Reproduced with permission from Bettschart V, Rahman MQ, Engleken FJ, et al. Presentation treatment and outcome in patients with ampullary tumors. *Br J Surg.* 2004;91:1600–1607.)

No. at risk							
Ampulla	88	78	67	57	49	45	37	32
Distal bile duct	41	30	17	13
Duodenum	13	7	5	3
Pancreas	419	207	95

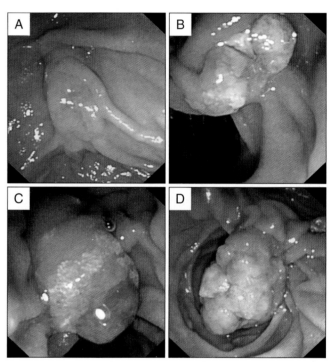

FIG 38.2 Different appearances of ampullary adenomas. **A,** Nearly normal macroscopic papilla. **B,** Adenoma with granular surface. **C,** Exposed protrusion of a villous adenoma. **D,** Large polypoid mass. (Redrawn from Bettschart V, Rahman MQ, Engleken FJ, et al. Presentation treatment and outcome in patients with ampullary tumors. *Br J Surg.* 2004;91:1600–1607.)

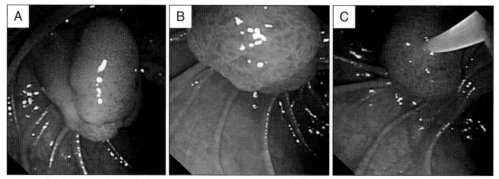

FIG 38.3 Prominent ampullary tumor. Biopsies revealed only adenoma, but the ampullectomy specimen revealed malignancy and the patient subsequently underwent pancreaticoduodenectomy.

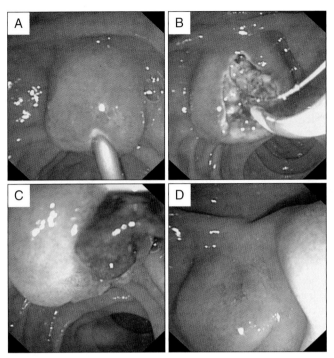

FIG 38.4 Inflamed papilla caused by gallstones. **A,** Swollen papilla with stent in situ and normal-appearing overlying mucosa. **B,** Sphincterotomy performed to permit biopsies from within the ampulla. **C,** Gallstones removed. **D,** Appearance 2 months later.

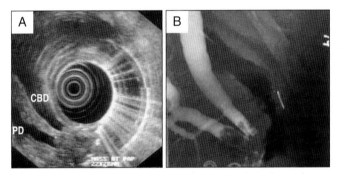

FIG 38.5 Endoscopic retrograde cholangiopancreatography and corresponding endoscopic ultrasonography images of a large ampullary mass. Note that both modalities demonstrate intraductal tumor extension. *CBD,* Common bile duct; *PD,* pancreatic duct.

drainage, often accompanied by diagnostic biopsy. Biliary sphincterotomy permits deeper tissue sampling and targeted biopsies, avoiding the pancreatic orifice. Sphincterotomy is also used as part of the ampullectomy technique, either to inferiorly displace a small lesion away from the ductal orifice before snare removal or to prevent subsequent papillectomy stenosis. Cholangiography remains an important tool to assess intraductal extension of a tumor (Fig. 38.5).[13]

Forceps Biopsy

Endoscopic forceps biopsy, taken from the surface of an ampullary lesion, is the usual mode of diagnosis. However, these biopsies can have a significant false-negative rate for malignancy.[9] To reduce sampling error, it is recommended that multiple biopsies should be obtained, taking care to avoid the pancreatic orifice. Malignant change within an ampullary adenoma may be seen in up to 30% (up to 50% in older

series).[9,14] Despite these limitations, recent series of endoscopic management of ampullary adenomas have quoted a malignancy rate of only 6% to 8% of ampullectomy specimens presumed to have benign disease.[13,15] This change is probably related to improved staging before endoscopic papillectomy and surgical ampullectomy. As mentioned previously, biopsies obtained from within a sphincterotomy may have a higher yield for malignancy. The best yield of biopsy is seen when the sample is obtained more than 10 days after sphincterotomy when diathermy artifact has cleared.[16] EUS-guided fine-needle aspiration may be useful in the assessment of ampullary masses, with reported sensitivity and specificity of 82% and 100%, respectively,[17] though further data on the role of EUS tissue sampling are required.

Transabdominal Ultrasonography, Computed Tomography, and Magnetic Resonance Imaging

Obstructive jaundice is often initially investigated with transabdominal ultrasonography (US) because of its accessibility, cost, and safety. In the case of obstruction caused by an ampullary lesion, the common finding is dilation of the entire biliary tree down to the duodenal wall. The tumor itself is not usually visualized. Similarly, the overall sensitivity for computed tomography (CT) is relatively low at 20% to 30% but is higher in the presence of larger tumors.[18–20] If a mass is not seen, EUS may be considered, with or without ERCP, depending on whether there is a need to relieve biliary obstruction. CT is a useful staging tool both for local staging (e.g., vascular involvement) and for distant metastases.[21] Magnetic resonance imaging (MRI) and MRCP have not been extensively investigated for ampullary lesions but appear to be promising alternatives to EUS.[22] CT cholangiography has recently been shown to be equivalent to MRCP in the evaluation of periampullary masses.[23]

Endoscopic Ultrasonography

EUS may be used for different purposes in the setting of ampullary neoplasia:

1. *Diagnosis.* EUS has a role in diagnosing patients with obstructive jaundice without a visible mass by transabdominal US or CT. For the detection of ampullary lesions, EUS (95%) has been shown to be superior to US (15%) and CT (20% to 30%).[18–20] However, the normal ampulla is usually hypoechoic and small lesions (<10 mm) may be missed with EUS.[19] EUS can be used in the investigation of an abnormal-appearing ampulla seen at endoscopy. The limited literature on this subject suggests that the specificity of EUS in this setting is about 75%.[24] False positives arise from an inflamed and swollen ampulla, possibly because of the recent passage of a calculus (see Fig. 38.4). In summary, EUS should be considered an important tool for clarifying the presence of an abnormal-appearing ampulla, but the diagnosis rests on tissue confirmation.

2. *Staging advanced ampullary cancer.* EUS is helpful in staging ampullary malignancy according to the TNM staging system (Box 38.1). Compared with CT and MRI, EUS is the most accurate tool for preoperative T-staging.[20,25] In a series of 50 patients, EUS was found to be more accurate (87%) than CT (24%) and MRI (46%) based on surgical and pathologic T-staging. The main limitation of EUS is in differentiating T2 and T3 lesions. Peritumoral pancreatitis may lead to overstaging a T2 lesion. Similarly, the presence of a biliary stent may lead to inflammatory changes that make T-staging more difficult. From a clinical perspective this is not a critical issue, because the surgical management of T2 and T3 lesions is identical (pancreaticoduodenectomy). N-stage accuracy has not been reported to be different between EUS, CT, and MRI. Metastatic regional nodes are detected by EUS with an accuracy of about 65% (Fig. 38.6).[25,26] Locoregional lymph node involvement usually does not influence surgical management. Surgical resectability depends mainly on

BOX 38.1   TNM Staging System for Ampullary Carcinomas

T1	Tumor limited to the ampulla of Vater*
T2	Tumor invades duodenal wall (muscularis propria)
T3	Tumor invasion into the pancreas <2 cm
T4	Tumor invasion into the pancreas >2 cm or into adjacent organs or vessels
N0	No regional lymph node metastasis
N1	Regional lymph node metastasis
M0	No distant metastasis
M1	Distant metastasis

*Some divide T1 tumors into d0 (limited to Oddi's sphincter) and d1 (tumor invading the duodenal submucosa).

From Sobin LH, Wittekind CH, eds. *International union against cancer (UICC): the TNM classification of malignant tumors.* 6th ed. New York: Wiley; 2002.

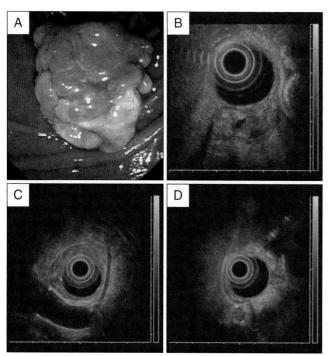

FIG 38.6 T2 N1 adenocarcinoma of the ampulla of Vater. **A**, Endoscopic appearance. **B**, Endoscopic ultrasonography showing polypoid tumor. **C**, Dilated common bile duct and pancreatic duct. **D**, Lymph node involvement.

vascular involvement and the presence of distant metastases. Because of the early presentation of ampullary tumors and relative distance from the mesenteric vessels, vascular involvement is uncommon. EUS is an accurate means of assessing vascular involvement[27,28] and can allow imaging of the portal venous system from the proximal duodenum and of the celiac vessels from the gastric fundus.

3. *Staging early ampullary lesions.* When local endoscopic or surgical intervention is being considered, accurate T-staging is of vital importance. Endoscopic resection is generally limited to premalignant lesions because early cancers have a 10% to 45% risk of lymph node metastasis[29] and should be managed with radical resection (Whipple procedure) in operable patients. EUS relies on infiltration and destruction of normal tissue planes to differentiate benign from malignant disease. In the case of benign biopsies, the role of EUS is to exclude an infiltrative lesion deep to the endoscopically visible part of the lesion. The accuracy of EUS to distinguish lesions >T1 stage is high, between 87% and 95%.[19,25,27,30] T1 tumors have further been subclassified into T1d0 (limited to the sphincter of Oddi) and T1d1 (invasion of the duodenal mucosa). Local resection is appropriate if the lesion is T1d0 and there is no evidence of malignancy. For the d0/d1 subgrouping, intraductal ultrasonography (IDUS) appears to have the best accuracy (see the following section) but is not readily available.

4. *Extension of tissue into the distal bile duct or pancreatic duct is a relative contraindication for endoscopic resection.* This may be assessed by carefully performed ERCP or EUS (see Fig. 38.5).

Intraductal Ultrasonography

IDUS is a promising tool for the staging of ampullary and biliary tumors. After cannulation of the bile duct at ERCP, a 7-Fr ultrasonography catheter is advanced over a guidewire into the ductal system. These catheters are reusable rotating mechanical probes that operate at relatively high frequency (12 or 20 MHz) to produce high-quality near-field images but with limited depth. In the largest prospective study on this subject, IDUS was superior to CT and EUS in terms of tumor visualization, especially in detecting small lesions.[19] Another recent study showed that IDUS had a 94% sensitivity for detecting ampullary neoplasia and 80% T-stage accuracy.[31] IDUS is the only imaging modality that demonstrates the sphincter of Oddi as a distinct structure.[30] Furthermore, IDUS has been shown to improve the sensitivity of malignancy in early lesions compared with forceps biopsy.[32] Clearly IDUS has the potential to play a large role in the selection of patients for endoscopic resection, but further prospective studies are required.

Colonoscopy

Ampullary adenoma may be the presenting feature of attenuated FAP syndrome. Furthermore, there are reports of patients with ampullary adenomata being at increased risk of colonic neoplasia, even in the absence of FAP syndrome.[33–35] Ponchon's group has described colonic polyps in 50% of their patients with sporadic ampullary adenomas, including one with eight polyps and another with a sigmoid malignancy.[36] Although these studies are small, it seems prudent to perform colonoscopy in all patients diagnosed with ampullary adenomas and carcinomas, especially before surgical resection of the ampullary lesion.

PATHOLOGY

Ninety-five percent of neoplasms of the ampulla consist of adenomas or adenocarcinomas. Ampullary tumors are increasingly recognized as sporadic lesions (i.e., not associated with hereditary neoplastic condition; see Fig. 38.2 and Box 38.2), and these probably account for more than 50% of ampullary adenomas and carcinomas. There is a wide range of other benign and malignant neoplastic conditions that can affect the ampulla of Vater. These are listed in Boxes 38.3 and 38.4 (see also Chapter 25). In the following sections, the most common conditions are described in further detail.

Adenoma

The ampulla of Vater is anatomically complex and in most patients is composed of the common channel, the intraduodenal segment of the bile duct and pancreatic duct, and the duodenal mucosa (Fig. 38.7). The common channel, bile duct, and pancreatic duct are all surrounded by smooth muscle fibers. The common channel is probably the site from which most ampullary tumors arise, as shown by histologic and autopsy series.[37]

BOX 38.2   Cancer Syndromes Associated With Ampullary Carcinoma

Familial adenomatous polyposis
HNPCC*
Neurofibromatosis type 1[†]
Muir-Torre syndrome[‡]

*Hereditary nonpolyposis colorectal carcinoma (HNPCC) is weakly associated with ampullary carcinoma.
[†]Neurofibromatosis seems to be a predisposition of both somatostatinomas and carcinomas of the ampulla of Vater.
[‡]Muir-Torre syndrome is a condition characterized by the association of multiple sebaceous tumors and keratoacanthomas with internal malignancies, including ampullary carcinomas.

BOX 38.3   Differential Diagnosis of Tumors and Pseudotumors of the Ampulla of Vater

Benign Disease
- Adenoma
- Carcinoid
- Gastrointestinal stromal tumor
- Lipoma
- Leiomyoma
- Hamartoma (Peutz-Jeghers polyp)
- Schwannoma
- Lymphangioma
- Hemangioma
- Fibroma
- Neurofibroma
- Granular cell tumor
- Adenomyoma
- Eosinophilic gastroenteritis
- Duodenal duplication
- Choledochocele
- Heterotopic pancreas
- Brunner gland hyperplasia
- Heterotopic gastric mucosa
- Inflammatory nonneoplastic lesions: odditis/papillitis (e.g., caused by lithiasis)
- Large but normal variant ampulla

BOX 38.4   Differential Diagnosis of Malignant Tumors and Pseudotumors of the Ampulla of Vater

Malignant Disease
- (Adeno)carcinoma*
- Neuroendocrine carcinoma
- Malignant gastrointestinal stromal tumor
- Lymphoma
- Pancreatoblastoma
- Leiomyosarcoma
- Neurofibrosarcoma
- Kaposi sarcoma
- Angiosarcoma
- Malignant schwannoma
- Rhabdomyosarcoma (only described in children)
- Metastasis to the ampulla

*Mixed cellular populations of carcinoma have been described, such as sarcomatoid carcinomas (an intermixture of carcinomatous and sarcomatous elements); adenocarcinoid tumors (an intermixture of adenocarcinoma and carcinoid tumor); and ampullary carcinomas with unusual patterns of differentiation (e.g., papillary carcinomas, Paneth cell carcinomas, and signet-ring cell carcinomas).

The periampullary region is the site of the vast majority of significant small intestinal adenomas in both sporadic and FAP patients. These lesions seem to parallel mucosal exposure to bile (see the section, "Ampullary Adenoma and FAP Syndrome"), particularly with regard to the characteristic inferior extension of early adenomas ("goatee" appearance; Fig. 38.8). Ampullary adenomas are histologically similar to their colonic counterparts and are classified as tubular, tubulovillous, or villous, in order of increasing dysplasia and malignant potential. As in the colon, progressive genetic changes and increasing dysplasia may lead to malignant transformation. Several lines of evidence support this hypothesis:

- Adenomatous remnants have been found adjacent to malignancy.[10,38,39]
- Histologic progression from adenoma to malignancy has been seen in patients followed longitudinally.[40]
- A retrospective study by Bleau and Gostout supported the temporal progression of periampullary adenomas to carcinoma, with mean diagnosis of adenoma at age 39, high-grade dysplasia at age 47, and malignancy at age 54.[7]

- A genetic alteration model describing change to malignancy has been described, analogous to that seen in the colonic adenoma-carcinoma sequence.[41]

Autopsy series have also demonstrated cancer without evidence of adjacent adenoma, suggesting that either the cancer has replaced all adenomatous tissue or some lesions may progress to cancer without an adenomatous precursor.[37]

Carcinoma

Adenocarcinoma of the ampulla can be categorized histologically and immunohistochemically as either intestinal type or pancreaticobiliary type.[42] The intestinal type resembles colonic neoplasia and arises from the mucosa; the pancreaticobiliary type arises from the ductal epithelium of the ductal system, thought usually to originate from the common channel. There are conflicting reports on whether the prognosis differs between these two forms of malignancy.[38,42]

Neuroendocrine Tumors

Neuroendocrine tumors (NETs) are morphologically and biologically diverse, with a broad spectrum of subtypes. Ampullary NETs are rare, with fewer than 200 cases reported worldwide. Most reported cases are somatostatinomas, but gangliocytic paragangliomas and other NETs have been reported (Figs. 38.9 and 38.10). Most ampullary NETs are nonfunctional in that they may produce specific hormones detected on immunostaining of the lesion but do not lead to raised serum peptide levels or clinical neuroendocrine syndromes.[43]

There is a strong relationship between ampullary NETs and von Recklinghausen disease; approximately 25% of reported NETs occur in the setting of neurofibromatosis.[44]

Presentation is usually with jaundice. The diagnosis is often made after surgical resection because of the submucosal location of the tumor hindering mucosal-based biopsies.[45] The size of the tumor correlates poorly with metastatic potential and prognosis.[44,45] In addition to the imaging modalities discussed previously, somatostatin receptor scintigraphy may be helpful.[43] Pancreaticoduodenectomy is the recommended management for ampullary NETs >2 cm.[45] Local resection or endoscopic removal may be considered for small lesions after thorough investigation

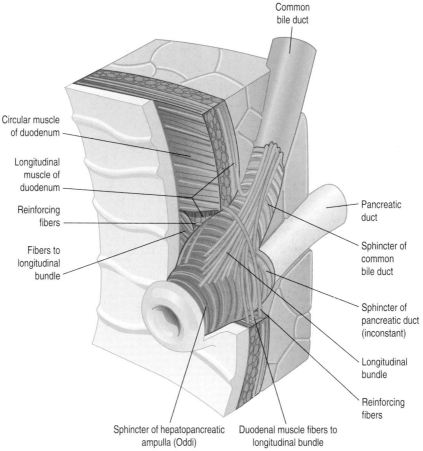

FIG 38.7 Illustration of the anatomy of the ampulla of Vater. Note the distinct muscle components of the papilla, choledochus, and pancreatic duct.

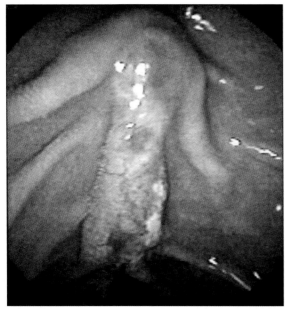

FIG 38.8 Ampulla of Vater in a patient with familial adenomatous polyposis syndrome. Note the goatee-like extension of adenomatous tissue inferior from the papillary os.

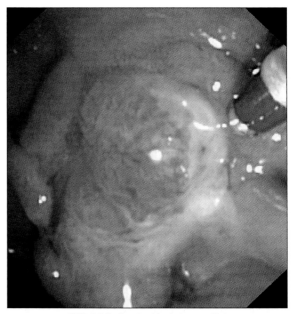

FIG 38.9 Carcinoid of the papilla.

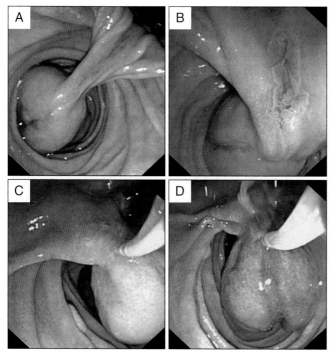

FIG 38.10 Periampullary gangliocytic paraganglioma. **A,** Large stalked polyp. **B,** Papillary orifice. **C,** Cannulation. **D,** Snare resection under the orifice after placement of an endoloop.

TABLE 38.1   Staging System for the Severity of Duodenal Polyposis in Familial Adenomatous Polyposis: The Spigelman Classification

Points	1	2	3
Polyp number	1–4	5–20	>20
Polyp size (mm)	1–4	5–10	>10
Histology	Tubular	Tubulovillous	Villous
Dysplasia	Mild	Moderate	Severe

0 points = stage 0; 1–4 = stage I; 5–6 = stage II; 7–8 = stage III; 9–12 = stage IV.
From Spigelman AD, Williams CB, Talbot IC, et al. Upper gastrointestinal cancer in patients with familial adenomatous polyposis. *Lancet.* 1989;2:783–785 (with permission).

for metastatic disease. Generally the prognosis is good, with a 5-year survival of 90%.[45] However, poorly differentiated lesions may have an aggressive clinical course with early metastasis and fatal outcome.

Lymphoma

Lymphoma affecting the ampulla is very rare. Four types of lesions have been described:

1. *Primary ampullary mucosa–associated lymphoid tissue (MALT) lymphoma arising from the ampullary mucosa.* These are similar in appearance and behavior to gastric MALT lymphoma and often regress after treatment of *Helicobacter pylori.* If this fails, aggressive treatment with chemoradiation is usually successful.[46]
2. *Diffuse large B-cell lymphoma (DLBL).* Among the ampullary lymphomas, these are relatively common and are treated in the same way as DLBL elsewhere.[47]
3. *Follicular lymphoma.* These are often relatively diffuse and therefore are better treated with chemotherapy than surgery.[48]
4. *T-cell lymphoma.* These are very rare and may be associated with underlying celiac disease.

Gastrointestinal Stromal Tumor

There are several case reports of gastrointestinal stromal tumors (GISTs) arising in the ampullary complex. The lesions were generally treated with pancreaticoduodenectomy. Treatment with imatinib has been found useful in patients with metastatic disease or in those unfit for surgery.[49,50]

Ampullary Adenomas and FAP Syndrome

Asymptomatic adenomatous change of the ampulla is extremely common in FAP patients, occurring in up to 100% of subjects.[7] FAP syndrome and its variants (Gardner and Turcot syndromes) occur in about 1 in 2000 Europeans.[51] Duodenal cancer is the most common cause of cancer death in these patients after colectomy.[51] The incidence

of FAP-related duodenal and periampullary adenomas depends on the intensity of surveillance (see the section, "Diagnostic Workup and Evaluation"). A review of the Johns Hopkins FAP registry indicated that in patients with FAP, the relative risks of developing duodenal and ampullary cancer compared with the general population were 330 and 123, respectively.[52] The combined absolute risk of duodenal cancer in FAP patients was, however, only 1 per 1698 years. Because follow-up was incomplete and most cancers occur later in life, this risk of malignancy may be an underestimate. A study from the United Kingdom reported development of malignancy in 3 of 70 patients followed for more than 40 months[53]; therefore, although adenomatous change in the duodenum may be almost universal in FAP, only a minority of patients develop cancer. Several studies have indicated that the median age at onset of periampullary malignancy complicating FAP is in the sixth decade.[52,54,55] The literature on this subject has often not adequately differentiated sporadic from FAP-related periampullary adenomas. In an attempt to prevent duodenal malignancy in patients with FAP syndrome, various screening strategies have been developed. Spigelman and co-workers developed a staging system for ampullary adenomas in FAP patients to stratify their risk of developing cancer (Table 38.1).[56–58] Patients with stage IV disease have between 10 and 30 times the risk of developing cancer compared with patients with a low score. However, the best treatment approach for patients with a high score remains controversial. Although an early Scandinavian study showed that 25% of patients with stage IV disease developed cancer,[56] it is our current belief that better endoscopic examination of the ampulla is leading to upstaging of these lesions, and so the malignant risk of a given stage may not be as high as originally believed. Nonetheless, there is little doubt that these patients should be surveyed periodically in a structured way using a duodenoscope. It has been suggested by some that surveillance should occur at least every 3 years in patients with low-stage disease and every 6 months to 1 year in patients with stage IV disease.[59] Interestingly, ampullary adenomas are more likely to have malignant potential than lesions occurring elsewhere in the duodenum.[33,40,58] A normal-appearing ampulla is seen in at least 50% of cases harboring adenomatous change (see Fig. 38.2, *A*). The role of endoscopic treatment is not well defined because of the lack of prospective data. Nonetheless, the endoscopic intervention appears to be a viable alternative to surgery.[4,15,60,61]

Pathogenesis of Ampullary Adenoma and FAP Syndrome

It is of interest that the ampulla and periampullary region are by far the most likely sites of adenomatous change in the small bowel. Bile has been shown to have proliferative[62–64] and mutagenic[65] effects on gut mucosa. Furthermore, bile from patients with FAP has been shown to form more DNA adducts both in vitro and in vivo than bile from controls,[39,61] particularly at low pH (as found in the proximal duodenum).[66] These DNA adducts have the potential to give rise to mutagenesis. As an autosomal-dominant condition, all nucleated cells in FAP patients contain one normal and one abnormal *APC* gene (a germline mutation). In the colon, a somatic mutation in the previously normal (wild-type) *APC* allele is generally an early event in carcinogenesis. Accumulation of other somatic mutations (in genes such as *p53* and *K-ras*) drives the progression toward malignancy.[67] The situation with respect to periampullary malignancy appears to be similar, except that somatic *APC* mutations may be relatively less frequent and *K-ras* mutations relatively more frequent.[68] Another study has demonstrated p53 mutations associated with high-grade or malignant change in periampullary tumors.[69] A recent paper has suggested that other familial factors, possibly unidentified modifier genes, may influence the development of periampullary adenomas in FAP kindreds, which explains at least in part the familial segregation of periampullary disease observed in FAP families.[55] This segregation is independent of the kindreds' specific *APC* mutation. Spigelman and co-workers have reported a correlation between severity of duodenal polyposis and rectal polyposis after colectomy and ileorectal anastomosis.[70] They have suggested that other factors, possibly environmental, may be synergistic in some patients, resulting in more severe polyposis at both sites. The authors of this study caution, however, that paucity of rectal polyps does not eliminate the need for periampullary surveillance.

TREATMENT

Adenomas

Twenty years ago the treatment of ampullary adenoma was by pancreaticoduodenectomy. This effectively removed all adenomatous tissue but at the cost of significant morbidity and potential mortality. Transduodenal resection of the ampulla has significantly less morbidity but at the cost of significant risk of recurrent adenoma (5% to 30%), which requires subsequent endoscopic surveillance.[9,59,71] The current aim of treatment of adenomas differs between FAP patients and those with sporadic lesions. In those with a sporadic lesion, the aim is the same as that in the colon, which is complete excision of all adenomatous tissue. The aim with FAP patients is to "control" the disease through the removal of all significant-sized tissue (lesions greater than several millimeters).

Since 1983, series and reports have been published describing endoscopic management of periampullary adenomas using snare resection and laser photocoagulation.[72–74] Later, snare excision of the entire ampulla was described by Binmoeller et al. (Figs. 38.11 and 38.12).[75] Considerable literature demonstrates endoscopic therapy as an effective alternative to surgery in selected patients (Table 38.2). A recent large retrospective series comparing surgical and endoscopic resection concluded that there was no significant difference in recurrence between the two strategies, but that lesions larger than 3.6 cm or those extending into the ductal system should be managed surgically.[76] Although it has been traditionally thought that lesions extending into the ductal system cannot be removed endoscopically, recent literature suggests that selected lesions can be successfully removed.[77] One technique to facilitate this is the use of an intraductal balloon to prolapse proximal tissue into a snare.[78] (See Chapter 25 for a detailed discussion of endoscopic management of ampullary adenoma.)

Nonampullary duodenal adenomas can also be successfully removed using endoscopic mucosal resection (EMR) techniques developed for the removal of large colonic polyps. The duodenal wall is extremely

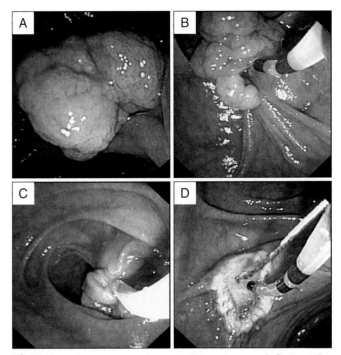

FIG 38.11 En bloc resection of a tubulovillous adenoma. **A,** Periampullary mass. **B,** Cannulation of the papilla. **C,** Snare resection. **D,** Result after ampullectomy and sphincterotomy.

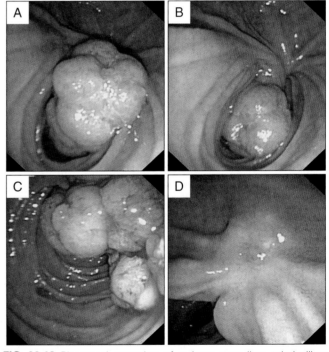

FIG 38.12 Piecemeal resection of a large ampullary tubulovillous adenoma. **A,** Large polyp with orifice of the papilla on top; note that with many of these large lesions the attachment to the duodenal wall is often quite small. **B,** Twisted stalk. **C,** Piecemeal resection. **D,** The result 2 months after resection.

TABLE 38.2 Summary of the Literature on Endoscopic Resection of Ampullary Tumors[a]

First Author	Year of Publication	Number of Patients Included	Retrospective or Prospective	Technique	Intraductal Growth	Adverse Event Rate[b]	Histology	Follow-up	Complete Endoscopic Resection[c]	Surgery[d]	Recurrence[e]
Katsinelos[88]	2006	14	Retrospective	Snare excision	0	Pancreatitis 7%, bleeding 7%	11 adenoma, 3 carcinoma	28 months	79%	21%	18%
Harewood[89]	2005	19	Prospective	Snare excision (RCT of prophylactic pancreatic stent placement)	0	Pancreatitis 33% without PD stent vs 0% with PD stent, cholestasis 5%	NR	NR	NR	NR	NR
Bohnacker[13]	2005	106 (109 lesions[f])	Prospective	Snare excision and/or electrocoagulation	31	Pancreatitis 12%, bleeding 3%	92 adenoma (18 with HGD), 4 carcinoma, 12 inflammatory lesion, 1 lymphangioma	43 months	73%	19%	18%
Han[90]	2005	22	Retrospective	Snare excision	0	Bleeding 5%, perforation 5%, papillary stenosis 5%, cholangitis 5%, cholestasis 5%	15 adenoma (3 with HGD), 2 carcinoma, 1 carcinoid, 3 inflammatory lesion, 1 lymphangioma	8 months	86%	NR	5%
Moon[91]	2005	6	Prospective	Snare excision (wire-guided endoscopic papillectomy)	0	Late-onset pancreatitis 17%, cholangitis 17%	6 adenoma (1 with HGD)	7 months	100%	0%	0%
Cheng[4]	2004	55	Retrospective	Snare excision	6	Pancreatitis 9%, bleeding 7%, perforation 2%	45 adenoma (7 with HGD), 5 carcinoma, 2 carcinoid, 1 gastric heterotopia, 2 normal histology	30 months	74%	13%	33%
Catalano[15]	2004	103	Retrospective	Snare excision	0	Pancreatitis 5%, bleeding 2%, papillary stenosis 3%	97 adenoma (14 with HGD), 6 carcinoma	36 months	80%	16%	20%

Continued

TABLE 38.2 Summary of the Literature on Endoscopic Resection of Ampullary Tumors—cont'd

First Author[e]	Year of Publication	Number of Patients Included	Retrospective or Prospective	Technique	Intraductal Growth	Adverse Event Rate[b]	Histology	Follow-up	Complete Endoscopic Resection[c]	Surgery[d]	Recurrence[e]
Saurin[36]	2003	24	Retrospective	Mainly laser photodestruction[g]	0	Pancreatitis 17%, bleeding 13%, perforation 4%	Forceps biopsies: 24 adenoma (10 with HGD)	81 months	67%	17%	6%
Norton[61]	2002	26 (28 lesions[f])	Retrospective	Snare excision	0	Pancreatitis 15%, perforation 4%, pancreatic duct stenosis 8%	25 adenoma, 1 carcinoma, 1 inflammatory lesion, 1 normal histology	9 months	96%	4%	10%
Desilets[92]	2001	13	Retrospective	Snare excision (piecemeal)[g]	0	Pancreatitis 8%	13 adenoma (1 with HGD)	19 months	92%	8%	0%
Zádorová[93]	2001	16	Retrospective	Snare excision	NR	Pancreatitis 13%, bleeding 13%	16 adenoma	NR	100%	6%	19%
Vogt[94]	2000	18	Retrospective	Snare excision	NR	Pancreatitis 11%, bleeding 11%, stent dysfunction 6%	18 adenoma	75 months	100%	17%	44%
Park[95]	2000	6	Retrospective	Snare excision	NR	Pancreatitis 33%	4 adenoma, 2 carcinoma	21 months	67%	17%	0%
Binmoeller[75]	1993	25	Prospective	Snare excision	2	Pancreatitis 12%, bleeding 8%	25 adenoma (1 with HGD)	37 months	92%	12%	26%

HGD, High-grade dysplasia; NR, not reported; PD, pancreatic duct; RCT, randomized controlled trial.

[a]Inclusion: Studies published from 1990, and with more than five patients included, on endoscopic treatment of ampullary tumors with benign features.

[b]Adverse event rate (percentage per total number of patients): Only clinically evident bleeding that occurred after completion of the procedure was regarded as an adverse event. Pancreatitis and perforation were managed conservatively in the majority of patients.

[c]Complete endoscopic resection (percentage per total number of patients): Total clearance of adenoma in one or more treatment sessions, without the need for surgery (this includes recurrences that could be treated endoscopically).

[d]Surgery (percentage per total number of patients): Includes the need for surgery for malignant disease, for persistent adenoma, for adverse events, and for recurrences that could not be treated endoscopically.

[e]Recurrence: Recurrence of adenoma (or adenocarcinoma) after complete endoscopic resection (patients lost to follow-up are excluded).

[f]Synchronous tumors of the major and minor papillae.

[g]Median number of three therapeutic sessions to achieve complete destruction of adenomatous tissue.

thin and EMR requires submucosal injection with saline or other solution. Analogous to the colon, the size of lesions removed endoscopically is increasing with increased experience.[79]

Carcinomas

Standard surgical management of invasive ampullary cancer is with pancreaticoduodenectomy. Local surgical resection is not recommended, as the resection margin may be inadequate[80] and lymph node involvement is common. This is further supported by poorer outcomes in patients treated with local resection compared with Whipple procedure.[81] A recent study of 106 patients with ampullary cancer reported 45% lymph node invasion in T1 cancers.[29] Another large study demonstrated a close correlation between lymph node metastasis and T stage (28%, 51%, 70%, and 78% for T stages I, II, III, and IV, respectively).[82] An alternative strategy may be to commence with a local resection and convert to a pancreaticoduodenectomy if the resected specimen is shown to be inadequately resected, either macroscopically or by frozen section.[83] This strategy does not appear to compromise patient outcomes compared with initial pancreaticoduoenectomy.[83] In the event of a surgical or endoscopic resection demonstrating high-grade dysplasia (carcinoma in situ), there is inadequate evidence to support subsequent radical resection with lymphadenectomy.[84]

Survival after resection is closely related to T stage (see Table 38.1).[2] Operative mortality has improved over time and in high-volume centers should be ≤5%. Various factors that influence survival include R0 resection, lymph node status, differentiation of the tumor, and local invasion (pancreatic, perineural, or perivascular).[2,80] Those lesions with an intestinal origin may do better than those of pancreaticobiliary type.[85]

A recent meta-analysis suggested that patients with ampullary cancer may benefit from adjuvant chemoirradiation, including those with locally advanced disease or nodal metastases.[86]

Palliative treatment is determined on an individual basis. There is some evidence that biliary sphincterotomy, local resection,[84] and snare papillectomy[87] may be reasonable strategies. Other endoscopic approaches include placement of a self-expandable metal biliary stent. Occasionally, placement of a duodenal stent is required to relieve gastric outlet obstruction.

CONCLUSIONS

Ampullary tumors are relatively uncommon but are regularly seen in clinical practice, especially in referral institutions. The prognosis is better than that for pancreatic cancer. Early lesions are usually treated with endoscopic resection, and more advanced lesions and cancers are usually treated with pancreaticoduodenectomy. The diagnostic workup of these lesions is challenging. Close inspection of the ampulla is important and must be done with a duodenoscope. Care should be taken with biopsy of the ampulla, especially in patients who have not had a previous biliary sphincterotomy. Patients with FAP should be enrolled in a surveillance program. Endoscopic ultrasonography may be useful in the local staging of the lesion, and CT may be useful to assess metastatic spread in advanced lesions.

The complete reference list for this chapter can be found online at www.expertconsult.com.

39

Malignant Biliary Obstruction: Distal

Meir Mizrahi, Jonah Cohen, João Guilherme Guerra de Andrade Lima Cabral, and Douglas Pleskow

Malignant strictures of the pancreaticobiliary tree are often difficult to diagnose and treat. Therefore the majority present in more advanced stages of disease, contributing to poor prognosis and outcome. Jaundice is the most common presenting sign and symptom of malignant biliary obstruction. Different etiologies cause distal malignant biliary obstruction and include pancreatic cancer, carcinoma of the ampulla of Vater, distal cholangiocarcinoma (CCA), and metastatic disease that involves the head of the pancreas or the common bile duct (CBD) (Table 39.1). Obstructive jaundice often presents in the context of advanced disease and negatively affects the patient's quality of life. This chapter reviews the role of endoscopic retrograde cholangiopancreatography (ERCP) in the management of malignant distal biliary obstruction. Management of biliary obstruction in the setting of proximal biliary obstruction is discussed in Chapter 40.

EPIDEMIOLOGY

The most common cause of malignant distal biliary obstruction is pancreatic cancer. During 2014 there were more than 40,000 deaths from pancreatic cancer, which ranks as the fourth most common cause of overall cancer mortality.[1] The number of pancreatic cancer–related deaths is expected to increase in the United States, and pancreatic cancer may soon become the second leading cause of cancer-related deaths.[2] Worldwide, pancreatic cancer is a leading cause of cancer mortality, with more than 330,000 new cases and similar number of deaths annually.[3–7] In 2017 it is estimated that the overall pancreatic cancer mortality will level off in US and European men but will increase in Japan. Unfortunately, in women, pancreatic cancer–related mortality will continue to rise in most countries except the United States.[2] Based on evidence that the occurrence of pancreatic cancer varies greatly across different global areas, lifestyle and environmental factors have been implicated in its pathogenesis. Various risk factors have been found to play a pathogenic role. Advanced age is the most significant risk factor for pancreatic cancer. The median age at diagnosis of pancreatic cancer in the United States is 72 years. About 5% to 10% of patients develop pancreatic cancer before the age of 50 years, but this group is more likely to include those with predisposing genetic disorders[8] or those who have previously undergone cancer treatments, such as radiation.[2,3] Cigarette smoking has been strongly associated with pancreatic cancer, and the risk increases 70% to 100% compared with nonsmokers.[9–11] Daily alcohol consumption (≥3 drinks or equal to 30 to 40 g of alcohol per day) is associated with a 22% increase in the risk of pancreatic cancer incidence.[12] Underlying chronic pancreatitis also increases the risk for developing pancreatic cancer.[13] Other implicated risk factors for pancreatic cancer include vitamin D and ultraviolet B (UVB)

radiation, occupational exposure, and obesity.[14–17] A family history of pancreatic cancer is associated with a twofold increase in pancreatic cancer risk.[18] Genetic factors that increase the risk of pancreatic cancer include familial atypical multiple mole melanoma (FAMMM) syndrome, hereditary pancreatitis, Peutz-Jeghers syndrome, familial pancreatic cancer, cystic fibrosis, familial adenomatous polyposis, and hereditary nonpolyposis colorectal cancer (HNPCC) syndrome.

Malignant distal biliary obstruction can also be caused by CCA. CCA can originate either within the liver or in the extrahepatic bile ducts. Worldwide, CCA is the second most common primary hepatic malignancy after hepatocellular carcinoma.[19] Recent epidemiologic studies show that the incidence and mortality rates of intrahepatic CCA are increasing, whereas those of extrahepatic CCA are falling globally.[20–25] The peak age for CCA is the seventh decade of life and the overall incidence is higher in men.[20] The majority of cases are sporadic, and specific risk factors are identified only in a minority of patients. Various factors causing ongoing chronic inflammation of the biliary system are often implicated. These risk factors include advanced age; male gender; and underlying conditions such as primary sclerosing cholangitis (PSC), fibropolycystic liver disease, Caroli's disease, choledochal cysts (see Chapter 35), HNPCC, and bile duct adenomas.[20] PSC (see Chapter 48) in particular is associated with earlier onset of CCA.[20] CCA has been associated with diabetes, obesity, viral hepatitis (hepatitis C and possibly hepatitis B); lifestyle factors such as smoking and alcohol use; and exposure to toxins such as asbestos, dioxins, nitrosamines, and thorotrast.[26–29] In Asia, especially Thailand and China, infestation with liver flukes *Clonorchis sinensis* and *Opisthorchis viverrini* is strongly associated with CCA.[30]

Adenocarcinoma of the gallbladder is another cause of distal biliary obstruction. In the United States, gallbladder cancer is the fifth most common gastrointestinal cancer and the most common cancer involving the biliary tract. Over 5000 new cases are diagnosed each year in the United States. Among Southwestern Native Americans and Mexican Americans, gallbladder cancer is the most common gastrointestinal malignancy.[31] Cholelithiasis is a well-described and strong risk factor for gallbladder cancer. Most of the patients diagnosed with gallbladder cancer will be diagnosed incidentally during investigation for cholelithiasis.[32–34] Other risk factors for gallbladder malignancy include advanced age, female gender, and specific geographic areas. In South American countries such as Chile, Ecuador, and Bolivia and in Asian countries such as India, Pakistan, Japan, and Korea, the incidence of gallbladder cancer is higher.[35–38] Underlying gallbladder conditions such as porcelain gallbladder, gallbladder polyps, congenital biliary cysts, and abnormal pancreaticobiliary duct junction are associated with higher risk of cancer of the gallbladder.[6] Smoking and obesity have also been implicated, although the evidence linking them to gallbladder cancer is weak. Risk factors for pancreaticobiliary malignancies are summarized in Table 39.2.

Video for this chapter can be found online at www.expertconsult.com.

NATURAL HISTORY

Malignant distal biliary obstruction may occur as a consequence of extrinsic bile duct compression or may involve the duct intrinsically either through a primary process or from metastasis directly to the bile duct. The most frequent cause of malignant biliary obstruction is adenocarcinoma of the pancreas located at the head or uncinate process, which accounts for more than 90% of cases.[39] Other cancers include gallbladder cancer, cancer of the ampulla of Vater, CCA, metastatic cancers, and malignant lymphadenopathy. In most cases, advanced disease is detected at the time of detected biliary obstruction.

The role of the endoscopist in the management of these conditions extends to providing both diagnostic and therapeutic/palliative solutions depending on the type and stage of cancer. Endoscopic diagnostic procedures include endoscopic ultrasonography (EUS) with fine-needle aspiration (FNA) and fine-needle core biopsy (FNB) and ERCP with brush cytology. Alternatively, therapeutic endoscopic procedures such as ERCP with biliary stenting, placement of duodenal/pyloric stenting, EUS-guided fiducial placement to facilitate radiotherapy, and EUS-guided celiac plexus neurolysis for pain control can become part of overall management. Despite current advances in the diagnostic and therapeutic aspects of pancreaticobiliary cancers, the majority of patients have unresectable disease at presentation, with a median survival of 4 months without treatment.

CLINICAL FEATURES AND INITIAL EVALUATION

The most common clinical presentations of pancreatic and biliary malignancies include painless jaundice, weight loss, and anorexia.[40] Biliary obstruction leads to scleral icterus, clay-colored stools, dark urine, pruritus, nausea, and emesis. Advanced forms of pancreatic cancer can present with epigastric pain radiating to the back, suggesting pancreatic duct obstruction and infiltration of retroperitoneal structures,[41,42] palpable gallbladder, dyspepsia, early satiety because of gastric outlet obstruction, new-onset glucose intolerance or diabetes mellitus, and acute pancreatitis. CCA presents with abdominal pain mostly in the right upper quadrant, jaundice, pruritus, and weight loss.[43–45]

Risk factors for pancreaticobiliary malignancies should be evaluated during history taking. For pancreatic cancer, these include a history of tobacco smoking and smokeless tobacco usage, family history of pancreatic cancer, and personal history of diabetes, pancreatitis, and obesity.

For CCA, a history of previously known conditions should be obtained. Relevant conditions include inflammatory bowel disease; PSC; cholelithiasis; choledochal cysts; Caroli's disease; HNPCC; human

TABLE 39.1 Causes of Malignant Biliary Obstruction	
Primary Cancer	**Metastatic Cancer**
Pancreatic cancer	Gastric cancer
Carcinoma of ampulla of Vater	Colon cancer
Cholangiocarcinoma	Breast cancer
Gallbladder carcinoma	Lung cancer
	Renal cell carcinoma
	Melanoma
	Hepatocellular cancer
	Malignant lymphadenopathy

TABLE 39.2 Risk Factors for Pancreaticobiliary Cancers		
Pancreatic Cancer	**Cholangiocarcinoma**	**Gallbladder Cancer**
• Demographic	• Demographic	• Cholelithiasis
Age	Age	• Demographic
Male gender (slightly higher)	Male gender	Age
Race: highest for African Americans	• Underlying conditions	Female gender
• Lifestyle	Primary sclerosing cholangitis	Race/ethnicity
Smoking	Fibropolycystic liver disease	Caucasian
Alcohol (3 or more drinks per day)	Caroli's disease	Southwestern Native American
• Occupational exposure	Choledochal cysts	Mexican American
Chlorinated hydrocarbons	Lynch syndrome	• Geographic pattern
Formaldehyde	Bile duct adenoma	South America
• Underlying conditions	Obesity	Chile
Chronic pancreatitis	• Infections and parasitic infestations	Bolivia
Diabetes	Liver fluke	Ecuador
Periodontal disease	*Clonorchis*	Asia
• Infections	*Opisthorchis*	India
Hepatitis C	HIV	Pakistan
Helicobacter pylori	Hepatitis C	Japan
• Genetic susceptibility	• Lifestyle	Korea
FAMMM syndrome	Smoking	• Porcelain gallbladder
Hereditary pancreatitis	Alcohol use	• Gallbladder polyps
Peutz-Jeghers syndrome	• Occupational exposure	• Congenital biliary cysts
Familial pancreatic cancer	Asbestos	• Abnormal pancreaticobiliary duct junction
Cystic fibrosis	Nitrosamines	• Occupational exposure
Lynch syndrome		Thorotrast
Familial adenomatosis polyposis		
Li-Fraumeni syndrome		

FAMMM, Familial atypical multiple mole melanoma; *HIV,* human immunodeficiency virus.

TABLE 39.3 Common Symptoms Associated With Pancreaticobiliary Malignancies

Symptoms	Signs

• Symptoms of biliary obstruction
  Jaundice
  Pale stools
  Steatorrhea
  Dark urine
  Generalized pruritus
  Nausea
• Constitutional symptoms
  Weight loss
  Anorexia
• Pain
  Epigastric or right-upper-quadrant
    abdominal pain
  Back pain (mostly advanced disease)
• Nausea, vomiting, early satiety
  From gastric outlet or duodenal
    obstruction
	• Scleral icterus
	• Organomegaly
	  Liver
	  Gallbladder
	  Lymph nodes
	• Trousseau sign: swollen
	  blood vessels

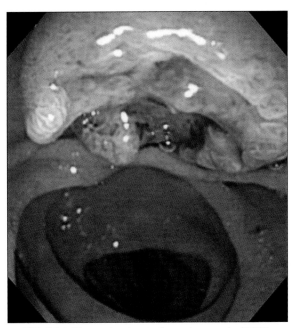

FIG 39.1 Diagnosis of ampullary adenoma by ERCP.

immunodeficiency virus (HIV); hepatitis C and hepatitis B exposure; diabetes; and exposure to toxins such as asbestos, dioxins, nitrosamines, and thorotrast. A complete physical examination should include identification of icterus and palpation to identify organomegaly, including liver, gallbladder, and lymph nodes. Migratory thrombophlebitis can be recognized via positive Trousseau sign or swollen visible blood vessels that resolve and then appear at another area of the body. The various symptoms and physical examination findings of pancreaticobiliary malignancies are summarized in Table 39.3.

Laboratory tests should include total bilirubin, fractionated bilirubin, alkaline phosphatase, alanine aminotransferase (ALT), aspartate aminotransferase (AST), and tumor markers such as cancer antigen (CA) 19-9 and carcinoembryonic antigen (CEA). Further testing with imaging studies such as transabdominal ultrasonography (TUS), pancreas protocol computed tomography (CT), or magnetic resonance cholangiopancreatography (MRCP) should be based on the initial suspicion of pancreaticobiliary malignancy from the history, physical examination, and initial laboratory test results.

DIFFERENTIAL DIAGNOSIS OF DISTAL BILIARY MALIGNANCIES AND IMAGING TECHNIQUES

Ampullary Carcinoma

Ampullary carcinoma often presents with obstructive jaundice and is suspected if imaging studies detect dilation of the pancreaticobiliary ducts. TUS should be the first imaging test, based on its ability to detect intrahepatic and extrahepatic bile duct dilatation and to confirm the presence of gallstones. However, TUS has poor sensitivity for detection of ampullary carcinoma because of the small size of the tumor and overlying bowel gas that limits views of retroperitoneal structures.[46,47] CT scan provides more accuracy than ultrasonography in this regard. Water may be used as oral contrast to distend the duodenal wall. Even though CT is more sensitive than TUS, a substantial number of ampullary lesions can be missed, especially small lesions.[48] Skordilis et al. reported CT scan to have an overall accuracy of 20% in detecting ampullary carcinoma.[47] MRCP is also a noninvasive technique and superior to CT in detecting biliary obstruction. Ampullary carcinomas appear as

filling defects protruding into the duodenal lumen, with characteristic delayed enhancement and hyperintensity on diffusion-weighted imaging.[49] Domagk et al. reported 76% overall accuracy of MRCP in detecting ampullary carcinoma.[50] However, MRCP cannot differentiate between tumors and other benign causes of ampullary obstruction such as stones and benign strictures.[51]

ERCP can be both diagnostic, by detecting an ampullary mass and providing tissue samples (Fig. 39.1), and therapeutic, for relieving obstructive jaundice. Overall diagnostic accuracy of ERCP for detecting ampullary carcinoma is up to 88%, with tissue acquisition performed at least 48 hours after sphincterotomy, which includes multiple biopsies and the use of polymerase chain reaction or immunohistochemical staining to detect *p53* or *K-ras* gene mutations.[50,52–56]

EUS and ERCP are comparable in terms of detecting ampullary cancers. EUS is the most accurate imaging modality to provide local tumor staging for ampullary neoplasms.[57,58] The choice of surgery performed as local resection versus pancreaticoduodenectomy is determined by the staging information obtained from the previously mentioned techniques (see Chapter 38).

Pancreatic Cancer

The pancreatic malignancies that cause distal biliary obstruction involve the head or uncinate process of the pancreas, although large lesions involving other areas of the pancreas can also obstruct the biliary system. Metastasis to the porta hepatis can cause more proximal obstruction. The workup for suspected pancreatic cancer often begins with one or more of the following, depending on clinical and institutional protocols: TUS, CT scan, magnetic resonance imaging (MRI), EUS, and ERCP. These options enable cancer diagnosis and staging, determine tumor resectability, and provide a histopathologic diagnosis. TUS with and without contrast has a diagnostic accuracy of about 82% to 86% for diagnosing pancreatic head malignancies.[59] The diagnostic accuracy of TUS is lower for pancreatic head cancers less than 3 cm in diameter.[60–62]

CT scan improves tumor detection and provides information about local staging and invasion of vascular structures. Dynamic contrast-enhanced multidetector CT scan has significantly improved pancreatic cancer imaging, with an ability to provide enhanced three-dimensional

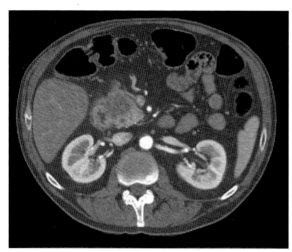

FIG 39.2 Computed tomography scan showing a mass at the head of the pancreas obstructing the common bile duct without adjacent major vascular involvement.

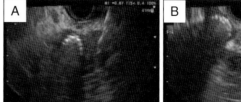
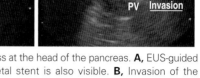

FIG 39.3 EUS showing mass at the head of the pancreas. **A,** EUS-guided FNA of mass. A biliary metal stent is also visible. **B,** Invasion of the portal vein by the mass. The FNA results confirmed malignancy. *EUS,* Endoscopic ultrasonography; *FNA,* fine-needle aspiration; *PV,* portal vein.

reconstructions of pancreatic tumors and their vascular involvement (Fig. 39.2). The sensitivity of multidetector CT ranges from 89% to 97%, and this is currently the preferred modality for preoperative staging and assessment of resectability of patients with pancreatic malignancy.[63,64]

MRI with either gadolinium-enhanced or mangafodipir-enhanced sequences is as sensitive as CT in detecting pancreatic cancers. MRI for the pancreas includes conventional MRI, MRCP, and magnetic resonance angiography. In a recent study Fusari et al. compared the diagnostic accuracy of multidetector CT scan and MRI and reported comparable diagnostic accuracies for tumor identification and resectability between the two techniques.[65] Rao et al. showed comparable results of CT and MRI for characterization of small pancreatic tumors ≤2 cm.[66] A recent study of multidetector (64-detector row) CT scan compared with gadobenate dimeglumine–enhanced 3.0-T MRI imaging (compared with previously used 1.5-T MRI imaging) also showed similar sensitivities and specificities for the two techniques in detecting pancreatic cancer.[67] Although in routine practice it is common to use both CT and MRI in the evaluation of patients with known or suspected pancreatic cancer, MRI is especially useful in cases where iodinated contrast material cannot be administered because of contrast allergy or renal insufficiency.

EUS allows the ability to place a high-frequency transducer in close proximity to the tumor and provides high-resolution images and enhanced detection of pancreatic cancer. Dewitt et al. published a systematic review comparing the diagnostic sensitivity of CT scan and EUS in the detection of pancreatic cancer; this publication included 11 studies and 678 patients and concluded that EUS had higher sensitivity than CT scan in detecting pancreatic tumors.[68] Another study that evaluated the accuracy of EUS, dynamic CT, and MRI in detecting pancreatic tumors <3 cm in diameter found sensitivities of 93%, 53%, and 67%, for EUS, CT, and MRI, respectively.[69] However, multidetector CT scanning was developed and introduced to clinical use after most of the previously mentioned studies were published.

Recently, multiple studies comparing different modalities for the staging of pancreatic cancer based on the tumor, node, metastasis (TNM) staging proposed by the American Joint Committee on Cancer (AJCC) were published. Dewitt et al.[70] and Soriano et al.[71] found that EUS was superior to multidetector CT in terms of T-staging, with an overall lower rate of overstaging compared with CT and MRI.

Comparing the accuracy of EUS and CT scan for N-staging, different reports have not conclusively established the superiority of one technology over the other.[70,72]

For M-staging, the advantage of multidetector CT scan over EUS rests with the fact that, in addition to local spread, CT scan also provides information about distant metastasis. Therefore CT scan currently is more commonly used for the initial staging of pancreatic cancer. EUS becomes a valuable staging tool in situations where CT scan provides equivocal results about surrounding lymph nodes or when small solid tumors less than 3 cm are detected on CT scan.[73]

With improvements in cross-sectional imaging and EUS in the last decade, the role of ERCP in the diagnosis and staging of pancreatic cancer has greatly diminished. Nevertheless, certain signs, such as combined dilation of the CBD and the main pancreatic duct (double-duct sign) and abrupt cutoff of the pancreatic duct or a single long stricture (>1 cm) of the pancreatic duct observed during ERCP, should alert the clinician to the possibility of pancreatic cancer.

If the initial imaging studies are suggestive of pancreatic malignancy and the patient is an appropriate operative candidate, it is rational to refer the patient for surgical resection with the hope of curative intent. Currently, select medical centers in the United States use multidisciplinary clinics (MDCs) for their pancreatic cancer care. The MDC model enables convenience and improves communication by having patients assessed during their initial visit by each main member of the care team, including surgical oncology, medical oncology, gastroenterology, radiation therapy, and genetics.

Because of late presentation of this disease, only a small proportion of patients are considered to be surgical candidates (15% to 20%). More frequently, cytologic diagnosis of pancreatic cancer is obtained by performing FNA/FNB (ultrasonography-guided, CT-guided, or EUS-guided) and brush cytology (obtained during ERCP). A recent meta-analysis published by Chen et al. of EUS-guided FNA in the diagnosis of pancreatic cancer showed a sensitivity of about 92% and a specificity of about 96%.[73] A second meta-analysis including 41 papers was published by Puli et al. and found that EUS-guided FNA has a sensitivity of 89% and a specificity of 96%.[74] The accuracy (calculating true-positive cases plus true-negative cases) was found to be lower in the setting of chronic pancreatitis.[75] Therefore a negative EUS-FNA result does not exclude the presence of cancer. A recent randomized trial published by Horwhat et al. comparing EUS-guided FNA with other modalities for tissue acquisition, such as CT-guided FNA, found no significant differences in the sensitivities of the two techniques.[76] However, EUS is the test of choice when tumor size is <3 cm (Fig. 39.3).

The adverse events of EUS-FNA include bleeding, pancreatitis, perforation, and tumor seeding. In a prospective study from high-volume centers, 355 patients with solid pancreatic tumors underwent EUS-FNA with an overall adverse event rate of 2.54% (3 cases of pancreatitis), with 1.9% of patients requiring hospitalization.[77] The same group found that even when performed by less experienced operators, the adverse event rate with EUS-FNA was reported to be as low as 1.1%.[78] There have been three reports of tumor seeding into the gastrointestinal wall as a result of EUS-FNA.[79] There have also been reports of development of peritoneal carcinomatosis. However, compared with TUS-guided or CT scan–guided percutaneous biopsy, the risk of peritoneal tumor seeding can occur and is greater than that seen with EUS-FNA (16.3% vs 2.2%).[80]

Ikezawa et al. found that peritoneal carcinomatosis ultimately developed during the course of disease in patients who had undergone EUS-guided FNA for pancreatic cancer in 17.9% compared with 14.9% when ERCP with brush cytology was performed, suggesting that EUS-FNA is not a risk factor for peritoneal seeding.[81]

In the process of improving diagnostic yield and tissue acquisition, newer biopsy needles have been developed. Mizrahi et al. showed that the use of a forked-tip FNB needle had a higher diagnostic yield for pancreatic cancer compared with FNA.[82]

In addition to obtaining tissue by EUS-guided FNA/FNB, cytology specimens can be taken at the time of biliary decompression during ERCP. Brush cytology has a sensitivity that ranges from 30% to 60%. Increasing the number of samples by obtaining multiple brush cytology samples before and after stricture dilation and sending the entire brush for analysis can increase diagnostic yield.[83,84] Brush cytology has a high positive predictive value but poor negative predictive value. Ramchandani et al. showed that, when brush cytology was nondiagnostic, cholangioscopy-guided biliary duct biopsies were accurate in up to 82%.[85]

Cholangiocarcinoma

Intrahepatic CCA may present as one or more mass lesions on imaging studies. Hilar and distal CCA are suspected in patients presenting with biliary obstruction, right-upper-quadrant abdominal pain, and cholangitis. Noninvasive biliary imaging with MRCP is the radiologic modality of choice to determine the extent of the disease. In addition, obtaining MRCP before ERCP may offer additional information to serve as a road map to direct placement of biliary stents (see Chapter 40).[86] ERCP with brush cytology and/or cholangioscopy with bile duct biopsies may be required. Newer cytologic techniques, such as digital image analysis (DIA) and fluorescence in situ hybridization (FISH), have been incorporated into the cytologic evaluation of bile duct brushings to enhance the sensitivity of cytology (Fig. 39.4; see also Chapter 41).[87,88] Both techniques identify aneuploidy, which is a hallmark of chromosomal instability and cancer. Malhi and Gores found that the combination of DIA and FISH offers the highest sensitivity for the diagnosis of malignant biliary strictures in patients both with and without PSC.[89] EUS might be valuable in determining the extent of disease and when sampling regional lymph nodes for staging is needed. Choice of surgical resectability and type of surgery can be aided by the Bismuth-Corlette classification of hilar CCA (Fig. 39.5). Although surgical resection is the mainstay of curative treatment for CCA in the absence of PSC, surgery is not recommended in patients with PSC because of multifocality of the disease. There is a poor impact on overall disease mortality after surgery. In patients with PSC with early CCA, liver transplantation has been

considered as a curative option.[89] Surgical resection for distal CCA requires pancreaticoduodenectomy, as for pancreatic cancer. Factors that may influence surgical decision include poor performance status, presence of cirrhosis, and other comorbidities. Five-year survival in patients with distal bile cancers is 37%.[90,91]

Metastatic Disease

Multiple GI and non-GI malignancies may metastasize and cause malignant biliary tract obstruction. Cancer types in order of frequency are gastric, colon, breast, and lung. Others include renal cell carcinoma, melanoma, and hepatocellular cancer. Infrequently, malignant lymphadenopathy can cause malignant biliary obstruction (see Table 39.1). These lesions may cause either extrinsic or intrinsic compression of the bile duct.

AN APPROACH TO THE MANAGEMENT OF PATIENTS WITH DISTAL BILIARY MALIGNANCIES

The initial step in the approach to pancreaticobiliary malignancy is to establish a diagnosis and stage the disease. As mentioned earlier, CT and MRI scans may establish the location and extension of disease, vascular involvement, and the presence or absence of distal metastatic disease. Tissue samples can be obtained for histopathologic assessment by EUS if the lesion is within the pancreas, distal CBD, or a surrounding lymph node. ERCP with brush cytology with or without the additional use of DIA and FISH methods or directed intraductal biopsies may reveal the diagnosis in both pancreatic and biliary malignancies. Rarely, given the strong suspicion of cancer from imaging studies and fairly high accuracy of staging offered by these

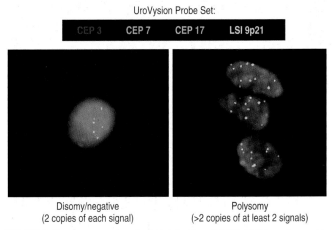

FIG 39.4 Fluorescence in situ hybridization (FISH). FISH performed in a patient with cholangiocarcinoma demonstrating chromosomal instability. (Courtesy Gregory J. Gores, MD.)

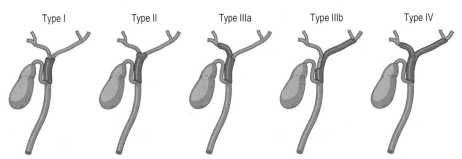

FIG 39.5 Bismuth-Corlette classification of hilar cholangiocarcinoma.

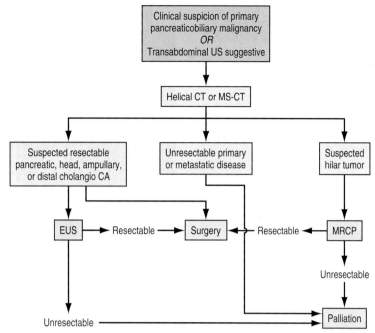

FIG 39.6 A proposed algorithm by the American Society for Gastrointestinal Endoscopy for diagnosis and management of suspected pancreaticobiliary malignancy. *CA,* Carcinoma; *CT,* computed tomography; *EUS,* endoscopic ultrasonography; *MRCP,* magnetic resonance cholangiopancreatography; *MS-CT,* multislice computed tomography; *US,* ultrasonography. (Redrawn from Baron TH, Mallery JS, Hirota WK, et al. The role of endoscopy in the evaluation and treatment of patients with pancreatobiliary malignancy. *Gastrointest Endosc.* 2003;58:643–649.)

imaging modalities, a patient is referred directly for surgery and tissue diagnosis, and surgical staging may be achieved. Staging is critical to determining whether curative surgery is possible and whether adjuvant or neoadjuvant therapies are required. The best management approach for obstructive jaundice may also vary according to the level of biliary obstruction. An algorithm proposed by the American Society for Gastrointestinal Endoscopy for the diagnosis and management of patients with suspicion for pancreaticobiliary malignancies is shown in Fig. 39.6.

Curative Surgery

Despite significant improvements in the field of diagnosis and treatment, pancreaticobiliary malignancy is still associated with overall poor prognosis. At the time of diagnosis, only 15% to 20% of patients are considered candidates for curative resection.[92,93] The presence of one or more conditions such as advanced disease or poor performance status because of comorbid conditions may influence the classification of a patient as a good or poor surgical candidate. For cancer that involves the head of the pancreas, the curative surgical procedure is a classic Whipple procedure (pancreaticoduodenectomy), which involves removal of the head of the pancreas, gallbladder, CBD, duodenum, antrum of the stomach, and the proximal 10 to 15 cm of jejunum.[94] The most common postoperative complications include delayed gastric emptying (7% to 18%), pancreatic leak/fistula (10%), and wound infection (6%). The incidence of cardiopulmonary events varies significantly (3% to 15%).[95,96] A more recent surgical approach is a modification of the classic Whipple procedure, the pylorus-preserving pancreaticoduodenectomy, in which the stomach is retained, potentially improving postsurgical problems such as bile reflux, dumping, and marginal ulceration. In a recently published meta-analysis of classic and pyloric-sparing, comparable mortality, morbidity, and overall survival were seen.[97] Pancreatic cancers found at the level of the pancreatic

body and tail are less common and tend to have a worse prognosis compared with cancers at the pancreatic head, as jaundice does not appear until hepatic metastases develop.[98] Cancers of the body and tail are generally treated with distal pancreatectomy, often performed with concomitant splenectomy. These surgeries do not involve biliary reconstruction.

The surgical options for patients with distal CCA are the same as those for pancreatic head cancer, with 5-year survival ranging from 20% to 30%.[99,100] Even with extensive hepatobiliary resection, recurrence is frequent (46%).[101] Similarly, recent data for ampullary cancers treated with pancreaticoduodenectomy show a morbidity rate of 38% and mortality rate of 0%, with 5-year survival of 38%.[102] Diagnostic laparoscopy with peritoneal washings for cytology before open resection or exploratory laparoscopy can also prevent unnecessary pancreaticoduodenectomy.

Palliation

Palliation in patients with pancreaticobiliary malignancy is for obstructive jaundice with or without cholangitis, pain, and duodenal obstruction. Palliation of jaundice stemming from distal malignant biliary obstruction is accomplished by one of three means: endoscopic stent placement, percutaneous transhepatic biliary drainage, or surgical biliary bypass (Table 39.4).

Endoscopic Stenting

In patients with malignant biliary obstruction, relieving obstructive jaundice through palliative biliary decompression has been shown to improve quality of life.[103] The role of ERCP in biliary decompression is discussed later in this chapter. Technical aspects of endoscopic biliary stenting and the equipment are discussed in Chapter 23.

Background. The placement of a plastic stent (see Chapter 22) is inexpensive and effective, and the stent can be easily removed or

TABLE 39.4 Techniques of Palliative Biliary Drainage

Type of Intervention	Type of Procedure	Type of Drainage
Surgical	Choledochojejunostomy	Internal
	Choledochoduodenostomy	
	Cholecystojejunostomy	
	Cholecystogastrostomy	
	Cholecystoduodenostomy	
	Hepaticojejunostomy	
Percutaneous (image-guided)	Percutaneous internal biliary drainage	Internal, external, or both
	Percutaneous external biliary drainage	
	Percutaneous external-internal biliary drainage	
Endoscopic	Transpapillary biliary drainage	Internal
	Nasobiliary drainage	

exchanged. The earliest study reporting endoscopic biliary stenting using 7-Fr stents for nonresectable pancreatic cancer was published by Soehendra in the late 1970s.[104] The majority of patients developed recurrent biliary obstruction, and the need for larger-diameter stents was quickly recognized. Therefore, side-viewing endoscopes that allow insertion of stents up to 12 Fr were developed. The placement of large-caliber (10-Fr) plastic stents improved patency to an average of 3 to 4 months. Placement of 11.5-Fr biliary stents is technically more challenging but does not offer significant improvement in stent patency. As a means to overcome the limitations of size and therefore stent patency, self-expandable metal stents (SEMS) were developed during the late 1980s.[105,106]

Indications for biliary stenting. Obstructive jaundice is often associated with symptoms of loss of appetite, nausea, pruritus, recurrent cholangitis, delayed wound healing, and renal failure. Biliary drainage is recommended in patients who have advanced cancer and are deemed nonsurgical candidates. In this setting palliative biliary stenting relieves symptoms and improves quality of life.[103] Stenting is also indispensable before initiating chemotherapy to avoid potential hepatotoxic effects of chemotherapeutic drugs. However, preoperative stenting in obstructed patients who are otherwise asymptomatic is an area of controversy. There are studies that have shown stenting to be beneficial before surgery, whereas other studies reported higher rates of serious complications within 120 days postsurgery (74% in the biliary-drainage group compared with 39% in the early-surgery group). No improvement in any outcome was seen in the biliary-drainage group.[107-110] The current consensus is that if surgical resection is planned within 1 to 2 weeks, drainage is usually not recommended in an otherwise asymptomatic patient. However, Lee showed that when surgical intervention is planned beyond 3 weeks or if the patient becomes symptomatic, stent placement should be undertaken.[111] Cholangitis is an accepted indication for stenting. Patients undergoing neoadjuvant chemoradiation also benefit from SEMS placement.[112] If ERCP is done for diagnostic purposes, drainage is performed during the same procedure.

Plastic stents. Plastic stents are usually composed of polyethylene or polytetrafluoroethylene (Teflon), are relatively inexpensive, and can be removed without difficulty if future surgical resection is planned. It has been shown that a stent with the lowest coefficient of friction has the least potential for clogging.[113] Although Teflon has the lowest

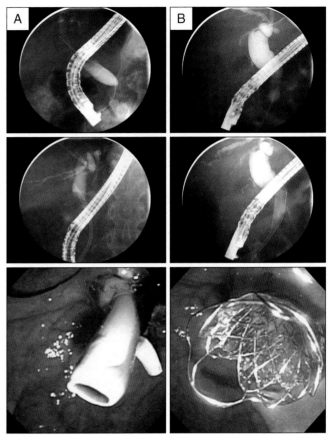

FIG 39.7 Stents in the management of biliary obstruction. **A,** The *upper panel* shows a malignant distal common bile duct (CBD) stricture with postobstructive dilation of the proximal CBD. A single straight plastic stent was placed to relieve biliary obstruction, as demonstrated by the fluoroscopic image in the *middle panel* and endoscopic image in the *lower panel.* **B,** The *upper panel* shows a malignant distal CBD stricture with severe postobstructive dilation of the proximal CBD. A single self-expandable metal stent was placed to relieve biliary obstruction, as demonstrated by the fluoroscopic image in the *middle panel* and the endoscopic image in the *lower panel.*

coefficient of friction, Teflon stents are stiffer and may increase the chance of perforation at the opposite duodenal wall if migration occurs. Polyurethane stents tend to fragment during attempted retrieval. Therefore, currently polyethylene remains the preferred material, as it is relatively pliable (Fig. 39.7, *A*).[114,115]

A large variety of plastic biliary stents are available, with internal diameters that range from 5 to 11.5 Fr and in lengths ranging from 5 to 19 cm. The most common type of plastic stent used is a straight stent with side holes and flaps at both ends that are designed to minimize the risk of stent migration. A pigtail stent offers the advantage of lower risk of migration, as its curves allow better positioning and anchoring within the bile duct and the duodenum (Fig. 39.8). The length of the stent is selected to minimize the length within the biliary tree and the duodenum and at the same time to ensure effective biliary drainage. Usually stents are inserted such that their ends extend 1 to 2 cm above the proximal end of the biliary obstruction and about 1 cm in the duodenum.

Adverse events associated with plastic stents include the following:

1. *Stent occlusion:* Obstruction of a plastic stent usually occurs within a few months of insertion and therefore requires repeated stent

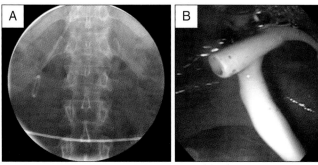

FIG 39.8 Pigtail plastic biliary stent. **A,** Radiographic image of pigtail biliary stent with distal end in the duodenum. **B,** Endoscopic image from same patient.

exchanges because of the risk of obstructive jaundice and cholangitis. The mechanism of obstruction of a plastic stent involves absorption of proteins from bile by the stent, attraction by bacterial adherence to these proteins, and formation of a biofilm of bacterial glycoproteins that shield the bacteria from the mechanical forces of bile flow, antibiotics, and cells of the immune system.[116,117] Ultimately, enzymatic activity of bacterial enzymes induces precipitation of deconjugated bilirubin and crystals of fatty acid and calcium salts, which result in the formation of sludge. Confocal laser scanning and scanning electron microscope studies have also shown that large networks of dietary fibers that reflux from the duodenum contribute to stent occlusion.[118] Removal of an occluded stent can be performed using a snare, Dormia basket, or Soehendra stent retrieval device (see Chapter 24).

Several strategies have been adopted in an attempt to prevent stent occlusion. Plastic biliary stents with larger diameter have prolonged patency.[119] The presence or absence of side holes has also been considered as a stent occlusion prevention strategy. Studies have shown that considerable sludge formation occurs around the side holes of stents. The Tannenbaum stent (Cook Medical Inc., Bloomington, IN), a straight Teflon stent without side holes, was introduced for this purpose. However, studies failed to show a significant difference in stent patency.[120,121] In a randomized trial a DoubleLayer stent (Olympus Corp., Tokyo, Japan) without side holes had a significantly longer duration of patency and decreased risk of occlusion compared with a standard polyethylene stent with side holes in patients with malignant strictures.[122] However, a recent prospective randomized trial showed comparable patency for the DoubleLayer and Tannenbaum stents.[123]

Attempts to improve the duration of stent patency by countering duodenobiliary reflux led to the development of antireflux stents with a unidirectional valve mechanism that allows only anterograde bile flow. A randomized trial showed the median patency of the antireflux plastic stents to be significantly higher (145 days) than conventional plastic biliary stents (101 days), and they displayed equal efficacy in improving liver tests, with comparable adverse event rates.[124] However, a more recent study was terminated early because of valve malfunction and early stent occlusion.[125]

The utility of agents such as ursodeoxycholic acid (UDCA) and antibiotics to increase stent patency has been studied. A meta-analysis of five randomized trials in 258 patients with malignant biliary strictures who had polyethylene stents placed and were treated with either a combination of UDCA and antibiotics or no treatment showed no significant effects on stent patency.[126] Those findings were confirmed in a more recent publication.[127]

2. *Stent migration:* Migration of a stent may occur in up to 10% of patients.[128] Stent migration can be either proximal or distal to the site of insertion. A migrated stent may become dysfunctional, can become a focus of infection, or can result in perforation of the biliary tree or duodenum. Management of migrated stents is discussed in Chapter 24. Snares, baskets, and rat-tooth forceps are the most common tools used to remove migrated stents. Other techniques include using a stone extraction balloon by inflating it above the stent and slowly withdrawing the balloon. It may become necessary to use special devices such as a Soehendra screw extractor (Cook Medical Inc., Winston-Salem, NC). If a stent migrates above a stricture, extraction may require balloon dilation of the stricture.[114] If endoscopic approaches fail, either a percutaneous or surgical approach may be necessary to remove the stent.

3. *Stent fracture:* A rare adverse event with plastic stents is prosthesis fracture. Since the introduction of polyethylene stents, breakage of stents has become extremely rare. The distal portion of the stent is susceptible to fracture, possibly as a consequence of repeated peristalsis.

Self-expandable metal stents. SEMS were developed for palliative treatment of malignant biliary obstruction in an attempt to prolong the duration of patency by increasing the stent diameter while simultaneously overcoming the limitation of the diameter of the working channel of the duodenoscope. SEMS have a tubular structure consisting of a braided or laser-cut form of a metal alloy such as stainless steel, nitinol, Platinol, or Elgiloy. These stents are constrained by a sheath onto a 6-Fr to 8.5-Fr delivery catheter with radiopaque markers to ease their precise release within the bile ducts. After the desired location of the stent is reached, the sheath is slowly withdrawn distally, leaving behind the stent, which then expands to assume its original configuration within the bile duct, spanning the stricture (see Fig. 39.7, *B*). In their fully expanded state, SEMS have a lumen diameter that is three to four times that of plastic stents (Table 39.5).

Since the initial reports of SEMS to relieve biliary strictures in 1989,[105,106] SEMS have been widely used in the treatment of malignant distal biliary obstruction. Initial SEMS were uncovered bare-metal stents that imbedded in the surrounding tissue in a short period, making retrieval almost impossible. Partially covered and fully covered stents were developed to overcome the barrier of stent occlusion via tumor ingrowth and reactive tissue hyperplasia through the stent meshwork. The covering of the stent prevents imbedding into the tissue and theoretically permits removal, especially if the distal end of the stent extends into the duodenum. Currently, SEMS composed of a variety of metals that are uncovered, partially covered, or fully covered are available. These stents have lengths ranging from 40 to 120 mm and diameters ranging from 6 to 10 mm. The median patency durations for SEMS have been reported to be in the range of 9 to 12 months when used for palliation of malignant distal obstruction.[129–131] Existing data do not favor one type of SEMS over another.[132–136] Thus their use is generally based on endoscopist preference.

SEMS are placed during ERCP after cannulation of the bile duct, often with a sphincterotome and a guidewire (see Chapter 14). The least amount of contrast should be injected to define the anatomy of the bile duct and to confirm the location of the stricture, which is often known by prior imaging studies. Most SEMS have radiopaque markers located at the proximal and distal ends and some in the midportion. Stents should be placed such that the proximal marker lies above the proximal edge of the stricture. After determining the final position of the stent, the outer constraining sheath of the stent is slowly withdrawn (or, in some cases, unwoven) with simultaneous traction on the stent to maintain its position within the bile duct as the stent moves away from the papilla as it is "pushed" from the sheath. Flow of bile is a

TABLE 39.5   **Specifications of Various Biliary SEMS**

Stent	Manufacturer	Metal Design Coating	Covering Options	Length (mm)	Diameter (mm) Options	Radiopacity/ No. Markers	Reconstrainability	Delivery Catheter (Fr)	Shortening (%)	Cell Size	Axial Force	Radial Force	Ends
Flexus	ConMed	Nitinol	UC only	40, 60, 80, 100	8, 10	++ (tantalum)/4	No	7.5	<1	+++	++	++	Flared
Niti-S*	Taewoong Medical	Nitinol, hand-woven	FC, UC	40, 50, 60, 70, 80, 90, 100, 110, 120	8, 10	++/10	Yes (30%–40%)	8.5	No	++	+	++	Looped, flared
X-Suit NIR	Olympus Medical	Nitinol	UC	40, 60, 80	8, 10	++/4	No	7.5	No	++	N/A	N/A	Rounded
Viabil	Gore Medical	Nitinol, laser cut, ePTFE	FC	40, 60, 80, 100	8, 10	++/2	No	10	No	N/A	+	++	Flared
WallFlex RX	Boston Scientific	Platinol, braided, silicone	UC, PC, FC	40, 60, 80, 100	8, 10	+++/4	Yes (80%)	7.5	40	+	+++	+	Looped, flared
Wallstent RX	Boston Scientific	Elgiloy, braided	UC, FC, PC	40, 60, 80, 100	8, 10	+++/4	Yes (80%)	7.5	40	+	+++	+	Open, flared
Ziver	Cook Medical Endoscopy	Nitinol	UC	40, 60, 80	6, 8, 10	++/4	No	7	No	+++	+	+	Flared

ePTFE, Polytetrafluoroethylene; *FC*, fully covered; *N/A*, not applicable; *PC*, partially covered; *UC*, uncovered.
*Widely available outside the United States.
Adapted from Lee JH. Self-expandable metal stents for malignant distal biliary strictures. *Gastrointest Endosc Clin N Am.* 2011;21:463–480.

good indicator of successful stent placement. If poor drainage of bile is noted because of failure of SEMS to expand, dilation of the waist of the stricture using a balloon up to the maximal diameter of the stent can be performed. Complete expansion of SEMS may take up to 72 hours.

Involvement of the distal bile duct by malignancy often distorts local anatomy and prevents biliary access. In those cases, other endoscopic techniques for biliary access should be considered for SEMS placement. A precut needle-knife sphincterotomy (see Chapter 15) after placement of a pancreatic duct stent may be possible. EUS-ERCP rendezvous technique, EUS-guided transhepatic SEMS placement, and EUS-guided transluminal SEMS placement are also options (see Chapter 32). The EUS-ERCP rendezvous technique involves accessing the bile duct using a 19-gauge or 22-gauge needle under EUS guidance at a point proximal to the papilla. A guidewire is then passed through the needle into the bile duct and passed antegrade through the papilla. Conventional ERCP is then performed to place the SEMS. Successful biliary drainage using EUS rendezvous ranges from 80% to 100%.[137–139] In EUS-guided transhepatic SEMS placement, a needle is passed through the stomach wall, liver, and finally the papilla under EUS guidance and a guidewire is passed through the needle. The tract can then be dilated using a catheter or balloon and the SEMS placed over the guidewire through the papilla.[140]

Adverse events of SEMS placement (see Chapter 8) include stent occlusion, stent migration, and pancreatitis. Occlusion of the cystic duct can lead to cholecystitis. Occlusion of the pancreatic duct can theoretically lead to pancreatitis. The mechanism of uncovered SEMS occlusion includes tumor ingrowth, tumor overgrowth, and mucosal hyperplasia. SEMS that are occluded by sludge can be cleared by performing balloon sweeps. If the occlusion is secondary to tumor ingrowth, as seen with uncovered stents, the management strategy involves placing a second SEMS (covered or uncovered) or a plastic stent (Fig. 39.9) inside the original stent. Comparative studies of SEMS and plastic stents have shown longer duration of patency with SEMS.[141,142] Occluded SEMS may be managed by placing additional SEMS or plastic stents within the original stent, with one study showing similar outcomes.[143] When considering only the initial placement, covered SEMS may provide longer patency than uncovered SEMS.[141]

Post-ERCP pancreatitis has been reported to occur more commonly after SEMS placement than plastic stent placement.[144] However, when comparing covered SEMS and uncovered SEMS, rates of pancreatitis and cholecystitis have been conflicting.[144,145]

Stent migration is an uncommon adverse event (Fig. 39.10). Migration of covered SEMS is more common than of uncovered SEMS. In the case of incomplete stent migration, removal of an uncovered stent can be very difficult. The mesh of an uncovered stent becomes imbedded in the wall and attempted removal may lead to bile duct injury. Because of the membrane coating, covered stent tissue ingrowth does not develop (unless partially covered SEMS are used). Fully covered stents are easily removed using a snare or rat-tooth forceps.[146]

Stent choices for palliation of malignant biliary obstruction. Several aspects must be considered before determining the choice of stent in a given patient. These factors include choosing the type of stent to be used (plastic vs SEMS) and, if a SEMS is chosen, whether to use uncovered or covered. The decision requires consideration of technical, economic, and patient factors. Technical factors include the ease of stent placement, stent efficacy, duration of patency, anticipated need for reintervention, and whether removal of the stent could be required. Economic factors include costs of stents and costs associated with reintervention. Patient factors include socioeconomic status, expected length of survival, and the level of obstruction of the biliary tree.

Both plastic stents and SEMS have similar rates of successful placement for distal malignant biliary obstruction. The mean patency of plastic stents is approximately 3 to 4 months, compared with 9 to 12 months for SEMS.[129–131,147] A meta-analysis of seven randomized controlled trials showed no difference between plastic stents and SEMS in terms of technical success, therapeutic success, 30-day mortality, or adverse events. However, SEMS were associated with higher patency rates compared with plastic stents at 4 months.[148]

The choice of using covered SEMS over uncovered SEMS for palliation of distal malignant obstruction remains controversial. Although covered SEMS were developed in an attempt to prolong stent patency, this has not been definitively demonstrated. Earlier retrospective studies demonstrated superior patency of covered SEMS over uncovered SEMS. A meta-analysis that included five randomized trials comparing covered and uncovered SEMS for palliation of distal malignant biliary obstruction found that covered SEMS had a significantly longer duration of patency by a mean of 61 days during a median follow-up of 212 days.[149] Although both covered and uncovered SEMS showed similar rates of stent dysfunction, there was a trend toward delayed time to

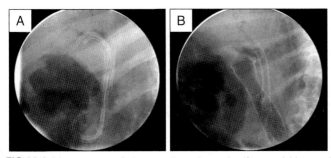

FIG 39.9 Management of obstructed or migrated self-expandable metal stent (SEMS). **A,** Multiple plastic stents placed to relieve SEMS obstruction. **B,** Placement of SEMS within a distally migrated SEMS. The first step was to create an opening within the wall of a previously placed duodenal SEMS, followed by creating an opening within the wall of the migrated SEMS using a Soehendra screw stent retriever. This was followed by cannulating the bile duct through the wall of the migrated stent, followed by placing the new SEMS.

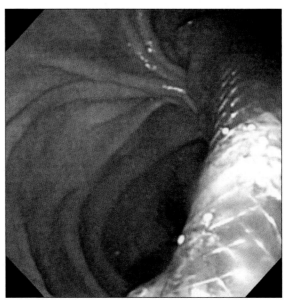

FIG 39.10 Endoscopic image of a distally migrated covered self-expandable metal stent.

reobstruction (stent survival) with covered SEMS. Stent migration, tumor overgrowth, and sludge formation were found to be significantly higher with covered SEMS, whereas tumor ingrowth was the most common cause of obstruction with uncovered SEMS. Additionally, covered SEMS did not appear to increase the risk of cholecystitis. However, most of the studies incorporated measures to prevent cholecystitis, such as the use of stents with transmural drainage holes or placement of the stents below the level of the cystic duct in patients with an intact gallbladder, which are strategies that may not be applicable or successful in routine clinical practice.[149] Furthermore, the rate of pancreatitis was similar between covered and uncovered SEMS. A subgroup analysis in this study showed no difference in stent patency and rate of migration between fully covered and partially covered SEMS. Major limitations of this meta-analysis include that two of the included studies were from a single institution and in two of the studies SEMS were placed percutaneously.

Different circumstances warrant removal of stents, including migration or irreversible occlusion and, in rare instances, remission of tumor (e.g., if the obstruction is from lymphoma that responds to chemotherapy). Plastic stents and covered SEMS are easily removable. Uncovered SEMS can be impossible to remove and attempts at removal may induce perforation of the bile duct. In a retrospective study that compared removal of uncovered and covered SEMS in patients with migrated or malfunctioning stents, covered SEMS could be removed in 92% of cases, whereas only 38% of uncovered stents could be removed.[146]

Patient-related factors such as cost, expected length of survival, and level of biliary obstruction can also influence the choice of stents. SEMS may be up to 40 times more expensive than plastic stents. The lower cost of plastic stents is offset by the need for repeat interventions because of stent occlusion. Two factors found to influence overall cost were the local cost of ERCP and patient survival. The general consensus is that SEMS are preferred to plastic stents when patient survival is expected to be beyond 4 to 6 months.[129,130,147,148,150] Although it is difficult to predict patient survival, two different studies reported that tumor size and presence of liver metastasis were independent indicators of shorter survival,[131,151] and these prognostic factors may be used to establish the choice of stent.[114] However, a recent study suggested that SEMS placement was cost-effective regardless of patient survival and is considered a superior choice in almost all instances.[152,153]

After stent placement, a follow-up plan is needed that considers the limitations of the chosen stent type. If a plastic stent is chosen for initial stenting, a decision should be made as to elective scheduled replacement before occlusion or replacement "on demand" when occlusion occurs. A randomized trial that compared prophylactic plastic stent exchange every 3 months and on demand showed that the scheduled replacement patients had a longer adverse event–free survival, although overall survival was not different.[129]

Percutaneous Approach to Biliary Drainage

In some patients, endoscopic biliary drainage may be unsuccessful or impossible. This group includes the following: patients with duodenal stenosis, altered anatomy because of previous surgery (e.g., Roux-en-Y gastric bypass or previous creation of bilioenteric anastomosis), difficulty traversing the biliary stricture, and unsuccessful cannulation of the papilla because of tumor involving the papilla or as a result of its location within a duodenal diverticulum. For such patients, percutaneous transhepatic cholangiography (PTC) is a relatively safe and effective option. This approach involves transhepatic access of the biliary system with a thin needle and a guidewire under radiologic guidance, placing a sheath over the guidewire and negotiating the strictures using a catheter,

thus achieving an internal-external drainage system. In a two-step approach, the stent is subsequently internalized. This approach, termed *secondary percutaneous stent placement*, may require that the percutaneous drain remain in place for 2 to 6 weeks before complete internalization with a metal stent to allow maturation of an epithelialized tract from the biliary tree to the skin and thus minimize the risk of intraperitoneal bile leakage when the catheter is removed.[154] Internal drains are preferred because they are more physiologic, as the enterohepatic circulation of bile is maintained. Animal model studies have demonstrated that internal drainage is superior to external drainage in preserving intestinal immunity and preventing bacterial translocation, although such results have not been validated in humans. In addition, internalization of the drainage tube helps avoid lifestyle limitations and potential adverse events associated with external drains, such as catheter dislodgement, pain at the insertion site, and infection and leakage of bile around the catheter. In some centers primary percutaneous stenting of malignant bile duct obstruction using a one-step approach to a percutaneous internal drainage system is used. With this approach, the external catheter was removed as early as 24 hours after percutaneous biliary stent placement in the majority of patients.[155]

Percutaneous biliary drainage has been found to be as effective as surgery at relieving biliary obstruction. However, a Cochrane database systematic review that compared benefits and harms of preoperative biliary drainage and included four randomized clinical trials that compared percutaneous transhepatic biliary drainage with direct surgery found no significant difference in mortality or morbidity between the two groups.[156]

For the purpose of percutaneous transhepatic biliary stenting, SEMS have become the standard of choice. They are preferred over percutaneously placed plastic stents owing to their higher patency rates and because they avoid the need for repeat procedures. Moreover, if re-obstruction occurs, a new stent can be inserted within the occluded metal stent without having to remove it.

Two older randomized trials compared PTC and endoscopic biliary drainage. Speer et al. showed that ERCP was significantly more effective at relieving jaundice compared with PTC (81% vs 61%), with significantly lower 30-day mortality (15% vs 33%). The higher mortality after percutaneous stents is attributed to hemobilia and bile leakage. However, the use of rigid plastic drainage tubes for PTC may not be generalizable to modern settings where SEMS placement has become the norm. In another trial, Pinol et al. compared placement of PTC with SEMS with endoscopic placement of polyethylene stents. They observed that although the technical success rates of both procedures were similar, therapeutic success was significantly higher in the PTC group (71% vs 42%).[157] However, major adverse events were more commonly observed in the PTC group (61% vs 35%). Despite this observation, the 30-day mortality rates were comparable. The overall median survival was noted to be significantly higher in the PTC group than in the endoscopic group (3.7 vs 2.0 months). The study concluded that PTC with placement of SEMS is an alternative to placement of endoscopic plastic stents. It must be noted that the two studies discussed here included patients with both distal and proximal bile duct obstruction. Considering that PTC is easier to perform in proximal bile duct obstruction than distal obstruction, the studies' results should be viewed with caution, as the success rates of ERCP and stent placement for distal obstruction should be at least 80% to 90%. In addition to these studies, data from several noncomparative studies suggest no significant differences in technical success rates, adverse event rates, and mortality rates between the two techniques. However, the types of adverse events differ between the groups. Thus, although bile leak is more frequently observed after PTC, pancreatitis is more frequently seen with endoscopic drainage.

To summarize, PTC is reserved primarily for unsuccessful endoscopic biliary drainage or when the papilla or biliary tree is inaccessible. However, institutional preferences and operator skills and experience factor into the decision to use one technique over the other. With the advent of EUS-guided drainage techniques, it is anticipated that the need for percutaneous drainage will diminish.

Surgical Palliation

Surgical palliation was the mainstay option for palliation of distal malignant biliary obstruction. With advancements in percutaneous and endoscopic approaches, surgical palliation has diminished. Surgical palliation can be achieved using cholecystojejunostomy, choledocho-duodenostomy, or hepaticojejunostomy. Hepaticojejunostomy has been shown to be superior to both cholecystojejunostomy and cholecysto-enterostomy.[158,159] Surgery in good operative patients allows concomitant gastric bypass for duodenal obstruction and pain control via intraoperative celiac nerve block.[159]

Randomized trials of palliative surgery and endoscopic stent placement were performed between 1988 and 1994.[160–162] A meta-analysis of these studies concluded that the stent group had a higher likelihood of reintervention for biliary obstruction than the surgery group.[163] However, these studies were performed before the advent of SEMS. A randomized study in patients who underwent laparoscopic staging before pancreaticoduodenectomy and were found to be unresectable were randomized to uncovered SEMS placement versus surgical bypass. No difference was noted in mortality, morbidity, length of hospital stay, readmissions, or adverse events.[164] A 2007 meta-analysis of studies that compared surgery and ERCP-guided biliary stent placement showed that endoscopic stenting with plastic stents was associated with a lower risk of overall adverse events but a higher risk of recurrent biliary obstruction compared with surgical bypass. SEMS were found to be associated with a significantly lower risk of recurrent biliary obstruction at 4 months. Plastic and metal stents were comparable in terms of technical success, therapeutic success, mortality, and adverse events.[115] The major limitation of the previously cited studies and meta-analysis is that these studies were published almost 2 decades ago, and since then both surgical and endoscopic palliation have undergone remarkable advances. For example, laparoscopic cholecystojejunostomy has been developed as a minimally invasive approach to provide biliary drainage in distal malignant biliary obstruction. Similarly, stenting technology has also dramatically improved. It appears that the use of surgical palliation has dramatically declined and has been replaced by endoscopic and percutaneous biliary drainage.

Whether prophylactic gastrojejunostomy should be performed in the setting of unresectable cancer remains controversial because up to 20% of cases will develop late gastric outlet obstruction (GOO). GOO is commonly treated by endoscopic enteral stent placement (see Chapter 42). A recent study showed that patients with GOO with obstruction of the third portion of the duodenum may be at higher risk for stent malfunction and migration.[165] If stent placement fails or is not available, surgical gastrojejunostomy is an option. A systematic review of two randomized controlled trials and six studies that compared gastrojejunostomy with enteral stent placement for patients with malignant GOO found that technical success rates, adverse events, and symptom relief were comparable. The authors concluded that stents are preferred in patients with relatively short life expectancy and that gastrojejunostomy should be reserved for patients with a more prolonged survival prognosis based upon functional status.[166] Thus surgical biliary bypass is a viable option in patients who are not good candidates for biliary stenting, who are found to have an unresectable tumor at the time of laparotomy, and who have anticipated survival ≥6 months, and in a subset of patients who undergo laparotomy for surgical ablation of the celiac nerves for refractory pain.

Adjuvant Chemotherapy

Although surgery has the potential to provide definitive cure for patients with pancreatic cancer, 5-year survival after pancreaticoduodenectomy is only about 10% for node-positive disease[167] and 25% to 30% for node-negative disease.[168] Recognizing the need to improve survival in these patients, the impact of concomitant adjuvant chemotherapy has been explored. Studies have shown a definite improvement in quality of life after adjuvant therapy irrespective of the mode of treatment.[169–171] In early studies that randomized patients to receive chemoradiation that included radiation plus 5-fluorouracil (5-FU) versus surgery alone, the median 2-year survival was found to be significantly increased in the chemoradiation group compared with the surgery-alone group (42% vs 15%).[170] Similar trials in Europe showed survival benefit in the chemotherapy group but not in the chemoradiation group.[171] A randomized trial also showed survival advantage for combination chemotherapy using 5-FU, doxorubicin, and mitomycin C.[172] Although these agents improved 5-year survival rates, they also had significant systemic toxicity profiles. In this context the introduction of gemcitabine is considered a significant milestone. Studies have shown significant increases in disease-free survival after gemcitabine treatment compared with surgery alone.[173] The ESPAC-3 trial, which represents the largest randomized controlled trial in pancreatic cancer treatment and included centers in Europe, Australasia, Japan, and Canada, found no difference between the 5-FU and folinic acid combination group and the gemcitabine group, although gemcitabine had an improved safety profile.[174]

Recent advances in palliative radiotherapy for pancreatic cancer include the development of imaging-guided radiation therapy (CyberKnife stereotactic radiation) and have produced promising palliative results, good local control, and control of metastatic disease and recurrent cancer. Radiopaque gold fiducials placed in or around the tumor site enable real-time tumor tracking to maintain special precision and thus facilitate delivery of focused radiation. Until recently, gold fiducials were placed in or near the tumor site percutaneously under image guidance or during surgery. EUS-guided fiducial placement in or near the pancreatic tumor site has become a newer alternative. The safety of this approach has been demonstrated.[175,176]

Irrespective of adjuvant therapy selected, the management of symptoms arising from distal biliary obstruction requires endoscopic, percutaneous, or surgical intervention. Biliary drainage helps subvert potential hepatotoxic effects of chemotherapeutic agents. The improved survival profiles provided by adjuvant chemotherapy affect the choice of biliary drainage. It is clear that SEMS (either short uncovered or longer covered) is superior to plastic stents during the time neoadjuvant therapy is delivered and the time the patient undergoes pancreaticoduodenectomy, with decreased stent occlusion and decreased need for reintervention, especially when the patient is vulnerable from cytotoxicity (leukopenia).[177] Although the patency of plastic stents is unaffected by chemotherapeutic agents, SEMS patency may be prolonged. In this regard, local delivery of chemotherapeutic agents via drug-eluting stents (DES) is a new area of interest. In a multicenter pilot study, the technical feasibility and safety of using metal stents covered with a paclitaxel-incorporated membrane was demonstrated.[178] In 21 patients with malignant biliary obstruction who received DES, cumulative stent patency rates at 3, 6, and 12 months were 100%, 71%, and 36%, respectively. Of the nine patients who developed stent occlusion, four had biliary sludge, three had tumor overgrowth, and two had tumor ingrowth. The serum level of paclitaxel was highest between 1 and 10 days after DES insertion.

SUMMARY

Malignant distal biliary obstruction most frequently occurs in the context of an unresectable tumor that requires effective therapeutic strategies to provide palliative biliary drainage. Significant recent advances in the field of endoscopic stenting have resulted in a shift in the focus of treatment from surgery to endoscopic intervention to manage biliary obstruction. However, the complex nature of these conditions warrants a multidisciplinary approach to treatment that involves surgeons, radiologists, and gastroenterologists. Anticipated improvements in the fields of early cancer detection and chemotherapy are expected to increase the length of survival of patients with pancreaticobiliary malignancies and increase the demand for improved strategies for biliary decompression.

The complete reference list for this chapter can be found online at www.expertconsult.com.

40

Malignant Biliary Obstruction of the Hilum and Proximal Bile Ducts

Alexander M. Sarkisian and Reem Z. Sharaiha

Malignant biliary obstruction of the hilum and proximal intrahepatic bile ducts can result from primary pancreaticobiliary cancers, primary liver cancers, portal lymphadenopathy, or metastatic disease. Primary pancreaticobiliary cancers affecting the proximal bile ducts and hilum include cholangiocarcinoma (CCA) and gallbladder cancer. CCA can cause obstruction at any level of the biliary tract. Cancer of the gallbladder can present with hilar or right intrahepatic duct obstruction caused by local tumor extension, extrinsic compression from portal adenopathy, or Mirizzi's syndrome. This chapter will focus on the diagnosis and management of biliary obstruction from hilar and proximal bile duct cancers. Refer to Table 40.1 for a differential diagnosis of hilar strictures.[1–4] This chapter also features a discussion of recent developments in local ablative therapy for CCA and a comparison of endoscopic to percutaneous drainage in the setting of malignant biliary obstruction. Malignant biliary obstruction of the distal bile ducts, including distal CCA, is discussed in Chapter 39.

CHOLANGIOCARCINOMA

CCA arises from cholangiocytes, the epithelial cells of the bile ducts. CCA accounts for approximately 3% of all gastrointestinal malignancies. CCA can be divided into three unique subtypes: proximal (intrahepatic), hilar, and distal (extrahepatic) cancers. Most CCA is located in the hilar region (60% to 70%), whereas 20% to 30% are distal tumors and CCA originating from the intrahepatic ducts accounts for only 5% to 10%.[5] Cancers arising in the hilar region have been further classified according to the pattern of involvement of the hepatic ducts (see the section, "Bismuth-Corlette Classification"). There have been a number of studies reporting an increased incidence of intrahepatic CCA over the past few decades in several countries worldwide. Everhart and Ruhl reported that, between 1979 and 2004, the incidence of CCA increased by 22% in the United States, with increasing incidence of intrahepatic CCA responsible for all of this increase.[6] Over this same period, the 5-year survival rate did not change, remaining near 10%.[6] There is evidence supporting that misclassification of the location of CCA in SEER data and changes in the ICD coding practice may be responsible for a portion of the observed increase in intrahepatic CCA.[7] Independent of the impact of classification errors, a real increase in the incidence of intrahepatic CCA has been reported in many nations worldwide, an issue that warrants further investigation.[8,9] The majority of CCAs (>90%) are adenocarcinomas. Squamous cell carcinomas account for most of the remaining cases. Adenocarcinomas are divided into the sclerosing (>70%), nodular (20%), and papillary (5% to 10%) types.[10] Both nodular and sclerosing (scirrhous) tumors have lower resection and cure rates.[11]

Risk Factors

The single most important risk factor for the development of CCA is primary sclerosing cholangitis (PSC). Almost one-third of CCAs are diagnosed in patients with primary PSC, with or without associated chronic ulcerative colitis.[12] Other notable risk factors associated with CCA include biliary tract disease (e.g., hepatolithiasis, choledochal cysts), non–PSC-related cirrhosis, hepatitis B viral infection, parasitic infection (e.g., with *Clonorchis sinensis* or *Opisthorchis viverrini*), polycystic liver disease, toxic exposures (e.g., to thorotrast and rubber), and genetic disorders (e.g., Lynch syndrome and biliary papillomatosis).[13–16] Each CCA subtype (proximal, hilar, or distal) is a unique pathologic entity and consequently each risk factor confers a different amount of risk for each of the CCA subtypes, although the subtypes share most known risk factors.[16]

Conversely, there is evidence from case-control studies that aspirin use is associated with a roughly threefold decrease in the risk of developing CCA.[16] Moreover, preclinical evidence in mice and correlative data from case-control studies indicate that metformin has a protective effect in CCA, which warrants further investigation.[17,18]

ANATOMY OF THE BILE DUCTS

Understanding segmental liver anatomy and variations in the relationships of the major sectoral ducts is of paramount importance in performing safe and appropriate drainage and decreasing endoscopic retrograde cholangiopancreatography (ERCP)–related adverse events (see Chapter 8) in patients with hilar obstruction. It is a common misperception that the bile ducts are simply shaped like a "Y," with the right and left ducts joining together to form the common hepatic duct. In reality, the anatomic pattern of the biliary tree can be quite variable and includes eight segments (Fig. 40.1). Knowledge of this anatomy, as well as the common variations of the segmental intrahepatic ducts and biliary confluence (Figs. 40.2 and 40.3), is essential for successful endoscopic management of complex proximal and hilar CCA. Segment I (caudate lobe) is typically drained by several small ducts into both the right and left ductal systems. These branches are generally not seen on ERCP. Segments II, III, and IV comprise the left lobe. Segment II/III is usually drained by the large left intrahepatic duct that is targeted on endoscopic therapy. Segment IV is further divided into two smaller segments, IVa and IVb, which are typically not targets of endoscopic drainage given the small portion of hepatic parenchyma they drain. The right hepatic ducts are divided into the right anterior sectoral duct, which drains segments V and VIII, and the right posterior sectoral duct, which drains segments VI and VII.[19,20]

Bismuth-Corlette Classification

Cancers arising in the perihilar region have been classified according to their pattern of involvement of the hepatic ducts. The Bismuth classification[21] for CCA is useful for determining and planning surgical resection and endoscopic stent placement. Bile duct tumors that involve the confluence of the major ducts are referred to as Klatskin tumors or hilar CCA (Fig. 40.4).

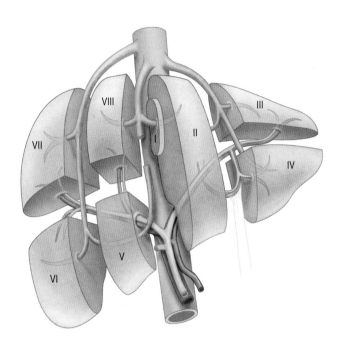

FIG 40.1 Functional division of the liver into segments, according to Couinaud's nomenclature. (Redrawn from Blumgart LH, Fong Y, eds. *Surgery of the Liver and Biliary Tract.* 3rd ed. Philadelphia: W.B. Saunders; 2000.)

TABLE 40.1   Differential Diagnosis of Hilar Strictures

Malignant	Benign
Cholangiocarcinoma	Primary sclerosing cholangitis
Gallbladder cancer	Choledocholithiasis/hepatolithiasis
Nodal metastases at porta hepatis	Inflammatory stricture
	Postoperative stricture
Hepatocellular carcinoma	Extrinsic compression (Mirizzi syndrome)
Hepatic metastases	Benign fibrosing/sclerosing cholangitis
Metastases to biliary tree	Radiation-induced stricture
Lymphoma	Caroli disease
	Ischemic stricture
	Infectious associated
	IgG4-associated cholangitis

Data from Wetter LA, Ring EJ, Pellegrini CA, et al. Differential diagnosis of sclerosing cholangiocarcinomas of the common hepatic duct (Klatskin tumors). *Am J Surg.* 1991;161:57. Verbeek PC, van Leeuwen DJ, de Wit LT, et al. Benign fibrosing disease at the hepatic confluence mimicking Klatskin tumors. *Surgery.* 1992;112:866. Chapman R, Fevery J, Kalloo A, et al. Diagnosis and management of primary sclerosing cholangitis. *Hepatology.* 2010;51:660. Zaydfudim VM, Wang AY, de Lange EE, et al. IgG4-associated cholangitis can mimic hilar cholangiocarcinoma. *Gut Liver.* 2015;9:556–560.

- *Type I:* Tumors below the confluence of the left and right hepatic ducts
- *Type II:* Tumors reaching the confluence of the right and left hepatic ducts
- *Type III:* Tumors occluding the common hepatic duct and either the first radicals of the right (*IIIa*) or left (*IIIb*) intrahepatic system

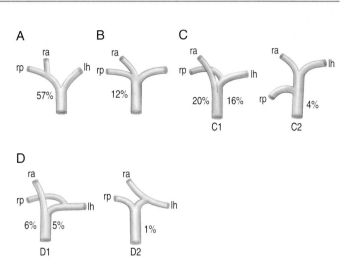

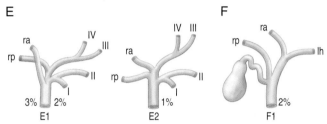

FIG 40.2 Common variations of biliary confluence anatomy. **A,** Typical anatomy. **B,** Triple confluence. **C,** Ectopic drainage of right sectoral duct into common hepatic duct. **D,** Ectopic drainage of right sectoral duct into left hepatic duct. **E,** Absence of confluence. **F,** Ectopic drainage of right posterior sectoral duct into cystic duct. *lh,* Left hepatic duct; *ra,* right anterior; *rp,* right posterior. (Redrawn from Blumgart LH, Fong Y, eds. *Surgery of the Liver and Biliary Tract.* 3rd ed. Philadelphia: W.B. Saunders; 2000.)

- *Type IV:* Tumors that are multicentric or involve the confluence of the major ducts and radicals of both right and left intrahepatic ducts

DIAGNOSTIC EVALUATION

The necessity of obtaining a definitive tissue diagnosis of malignancy preoperatively is debated. There is concern that preoperative tissue acquisition via endoscopic ultrasonography (EUS) or computed tomography (CT)–guided fine-needle aspiration (FNA) can result in peritoneal seeding of tumor cells and should be avoided in patients with potentially curable tumors.[22] Acquisition of these biopsies can be challenging, and even after extensive diagnostic evaluation many patients will require surgical exploration to confirm the diagnosis and determine resectability of suspected malignant lesions.

Serologic Testing

Although nonspecific, serum liver chemistry is usually consistent with a pattern suggestive of biliary obstruction; the degree of elevation depends on the location, severity, and chronicity of the obstruction. A proximal lesion can be associated with an isolated alkaline phosphatase elevation. A prolonged prothrombin time may be seen in patients with chronic biliary obstruction because of vitamin K malabsorption.[23] Carcinoembryonic antigen (CEA) and cancer antigen (CA) 19-9 are the two markers that have been most widely used, but neither is highly sensitive or specific to be used alone for diagnosis. CEA and CA 19-9 may be elevated in a wide array of conditions, both benign and malignant.[24]

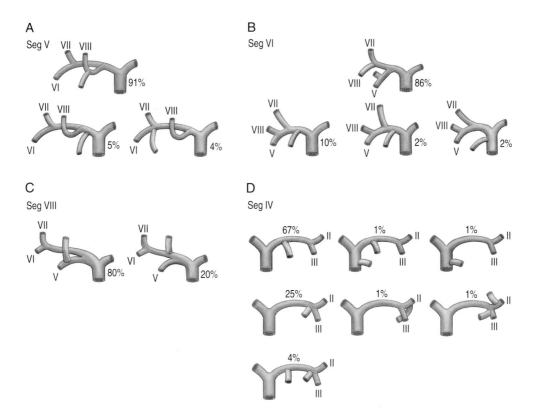

FIG 40.3 Common variations of the segmental intrahepatic ducts. **A,** Segment V. **B,** Segment VI. **C,** Segment VIII. **D,** Segment IV. (Redrawn from Blumgart LH, Fong Y, eds. *Surgery of the Liver and Biliary Tract.* 3rd ed. Philadelphia: W.B. Saunders; 2000.)

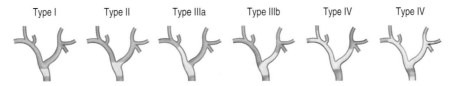

FIG 40.4 Schematic representation of Bismuth classification of hilar cholangiocarcinoma. *Type I:* tumors below the confluence of the left and right hepatic ducts (ceiling of the biliary confluence is intact; right and left ductal systems communicate); *type II:* tumors reaching the confluence but not involving the left or right hepatic ducts (ceiling of the confluence is destroyed; bile ducts are separated); *type III:* tumors occluding the common hepatic duct and either the right (*IIIa*) or left (*IIIb*) hepatic duct; *type IV:* multicentric tumors or tumors involving the confluence and both right and left hepatic ducts.

The use of CA 19-9 and CEA in concert with a host of novel markers identified with ELISA has the potential to improve the specificity of serologic testing for CCA. One marker, IL-6, has been studied for several years and has been shown to have specificity of approximately 90% to 92% and sensitivity ranging from 71% to 100% for detecting CCA.[24] IL-6 may also be elevated in benign biliary disease and hepatocellular carcinoma as well as metastatic disease.[24] This is an active area of research, and it will be of the utmost importance to identify reliable, validated markers to facilitate more timely detection of CCA in at-risk groups and in the general population.

Cytology

Bile aspirated during ERCP will result in positive cytology in only 30% of CCAs. Brush cytology also has a limited sensitivity of 35% to 69% and a specificity of 90%.[25] The yield is increased if the stricture is disturbed by performing brushings (Fig. 40.6) or biopsies of the lesion.[26] A plastic stent placed during a prior ERCP can be sent for cytologic evaluation at the time of removal or exchange. Combining brushings, biopsies, FNA, and stent cytology can result in a positive diagnosis in approximately 80% of patients.[27]

Assessment of DNA proliferation by both fluorescence in situ hybridization (FISH) and digital image analysis may further improve the specificity of cytology (see Chapter 41).[28–30] FISH uses fluorescence-labeled DNA probes to detect abnormal loss or gain of chromosomes or chromosomal loci on cytologic analysis. Digital image analysis quantifies cellular DNA by measuring the intensity of nuclei stained with a dye that binds to nuclear DNA. Although both tests show promise in improving diagnostic yield, further studies are needed. Patients with PSC may have benign strictures that yield abnormal FISH results (see Chapter 48). In the setting of PSC, the positivity of FISH for trisomy/tetrasomy on multiple samples of the biliary tree is more specific for CCA.[31]

Pathology

During ERCP, two methods can be used to obtain biopsies: targeted biopsies using direct visualization during cholangioscopy (see Chapters

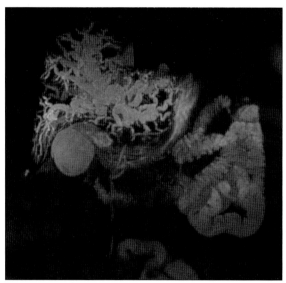

FIG 40.5 MRI-MRCP of diffuse biliary dilation secondary to a large tumor at the confluence.

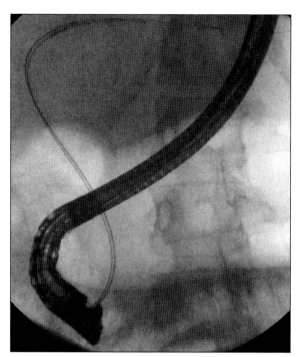

FIG 40.6 Fluoroscopic image of a left hepatic duct lesion undergoing brushing.

27 and 41) or biopsy forceps using fluoroscopy to target the site. The cumulative diagnostic yield for bile duct strictures is increased to 63% when biopsies are obtained in addition to brush cytology.[32] It has been proposed that biopsies performed with direct visualization during cholangioscopy may have a higher yield than biopsies obtained using fluoroscopic guidance without cholangioscopy.[33] Genotyping of CCA tumor cells has led to a number of prognostic and theranostic (individualized) markers currently under investigation, which will likely pave the way for effective and precise therapeutic options and prognostication.[34]

Radiologic Evaluation

In a patient with painless jaundice, CT scan and magnetic resonance imaging (MRI) are the preferred imaging modalities (see Chapter 34). MRCP can create three-dimensional images of the biliary tree, which are very useful for anatomic mapping with the added advantage of not requiring biliary instrumentation; it is the modality of choice when CCA is suspected (Fig. 40.5).[35] MRI with intravenous gadolinium administration commonly demonstrates CCA as minimal enhancement in the tumor periphery in the early arterial phase, with subsequent increased central enhancement in the delayed phase as a result of the central fibrous composition.[35] Contrast-enhanced CT scans are also an excellent imaging tool for intrahepatic CCA. On contrast-enhanced CT scans, intrahepatic CCA is most often hypoattenuating or isoattenuating in relationship to healthy hepatic parenchyma throughout all phases of the study, except for enhancement seen in the delayed phase of the study.[35] Positron emission tomography (PET) scan has been shown to detect nodular CCA as small as 1 cm because of the high glucose uptake of bile duct epithelium.[35] PET is less helpful for detection of infiltrating tumors, and its sensitivity is also dependent on local expertise. Difficulty in distinguishing benign from malignant lesions makes the utility of PET scans limited as an independent imaging modality. PET may help in identifying distant metastatic disease, which may lead to adjustment of surgical planning.[35]

Endoscopic Evaluation
Endoscopic Ultrasonography With Fine-Needle Aspiration

EUS with FNA (EUS-FNA) can be performed to evaluate indeterminate hilar lesions and to evaluate and sample portal adenopathy and accessible lesions in the liver (particularly those located in the left lobe).[22,36] The potential advantage of EUS-FNA over ERCP is that it is less invasive and it provides information in patients who do not otherwise require biliary drainage. One concern, however, is the potential for tumor seeding from the needle tract during EUS-FNA,[37,38] a particular concern in patients who are candidates for curative surgical resection. In the case of indeterminate biliary strictures, EUS-FNA when added to MRCP substantially increases the positive predictive value of the tests and may help find masses missed on other imaging modalities.[39]

Intraductal Ultrasonography

Intraductal ultrasonography (IDUS) probes are approximately 2 mm in diameter and can be advanced over a guidewire without need for biliary sphincterotomy. IDUS can help determine the longitudinal tumor extent more accurately than cholangiography. IDUS can also be used to evaluate for tumor invasion into the portal vein and right hepatic artery.[40] With the advent of more user-friendly cholangioscopy systems, IDUS is performed less frequently.

Cholangioscopy

Of the previously mentioned tools, cholangioscopy (Fig. 40.7) is most frequently used because of its ability to visualize ducts and because it allows further characterization of strictures and acquisition of directly targeted biopsies.[41–43] Also, more current single-operator systems (SpyGlass; Boston Scientific, Marlborough, MA) are technically easier to use, and digital images provide much better resolution than previously available images, improving diagnostic accuracy.[42] Visual consensus criteria of malignancy are being developed.

Confocal Laser Endomicroscopy (see also Chapter 28)

More recently, confocal imaging has been added to the endoscopic armamentarium. Confocal laser endomicroscopy (CLE) illuminates tissues with a low-power laser and detects reflected fluorescent light, eliminating scattered light and increasing spatial resolution. Intravenous fluorescein is used to highlight the vasculature, lamina propria, and intracellular spaces of examined tissues. The smallest available confocal probe (CholangioFlex probe; Mauna Kea Technologies, Paris, France) has a diameter of 0.9 mm and can be advanced through the instrument channel of a cholangioscope or catheter (Fig. 40.8).[44] A multicenter trial using probe-based CLE (pCLE) found significantly higher accuracy when the combination of ERCP and pCLE was used compared with ERCP and tissue acquisition (90% vs 73%). The sensitivity, specificity, positive predictive value, and negative predictive value of pCLE for detecting cancerous strictures were 98%, 67%, 71%, and 97%, respectively, compared with 45%, 100%, 100%, and 69%, respectively, for routine pathology. One major limitation, however, was the lack of blinding to clinical information, which could potentially lead to bias.[45] In an international prospective multicenter study of 136 patients with indeterminate biliary structures, the addition of pCLE resulted in more favorable sensitivity and diagnostic accuracy than tissue sampling alone.[46]

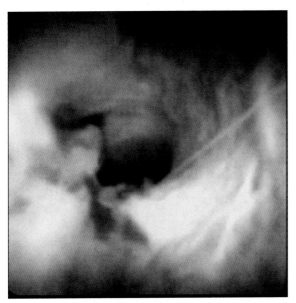

FIG 40.7 Choledochoscopy image of an intraductal lesion confirmed to be cholangiocarcinoma.

Narrow Band Imaging and Chromoendoscopy

Narrow band imaging (NBI) and chromoendoscopy are not routinely used during ERCP. To date, the published literature on NBI and chromoendoscopy during cholangioscopy is limited to case reports and small case series.[47–49]

MANAGEMENT

Surgical Resection

Surgery provides the only possibility for cure in patients diagnosed with CCA. However, as a result of the late presentation of most cases of CCA, approximately two-thirds of patients are not resectable at the time of diagnosis. The average 5-year survival rate for CCA is less than 10%. Even in patients who undergo a potentially curative resection, tumor-free margins are obtained in only 20% to 40% of patients with proximal and hilar CCA.[50] Attempts to increase the number of patients who are candidates for surgical resection include preoperative portal vein embolization,[51,52] orthotopic liver transplantation (OLT), and living related donor transplantation. Because of high recurrence rates and a limited number of donor organs, OLT cannot be recommended as standard therapy at this time.[53] The premise behind portal vein embolization is to cause atrophy of the affected lobe and hypertrophy of normal liver tissue in the contralateral lobe to potentially accomplish negative tumor margins and allow resection without postoperative liver failure. Neoadjuvant chemoradiation before transplant in the setting of very selected patients with unresectable hilar CCA has improved 5-year recurrence-free survival rates to 65%, which is favorable in comparison to the 75% 5-year survival rate of patients with other indications for orthotopic liver transplant.[54,55]

Preoperative Biliary Drainage

Whether patients with potentially resectable disease benefit from preoperative biliary drainage (PBD) remains controversial for many reasons, including the potential for delay in surgery and an increase in adverse events. Additionally, many of the data are from studies evaluating jaundiced patients with distal malignant biliary obstruction caused by cancers other than CCA. In a meta-analysis of 11 studies (10 retrospective

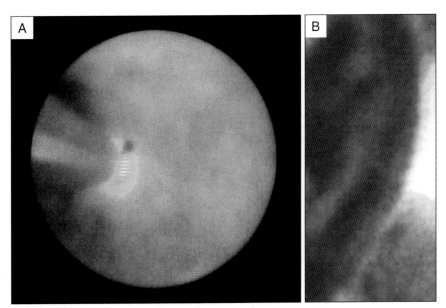

FIG 40.8 Probe-based confocal endomicroscopy. **A,** Confocal probe advanced under choledochoscopy visualization against lesion. **B,** Confocal images obtained during choledochoscopy of a cholangiocarcinoma.

and 1 prospective) evaluating the benefit of PBD (via ERCP and percutaneous transhepatic cholangiography) in jaundiced patients with hilar CCA, the following conclusions were made[56]:

- There was no difference in mortality.
- There was no difference in length of postoperative stay.
- The PBD group had higher postoperative adverse events and infections.
- PBD should not be routinely performed.

In practice, many surgeons prefer PBD in patients with renal impairment, cholangitis, pruritus, and serum bilirubin levels >10 mg/dL and before a major hepatic resection when the future liver remnant is predicted to be <30% of total liver volume.[57] If biliary decompression is performed, it should be undertaken by an experienced endoscopist after careful review of cross-sectional imaging, with selective contrast injection and drainage of healthy liver.

Surgical Drainage

In general, surgical bypass is reserved for those patients who were found to be unresectable during curative-intent surgery. Prolonged recovery and delay in chemotherapy administration postoperatively have limited the use of palliative surgical bypass.

Biliary Drainage in Patients With Hilar or Proximal Biliary Obstruction

For those patients who are not candidates for surgical resection, biliary drainage can be performed percutaneously, endoscopically (via ERCP or EUS-guided drainage), or by biliary-enteric bypass. Indications for biliary drainage in patients with obstructed bile ducts include intractable pruritus, a need to decrease bilirubin in preparation for chemotherapy, and treatment of cholangitis.

General Principles for ERCP in Hilar and Proximal Cholangiocarcinoma

The following rules should be adhered to (Box 40.1)[58–60]:

- Approximately 50% of the liver parenchyma needs to be drained (≥50% if there is underlying liver dysfunction).[61,62]
- Contrast injection should only be into segments intended to be drained. Guidewires should be placed in each segment where there is an intention to drain (Fig. 40.9, A and B).
- Antibiotics should be administered when performing ERCP for hilar or intrahepatic obstruction to avoid cholangitis.

- Attempt to drain only bile ducts that drain "healthy" segments of liver.
  - Segments that are "tumor-ridden" or atrophic should not be entered or drained.
  - Dilated bile ducts in healthy liver should be drained.
- Consider biliary sphincterotomy after initial biliary cannulation, particularly if more than one stent is placed across the level of the papilla (see Fig. 40.9, C, stent placement).
- Tissue sampling should be performed in all cases, with cytology as the minimum. Cholangioscopy should be considered to assess and sample the stricture, noting that the risk of cholangitis is increased, especially with water insufflation.
- Consider stricture dilation with balloon or dilating catheter, especially if more than one stent is placed.

Percutaneous versus Endoscopic Biliary Drainage

A great deal of controversy and debate have surrounded this topic since initial studies that compared ERCP to percutaneous biliary drainage

---

BOX 40.1 Key Points in Performing ERCP for Hilar or Proximal Biliary Obstruction

- Understand segmental liver anatomy and common variations of anatomy of the biliary confluence.
- ERCP should be performed only using image-guided biliary drainage.
- EUS-guided biliary drainage should be attempted under expert hands in patients who failed ERCP.
- Approximately 50% of the liver parenchyma needs to be drained to consistently relieve jaundice.
- Contrast injection should be limited to hepatic segments that are going to be drained.
- Attempt to drain only bile ducts that drain "healthy" liver segments.
- Antibiotics should be administered to avoid cholangitis.
- Tissue sampling should be attempted in all cases.
- Consider stricture dilation with balloon or dilating catheter.
- Consider biliary sphincterotomy after initial biliary cannulation.
- The choice between metal and plastic stents should be individualized based on potential resectability and eventual ablation therapy.

ERCP, Endoscopic retrograde cholangiopancreatography; *EUS,* endoscopic ultrasonography.

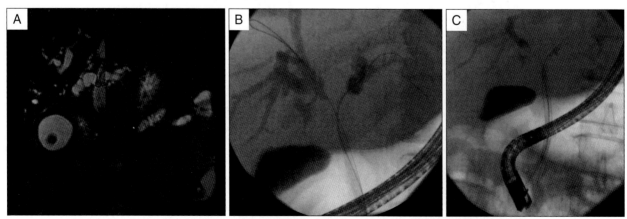

FIG 40.9 Imaging and drainage of a patient with a Bismuth IIIa lesion. **A,** MRI-MRCP demonstrating minimal dilation of radicals draining segments VI and VII. **B,** Fluoroscopic image with wires on each side to be drained (V–VIII and II–III). **C,** Fluoroscopic image of bilateral metal stent placement placed on each side (V–VIII and II–III).

(PTBD) found PTBD to be associated with a higher success rate and a lower rate of cholangitis.[63] These studies, however, were performed before implementation of imaging-targeted ERCP and did not include the use of self-expandable metal stents (SEMS), so they are therefore considered to be outdated and not applicable to current practice.

Advances in the understanding of biliary anatomy and techniques in cross-sectional imaging have improved outcomes for endoscopic biliary drainage in hilar CCA. ERCP-related cholangitis has decreased dramatically by avoidance of nonselective contrast injection with contamination of segments that cannot be drained.[64] In addition, the advent of larger-diameter SEMS has significantly decreased rates of stent occlusion. This in turn has also reduced the risk of cholangitis and the need for repeat interventions, which has therefore also reduced cost.[65,66]

Treatment should be considered on a case-by-case basis and weighed against the potential psychosocial impact of having an external drain when choosing the method for palliative drainage.

EUS-Guided Biliary Drainage

When ERCP is unsuccessful or not able to be performed because of altered anatomy, EUS-guided biliary drainage (EUS-BD; see Chapter 32) has become the preferred alternative to percutaneous-guided drainage and is safe and efficacious when performed by experienced endoscopists.[67] EUS-guided drainage can be performed at the time of the initial ERCP, thus avoiding the need for additional procedures and anesthesia. An additional advantage is that biliary drainage is internalized, reducing the potential for electrolyte and fluid disturbances. EUS guidance with Doppler provides an additional safety barrier to reduce the risk of puncturing blood vessels during stent insertion. Several recent retrospective studies[68] comparing patients who underwent EUS-BD or PTBD after failing conventional ERCP demonstrated technical success rates that were not statistically significant between the two groups.[68–70] The patients had a wide range of etiologies for biliary obstruction, so one should be cautious when extrapolating the results to patients with isolated proximal or hilar malignant obstruction. In the setting of failed ERCP, EUS-BD is associated with significantly lower postprocedural pain, fewer reinterventions, fewer late adverse events, and reduced cost compared with PTBD.[69–71]

SEMS versus Plastic Stents

Placement of SEMS versus plastic stents and the utility of unilateral versus bilateral stenting are topics of debate. In general, insertion of SEMS is preferred over plastic stent placement unless surgery or ablation therapy, such as photodynamic therapy (PDT) or radiofrequency ablation (RFA), is anticipated during subsequent procedures.[64] In comparison to plastic stents, SEMS have been shown to have prolonged patency, improved therapeutic success rates, and decreased cholangitis rates in hilar and distal CCA.[72–74] Although procedure costs vary widely, SEMS are more costly than plastic stents. The average price of the most commonly used SEMS is in excess of $1200, whereas the average plastic stent costs $75.[75] However, it is generally more cost-effective to use SEMS over plastic stents in patients with malignant biliary obstruction who are expected to survive longer than 4 months, because fewer reinterventions are required.[62,65,76,77] Placement of a plastic stent, however, may be more cost-effective if life expectancy is anticipated to be less than 4 months.[77]

Uncovered SEMS should be placed for hilar and intrahepatic lesions because of the potential for covered metal stents to obstruct contralateral and/or ipsilateral intrahepatic segments. Different stents and techniques can be used. One commonly employed technique is to leave a guidewire in each segment to be drained and sequentially deploy SEMS side-by-side over each guidewire one at a time. Alternatively, SEMS can be placed in a "Y" configuration at the hilum, with one stent deployed through the interstices of the other metal stent.[78] This has been used with US Food and Drug Administration–approved stents with a large cell width.[79] Fig. 40.10 shows a "Y" configuration stent designed specifically for hilar lesions. Another option for side-by-side placement is to place SEMS with 6-Fr delivery systems that can be passed side-by-side, predeployed through a standard 4.2-mm-diameter working channel with subsequent deployment.

SEMS occlusion remains a significant problem in patients with advanced CCA as a result of tumor ingrowth or overgrowth, tissue hyperplasia, and biliary sludge or debris. Current options for treatment of SEMS occlusion include placement of plastic stents within the SEMS and placement of another metal stent within the preexisting metal stent. Studies have demonstrated mixed results as to whether placement of a second metal stent within the previous metal stent is superior or similar in efficacy to placement of plastic stents within occluded metal stents.[80–82]

Local Ablative Techniques

In patients with unresectable CCA, tumor ablation is a means to provide local therapy, thereby potentially increasing both stent patency and life expectancy. Although these therapies may be associated with substantial

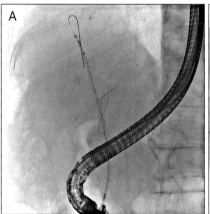 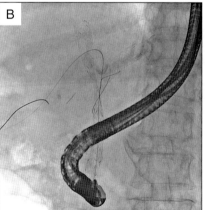 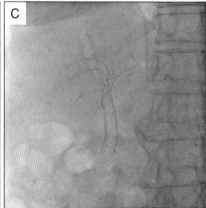

FIG 40.10 Fluoroscopy of metal stent deployed using the "Y" configuration. **A,** Fluoroscopic placement of two metal stents on the right and left (VI–VII and II–III). **B,** Fluoroscopic placement of the third stent draining segment V–VIII through a metal stent interstice. (Courtesy Dr. Moon, Department of Internal Medicine, Soon Chun Hyang University School of Medicine, Bucheon/Seoul, South Korea.)

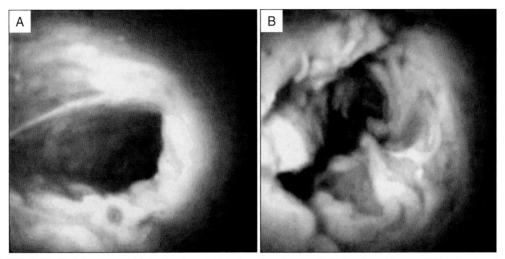

FIG 40.11 Radiofrequency ablation treatment of cholangiocarcinoma. **A,** Pretreatment image. **B,** Posttreatment image.

cost, they are justified based on the improvement in quality of life. These therapies can reduce stent occlusion, resulting in fewer complications such as cholangitis, hospitalization, and repeat endoscopic procedures to change stents.

Photodynamic Therapy

PDT involves the injection of an intravenous porphyrin photosensitizing agent followed by the endoscopic application of a specific wavelength of light to the tumor bed. This results in the generation of oxygen free radicals, which are tumoricidal, and/or an enhanced antitumor immunologic response, causing tumor cell death. In 2003 Ortner et al. reported that patients undergoing PDT with plastic stenting were found to have significantly longer survival time (median 493 vs 98 days), improved biliary drainage, and improved quality of life compared with patients who underwent stenting alone.[83] Several studies have demonstrated benefits of PDT.[84] Furthermore, PDT has demonstrated favorable results in a long-term follow-up of a case-control study investigating its utility as a neoadjuvant agent in patients who presented with unresectable hilar CCA.[85] The main adverse events from PDT are light sensitivity, cholangitis, and liver abscess.[86] The use of talaporfin sodium, which has a shorter period of light sensitivity than porfimer sodium, is an effective photosensitizing agent with minimal adverse effects.[87,88]

Radiofrequency Ablation

The effects of RFA have been described in the surgical literature in primary and metastatic tumors of the liver since at least the early 1990s. RFA acts by inducing tumor necrosis and cytoreduction resulting from local heat energy delivered by high-frequency alternating current via a radio frequency (RF) probe. Endoscopically, RFA, proven useful in Barrett's esophagus, has emerged as an option to apply local therapy for CCA using specifically designed endobiliary probes. Important parameters to consider in the application of RFA are the number of RFA sessions applied and the power settings and duration of application. Recent studies in which RFA was used before stenting employed a radiofrequency current of 7 to 10 W for 90 to 120 s, with a 1-minute to 2-minute resting period between each application.[89–91] Fig. 40.11 shows pretreatment and posttreatment images of a patient with CCA after RFA application. Another potential application of RFA is for recanalization of uncovered SEMS occluded by tumor ingrowth or tissue hyperplasia (Fig. 40.12).[30]

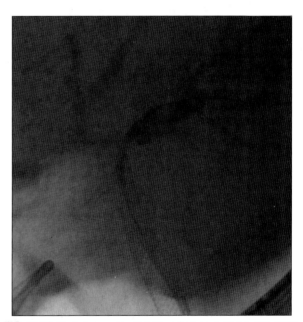

FIG 40.12 Radiofrequency ablation of an occluded metal stent.

A growing body of evidence supports the utility of wire-guided endobiliary RFA in the management of malignant biliary obstruction and occluded SEMS. Recent evidence has indicated that RFA applied to malignant strictures before stent deployment may improve survival.[89,92] The reported adverse event rates and types seem to be consistent with those reported from placement of biliary SEMS without RFA.[91,93] Rare adverse events include (in no particular order) portal vein thrombosis, cholangitis, rigors, acute pancreatitis, gastrointestinal bleeding, hemoperitoneum, intraabdominal abscess, abdominal fluid collections, and technical failure of biliary decompression.

CONCLUSIONS

Despite the availability of many endoscopic diagnostic tools, distinguishing benign and malignant bile duct strictures remains a challenge. Employing various radiographic and endoscopic imaging modalities can aid in this disambiguation. ERCP for hilar and proximal bile duct lesions is more complex than that for distal lesions and requires a comprehensive understanding of the hepatobiliary anatomy to achieve successful drainage and decrease the risk of infection. Image-guided biliary drainage is crucial for the important determination of which bile ducts are to be drained. After review of cross-sectional imaging, selective cannulation and contrast injection should be performed only in the segments that are intended to be drained. The choice of metal or plastic stents should be individualized based on potential resectability or the plan for subsequent ablation therapy. There is a growing body of evidence supporting the benefits of PDT and RFA in treating CCA.

ACKNOWLEDGMENTS

The authors would like to acknowledge Savreet Sarkaria and Michel Kahaleh for their work on the previous edition of this chapter.

The complete reference list for this chapter can be found online at www.expertconsult.com.

41

Indeterminate Biliary Stricture

Bret T. Petersen

Biliary obstruction results from diverse benign and malignant processes, and patients can present with acute or chronic signs and symptoms that vary greatly in severity (Table 41.1). The nature of an obstruction is often immediately clear at the time of initial investigation, whereas at other times obstruction is readily apparent but the nature of the pathologic process remains uncertain. No single definition exists for the term "indeterminate stricture," but it commonly refers to biliary strictures in patients in whom cross-sectional imaging is unrevealing, that is, without an associated mass lesion and without pathologic confirmation. Others describe the indeterminate lesion as one for which laboratory testing, imaging, and endoscopic retrograde cholangiopancreatography (ERCP) with cytology brushing fail to establish an etiology.[1,2]

When biliary obstruction is identified, an efficient approach to early diagnostic testing and management is important for reduction in morbidity and guidance of definitive therapy. Untreated obstructive cholestasis of even moderate degree can culminate in secondary biliary cirrhosis within several months.[3,4] In several studies patients with unresolved postcholecystectomy duct strictures developed secondary biliary cirrhosis in 15 to 62 months.[5,6] Key steps in the assessment and management of patients with indeterminate biliary strictures include characterization of the pathogenesis of the stricture, relief of biliary obstruction, and/or definitive treatment of the pathologic process employing medical, endoscopic, percutaneous, or surgical means. Stricture characterization and relief of obstruction are not independent pursuits but are typically accomplished in unison. Stricture characterization is based on historical features, laboratory testing, noninvasive and invasive imaging, and the use of various tissue sampling methods (Fig. 41.1).[7]

HISTORICAL FEATURES

Historical features may contribute to both the correct diagnosis and the management strategy for newly identified biliary strictures (Box 41.1). History of inflammatory bowel disease, complicated biliary surgery, or chronic pancreatitis suggests primary sclerosing cholangitis, postoperative strictures, or pancreatic compression of the common bile duct, respectively. An acute presentation in the early postoperative period or during an episode of pancreatitis suggests significant operative injury or stone-related obstruction, whereas subacute but early (<3 months) presentation suggests inflammatory processes that may resolve with time—hence minimally invasive and temporizing approaches may suffice. Presentation more than 3 months after a prior insult suggests a more fibrotic and rigid stricture that may require more aggressive or prolonged therapy. Strictures that present in an occult or delayed fashion and those presenting without known predisposing factors all raise the specter of a malignant etiology. A waxing and waning presentation is suggestive of benignity, whereas an inexorable progression of symptoms associated with weight loss suggests malignant etiologies.

A variety of systemic or typically nonbiliary diseases that rarely present with or develop cholangiopathy characterized by biliary strictures resembling sclerosing cholangitis can be suspected on the basis of the history or laboratory findings.

LABORATORY FEATURES

Laboratory features obtained at the time of presentation with a stricture may provide an assessment of the stricture's severity and chronicity, as well as the etiology. Isolated mild to moderate elevations of alkaline phosphatase, without transaminase or bilirubin elevations, imply modest impairment to bile flow caused by intrahepatic or extrahepatic etiologies. Enzyme fractionation should confirm the hepatobiliary source of the elevation, and cross-sectional imaging should identify when obstruction involves larger central or extrahepatic ducts. Concurrent elevations in the transaminases imply either a hepatitic process or relative acuity of onset of the obstruction. Total bilirubin values are not highly indicative of obstruction, but in the setting of complete obstruction with an otherwise healthy liver, bilirubin is said to generally peak under 20 mg/dL, whereas values beyond this imply hepatocellular injury, with or without obstruction. Chronic obstruction with deep jaundice can induce malabsorption of the fat-soluble vitamins, including vitamin K, thus leading to elevated prothrombin times. Hence a prothrombin time or an international normalized ratio (INR) should be checked before interventional techniques in these patients. Elevated pancreatic enzymes imply concurrent pancreatitis or pancreatic duct obstruction, commonly caused by biliary stone disease, pancreatic carcinoma, or advanced chronic pancreatitis.

Very few serologic markers contribute to characterization of the benign or malignant nature of indeterminate biliary strictures. Carbohydrate antigen 19-9 (CA 19-9) is a serum moiety that is elevated in the settings of pancreatic and biliary carcinoma, cholangitis, and, to a lesser degree, acute or chronic pancreatitis, obstructive jaundice of any variety, and miscellaneous other causes.[8] Marked CA 19-9 elevations above 1000 IU are seen only with cancer or florid cholangitis. Elevations above 100 IU are strongly suggestive of cancer in the absence of known pancreatitis or cholangitis, but CA 19-9 alone is not an accurate means of diagnosing malignant lesions of the bile duct.[9] When an elevated CA 19-9 is detected in the setting of cholangitis, it should be reassessed after appropriate therapy for the infectious process.

Immunoglobulin G subfraction four levels (IgG4) are often, but not invariably, elevated in autoimmune pancreatitis, which can cause distal biliary strictures that mimic those that occur with chronic pancreatitis of other etiologies or pancreatic cancer.[10] Such strictures are often rapidly responsive to therapy using corticosteroids, and short-term stent therapy is often not necessary. IgG4-related cholangitis can mimic sclerosing cholangitis with multifocal strictures in any location. Such patients are generally older (mean age, 62 years) men (85%), presenting with obstructive jaundice (77%) associated with autoimmune pancreatitis

TABLE 41.1 Differential Diagnosis of Biliary Strictures

Malignant	Benign
Primary Carcinoma	**Traumatic/Iatrogenic**
• Pancreatic	• Postoperative
• Biliary	• Anastomotic
• Hepatocellular	
• Ampullary	**Ischemic**
• Metastatic	• FUDR intraarterial chemotherapy
• Intrahepatic vs hilar nodes	• Post OLT anastomoses
Infrequent Types	**Inflammatory**
• Lymphoma	• Gallstone induced
• Sarcoma	• Mirizzi syndrome
	• Primary sclerosing cholangitis
	• Chronic pancreatitis
	• Papillary stenosis
	• IgG4 related
	• AIDS cholangiopathy
	• Sarcoidosis
	• Eosinophilic cholangitis
	Mechanical: Extrinsic Compression
	• Pancreatic pseudocyst

(92%), increased serum IgG4 levels (74%), and abundant IgG4-positive cells in bile duct biopsy specimens (88%).[11]

A variety of putative biomarkers for pancreatic or biliary cancer have been described in serum or bile but remain insufficiently studied.[1] These markers can be assayed from discarded supernatant obtained during cytologic or fluorescence in situ hybridization (FISH) samples.[12] Multicomponent fingerprinting of volatile organic compounds run on samples from the head of gas in vials of bile has yielded encouraging results in pilot studies.[14]

NONINVASIVE CROSS-SECTIONAL IMAGING

Ultrasonography (US), computed tomography (CT), and magnetic resonance imaging (MRI) play a primary role in the confirmation of biliary obstruction (based on findings of duct dilation or mass lesions), the identification of associated complications such as abscess or bowel obstruction, and the initial characterization of the pathologic process. Settings in which ductal dilation proximal to a stricture may not be present include early or fluctuating processes that are inadequately advanced to cause obstruction and diseases in which the ducts and/or the liver are fibrosed and cannot dilate easily, as in sclerosing cholangitis.

Transabdominal ultrasonography (TUS) is usually the first study employed in jaundiced patients to identify the presence and level of duct dilation and to look for bile duct or gallbladder stones or masses. Although US is extremely sensitive for duct dilation and gallbladder stones, it is less so for bile duct stones or for identifying the specific etiology of a stricture.

Once a stricture is localized by cross-sectional imaging with US (or CT scanning), the next step in evaluation is highly dependent on clinical judgment as to whether the setting favors a benign or malignant process, the patient's fitness for surgery, and the apparent resectability of the lesion based on initial studies. Ultrasonographic evidence of a stricture, without evidence of advanced cancer, is *usually* followed by abdominal CT scanning to define whether a mass exists and to provide initial staging information. If US demonstrates a distal unresectable mass, based on local-regional extension, hepatic metastasis, or associated ascites, then CT is usually performed for more formal staging, and ERCP, with or without endoscopic ultrasonography (EUS), is performed for both palliation of obstructive jaundice and tissue acquisition. If US suggests hilar obstruction, with or without evidence of a mass or unresectability, then MRI with magnetic resonance cholangiopancreatography (MRCP) is helpful to better define the level and etiology of the obstruction, assist with assessment of resectability, and guide the subsequent approach to invasive cholangiography, tissue sampling, and palliative stenting.[15] Extrahepatic biliary obstruction without a mass in the setting of fever, apparent biliary pancreatitis, or gallbladder stones can usually be evaluated directly with ERCP in anticipation of identifying an obstructing duct stone.

Abdominal CT scanning is commonly employed in patients with associated weight loss, fever, or significant pain, as it is particularly useful for identification and staging of extraductal mass lesions, inflammatory processes, and bile collections or leaks (Fig. 41.2). CT, however, is less specific than MRI/MRCP for benign versus malignant characterization and staging of cholangiocarcinoma (CCA) and other biliary strictures without associated mass lesions.[16] CT is preferred over US in obese subjects.

Abdominal MRI yields cross-sectional information analogous to CT scanning plus noninvasive relatively sensitive cholangiographic images that usually allow determination of stricture location and extent (Fig. 41.3). MRCP is the most sensitive noninvasive imaging test for biliary obstruction, duct stones, and strictures. It approaches the sensitivity of ERCP for identification of biliary strictures.[17] Although complementary, studies differ as to whether it is equivalent to ERCP for the differentiation of benign from malignant lesions.[17,18] Extraductal pathology or extent of disease tends to be less readily interpreted by the nonradiologist when it is acquired and displayed by standard cross-sectional MRI images, as opposed to CT images. MRCP has largely replaced diagnostic endoscopic cholangiography when there is not a need for tissue acquisition or therapy. The primary benefits of MRCP over ERCP are the avoidance of intubation, sedation, and the risk of pancreatitis and cholangitis. Other advantages of MRI include the ability to assess periductal anatomy, to display the anatomy of the ducts and the liver above a stricture without contamination (as occurs with contrast injection during ERCP) and when complete obstruction is present, and to generate multiple perspectives or angles of view for the same lesion. A disadvantage of MRI is that the cholangiographic display includes all ducts, without the ability to localize images to the region of interest around a stricture, as is done with "early films" acquired during initial contrast instillation during ERCP. This sometimes makes interpretation of a central or a complex stricture difficult because of overlapping peripheral ducts that are of little consequence. Several studies have demonstrated the utility of MRCP as a guide to subsequent ERCP and palliative stent placement for hilar lesions[15] (Fig. 41.4).

INVASIVE IMAGING TECHNIQUES

Invasive techniques for evaluation of the biliary tree include EUS and traditional contrast-based cholangiography via percutaneous transhepatic (PTC) or endoscopic retrograde (ERCP) routes. Intraductal ultrasonography (IDUS) and peroral cholangioscopy are specialized techniques employed during performance of ERCP, which will be discussed in subsequent sections.

Endoscopic ultrasonography (EUS) is becoming indispensable for both diagnosis and staging of malignant biliary strictures when ERCP and MRI have not yielded a diagnosis.[19] EUS is accomplished from the duodenal bulb and/or the antrum, depending on the patient's anatomy.

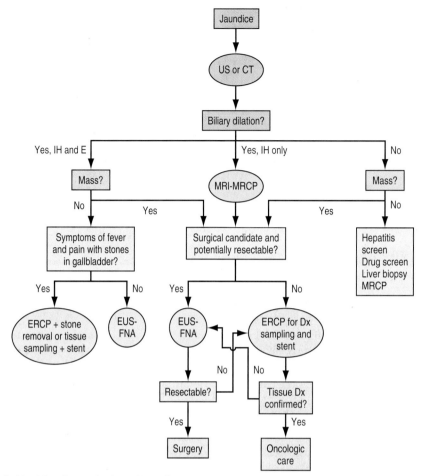

FIG 41.1 Algorithm for evaluation of jaundice and suspected biliary obstruction. See text for discussion. Biliary obstruction associated with pancreatic mass lesions with clinical or radiographic (CT) suspicion for autoimmune pancreatitis warrants further characterization and possibly steroid trials before entertaining surgery. *CT,* Computed tomography; *Dx,* diagnosis; *E,* extrahepatic; *ERCP,* endoscopic retrograde cholangio-pancreatography; *EUS,* endoscopic ultrasonography; *FNA,* fine-needle aspiration; *IH,* intrahepatic; *MRCP,* magnetic resonance cholangiopancreatography; *MRI,* magnetic resonance imaging; *US,* ultrasonography. (Adapted with permission from ASGE Standards of Practice Committee. An annotated algorithmic approach to malignant biliary obstruction. *Gastrointest Endosc.* 2001;53:849–852.)

BOX 41.1   Historical Features and Character of Biliary Strictures

A. Historical Features Suggestive of Benign Etiologies
- History of right-upper-quadrant surgery
- Trauma
- Ulcerative colitis or Crohn's disease
- Chronic pancreatitis
- Difficult biliary stone disease
- Stable weight
- Fluctuating labs

B. Historical Features Suggestive of Malignant Etiologies
- Never-operated abdomen
- Absent history of abdominal illness
- Weight loss
- Short course without antecedent illness
- Decompensation of known primary sclerosing cholangitis

Radial or linear technology can be employed, but the frequent use of fine-needle aspiration (FNA) and fine-needle biopsy is driving an evolution toward predominantly linear imaging. Malignancies are identified as hypoechoic masses or thickening of the bile duct wall. In one study of 40 indeterminate biliary strictures (24 malignant and 16 benign), EUS findings of a pancreatic head mass and/or an irregular bile duct were more sensitive than concurrent FNA sampling.[20] Wall thickness >3 mm was 79% sensitive and 79% specific for malignancy. In a comparative study of several modalities, EUS sensitivity and specificity (79% and 62%) were less than those of ERCP or MRCP but complementary to them.[17] In contrast, a study evaluating EUS with FNA in 28 patients with nondiagnostic sampling of biliary strictures obtained during ERCP, PTC, or CT demonstrated 86% sensitivity, 100% specificity, 100% positive predictive value, 57% negative predictive value, and 88% accuracy for malignant lesions.[21] Importantly, management was influenced in 84% of patients. Most studies note a greater sensitivity of EUS/FNA for pancreatic lesions, particularly with presence of a demonstrable mass, than for extrahepatic CCA.[22,23]

A prospective observational study from a large tertiary hospital compared EUS versus CT and MRI for the detection of tumor and prediction of unresectability among 228 patients with biliary strictures,

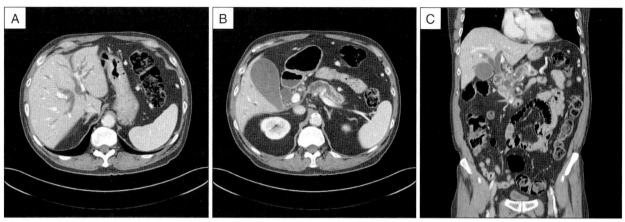

FIG 41.2 Abdominal computed tomography scan shows distal extrahepatic obstruction, based on traditional cross-sectional views showing dilation of the intrahepatic ducts (**A**) and proximal extrahepatic ducts (**B**) and similar dilation plus pancreatic duct dilation and a distal mass seen on the coronal view (**C**).

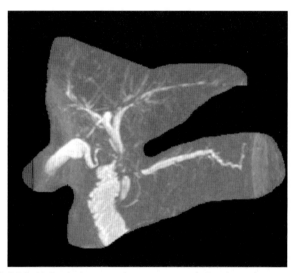

FIG 41.3 Abdominal magnetic resonance cholangiopancreatography demonstrating a distal extrahepatic stricture with a "double-duct" sign, analogous to that seen on computed tomography in Fig. 41.2.

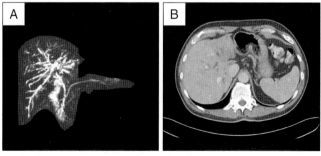

FIG 41.4 Cross-sectional imaging with MRCP or CT provides guidance to the preferred lobe for palliative biliary drainage during ERCP in patients with proximal biliary obstruction. **A,** MRCP suggests that access should be pursued toward the dominant right lobe. **B,** CT in the same patient demonstrates left lobe atrophy, also suggesting that access should be to the right lobe. *CT,* Computed tomography; *ERCP,* endoscopic retrograde cholangiopancreatography; *MRCP,* magnetic resonance cholangiopancreatography.

81 of whom had CCA. For those with available imaging, tumor detection was superior with EUS compared with triphasic CT (94% vs 30%, respectively; $p < 0.001$). MRI identified the tumor in 42% ($p = 0.07$ vs EUS). EUS identified CCA in 100% of distal and 83% of proximal tumors ($p < 0.01$). The overall sensitivity of EUS-FNA for the diagnosis of CCA was 73% (95% confidence interval, 62% to 82%). This was significantly higher in distal compared with proximal CCA (81% vs 59%, respectively; $p = 0.04$). EUS correctly identified unresectability in 8 of 15 and correctly identified the 38 of 39 patients with resectable tumors (53% sensitivity and 97% specificity for unresectability). CT and/or MRI failed to detect unresectability in six of these eight patients.[23]

Percutaneous and EUS-guided FNA of bile duct lesions preclude subsequent management of CCA with regimens that employ liver transplantation because of the risk for seeding of the extraductal needle track.[24] In this potential setting, EUS-guided FNA is used to sample only periductal or hilar lymph nodes or other distant lesions to diagnose metastases that would independently exclude the use of transplantation, if present. Hence, although not a primary imaging modality for biliary strictures, EUS with FNA is an important ancillary technique when diagnosis remains elusive and when staging for determination of resectability or transplant therapy is sought.

Cholangiography is the mainstay for diagnosis and characterization of extrahepatic biliary lesions of all types. Endoscopic and percutaneous approaches to cholangiography are complementary and on occasion, both will be necessary to characterize and treat difficult biliary lesions (Box 41.2). In general, proximal lesions that appear to involve the hilar region are best investigated initially with noninvasive MRCP, as this study provides directional guidance for subsequent invasive imaging and palliation[15] and avoids the risk of cholangitis that occurs with ERCP when contrast is injected into areas that may not be drainable. However, preoperative planning for hilar lesions may still require the clarity of contrast-based cholangiography (ERCP or PTC).

The cholangiographic appearance of strictures is generally inadequate for interpretation of malignancy, and many strictures that are interpreted as benign prove to be malignant.[25] Features suggestive of malignancy include progressive focal stricturing over time, abrupt shelf-like borders, length greater than 14 mm, intrahepatic duct dilation, and presence of intraductal polypoid or nodular areas.[25,26] In the setting of background sclerosing cholangitis with dominant strictures, malignant lesions are more likely to exceed 1 cm in length, be located at the bifurcation as opposed to the common bile duct, and have irregular margins.[27] Despite these criteria, cholangiography alone correctly identified only 8 of 12

(66% sensitivity) malignant lesions and 21 of 41 (51% specificity) benign lesions in sclerosing cholangitis.[27]

Endoscopic retrograde cholangiopancreatography (ERCP) has become the primary nonoperative modality for both investigation and palliation of biliary strictures because it provides high-quality contrast-based images of the ductal systems, access for tissue sampling, and means of therapy via internal drainage. ERCP is preferred over percutaneous routes when biliary stenting or decompression appears indicated if there is a likely need for stone extraction, when coagulopathy or ascites is present, and when the bile ducts are not dilated. It should be undertaken only by endoscopists with the experience and ability to proceed with appropriate imaging, tissue sampling, and therapies. In inexperienced hands, initial studies often yield poor stricture definition, inadequate drainage, or procedural complications.

Endoscopic cholangiography in the setting of obstructive jaundice should be performed with periprocedural antibiotic coverage when complete drainage is not anticipated and continuing antibiotics if complete drainage is not achieved. Stent placement should be performed whenever significant contrast is instilled above a lesion that prevents spontaneous drainage. In the setting of hilar strictures, intrahepatic filling of contrast should be avoided until deep wire and cannula access allows instillation from above the stricture, thus ensuring the ability to provide subsequent palliative drainage of the imaged segments. As noted, prior high-quality CT or MRCP imaging can guide selection of optimal intrahepatic systems for wire access and stent placement.

Optimal characterization and successful access for sampling and treatment require attention to imaging principles that are often not appreciated by nonradiologists. The following points apply equally to imaging of benign or malignant strictures (Box 41.3):

1. Strictures, unlike large dilated systems, are best imaged with full-strength contrast.
2. Multiple early films should be taken as contrast is first crossing the lesion, continuing the injection until the image has been obtained (Fig. 41.5). This allows later reference back to the minute details of angles or bifurcations, which may not be evident when the ducts are completely filled.
3. Coning down on an area of interest will sharpen the detail seen on static images. This requires at least some larger views to maintain anatomic reference.
4. Tissue sampling and therapy should be performed with the least contrast filling required to adequately demonstrate the anatomy. Excessive filling of peripheral intrahepatic ducts often obscures the strictures at the bifurcation.
5. The proximal extent of duct involvement must be well demonstrated for surgical or endoscopic decision making. After deep wire access, marked filling from above within the obstructed sector may be required to delineate the proximal end of the stricture.
6. Head-up and head-down positions on a tilt table can facilitate imaging of stricture extent by employing gravity to shift contrast to the area of interest.
7. An open view of the hilum, without overlapping ducts, is best seen in an oblique position, which is achieved with use of a C-arm or by rolling the prone patient rightward toward the endoscopist (Fig. 41.6).
8. After demonstrating a distal extrahepatic stricture, the central intrahepatic ducts and hepatic confluence should be filled adequately to exclude additional proximal strictures (e.g., adenopathy) within reach of endoscopic management.
9. Some lesions can be well characterized only by percutaneous cholangiography (Fig. 41.7).
10. Limited pancreatography may aid in demonstrating or excluding a pancreatic primary lesion when biliary strictures involve the distal third of the duct.

Stricture access with guidewires and subsequently other over-the-wire accessories is required to accomplish optimal and safe imaging, cytology brushing, dilation, and palliative or definitive endoscopic stent therapy. Access is usually gained with multipurpose plastic-coated guidewires or angled specialty hydrophilic wires that are extremely slippery, flexible, and torqueable.[28] Manipulation of angled wires using simultaneous torque and advancement can be performed by the assistant or by the endoscopist using any of several recently designed short-wire systems. This is best done with two hands to facilitate fine wire control and maintenance of position (Fig. 41.8).

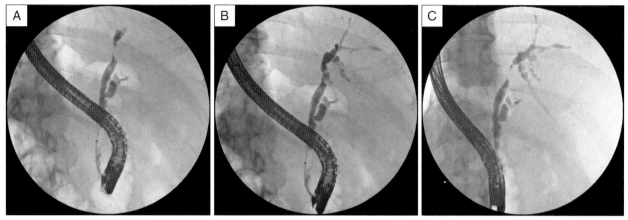

FIG 41.5 Early (A) vs later (B) images acquired during endoscopic retrograde cholangiopancreatography. Note that detail evident on early image is obscured by intrahepatic filling overlapping the area of interest in the subsequent view. Note improved view (C) with oblique imaging.

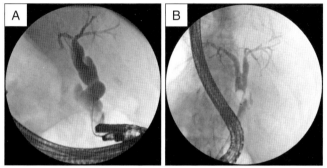

FIG 41.6 A and B, Overlapping and open views of the ducts at the hilum. B is obtained by rolling the patient rightward 15 ± 20 degrees or by leftward rotation of a C-arm.

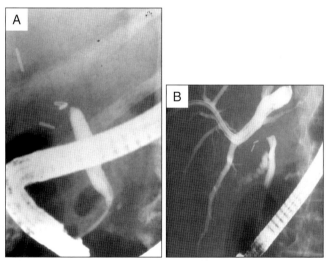

FIG 41.7 Benefit of percutaneous transhepatic cholangiography (PTC) for proximal evaluation of selected duct lesions. A, Partial endoscopic cholangiogram demonstrating complete duct obstruction after laparoscopic cholecystectomy. B, PTC-placed hepatic drain showing intrahepatic ducts, confirming complete duct disruption.

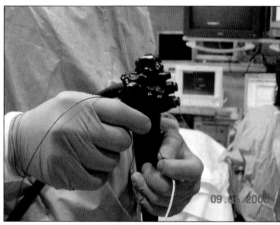

FIG 41.8 A view of the endoscopist's hands during manipulation of a slippery guidewire through difficult strictures. Note that two hands are used to hold and move the wire while the base of one hand holds the control section of the endoscope.

Stricture dilation should be performed before passage of larger-caliber devices. In the case of benign lesions, this constitutes the first step in therapy. For the tightest strictures that will not accept anything beyond 0.035-inch guidewires, initial dilation can be accomplished with angioplasty balloons that traverse 0.018-inch wires and expand up to 4 mm from their deflated 0.035-inch caliber (Fig. 41.9). Rigid 4-Fr–5-Fr–7-Fr dilators can be passed over a 0.025-inch guidewire. Standard balloon dilators can then be used to expand to larger calibers. Balloon selection is based on the size of the nonobstructed duct just distal to the stricture. Most often this calls for balloons with a diameter of 4, 6, or 8 mm. Tight chronic strictures carry some risk for rupture or tear during dilation. Should this occur, adequate stenting for drainage is mandatory and addition of a nasobiliary drain may be useful during a several-day hospital stay for parenteral antibiotics.

Percutaneous transhepatic cholangiography (PTC) has similar capabilities of duct imaging, access, and palliative drainage as does ERCP; however, it is performed through a sterilely prepped cutaneous field and hence cholangitis risks are lessened and drainage of filled segments is less critical. PTC is indicated only when the proximal end of a stricture has not been adequately characterized by MRCP or retrograde methods (if this information will change management), endoscopic routes fail

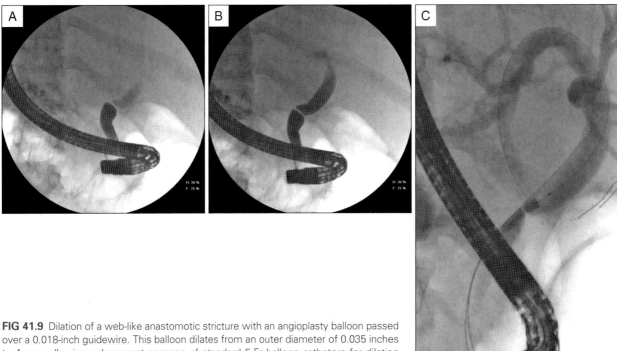

FIG 41.9 Dilation of a web-like anastomotic stricture with an angioplasty balloon passed over a 0.018-inch guidewire. This balloon dilates from an outer diameter of 0.035 inches to 4 mm, allowing subsequent passage of standard 5-Fr balloon catheters for dilation to 6 or 8 mm.

to access and decompress an obstructed system, or altered anatomy dictates that percutaneous routes be used. When an extrahepatic stricture cannot be accessed from below, a guidewire can be advanced via PTC for subsequent retrograde access. Use of this so-called "combined procedure" to enable stent placement and decompression should have less morbidity than conversion of the entire management plan to a percutaneous approach. Similarly, internal combined or rendezvous approaches can be accomplished via EUS-guided puncture of the intrahepatic biliary tree and antegrade delivery of a guidewire through the stricture.[29]

TISSUE ACQUISITION AND PATHOLOGIC INVESTIGATIONS

Methods of tissue acquisition and analysis for cholangiography include performance of transpapillary FNA and mucosal brushing for thin preparation cytologic examination, mucosal biopsy for standard histologic analysis, evaluation of both cytology and biopsy specimens using a variety of specialized tests for nucleic abnormalities or byproducts of neoplasia, and in situ histologic examination via endoscopically positioned probes. Tissue acquisition is a key element of all but the last of these techniques.[30] Overall, the results for pathologic examination of tissues acquired by brush cytology and pinch biopsy at ERCP remain frustratingly low.[31,32] This is attributable to several factors, including the scirrhous nature of many tumors, the small tissue samples acquired, and the difficulty in targeting the abnormality in question. During cholangiography, spot film radiographic documentation should be obtained of all sampling techniques and locations.

Brush Cytology

The yield of brush cytology for the diagnosis of strictures varies widely, with confirmation of malignancy in 15% to 65% of biliary strictures secondary to pancreatic cancer and in 44% to 80% of strictures because of CCA.[31,32] Combined results in over 800 patients reported sensitivity

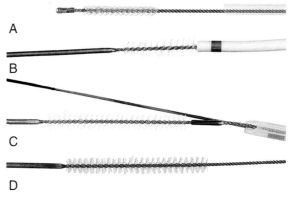

FIG 41.10 Various cytology brush designs include **(A)** metal-tipped brush, **(B)** brush with flexible wire leader in single-lumen catheter, **(C)** brush with leader and guidewire in dual-lumen catheter, and **(D)** large-caliber brush. (From Ginsburg GG, Kochman ML, Norton ID, Gostout CJ, eds., *Clinical Gastrointestinal Endoscopy*, ed 2, 2011, Philadelphia, Elseiver.)

of 42%, specificity of 98%, and positive predictive value of 98% among patients with confirmed cancer.[31] Studies pertaining to sampling technique note that cellular yield is improved by using a minimum of five brush passes through the stricture, removing the catheter and brush together to avoid brush withdrawal through the length of the catheter, and flushing residual cells from within the catheter into the sample vial after removal of the brush.[30] It is unclear whether stricture dilation improves sample cellularity. Including washings from the barb or lumen of removed plastic stents may also enhance cytology yield. A variety of brushes are available but little comparative data exist among them (Fig. 41.10).[33]

Biliary cytology brushing is accomplished using wire-guided devices (Fig. 41.11). The technique involves first establishing wire access through the stricture, advancing the cytology device over the guidewire across

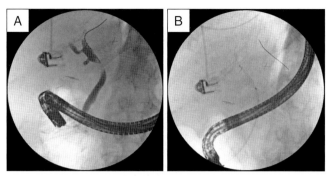

FIG 41.11 **A,** Cholangiogram demonstrating an indeterminate biliary stricture. **B,** Wire-guided brush cytology device within the stricture.

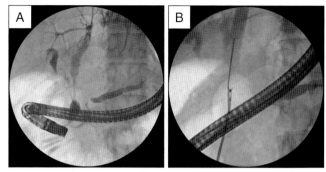

FIG 41.12 **A,** An indeterminate biliary stricture with a neighboring pancreatic stricture representing a double-duct sign, suspicious for pancreatic carcinoma. **B,** Forceps biopsy being performed parallel to a guidewire.

the stricture, advancing the brush beyond the end of the sheath, and withdrawing the two together until the brush is within the stricture. The brush is then passed up and down through the stricture at least five times, using either combined movement of the sheath and the brush by the endoscopist, or movement of the brush itself by the assistant as the sheath is held in place. Some tight or angled strictures can be brushed only with a downward movement or brush withdrawal, requiring repeated access with the entire assembly for each brush pass. The risks of cytology brushing are low but include cholangitis, ductal perforation, and rare instances of device disassembly and retained foreign body within the bile ducts.

Intraductal Transmucosal Fine-Needle Aspiration

This transpapillary ERCP-FNA method was reported to yield positive or suspicious cytology in 67% of cancers in the hands of one proponent,[34] but cumulative data from over 220 patients in five series yielded a sensitivity of only 34%, with 100% specificity and 100% positive predictive value.[30] The technique has not gained favor as it is difficult and is optimally performed with an on-site pathologic assessment.

Intraductal Forceps Biopsies

Intraductal biopsies provide the greatest yield for detection of malignancy among the ERCP-based modalities, with a cumulative sensitivity of 56%, specificity of 97%, and positive predictive value of 97% based on 500 patients in five cumulative studies.[30,31] A recent systematic review and meta-analysis identified nine studies providing a direct comparison between brushing and intraductal fluoroscopically guided biopsies.[35] Among 730 patients, the pooled sensitivity and specificity for brush cytology (45% and 99%) were similar from those for intraductal biopsy (48.1% and 99.2%). A variety of straight, angled, and malleable forceps are available in adult and pediatric calibers for intraductal use. Passage of these devices typically requires performance of a biliary sphincterotomy; however, passing the forceps alongside a guidewire without sphincterotomy is possible. There are limited data comparing different biopsy devices.

The technique of passing a biopsy forceps into the bile duct involves impacting the rigid leading end of the biopsy cable into the papillary os or the sphincterotomy opening from a short scope position and then advancing the endoscope several centimeters while simultaneously flexing the large ratchet backward to look upward from below the papilla, followed by upward advancement of the cable (Fig. 41.12). Alternatively one can occasionally advance the biopsy cable directly into the papilla from a slightly longer flexed position, looking upward from below the papilla.

One single-center retrospective study described the use of a novel sampling and processing technique for biliary biopsies obtained at the time of ERCP.[36] In the "smash" protocol, serial forceps biopsy specimens

are crushed between two dry glass slides, immediately fixed, stained with a rapid Papanicolaou technique, and interpreted by an on-site pathologist. Among 133 patients with suspicious biliary strictures, 117 were proven to have cancer. The smash technique alone had an overall sensitivity of 76% for all cancers, with 100% specificity and no adverse events. True-positive smash preps included pancreatic cancer in 49/66 (74%), CCA in 23/29 (79%), metastatic cancer in 8/15 (53%), and other neoplasms in 4/7 (57%). Suspicious or atypical results were considered to be negative. The median number of smash biopsies to diagnosis was 3 (range 1 to 17). When combined with intraductal FNA by ERCP and routine histology of forceps biopsies, the smash prep protocol yielded a true-positive diagnosis for primary pancreaticobiliary cancers in 77/95 (81%).

The highest diagnostic yield for tissue sampling during ERCP is obtained when two or more of the standard modalities are combined at the same procedure.[37,38] Ponchon increased the cumulative yield to 63% by combining brush cytology (43% sensitivity) and intraductal biopsy (30%).[37] In a recent meta-analysis of directly comparative studies, six provided data on the combination of brushing (sensitivity 45%) and biopsy (sensitivity 48.1%), showing only modest improvement in sensitivity (59.4%).[35]

Given the suboptimal diagnostic yield from standard analyses of brush cytology and tissue biopsy samples, a variety of advanced analytic techniques have been investigated. They include flow cytometry, digital image analysis (DIA), and FISH. In a limited number of studies, flow cytometry for DNA assessment of large cellular populations yielded improved sensitivity at the expense of significantly reduced specificity.[39] DIA uses a computerized assessment of cellular DNA ploidy within a smaller number of individual cells identified on a cytology slide to estimate the relative proportion with aneuploidy, which serves as a marker of malignancy. In a prospective study of 100 patients with mixed benign and malignant strictures, the sensitivity, specificity, and accuracy of DIA of biliary brush cytology samples were 39.3%, 77.3%, and 56%, compared with 17.9%, 97.7%, and 53% for standard cytology, respectively.[40] False-positive results from DIA (10 of 44 [22.7%]) and routine cytology (1/44 [2.3%]) occurred only in patients with primary sclerosing cholangitis.

FISH employs fluorescent probes that label specific portions of selected chromosomes, allowing for determination of cellular ploidy via fluorescent microscopy of specific cellular samples (Fig. 41.13). Most studies employ chromosomal probes designed for identification of urothelial cancers (centromeres to chromosomes 3, 7, and 17 plus chromosomal band 9p21).[41] Detection of more than five cells with polysomy is considered evidence of malignancy. In preliminary studies, the FISH technique increased the sensitivity of brush sampling for

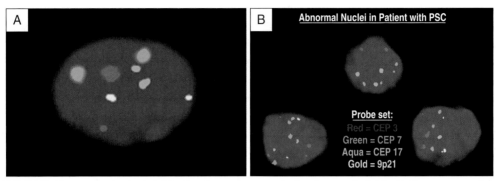

FIG 41.13 Fluorescent in situ hybridization demonstrates a single microscopic field with fluorescent probes of different colors attached to specific chromosomal loci. Two copies of each probe should be present. Presence of more than two copies represents aneuploidy in a cell. **A,** A normal cell. **B,** A cell from a malignant stricture in a patient with primary sclerosing cholangitis (*PSC*).

detection of malignancy from 15% to 34% ($p < 0.01$), with corollary nonsignificant reduction in specificity from 98% to 91% ($p = 0.06$).[41] In a retrospective comparison of data from 498 consecutive patients with biliary strictures evaluated by routine cytology plus DIA and FISH on clinical brushing specimens, the sensitivity of polysomy FISH (42.9%) was significantly higher than routine cytology (20.1%) when equivocal cytology results were considered negative ($p < 0.001$) with identical specificity (99.6%). DIA was not a significant independent predictor of malignancy. Logistic regression analysis revealed that polysomy FISH, trisomy FISH, suspicious cytology, primary sclerosing cholangitis status, and age were associated with carcinoma ($p < 0.05$).[42] In a prospective study of 81 patients with biliary or pancreatic strictures, compared with routine cytology, FISH improved the sensitivity (35.2% vs 51.9%) but not the specificity (100% vs 88.9%).[43] A pooled meta-analysis of FISH in 8 studies encompassing 828 patients with primary sclerosing cholangitis noted sensitivity and specificity of 68% and 70%, respectively.[44] Combined triple assessment with standard cytology brushing, intraductal biopsy for histology, and FISH analysis yielded a sensitivity of 0.82, specificity of 1.0, and positive and negative predictive values of 1.0 and 0.82.[45] Studies designed to identify products of other genetic mutations (p-53, k-ras, etc.) in bile or tissues continue but have not yet achieved clinical utility.

Confocal laser endomicroscopy (CLE) is a Food and Drug Administration–approved technology that enables in situ assessment of histology at the cellular level during endoscopy.[46] For ERCP applications a reusable miniprobe (CholangioFlex, Cellvizio; Mauna Kea Technologies, Paris, France) is delivered through the duodenoscope after administration of 2.5 to 5.0 mL of 10% intravenous fluorescein dye. Visualization is based on tissue illumination with a low-power laser (488 or 660 nm) and subsequent detection of reflected fluorescence light. Probe-based CLE (pCLE) generates 12 images per second with a tissue depth of imaging of 40 to 70 mm and lateral resolution of 3.5 mm, providing real-time "optical biopsy" of imaged tissues.[47]

From a longitudinal registry of 89 patients (40 cancers) at 5 centers, application of standardized "Miami" criteria for interpretation of pCLE findings in pancreatobiliary malignancy yielded impressive sensitivity of 98% at the expense of specificity of 67%, attributed to challenges with recognizing inflammation.[48] Using the Paris criteria (developed from prior "Miami" datasets to improve specificity by enhancing the criteria for inflammation) in a prospective multicenter validation study in 112 patients, tissue sampling alone was 56% sensitive, 100% specific, and 72% accurate; pCLE via ERCP was 89% sensitive, 71% specific, and 82% accurate.[49] The combination of cytology and pCLE enabled reclassification of some cases, yielding 88% accuracy for stricture

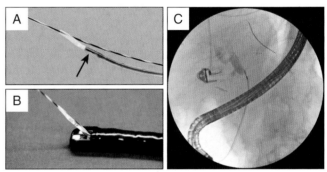

FIG 41.14 A, Leading end of 5-Fr wire-guided intraductal ultrasonography (IDUS) probe. The mechanical radial ultrasound crystal is noted with an arrow. **B,** IDUS catheter exiting from the duodenoscope. **C,** IDUS probe within stricture in Fig. 41.11.

characterization. Although encouraging, pCLE assessment of indeterminate strictures remains short of the goal of definitive in situ histology results. Given the current expense and training requirements of this technology, its role in clinical decision making amid the various corollary tests remains undefined, and it is best practiced in high-volume centers dedicated to its performance and evaluation.

ANCILLARY TECHNIQUES

IDUS employs a 12-MHz or 20-MHz radial ultrasound probe on the leading end of a 7-Fr catheter that can be passed over a guidewire into the biliary and pancreatic ducts during ERCP (Fig. 41.14). IDUS has been employed for identification of residual duct stones, characterization of strictures, and staging of local cancer involvement. After performance of cholangiography, a 0.035-inch guidewire is left in the duct and the ultrasound probe is advanced over the wire with the radial crystal stationary. To limit trauma to the mechanical drive of the probe, imaging is performed primarily during catheter withdrawal. Acquisition of IDUS skills is less involved than acquisition of EUS skills, and most experienced endoscopists should be able to adopt IDUS for the management of stone disease with limited training and for stricture assessment with slightly greater experience.

Ultrasonographic features of malignant strictures include hypoechoic asymmetric wall thickening, poorly demarcated borders, and abrupt shoulders (Fig. 41.15). Benign lesions tend to be hyperechoic and have greater symmetry, sharper demarcation with surrounding tissues, preserved tissue planes, and smooth edges. IDUS interpretation is more

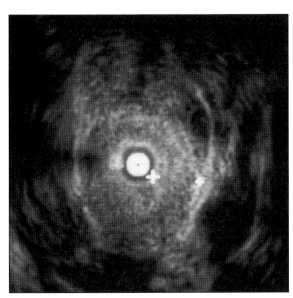

FIG 41.15 Intraductal ultrasonography images from an extrahepatic cholangiocarcinoma. Note the asymmetry of wall thickening and its irregular outer boundary.

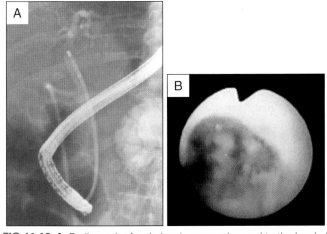

FIG 41.16 A, Radiograph of a cholangioscope advanced to the level of the proximal extrahepatic duct. **B,** Cholangioscopic view of hepatic confluence with open left hepatic duct and tumor-occluding right hepatic duct.

difficult in the setting of primary sclerosing cholangitis, where widespread background inflammation and duct thickening are present. Similarly, prolonged stenting can induce more widespread duct abnormalities than were originally present at the level of the index stricture.

Multiple retrospective and prospective studies have demonstrated the superior sensitivity and accuracy of IDUS for characterization of strictures as malignant (sensitivity >90%; accuracy 88% to 92%) compared with EUS (~75% accuracy) and standard cholangiography, with or without cytology and biopsy sampling (sensitivity 48% to 57%; accuracy 73% to 78%).[50–55] In a prospective study of 87 patients, elevated serum CA 19-9 (>100 units), routine cytology, and intraductal biopsy were compared with advanced cytologic assessment with DIA and FISH and stricture assessment with IDUS. IDUS showed the greatest sensitivity (87%) and accuracy (90%), and the combination of IDUS, DIA, and FISH allowed diagnosis of malignancy in 87% of those with false-negative routine cytology.[53] Studies of IDUS for tumor staging also report utility

for defining longitudinal extent, as well as the extent of invasion to the pancreatic parenchyma, portal vein, and right hepatic artery.[56] Tissue acquisition using IDUS guidance is currently not feasible. Periductal, nodal, and distant spread is not adequately assessed by IDUS.

Cholangioscopy, or direct visual evaluation of the biliary tree, is increasingly used for visually directed sampling of indeterminate strictures, electrohydraulic and laser lithotripsy therapy of intractable stones, and visually directed placement of guidewires[57] (Fig. 41.16). Cholangioscopy can be performed with dual-operator reusable baby endoscopes passed through a mother therapeutic duodenoscope, single-operator single-use baby endoscopes also passed through the duodenoscope, or directly via passage of ultraslim transnasal or pediatric-caliber upper endoscopes. Cholangioscopy with dedicated reusable instruments is usually performed with the assistance of a second endoscopist to manipulate the cholangioscope controls and biopsy cables while the primary endoscopist controls the duodenoscope and the insertion of the cholangioscope. Some centers employ custom endoscope holders for the cholangioscope to enable studies by a single operating physician.[58] Cholangioscopy techniques are discussed in Chapter 27.

Recent series demonstrate improved sensitivity and accuracy for diagnosis of malignant obstruction when cholangioscopy is employed.[59,60] In one study, ERCP with fluoroscopically guided tissue sampling had a sensitivity of 58% and accuracy of 78% for malignancy, whereas addition of cholangioscopy raised these values to 100% and 94%, respectively.[59] Cholangioscopy may be particularly useful in differentiating benign from malignant strictures in the setting of primary sclerosing cholangitis. One study showed improved sensitivity (92% vs 66%, $p = 0.25$), specificity (93% vs 51%, $p < 0.001$), and accuracy (93% vs 55%, $p < 0.001$) for cholangioscopic characterization compared with radiographic characterization.[27] The endoscopic criterion for suspicion of malignancy in this study was the presence of an associated polypoid or villous mass or irregularly shaped ulceration. Another study of the utility of narrow-band imaging in a digital cholangioscope showed no further enhancement in the diagnosis of malignancy complicating primary sclerosing cholangitis.[61]

A disposable technology employing a single-use 10-Fr multichanneled sheath has been designed for single-operator cholangioscopy. The original, partially disposable fiberoptic version (SpyGlass Direct Visualization System; Boston Scientific, Marlborough, MA; now referred to as SpyGlass Legacy) has now been upgraded to a fully digital version (SpyGlass DS) with markedly enhanced visualization, greater ease of setup, and improved flushing and aspiration capabilities. The disposable endoscope attaches to the head of the duodenoscope just below the biopsy port and advances through the accessory channel for insertion into the duct (Fig. 41.17). It provides four-way steering of the tip, illumination, water flushing, and a channel for passage of guidewires or of therapeutic or sampling devices (e.g., an electrohydraulic probe, biopsy cables [SpyBite], or cytology brushes).[62] Most published case series employed the original fiberoptic SpyScope. A large prospective observational study performed in 15 tertiary centers reported on direct visualization with the SpyGlass system for characterization of biliary lesions or treatment of large duct stones in 297 patients.[63] Visualization of nonstone target lesions and performance of directed biopsy were adequate for histologic examination in 88% of 140 patients. Visualization alone was 78% sensitive and 82% specific for malignancy, whereas directed biopsy was 49% sensitive and 98% specific. Single-operator diagnostic cholangioscopy altered subsequent clinical management in 64% (95% confidence interval, 57% to 70%) of cases. Overall, 7.5% of patients experienced a serious adverse event related either to ERCP or to the performance of cholangioscopy, including cholangitis in 7/17 events, bacteremia, hypotension or distention with pain in 2 cases each, and an individual case of pancreatitis. One patient with cholangitis required subsequent stent placement; the

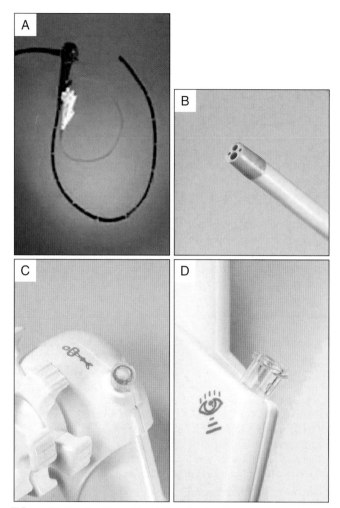

FIG 41.17 The SpyGlass Direct Visualization System attached to the duodenoscope and advanced into the accessory channel. Close-up demonstrates ratchets for steering and ports for passage of guidewire, biopsy forceps, and 0.035-inch SpyGlass fiberoptic probe.

others resolved with medical management alone. At least six additional prospective studies and seven retrospective studies of SpyGlass visualization have been published.[1] A recent systematic review of single-operator cholangioscopy in 10 studies encompassing 456 patients with indeterminate biliary strictures reported a pooled sensitivity of 60.1% and specificity of 98%.[64]

Direct peroral cholangioscopy employs standard pediatric-caliber (ultraslim) gastroscopes. Biliary access is gained over a guidewire or a tethering guide/balloon catheter via acute retroflexion in the duodenum or after initial access with a duodenoscope. Success is highest with a tethering balloon, but one such device was withdrawn from development after several cases of air embolism related to insufflation within a closed or obstructed biliary tree. The 5-mm to 6-mm caliber of the instruments requires a prior generous sphincterotomy but also enables greater visualization, sampling, and therapeutic capabilities. Risks of direct cholangioscopy, in addition to rare cases of air embolism resulting in stroke or death, are primarily related to cholangitis, sedation, and aspiration. The benefits of the enhanced capabilities of larger dedicated endoscopes will undoubtedly generate improvements in access tools and safety in coming years.[65]

Stent placement for biliary decompression is the major therapeutic modality used for patients with indeterminate strictures. Stenting as palliative therapy for distal (see Chapter 39) and proximal (see Chapter 40) malignant biliary obstruction and as definitive therapy for benign lesions (see Chapter 43) is discussed elsewhere. Plastic stents or fully covered metal stents are usually employed for palliation of indeterminate strictures to ensure the ability to remove them at a later endoscopic or surgical procedure. If the patient is not a surgical candidate regardless of the diagnosis, it is preferable to palliate the indeterminate lesion with larger-caliber 10-Fr stents or self-expandable metal stents (SEMS), which remain patent longer and may minimize the number of subsequent procedures. In the patient with an indeterminate stricture, bare SEMS are typically avoided because of both their permanence and their expense. Partially coated SEMS are generally removable when they are left extending into the duodenum; however, proximal ingrowth can complicate their removal. Fully coated SEMS designed to prevent ingrowth are easily removed, especially if positioned extending into the duodenum. Their use can be entertained in the indeterminate lesion if prolonged stenting for either treatment of benign stricture or palliation of cancer is desirable.

Modern imaging and new analytic techniques are advancing our ability to characterize indeterminate biliary strictures. Nevertheless, in some patients with indeterminate strictures, a definitive diagnosis via minimally invasive approaches remains elusive. In these instances, surgical exploration with a goal of diagnosis and resection should be considered in operable patients. Evolving and future techniques for assessment of molecular markers will likely further reduce the need to opt for biopsy via resection.

The complete reference list for this chapter can be found online at www.expertconsult.com.

42

Endoscopic Approaches to Concomitant Malignant Biliary Obstruction and Gastric Outlet Obstruction

Yen-I Chen, Todd H. Baron, and Mouen A. Khashab

Gastric outlet obstruction (GOO) and biliary obstruction (BO) occur commonly in patients with primary or metastatic periampullary malignancies. In pancreatic cancer, for example, GOO occurs in up to 10% to 25% of patients, whereas 70% of the patients present with BO.[1–4] Clinically, BO and GOO are accompanied by debilitating symptoms, and GOO is also generally associated with poor prognosis.[5,6] As such, one of the main goals in therapy is to reinstitute patency of both the biliary and gastrointestinal lumens. Traditionally this is achieved with surgical bypasses through two anastomosis: a gastrojejunostomy and a hepaticojejunostomy. This approach, however, is invasive and can be associated with significant surgical morbidity.[7–11] The advent of endoscopically placed enteral stents (ES) has led to their widespread application for nonsurgical management of GOO,[1,5,9,12,13] but endoscopic retrograde cholangiopancreatography (ERCP) remains the current standard approach for BO. Both ES and ERCP, however, have important limitations, such as risk for stent obstruction from tumor overgrowth or ingrowth.[13] In addition, ERCP may be difficult or impossible in the setting of GOO and can be very difficult in the setting of an in situ ES placed across the papilla.[14]

Endoscopic ultrasonography–assisted gastroenterostomy (EUS-GE) and biliary drainage (EUS-BD) are two of the most important techniques that have emerged from the evolving field of interventional EUS. Endoscopic bypass is a novel concept that can potentially provide sustained luminal patency of a surgical bypass through a minimally invasive endoscopic approach. EUS-GE was first described in 1991 in an animal model.[15] However, it became a reality in humans only after the advent of lumen-apposing metal stents (LAMS), which allowed for a safer and more secure bypass.[16] A recent multicenter prospective study demonstrated excellent technical and clinical success rates with endoscopic GE of 92% and 85%, respectively, in 26 patients through either the EUS-GE or natural orifice transluminal endosurgery (NOTES) technique.[17] EUS-BD, on the other hand, was first suggested as an option when Wiersema described EUS-guided cholangiography in 1996 and has evolved to become an accepted and effective alternative to ERCP and percutaneous BD.[18–21] Recently, Khashab et al. demonstrated the feasibility of performing both EUS-GE and EUS-BD in a single session in patients presenting with concomitant GOO and BO.[22]

The aim of this chapter is to describe the endoscopic approaches to combined biliary and duodenal obstruction with the use of ES and ERCP, as well as EUS-GE and EUS-BD, in malignant GOO and BO. This will include a detailed description of the different techniques involved, indications and contraindications, current literature on the clinical outcome, and potential procedure-related adverse events and their management.

ANATOMIC AND CLINICAL SCENARIOS

Anatomic and clinical scenarios determine the endoscopic approach to the palliative management of patients with both biliary and duodenal obstruction when approached using traditional luminal stents and ERCP.

Anatomic Scenarios of Biliary and Duodenal Obstruction

The location of the duodenal obstruction in relation to the major papilla is the major determinant for successful endoscopic simultaneous palliation of biliary and duodenal obstruction using ERCP techniques, because duodenal obstruction can limit access to the bile duct. Mutignani et al.[23] proposed a classification system for the three anatomic scenarios of duodenal obstruction in relation to the major papilla that determine the endoscopic approach to and technical success of combined palliation of biliary and duodenal obstruction. The classification system is as follows (Fig. 42.1):

Type I stenosis occurs at the level of the duodenal bulb or upper duodenal genu but without involvement of the papilla.

Type II stenosis affects the second part of the duodenum with involvement of the major papilla.

Type III stenosis involves the third part of the duodenum distal to and without involvement of the major papilla.

Of the three types of biliary-duodenal stenoses, technical difficulty in achieving successful combined biliary and duodenal palliation is least in patients with type III duodenal stenosis, whereas type I is intermediate and type II is the most technically difficult.

The approach to type I cases is to pass the duodenoscope through the duodenal stricture to the major papilla, if possible. This may require balloon dilation of the stricture to a diameter of 15 to 18 mm (Fig. 42.2, *A*) and/or passing the balloon to the third duodenum to be used as an anchor to pull the endoscope across the stricture.[24] Once the major papilla is reached, the biliary tree is cannulated and an expandable metal biliary stent is placed (Fig. 42.2, *B*). A guidewire is then advanced through the channel of the endoscope and passed into the fourth portion of the duodenum; the duodenoscope is withdrawn into the stomach and a duodenal stent that passes through the working channel of the endoscope is deployed across the duodenal stricture as previously described[25] (Fig. 42.2, *C*). It is usually necessary to place the proximal end of the stent into the stomach to allow enough stent coverage of the duodenal stricture because type I strictures tend to be in the proximal duodenal bulb. If the duodenoscope cannot be advanced through the stricture despite balloon dilation, a duodenal stent can be placed across the stricture. Because the luminal diameter of commercially available duodenal stents is 20 to 22 mm and duodenoscopes are approximately

11 mm, the endoscope can usually be passed through the stent during the same procedure to allow the biliary system to be accessed with placement of biliary self-expandable metal stents (SEMS). However, this may require balloon dilation of the duodenal stent. It is important that the duodenal stent be placed with the distal end positioned proximal to the level of the major papilla to allow the bile duct to be accessed (Fig. 42.3, *A* and *B*). The location of the major papilla can be estimated fluoroscopically in the presence of a prior biliary stent or by passing a smaller-caliber forward-viewing endoscope to the papilla and obtaining a radiographic image with the endoscope positioned at the level of the papilla for later reference. If the duodenoscope cannot be passed through the duodenal stent lumen because of inadequate stent expansion despite balloon dilation, there are three options: Option 1 is to repeat the ERCP after waiting at least 48 to 72 hours, at which time the duodenal stent is almost always fully expanded and allows passage of the duodenoscope to the second duodenum. Option 2 is percutaneous access to the biliary tree, and option 3 is EUS-guided entry into the biliary tree to palliate BO as described in the following paragraphs.

The approach to type II cases is most difficult. The second duodenum is strictured and involves the major papilla. Unless the patient has had a prior transpapillary biliary stent placed, bile duct cannulation is often not successful because the major papilla is not endoscopically identifiable due to extensive tumor infiltration. In addition, the lumen is narrowed and there is little working room between the tip of the endoscope and the major papilla. Nonetheless, one should first attempt placement of an expandable metal biliary stent. If successful, the duodenal stent is then placed across the stricture and overlies the biliary stent. If identification and/or cannulation of the major papilla cannot be achieved, then a duodenal stent is placed across the stricture. Unfortunately, the stent will invariably further impair endoscopic visualization of the major papilla. In some cases, however, the major papilla can be identified through the interstices of the duodenal stent and the bile duct accessed with placement of a biliary SEMS. If the bile duct cannot be accessed through a transpapillary approach after duodenal stent placement, then biliary access can be achieved using a percutaneous or EUS approach.[26] Typically, in either of the two approaches the bile duct is accessed through the liver (when EUS is used, a transgastric approach is most often used). In addition, with either approach there are two options: a rendezvous (RV) approach or completion alone using a percutaneous or EUS approach. When the RV approach is used, a guidewire is passed into the biliary tree across the stricture and through the interstices of the stent into the stent lumen (Fig. 42.4, *A* and *B*); if the EUS approach is used, the echoendoscope is removed. A duodenoscope is advanced into the lumen of the duodenal stent and the guidewire is grasped with a snare and withdrawn into the channel of the endoscope. A biliary stent is advanced through the endoscope channel over the guidewire into the biliary tree and deployed. The distal end of the biliary stent resides within the lumen of the duodenal stent (Fig. 42.4, *C*). When the biliary stent is placed entirely using the percutaneous approach, the stent is passed antegrade and the distal end is positioned into the duodenal lumen as described earlier (Fig. 42.5, *A–C*). When the EUS approach is undertaken, the distal end of the biliary stent can reside within the biliary tree proximal to the biliary stricture and with the proximal end deployed into the gastric lumen to create a hepaticogastric anastomosis as described later. The latter EUS-guided approach is similar to the percutaneous approach in which the guidewire is passed antegrade into

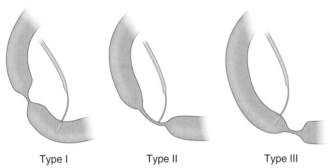

Type I   Type II   Type III

FIG 42.1 Classification of duodenal obstruction in relation to the major papilla as proposed by Mutignani et al.[23] Type I stenosis is at the level of the duodenum proximal to and without involvement of the papilla. Type II stenosis affects the second part of the duodenum with involvement of the major papilla. Type III stenosis involves the third part of the duodenum distal to and without involvement of the major papilla.

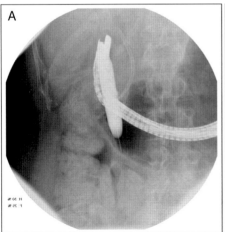
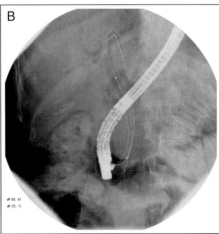
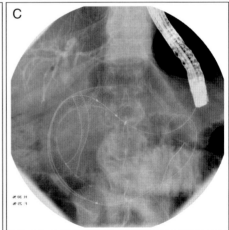

FIG 42.2 Palliation of biliary and duodenal obstruction in type I stenosis. **A,** The duodenal stricture is balloon dilated to allow passage of the duodenoscope to the level of the major papilla (note prior placement of plastic biliary stent). **B,** After the endoscope is passed to the major papilla, the plastic stent is removed and an expandable metal biliary stent is deployed. **C,** After deployment of the biliary stent, an expandable metal duodenal stent is placed. (From Baron TH. Management of simultaneous biliary and duodenal obstruction: the endoscopic perspective. *Gut Liver.* 2010;4 Suppl 1:S50–S56.)

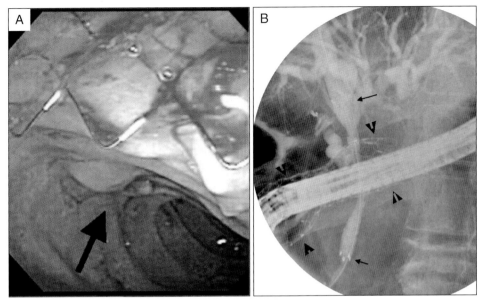

FIG 42.3 Type I duodenal stenosis with duodenal stent placement to allow access to the bile duct. **A,** The duodenal stent is positioned with the distal end proximal to the major papilla (*arrow*) as seen with an upper endoscope. **B,** In the same patient, the endoscope has been passed through the duodenal stent (*arrowheads*) lumen, and an expandable metal biliary stent (*arrows*) is placed. (From Baron TH. Management of simultaneous biliary and duodenal obstruction: the endoscopic perspective. *Gut Liver.* 2010;4 Suppl 1:S50–S56.)

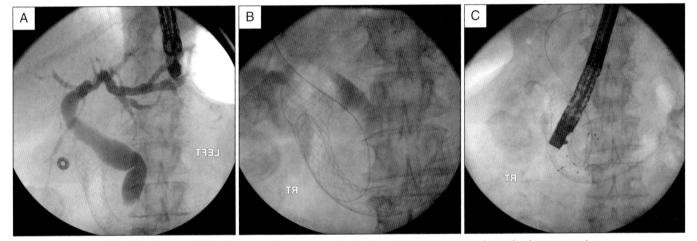

FIG 42.4 Successful simultaneous biliary and duodenal stent placement using endoscopic ultrasonography (EUS) rendezvous in type II duodenal stenosis. **A,** After placement of a duodenal self-expandable metal stents (SEMS) the bile duct could not be cannulated. A transgastric EUS-guided puncture was performed. **B,** A guidewire was passed into the lumen of the duodenal stent. **C,** After the echoendoscope was withdrawn a duodenoscope was advanced into the duodenal stent lumen, the guidewire grasped, and a biliary SEMS deployed. (From Baron TH. Management of simultaneous biliary and duodenal obstruction: the endoscopic perspective. *Gut Liver.* 2010;4 Suppl 1:S50–S56.)

the duodenum across the duodenal stricture. The stent is then passed through the echoendoscope and deployed across the stricture with the distal end into the duodenum.[27] Finally, in a recent case report, an EUS-guided approach was performed where the echoendoscope was passed into the lumen of a previously placed duodenal stent in a type II stenosis in which the papilla could not otherwise be endoscopically visualized. The bile duct opening was identified and a transpapillary biliary SEMS placed.[28]

Type III cases are the least common and often result from pancreatic cancer that arises from the uncinate process. The tumor encases the bile duct, causing BO, and extends inferiorly, causing duodenal obstruction

below the level of the major papilla. These cases are the least technically difficult because the duodenoscope can be passed to the major papilla and to the level of the stricture. In addition, it is not necessary to pass the endoscope beyond the duodenal stricture and thus balloon dilation of the stricture is not necessary. The sequence of SEMS placement (biliary stent first and then duodenal stent, or vice versa) is usually not critical when the major papilla and the proximal portion of the biliary stricture are not in close proximity (Fig. 42.6, *A–C*). However, if the proximal level of the duodenal obstruction is very close to the major papilla, it is best to place the biliary stent first because the proximal end of the duodenal stent may need to be placed across the level of

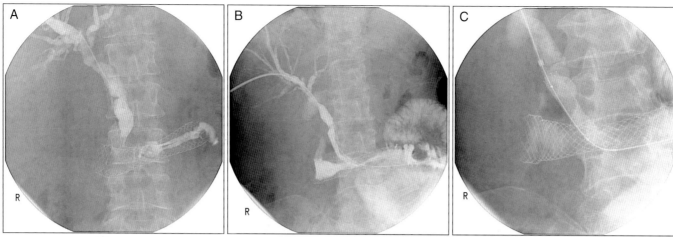

FIG 42.5 Successful combined biliary and duodenal stent placement using a percutaneous approach in type II duodenal stenosis. A duodenal stent was endoscopically placed and the duodenum was involved with tumor, precluding endoscopic bile duct cannulation. **A,** Percutaneous cholangiography demonstrates a tight distal bile duct stricture. **B,** A guidewire was passed into the lumen of the duodenal stent. **C,** After balloon dilation of the stent interstices, a biliary self-expandable metal stent was deployed percutaneously as a one-step procedure. (From Baron TH. Management of simultaneous biliary and duodenal obstruction: the endoscopic perspective. *Gut Liver.* 2010;4 Suppl 1:S50–S56.)

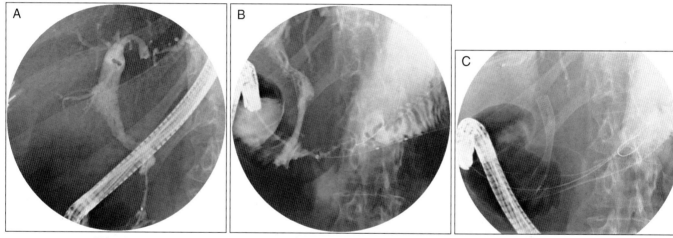

FIG 42.6 Successful combined endoscopic biliary and duodenal stent placement in type III duodenal stenosis. **A,** The bile duct is cannulated, showing a distal bile duct stricture. **B,** After placement of the biliary self-expandable metal stent (SEMS), the duodenal stricture is delineated with contrast. **C,** The duodenal SEMS is deployed across the duodenal stricture with the proximal end just distal to the biliary SEMS. (From Baron TH. Management of simultaneous biliary and duodenal obstruction: the endoscopic perspective. *Gut Liver.* 2010;4 Suppl 1:S50–S56.)

the major papilla to allow adequate coverage of the duodenal stricture. Whatever sequence of stent placement is chosen, it is best to avoid placing the duodenal stent across the biliary opening so that biliary access is preserved both at the time of the initial procedure and in the future should biliary stent occlusion occur.

Clinical Scenarios

In addition to the relationship of the duodenal obstruction to the major papilla, other factors influence the endoscopic approach. These include prior surgical palliation (gastrojejunal bypass) and clinical scenarios. The most common clinical scenario is the initial development of BO followed by later onset of duodenal obstruction. Many patients with duodenal obstruction have already undergone a palliative intervention for relief of BO—endoscopic, percutaneous, or surgical.

If a transpapillary stent was previously placed, then the type of stent and timing of stent placement need to be determined. For example, if a plastic biliary stent was previously placed, it is likely occluded or will become occluded and needs to be replaced. In such patients it is recommended that a metal biliary stent be placed at the time of duodenal stent placement, especially in type II patients (see Fig. 42.2) because the duodenal stent must cross the level of the major papilla, making subsequent biliary stent placement difficult, if not impossible, since it may not be accessible through the interstices of the duodenal stent.

Another scenario is simultaneous presentation of gastric and duodenal obstruction without prior intervention. In this scenario it is recommended that placement of a biliary SEMS be performed during the same procedure as placement of the duodenal SEMS, if possible.

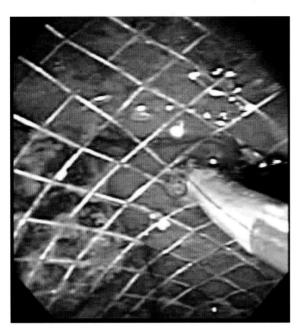

FIG 42.7 Endoscopic photograph demonstrates successful cannulation of the bile duct in a type I patient in whom a gastroduodenal self-expandable metal stent (SEMS) was placed across the papilla 3 days prior. A biliary SEMS was placed. (From Baron TH. Management of simultaneous biliary and duodenal obstruction: the endoscopic perspective. *Gut Liver.* 2010;4 Suppl 1:S50–S56.)

An additional clinical scenario is duodenal obstruction followed by later BO. This is uncommon and could be difficult to treat endoscopically because the papilla is usually inaccessible if the duodenal stent was placed across the papilla. If the stent does not cross the papilla, the endoscope can be passed through the metal stent and ERCP performed as usual. If the stent has crossed the papilla in a type I duodenal stenosis, it may be possible to identify a normal papilla through the interstices of the stent, followed by successful cannulation of the bile duct (Fig. 42.7), or to create a window within the stent at the level of the papilla using rat-tooth forceps or argon plasma coagulation.[23,29] If these maneuvers fail, then either a percutaneous or EUS-guided approach to placement of a metal biliary stent is usually required, as described earlier.

Finally, when considering endoscopic management of duodenal obstruction in the patient without clinically overt BO, prophylactic placement of a biliary SEMS should be considered, especially if there is any evidence of biliary ductal dilation by noninvasive imaging or in the presence of abnormal liver function tests that cannot be explained by other processes such as medications or presence of liver metastases.

RESULTS

There are several series describing successful combined biliary and endoscopic drainage.[23,30–32] In an early study[30] 18 patients underwent simultaneous biliary and duodenal self-expandable metal stent placement. Ten patients had prior plastic biliary stents in place. Combined metal stenting was technically successful in 17 patients. All the patients had relief of BO and 16 had a relief of gastric outlet obstructive symptoms. No immediate stent-related adverse events occurred. Median survival time was 78 days. The authors who devised the duodenal stenosis classification[23] (see Fig. 42.1) achieved technically successful combined biliary and duodenal stent placement in the vast majority of patients with all three types of duodenal stenosis, though the majority of patients

(46/64) had biliary stents placed at a mean interval of 107 days before duodenal stent placement; prior biliary stent placement greatly facilitates successful combined stenting in type II duodenal stenoses. However, some of these patients required RV procedures. Early adverse events occurred in 6% of patients and late complications occurred in 16%. The median survival after combined stenting was 81 days. In another series of 23 patients who had both biliary and duodenal stenoses, successful combined stenting was achieved in 91% of cases.[31] More recently, the use of a dedicated duodenal stent with a central portion designed to facilitate passage of a biliary stent through the interstices was reported in a small number of patients.[32] Endoscopic placement of duodenal SEMS was achieved in all, and placement of a self-expandable metal biliary stent through the mesh of the duodenal stent was technically successful in 7 (87.5%) of 8 patients. However, two of three patients with type II duodenal strictures failed bile duct cannulation and required an RV procedure. Early adverse events occurred in one patient. Median survival after combined stenting was 91 days (range 36 to 314 days).

In summary, the results of these series suggest that in experienced centers, combined biliary and duodenal stent placement for palliation can be achieved in the majority of patients, though an RV approach is required more often in type II patients. Overall survival from the time of combined biliary and duodenal stent placement is relatively short.

EUS-GUIDED GASTROENTEROSTOMY

Technical Approaches

Since the first description of EUS-guided GE by Fritscher-Ravens et al.[33] and the advent of the lumen-apposing stent,[16] three EUS approaches have been developed for stent insertion: (1) direct EUS-GE, (2) balloon-assisted EUS-GE, and (3) EUS-guided double-balloon-occluded gastrojejunostomy bypass (EPASS) (Table 42.1). In patients with concomitant GOO and BO, we suggest performing both EUS-GE and EUS-BD in a single session.

Direct EUS-GE

Direct Technique With a Non–Cautery-Tip-Assisted LAMS. The direct approach entails direct puncture of a small-bowel loop adjacent to the gastric wall using a therapeutic echoendoscope.[34–36] Locating the appropriate small-bowel loop can be difficult, especially if the lumen is collapsed. Infusion of water into the small bowel may be helpful for better sonographic visualization while facilitating needle puncture. Water infusion can be performed by first passing a guidewire across the obstruction, followed by a standard ERCP catheter, which can then be used to infuse water, saline, contrast, and/or methylene blue. Care must be taken to avoid infusion of more than 500 mL of water, which can lead to the development of hyponatremia. As such, normal saline may be the preferred solution. The infusion of contrast agent has the added benefit of facilitating fluoroscopic visualization of the small bowel, and the addition of methylene blue can help with proper puncture site confirmation when blue-tinged fluid is aspirated from the fine-needle aspiration (FNA) needle. For the puncture, a 19-gauge needle should be used to allow passage of a 0.025-inch-caliber or 0.035-inch-caliber guidewire. Large-caliber guidewires are essential to provide adequate traction for GE tract dilation and subsequent stent insertion. After confirmation of puncture position via enterogram, the GE tract is dilated to facilitate stent insertion. Dilation can be performed with a variety of instruments, including bougie, balloon, needle knife, and/or cystotome. When choosing the dilation size, it is important to remember that most LAMS insertion catheters measure 10.8 Fr in diameter and over-dilation must be avoided to minimize gastroenteric leakage. Once dilation is complete, a lumen-apposing stent

TABLE 42.1 Endoscopes and Accessories for EUS-GE

	Direct EUS-GE	Balloon-Assisted EUS-GE	EPASS
Endoscope	• Gastroscope • Pediatric colonoscope if more distal obstruction • Therapeutic linear echoendoscope	• Enteroscope with overtube • Therapeutic linear echoendoscope	• Enteroscope with overtube • Therapeutic linear echoendoscope
Use of electrocautery tip–assisted LAMS (Axios or Spaxus)	• 0.035-inch guidewire (to help traverse the obstruction) • ERCP catheter • Multiple 60-mL and 10-mL syringes filled with saline, contrast, and methylene blue • 19-gauge FNA needle • Dilating balloon 12–15 mm	• 0.035-inch guidewire • Stone retrieval balloon +/– snare or dilating balloon • 19-gauge FNA needle • Dilating balloon 12–15 mm	• 0.89-inch guidewire • Specialized double-balloon enteric tube • Dilating balloon 12–15 mm
Use of non–electrocautery-tip-assisted LAMS	• 0.035-inch guidewire • ERCP catheter • Multiple 60-mL and 10-mL syringes filled with saline, contrast, and methylene blue • 19-gauge FNA needle • Biliary balloon dilator, boogie, and/or cystotome • Dilating balloon 12–15 mm	• 0.035-inch guidewire • Stone retrieval balloon +/– snare or dilating balloon • 19-gauge FNA needle • Biliary balloon dilator, boogie, and/or cystotome • Dilating balloon 12–15 mm	• N/A

EPASS, Endoscopic ultrasonography-guided double-balloon-occluded gastrojejunostomy bypass; *ERCP,* endoscopic retrograde cholangiopancreatography; *EUS-GE,* endoscopic ultrasonography–assisted gastroenterostomy; *FNA,* fine-needle aspiration; *LAMS,* lumen-apposing metal stents; *N/A,* not applicable.

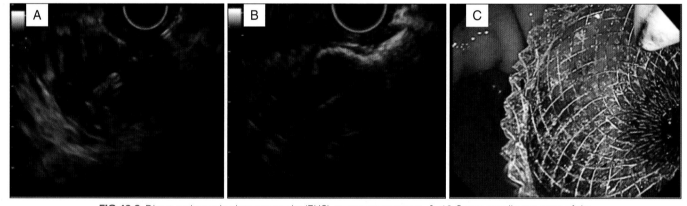

FIG 42.8 Direct endoscopic ultrasonography (EUS)–gastroenterostomy. **A,** 19-Gauge needle puncture of the small bowel. **B,** Lumen-apposing stent insertion with distal flange seen on EUS. **C,** Endoscopic view of the deployed stent.

is inserted over the wire and deployed with sonographic and fluoroscopic guidance.

Direct Technique With an Electrocautery Tip–Assisted LAMS. Recently LAMS with a cautery tip to facilitate catheter insertion has been developed (electrocautery-enhanced Axios stent [Boston Scientific, Marlborough, MA] or Niti-S Spaxus stent [Taewoong Medical, Ilsan, Korea]). These devices have cautery-enabled delivery catheter tips, meaning that electrocurrent can be applied as the catheter is advanced through the stomach and small-bowel wall. These stents obviate the need for wire guidance and tract dilation, which can greatly facilitate the performance of EUS-GE while potentially shortening procedure time.

Optimal small-bowel distension with fluid infusion is of utmost importance when using this approach. In addition, it is important to use methylene blue along with isotonic saline and contrast in order to confirm appropriate puncture into the small bowel. Once the small

bowel is optimally distended with a forward-viewing endoscope, the endoscope should then be quickly exchanged for an echoendoscope. The distended small-bowel loops are then located from the stomach using EUS and fluoroscopy. A 19-gauge FNA needle is then used to puncture the small bowel distal to the obstruction (Fig. 42.8). Proper puncture into the small bowel is then confirmed by aspirating methylene blue through the FNA needle (Fig. 42.9). Note that differentiating small-bowel loops from colon can be very difficult on EUS and fluoroscopy and that aspiration of blue-tinged fluid from the FNA needle is imperative to confirm the puncture site within the small bowel. Once the proper puncture site is confirmed, further infusion of fluid can be achieved to distend the small bowel by injecting through the 19-gauge needle. The 19-gauge needle is then withdrawn while keeping the echoendoscope in a stable position. An electrocautery tip–assisted LAMS delivery catheter is then introduced through the endoscope and cautery-assisted puncture performed of the stomach and the distended small-bowel loop. The LAMS can then be deployed under EUS and/or endoscopic visualization. However, using a cautery-enhanced catheter tip also has the potential to damage the contralateral wall of the small bowel as the catheter is advanced. As such, care must be taken to ensure that the small bowel is appropriately distended before stent insertion.

Balloon-Assisted EUS-GE

The major challenge with the direct EUS-GE technique is the difficulty in locating the appropriate small-bowel loop for puncture. Differentiating colon and small bowel and ensuring puncture distal to the obstruction can be difficult. In addition, if a non–cautery-assisted LAMS is used, maintaining proper wire traction for dilation and stent insertion can

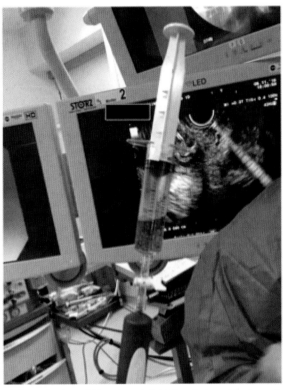

FIG 42.9 Aspiration of blue-tinged fluid (methylene blue) confirming small-bowel puncture with a 19-gauge fine-needle aspiration needle.

also be precarious with the direct method. Balloon-assisted EUS-GE has been developed in hopes of improving both the small-bowel access and possibly the subsequent GE tract wire traction and tension for dilation and stenting.[34,35,37]

The balloon-assisted technique is best initiated with an enteroscope fitted with a single- or double-balloon overtube. A stiff guidewire is then inserted across the obstruction and advanced deep into the small bowel. The endoscope is then removed via exchange over the wire while keeping the overtube in place (across the obstruction or just proximal to the obstruction). A stone retrieval or dilating balloon is then inserted through the overtube and over the wire. The primary role of the overtube is to facilitate balloon catheter insertion by preventing looping in the stomach. After insertion beyond the obstruction and inflation of the balloon with contrast fluid, EUS-guided puncture of the balloon is performed transgastrically with a 19-gauge needle (Fig. 42.10). Bursting of the balloon confirms the correct location of the puncture. The advantage of using a large dilating balloon is the ability at times to curl the distal end of the guidewire within the balloon after puncture. As such, when the balloon catheter is withdrawn from the patient, it brings along the distal end of the guidewire within the collapsed balloon. This provides access to both the proximal and distal ends of the guidewire from the patient's mouth. By having access to both ends of the wire, optimal traction and wire tension can be provided to enable safer and easier GE tract dilation and stent insertion or direct stent insertion with an electrocautery tip–enhanced LAMS. If a stone retrieval balloon is used, curling the wire within the balloon is usually not feasible. A novel technique has also been described where a snare is secured alongside the balloon catheter and opened when the balloon is inflated.[37] Once puncture occurs, the guidewire is then advanced through the snare, which is then closed onto the wire and withdrawn through the patient's mouth, giving the endoscopist access to both ends of the wire.

EUS-Guided Double-Balloon–Occluded Gastrojejunostomy Bypass

Despite facilitating small-bowel access and wire traction, balloon-assisted EUS-GE, as with direct EUS-GE, is associated with the risk for cautery damage to the contralateral small bowel when inserting an electrocautery-enhanced LAMS. In addition, even with the ability to apply traction to both ends of the inserted guidewire, the small bowel tends to move away with dilation and/or stent insertion. To overcome this problem, a specialized double-balloon enteric tube (Tokyo Medical University Type; Create Medic, Yokohama, Japan) has been introduced.[38,39] The balloon delivery catheter is inserted over a stiff wire through an overtube

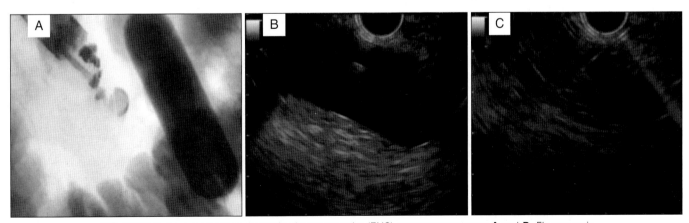

FIG 42.10 Balloon-assisted endoscopic ultrasonography (EUS)–gastroenterostomy: **A** and **B,** Fluoroscopic and EUS view of a dilating balloon within a jejunal loop. **C,** Puncture of the balloon with a 19-gauge fine-needle aspiration needle.

to prevent looping in the stomach and facilitate passage across the malignant obstruction. Dilute contrast is then used to inflate both balloons to anchor and seal the small bowel at two ends. Saline is then infused generously between the two balloons. This fluid insufflation allows for approximation of small-bowel loop to the gastric wall, leading to easier and safer transgastric EUS puncture and stent insertion with the cautery-tipped Axios or Spaxus system. This technique has the potential to greatly facilitate small-bowel access and keeps the enteric wall close to the stomach during stent insertion while ensuring optimal luminal distension to prevent cautery damage to the contralateral small intestinal wall. With experience, some experts have adapted direct specialized enteric balloon-assisted electrocautery-enhanced LAMS insertion without the need for needle puncture or wire insertion.[38] This may further shorten procedure time and may actually decrease the risk for stent misdeployment, as the authors have noticed that the small bowel tended to move away from the stomach during advancement of the wire through the needle into the small bowel.

The major limiting factor for successful EPASS is high-grade luminal obstruction where the specialized enteric balloon cannot traverse the tumor. Moreover, the accessibility of this balloon is currently limited and is not available in North America.

Indications and Contraindications to EUS-GE

EUS-GE can be considered in histologically established malignant GOO. It can be performed as the primary approach (e.g., for patients with expected survival >3 months) or after failure of enteral stenting (e.g., technical failure or stent obstruction during follow-up).[40] Patients may have gastroparesis after enteral stenting, and EUS-GE should be considered only if recurrent or persistent GOO symptoms are truly from stent occlusion. EUS-GE should not be performed if there is evidence of distal small-bowel obstruction beyond the ligament of Treitz. Furthermore, tissue diagnosis should be obtained before EUS-GE, because tissue acquisition after stent insertion can be challenging. Other contraindications include uncorrectable thrombocytopenia (platelet count $<50 \times 10^9$/L) and/or coagulopathy (international normalized ratio [INR] >1.5).

Clinical Data on EUS-GE

Although promising, the data supporting EUS-GE have come from animal studies, case reports, and retrospective series. Khashab et al.[35] reported the first EUS-GE case series performed in the United States. Overall, 10 patients underwent EUS-GE for benign and malignant GOO. Direct EUS-GE was performed in one patient, with the remaining patients undergoing balloon-assisted EUS-GE. Technical success was 90%, whereas clinical success was achieved in all patients with successful stent insertion. No adverse events occurred and there were no cases of stent obstruction

or need for reintervention. More recently, a multicenter prospective series involving 26 patients (17 malignant and 9 benign GOO) who underwent endoscopic GE either through EUS-guided GE or NOTES-GE also demonstrated excellent technical and clinical success of 92% and 85%, respectively.[17]

In terms of comparative data between EUS-GE and ES, only one retrospective comparative trial has been published.[41] In this multicenter international study, clinical outcomes in 30 patients who underwent EUS-GE were compared with those of 52 patients who underwent ES for malignant GOO. In terms of technique, EPASS, balloon-assisted EUS-GE, and direct EUS-GE were performed in 73.3% ($n = 22$), 20% ($n = 6$), and 6.7% ($n = 2$) of the patients, respectively. Similar technical and clinical success rates were achieved in the EUS-GE and ES cohorts (86.7% vs 94.2%, $p = 0.2$; 83.3% vs 69.9%, $p = 0.2$); however, the former was associated with fewer stent obstructions (3.3% EUS-GE vs 26.9%) and less requirement of reintervention. In addition, no difference in terms of adverse events was noted between the two groups.

Overall, preliminary data on EUS-GE in GOO are promising. It appears to be associated with excellent technical success and clinical success. Compared with ES, it may offer a more sustainable clinical response with fewer requirements for reintervention because of stent obstruction. Currently, the major limiting factor for the widespread use of EUS-GE is the difficulty involved in performing the procedure, which requires expert EUS and fluoroscopic skills with nuanced knowledge of the required accessories and patient anatomy. The lack of dedicated accessories to perform the procedure is also a major impediment to its implementation at most centers. However, progress has been made in facilitating the procedure with the introduction of LAMS and specialized enteric balloons. As EUS endoscopes and accessories continue to evolve, uses of EUS-GE will likely disseminate further. Prospective data are also needed to further validate this treatment modality.

EUS-BD Technical Approaches

In general, EUS-BD can be performed using three approaches: (1) RV, (2) direct transluminal (TL), and (3) antegrade transpapillary (Table 42.2). We generally suggest reserving EUS-BD as a salvage modality after failure with ERCP. Note, however, that if enteral stenting is needed for concomitant GOO to allow passage of a duodenoscope, then ERCP in this setting is extremely difficult and associated with high failure rates.[14] In this instance, EUS-BD may be considered as a primary modality.

Rendezvous

The RV technique starts with advancement of a linear echoendoscope into the stomach or duodenal bulb, where the extrahepatic or intrahepatic bile duct can be located. The extrahepatic bile duct approach may be

TABLE 42.2 Endoscopes and Accessories for EUS-BD

	Rendezvous	Direct Transluminal (CDS or HGS)	Antegrade Stenting
Endoscope	• Therapeutic linear echoendoscope • Side-viewing duodenoscope	• Therapeutic linear echoendoscope	• Therapeutic linear echoendoscope
Accessories	• 19-gauge FNA needle • 0.025-inch or 0.035-inch guidewire • Snare or biopsy forceps • Traditional ERCP accessories for cannulation • Metal or plastic biliary stents	• 19-gauge FNA needle • 0.025-inch or 0.035-inch guidewire • Biliary dilating balloon, bougie or cystotome • Biliary fully covered metal stent • CDS can be performed with LAMS with electrocautery-assisted tip • One-step EUS-BD stent system if available	• 19-gauge FNA needle • 0.025-inch or 0.035-inch guidewire • Biliary dilating balloon, bougie or cystotome • Biliary fully covered metal stent or plastic stent

CDS, Choledochoduodenostomy; *ERCP,* endoscopic retrograde cholangiopancreatography; *EUS-BD,* endoscopic ultrasonography–assisted biliary drainage; *FNA,* fine-needle aspiration; *HGS,* hepatogastrostomy; *LAMS,* lumen-apposing metal stents.

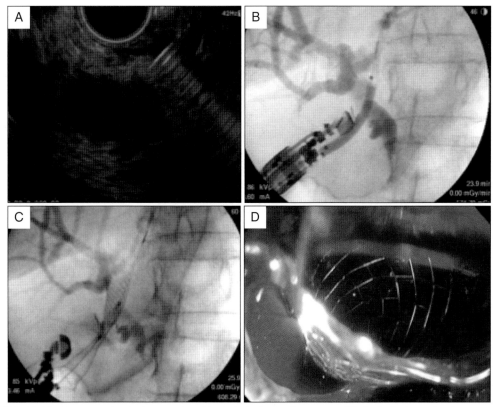

FIG 42.11 Direct transluminal approach with choledochoduodenostomy (CDS). **A,** Endoscopic ultrasonography–guided puncture of the dilated extrahepatic bile duct from the duodenal bulb with a 19-gauge needle. **B,** Dilation of the CDS tract with a biliary dilating balloon to 4 mm. **C** and **D,** Fluoroscopic and endoscopic images of deployed CDS fully covered metal stent.

preferred, given that it may be associated with shorter procedure time and potentially lower risk for postprocedure bile leak[42]; however, this may not be possible if there is tumor involvement of the duodenal bulb. Regardless of the approach, puncture of the bile duct should be performed with a 19-gauge needle. In general, larger needles are preferred to accommodate 0.035- or 0.025-inch guidewires, which are essential in providing enough traction for tract dilation or stent insertion (may be less important in RV). Once the needle puncture is performed, bile aspiration followed by contrast injection can be done to confirm appropriate location within the biliary system. A 0.035-inch or 0.025-inch guidewire is then advanced through the needle and directed in an anterograde fashion through the papilla and curled into the small-bowel lumen. The echoendoscope is then removed from the patient via exchange over the guidewire. A side-viewing duodenoscope can then be inserted and advanced to the papilla where standard ERCP can be performed either next to the EUS inserted wire or by grasping the wire with a snare or biopsy forceps and performing standard biliary cannulation over wire. Although often considered the safest approach to EUS-BD, the RV approach is not possible if there is GOO proximal to the ampulla.

Direct Transluminal Approach

The TL approach is performed to establish a choledochoduodenostomy (CDS) or hepatogastrostomy (HGS). Biliary puncture is performed as described earlier; however, instead of transpapillary stenting, biliary drainage is achieved through a neofistula between the duodenum and the extrahepatic bile duct (CDS) or the stomach and the intrahepatic bile duct (HGS).

Choledochoduodenostomy. With CDS the echoendoscope is advanced to the duodenal bulb in a long and stable position (Fig. 42.11). Contrary to the RV approach, the trajectory of the needle puncture of the bile duct should be retrograde toward the hilum, which then allows the passage of a guidewire followed by stent insertion in the same direction. Once the guidewire (0.025 or 0.035 inch) is in place, the neofistula needs to be dilated with a bougie biliary dilating balloon, cystotome, or needle knife to allow passage of a stent. Overdilation should be avoided and the size of the dilation should be just enough to accommodate the caliber of the stent catheter to minimize risk for bile leakage. A biliary fully covered self-expanding metal stent (FCSEMS) can then be inserted over the wire, which is generally preferred over a plastic biliary stent given its ability to provide a tighter seal to prevent bile leak.

Hepatogastrostomy. To perform HGS, there must be intrahepatic dilation of the left biliary system. The left hepatic bile duct can then be accessed through segment II or III of the liver from the proximal gastric body or cardia of the stomach. Needle puncture is performed in similar fashion as the RV approach, and the wire is advanced toward the hilum (Fig. 42.12). Tract dilation is then performed judiciously as described earlier. As with CDS, an FCSEMS is preferred to minimize risks of bile leak. However, unlike the stable and relatively static environment of CDS, the stomach and the liver tend to move independently from each other during respiration, which can lead to dislodgment of the stent. As such, care must be taken to ensure at least 3 cm of stent within the gastric lumen. A partially covered stent may also be considered to prevent occlusion of secondary ducts and minimize risk of stent migration.

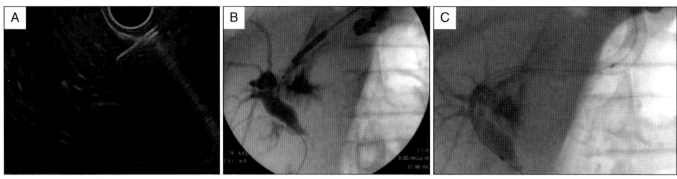

FIG 42.12 Direct transluminal approach with hepatogastrostomy (HGS). **A,** Endoscopic ultrasonography–guided puncture of the dilated intrahepatic bile duct from the proximal gastric body with a 19-gauge needle. **B,** Dilation of the HGS tract with a biliary dilating balloon. **C,** Fluoroscopic image of the deployed HGS fully covered metal stent.

Antegrade Stenting

Biliary access, wire passage, and tract dilation are performed in a similar fashion as described earlier for antegrade stenting. Note that the trajectory of the needle puncture and wire passage should be anterograde and across the BO and papilla in a similar fashion as the RV procedure. A biliary plastic or FCSEMS can then be advanced over the wire and through the obstruction and papilla for transpapillary stenting. The choice of stent type depends on patient factors and tumor resectability.

Indications for and Contraindications to EUS-BD in Malignant Obstruction

In malignant BO, EUS-BD can be considered after failure of conventional ERCP or as the primary modality, especially if there is concomitant GOO and in patients with altered anatomy. In the setting of GOO, EUS-BD can be performed during the same session as EUS-GE.[22] The CDS approach should be avoided in potentially resectable cancer, given that it may render the surgical procedure more difficult. EUS-BD with hepatogastrostomy should be undertaken only if there is evidence of intrahepatic biliary dilation. As with EUS-GE, uncorrectable thrombocytopenia (platelet count $<50 \times 10^9$/L) and/or coagulopathy (INR >1.5) are contraindications to EUS-BD.

Selecting the Optimal Technical Approach to EUS-BD in Malignant Biliary Obstruction With Gastric Outlet Obstruction

Although many endoscopists favor the RV method to avoid tract dilation and potential risk for bile leak, this method is often not possible in the setting of GOO. In addition, transpapillary drainage may be associated with higher risk for stent obstruction with tumor overgrowth or ingrowth compared with CDS or HGS.[43] Therefore, the direct TL approach is likely the optimal technique in achieving sustained biliary drainage in patients with concomitant malignant GOO. In choosing between CDS and HGS with the direct TL technique, there are data (although limited) suggesting greater safety with the extrahepatic approach.[44,45] In fact, a multivariable analysis by Dhir and colleagues[44] found the intrahepatic approach to be the only independent predictor for procedure-related adverse events. Postulated reasons for higher adverse events with the intrahepatic approach include the need for a transperitoneal puncture and the aforementioned movement of the stomach and liver with respiration, increasing the risk for stent migration and leak.[18] As such, when performing EUS-BD with the direct TL technique, CDS should be performed whenever possible; however, in patients with malignant GOO

this may not be possible if there is tumor involvement or obstruction of the proximal duodenum. In such instances, HGS should be the technique of choice.

Clinical Outcome With EUS-Biliary Drainage in Malignant Biliary Obstruction

EUS-BD has been well established as an alternative to ERCP. Unfortunately, however, most of the data on EUS-BD are from retrospective series, with very few well-designed controlled trials. In a systematic review of 42 studies and 1192 patients, EUS-BD was shown to have technical success, functional success, and adverse event rates of 94.7%, 91.7%, and 23.3%, respectively.[20] In an international multicenter prospective series involving 96 patients who underwent EUS-BD, technical and clinical success were 95.8% and 89.5%, respectively, with an adverse event rate of 10.5%.[21] Given the significant rates of adverse events and paucity of controlled data, ERCP remains the standard of care for the management of BO. Where available, EUS-BD is generally reserved as a salvage modality at most centers after failure with ERCP.

In malignant BO with concomitant GOO, however, ERCP may not be possible given the inability to reach the papilla.[46] Therefore, in this setting, EUS-BD or percutaneous transhepatic biliary drainage (PTBD) may be considered as the first-line treatment. Traditionally, at most centers, PTBD would be the favored approach given the lack of EUS-BD expertise; however, there are accumulating data that EUS-BD may attain similar technical and clinical success as PTBD while being associated with fewer adverse events, less need for reintervention, and potentially better cost-effectiveness.[47,48] Most recently a noninferiority randomized controlled trial comparing EUS-BD with PTBD in the management of malignant BO showed similar technical and clinical success rates of 94.1% EUS-BD versus 96.9% PTBD and clinical success of 87.5% EUS-BD and 87.1% PTBD. More importantly, EUS-BD appeared to be associated with fewer adverse events (8.8% EUS-BD vs 31.2% PTBD; $p = 0.022$) and less need for unscheduled reintervention, with a mean frequency of 0.34 in EUS-BD and 0.93 in PTBD ($p = 0.02$).[49] However, all EUS-BDs in this trial were performed with the use of the one-step EUS-BD stent system (DEUS; Standard Sci Tech, Inc., Seoul, Korea). This one-step system allows for insertion of a partially covered metal stent without the need for tract dilation and is currently not available in North America. Other technologic developments such as the LAMS (6 mm or 8 mm in diameter) have also been described with the CDS approach to establish a bypass that is stable and potentially safer by decreasing the risk for stent migration and leak.[50–53] Data on these novel technologies, however, cannot be extrapolated to the traditional method of EUS-BD where tract dilation is required before insertion of a traditional metal or plastic stent. Nevertheless, overall comparative studies between the two modalities appear to favor EUS-BD.[47,48] In addition, other advantages of EUS-BD compared with PTBD include the ability to perform the procedure during the same session as a failed ERCP and the potential to concomitantly relieve GOO with EUS-GE.[22]

Overall, EUS-BD appears to be an important therapeutic option in the management of malignant BO, especially if there is concomitant GOO, with preliminary data favoring its use over PTBD. Current limitations to the dissemination of EUS-BD include the lack of available expertise and dedicated accessories. Recent advances such as the LAMS and the one-step EUS-BD stent system are promising and may make the procedure easier and safer. Further developments of dedicated endoscopes and accessories along with well-designed prospective trials are needed to further validate the role of EUS-BD.

Adverse Events and Their Management
EUS-GE

Although EUS-GE appears to be safe, the published experience remains very small. In the largest published retrospective series thus far, involving 26 patients, 3 patients experienced adverse events.[17] One patient had postprocedure abdominal pain and two patients had misdeployment of the LAMS into the peritoneal cavity. Itoi et al. also described two cases of similar misdeployment of the distal flange in a series of 20 patients who underwent EPASS.[38] Overall, in the four reported cases of misdeployed stents, one patient developed peritonitis, one patient was salvaged successfully by stent removal and insertion of a biliary FCSEMS, and two patients were successfully treated with conservative management without need for endoscopic or surgical rescue after stent removal.

In general, rescue stenting with a LAMS or an FCSEMS should be attempted after initial stent misdeployment whenever possible in order to minimize leakage of gastric and small-bowel content into the peritoneal cavity. If a guidewire is used for initial stent insertion, then rescue stenting can easily be performed over the same wire. However, if the initial stent insertion is performed without wire guidance, then rescue stenting can be very difficult. Anecdotally, we have rescued misdeployed EUS-GE LAMS with the NOTES approach. This entails removal of the LAMS from the stomach, followed by dilation of the gastric puncture defect to 12 mm with a controlled radial expansion (CRE) balloon. This then allows for peritoneoscopy to occur, where the endoscope is advanced through the stomach defect and into the peritoneal cavity (Fig. 42.13). From the peritoneal cavity, the small-bowel puncture site can then be located under direct endoscopic visualization. A guidewire

can then be inserted through the defect, followed by insertion of another LAMS with the deployment of the distal flange into the small bowel. The endoscope and LAMS insertion catheter can then be pulled back proximally into the stomach, followed by deployment of the proximal flange, essentially sealing the defect while achieving a successful endoscopic bypass. If recue stenting is not possible, then efforts should be made to close the stomach defect with a closure device such as an over-the-scope clip or endoscopic suturing. Note that this approach is likely suboptimal, given that the puncture defect of the small bowel will remain unrepaired. All patients should be placed on intravenous broad-spectrum antibiotics regardless of the approach and hospitalized for observation. Surgical consultation should be sought, as emergent surgery may be required.

Significant gastrointestinal bleeding can also occur with EUS-GE. This usually stems from the gastric feeding vessels with stent insertion and/or dilation but can also occur from the small bowel, especially with contralateral wall injury with the electrocautery tip–assisted LAMS insertion. Anecdotally, the first step in the management of these bleeds is to identify the exact source with good water irrigation and examine both the gastric end of the stent and the small-bowel lumen. The small-bowel lumen can be examined through the stent if dilation was performed. Otherwise, enteroscopy can be performed if the GOO is not traversable with the endoscope. If the bleed stems from the gastric feeding vessels, then balloon tamponade through the stent with a dilating balloon would be the best initial approach. If hemostasis is achieved during the tamponade, then the balloon should be kept inflated for several minutes. Sustained hemostasis should be ascertained during balloon deflation. If there is ongoing bleeding during deflation of the balloon, reinflation and repeat tamponade can be performed. If bleeding remains refractory to these maneuvers, then consultation with interventional radiology (IR) for embolization can be considered. Note that, if necessary, balloon tamponade can be maintained until embolization is performed. Bleeding from the small bowel with cautery injury can usually be controlled with standard hemostatic modalities, including through the scope clips, injection of dilute epinephrine, and/or thermal therapy. The challenge, however, is to reach the bleeding site with the endoscope. If traversing the stent or enteroscopy is not possible, then IR and surgery consultation should be considered.

EUS-BD

In a systematic review of prospective and retrospective series of 1192 patients who underwent EUS-BD, the pooled adverse event rate was

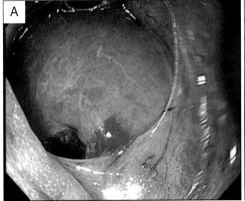
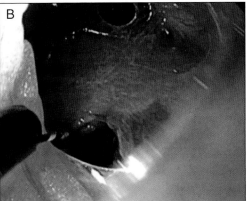

FIG 42.13 A, Peritoneoscopy with direct endoscopic visualization of the omental/peritoneal defect secondary to a misdeployed lumen apposing stent. **B,** Advancement of an ERCP catheter and guidewire through the defect for salvage stenting.

23.3%, including bleeding 4.03%, bile leakage 4.03%, pneumoperitoneum 3.02%, stent migration 2.68%, cholangitis 2.43%, abdominal pain 1.51%, and peritonitis 1.26%.[20] In general, the biggest concern specific to EUS-BD is the risk of bile leak, which can result in peritonitis. To minimize this risk, overdilation of the CDS or HGS tract should be avoided before stent insertion. In addition, needle-knife dilation should be avoided whenever possible, as it has been shown to be associated with increased risk for bile leak.[54] The advent of LAMS and the one-step EUS-BD stent system is promising for increasing the safety EUS-BD. Notably in the largest retrospective series of LAMS EUS-BD and the largest randomized controlled trial involving the DEUS one-step system, there were no reported cases of bile leak, with overall adverse events as low as 7% and 8.8%, respectively.[49,52] In the event of a bile leak, management should include broad-spectrum intravenous antibiotics and drainage of any collection via IR with surgical consultation in case of clinical deterioration. Stent migration is another potential serious adverse event of EUS-BD, especially in the setting of HGS. This risk can be minimized by ensuring proper stent length of at least 3 cm within the stomach and/or using a partially cover metal stent. If stent migration occurs, any collection should be drained via the IR approach, along with

consideration of PTBD and endoscopic or surgical removal of the inserted stent. Finally, patients with cholangitis or bleeding after EUS-BD should also be managed in a multidisciplinary fashion, including PTBD for cholangitis and IR embolization with surgical backup for refractory bleeding.

CONCLUSIONS

Malignant GOO with concomitant BO is a challenging endoscopic dilemma in patients with periampullary cancer. Traditional palliating options such as surgical bypass, enteral stenting, and ERCP have important limitations. EUS-GE and EUS-BD are promising modalities in providing the ideal treatment to reinstitute luminal and biliary patency in a sustained and minimally invasive fashion. As endoscopic technology continues to evolve, EUS-GE and EUS-BD are likely to become first-line treatment options that will provide effective and safe palliation for this frail patient population.

The complete reference list for this chapter can be found online at www.experconsult.com.

Benign Biliary Strictures

Guido Costamagna, Ivo Boškoski, and Pietro Familiari

Benign biliary strictures (BBS) are most commonly caused by iatrogenic surgical injury, usually after cholecystectomy, or may occur at the site of biliary anastomosis after hepatic resection or liver transplantation (LT). Other causes of BBS include primary sclerosing cholangitis (PSC), chronic pancreatitis (CP), immunoglobulin G4 (IgG4)–related cholangiopathy, and a variety of other causes (Box 43.1).

Endoscopic retrograde cholangiopancreatography (ERCP) has a pivotal role in the treatment of the vast majority of patients with BBS.

CLINICAL FEATURES AND DIAGNOSIS

Approximately 80% of patients with postoperative BBS present within 6 to 12 months after surgery with symptoms of jaundice, pruritus, abdominal pain, alterations of liver function tests, and recurrent cholangitis.[1] It is very important to promptly recognize these symptoms, as long-standing cholestasis can lead to secondary biliary cirrhosis.[2] About 10% of BBS patients present within 1 week of surgery, and the condition may be associated with biliary leaks.[1]

ERCP has primarily a therapeutic role in BBS. Nevertheless, the diagnostic (cholangiographic) phase of ERCP is essential to determine the morphologic type of the stricture. The classification of Bismuth and Lazorthes[3] is a morphologic classification developed before the advent of laparoscopy. This classification was intended to guide surgical repair of postoperative BBS.[4] Today it is widely used to classify lesions according to the cholangiographic appearance and classifies BBS into five types[3]: type 1, low common hepatic duct (CHD) or bile duct (CHD >2 cm); type 2, mid-CHD (CHD <2 cm); type 3, hilar stricture; type 4, involvement of the main hilar confluence (right and left hepatic ducts separated); type 5, involvement of a right hepatic branch alone or with common duct.

The clinical presentation of biliary strictures is somewhat different in patients with CP.[5] In a retrospective review of 78 patients with CP, overt jaundice was found in only a minority of patients.[6] No relationship was found between features of the common bile duct (CBD) and severity of pancreatitis or disease duration. Up to one-third of patients with advanced CP develop symptomatic biliary stenosis.[7,8] Biliary obstruction caused by compression from an edematous pancreatic head or a pseudocyst usually resolves when the inflammation subsides or after resolution of the pseudocyst. However, obstruction caused by a fibrotic stricture does not resolve spontaneously and requires therapeutic intervention.

The preferred noninvasive method for diagnostic cholangiography in BBS is magnetic resonance cholangiopancreatography (MRCP).[9] MRCP is extremely useful in providing a roadmap for endoscopic drainage. MRCP is also used to distinguish between anastomotic (extrahepatic) and ischemic (intrahepatic) strictures after LT.[10]

Ruling out underlying malignancy is especially important in the presence of BBS in patients with underlying CP and those with PSC. MRCP, computed tomography scan, endoscopic ultrasonography with fine-needle aspiration (EUS/FNA), and ERCP with biliary brush cytology and/or intraductal biopsies are the first-line diagnostic modalities in these situations. EUS/FNA is widely used in ruling out malignancy in patients with mass-forming CP. This method can also be used for rendezvous EUS/ERCP procedures in case of failed transpapillary access to the bile ducts (see Chapter 32). Cholangioscopy with targeted biopsy (see Chapter 27) is useful in selected cases where other diagnostic methods have failed to confirm malignancy, especially in patients with autoimmune (IgG4-related) cholangiopathy and PSC.[11]

ENDOSCOPIC TECHNIQUE

Endoscopic treatment of BBS involves two technical steps: (1) negotiating the stricture and (2) dilating the stricture. Negotiating the stricture requires continuity of the CBD. In cases of complete transection or ligation of the CBD, a guidewire cannot be passed across the lesion and thus endotherapy alone is not feasible. Although surgical reconstruction is indicated in complete transection or ligation of the CBD, in some reports a combined percutaneous/endoscopic technique has been adopted, aiming to bring together the two stumps of a transected bile duct.[12,13]

After deep bile duct access, a cholangiogram is performed to determine the type and features of the BBS. Performing a complete biliary sphincterotomy is important because repeated stent exchanges and insertion of multiple stents are required in most cases.

BBS are generally short, asymmetric, and rich in fibrous tissue, which makes them more difficult to negotiate compared with neoplastic strictures. These strictures are more complex and negotiation is more difficult when the hepatic hilum is involved. It is therefore often necessary to use thin hydrophilic guidewires (0.021-inch or 0.018-inch diameter) with a straight or curved (J-shaped) tip to traverse the stricture. Guidewire manipulation requires patience, skill, and optimal fluoroscopic imaging. Forceful maneuvers may create false passages and should be avoided. Using an inflated stone retrieval balloon positioned just distal to the stricture and applying downward traction results in stretching the bile duct and modifying the axis of the guidewire and stricture. Steerable catheters or papillotomes may also be used to negotiate the stricture. Once the stricture is traversed, the hydrophilic guidewire can be exchanged for a stiffer wire to facilitate dilation.

Stricture dilation has two objectives: (1) to reopen the CBD to achieve bile drainage and (2) to keep the stenosis open and avoid restricturing.

Insertion of the guidewire through the stricture is followed by placement of a 5-Fr or 6-Fr catheter over the guidewire. Dilation can be done mechanically or with balloons. Mechanical dilation is usually done with dilation catheters (e.g., 6- to 9.5-Fr Cunningham-Cotton sleeve; Cook Endoscopy, Winston-Salem, NC) to test the caliber of the stricture before attempting stent insertion. Hydrostatic balloon dilation is generally done with 4-mm, 6-mm, and 8-mm low-profile balloons,

BOX 43.1   **Causes of Benign Biliary Strictures**

- Postoperative
- Anastomotic
- Nonanastomotic
- Ischemia (including polyarteritis nodosa)
- Primary or secondary sclerosing cholangitis
- Autoimmune cholangitis
- Scar after endoscopic sphincterotomy
- Chronic pancreatitis
- Radiation therapy
- Portal bilopathy
- Tuberculosis
- Abdominal trauma
- Radiofrequency tumor ablation
- Endoscopic sclerotherapy for bleeding duodenal ulcer

particularly in cases where the stricture is not amenable to mechanical dilation. Balloon dilation is usually performed to a size 1 to 2 mm larger than the downstream bile duct diameter. Although immediately effective, endoscopic and percutaneous balloon dilation alone, whether in a single session or multiple sessions, is considered inadequate and associated with a high restenosis rate (up to 47%).[14–16]

Stent placement in addition to dilation maintains stricture patency for a prolonged period to allow scar remodeling and consolidation.[17] When mechanical and/or balloon dilation is unsuccessful in allowing large-bore stent placement, leaving a 5-Fr or 6-Fr nasobiliary drainage tube in situ for 24 to 48 hours may increase the chances of subsequent endoscopic stent placement. Alternatively, screw-type stent extractors (Soehendra stent extractor; Cook Endoscopy) and angioplasty balloons mounted on 3-Fr catheters can allow for passage of balloon dilators mounted on 5-Fr catheters and subsequent stent placement.

Placement of a single plastic stent leads to unsatisfactory long-term outcomes.[18] Currently, the most effective method for calibration of postoperative BBS is the temporary simultaneous placement of a progressive number of plastic stents, over a period of 1 year (with stent exchanges every 3 to 4 months). This "aggressive multistenting strategy" is highly effective but requires multiple ERCP sessions and is dependent on patient compliance (Fig. 43.1).[12,19,20]

Removable fully covered self-expanding metal stents (SEMS) have emerged as an alternative to multiple plastic stents to avoid multiple ERCP sessions with need for upsizing and plastic stent exchanges. When SEMS are used, theoretically only two ERCP procedures are needed: one for stent placement and one for removal. Placement of uncovered SEMS should be avoided in all types of BBS, because stent imbedding and ingrowth of reactive tissue through the mesh of the stent makes them irretrievable.[12,21]

Candidates for fully covered SEMS should be selected very carefully. Bismuth type I postcholecystectomy strictures, selected cases of biliary anastomotic strictures in LT patients, and CP-related BBS are the best candidates. Placing fully covered SEMS in strictures of the hepatic hilum should be avoided, mainly because of the risk of impaction and occlusion of intrahepatic branches that can lead to sepsis.[12]

Biodegradable biliary stents could be used in the future for endoscopic management of BBS. The potential advantages of these stents are that only one ERCP session is needed for placement and removal is unnecessary. Different biodegradable materials have been tested to date (polylactide, polycaprolactone, and polydioxanone) but are still under investigation. The main disadvantages of these stents are that the expansive radial force decreases with the degradation of the stent and there is a potential inflammatory foreign body reaction leading to hyperplasia. Additionally, there are scarce data to support their use.[22] Currently, the only data available in humans were published recently by Siiki et al.[23] The authors placed two biodegradable stents in two patients with excellent stricture resolution at 6 months, with biodegradability confirmed on magnetic resonance imaging. Before this report, the efficacy of biodegradable stents had been proven only in animal models.[24] This promising new treatment requires further investigation.

OUTCOMES OF ENDOTHERAPY

Postcholecystectomy Strictures

The incidence of BBS has increased up to three times with the advent of laparoscopic cholecystectomy.[25,26] Misidentification of anatomic structures during dissection, anatomic variations of the biliary tree, presence of acute inflammation or fibrous adhesions in the gallbladder fossa, excessive use of electrocautery to control bleeding, inaccurate placement of clips, sutures, ligation, and excessive traction on the gallbladder neck are all causes that can lead to BBS and injuries.[25,26] Historically, surgery was the treatment of choice, and ERCP was limited to diagnosis. Today ERCP is the first-line treatment for BBS, because it is safe and repeatable, with fewer adverse events compared with surgery, and has high treatment success rates.[19,27]

As already mentioned, endoscopic placement of one biliary stent is not sufficient to appropriately dilate a postcholecystectomy BBS.[18] Today, placement of a progressive number of plastic stents exchanged every 3 to 4 months over a period of 12 months is established as the gold-standard treatment for BBS.[19,20,27,28] At every stent exchange, all previously placed stents are removed and a maximum number of large-diameter plastic stents are reinserted, inducing progressive stretching of the fibrotic biliary stricture. ERCP with plastic stent placement is repeated until complete morphologic disappearance of the stricture is confirmed at cholangiography, which usually takes 1 year, and is associated with good long-term results that range from 80% to 100%.[12,14,19,20,27,29] These results are maintained after more than 10 years of follow-up.[20]

There are fewer data concerning the use of fully and partially covered SEMS in patients with postcholecystectomy strictures. SEMS placement in patients with postcholecystectomy biliary strictures might be an inappropriate treatment when the stricture is located close to the hilum and the bile duct below the stricture is of normal caliber.

Deviere et al. published a large multicenter trial in which fully covered SEMS were placed in 187 patients with BBS of different etiologies. In this trial, only 18 patients had postcholecystectomy strictures, of whom 14 were previously treated with plastic biliary stents. Of these 18 patients, 13 (72%) had stricture resolution after 10 to 12 months without need for further treatments. Furthermore, stent migration occurred in two-thirds of the patients, and 6 patients (33%) suffered from cholangitis, pancreatitis, or fever.[30]

Recently Cote et al. conducted a randomized trial showing that fully covered metal stents were not inferior to multiple plastic stents in achieving resolution of BBS of different etiologies.[31] In this trial the majority of patients (108) had BBS related to LT and CP, whereas only 4 patients (3.6%) had postoperative biliary injury, probably because of cholecystectomy (the authors did not clearly specify).

Given the scarcity of data in this field, covered SEMS are not recommended as a routine treatment for postcholecystectomy strictures but can be used in carefully selected cases.[12,30] Nonforeshortening fully covered SEMS are ideally suited for strictures located close to the bifurcation.

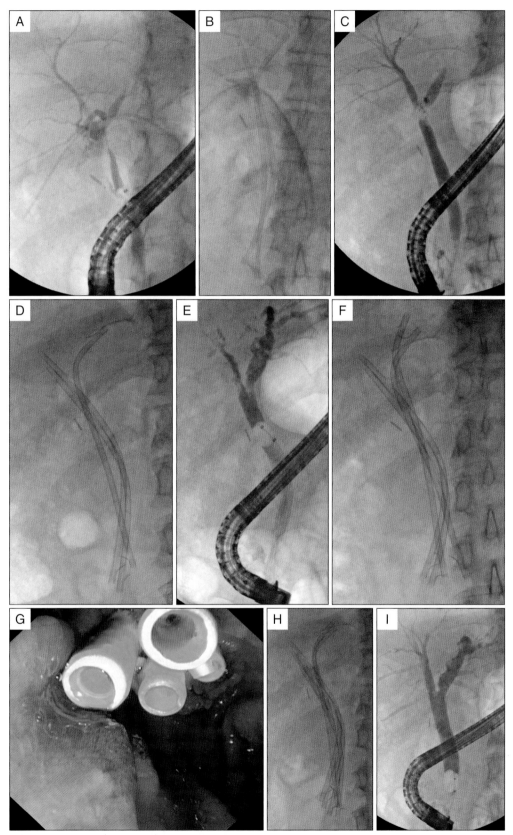

FIG 43.1 Bismuth type 3 stricture after laparoscopic cholecystectomy with associated bile leak **(A)** and two 8.5-Fr stents placed during the first treatment **(B)**. Cholangiogram at 3 months after stent removal shows clearly the Bismuth type 3 stricture **(C)** and three 10-Fr stents placed at endoscopic retrograde cholangio-pancreatography **(D)**. Cholangiogram at further 3 months after stent removal **(E)** and four 10-Fr stents placed **(F)**. **G,** Endoscopic appearance of the four plastic stents. **H,** Radiograph with five 10-Fr stents. **I,** Final cholangiogram at stent removal after 1 year of treatment.

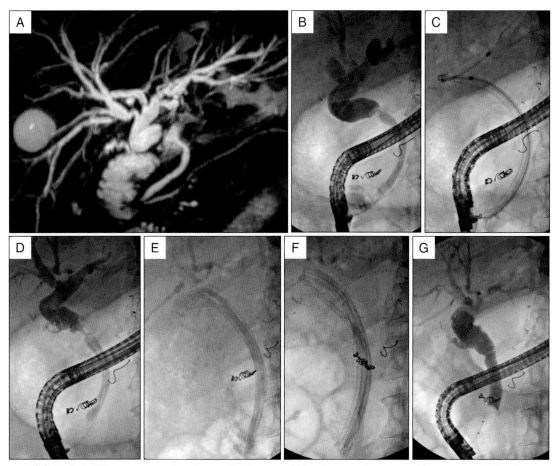

FIG 43.2 A, Biliary anastomotic stricture after liver transplantation noted at magnetic resonance cholangio-pancreatography. **B,** Cholangiographic appearance of the anastomotic biliary stricture at endoscopic retrograde cholangiopancreatography (ERCP). **C,** Two 10-Fr plastic stents placed during the first ERCP session; also a pancreatic plastic stent was placed. Cholangiographic appearance after removal of the two biliary stents at 3 months **(D)** and four 10-Fr plastic stents placed **(E)**. **F,** Five plastic stents placed at third ERCP. **G,** Chol-angiogram after stent removal shows complete stricture resolution after 1 year of treatment.

Anastomotic Strictures After Liver Transplantation (See Also Chapter 44)

Post-LT strictures can be anastomotic biliary strictures (ABS) or nonanas-tomotic biliary strictures (NABS; arising elsewhere in the biliary tree). Biliary stricture formation is one of the most common complications after LT, with an incidence of 5% to 32%.[32–34] ERCP is the first-line treatment modality for ABS. ERCP also plays a role in selected cases of NABS. ABS are the vast majority (80%) of all post-LT biliary strictures and arise at the site of the choledochocholedochostomy.[35]

Endotherapy with placement of multiple plastic stents is the first-line treatment for ABS, with long-term success rates ranging from 90% to 100% (Fig. 43.2).[32,36–39] Similar results were found by Tringali et al. in a recent study of 56 patients with biliary strictures after LT.[40] The success rate was 98% with a mean follow-up of 5.8 years.

Partially covered SEMS were placed by Chaput and colleagues[41] in 22 patients with anastomotic biliary strictures after LT, remaining in place for 2.2 months. There were two distal migrations and five partial dislocations. At the end of treatment 3 patients (13.6%) had persistence of the stricture, and recurrence occurred in 9 of 19 patients (47.4%) within 3.5 ± 2.1 months. Sustained stricture resolution was reported in only 10 of 19 patients (52.6%). Better results have been obtained in this setting with fully covered SEMS, with success rates ranging from 92% to 100% and a migration rate of 24%.[42–45]

NABS represent 10% to 25% of post-LT biliary strictures[46,47] and are a consequence of hepatic artery thrombosis, prolonged graft ischemic time, and ABO incompatibility of the donor and recipient.[48] Their appearance is unifocal but they can also be found anywhere in the biliary tree.

The role of ERCP in patients with NABS is limited to graft preserva-tion until surgery with hepaticojejunostomy or retransplantation.[49–51] In selected cases plastic stents can be useful but with lower long-term success rates that range from 50% to 75%.[49,52]

Chronic Pancreatitis (See Also Chapter 45)

Compared with postcholecystectomy and post-LT biliary strictures, endotherapy in BBS related to CP has lower success rates, mostly because of fibrosis of the pancreatic parenchyma and chronic inflammatory processes.[53] The outcome of endotherapy is negatively influenced in the presence of stones in the region of the pancreatic head (chronic calcifying pancreatitis).[54–57] The success rates of treatment with multiple plastic stents in these patients range from 44% to 92%.[54–56]

Because the stricture is typically located in the distal (intrapancreatic) bile duct, covered SEMS have been widely used in this setting. Overall, the success rates range from 43% to 77% but with high migration rates.[57–60] To overcome migration, SEMS with antimigration flaps have been adopted.[57,61,62] Park and colleagues used covered stents with either an anchoring flap or a flared end at the proximal part.[62] These stents were placed in 43 patients with biliary strictures of different etiologies, including CP (11 patients). No migration was seen in stents with anchoring flaps, and a 33% migration rate was found in flared-end SEMS after 6 months of placement on average. There was a 100% removal rate in both groups with few endoscopic sessions and no complications. Indeed, there is now one fully covered SEMS (Wallflex RMV; Boston Scientific, Marlborough, MA) approved by the European Union and the US Food and Drug Administration.

In the setting of CP-related BBS that are unresponsive to endoscopic treatment, hepaticojejunostomy remains the procedure of choice.

Primary Sclerosing Cholangitis (See Also Chapter 55)

The etiology of PSC is idiopathic and it is characterized by periductal inflammation and fibrosis that can occur anywhere in the biliary tree, leading to stricture formation. Strictures in PSC can be dominant or multiple (intrahepatic). Dominant strictures occur in 50% of patients with PSC and are defined as stenosis of the CBD that is ≤1.5 mm in diameter or of the hepatic duct ≤1 mm in diameter.[63,64]

With the advent of MRCP, the diagnostic role of ERCP in PSC has become obsolete. Furthermore, considering the high risk of cholangitis, the diagnostic role of ERCP should be limited to tissue acquisition in dominant strictures where there is a concern for underlying cholangiocarcinoma,[65,66] which can occur in up to 20% of patients with PSC.[67]

Brush cytology and cholangioscopy with endoscopic tissue sampling are both useful tools for distinguishing between malignant and benign dominant strictures. The goal of endoscopy in PSC patients with dominant strictures is to improve symptoms and sequelae of biliary obstruction. Balloon dilation of dominant strictures is the preferred treatment method, as stent placement alone is associated with higher rates of complications in the long term (e.g., cholangitis caused by plastic stent occlusion).[66,68,69] In some patients, to achieve maximal clinical benefit, repeated dilation sessions may be necessary.[70]

Short-term stenting can be taken into consideration in cases of failed balloon dilation of dominant strictures.[70]

Autoimmune Cholangiopathy

IgG4-associated cholangiopathy may affect any part of the biliary tree. The disease can mimic hilar tumors, CBD tumors, pancreatic cancer, or PSC.[11,71] IgG4-associated cholangiopathy can also be associated with autoimmune pancreatitis.[24,72]

Elevated serum IgG4 has a low sensitivity for diagnosis, and in many cases the serum levels are normal.[11,71] Cholangioscopy and tissue acquisition during ERCP and/or EUS are currently the preferred diagnostic methods.[24] Histology with IgG4 immunostaining is characteristic with hematoxylin and eosin staining and extensive infiltration by IgG4 plasma cells.[24,72] Biopsies of the ampullary region have also been proposed for histologic diagnosis.[73]

IgG4-associated cholangiopathy responds very well to steroid therapy, and in some instances steroid therapy can confirm the diagnosis "ex adiuvantibus."[24,74] Stenting can be useful in patients with jaundice in the acute phase before institution of corticosteroid therapy.[24,75]

CONCLUSIONS

Endoscopic diagnosis and management of BBS have significantly advanced in the past 2 decades. Endoscopy is minimally invasive, repeatable, and a safe diagnostic and therapeutic management option for most patients with BBS. Currently, the multistenting protocol with plastic stents is the standard of care for postcholecystectomy strictures and post-LT biliary anastomotic biliary strictures. Covered SEMS are a good alternative to plastic stents in many situations, but larger trials are needed to better understand their place in the therapeutic algorithm. The evolution of biodegradable stents could lead to better clinical outcomes, and more studies are awaited in this field. The biggest challenge for endoscopists today is defining the etiology of and excluding malignancy in certain types of BBS.

The complete reference list for this chapter can be found online at www.expertconsult.com.

44

Biliary Surgery Adverse Events, Including Liver Transplantation

Ilaria Tarantino, Todd H. Baron, and Dario Ligresti

Iatrogenic bile duct injury (BDI) continues to be an important clinical problem after biliary surgery, resulting in serious morbidity and occasional mortality. The management, operative risk, and outcome of BDIs vary considerably and are highly dependent on the type of injury, the severity, and location. Although perioperative complications are frequent, nearly all can be managed nonoperatively. Early referral to a tertiary care center with experienced hepatobiliary surgeons, skilled therapeutic endoscopists, and interventional radiologists is necessary to assure optimal results.

Endoscopic interventions, including endoscopic sphincterotomy and stent placement, have essentially replaced surgery as the first-line treatment option for most postsurgical biliary injuries (Box 44.1). These nonsurgical interventions decrease or eliminate the pressure gradient between the bile duct and duodenum, allowing preferential flow of bile from the duct into the duodenum rather than extravasation via the leak, allowing the defect to heal. They also promote healing of strictures, through the placement of prostheses that dilate and maintain biliary patency. The frequency of biliary injury, from lowest to highest, is laparoscopic cholecystectomy (LC), liver resection, and liver transplantation (LT) (Box 44.2).

LAPAROSCOPIC CHOLECYSTECTOMY

LC is currently the preferred treatment approach to symptomatic or complicated cholelithiasis. By the early 1990s, LC had supplanted open cholecystectomy in the operative management of gallstone disease. The laparoscopic approach is preferred because it results in less postoperative pain, shorter hospital stay, and faster return to normal activity. However, the widespread application of LC led to a concurrent rise in the incidence of BDIs. Reports estimate that the incidence of BDI rose from 0.1% to 0.2% during the era of open cholecystectomy to 0.4% to 0.6% between the era of open cholecystectomy[1] and the age of LC.

BDI can occur even in experienced hands, when one is beyond the learning curve of laparoscopic surgery. Recently a large observational study examined long-term mortality rates after common bile duct (CBD) injury after LC.[2] In total, 125 patients with CBD injuries were identified after 156,958 laparoscopic cholecystectomies for cholelithiasis performed in New York State from 2005 to 2010. This study revealed a significantly higher all-cause mortality rate after CBD injury compared with previous studies at 20.8%. This was an increase of 8.8% above the cohort's expected age-adjusted death rate. This high rate is associated with common BDIs requiring operative intervention. The mortality rate appears appreciably higher than that quoted previously.

Large studies published in the last decade have demonstrated incidences of major and minor biliary injury of 0.25% to 1.90% and 0.38% to 1.20%, respectively. This is mostly attributable to misidentification of anatomic structures during laparoscopic surgery, acute inflammation or fibrous adhesions in the gallbladder fossa, excessive use of electrocautery, and inaccurate placement of clips, sutures, and ligatures.

A classic laparoscopic injury occurs when the CBD is mistaken for the cystic duct and is caused by excessive cephalad retraction of the fundus of the gallbladder, in which the cystic and common ducts become closely aligned. The surgeon, erroneously thinking that the cystic duct has been successfully divided, continues to dissect the common duct proximally and eventually transects the common hepatic duct. The right hepatic artery is also typically injured or ligated because of its proximity.

Demonstration of the critical view of safety as described by Strasberg et al.[2a] allows identification of the cystic duct and artery as they enter the gallbladder and permits safe clipping and division of these structures. Unfortunately, only about 20% to 30% of injuries are diagnosed at the time of initial surgery. Initial symptoms may be delayed and nonspecific; patients are frequently discharged from the hospital only to present a few days later (usually within the first postoperative week) with jaundice, biliary drainage from an existing drain, biliary ascites, and/or bile peritonitis.

Despite the presence of various classification systems for BDI, the Strasberg system remains the most popular and widely used (Table 44.1).[3] Continuity of the injured bile duct with the CBD is the most important factor in relation to endoscopic management (Fig. 44.1).

BOX 44.1 Indications for ERCP After Biliary Surgery

- BDI diagnosed after surgery
- BDI without loss of CBD continuity:
  - Strasberg type A
  - Strasberg types B and C with communication with CBD
  - Strasberg type C with small tears/burn of the CBD
  - Strasberg type E if there is an incomplete transection

BDI, Bile duct injury; *CBD,* common bile duct; *ERCP,* endoscopic retrograde cholangiopancreatography.

BOX 44.2 Type of Biliary Surgery and Bile Duct Injury Rate

- Laparoscopic cholecystectomy, 0.4% to 0.6%
- Liver resection, 10%
- Liver transplantation, 8% to 35%

TABLE 44.1	Strasberg Classification and Subsequent Treatment of Bile Duct Injury		
Strasberg Classification	**Type of Injury**		**Treatment**
Type A	Leak from the cystic duct/duct of Luschka		ERCP
Type B	Ligation of a sectorial duct with obstruction	Communication with CBD branches	ERCP
		No communication with CBD branches	Surgery
Type C	Leak from a nonligated sectorial duct	Communication with CBD branches	ERCP
		No communication with CBD branches	Surgery

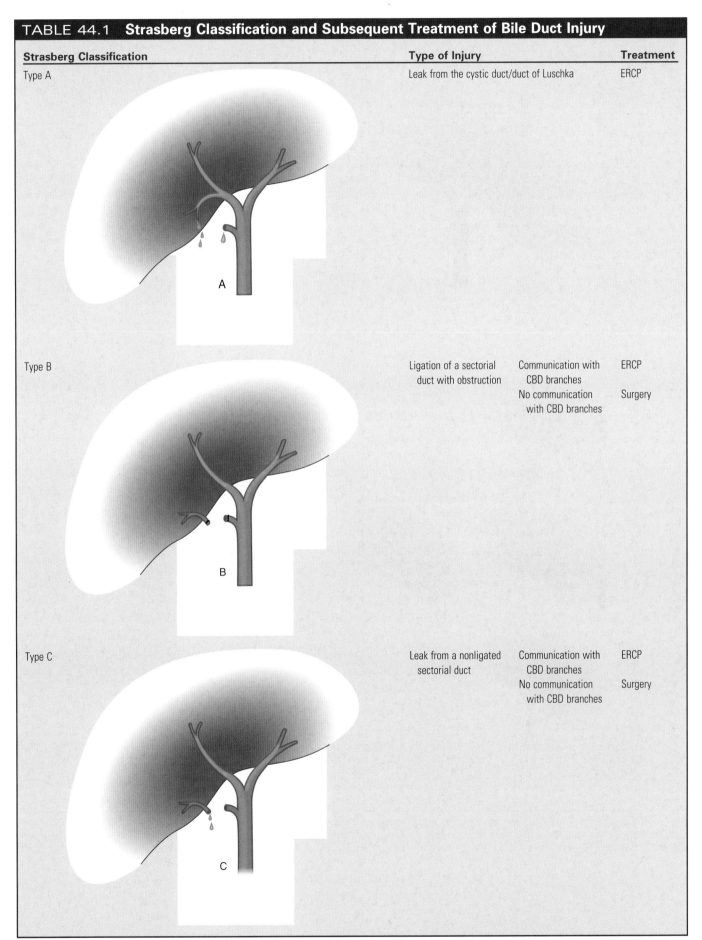

Continued

TABLE 44.1 Strasberg Classification and Subsequent Treatment of Bile Duct Injury—cont'd

Strasberg Classification	Type of Injury		Treatment
Type D	Lateral injury to extrahepatic duct	Small tear/burn of the CBD	ERCP
		Significant loss of substance of the CBD	Surgery
Type E	CBD transection	Incomplete (continuity maintained)	ERCP
		Complete	Surgery
	CBD resection	No continuity	Surgery

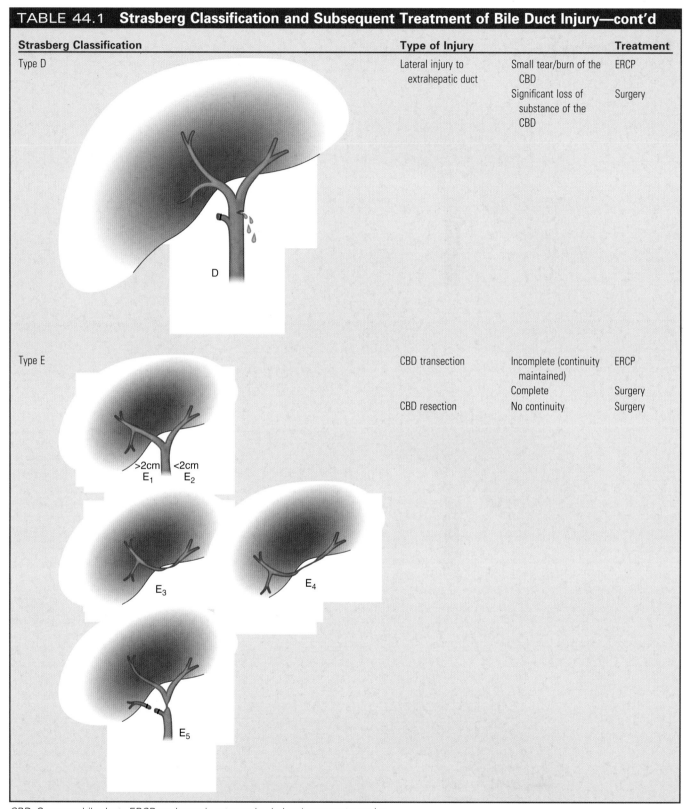

CBD, Common bile duct; *ERCP,* endoscopic retrograde cholangiopancreatography.
Pictures redrawn from Strasberg SM, Hertl M, Soper NJ. An analysis of the problem of biliary injury during laparoscopic cholecystectomy. *J Am Coll Surg.* 1995;180:101–125. Reproduced with permission from the *Journal of the American College of Surgeons.*

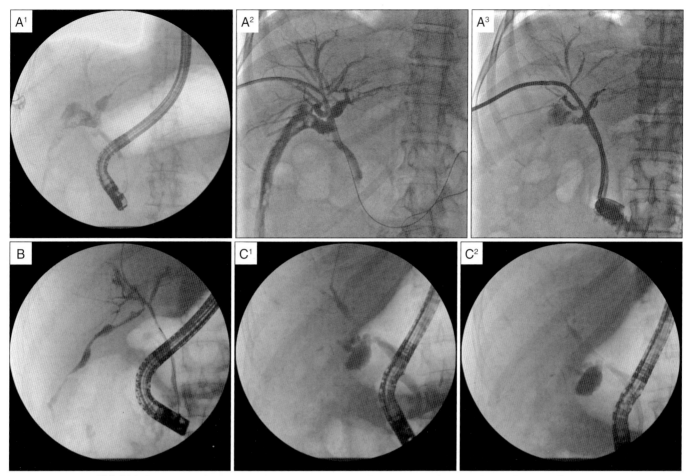

FIG 44.1 Post–laparoscopic cholecystectomy biliary leaks. **A1,** Leak at the hepatic hilum with no opacification of the right intrahepatic biliary system. Rendezvous in the same patient showing the leak (**A2**) and the positioning of a percutaneous transhepatic biliary drainage and an endoscopic biliary plastic stent (**A3**). **B,** Biliary leak at the right hepatic duct. **C1,** Biliary leak at the cystic duct. **C2,** Biliary plastic stent inserted in the common bile duct after sphincterotomy in the same patient.

If there is continuity of the injured duct (Strasberg type A), endoscopic retrograde cholangiopancreatography (ERCP) is considered the treatment of choice, with a 99% success rate.[4] Ligated sectorial ducts (Strasberg type B) may remain asymptomatic or present late with atrophy-hypertrophy complex and sectoral cholangitis requiring hepatectomy. For nonligated sectorial ducts (Strasberg type C), ERCP is the primary therapy only when there is connection between the leaking sectorial duct and CBD branches. If the injury cannot be detected by cholangiography using an appropriate amount of contrast under pressure to exclude small leaks, then there is likely a lack of communication between the injured duct and the biliary system (disconnection). In these patients magnetic resonance cholangiopancreatography (MRCP) is useful for detecting a biliary leak and the underlying anatomy. Percutaneous drainage of the isolated segment allows proximal control of the biliary leak in many cases.[5] In patients who require surgery, hepaticojejunostomy is the treatment of choice[6] and the percutaneous catheter can act as a guide at the time of reconstructive surgery. In cases of postoperative detection of a small tear or burning of the CBD (Strasberg type D), ERCP is the primary therapy. In patients with significant loss of duct, hepaticojejunostomy is the preferred option.

For injuries with complete bile duct transection/resection or lack of continuity between segments (Strasberg type E), endoscopic treatment is generally precluded. MRCP is helpful to define biliary anatomy, and surgery is needed to reestablish ductal continuity.

Bile Leak

Minor and clinically insignificant or unapparent bile leaks are common after cholecystectomy; they arise from ducts in the gallbladder bed and occur in up to 24% of patients. These are associated with low output through a surgical drain (if not unapparent) and usually resolve without intervention.

Significant and clinically relevant postoperative bile leaks occur in approximately 0.8% to 1.1% of patients. Bile leaks can be classified into two categories using an ERCP-based assessment of severity:

- Low-grade leaks are present if leakage from the biliary tract is observed only after complete filling of the intrahepatic bile ducts with contrast (i.e., injecting contrast under pressure).
- High-grade leaks are present if a large amount of contrast extravasation occurs before filling of the intrahepatic bile ducts.

Most low-grade leaks occur from the cystic duct or duct of Luschka (types A and C) and can be treated definitively by an endoscopic approach. The endoscopic approach to bile leaks has been reviewed.[7] The aim is to decrease the transpapillary pressure gradient; an increase in transpapillary bile flow diverts bile from the leak site.

Whether to perform biliary sphincterotomy alone without placement of a biliary stent for bile leaks remains debatable, but most endoscopists agree that sphincterotomy alone is not adequate unless there are obstructing stones as an additional factor or if a very large sphincterotomy can be done (which usually necessitates a dilated duct, often absent in the setting of a leak in a young patient). It is usually not necessary to place a stent beyond the site of leak, and we insert a 10-Fr plastic stent after biliary sphincterotomy.

Insertion of a biliary stent across the papilla without sphincterotomy is generally desirable to preserve the biliary sphincter in younger patients.[8] However, when 10-Fr stents are placed without sphincterotomy, it is associated with a higher rate of post-ERCP pancreatitis (PEP).[9] This study was published before the use of prophylactic measures to reduce PEP, such as pancreatic stent placement or administration of rectally administered nonsteroidal antiinflammatory drugs. After successful stent placement, the stent remains in place for approximately 4 to 6 weeks and is not replaced if follow-up ERCP shows resolution of the leakage. Some authors have shown that follow-up ERCP may be unnecessary for patients with cystic duct and duct of Luschka leaks when the initial ERCP is otherwise normal, and a standard upper endoscopy with stent removal can be safely performed.[3] The same approach can be used for minor lateral injuries of the right or CBD (type D). However, whenever the main duct is involved, follow-up ERCP is mandatory to assess complete leak closure and to detect development of a stricture, which occurs more often with main duct injuries.

When a percutaneous drain has been placed during management of the leak (e.g., patients who developed a biloma), the drainage output should be less than 10 mL/day (preferably the drain has been removed) before removing the stent. With minor bile leaks, we advise placing the external drain to gravity drainage rather than to suction, to decrease the resistance of flow through the leak site and promote bile flow through the stent into the duodenum.

An alternative approach is to combine biliary sphincterotomy with nasobiliary drainage (NBD). NBD allows for suction and irrigation and noninvasive cholangiograms, and it is easily removed. Unfortunately, NBD is uncomfortable and frequently becomes dislodged. Biliary stenting has advantages of larger-bore drainage and better comfort for the patient but does not allow for interval cholangiography and requires endoscopic removal.

In 10% of patients, bile leaks do not respond to sphincterotomy and/or placement of a single large-bore plastic stent: such cases can be managed by placement of multiple plastic stents or placement of a fully covered self-expandable metal stent (FCSEMS), which may be removed up to 6 months later.[10] In such cases biliary sphincterotomy is recommended to minimize the risk of PEP. In one nonrandomized trial, multiple plastic stents were found to be superior to an FCSEMS.[11] Refractory biliary leaks have been treated with injection at the distal takeoff of the leaking duct with cyanoacrylate glue.[12]

In patients with refractory bile leaks, one must always consider the possibility that the lesion is coming from transection of an anomalous aberrant right hepatic duct from which the cystic duct arose. Diagnosis may require MRCP; this lesion often requires surgical repair with hepaticojejunostomy. Injuries to main common bile or common hepatic ducts are the most serious and are similar to the injuries most commonly seen in open cholecystectomy. Clinical presentations are highly variable and the patient can deteriorate rapidly, depending on the type of injury: the main duct may be completely transected or clipped with or without bile leak. Patients with bile leak have early symptoms (sepsis, bile peritonitis) at a median of 3 days, whereas patients developing strictures without associated bile leak have a significant longer symptom-free interval. Early diagnosis can be obtained by computed tomography scan and transabdominal ultrasonography; MRCP is useful to define biliary anatomy, particularly in patients with complete biliary transection (type E) where the proximal extent of the injury cannot be assessed by ERCP. The presence of concomitant right hepatic artery cinjury should also be assessed, because it is a prognostic factor of late complications.

Primary surgical repair of the bile ducts in the presence of an acute local inflammatory response should be avoided because of the high rate of breakdown and stricture formation. Injuries involving the biliary bifurcation have a high risk of early and late complications; surgery involves a bilioenteric anastomosis in all cases, usually a proximal hepaticojejunostomy with Roux-en-Y for the prevention of ascending cholangitis. These operations can be difficult and time-consuming. A complex biliary injury recognized at the time of operation by a surgeon with minimal experience in complex biliary reconstruction should not be repaired at that time. Instead, the patient should be stabilized and transferred as soon as possible (ideally within 24 hours) to an institution with hepatobiliary expertise. Major damage to the bile ducts (e.g., complete transection) not amenable to treatment with endoscopic stent placement should be treated by a surgeon with sufficient experience in advanced biliary surgery.

In patients with severe gangrenous cholecystitis, subtotal cholecystectomy is often performed[13] because the severe inflammation prevents dissection down to the cystic duct. The patient is therefore left with an open cystic duct leading into surgical drains. In these cases, we believe that placement of a fully covered stent is preferable to placement of a plastic stent.

Biloma

In the case of an established biloma after successful endoscopic closure of a postcholecystectomy biliary leak, percutaneous drainage is the treatment of choice. Most patients will have rapid reabsorption, and only a small percentage of patients (up to 6%) require open surgical drainage. Endoscopic ultrasonography (EUS)–guided drainage of bilomas that are close to the gastric or duodenal wall is also an option.[14]

LIVER RESECTION

Although biliary complications after liver resection occur in approximately 10% of patients, they are responsible for approximately one-third of the postoperative mortality. Fortunately, the majority are amenable to nonsurgical treatment, but when reoperation is needed, mortality may reach up to 70%.

Preoperative assessment of biliary anatomy and possible variations in order to prevent intraoperative injury is mandatory. Preoperative imaging of the biliary branching pattern remains the only way to properly recognize and address the problem posed by variant biliary anatomy. MRCP offers reliable and noninvasive visualization of the biliary tree to allow for surgical planning, which can be adapted to prevent an injury in the setting of variant anatomy of the hepatic duct confluence. If a biliary variant is assumed to be injured intraoperatively, intraoperative cholangiography through the injured bile duct allows assessment of the type and extent of injury. In cases of a disconnected sectorial bile duct, the surgical approach is based on volume of the liver remnant and liver functional reserve, especially when additional hepatectomy is undertaken; otherwise a Roux-en-Y bilioenteric anastomosis is performed.

If the BDI becomes evident postoperatively, conservative treatment is the initial approach. Failure to resolve the leak with a conservative approach leads to a planned reoperation that includes either a bilioenteric anastomosis or a resection of the injured segment of the liver.

Bile Leak

Bile leaks still occur postoperatively in as many as 15% of liver resections and are associated with high mortality. Despite ongoing advances in hepatic surgical techniques, there has not been a significant decrease in the incidence of postoperative bile leak.

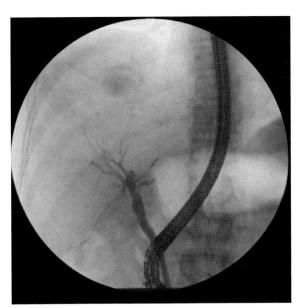

FIG 44.2 Post–hepatic resection biliary leak. Biliary leak in a patient who underwent left lobectomy.

Postoperative bile leaks can be classified into peripheral bile leaks, which arise from the surface of the cut liver (Fig. 44.2), and central bile leaks, which arise from the hilum or the hepatic ducts. Compared with peripheral bile leaks, central bile duct leakage is usually associated with a larger volume of bile flow and a worse prognosis. The clinical presentation and treatment are the same as those for leakage occurring after cholecystectomy.

Biliary sphincterotomy with or without plastic stent insertion is the first-line treatment option. In cases of persistent leakage, FCSEMS placement should be considered before endoscopic treatment is abandoned. Definitive surgery is considered the last option.

Strictures

Biliary strictures may present with pain, jaundice, cholangitis, or pruritus or with alteration of liver function tests. Dilatation of the intrahepatic biliary tree or of the CBD can be found on ultrasonography, but it is not always present. MRCP can accurately delineate the biliary anatomy, site, and length of the stenosis and is very useful for planning ERCP therapy (see Chapter 34). Endoscopic plastic stent placement is the first-line therapy for benign biliary strictures, allowing high stricture resolution rates to be achieved.

The standard endoscopic strategy for postoperative CBD strictures consists of placement of multiple large-bore (10 Fr) plastic stents, maintained over a period of up to 1 year.[15] Stent exchanges are usually performed every 3 months, though one study showed that premature stent occlusion did not occur when multiple stents were placed for nonhilar benign bile duct strictures, suggesting that a 6-month interval for stent exchange is possible.[16] Complete resolution of the stricture is shown by cholangiography after stent removal. Results from up to 10-year follow-up are excellent and stricture recurrences can usually be successfully retreated by ERCP.[17] Multiple plastic stent placement is believed to lead to stricture remodeling by progressive adaptation to the increasing number of stents. The main limitation of the multistent strategy is the need for multiple ERCP sessions over the 1-year period, where FCSEMS have a larger diameter compared with plastic stents and therefore a higher patency rate, with fewer interventions required.[18] Surgery is an option in cases of complete ligation of the CBD or strictures that do not respond to endoscopic treatment.

Sump Syndrome After Choledochoduodenostomy

Biliary sump syndrome is a rare complication of side-to-side choledochoduodenostomy. Perhaps with the increased use of EUS-guided choledochoduodenostomy (see Chapter 32) we might expect an increased incidence of this clinical presentation,[19] but there are as yet no data to support this speculation. Classically, the distal bile duct becomes obstructed by food, stones, or debris after choledochoenterostomy, where the segment of CBD between the anastomosis and the ampulla of Vater may act as a stagnant reservoir or sump. When food, stones, sludge, or debris accumulates in the sump, recurrent episodes of pain, fever, cholangitis, pancreatitis, biliary obstruction, or hepatic abscesses may develop.

Pathophysiologically, intraluminal contents reflux into the remaining distal duct through the anastomosis, whereas bile content drains through the duct. Consequently, sludge, stones, or food residue lodges and gets trapped in this nonfunctional reservoir above the papilla, resulting in bacterial infection, stasis, and de novo stone formation. Sump syndrome usually becomes evident only after a long postoperative delay.

Endoscopic biliary sphincterotomy with removal of debris and stones by a balloon catheter and/or Dormia basket is the primary and definitive treatment modality.[20] If the problem persists, surgical revision to hepaticojejunostomy may be needed.

The technical modalities and adverse events rate are the same as those of biliary stone removal in normal CBD stone removal (see Chapter 19).

LIVER TRANSPLANTATION

Biliary complications (bile duct strictures, leaks, and stones) after LT can be categorized as early (within 4 weeks) or late. Biliary strictures can be further divided into anastomotic, nonanastomotic, and diffuse intrahepatic. Other complications such as bile casts, sphincter of Oddi dysfunction, mucocele, and hemobilia are rare and most can be managed endoscopically. Despite continuous surgical improvement, biliary complications are a serious source of morbidity after orthotopic and living-related-donor LT (OLT and LRLT, respectively), and a number of studies on endoscopic treatment of these complications have been published. The type of biliary reconstruction, underlying ischemia and reperfusion injuries, hepatic artery thrombosis, cytomegalovirus infection, and primary sclerosing cholangitis are principal risk factors for the development of post-LT biliary morbidity.[21,22]

The rate of biliary complications in transplant recipients in published series ranges from 8% to 35%. This complication rate is higher for LRLT than for OLT patients.[23–25] Depending on the type of surgical biliary reconstruction (choledochojejunostomy or duct-to-duct anastomosis), biliary complications can be treated by percutaneous transhepatic cholangiography (PTC) and/or by ERCP.

The most common biliary complication is anastomotic stricture (AS), followed by bile leaks (8%), CBD filling defects (3% to 12%), sphincter of Oddi dysfunction (2% to 4%), and biliary cast syndrome (2% to 4%). Often patients develop more than one complication (Fig. 44.3). ERCP is currently considered the diagnostic gold standard for patients with duct-to-duct anastomosis because it allows a direct approach for interventional procedures. Several studies have evaluated endoscopic treatment of biliary complications in patients with duct-to-duct reconstruction and have shown a success rate of approximately 70% to 80% in cases of OLT and about 60% in LRLT cases. The current therapeutic options vary from sphincterotomy with stent placement for biliary leak (Fig. 44.4), with progressive balloon dilatation and multiple stent placement for treatment of strictures (Fig. 44.5), to biliary sphincterotomy alone for treatment of sphincter of Oddi dysfunction

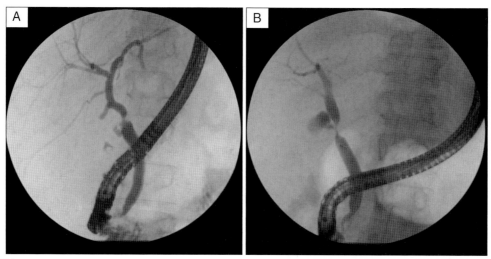

FIG 44.3 Post-OLT bile duct injury. **A,** Biliary stricture after orthotopic liver transplantation with duct-to-duct anastomosis. **B,** Post-OLT biliary anastomotic stricture and leak. *OLT,* Orthotopic liver transplantation.

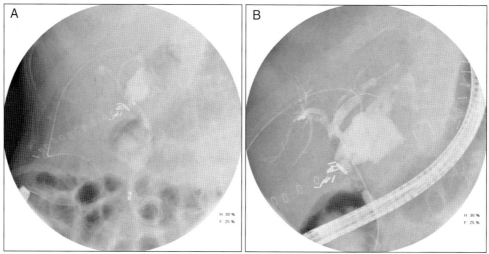

FIG 44.4 **A,** Cholangiogram from a patient with post-OLT biliary leak. A large amount of contrast extravasation can be seen. **B,** Fluoroscopic image after placement of bilateral intrahepatic plastic stents. The leak resolved and the stents were removed 12 weeks later without sequelae. *OLT,* Orthotopic liver transplantation.

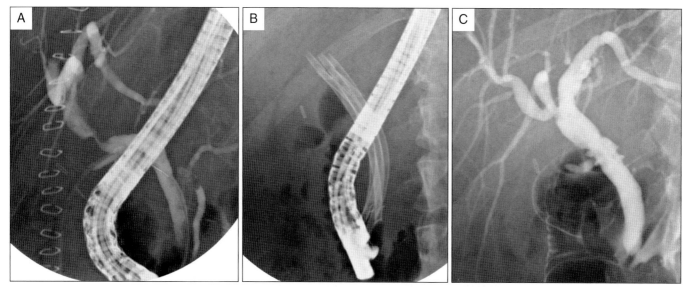

FIG 44.5 **A,** Cholangiogram from a patient with post-OLT anastomotic stricture. **B,** Fluoroscopic image after placement of five side-by-side 11.5-Fr plastic stents across the stricture. **C,** Cholangiogram after stent removal 4 months later shows complete resolution of stricture. *OLT,* Orthotopic liver transplantation.

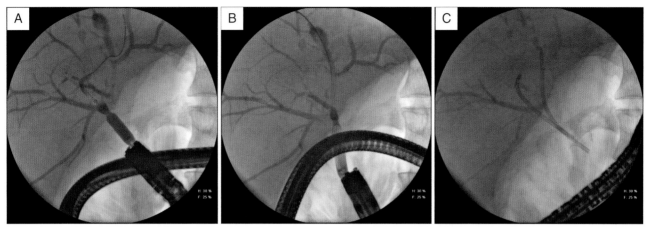

FIG 44.6 A, Cholangiogram from a patient with angulated post-OLT anastomotic stricture. **B,** Fluoroscopic image after placement of a 10-mm fully covered metal biliary stent across the stricture. **C,** Cholangiogram after stent removal 4 months later shows complete resolution of stricture. *OLT,* Orthotopic liver transplantation.

and removal of stones, if present. Evidence of continuous bile leakage despite endoscopic stent placement or the persistence of stenosis after 1 year despite multiple dilatations and stent placement is considered a criterion for switching to another type of treatment: PTC is usually the first choice, and surgery with biliary reconstruction is reserved for cases in which the PTC approach fails or there is a very large leak.

Strictures

The clinical presentation can range from severe acute manifestations (cholangitis) to asymptomatic abnormalities in liver function tests. Presence of a biliary complication should be suspected when there is unexpected increase in liver function tests (aspartate transaminase, alanine transaminase, gamma-glutamyl transferase, alkaline phosphatase, or bilirubin); patients may also report nonspecific symptoms, such as fatigue, abdominal pain (right-upper quadrant), or fever. No validated diagnostic algorithms have been proposed for the investigation of suspected biliary strictures; however, it is widely accepted to perform transabdominal ultrasonography with Doppler as the first-line test for the exclusion of hepatic artery stenosis and evaluation of biliary ductal dilation. Transabdominal ultrasonography carries low sensitivity because of the lack of intrahepatic biliary dilatation in the majority of transplanted patients with biliary stenosis. In the case of suspected vascular complication, a computed tomography scan with vascular reconstruction followed by therapeutic hepatic angiography is the next step. On the other hand, the patient should undergo liver biopsy to exclude rejection or recurrence of hepatitis C. After exclusion of both vascular and parenchymal conditions that could explain the clinical presentation, MRCP or even a cholangiogram through a T-tube, if present, is considered as a next step. Invasive approaches such as endoscopic retrograde cholangiography (ERCP) or PTC should be considered treatment options rather than diagnostic tools. The treatment approach is chosen based on local expertise and residual biliary tree anatomy: ERCP is preferred in the case of duct-to-duct biliary reconstruction, whereas percutaneous treatment (PTC) should be reserved for patients with Roux-en-Y choledochojejunostomy when endoscopic expertise is not available or after failure of endoscopic attempts (see Chapter 31). Surgery is considered a rescue therapy after failure of all other treatment options.

For anastomotic biliary strictures, standard endoscopic treatment consists of sphincterotomy plus progressive pneumatic dilation with multiple stent placement (see Fig. 44.5); ERCP should be repeated and stents exchanged every 3 to 4 months. Several studies have evaluated this endoscopic treatment approach and have shown success rates of approximately 70% to 80% in cases of OLTx and about 60% in LRLTx cases.[4–8] In patients successfully responding to endoscopic therapy, there is still the risk of biliary stricture recurrence. In a study by Alazmi et al.[26] the rate of cholestasis recurrence with evidence of biliary stricture after initial success with endoscopic therapy was approximately 18%. Other endoscopic approaches have recently been described: the multistenting technique and FCSEMS placement. The first consists of insertion of an increasing number of plastic biliary stents until morphologic benign biliary stricture resolution (Video 44.1 and Fig. 44.5); this approach provides good results during long-term follow-up but with disadvantages: the need for repeated ERCPs, good patient compliance, and a recall system to reduce the risk of adverse events (mainly cholangitis) secondary to retained stent.

The second option consists of placement of one fully covered metal stent (FCSEMS) across the stricture (Fig. 44.6). Placement of a single FCSEMS results in radial dilation of a stricture equivalent to that of at least three side-by-side plastic stents (which cannot generally be placed during the initial ERCP). Clinical trials support the hypothesis that deployment of FCSEMS is effective in patients with benign strictures.[27–29] The use of FCSEMS can shorten the duration of endoscopic treatment. The stent is removed 3 to 6 months after initial insertion, requiring only two procedures. The technique has been shown to be safe, but FCSEMS migration rate is high and stricture recurrence occurs in 9% to 47% during 5 years of follow-up.[30–32] Removal of FCSEMS is usually successful, but the need for a "SEMS-in-SEMS" technique has been reported in cases where removal was difficult.[33]

Nonanastomotic strictures (NAS) result mainly from hepatic artery thrombosis or other forms of ischemia. Less commonly, they can be caused by recurrence of an underlying disease such as primary sclerosing cholangitis. They account for 10% to 25% of all strictures occurring after LT, with an incidence in the range of 0.5% to 10%. There may be multiple strictures involving the hilum and intrahepatic ducts, causing a cholangiographic appearance that resembles primary sclerosing cholangitis (Fig. 44.7). Biliary ischemia leading to sloughing of mucosa can lead to the formation of casts. This may predispose to development of recurrent episodes of cholangitis. NAS are more difficult to treat than AS. Endoscopic therapy of NAS typically consists of 4-mm to 6-mm balloon dilation (compared with 6 to 8 mm for AS) followed by sphincterotomy and placement of plastic stents, which are replaced every 3 months, similar to the management of AS. However, time to response with NAS is more prolonged than with AS.

The outcomes of NAS are not as favorable as AS. Only 50% of patients have a long-term response with endoscopic therapy using dilation and stent placement.[34,35] Furthermore, up to 50% of patients undergo retransplantation or die as a consequence of this complication despite endoscopic therapy.[36,37] As a general rule, ischemic events that lead to diffuse intrahepatic bile duct strictures are associated with poor graft survival and in most instances will require retransplantation in suitable operative candidates.

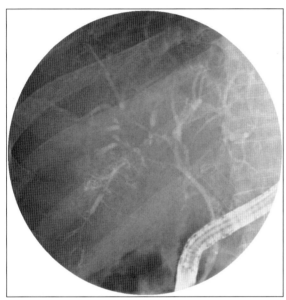

FIG 44.7 Cholangiogram of typical ischemic, nonanastomotic strictures in OLT patient. Note that the intrahepatic ducts appear narrowed and irregular. *OLT*, Orthotopic liver transplantation.

Bile Leak

Bile leakage in early post-LT can arise from the anastomosis, from the cystic duct stump, from the insertion of the T-tube, or, in the case of living-donor LT or split-LT, from the cut surface of the liver graft (Fig. 44.8). The overall estimated incidence is about 10%.

In the case of early occurrence in patient with a T-tube in situ, bile leaks can be managed conservatively by leaving the T-tube open without further intervention. In the case of small leaks, ERCP with biliary sphincterotomy may resolve the leak. In the case of larger leaks, placement of the biliary plastic stent resolves more than 90% of early bile leaks. Usually, the biliary stent is removed after 6 to 8 weeks (a shorter period is generally not adequate for healing because of immunosuppressive therapy).

LIVING-RELATED-DONOR TRANSPLANTS

Patients with living-related-donor transplants are more technically difficult to treat endoscopically than patients with orthotopic living donors for two reasons. First, these patients are more likely to have Roux-en-Y reconstruction, and second, the anastomosis is often intrahepatic, sometimes with multiple biliary anastomoses. Thus the anatomy is less predictable. It is important to meticulously review the operative note, discuss with the transplant surgeon, and carefully review any imaging.

Retained Surgical Stents

Some surgeons prefer to place stents across the duct-to-duct or hepaticojejunal anastomosis. Such "stents" may actually be modified pediatric feeding tubes and are difficult to detect by plain radiographs and nondetectable by MRCP. Thus, in a patient who had such stents placed, the endoscopist should be aware of this entity when faced with posttransplant cholangitis or biliary obstruction.

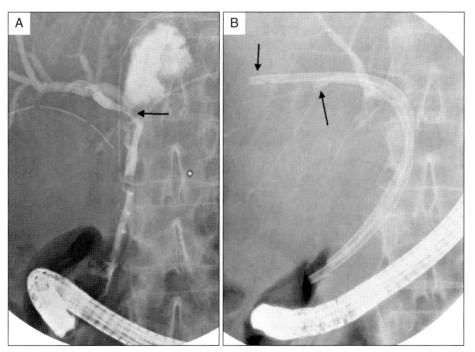

FIG 44.8 A, Cholangiogram of leak after living related donor from anastomosis and/or cut surface of liver. **B,** Fluoroscopic image after placement of one stent in the right anterior and one in the right posterior intrahepatic duct. The leak resolved uneventfully.

SUMMARY

Endoscopic intervention should be regarded as an initial treatment of choice in patients with postoperative BDI, including leak and stricture.[38] In the past, surgery was the treatment of choice for postoperative biliary strictures and ERCP was limited to the diagnosis and definition of the level and extent of the stricture. Today, ERCP is preferred over surgery and percutaneous approaches because it is less invasive, well tolerated, and safe and can repeated as often as necessary without precluding subsequent surgery, if needed. Surgery is a reasonable option in cases of complete transection or ligation of the CBD and in poorly compliant patients. The percutaneous approach is generally limited by the adverse event rates, discomfort caused by indwelling catheters, and high stricture recurrence rates. Still, the percutaneous approach can be useful in cases of failed ERCP for rendezvous techniques, and in patients with surgically altered anatomy and nonaccessible papilla. Postoperative BDI is a very complex condition that requires a multidisciplinary approach. An important factor in the management of biliary complications after surgery is the time-to-diagnosis interval. Delayed detection of biliary complications may lead to increased morbidity, increased severity of the injury, treatment failure, and even death. In any case, endoscopy should always be attempted, because it is safe and repeatable. Finally, endoscopists should bear in mind that patients who do not present for ERCP on scheduled dates must be contacted to avoid the risk of potentially fatal septic complications due to retained endoscopically placed stents.

The complete reference list for this chapter can be found online at www.expertconsult.com.

45

ERCP and EUS for Acute and Chronic Adverse Events of Pancreatic Surgery and Pancreatic Trauma

Prabhleen Chahal and Todd H. Baron

Chronic pancreatitis, cystic neoplasms, and suspected or established malignancy are the main indications for pancreatic surgery. The various types of pancreatic surgery are outlined in Box 45.1. This chapter focuses on types of pancreatic surgery, their associated adverse events, and the role of endoscopy in management of adverse events. Finally, we highlight the role of endoscopic retrograde cholangiopancreatography (ERCP) in the treatment of pancreatic trauma. ERCP in postsurgical anatomy is also addressed in Chapter 31.

PANCREATICODUODENECTOMY (WHIPPLE OPERATION) WITH AND WITHOUT PYLORUS PRESERVATION

Anatomy

The classic Whipple operation involves removal of the pancreatic head, pancreatic neck, gastric antrum, duodenum, 20 cm of proximal jejunum, gallbladder (if present), distal common bile duct, and regional lymph nodes. There are two side-to-side enteroenterostomies visible from the gastric remnant (Fig. 45.1). The afferent limb, which is usually 40 to 60 cm long, ascends superiorly and ends blindly with an end-to-end or end-to-side pancreaticojejunostomy. An end-to-side choledochojejunostomy is usually located 10 cm distal to the end of the afferent limb and along the antimesenteric border, often behind a mucosal fold.

Pylorus-preserving pancreaticoduodenectomy (modified Whipple surgery) is performed to maintain gastric function. The entire stomach is preserved and a cuff of the duodenal bulb remains (Fig. 45.2). Upon exiting the stomach, a duodenal stump is encountered with two end-to-side enteroenterostomies, with one leading to the afferent limb containing the biliary and pancreatic anastomoses (Fig. 45.3). The location of the afferent limb within the visual field is not uniform and also is dependent on the type of endoscope used (side-viewing vs forward-viewing).

Role of Endoscopy in the Management of Adverse Events

Endoscopy plays a very limited role in the management of acute postoperative adverse events after Whipple surgery. Pancreatic leaks, although reported to occur in up to 20% of Whipple surgeries, are managed by percutaneous drainage, administration of octreotide, and intravenous hyperalimentation. However, endoscopy plays a significant role in the management of delayed pancreaticobiliary strictures and/or stones (Box 45.2). The necessity of endoscopic intervention is decided with the aid of abdominal computed tomography (CT) or magnetic

resonance cholangiopancreatography (MRCP) with or without secretin.

Before embarking on endoscopy, it is imperative to plan, which includes choice of endoscope, accessories, patient position, and need for anesthesia support, so that optimal outcomes can be achieved in this subset of patients (Box 45.3; see also Chapter 10).

In classic Whipple anatomy, the biliary anastomosis can occasionally be reached with a standard duodenoscope. The side-viewing endoscope offers the technical advantages of an *en face* view of the anastomosis and presence of an elevator to assist with control of accessories. However,

> **BOX 45.1   Types of Pancreatic Surgery**
>
> - Classic Whipple operation (pancreaticoduodenectomy with antrectomy)
> - Modified Whipple operation (pylorus-preserving pancreaticoduodenectomy)
> - Distal pancreatectomy
> - Central pancreatectomy
> - Enucleation
> - Puestow procedure (longitudinal pancreaticojejunostomy)
> - Beger procedure (duodenal-preserving pancreatic head resection)
> - Frey procedure (duodenal-preserving pancreatic head resection with lateral pancreaticojejunostomy)

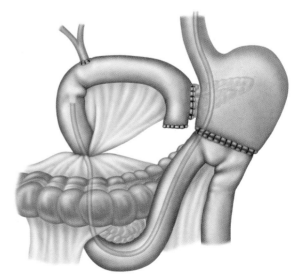

FIG 45.1 Illustration of a classic pancreaticoduodenectomy. Note the antrectomy with gastrojejunal anastomosis.

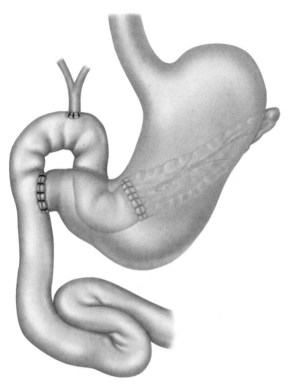

FIG 45.2 Illustration of a pylorus-preserving pancreaticoduodenectomy.

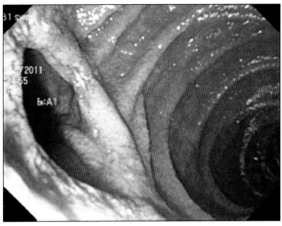

FIG 45.3 Endoscopic image of the afferent and efferent limbs taken from inside the duodenal stump of a pylorus-preserving pancreaticoduodenectomy.

BOX 45.2   Adverse Events of Pancreaticoduodenectomy and Pylorus-Preserving Pancreaticoduodenectomy

- Early adverse events
  - Pancreatic duct leak
  - Pancreatic fistula
  - Bile leak
  - Hemorrhage
  - Wound infection
  - Abscess
  - Afferent limb syndrome
  - Efferent limb syndrome
  - Delayed gastric emptying
- Delayed adverse events
  - Stenosis of choledochojejunostomy (presenting as cholangitis, jaundice)
  - Stenosis of pancreaticojejunostomy (presenting as abdominal pain, pancreatitis with or without pancreatic duct stones)
  - Recurrence of malignancy
  - Retained surgically placed pancreatic stent
  - Diabetes mellitus

BOX 45.3   Checklist Before Starting Endoscopy

- Choice of endoscope
  - Duodenoscope
  - Pediatric colonoscope with or without variable-stiffness feature
  - Adult (therapeutic channel) colonoscope with or without variable-stiffness feature
  - Prototype oblique-viewing endoscope with elevator
  - Single-balloon enteroscope
  - Double-balloon enteroscope (short vs long)
  - Curvilinear echoendoscope
- Accessories
  - Standard ERCP accessories
  - Straight and pigtail plastic stents
  - Fully covered metal stents, lumen-apposing metal stents
  - Long-length accessories
  - EUS-FNA needle
- Patient position
  - Prone
  - Supine
  - Left oblique
  - Left lateral
- Anesthesia
  - Moderate sedation
  - Monitored anesthesia care
  - General anesthesia

ERCP, Endoscopic retrograde cholangiopancreatography; *EUS,* endoscopic ultrasonography; *FNA,* fine-needle aspiration.

---

the success rate in accessing the pancreatic anastomosis is suboptimal at best.[1] A widely patent anastomosis is seen in Fig. 45.4.

Commonly the approach using a side-viewing endoscope results in failure to reach either the biliary or the pancreatic anastomosis because of the insertion tube length. This is especially true in patients with pylorus-preserving anatomy and longer afferent limbs. In these cases, the procedure may be accomplished with a colonoscope. Therapeutic channel colonoscopes allow placement of 10-Fr plastic biliary stents, though the rigidity can prevent negotiating angulated, fixed afferent limbs. Some biliary self-expandable metal stents can be passed through colonoscopes (both pediatric and adult).[2] Absence of an elevator can make it challenging to maneuver accessories and accomplish therapeutic interventions.

Various other techniques can be employed to gain access to the end of the afferent limb and the biliopancreatic anastomosis (Box 45.4).

There are now robust data on the use of single-balloon enteroscopes,[3–5] double-balloon enteroscopes,[6] and rotational overtube endoscopes[7] to allow technical success for accessing biliary and pancreatic anastomoses.

These procedures are most often performed by experienced endoscopists at tertiary care centers when ERCP failure is caused by inability to reach the anastomosis with standard endoscopes. Balloon-assisted ERCP is often time-consuming and difficult because of the limited availability of compatible accessories. On the contrary, endoscopic ultrasonography (EUS) has gained popularity in the management of delayed pancreatobiliary complications in post–pancreatic surgery patients.

BILIARY OBSTRUCTION

Bilioenteric Anastomotic Stricture

Bilioenteric anastomotic strictures can be benign or malignant as a result of recurrent disease such as pancreatic cancer, primary sclerosing cholangitis, or autoimmune disease. Distinguishing between the two can be extremely difficult because of submucosal tumor invasion. Treatment of these strictures is undertaken as for other benign (Fig. 45.5) and malignant strictures, although the options can be limited by the endoscope length and channel diameter. In some cases, needle-knife entry can be undertaken, though this carries risk of perforation.

In patients in whom the biliary anastomosis cannot be reached, EUS has been used for antegrade placement of plastic and self-expandable metal stents. More recently, lumen-apposing metal stents (LAMS) have been deployed under EUS guidance for management of bilioenteric anastomotic stricture.[8]

Afferent Limb Obstruction

Afferent limb obstruction is often caused by recurrent tumor, usually occurring at the ligament of Treitz, but can also occur from radiation therapy. Such downstream obstruction most commonly presents with obstructive jaundice or cholangitis. Other presenting symptoms include abdominal pain, nausea, and vomiting. The most common endoscopic findings are malignant or benign luminal stricturing of the afferent limb, severe angulation of or fixed afferent limb, and mucosal changes of friability, ulceration, and telangiectasia from radiation enteropathy. Endoscopic interventions performed for management include placement of plastic and self-expandable metal stents in the afferent limb and/or obstructed bile duct.[9,10] EUS-guided management of afferent limb obstruction using lumen-apposing stents is an alternative to traditional luminal stent placement in post–Whipple surgery patients.[11]

Efferent Limb Obstruction

Recurrent malignancy is the most common cause of efferent limb obstruction, followed by adhesions and radiation-induced strictures. The most common presenting symptoms are similar to afferent limb obstruction plus features of gastric outlet obstruction. Self-expandable

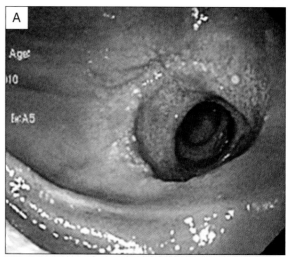
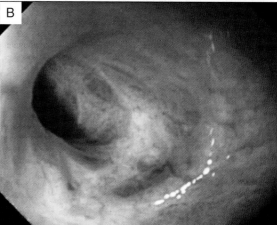

FIG 45.4 Endoscopic images of representative widely patent choledochojejunostomies after pancreaticoduodenectomy from two different patients.

metal stents (SEMS) can be placed for efferent obstruction alone or combined with stent placement in both the afferent and efferent limbs.[12] Although not reported, it may be feasible in some patients to perform EUS-guided gastrojejunostomy of the efferent limb using LAMS.

Miscellaneous

Miscellaneous causes of biliary obstruction include stones and sludge and retention or migration of surgically placed stents into the biliary tree.[13]

In patients with failed retrograde endoscopic access, EUS has been successfully used for management of biliary stones in the hepatic duct using an antegrade approach.[14]

Other Treatment Options for Biliary and Pancreatic Ductal Obstruction

More recently, there have been reports of use of combined modalities.

Interventional Radiology and ERCP

A combined interventional radiology (IR) and ERCP approach can be used to access the biliary tree. This is most useful when the endoscope can be passed to the area of the choledochojejunostomy but the opening cannot be identified or accessed. It can be decided to place an internal stent entirely by IR with subsequent management endoscopically or by

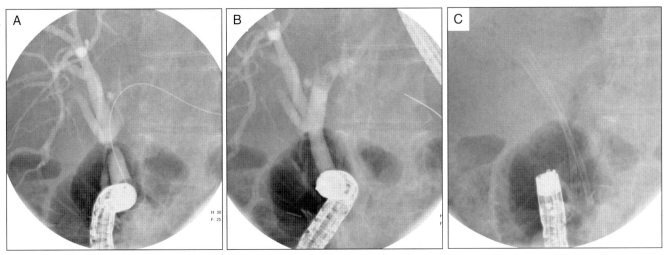

FIG 45.5 Endoscopic therapy for a choledochojejunal anastomotic stricture after pancreaticoduodenectomy.

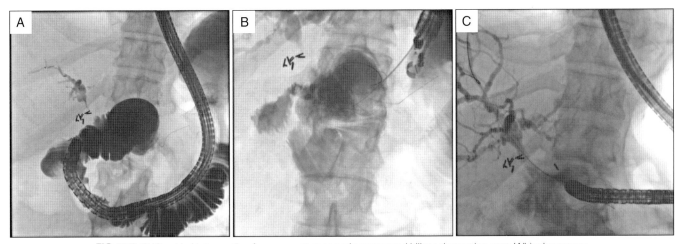

FIG 45.6 EUS-guided intervention for recurrent pancreatic cancer and biliary obstruction post–Whipple surgery. **A,** Attempts to reach the choledochojejunostomy with a colonoscope failed. **B,** EUS-guided gastrojejunostomy into the afferent limb was performed with a 15-mm LAMS. **C,** ERC was performed by passing a standard upper endoscope through the LAMS, and a biliary self-expandable metal stent was placed. *ERCP,* Endoscopic retrograde cholangiography; *EUS,* endoscopic ultrasonography; *LAMS,* lumen-apposing metal stent.

IR placement of a guidewire followed by endoscopic management by rendezvous. A percutaneous approach to pancreaticojejunal anastomotic strictures has been used at tertiary care centers by experienced endoscopists when the pancreatic anastomosis cannot be identified or accessed.[15] This combined approach is preceded by acquisition of detailed cross-sectional imaging such as CT or MRCP.[16] Administration of periprocedural antibiotics is recommended.

EUS-Guided Techniques for Biliary Obstruction

EUS can allow biliary drainage in post–Whipple surgery patients from a variety of approaches. These include EUS-guided rendezvous, EUS-guided antegrade stent placement, and EUS-guided transmural drainage (hepaticogastric) (Fig. 45.6).[17]

EUS-Guided Techniques for Pancreatic Duct Obstruction

Similar to access and management of biliary disease, EUS is useful for managing pancreatic duct obstruction. Although pancreatic duct obstruction often occurs after pancreaticoduodenectomy, it is not as clinically relevant as biliary obstruction because most patients are

asymptomatic or can be managed with oral pancreatic enzyme replacement for exocrine pancreatic insufficiency due to pancreatic duct obstruction. Endoscopic therapy is reserved for development of upstream leaks, which can result from ductal hypertension and blowout, and for patients with recurrent obstructive pancreatitis. The latter may be associated with pancreatic duct stones.

EUS-Guided Rendezvous

A combined EUS and ERCP technique has been described in cases with failed identification of or access to the pancreatic anastomosis (see Chapters 31–33). This can be performed by a single operator with expertise in both EUS and ERCP or by two endoscopists, one with expertise in interventional EUS and the other with expertise in advanced ERCP. Ideally, this should be undertaken at tertiary care centers with pancreaticobiliary surgical and IR backup. Under fluoroscopic guidance, the pancreatic duct is punctured transgastrically with a 19-gauge or 22-gauge fine-needle aspiration (FNA) needle under real-time EUS visualization. In some cases, ducts as small as 1 mm can be accessed. After contrast opacification of the pancreatic duct, a 0.018-inch to

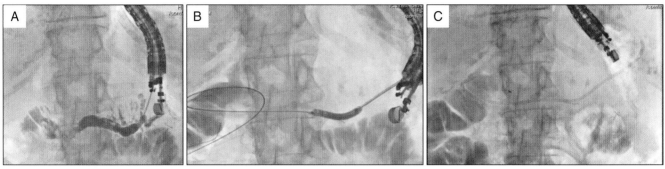

FIG 45.7 EUS-guided intervention for recurrent pancreatitis post–Whipple surgery with obstruction at the pancreaticojejunostomy; attempts to identify the pancreaticojejunostomy in a retrograde manner with a colonoscope failed. **A,** EUS-guided pancreatic injection shows a dilated duct with anastomotic obstruction. **B,** Balloon dilation of the stomach and pancreatic tissue is followed by **(C)** placement of a transgastric/transanastomotic double pigtail stent. *EUS,* Endoscopic ultrasonography.

0.035-inch guidewire is passed through the needle in an antegrade fashion into the pancreatic duct and across the anastomosis, if possible. This is then followed immediately by a rendezvous ERCP, most often using a colonoscope or balloon enteroscope.

EUS-guided antegrade drainage. More recently, with advances in therapeutic endosonography, pancreatic ductal access and therapeutic intervention are accomplished entirely with a linear array echoendoscope.[18–24] The initial technique of transanastomotic guidewire advancement into the jejunum is performed as described earlier in this chapter. The transgastric fistula is dilated with a 6-Fr cystotome, needle knife, or bougie, followed by 4-mm or 6-mm tract dilation, for eventual deployment of a 7-Fr or 10-Fr temporary plastic stent across the anastomosis. Two techniques of stent deployment have been described: long double-pigtail stents or straight stents with anchoring flaps on either end with the distal end of the stent across the anastomosis (transenteric anterograde) into the afferent limb distally and the proximal end in the stomach (Fig. 45.7). Some endoscopists prefer to place stents without side holes to prevent perigastric contamination with pancreatic secretions. The distal end of the stent is left in the pancreatic duct or across the anastomosis into the jejunum, and the proximal pigtailed end is left in the stomach (pancreatogastrostomy or transluminal technique). More recently, there have been reports of using fully covered 6 to 8 mm, 8-cm-long to 10-cm-long self-expandable metal stents for drainage, with a theoretical advantage of creating a seal to prevent perigastric leakage of pancreatic secretions.

The cumulative technical success rates and adverse event rates using these techniques are approximately 83% and 19%, respectively.[25] Adverse events reported in another series included pancreatitis, bleeding, stent dislocation, perforation, pseudocyst formation, transient fever, and "shaving" of the guidewire by the EUS-FNA needle.

A recent international multicenter retrospective study of 66 post–Whipple surgery patients compared 40 EUS-guided pancreatic duct drainage procedures to 35 enteroscopy-assisted endoscopic retrograde pancreatographies.[26] The transluminal technique was used in 21 patients, transenteric anterograde drainage performed in 16, and rendezvous in 3 patients.

EUS-guided drainage had superior technical and clinical success (88% to 93% vs 20% to 23%), although there was a greater number of adverse events (35% vs 3%). All adverse events were either mild or moderate, with 81% attributable to postprocedural pain and requiring hospitalization.[27]

Pancreatic antegrade needle knife. Pancreatic antegrade needle knife (PANK) is a modified version of EUS-guided rendezvous technique when the pancreatojejunostomy cannot be traversed with a guidewire.

After accessing the pancreatic duct with a wire, the tract is dilated and a wire-guided needle knife is advanced over the wire toward the anastomosis. Once the indentation of air-filled jejunum is visualized fluoroscopically, the antegrade needle-knife pancreatojejunostomy is performed by creating a "new" anastomosis. This is followed by advancement of wire across into the jejunum and balloon dilation of the fresh anastomosis, followed by placement of stent traversing the anastomosis with the proximal end in the stomach and the distal end in the jejunum.[28]

Retained stents. It is important to discuss the management of retained temporary plastic stents inserted during pancreaticoduodenectomy. Transanastomotic biliary stents and, more often, pancreatic stents (5 to 8 Fr) are used by some surgeons to decrease the risk of pancreatic leak and may prevent late adverse events such as stricture formation. Such stents are usually inserted 3 cm or less into the remnant duct. The stent can be externalized by bringing it out through the jejunum and through the abdominal wall or, more commonly, can be left in the bowel lumen for spontaneous dislodgment. Although they may be secured to the pancreas by absorbable suture to prevent early dislodgment, these stents may fail to migrate distally out of the duct. Such retained pancreatic stents have been reported to cause chronic and acute intermittent abdominal pain and steatorrhea, as well as acute recurrent and chronic pancreatitis.[27] Rarely, these prostheses migrate out of the pancreatic duct and into the biliary tree, causing biliary obstruction. Some stents are fashioned from pediatric feeding tubes and can be difficult to visualize radiographically but are easily recognized by EUS imaging. A careful review of the surgical note should prompt investigation into this clinical scenario in symptomatic patients. Such prostheses can be removed using conventional forward-viewing endoscopes and balloon enteroscopes,[29] particularly because the latter endoscopes are flexible and can be retroflexed in the proximal afferent limb (Fig. 45.8). In cases where EUS access is not available or not possible, IR can assist in stent removal (Fig. 45.9). In one case of inward migration and stent-related stricture, lateral pancreatojejunostomy was ultimately required.[30]

DISTAL AND CENTRAL PANCREATECTOMY

Anatomy

When distal and central pancreatectomies are performed, the gastric, duodenal, and ampullary anatomy is intact and thus ERCP is performed in standard fashion with a side-viewing endoscope.

Distal pancreatectomy (resection of the tail portion of the pancreas, anatomically a proximal pancreatectomy) involves variable lengths of resection from the neck and includes the pancreatic tail, often with splenectomy.

Central pancreatectomy includes removal of the pancreatic neck and body. There are two pancreatic remnants: the pancreatic head and tail. The tail is anastomosed either to a jejunal loop or to the posterior gastric wall. Access to the tail remnant after central pancreatectomy can be achieved if it is anastomosed to the gastric wall or to a short Roux-en-Y limb. In both scenarios, cannulation of the papillary orifice and contrast injection will reveal a surgically shortened pancreatic duct.

Adverse Events

The most common adverse event of distal and central pancreatectomy is the development of a postoperative pancreatic leak that may develop into a fistula or pancreatic fluid collection, usually a pseudocyst. Leaks occur in up to 30% of distal pancreatectomies and 54% of central pancreatectomies. The International Study Group on Pancreatic Fistula (ISGPF)[31] categorizes postoperative pancreatic fistulae into grade A (low grade) and grades B and C (clinically significant or high grade).

Most fistulae are low grade (grade A) and resolve promptly without intervention. However, approximately 40% of fistulae are clinically significant (grade B or C) and require medical, radiologic, or surgical intervention. These patients are clinically symptomatic, with abdominal pain, fever, signs and symptoms of systemic inflammatory response, abscess formation, delayed gastric emptying, bleeding, sepsis, wound dehiscence, and, at times, death.[32]

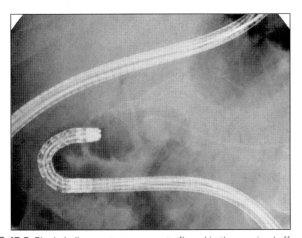

FIG 45.8 Single-balloon enteroscope retroflexed in the proximal afferent limb in search of pancreaticojejunostomy after pancreaticoduodenectomy. Note the long retained surgical stent.

Role of Endoscopy in Patients With Distal Pancreatectomy

There is currently no standardized management algorithm for patients with postoperative pancreatic fistulae. Usually a combination of *nil per os* status, intravenous hyperalimentation, octreotide, and placement of percutaneous drains leads to closure in the majority of cases. However, a very small proportion of grade C fistulae can be refractory to the these measures. ERCP with or without pancreatic sphincterotomy and transpapillary pancreatic stent placement have been shown to accelerate resolution of fistulae,[33–35] thus obviating further intervention or surgery. Transpapillary injection of cyanoacrylate glue has been used to close pancreatic fistulae, but because of potential adverse events it is not a widely accepted management strategy, especially as first-line therapy.

Treatment of symptomatic or enlarging pancreatic fluid collections can be achieved endoscopically by placement of transpapillary stents (Fig. 45.10) and/or via transmural drainage. Because the collections are nearly always noncontiguous from the duodenum (Fig. 45.11), transmural drainage is usually performed transgastrically (Fig. 45.12).[36,37] In one study, combined EUS and ERCP procedures were performed for management of chronic, persistent pancreatic fistulae with recurrent symptomatic peripancreatic fluid collection, using an inflated dilating balloon as a target for localization of chronic fistula tract followed by EUS-guided creation of transgastric pancreatic fistula anastomosis using plastic stents.[38] Endoscopic treatment of pancreatic fluid collections arising after distal pancreatectomy is at least as effective as percutaneous drainage.[39,40]

Limited data suggest that preoperative ERCP with pancreatic sphincterotomy and stent insertion significantly decreases the rate of postoperative pancreatic fistula in patients who undergo distal pancreatectomy,[41–44] although one randomized trial did not show a benefit.[45]

PUESTOW OR LONGITUDINAL PANCREATOJEJUNOSTOMY

Anatomy

This pancreatic ductal drainage procedure was commonly performed in patients with chronic pancreatitis and abdominal pain associated with ductal obstruction; most pancreatic surgeons now prefer resective surgery. In a Puestow procedure, the pancreatic duct is opened from the pancreatic head to the tail and a side-to-side anastomosis is created between the open margins of the pancreatic duct and a loop of jejunum (pancreaticojejunostomy). The gastric, duodenal, and pancreatobiliary anatomy remains intact, and ERCP is performed in the usual fashion

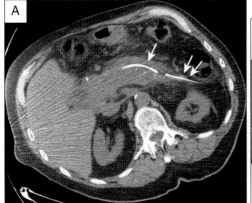
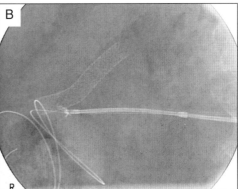

FIG 45.9 Interventional radiology approach to the patient shown in Fig. 45.8.

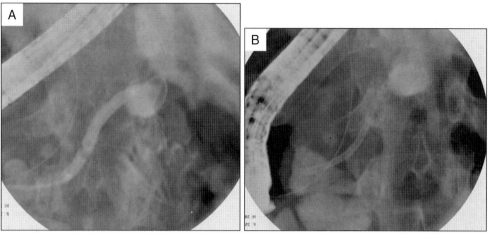

FIG 45.10 **A,** Endoscopic retrograde cholangiopancreatography showing a pancreatic duct leak with cyst formation after a distal pancreatectomy for chronic pancreatitis. **B,** Pancreatic duct stenting with a 7-Fr pancreatic duct stent for management of pancreatic duct leak after distal pancreatectomy.

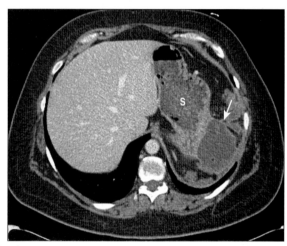

FIG 45.11 Computed tomography scan of infected pancreatic fluid collection (*arrow*) after distal pancreatectomy and splenectomy. The fluid collection occupies the splenic bed and is adjacent to the stomach (*S*).

to assess patency of the pancreaticojejunostomy (most often for recurrent pain) and to treat biliary strictures (see Chapters 43 and 55).

Adverse Events

Apart from usual postsurgical adverse events, delayed anastomotic strictures at the pancreaticojejunal anastomosis have been reported to occur in up to 10% of Puestow procedures.[46,47]

There are no large series on the role of ERCP in management of postsurgical adverse events in these patients.

ENUCLEATION

Enucleation of the pancreas is a viable option to major resective surgery, especially for cystic lesions and low-grade malignant or premalignant lesions.[48]

Adverse Events

The main adverse event after enucleation is injury to the main pancreatic duct, uncinate branch, or side branches, with development of a leak and/or fistula. Endoscopic therapy involves stent placement across the leak, if possible,[49] and transmural drainage of collections, as indicated for pseudocysts and other fluid collections. There is one case of placement of a covered self-expandable biliary stent into the main pancreatic duct for treatment of a fistula refractory to plastic stent placement (Fig. 45.13).[50]

Role of ERCP in Pancreatic Trauma

Pancreatic injury occurs in 1% to 5% of patients with blunt abdominal trauma and in up to 12% of patients with penetrating trauma.[51,52]

The American Association for the Surgery of Trauma (AAST) published a pancreas organ injury scale in 1990 (Table 45.1).[53] The scale organizes injury patterns into five grades, which are determined by the presence or absence of ductal disruption and by the anatomic location of the injury.

A multidetector CT scan has poor sensitivity for the diagnosis of pancreatic trauma in the acute setting.[54] Secretin-MRCP is superior in delineating the ductal anatomy when there is a high index of clinical suspicion for underlying pancreatic trauma and ductal injury (Fig. 45.14).[55–57]

Isolated pancreatic injury can present with minimal symptoms, physical findings, and laboratory data, including amylase levels, that can be normal in up to one-third of patients with complete pancreatic duct transection.[58] Early ductal injuries may manifest as a pancreatic fistula, "smoldering" pancreatitis, inability to eat, and symptomatic pancreatic pseudocyst or infected fluid collection. Patients with an unrecognized pancreatic injury can present with recurrent pancreatitis because of an underlying pancreatic duct stricture.

The role of early ERCP in the management of pancreatic trauma has not been established. In a few series, the utility of emergency intraoperative "on table" ERCP to assess ductal integrity has been shown to influence surgical management.[59] Associated potential risks and lack of widespread availability of expertise make this a less attractive approach in critically ill patients.

ERCP is now reserved as a third intent test after CT and MRCP in the setting of pancreatic trauma. However, ERCP is useful when there is a high suspicion of pancreatic duct injury in which there is the likelihood that a therapeutic intervention will be performed.[60]

Its role in the management of stable patients with pancreatic ductal disruption has been substantiated in the adult and pediatric literature.[52,59,61–63] For treatment of traumatic pancreatic fistula and ductal disruption, endoscopic pancreatic sphincterotomy and temporary stent

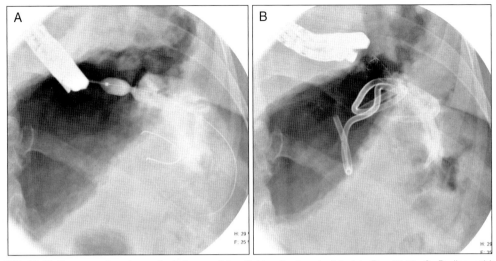

FIG 45.12 Transmural endoscopic drainage of the fluid collection depicted in Fig. 45.11. **A,** Radiographic image of balloon dilation of transgastric tract over guidewire. **B,** Radiographic image immediately after placement of two 10-Fr double-pigtail stents into collection.

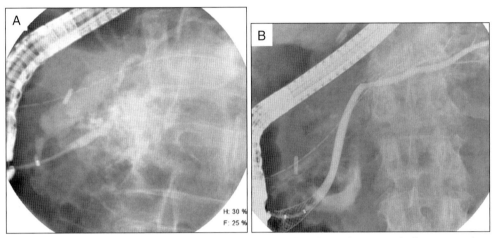

FIG 45.13 Placement of covered self-expandable metal stent into the main pancreatic duct to treat large disruption of duct after surgical enucleation of a pancreatic head islet cell tumor. **A,** Radiographic image of pancreatogram showing large disruption in pancreatic head. Upstream duct can be seen. **B,** Radiographic image immediately after placement of covered metal stent. Contrast injection shows closure of the leak.

TABLE 45.1   AAST Classification of Pancreatic Injury

Grade	Injury	Description
I	Hematoma	Minor contusion without duct injury
	Laceration	Superficial laceration without duct injury
II	Hematoma	Major contusion without duct injury or tissue loss
	Laceration	Major laceration without duct injury or tissue loss
III	Laceration	Distal transection or parenchymal injury with duct injury
IV	Laceration	Proximal transection or parenchymal injury involving ampulla
V	Laceration	Massive disruption of pancreatic head

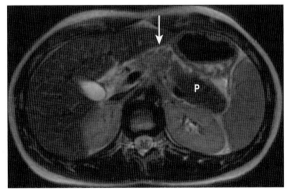

FIG 45.14 Magnetic resonance cholangiopancreatography after pancreatic trauma. *Arrow* indicates pancreatic duct disruption from injury. *P,* Pancreas.

placement is an effective nonoperative strategy that may obviate the need for surgical intervention (Fig. 45.15).[61,62] Its role in grade III pancreatic injury is controversial and surgery is considered the mainstay of treatment, although some of these have been managed endoscopically.[64] Reservations and widespread acceptance of ERCP in this patient subset are partly attributed to the stent-related and procedure-related risks of sepsis, stent migration, ductal stenosis, and acute and chronic pancreatitis. However, it appears that endoscopic therapy is becoming more accepted.[65,66] EUS may play a role in assisting therapy in acute trauma.[67] Late presentation (after weeks to months and up to years later) is often caused by stricture formation, with acute recurrent pancreatitis and/or pain. The role of ERCP in the management of symptomatic post-traumatic pseudocysts is similar to that of nontraumatic pseudocysts, and ERCP is successful in 90% of patients, with low recurrence rates (see Chapters 34, 54, and 56).[63]

Management of pancreatic pseudocysts depends on symptoms, size of the cyst, location, type of duct injury, and maturity of the cyst wall. The assessment of concomitant ductal injury and communication with the cyst can be made by secretin-MRCP. Pseudocysts that are in direct apposition to the gastric or duodenal wall can be drained transmurally. If there is communication of the cyst with the main pancreatic duct, transpapillary stent insertion can be accomplished along with treatment of underlying ductal abnormalities.

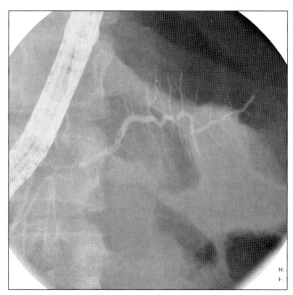

FIG 45.15 Endoscopic therapy for pancreatic trauma.

SUMMARY

ERCP plays a substantial role in the management of delayed adverse events resulting from pancreatic surgeries. Significant advances have been made in the realm of therapeutic echoendosonography, single-balloon endoscopy, and double-balloon endoscopy, and their clinical role and applicability continue to be explored and defined in post–pancreatic surgery patients.

The available literature substantiates the role of ERCP in the management of stable postpancreatic trauma resulting in ductal leaks and pseudocysts.

The complete reference list for this chapter can be found online at www.expertconsult.com.

Choledocholithiasis

John C.T. Wong, James Y.W. Lau, and Joseph J.Y. Sung

Gallstones and their related complications have a prevalence ranging from 7% to 10% in developed countries to more than 70% among high-risk groups such as Pima Indians.[1] Direct and indirect costs related to gallstones in the United States in 2004 amounted to more than 6 billion dollars.[2] Gallstones have also been associated with increased overall and cardiovascular-specific mortality, even after adjustment for demographics and cardiovascular risk factors.[3] Advanced age; female sex; Native Indian ethnicity; dyslipidemia; obesity; pregnancy; medications such as octreotide, ceftriaxone, thiazide diuretics, and oral contraceptives; prolonged fasting; rapid weight loss; and total parenteral nutrition are recognized risk factors for cholesterol gallstone development, whereas biliary infections, ileal Crohn's disease, cystic fibrosis, chronic hemolysis, and cirrhosis predispose to pigmented stone formation.[1,4]

In the West, migration of gallstones into the common bile duct is largely responsible for complications such as biliary colic, choledocholithiasis, cholangitis, and biliary pancreatitis. In a cohort of 664 Danes with asymptomatic gallstones followed for a median of 17 years, 20% developed clinical events. Identified predisposing factors included young age, female sex, >2 gallstones, and gallstones >1 cm.[5] Another study reported that gallstones causing cholecystitis (8 mm) tended to be larger on transabdominal ultrasonography (TUS) than those found in obstructive jaundice and pancreatitis (3 to 4 mm).[6] The natural history of bile duct stones has also been explored. In a study of 92 patients with bile duct stones on endoscopic ultrasonography (EUS), 21% had passed them within 1 month as noted during endoscopic retrograde cholangiopancreatography (ERCP).[7] Stone size <5 mm was an independent predictive factor for spontaneous passage. Conversely, a positive intraoperative cholangiogram coupled with elevated serum bilirubin count best predicted the presence of bile duct stones after cholecystectomy.[8] Smaller stones may therefore pass asymptomatically and spontaneously into the duodenum, whereas larger stones can become impacted at the distal bile duct, causing biliary obstruction, cholangitis, and pancreatitis. Stone passage through the ampulla of Vater may cause bile reflux into the pancreatic duct, with resultant acute biliary pancreatitis. In patients with acute biliary pancreatitis undergoing early ERCP, bile duct stones can be found in up to 47%.[9] Although uncommon, chronic obstruction by stones can also lead to secondary biliary cirrhosis and portal hypertension. Therefore patients with suspected bile duct stones should be investigated and have stones extracted when identified.

EVALUATION OF PATIENTS WITH SUSPECTED CHOLEDOCHOLITHIASIS

Roles of Liver Biochemistry and Transabdominal Ultrasonography

Initial investigations in patients suspected to have bile duct stones should include liver biochemical tests and TUS. Normal liver function and biochemical tests are useful in excluding bile duct stones. In 1002 patients undergoing laparoscopic cholecystectomy, normal liver biochemistry accurately predicted the absence of bile duct stones.[10] The negative predictive values (NPVs) of gamma glutamyl transferase (GGT), alkaline phosphatase, total bilirubin, alanine, and aspartate aminotransferases were all high and ranged from 94.7% (for total bilirubin) to 97.9% (for GGT). Unfortunately, the positive predictive value of only one abnormal liver biochemical test was just 15%.

TUS has a sensitivity of <50% in diagnosing bile duct stones. However, a bile duct stone seen during TUS is highly specific for stones found at ERCP and surgery. TUS is sensitive in detection of bile duct dilation (>6 mm in diameter), which is associated with the presence of bile duct stones. Mild biliary ductal dilation can be seen, however, in the elderly and in those with prior cholecystectomy. A TUS finding of a normal-sized bile duct has a 95% NPV of finding bile duct stones at ERCP.[11]

No single parameter accurately predicts presence of bile duct stones in patients with gallstones. Most predictive models are based on a combination of clinical, biochemical, and TUS findings. For example, a patient older than 55 years with a serum bilirubin >30 μmol/L (1.8 mg/dL) and a dilated bile duct on TUS has a 72% probability of having bile duct stones found at ERCP.[12] In 2010, the American Society for Gastrointestinal Endoscopy (ASGE) Standards of Practice Committee proposed stratification of symptomatic patients with gallstones into those at low (<10%), intermediate (10% to 50%), and high (>50%) risk of harboring bile duct stones.[13] Very strong predictors include clinical cholangitis, bilirubin >4 mg/dL, and bile duct stone on TUS. Strong clinical predictors are a serum bilirubin of 1.8 to 4 mg/dL or a dilated bile duct on TUS (>6 mm with an intact gallbladder). The presence of any one very strong predictor or both strong predictors categorizes a patient at high risk of having a bile duct stone. Age greater than 55 years, clinical gallstone pancreatitis, and abnormal liver function tests other than a raised serum bilirubin are intermediate predictors of choledocholithiasis. The absence of any of these predictors is considered low risk. Those at high risk of harboring a bile duct stone should undergo preoperative ERCP and stone extraction. Patients at low risk should undergo cholecystectomy without further investigation. Patients at intermediate risk should be offered preoperative imaging, such as magnetic resonance cholangiography (MRC) or EUS to minimize diagnostic ERCP and the associated risk of post-ERCP pancreatitis (PEP).

Multiple groups recently prospectively applied the approach described earlier to patients with suspected bile duct stones and showed that the diagnostic accuracy for choledocholithiasis in the ASGE-designated high-risk group was only 59% to 69%.[14–16] More refined stratification tools are needed to avoid unnecessary ERCPs. Among patients at intermediate risk of bile duct stones, a pooled analysis of 213 patients in 4 trials comparing an EUS-first versus direct ERCP approach found that initial use of EUS could reduce the need for ERCP in 67% of patients and the risk of PEP (relative risk [RR] 0.21; 95% confidence interval [CI] 0.06 to 0.83).[17]

Roles of Magnetic Resonance Cholangiography and Endoscopic Ultrasonography

A meta-analysis found both high sensitivity (92%; 95% CI 80% to 97%) and high specificity (97%; 95% CI 90% to 99%) of MRC in the detection of bile duct stones.[18] The sensitivity of MRC appears to be related to stone size. In one study, the sensitivity was 100% for stones approximately 1 cm in diameter and decreased to 71% for stones <5 mm in diameter.[19] Another study, in which bile duct stone diameter >4 mm as cutoff on MRC was an indication for ERCP, had the best sensitivity (83%; 95% CI 78% to 88%) and specificity (66%; 95% CI 53% to 77%) for a positive ERC.[20] False positives can also occur and are mostly related to air bubbles or bilioenteric anastomosis, such as a choledochoduodenostomy. MRC has the distinct advantages of being entirely noninvasive, usually not requiring sedation, and being unaffected by altered anatomy; it is contraindicated in patients with pacemakers, defibrillators, or other indwelling metallic objects.

EUS is an alternate modality to evaluate the bile duct among intermediate-risk patients. With the patient in the left lateral decubitus position and the transducer at the apex of the duodenal bulb, the second portion of the duodenum, and the papilla, the bile duct can be well visualized from the biliary hilum down to the ampullary region. Both radial and linear EUS have high sensitivity (~90%) and specificity (>93%) for the diagnosis of bile duct stones, though direct comparisons have not been performed (Fig. 46.1).[21,22] Importantly, sensitivity does not seem to be affected by stone size or bile duct diameter, though EUS is subject to operator variability.[23] If bile duct stones are detected on EUS, ERCP can be performed during the same endoscopy session, reducing the need for an additional procedure and sedation and minimizing the risk of interval cholangitis.[24]

A 2016 systematic review of eight prospective blinded studies that compared MRC and EUS against a gold standard of ERCP and/or intraoperative cholangiography identified 538 patients with intermediate probability of choledocholithiasis. The sensitivity of EUS (94%) was numerically superior to MRCP (84%). MRCP had a numerically higher specificity at 92% compared with EUS (89%), though statistical significance was not reached.[25] For small stones and biliary

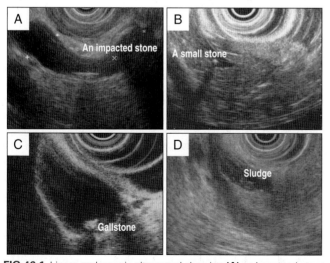

FIG 46.1 Linear endoscopic ultrasound showing **(A)** an impacted stone at the distal bile duct, **(B)** a small stone at the bile duct, **(C)** sludge, and **(D)** a gallstone.

sludge, EUS is likely more sensitive. Ultimately, the choice between MRC and EUS is often determined by resource availability and patient preference.

EXTRACTION OF BILE DUCT STONES (SEE CHAPTER 19)

Patient Preparation

Patients with an indication for ERCP and endoscopic sphincterotomy (ES) for stone extraction should be evaluated for fitness for the procedure. Patient age is one of the first considerations, but procedural technical success and adverse events, including cardiopulmonary complications and PEP, were comparable between octogenarians and a younger patient group in a Korean multicenter review of over 600 patients.[26] With the wider use of novel oral anticoagulant drugs and antiplatelets, endoscopists must become familiar with their indications (see Chapter 10). An updated ASGE guideline on the management of antithrombotic agents for patients undergoing gastrointestinal endoscopy outlined an approach weighing clinical urgency, bleeding risk of ERCP, and cardiovascular risk of withholding antithrombotics.[27] In patients with sepsis mandating urgent ERCP, the use of anticoagulation should not defer the procedure, as waiting for ERCP >48 hours after hospitalization was associated with a threefold risk of persistent organ failure on a retrospective review of 203 patients with cholangitis.[28] A short-length plastic biliary stent can be safely inserted for drainage without the need for ES. Otherwise, in nonurgent situations, ES is considered to be a procedure at high risk for bleeding, whereas endoscopic papillary balloon dilation (EPBD) without ES is categorized as low bleeding risk, and antithrombotics can be maintained. In patients at low cardiovascular risk with planned ES, anticoagulation can likely be held, but anticoagulation bridging should be considered in higher-cardiovascular-risk patients. The value of bridging therapy has, however, been questioned, as a recent multicenter randomized controlled trial of atrial fibrillation patients with a mean CHADS$_2$ score of 2.3 showed that low-molecular-weight heparin bridging resulted in more major and minor bleeding but similar incidence of thromboembolism compared with no bridging.[29] As 90% of the procedures in this trial were low risk for bleeding, the increased bleeding observed in the bridging group is likely even greater for high-bleeding-risk procedures like ES. Patients on dual-antiplatelet therapy at low and high cardiovascular risk anticipating ES should continue aspirin/nonsteroidal anti-inflammatory drugs, while holding thienopyridines for at least 5 days before endoscopy. On the use of preprocedural antibiotic prophylaxis (see Chapter 10), ASGE guidelines from 2015 recommend it in liver transplant patients and patients with biliary obstruction in whom incomplete biliary drainage is anticipated (those with multiple stones or with complex strictures).[30] In those with biliary obstruction in the absence of cholangitis and in whom complete biliary drainage is likely after ERCP, it has not been shown conclusively that preprocedural antibiotics decrease post-ERCP cholangitis. We recommend routine use of antibiotics in immunocompromised patients. Recently a multicenter randomized controlled trial of over 2500 Chinese patients undergoing ERCP mostly for bile duct stones showed routine use of 100 mg rectal indomethacin 30 minutes before ERCP in an unselect group of patients was superior to post-ERCP rectal indomethacin given selectively to high-risk patients for reducing PEP (RR 0.47; 95% CI 0.34 to 0.66; $p < 0.0001$).[31] Adverse events, specifically bleeding and perforation, were similar in both groups. Patients with sepsis who have unstable hemodynamics or potential airway problems should be resuscitated and endotracheally intubated for the procedure, which can be performed in the supine or left lateral decubitus position. We prefer to perform ERCP with the use of anesthesia-administered propofol.

Biliary Cannulation, Cholangiography, and Sphincterotomy (see Chapters 14 and 17)

ERCP with ES and stone extraction is a time-honored technique with a pooled success rate of ~90%, according to a 2013 meta-analysis of ERCP intraprocedural performance and quality.[32] We recommend wire-guided biliary cannulation because injection of contrast can increase hydrostatic pressure and cause mechanical trauma to the pancreatic duct. In a pooled analysis of controlled trials that compared contrast versus wire-guided techniques of biliary cannulation, primary cannulation success was significantly higher and PEP was significantly lower with wire-guided cannulation (RR 0.19; 95% CI 0.06 to 0.58).[33] We use a pull-type sphincterotome, typically with a 25-mm cutting wire preloaded with a 0.025-inch or 0.035-inch guidewire that has a hydrophilic terminal portion. Flexing of the sphincterotome provides additional angulation for cannulation. Upon deep cannulation of the bile duct, the sphincterotome is advanced above the cystic duct junction. Bile should first be aspirated, followed by injection of half-strength contrast for better visualization of stones. In patients with cholangitis, frank pus may be aspirated, and overdistension of the bile duct with contrast should be avoided as an increase in biliary pressure can induce bacteremia. Prompt biliary drainage can be accomplished by insertion of a 7-Fr nasobiliary drain or a short plastic stent to prevent calculous impaction. Although several randomized controlled trials showed no difference in biliary drainage and adverse events, we prefer to use a short plastic stent, as nasobiliary drains can kink at the back of the oropharynx, can be a source of discomfort, and are prone to accidental dislodgment, particularly in delirious or elderly patients.[34,35]

When stone extraction is permitted by the patient's clinical status, an optimal cholangiogram should be performed to highlight stone characteristics such as size, shape, location, number, and presence of impaction, and duct characteristics, including distal bile duct diameter and the presence of strictures, as they will influence the approach to stone extraction. An occlusion cholangiogram may be needed to prevent contrast drainage if prior sphincterotomy was performed. However, the sensitivity of cholangiography in diagnosing bile duct stones is imperfect, ranging from 67% to 94%.[36] In particular, small stones can be missed in a spacious and dilated bile duct. To visualize the bile duct behind the duodenoscope, the endoscope should be advanced into a semilong position. When a cholangiogram is obtained but no apparent stones are identified, the decision to perform an empiric ES is influenced by the pretest probability of finding a bile duct stone. When the clinical suspicion is high (e.g., stone seen on TUS or for a patient with clinical cholangitis), we advocate a more liberal policy of performing empiric ES. This is consistent with results of a randomized study showing that in patients with clinical cholangitis and cholelithiasis but no bile duct stones on ERCP, empiric ES led to a reduction in recurrent stones and sepsis (hazard ratio [HR] 0.305; 95% CI 0.095 to 0.975; $p = 0.045$) at a mean follow-up of 22 months compared with no ES.[37] In most circumstances, the risk of missing a bile duct stone outweighs that of empiric ES. When expertise is available, ancillary techniques like intraductal ultrasonography or EUS may aid in resolving the dilemma.

ES should be performed in a stepwise manner with the distal portion of the cutting wire in the duct and with minimal wire tension (see Chapter 17). Excessive wire tension during ES can otherwise result in a zipper cut with coagulated tissue being forced open, resulting in perforation and bleeding. We prefer to use a blended current in a pulsed mode, such as ENDO CUT (Erbe Elektromedizin GmbH, Tuebingen, Germany). A meta-analysis of 4 randomized studies with over 800 patients showed that ES with pure-cut mode resulted in more intraprocedural bleeding, with no difference in PEP, compared with mixed current.[38]

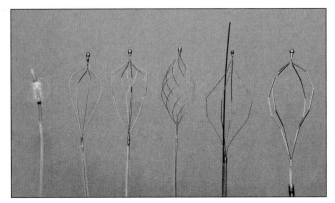

FIG 46.2 Biliary stone extraction devices. Starting from the *left:* soft extraction balloon, standard Dormia basket, flower and spiral baskets, and two lithotripter baskets: Trapezoid RX wire-guided basket (Boston Scientific, Marlborough, MA) and through-the-scope mechanical lithotripter basket (Olympus, Tokyo, Japan).

The diameter that a sphincterotomy can be created depends on the shape of the papilla and diameter and configuration of the distal bile duct. In the presence of a prominent papilla and a dilated bile duct with a flat and square distal end, a full ES to the top of the overlying transverse fold is possible. In a patient with a small papilla and a narrow, tapering distal bile duct, only a limited ES is possible. As muscle fibers to the biliary sphincter are severed, one should see free bile flow. Another sign of an adequate sphincterotomy is free passage of a fully bowed sphincterotome with a 25-mm cutting wire through the sphincterotomy orifice.

Devices and Techniques for Stone Extraction and Biliary Drainage

The choice of extraction device is dependent on the size and type of stones and the configuration of the distal bile duct (Fig. 46.2). Stone and duct diameters can be estimated by comparing to the width of the duodenoscope. Stone extraction devices available include soft Fogarty-type extraction balloons, wire baskets, and basket mechanical lithotripters (BML).[39] A duodenoscope with a 4.2-mm instrument channel is required for through-the-scope BML. When multiple stones are present, removal should start with the most distal stone, as starting extraction of more proximal stones can cause impaction at the distal bile duct. Furthermore, it is imperative that an ES commensurate with the size of the stone is made before attempted removal.

For small stones, a soft retrieval balloon catheter can be used. Many extraction balloons are triple-lumen devices, allowing passage over a guidewire, which can provide directional control and injection/aspiration of air for balloon inflation to preset sizes/deflation and for contrast injection. The balloon is advanced proximal to the target stone and inflated to the size of the bile duct as judged on the cholangiogram. An overinflated balloon can cause patient discomfort and resistance during trawling. The balloon and stone are then gently pulled to the level of the papilla. The tip of the duodenoscope is first deflected upward close to the ES. Then, with the extraction balloon fixed in position at the working channel valve, the scope tip is turned downward, along with slight advancement of the duodenoscope, to extract the stone. Sweeping using a soft balloon is least traumatic to the bile duct and avoids the risk of stone and device entrapment in the distal bile duct. An occlusion cholangiogram using the same balloon can be obtained at the end of the procedure.

Stones can also be removed using wire baskets. Types include Dormia baskets (which are made of four wires and open to the shape of two perpendicular hexagons) and spiral or flower baskets (which are made of eight wires with closer mesh for better engagement of small stones). The maneuver to advance a wire basket across the papilla is called the "kissing" technique. The tip of the closed basket is first impacted against the roof of the ES opening. Upward deflection followed by slight forward advancement of the duodenoscope aligns the shaft of the basket with the bile duct axis, facilitating cannulation. Once a target stone has been selected, the basket should be advanced from the catheter and opened proximal to that stone, preferably in a more dilated portion of the bile duct. Opening the basket distal to the stone may push it proximally into the intrahepatic ducts and should be avoided. Contrast can be injected to outline the stone if necessary. The stone is then captured within the wire mesh by jiggling the basket by gentle wrist rotation, with a rapid in-and-out movement of the catheter. Once engaged, the wire basket should be closed just enough to trap the stone, as excessive closure may result in the wires grinding into the stone. With a stone captured, downward scope tip deflection along with gentle scope advancement in line with the axis of the bile duct allows extraction of the stone. If the engaged stone is not easily withdrawn, the basket should be returned to the mid-bile duct and the stone disengaged. Forceful traction of the basket in an axis perpendicular to that of the bile duct can result in avulsion of the pancreatic head and should never be practiced. Extension of the sphincterotomy or EPBD or the use of mechanical or laser lithotripsy is often required. Should the stone fail to disengage from the basket, resulting in entrapment, a Soehendra lithotriptor (Cook Medical, Winston-Salem, NC) can be used for rescue (Fig. 46.3). The handle of the wire basket is cut outside the patient's mouth. The duodenoscope is carefully withdrawn from the patient under fluoroscopy. The plastic sheath surrounding the basket wires is then removed. The Soehendra lithotripsy cable is passed over the wires until the level of the stone. The cut wires are then fed through the Luer lock and the hole in the central rotating rod of the lithotripter. By slowly turning the crank handle to avoid wire fracture, the basket and trapped stone are crushed against the metal cable under fluoroscopy. Alternatively, digital single-operator cholangioscopy-guided laser lithotripsy can also resolve an impacted stone and basket device (Video 46.1).[40]

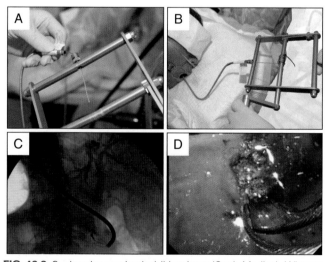

FIG 46.3 Soehendra mechanical lithotripter (Cook Medical, Winston-Salem, NC) for rescue of an entrapped basket with a stone. **A,** After the basket wires have been cut at the handle and the plastic sheath removed, the wires are passed over the lithotripsy cable and fed through the Luer lock and **(B)** the hole in the central rotating rod of the lithotripter. **C,** Slow rotation of the handle tightens the wires against the metal cable under fluoroscopy. **D,** Residual stone fragments are removed by conventional techniques.

Large (>15 mm) bile duct stones, as well as smaller stones with stone/distal duct size mismatch, are particularly challenging to treat, often requiring mechanical lithotripsy. As mentioned, the sphincter should be sufficiently large, and if necessary, enlargement by EPBD can be performed. There are several mechanical lithotriptor devices available, such as the LithoCrushV lithotriptor (Olympus, Tokyo, Japan), Trapezoid RX basket (Boston Scientific, Marlborough, MA), and Fusion basket (Cook Medical).[41] BML baskets in general consist of several parts: a basket with four wires attached to the control section via a Teflon catheter, over which a metal sheath can extend. With the basket closed, the Teflon catheter is used to cannulate the bile duct. Opening the basket within the bile duct advances the entire device deeper into the biliary tree. With the basket opened, contrast can be injected through the tip of the Teflon catheter to outline the stone. The stone is then engaged, and the wires slowly closed over it to avoid stone slippage (Fig. 46.4). The metal sheath is then advanced over a stretched-out Teflon catheter to the level of the stone and locked into a notch on the metal handle. As the control knob at the crank handle is turned, the wires tighten and the stone is crushed against the tip of the metal sheath. This should be done slowly, allowing for gradual grinding of the wires into the stone. Otherwise, a very hard stone can slip through the wire mesh. The Trapezoid RX basket (Boston Scientific) has an emergency release feature to avoid basket entrapment. In patients with multiple stones or large bile duct stones, complete removal cannot be assured. Adequate biliary drainage, however, must be secured at the end of ERCP. The temporary insertion of a short biliary stent or a nasobiliary drain can prevent impaction of residual fragments and subsequent cholangitis.

Endoscopic Papillary Balloon Dilation

Endoscopic balloon dilation of the biliary sphincter using a small-diameter (<10 mm) balloon-tipped catheter has been proposed as an alternative to ES in patients undergoing stone extraction for small stones. Conceptually, the bleeding and perforation risks associated with sphincter dilation should be less. Although less bleeding was confirmed in a 2004 meta-analysis of 8 randomized controlled trials involving >1000 patients comparing EPBD versus ES, PEP (7.4% vs 4.3%; $p = 0.05$) and need for mechanical lithotripsy (20.9% vs 14.8%; $p = 0.01$) were more frequent in the EPBD group.[42] As the mean patient age across the studies was ~65 years, this meta-analysis does not address PEP risk in younger patients, for whom sphincter preservation is proposed to be most beneficial but who are also at higher risk for PEP. A prospective American multicenter randomized trial of EPBD versus ES, not included in the meta-analysis, was stopped prematurely as EPBD showed not only more PEP but also significantly more morbidity (17.9% vs 3.3%; $p < 0.001$), including two deaths from necrotizing pancreatitis.[43] Notably, this study was performed before the advent of prophylactic pancreatitis stents and rectally administered nonsteroidal agents to prevent PEP. Interestingly, the risk of PEP may be related to the duration of EPBD. A randomized controlled trial that aimed to compare complete stone clearance rates by 1-minute versus 5-minute EPBD with a 10-mm balloon demonstrated that longer dilation was associated not only with fewer failed stone extractions but also with significantly fewer episodes of PEP (RR 0.32; $p = 0.038$).[44] Investigators proposed that short duration of dilation may cause insufficient loosening of the sphincter complex, paradoxically exacerbating pancreatic duct obstruction and increased ductal pressure induced by EPBD sphincter edema and spasm, as in compartment syndrome. This was confirmed in a subsequent network analysis, where dilation longer than 1 minute conferred a comparable risk of PEP as ES, whereas EPBD less than 1 minute had the highest PEP incidence of the three groups.[45] Nevertheless, EPBD alone should likely be restricted to select situations such as stones <10 mm in patients with difficult bile duct access, as seen after Billroth II gastrectomy or intradiverticular

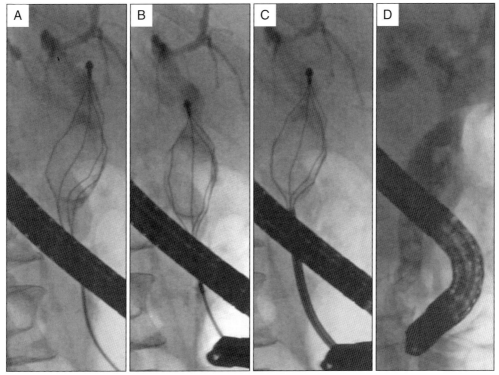

FIG 46.4 Basket mechanical lithotripsy. **A,** A large biliary stone is first trapped with wire basket. **B** and **C,** The metal sheath is progressively advanced over the Teflon catheter until it is at the level of the stone, at which point the stone is slowly crushed, **(D)** leaving smaller stone fragments for removal by conventional extraction techniques.

papilla, in cirrhotics with coagulopathy (particularly Child Pugh Class C patients), those who require anticoagulation soon after stone extraction, and patients at lower risk of PEP.[46,47]

Endoscopic Papillary Large Balloon Dilation (see Chapter 18)

Ersoz et al. first reported in 2003 the technique of endoscopic papillary large balloon dilation, ranging from 12 to 20 mm, after ES in managing large bile duct stones.[48] After ES, a balloon catheter, such as a CRE wire-guided esophageal/pyloric balloon dilator (Boston Scientific) with maximum diameter ranging from 12 to 20 mm and 5.5 cm in length, is positioned with its midpoint across the sphincterotomy (Fig. 46.5). The balloon is then slowly filled with half-strength contrast under fluoroscopic and endoscopic guidance to a maximal diameter not exceeding the diameter of the distal bile duct. In practice, we seldom dilate beyond 15 mm. Careful attention should be paid during balloon inflation, as the presence of a distal bile duct stricture is a major risk factor (odds ratio [OR] 17; 95% CI 3 to 74; $p < 0.001$) for endoscopic papillary large balloon dilation (EPLBD)–related perforation.[49] Resistance during balloon inflation or failure to obliterate balloon waisting was encountered in all three cases of fatal perforation after EPLBD in a retrospective review of over 900 patients from 12 centers in Korea and Japan. Caution should also be exercised in patients with portal hypertensive biliopathy, as massive hemobilia from rupture of anomalous varices around the bile duct because of EPLBD can occur. Most endoscopists leave the balloon inflated for 30 to 60 seconds after waist disappearance. Upon balloon deflation, mucosal bleeding from the edge of the papillary orifice is commonly observed but usually stops without the need for intervention. Risk factors of EPLBD-associated bleeding include cirrhosis (OR 8; 95% CI 2 to 31; $p = 0.003$), a preceding full-length

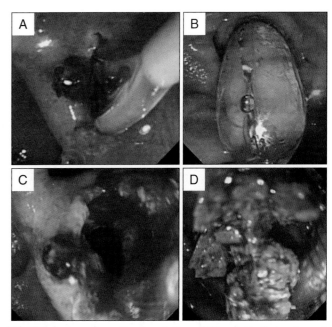

FIG 46.5 Endoscopic papillary large balloon dilation. **A,** Limited endoscopic sphincterotomy, **(B)** followed by endoscopic papillary large balloon dilation using a 15-mm-wide, 5.5-cm-long CRE balloon (Boston Scientific, Marlborough, MA). **C,** Self-limited bleeding is observed. **D,** Conventional stone extraction is performed.

ES (OR 6; 95% CI 2 to 16; $p < 0.001$), and bile duct stones >16 mm (OR 4; 95% CI 2 to 8; $p < 0.001$).[49] Variable-length ES followed by EPLBD has been compared with ES alone by multiple groups. Although the combined technique shows similar overall success in stone extraction, ES followed by EPLBD can reduce the need for mechanical lithotripsy, fluoroscopy time, hospitalization costs, and post-ERCP cholangitis and pancreatitis.[50-53] Initial ES separates the pancreatic orifice and controls the direction of muscle disruption during subsequent balloon dilation, perhaps accounting for the lower rate of PEP in the combined technique group.

The need for a limited ES before EPLBD was recently evaluated retrospectively in three Asian nonrandomized comparative studies of patients with native papilla undergoing ERCP for stone extraction. In all studies, complete stone clearance rates, need for mechanical lithotripsy, median procedure time, and overall adverse events, including PEP specifically, were comparable in patients with and without a preceding ES.[54-56] On the other hand, a review of 32 published studies suggested that initial success was lower (76% vs 84%, $p < 0.001$) and the need for BML was higher (22% vs 14%, $p < 0.001$) with EPLBD alone.[57] Recently, an international consensus meeting proposed a number of indications for EPLBD.[58]

Biliary Stents

In patients with cholangitis, especially those with suppurative cholangitis, insertion of a biliary stent can be a temporizing measure (Fig. 46.6). This allows time for sepsis to resolve and the patient's condition to be optimized while definitive treatment is planned. The purpose of stent placement is to prevent calculous impaction in the distal bile duct. There is also evidence suggesting that stones become smaller with a period of stenting.[59] This is probably because of friction of the stones onto the stent itself, especially in the case of pigmented stones. For this reason, placement of a biliary stent can also be considered for patients with large stones when initial extraction fails. Traditionally, plastic biliary stents, such as a 7-Fr, 7-cm-long double-pigtail stent, are used. As plastic stents invariably block over time, use of biliary stenting as long-term or even definitive treatment is discouraged. In two series of elderly patients in whom biliary stenting was used as definitive treatment, adverse events from stent occlusion developed in 34% to 40% of patients at a mean of 12 months after stent placement.[60,61] The most common adverse event was cholangitis. In one of these series, there

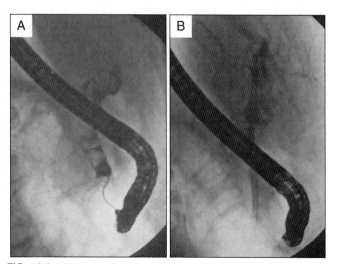

FIG 46.6 Biliary stenting. **A,** Clinical cholangitis caused by multiple common bile duct stones, **(B)** managed temporarily by placement of a 10-Fr plastic biliary stent.

was also a 15% mortality rate.[60] The rate of adverse events is higher in those with gallbladder in situ. Long-term stenting should therefore be restricted to select patients with limited lifespan or prohibitively high risk of needing repeat ERCP. Two series described temporary placement of 10-mm-wide partially or fully covered metal biliary transpapillary stents for difficult bile duct stones.[62,63] When stents were removed at a mean of 6 to 8 weeks later, duct clearance rates were achieved in ~83% of patients. Clinically insignificant stent migration rates between 10% and 22% were observed. As metal stent placement duration was relatively short, the long-term outcome of this approach remains undefined.

DIFFICULT BILE DUCT STONES

Clinical Scenarios

In 5% to 10% of patients, ERCP is unsuccessful at removing bile duct stones, which are termed *difficult bile duct stones*. ERCP may fail because of several reasons. The route to the ampulla may be altered, such as after a Billroth II gastrectomy or a Roux-en-Y jejunal limb reconstruction. The ampulla may be hidden within a periampullary diverticulum, which is associated with stone disease and commonly seen in elderly patients. A stone may be impacted at the papilla, preventing conventional biliary cannulation. A stone may be located proximal to a biliary stricture or in the intrahepatic duct. A stone may be difficult to capture by BML because of its size, shape, or location, or the lack of room in a narrow bile duct and because of calculous impaction, such as in Mirizzi syndrome. Even after capture, BML failure because of wire fracture, handle fracture, or impaction can occur, necessitating lithotripsy.

Surgically Altered Anatomy of the Upper Gastrointestinal Tract (see Chapter 31)

It is crucial that endoscopists understand the type of reconstruction and the postsurgical anatomy to plan for the types of endoscope and accessories to be used. As technical efficacy is lower and adverse events of ERCP are higher in the setting of surgically altered anatomy, alternate approaches should be considered and discussed with patients.

For patients with a Billroth II gastrojejunostomy, we prefer to use a side-viewing endoscope, because of better visualization of the papilla and because the elevator will ease biliary cannulation. In an isoperistaltic anastomosis, the afferent limb is anastomosed to the lesser curvature of the stomach and the more angulated limb to enter. Often, as the endoscope is advanced into the afferent limb, it forms a hockey stick configuration and backs away from the limb itself. Instead, the afferent limb opening can be engaged with the scope tip, which is then deflected downward and to the right for intubation. At the fixed retroperitoneal portions (third and fourth parts of the duodenum) along the path to the papilla, forceful advancement may result in perforation. With the papilla slightly away from as opposed to close to the scope tip, we prefer to use a straight ball-tip cannula with a preloaded hydrophilic wire for biliary cannulation (Fig. 46.7). A rotatable sphincterotome, such as Autotome RX (Boston Scientific), can also be useful. Upon deep cannulation of the bile duct, a short stent is inserted, and needle-knife sphincterotomy over the stent can be safely performed (Fig. 46.8). In a review of the 30-year experience at one highly specialized tertiary center in Italy, where ERCP in Billroth II patients predominantly used a duodenoscope, clinical success in 713 patients was over 94%, with 1.8% perforation and 0.3% mortality rates.[64] Outcomes are likely less favorable at lower-volume centers.

In patients with Roux-en-Y gastrojejunostomy, a standard endoscope is often not long enough to reach the papilla, requiring balloon-assisted enteroscopy. A 2014 systematic review of 945 single-balloon,

CHAPTER 46 Choledocholithiasis

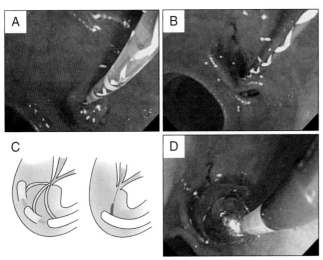

FIG 46.7 Biliary cannulation in Billroth II gastrojejunostomy with a side-viewing endoscope. **A,** The major papilla, located near the 12 o'clock position, is cannulated with a straight ball-tip catheter, **(B)** which is exchanged out, leaving a hydrophilic guidewire. Note the bile duct axis toward the 7 o'clock position. **C,** To align with the bile duct axis for cannulation, the scope can be pulled back for adjustment as shown. **D,** Primary endoscopic papillary balloon dilation is performed instead of endoscopic sphincterotomy.

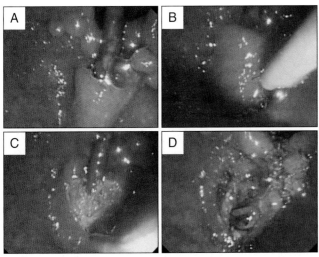

FIG 46.8 Endoscopic sphincterotomy in Billroth II gastrojejunostomy. **A,** A straight plastic biliary stent is inserted, **(B)** followed by needle-knife sphincterotomy over the stent, **(C)** which exposes the sphincter muscles, **(D)** permitting stone extraction.

double-balloon, and spiral enteroscopies for surgically altered anatomy showed successful ERCP in 76% of cases of Roux-en-Y with pancreaticoduodenectomy, pylorus-preserving pancreaticoduodenectomy, or hepaticojejunostomy and 70% of Roux-en-Y gastric bypass cases.[65] For Roux-en-Y gastric bypass, alternate approaches include laparoscopy-assisted ERCP via a 15-mm or 18-mm trocar, and EUS-guided transgastric ERCP via a gastrogastric or jejunogastro anastomosis created with a lumen-apposing metal stent has been reported.[66,67] EUS-guided antegrade management of bile duct stones in patients with surgically altered anatomy is also a promising technique but can be limited by unsuccessful bile duct puncture and guidewire manipulation (see Chapter 33).[68]

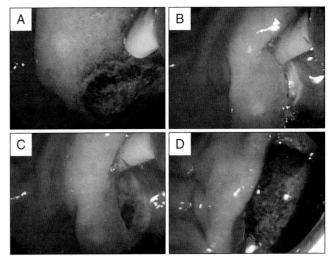

FIG 46.9 Biliary stone visualized impacted at papilla. **A–C,** Needle-knife sphincterotomy is progressively extended over the bulging papilla, **(D)** which disimpacts the stone.

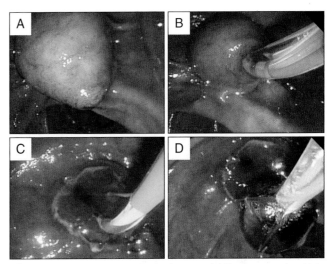

FIG 46.10 Bulging papilla. **A,** An impacted biliary stone should be suspected. **B,** Cannulation successfully disimpacts the stone. **C,** Full sphincterotomy is performed. **D,** The stone is captured with a Dormia basket.

Biliary Stone Impaction

Occasionally, a stone can be directly visualized impacted at the papillary orifice. Wire-guided cannulation can be particularly challenging, but needle-knife sphincterotomy on a bulging papilla is safe, as the stone protects the posteriorly located pancreatic orifice and often disimpacts, with dramatic relief of the obstruction (Fig. 46.9). Another technique involves gently closing a polypectomy snare above a small impacted papillary stone for expulsion.[69] Patients with a bulging intraduodenal portion of the papilla should also be suspected of harboring stones impacted at the distal common bile duct. The stone may disimpact on cannulation (Fig. 46.10). Alternatively, a balloon-tipped catheter can be positioned and inflated distal to the stone. Injection of contrast under pressure may then dislodge the stone proximally.

Biliary Stricture

When bile duct stones are upstream of a biliary stricture, stricture evaluation and management need to take place before stone extraction.

In cases where the stricture is suspected to be benign, balloon dilation up to the diameter of the normal-caliber bile duct can be considered, followed by attempted stone extraction. BML to crush the stones into much smaller fragments can facilitate complete stone removal. Often, however, placement of multiple plastic stents or a fully covered metal biliary stent to first dilate a downstream biliary stricture is needed before definitive stone management can be undertaken. As discussed, stent placement itself can facilitate future stone extraction by making stones smaller, most likely by a friction effect.[59]

Peroral Extracorporeal or Intracorporeal Lithotripsy

Large, hard biliary stones may fail extraction by conventional techniques for various reasons. The BML may not be able to fully open in a narrow duct or the stone exceeds the size of an open lithotriptor. Even after stone capture, BML wire or handle fracture may occur rarely. In such cases, shock wave lithotripsy delivered either extracorporeally (ESWL) or intracorporeally is needed. ESWL is performed with a prior endoscopically placed nasobiliary drain through which contrast injection for stone visualization and targeting are possible under fluoroscopy. In contemporary series, bile duct clearance can be achieved in 85% to 90% of patients over three sessions.[70,71] Adverse events include pain, hemobilia, and cholangitis in up to 35% of patients.

Alternatively, lithotripsy can be guided by direct peroral cholangioscopy (see Chapter 27) so that stones are fragmented under direct visualization to avoid ductal injury. A variety of cholangioscopes are available, such as the traditional mother-baby videocholangioscope, an ultraslim upper endoscope (direct peroral cholangioscopy), and a digital single-operator cholangioscope called SpyGlass DS direct visualization system (Boston Scientific). Each device has its inherent advantages and pitfalls, such as degree of tip deflection control, ease of biliary duct cannulation, visual resolution, enhanced imaging function, durability, and cost. Both holmium:YAG laser and electrohydraulic lithotripsy (EHL) fibers are effective at fragmenting large bile duct stones (Video 46.2). Often during lithotripsy, large amounts of stone fragments are created, necessitating generous duct irrigation, which, however, may result in a showering effect of small stones throughout the biliary tree and transient cholangitis. Judicial use of irrigation with regular aspiration is therefore recommended. Overall clearance rates of stones ≥15 mm ranging from 85% to 100% and adverse events rates between 1% and 7% have been reported using a variety of cholangioscopes for guidance of EHL and laser lithotripsy.[72–74]

Direct comparisons between ESWL and intraductal lithotripsy are few, but in one randomized trial of 60 patients, intraductal lithotripsy achieved higher overall bile duct clearance rates requiring fewer numbers of sessions, while the incidence of adverse events was comparable.[75] We also favor the use of intraductal lithotripsy, which can also be useful in patients with Mirizzi syndrome, where a large stone has eroded through the gallbladder neck into the bile duct. In these cases, the distal bile duct is often small and the stone too big to be engaged by BML.

Hepaticolithiasis

Intrahepatic duct stones, in association with biliary strictures from either recurrent pyogenic cholangitis (see Chapter 50) or post–liver transplantation (see Chapter 44), are prevalent in Southeast Asia in comparison to the West. They are technically challenging to treat, with complications including stone recurrence, cholangitis, liver abscess, secondary biliary cirrhosis, and cholangiocarcinoma. Management should be multidisciplinary. From a Japanese nationwide survey encompassing 40 years of experience and another single-center Korean study, stone extraction by ERCP resulted in more residual and recurrent stones than after percutaneous transhepatic cholangioscopic lithotripsy, which was in turn inferior to surgery.[76,77] Specifically, presence of biliary strictures was a significant risk factor (OR 4.43; $p = 0.02$) for stone recurrence after ERCP stone extraction. In the percutaneous approach, several days after access is achieved, single-stage or multistage dilation to accommodate various devices, including cholangioscopes, into the bile duct can be performed. After allowing for ~7 to 10 days for tract maturation, small stones can be grasped and removed by Dormia baskets, whereas larger ones can be directly visualized and fragmented by intraductal EHL or laser lithotripsy, with stone clearance rates between 60% and 85% and recurrence rates of hepaticolithiasis and/or cholangitis between 20% and 60%.[77,78] Another percutaneous approach through a mature T-tube tract for patients with retained stones after an operative bile duct exploration is also feasible. A novel method obviating the need for tract dilation and therefore useful in patients at risk for bleeding involves using an 8-Fr triple-lumen catheter to pass a fiberoptic probe to visualize lithotripsy of a target stone by a holmium:YAG laser fiber (Video 46.3).[79] Finally, although more invasive, hepatic resection is a more durable treatment and should be considered, particularly in cases with frequent recurrences, if strictures and stones are confined to one liver segment or lobe when the involved liver has become atrophic and when cholangiocarcinoma is suspected or diagnosed. In comparison to a historical cohort of open liver resections, robotic liver resections for primary hepaticolithiasis were recently shown to have shorter duration of hospitalization, with no differences in residual or recurrent stone rates.[80] An algorithm for managing hepaticolithiasis taking into consideration patient comorbidities, liver function status, and distribution of stones and strictures has been proposed by Cheon et al.[77]

CONCLUSIONS

Diagnostic evaluation of the biliary tract has expanded to highly accurate noninvasive modalities such as MRC and EUS. For the majority of bile duct stones, conventional extraction devices and techniques are highly successful and safe for complete stone extraction. For stones that are difficult to remove due to challenging access or unique stone or duct characteristics, advanced techniques continue to be refined. Failure to completely clear bile duct stones by endoscopic means is becoming exceedingly rare.

The complete reference list for this chapter can be found online at www.expertconsult.com.

47

Pancreaticobiliary Pain and Suspected Sphincter of Oddi Dysfunction

Paul R. Tarnasky and Robert H. Hawes

The diagnosis and treatment of sphincter of Oddi dysfunction (SOD) presents a significant challenge. This chapter is intended to provide readers with a practical guide to the evaluation and management of patients with pancreaticobiliary-type pain and suspected SOD by providing a pragmatic approach to the clinical evaluation and decisions regarding treatment. The specific goals are to (1) describe pancreaticobiliary pain patterns; (2) define SOD and the clinical presentations in which SOD should be considered; (3) describe a rational initial evaluation for patients with suspected SOD; (4) provide guidance for physician decisions regarding management of SOD; (5) describe techniques of sphincter of Oddi manometry (SOM) and endoscopic treatment of SOD; and (6) reinforce the risks inherent to the patient undergoing endoscopic evaluation of SOD and how these risks can be minimized. It should be emphasized that until recently, there has been a paucity of quality data to guide clinicians in this arena, especially on type III patients. There are now more robust data available to derive evidence-based recommendations.

Clinical syndromes that may be attributed to SOD range from functional disorders with purely subjective symptomatology to structural disorders having objective pathologic features. Functional and structural SOD diagnoses are widely divergent with regard to their presentation and management. Unexplained upper abdominal pain and idiopathic acute recurrent pancreatitis represent the most important examples at each end of this spectrum; this review will focus on unexplained upper abdominal pain, a functional disorder. Other clinical scenarios that may be associated with SOD include chronic acalculous cholecystitis, early chronic pancreatitis, biliary pancreatitis, postoperative bile leak, and pancreatic fistula.

DEFINITIONS

Confusing terminology and varied clinical presentations partly explain the complexity regarding SOD. *Biliary dyskinesia* is the encompassing term for a group of disorders with acalculous biliary-type pain. Subgroup diagnoses include chronic acalculous cholecystitis, gallbladder dyskinesia, cystic duct syndrome, and SOD. SOD may occur in patients with or without a gallbladder but is most commonly diagnosed in patients with postcholecystectomy symptoms.

Attempts have been made to develop consensus on defining the signs and symptoms of SOD, culminating in the latest iteration of the Rome criteria (Rome IV).[1] Diagnostic criteria for biliary pain and functional gallbladder disorders are listed in Box 47.1. The Rome criteria are meant to provide a general framework for clinicians but obviously do not describe all patients. A unifying symptom, present in all patients

Video for this chapter can be found online at www.expertconsult.com.

with SOD, is pain. When evaluating a patient with possible SOD, the most important aspect of the evaluation is the history. It is imperative that the clinician gain a clear understanding of the nature, location, and timing of pain. The Rome criteria specify that the pain should be intermittent, with pain-free intervals. Although typical biliary pain is classically intermittent, in some cases patients will have constant low-grade discomfort with exacerbations. The concept of chronic biliary pain is thought to be related to heightened visceral hypersensitivity, altered central nervous system processing, and/or generalized motility disorders.[2] Patients with more persistent pain should undergo careful review and extensive evaluation for other causes of pain (Box 47.2) but should not be arbitrarily excluded from evaluation for SOD based solely on there being a constant component to their pain. However, if associated symptoms such as nausea, vomiting, abdominal distension, or bowel dysfunction are dominant, the patient likely does not have SOD. Based on observations and after developing correlations between patients' presentations and outcomes after endoscopic sphincterotomy, Joseph Geenen, Walter Hogan, and Wylie Dodds published what have come to be known as the Geenen-Hogan (G-H) criteria (Table 47.1).[3] These have been modified over the years but provide a guide for clinicians to direct their evaluation and decision making. The original criteria were applied to patients who had previously undergone cholecystectomy

BOX 47.2 Diagnoses to Consider (Other Than Sphincter of Oddi Dysfunction) for Unexplained Upper Abdominal Pain

- Esophageal
  - Spasm or other motility disorder
  - Esophagitis
- Gastric
  - Gastroparesis
  - Ulcer
  - Hiatal hernia
  - Volvulus
  - Pyloric stenosis
- Duodenal
  - Stricture
  - Ulcer
  - Diverticulitis
  - Ampullary neoplasm
- Biliary
  - Stone
  - Benign stricture
  - Sump syndrome
  - Neoplasm
- Pancreatic
  - Chronic pancreatitis
  - Neoplasm
- Abdominal wall
  - Neuroma
  - Myopathy/myositis
- Irritable bowel syndrome

BOX 47.3 Important History Questions for Suspected Sphincter of Oddi Dysfunction

- When did the attacks begin?
- When do the attacks occur?
- Where is the pain?
- Where does the pain radiate?
- What is associated with the attacks?
- What has been done to investigate the cause?
- What has been done to treat the attacks?
- What are the consequences of the attacks?

BOX 47.4 Clinical Details Pertinent to Sphincter of Oddi Dysfunction

Laboratory and Pathology
- Serum liver and pancreas chemistries
- Serum fasting triglyceride
- Gallbladder pathology

Imaging
- Transabdominal ultrasonography
- Computed tomography
- Magnetic resonance cholangiopancreatography
- Biliary scintigraphy
- Endoscopic ultrasonography
- Intraoperative cholangiography

Previous Treatment
- Surgical
  - Cholecystectomy
  - Biliary bypass
  - Pseudocyst drainage
  - Pancreatic bypass or resection
  - Partial gastrectomy
  - Gastric bypass
- Endoscopic
  - Biliary sphincterotomy
  - Pancreatic sphincterotomy
- Stenting

TABLE 47.1 Geenen-Hogan Classification for Sphincter of Oddi Dysfunction

Type	Typical Pain	LFT >2X Normal	BD Diameter >10 mm
I	+	+	+
II	+	+	−
II	+	−	+
III	+	−	−

BD, Bile duct; *LFT*, liver function test.

and were based on three factors that could be assessed without endoscopic retrograde cholangiopancreatography (ERCP): (1) presence of "typical" pancreatic-type or biliary-type pain, (2) presence or absence of elevated liver or pancreas tests during or shortly after an episode of pain (that returned to normal when the pain subsided), and (3) presence or absence of bile and/or pancreatic duct dilation. The original criteria also included measurement of pancreatic and biliary drainage times, but these are no longer considered valid.[4,5]

The G-H criteria defined three subtypes and are important because they represent a framework around which a clinician can plan patient evaluation. If one obtains an appropriate history of pain, bile duct imaging should be obtained and the patient should be given a prescription directing health care providers (in an emergency room, hospital laboratory, or clinic) to obtain a liver panel and pancreatic tests (amylase and/or lipase) during or shortly after a pain episode. These data then can be used to stratify patients as to their likelihood of having SOD.

CLINICAL EVALUATION IN PATIENTS WITH SUSPECTED SOD

The first step is a detailed review of prior health care encounters pertinent to the clinical presentation, with a focus on questions of when, where, and what (Box 47.3). A complete history and thorough review of records will define the clinical symptoms, reveal what tests have been done, what treatments (surgical, endoscopic, medical) have been tried, and what the impact has been on the patient. Patients with unexplained symptoms that may be attributed to SOD often end up undergoing a

massive assault, which may diagnostic and therapeutic. It can be helpful to organize objective data regarding prior laboratory testing, imaging, and treatments (Box 47.4).

Some historical details may indicate that SOD is likely. It is common for SOD patients to have undergone cholecystectomy because of a "diseased" or "dysfunctional" gallbladder in the absence of documented cholelithiasis, preoperatively or postoperatively. Symptomatic patients who have a history of common bile duct exploration, postoperative bile leak, and/or post-ERCP pancreatitis (PEP) are at times discovered to have SOD.

Pain is a subjective complaint, especially the severity. Nevertheless, important information can be obtained by carefully defining the character of the pain. SOD should be considered only when there is typical biliary pain with classic features as follows: spontaneous in nature, epigastric or right upper quadrant in location, and intermittent with pain-free intervals lasting 30 minutes or longer. Patients may be awakened from sleep because of pain. It is common for postcholecystectomy patients to describe their symptoms as "my gallbladder pain" and even describe symptoms that are "worse than my gallbladder attacks."

Transient elevations of serum liver and/or pancreas enzymes drawn hours after pain onset may suggest SOD. The key to this criterion is documentation of normal tests before and/or after the elevation associated with a pain episode. In this era of an "obesity epidemic," one must be careful to evaluate patients with abdominal pain and "abnormal" liver tests. Persistently elevated liver tests in an obese patient with upper abdominal pain is more likely to be related to fatty liver; the pain is caused by capsular tension and patients are often seen splinting and/ or leaning to the side to relieve it.

The criterion of bile duct dilation also has pitfalls. Bile duct dilation associated with persistently abnormal liver tests should raise a suspicion for neoplasia or bile duct stones and prompt endoscopic ultrasonography (EUS) and/or magnetic resonance cholangiopancreatography (MRCP). Alternatively, a dilated bile duct with normal liver tests in a patient with intermittent pain should raise suspicion for SOD. Patients with a history of chronic narcotic analgesic use may develop a dilated bile duct, but these patients generally have chronic pain, not typical biliary colic. In summary, a careful symptom history and diagnostic testing should be directed at the comprehensive list of differential diagnoses for upper abdominal pain listed in Box 47.2 before considering SOD.

Patients with unexplained upper abdominal pain and suspected SOD should be categorized as to the likelihood of having SOD and the likelihood of having a favorable response to endoscopic treatment. The G-H classification (see Table 47.1) is the standard in this regard. Some experts further subtype SOD into biliary and pancreatic categories, but there may be some overlap. Type I SOD patients have objective evidence of impaired drainage and are more likely to have structural obstruction (papillary stenosis). In addition to characteristic pain, they have dilated ducts and transiently abnormal serum liver/pancreas enzymes during and/or shortly after episodes of pain.

Patients with type II SOD have characteristic pain and either a dilated duct or abnormal serum liver/pancreas enzymes with pain. Type III SOD patients have typical biliary or pancreatic pain but no objective evidence of impaired drainage. The G-H classification has been considered useful because it appears to predict the chance of finding an abnormal SOM and having a favorable outcome after sphincterotomy[6] (Table 47.2). Recently, a randomized trial directed specifically at G-H type III patients (Evaluating Predictors & Interventions in Sphincter of Oddi Dysfunction [EPISOD] study) has called into question whether type III SOD exists (see discussion of EPISOD trial in "Endoscopic" section).

Once a clinical impression of SOD is established, ideally a noninvasive test can confirm the clinical impression before proceeding to ERCP. Several tests have been studied and individual centers have reported good correlation with SOM and/or sphincterotomy. The problem is that when these tests are evaluated on a broader scale, their accuracy does not match previous single-center reports. The Hopkins group first reported on the accuracy of dynamic (quantitative) biliary scintigraphy.[7,8] The test was designed to measure delayed bile flow through the ampulla by assessing the time it takes for the radionuclide to reach the duodenum. These authors found a good correlation with SOM. Their results were supported by Corazziari et al.[9] This prompted the Hopkins group to suggest that scintigraphy could substitute for SOM.[10] However, when this test was evaluated in normal volunteers, it was found to have very poor specificity and little value in excluding SOD in patients suspected to suffer from this disorder.[11] Cicala et al. reported a small retrospective study in which biliary scintigraphy was superior to SOM for predicting favorable outcomes after biliary sphincterotomy.[12]

Another test hypothesized to detect SOD is fatty meal sonography (FMS). An abnormal test is defined as >2 mm dilation of the bile duct 45 minutes after ingestion of a standardized "fatty meal." Rosenblatt et al. compared SOM, FMS, and hepatobiliary scintigraphy (HBS) in a retrospective comparative study.[13] Poor correlation was observed between FMS and HBS with SOM. However, among the patients with abnormal SOM who had a good long-term response to sphincterotomy, 85% (11 of 13) had an abnormal FMS and HBS. Another small prospective study evaluated the utility of secretin-stimulated MRCP (ssMRCP) to diagnose and predict treatment responses in patients with suspected SOD.[14] Type II patients with a positive ssMRCP (a persistent increase in ductal diameter of ≥1 mm) were more likely to improve after sphincterotomy. Thus perhaps noninvasive tests should be further evaluated as to whether they predict response to sphincterotomy rather than whether they correlate with SOM.

UPPER ABDOMINAL PAIN WITH GALLBLADDER IN SITU

Management of patients with biliary-type pain without evidence of gallstones on standard imaging represents a challenge. Physicians (including surgeons) and patients usually prefer to identify some proof of gallbladder pathology before considering cholecystectomy. Biliary crystal analysis can be performed on bile collected from the duodenum or bile duct after cholecystokinin (CCK) stimulation. EUS is more sensitive for discovering biliary sludge and can also be used to assess for evidence of concomitant chronic pancreatitis that could explain the cause of pain.[15,16] If EUS and CCK-stimulated biliary drainage are performed and biliary crystals or gallbladder sludge is found, >90% of patients will have resolution of pain after cholecystectomy.[17] Also, good outcomes are reported when biliary scintigraphy reveals evidence of chronic acalculous cholecystitis (gallbladder ejection fraction <35%).[18] Empiric cholecystectomy, however, will benefit about three-fourths of those patients with classic biliary pain, independent of other testing.[19-23]

The exact role for SOM in this setting is not established. There has been limited study of the prevalence of SOD in patients with gallbladder in situ. Guelrud reported on 121 patients with biliary pain and a finding of gallstones but a normal-caliber bile duct by ultrasonography.[24] ERCP and SOM were performed, and elevated basal sphincter pressures were found in 14 patients (11.6%). Interestingly, 4% of patients in this group with a normal alkaline phosphatase had elevated basal sphincter pressures, whereas 40% with an elevated alkaline phosphatase were found to have SOD. Ruffolo et al. investigated 81 patients with typical biliary-type pain and a normal gallbladder ultrasonography.[25] When ERCP and SOM were performed, 53% of these patients had SOD, as diagnosed by elevated basal sphincter pressures. For the whole group, 49% had an abnormal ejection fraction on gallbladder scintigraphy, but the finding of SOD did not correlate with ejection fraction. All patients in this group with elevated sphincter pressures underwent biliary sphincterotomy and the short-term results for pain relief (1 year) were quite good.

TABLE 47.2   Correlation Between Geenen-Hogan Criteria, Results of Sphincter of Oddi Manometry, and Outcome With Sphincterotomy[6]

	Type I	Type II	Type III
Definition	Pain + 3 criteria	Pain + 1 or 2 criteria	Pain only
Baseline pressure >40 mm Hg	70% to 100%	40% to 86%	20% to 55%
Benefit from sphincterotomy	55% to 91%	p >40 mm Hg: 80% to 90% p <40 mm Hg: 30% to 35%	p >40 mm Hg: 8% to 56%

However, with longer-term follow-up, most patients ultimately required cholecystectomy.[26]

The recommended approach is to avoid SOM in patients with gallbladder in situ, because biliary dyskinesia is much more prevalent than SOD. Also, it is likely that SOM is unreliable at predicting response to sphincterotomy in patients with a normal-caliber bile duct and normal liver tests. However, ERCP with SOM may be reasonable where typical biliary pain is accompanied by transient elevations of liver enzymes.

INFORMED CONSENT FOR ERCP FOR SUSPECTED SOD

Most important to any discussion of suspected SOD is informed consent. Proper informed consent before ERCP in a patient with suspected SOD is in itself a complex venture. "Informed" means that both the physician and the patient have a thorough understanding of the clinical situation before determining the potential risks and benefits. The physician's role is largely limited to acquiring and sharing information. Information that is relayed to the patient includes a review of relevant data (if any) regarding efficacy and safety of endoscopic treatment. It may be just as important to disclose the fact that efficacy data are sparse. Fortunately, we do have reasonable data regarding adverse events of ERCP in suspected SOD (see section "Prevention of Post-ERCP Pancreatitis"). The physician should share his or her own adverse events data that are specific to that situation. For example, it is inappropriate to state adverse event data either for other endoscopists or for other clinical situations (e.g., bile duct stones). At present it remains particularly important that patients with purely functional symptoms who have no objective evidence of digestive duct obstruction understand that they are making a benefit–risk decision that pertains to a quality-of-life problem. Patients should understand that they are ultimately responsible for giving their consent and they should not depend solely on "physician advice."

SPHINCTER OF ODDI MANOMETRY: EQUIPMENT AND TECHNIQUE (SEE CHAPTER 16)

Traditionally, SOM can be performed with either a water-perfused or solid-state catheter. Cost and durability issues with the solid-state systems have limited their use, combined with a lack of values for "normal." Water-perfused systems require a catheter, water pump, and manometry system.

The primary catheter used consists of three lumens, two of which terminate in a side hole of the catheter, whereas the third lumen has both a side port and an end port (Cook Endoscopy, Winston-Salem, NC) (Fig. 47.1). The lumen with the end port accommodates a 0.018-inch or 0.021-inch guidewire. All three channels can be used for the manometry recording, but a randomized study showed that sacrificing the manometry recording lumen with side and end ports while using it for aspiration during a pancreatic manometry significantly reduced the postmanometry pancreatitis rate.[27] It was found that aspiration during manometry of the biliary sphincter was not necessary.[28]

The technique of SOM is relatively straightforward. A baseline is established (duodenal pressure). The catheter is then advanced deeply into the desired duct. The catheter is slowly withdrawn while continuously recording the pressures. A sustained elevation above 35 to 40 mm Hg in 2 or 3 leads is considered abnormal. One "weakness" in SOM is that interpretation of recordings is not standardized. Most people accept 40 mm Hg or greater as being abnormal, yet the largest study looking at normal values suggests that 35 mm Hg is a better figure.[29] Various systems are used to obtain an actual value for the basal sphincter pressure. The Indiana group advocates taking the nadir value for the four lowest nadirs over a 30-second run and then averaging those values.[30] There

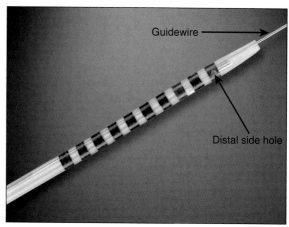

FIG 47.1 Distal tip of sphincter of Oddi manometry catheter. *Top arrow* points to the guidewire. *Bottom arrow* points to the distal side hole.

is consensus, however, that there should be a sustained time (most agree on 30 seconds) during which the nadir of the phasic waves does not dip below 40 mm Hg.

A controversial part of SOM has been the type of sedation and adjunctive medications used while performing it. In the past, "conscious" (moderate) sedation was employed for ERCP using a combination of narcotics and benzodiazepines. It is known that narcotics affect intestinal motility and sphincter recordings, and they were initially avoided during SOM. Sedation for ERCP/SOM with benzodiazepines alone was often suboptimal, and credit should be given to Grace Elta and her colleagues at the University of Michigan, who challenged the need to avoid narcotics.[31] In a small, limited study they found that basal sphincter pressures (the values used to determine whether manometry is normal or abnormal) were not affected by meperidine at a dose of 1 mg/kg. This finding was confirmed by a larger study done at Indiana University.[32] Currently, virtually all ERCPs are done with deep sedation using propofol. Several animal studies have demonstrated that propofol does not affect SOM in dogs and sheep.[33,34] However, only one human study has been reported and it involved only 11 patients. This study concluded that propofol did not alter basal sphincter of Oddi pressures.[35] In some cases, duodenal motility can make cannulation very difficult. Although glucagon (Eli Lilly, Indianapolis, IN) is used routinely in standard ERCP to control duodenal movement, it cannot be used during SOM as it affects sphincter pressures. If it is impossible to cannulate without the aid of glucagon, it is recommended that 5 minutes pass between the dose of glucagon and manometry recording.

TREATMENT OF SOD

When considering treatment options for SOD and their associated outcomes, it is imperative to understand several concepts:
1. The measured outcomes should be validated and the principal outcome should include an assessment of the principal problem, that is, pain.
2. Treatment and assessment of outcomes should be considered only for patients who are strongly considered to have SOD symptoms.
3. The expected outcomes should be realistic, as rarely do medical interventions achieve a "cure" in the majority of patients. If the desired outcome of cure is unlikely, other parameters such as patient satisfaction should be considered.

Medical

Medical therapy has not been widely studied as a treatment for SOD. Because the sphincter of Oddi is a smooth muscle structure, it makes some sense that pharmacologic therapy may be of benefit. If the theory is correct that SOD falls into functional and structural categories, medications would then be of benefit only for those with functional disease. Empiric pharmacologic trials are most reasonable in patients with relatively mild and infrequent episodes of pain. The drugs most studied in SOD are calcium channel blockers and nitrates. Khuroo et al. investigated nifedipine in a placebo-controlled crossover trial in 28 patients.[36] Endpoints for the study included reductions in pain scores, emergency room visits, and use of oral pain medication. Seventy-five percent of 28 patients responded to nifedipine. Sand et al. looked at the effects of three calcium channel blockers with differing smooth muscle selectivity (verapamil, nifedipine, and felodipine) on human sphincter of Oddi contractions.[37] Results showed that all three calcium channel blockers were potent inhibitors of contraction, and it was concluded that this category of drugs may be helpful in SOD. Sand et al. performed a 16-week double-blind crossover study using nifedipine in G-H type II patients and showed that it decreased the number of days that patients experienced pain.[38] A slow-release form of nifedipine was tested in a small pilot study in patients with SOD, with encouraging early results.[39] Although nitrates have been studied experimentally, there is very little human data regarding its use in SOD. Gocer et al. found that isosorbide dinitrate decreased rhythmic and tonic contraction in guinea pig–isolated sphincter of Oddi muscle.[40] Bar-Meir et al. described the disappearance of pain as well as a decrease in both basal and phasic sphincter activity on repeat manometry after nitrate therapy in a woman with manometry-proven papillary dysfunction.[41] Finally, Wehrmann et al. looked at topical application of nitrates onto the papilla of Vater and found that topically applied nitrates profoundly inhibited sphincter of Oddi motility.[42]

The new "drug" on the block may be nitric oxide (NO). NO plays an important role in the regulation of intestinal and pancreaticobiliary motility. Inhibition of NO synthase (NOS) increases intraluminal pressure within the gastrointestinal tract. Bak et al. investigated the effect of an inhibitor of NOS, NG-Nitro-L-arginine methyl ester (L-NAME), on the mean basal pressure of the sphincter of Oddi in an anesthetized pig.[43] It was found that L-NAME significantly increased mean sphincter of Oddi pressure in this animal model and the physiologic affect was sustained for the duration of the experiment (3 hours). Noting that topical administration of an NO donor induced sphincter of Oddi relaxation in humans, Niiyama et al. looked at the effect of intrasphincteric injection of sodium nitroprusside (SNP) on the pig sphincter of Oddi.[44] They found that intrasphincteric injection of SNP significantly reduced mean basal pressures, which lasted up to 45 minutes without inducing side effects or significantly lowering blood pressure. Research is ongoing to develop pharmaceutical agents that will generate NO, and these may serve as potential treatments for SOD.[45]

Despite some promising developments, medical therapy for sphincter of Oddi is still problematic for a number of reasons:
1. Current therapy, particularly nitrates, has a significant side effect profile (especially headache).
2. There is a lack of long-term data.
3. The variability of response may be because of our inability to differentiate between fixed stenosis and functional spasm.

To establish medical therapy for SOD, well-conducted, placebo-controlled, randomized trials with long-term follow-up will need to be performed. The ideal drug would be specific for the sphincter of Oddi, be long acting, and possess a low side effect profile.[46]

Endoscopic

Endoscopic therapy with sphincterotomy has been the most widely employed treatment for SOD. Endoscopic stenting as a trial and/or treatment was shown by some to have some predictive benefits but is not recommended because of an increased risk for PEP.[47,48] When assessing outcomes after endoscopic sphincterotomy, specifics of the patient population (subjective and objective criteria) and the exact nature of the intervention (biliary or dual sphincterotomy) must be taken into account.

There was only one study that focused on sphincterotomy solely in G-H type I patients.[49] This was a relatively small study population of 17 patients with biliary-type pain, dilated bile duct, and abnormal liver tests during episodes of pain. At ERCP, only 65% had abnormal basal sphincter pressures with SOM but all benefited from biliary sphincterotomy with a mean of 2.3 years of follow-up. There are other anecdotal reports of successful outcomes (85% improvement) with biliary sphincterotomy for type I SOD, most of which also suggested that SOM is not necessary.[50,51]

The strongest data supporting the efficacy of endoscopic intervention are contained in three randomized trials,[52–54] two of which[52,54] included only G-H type II patients who underwent either sham therapy or biliary sphincterotomy alone. In the landmark study by Geenen et al., all patients underwent ERCP with SOM and all were randomized to either sham therapy or biliary sphincterotomy (the endoscopist was blinded to the results of the manometry).[52] The results helped validate both the predictive capability of SOM and the benefit of sphincterotomy. The patients with normal SOM did not benefit from sphincterotomy, but those with abnormal basal sphincter pressures did. The important take-home points of this trial are:
1. Only type II patients were included.
2. Patients underwent biliary sphincterotomy alone.
3. Those patients with abnormal basal sphincter pressures treated with sphincterotomy benefited significantly more than those with normal sphincter of Oddi pressures treated with sham or sphincterotomy.

The Toouli et al. study[54] was designed somewhat similarly to the Geenen study. It included only G-H type II patients and involved randomization of all patients to sham therapy or biliary sphincterotomy. In this trial, however, if the manometry was initially normal, the patients were "provoked" with CCK in an effort to detect a subset of patients with "functional" SOD. The outcomes were similar to the Geenen study: 85% of patients (11 of 13) with elevated basal sphincter pressures benefited from sphincterotomy, whereas only 38% of patients (5 of 13) benefited from sham therapy ($p = 0.041$). The outcomes were similar for both the sphincterotomy and the sham group who had normal SOM.

The Indiana trial, however, was distinctive for several reasons: it had a three-group randomization—sham therapy, endoscopic biliary sphincterotomy, and surgical (dual) sphincteroplasty—and the trial involved G-H type II and III patients.[53] The latter characteristic of the Indiana trial is particularly important, because most centers that have expertise in SOD see a predominance of G-H type III patients. However, this trial did not randomize all patients, only those with abnormal SOM. The results with 3-year follow-up revealed that 69% of patients in the endoscopic sphincterotomy and surgical sphincteroplasty groups benefited, compared with only 24% of patients in the sham therapy group ($p = 0.009$). Although surgical sphincteroplasty (SSP) is reserved primarily for those who fail endoscopic intervention, a recent publication provided long-term outcomes on 17 patients who underwent SSP for SOD.[55] Strong conclusions cannot be drawn from this report, because it was a small retrospective study, but overall pain scores were significantly reduced after SSP and median satisfaction was quite high at 95%. Patient selection is critical, and SSP should be considered in patients with failed endoscopic treatment or possibly in those with altered anatomy (e.g., surgical bypass for obesity).

Until recently, the most serious void in the SOD literature was the lack of well-designed trials that address whether SOM predicts outcome and whether sphincterotomy is beneficial in G-H type III patients. The EPISOD trial evaluated only suspected type III SOD patients and randomized patients to sphincterotomy or sham therapy, irrespective of the SOM results.[56] This was a very well-designed study sponsored by the National Institutes of Health (NIH) and has had a significant influence on the approach to the endoscopic evaluation and management of patients with pancreaticobiliary pain. Before the EPISOD study, investigators developed and validated a new pain assessment tool, named RAPID (Recurrent Abdominal Pain Intensity and Disability).[57] The tool measures the reduction in productivity for various daily activities as a result of abdominal pain, and it was the principal outcome in the EPISOD study. RAPID scores are graded 1 to 4 according to the days of lost productivity because of pain in the last 90 days. Six days or fewer is scored as grade 1, whereas 20 days or more is scored as grade 4.

The EPISOD trial randomized patients with suspected type III SOD to sphincterotomy or sham therapy in a 2:1 fashion. Patients with pancreatic SOD were further randomized to biliary sphincterotomy alone or dual (biliary and pancreatic) sphincterotomy independent of SOM results. All patients (including sham) were treated with prophylactic pancreatic stents to reduce PEP. Patients and study coordinators were blinded to treatment groups. Patients who did not wish to be randomized were treated and followed prospectively (EPISOD2). Success was strictly defined as meeting all of the following criteria: RAPID score grade 1 at both months 9 and 12, no narcotics during months 10 to 12, and no reintervention.

Results from the EPISOD study were sobering for enthusiasts of the endoscopic evaluation and management of SOD. Overall, the RAPID scores decreased in all patients, but there was no difference in success between sham and patients treated with sphincterotomy (37% vs 23%). The end-of-study scores for physical and mental health, anxiety, and depression also improved compared with baseline, but to a similar degree for treatment and sham groups. No factors were found to be predictive for success; these included demographics, psychosocial comorbidities, clinical history, pain characteristics, SOM results, and whether biliary alone or dual sphincterotomy was performed in those with pancreatic SOD. Study outcomes were also similar between groups even after loosening the criteria for defining success.

In light of the negative study results in EPISOD, the potential risks are even more noteworthy. PEP occurred in 12% overall, of which nearly half were moderate to severe; 2 patients experienced perforation. There were no differences in adverse events between treatment and sham groups.

The EPISOD study was an extremely well-designed study, resulted in a landmark article, and has provided very important guidance with regard to the management of patients with postcholecystectomy pain but without any objective evidence of biliary obstruction. There is now a growing consensus that type III SOD does not exist.[58]

Clearly, the results of EPISOD argue strongly against the existence of SOD III. There are, however, as with any study, some weaknesses of the trial. At baseline, many of the patients studied had irritable bowel syndrome and a pain history that would be atypical for purely biliary pain; half had daily pain with pain overall in 69 of the prior 90 days. Also, a significant minority (40%) of patients had baseline psychological comorbidities. Regarding the measured outcomes, criteria for success were very strict, pain alone was not the primary outcome, and satisfaction was not evaluated. The negative results of EPISOD should not be surprising when considering the example of elective cholecystectomy for symptomatic gallstones. Predictors of postoperative pain relief include classic pain (e.g., infrequent, severe, steady pain), whereas IBS, GERD, atypical pain, poor health and/or physical function, psychiatric illness, and somatization are associated with poor outcomes.[59–62] Although elective cholecystectomy is accepted therapy for suspected symptomatic

gallbladder disease, a significant minority (20% to 30%) report persistent postoperative pain.[63,64] However, 94% of patients were satisfied with the outcome after cholecystectomy despite complete relief of pain in only two-thirds.[65] It should therefore not be surprising that outcomes after therapy for suspected SOD are unsatisfactory when the symptoms are atypical and/or associated with other disorders.

One could now argue that classifying patients with postcholecystectomy pain into subgroups is not useful. It is plausible that SOD is characterized subjectively by symptomatic biliary pain either without or with a spectrum of objective evidence to support the diagnosis.

An important issue regarding endoscopic therapy in all patients with suspected SOD concerns the efficacy of biliary sphincterotomy alone versus combined biliary and pancreatic sphincterotomy. It is known from reports in which dual manometry has been performed that there is generally a concordance between pancreatic and biliary sphincter pressures. In the majority of cases, pressures in both are normal or abnormal. There is, however, some discordance that suggests that about 10% of the time there is isolated biliary sphincter hypertension and about 20% of the time there is isolated pancreatic sphincter hypertension.[66,67]

As mentioned earlier, the EPISOD trial reported no statistical difference between biliary sphincterotomy alone versus dual sphincterotomy in patients with pancreatic SOD. In the randomized study there was a trend, however, toward improved outcomes with dual sphincterotomy (30% success) versus biliary sphincterotomy alone (20% success).[56] Similar results were reported in the nonrandomized EPISOD2 study. Dual sphincterotomy resulted in 31% success versus 24% for biliary sphincterotomy alone and only 17% for no therapy; this may be a more reliable expected outcome in clinical practice. An older study from the University of Iowa looked at a group of 26 patients who had not responded to biliary sphincterotomy despite abnormal sphincter of Oddi motility.[68] Twenty-five of 26 patients underwent repeat ERCP and pancreatic sphincterotomy, and 16 of these patients (64%) responded. A study by Kaw et al.[69] (abstract form only) looked at biliary versus dual sphincterotomy and related it to which sphincter had abnormal manometry. For those with abnormal biliary manometry alone, 80% responded to biliary sphincterotomy. However, if isolated pancreatic sphincter hypertension or combined biliary and pancreatic sphincter hypertension were found, only 7 of 23 patients (30%) responded if they underwent biliary sphincterotomy alone. For patients who had isolated pancreatic sphincter hypertension or combined biliary and pancreatic sphincter abnormalities, 11 of 16 patients (69%) responded to dual sphincterotomy. Because of reasonably good results with biliary intervention alone and the risks of pancreatic manipulations, our preference is to focus efforts on biliary investigation and intervention initially and consider pancreatic evaluation later if there are recurrent/persistent symptoms.

Some investigators have tried botulinum toxin (Botox; Allergan Inc., Irvine, CA) injections directly into the sphincter as a substitute for SOM,[70] as a permanent treatment for SOD,[71,72] or to prevent PEP.[73] The presumption with botulinum toxin is that the pain of SOD comes from the sphincter itself, and by preventing tonic contraction, symptoms can be relieved. Sand et al.[74] demonstrated that botulinum toxin inhibited pig sphincter of Oddi smooth muscle contractions, and Wang et al.[75] showed that in dogs it reduced contractile activity for a prolonged time. The first clinical report of its use in SOD was by Wehrmann et al.[71] They injected 100 international units of botulinum toxin in 22 patients with manometrically documented SOD (all were G-H type III patients). Six weeks later, 55% of patients (12 of 22) were symptom-free and 45% of patients (10 of 22) were not. The 10 nonresponders underwent ERCP and biliary sphincterotomy. Five of these 10 patients had normalized their sphincter pressure and did not respond to biliary sphincterotomy with longer-term follow-up. Eleven of 12 initial responders relapsed at a median of 6 months. Repeat manometry revealed sphincter hypertension in all 11 patients, and all 11 responded to endoscopic sphincterotomy. This initial report has not been followed by a prospective randomized study. Gorelick et al.[73] found botulinum toxin to be effective at decreasing the risk of PEP in manometrically positive SOD patients; however, the incidence of pancreatitis was 25%, which is unacceptable in the era of pancreatic stenting.[76] There are several drawbacks to this approach:

1. Botulinum toxin has not been subjected to a randomized study in the way that manometry has, at least in G-H type II patients.
2. When botulinum toxin is used as a treatment for SOD, it is logical that its effect will be transient, as has been seen when botulinum toxin is used in achalasia patients.
3. When used as a predictor of response to sphincterotomy, it requires a second procedure, which exposes patients with suspected SOD to additional risks, especially pancreatitis.

In summary, there are inherent drawbacks to botulinum toxin use in SOD. The most important factors are that overall experience is very small and botulinum toxin has not been subjected to well-designed randomized studies with sufficient follow-up to determine efficacy. Although data are scant, botulinum toxin does not appear to be as effective as short-term pancreatic stenting at preventing PEP.

PREVENTION OF POST-ERCP PANCREATITIS

It was originally thought that it was the actual performance of SOM that caused PEP. We have come to learn, however, that there are patient and procedural risk factors involved (see Chapter 8). This was outlined in a study published by Freeman et al.[77] This landmark article clearly outlined risk factors for PEP, and most are related to the patients themselves (Box 47.5). Performance of ERCP, with or without manometry, in a young female patient with suspected SOD carries a very high risk of PEP. To date, the best study performed to assess the role of manometry itself as a causative factor in PEP reviewed 76 patients with suspected SOD undergoing SOM.[27] The group was randomized to manometry in the standard fashion with all three ports perfused with 0.25 mL of water per minute versus perfusion through two channels with simultaneous aspiration through the third channel (as mentioned earlier). A prior study proved that aspiration during SOM did not affect the manometry results.[78] This study was important because the procedure

BOX 47.5 Patient Factors Correlated With Increased Risk of Pancreatitis[77]

The criteria used were the following:
1. ALT and alkaline phosphatase more than twice the upper limit of normal
2. Dilated bile duct on sonography
3. Delayed drainage of contrast material at ERCP

Multivariate Analysis	p
Suspected SOD	<0.001
Younger age	<0.001

Univariate Analysis	p
History of ERCP-induced pancreatitis	<0.001
Female sex	<0.001
History of pancreatitis	<0.001
Distal bile duct diameter	0.02

ALT, Alanine aminotransferase; *ERCP,* endoscopic retrograde cholangiopancreatography; *SOD,* sphincter of Oddi dysfunction.
Data from Freeman ML, Nelson DB, Sherman S, et al. Complications of endoscopic biliary sphincterotomy. *N Engl J Med.* 1996;335:909–918.

consisted only of SOM and the patients did not undergo ERCP after the manometry was complete. Thus the study isolated SOM and recorded the incidence of PEP. The results showed that in the group being perfused the pancreatitis rate was 23.5%, whereas in the group undergoing aspiration the pancreatitis rate was 3% ($p = 0.01$); however, notably no prevention for pancreatitis was used at that time (stents or nonsteroidal antiinflammatory drugs [NSAIDs]). The recorded rate of pancreatitis in the aspiration group is an acceptable rate for PEP in general, and well below the rate generally quoted for patients with suspected SOD.

Current data suggest that the most important factor in reducing the risk of PEP in patients with suspected SOD reported to date is stenting of the pancreatic duct. Manipulation of the ampulla while performing ERCP (with or without sphincterotomy) is thought to cause swelling, resulting in compromise of pancreatic juice flow leading to pancreatitis. In a landmark study, patients with manometrically documented SOD were randomized to short-term pancreatic stenting versus no stent after biliary sphincterotomy.[79] The results showed that the stented group had a PEP rate of 7% compared with a rate of 26% in the nonstented group ($p = 0.03$). A number of other single studies and meta-analyses have proven the benefit of pancreatic stenting to prevent PEP.[80–84] Pancreatic stenting is not without potential problems. The original prospective trials used short 5-Fr stents that required endoscopic removal. In an effort to avoid a second procedure to remove stents, stents with no flap on the pancreatic side have become the standard. Short pancreatic stents without a flap typically migrate within 1 to 2 weeks and are equally effective at preventing PEP.[85] Many experts favor the use of smaller-caliber (3 or 4 Fr), longer (8, 10, or 12 cm) pancreatic stents for this indication for the same reason. These stents have a pigtail on the duodenal side and no retention flap on the pancreatic side. These stents typically fall out within 2 to 3 weeks and can be checked by obtaining a "plain film of the abdomen to include the diaphragms" 3 weeks after the procedure. The main reason for using small-caliber stents is their softness and flexibility; moreover, they are associated with less iatrogenic ductal damage compared with larger stents.[86,87] Three-French stents also predictably stay in place for at least 72 hours, which is probably the time frame necessary to prevent PEP. The main drawback to the use of 3-Fr stents is the need for a 0.18-inch or 0.21-inch guidewire that must be passed to the tail of the pancreas. The ductal conformation ultimately determines the length of the stent one can use. If the main pancreatic duct makes a sigmoid-shaped or 360-degree turn (ansa loop), one should use a short (2 to 3 cm) 5-Fr stent with the internal (pancreatic side) flap(s) removed.

Although controversial and not yet subjected to a randomized trial, current retrospective data suggest that pancreatic stenting is helpful in preventing PEP in those patients found to have a normal SOM.[88] More recent data strengthen this position. A retrospective, nonrandomized review of 403 patients with suspected SOD but normal SOM was conducted.[89] One hundred and sixty-nine patients had a pancreatic duct stent placed (group 1) and 234 did not (group 2). The PEP rate was 2.4% in group 1 and 9% in group 2 ($p = 0.006$).

The reason for this is unknown, but the risk of PEP is inherent in patients *with suspected SOD* and not just in those proven to have SOD with abnormal manometry. Also, our data show that 42% of patients with suspected SOD who have a normal manometry at their index ERCP have an abnormal manometry if they return for a repeat examination, suggesting that the initial manometry may have been falsely negative.[90] Although current evidence is not robust, our recommendation is that a short-term pancreatic stent be placed in all patients deemed to be at high risk for PEP.

Multiple trials have been conducted to look at pharmacologic means to prevent PEP. With the exception of rectal administration of NSAIDs, these studies have been negative. A recent and somewhat controversial study has strengthened the position for use of rectal indomethacin to prevent PEP.[91] A multicenter, randomized, placebo-controlled, double-blind clinical trial randomized patients at high risk for PEP to a single 50-mg dose of indomethacin administered rectally immediately after ERCP or placebo. Approximately 80% of patients in both groups also underwent pancreatic stenting. The PEP rate in the treatment group was 9.2% compared with 16.9% in the placebo group ($p = 0.005$). The severity of the PEP was also less in the treatment group. The benefit of indomethacin was seen independent of whether or not a pancreatic stent was placed. These data, combined with a number of meta-analyses, have made administration of rectal indomethacin (before or after ERCP) in patients at high risk for PEP the standard of care.[92–96] The European Society of Gastrointestinal Endoscopy (ESGE) has gone so far as to put in its guidelines that rectal indomethacin should be administered to all patients undergoing ERCP.[97]

EVALUATION OF PATIENTS WITH RECURRENT PAIN AFTER ENDOSCOPIC INTERVENTION FOR SPHINCTER OF ODDI DYSFUNCTION

Little data exist and there are no randomized trials on the optimal management of patients who have recurrent pain after endoscopic intervention for SOD. Potential findings with reinvestigation include:

1. Incomplete prior biliary sphincterotomy
2. Residual pancreatic sphincter hypertension
3. Restenosis of the pancreatic sphincter
4. Completely normal examination
5. Evidence of early chronic pancreatitis

If patients experienced a long-term response to endoscopic therapy for SOD and re-present with significant pain, ERCP with SOM should be considered. In a study by Elton et al., pancreatic manometry was performed after biliary sphincterotomy in patients with SOD.[98] If pancreatic sphincter hypertension was found, pancreatic sphincterotomy was performed. The results showed that 73% of patients had complete resolution of symptoms after the index ERCP and an additional 18% showed partial or transient change. Only 8% of these G-H type I and II SOD patients had no change in symptoms. These results are somewhat better than other reports in the literature. Additionally, Eversman et al. looked at long-term follow-up after biliary sphincterotomy and correlated it with the SOM results.[99] In this study, 37 patients had isolated biliary sphincter hypertension and only 16% required reintervention. In a group of 62 patients who had elevated biliary and pancreatic basal pressures, 29% required reintervention. For the 33 patients who had isolated pancreatic sphincter hypertension (and underwent a biliary sphincterotomy alone), 39% required reintervention.

This concept of improved outcomes with dual sphincterotomy when pancreatic sphincter hypertension is present was further investigated by Park et al.[100] In this report, there was no significant difference in outcome when comparing dual sphincterotomy versus biliary sphincterotomy alone in patients with isolated biliary sphincter hypertension. Interestingly, there was also no difference between dual and biliary sphincterotomy alone in patients who had both abnormal biliary and abnormal pancreatic sphincter pressures. However, there was a significant difference in the rate of reintervention in patients with isolated abnormal pancreatic sphincter pressures (21% vs 39%, $p = 0.05$).

In summary, it does appear that outcomes can be improved if pancreatic sphincterotomy is performed in patients with documented pancreatic sphincter hypertension. However, definitive recommendations await appropriate randomized trials.

CONCLUSIONS

The evaluation and treatment of patients with suspected SOD remains a challenge. Obtaining a detailed history is a critical step, and evaluation for other causes of upper abdominal pain should be carefully undertaken. Empiric medical trials for endoscopically and radiologically negative diseases (gastroesophageal reflux disease, irritable bowel syndrome) should be tried. However, with an appropriate history and a failure to respond to empiric interventions, one should consider SOD. With current data, the caliber of the bile and pancreatic duct should be determined and a liver panel, amylase and/or lipase, should be obtained during or immediately after a severe attack.

With this information, the patient can be categorized into a G-H category (type I, II, or III). Because 90% of G-H type I respond to sphincterotomy and appear to have a low incidence of PEP, these patients should undergo sphincterotomy and do not require SOM. Type II patients should undergo manometry, because randomized trials have proven that manometry is an accurate discriminator of those who will respond to sphincterotomy. Patients with suspected SOD but without any objective evidence of biliary obstruction (type III) continue to be challenging. Recent data argue against ERCP in this setting, and any severe adverse events after ERCP might be legally challenged, because the ERCP might be considered "outside the standard of care," especially since publication of the EPISOD trial. Patients undergoing ERCP for suspected SOD are at high risk for PEP and should undergo short-term pancreatic stenting, and periprocedural NSAIDs should be considered, even if their manometry is normal. The need for dual manometry, combined with a potential need for pancreatic sphincterotomy and the mandatory expertise required for pancreatic stenting, dictates that patients be managed by endoscopists who have significant experience *and interest* in patients with SOD. Finally, patients with SOD who relapse after initial endoscopic intervention should be reevaluated if the severity of their recurrent symptoms warrants either endoscopic or surgical intervention.

The complete reference list for this chapter can be found online at www.expertconsult.com.

48

Sclerosing Cholangitis

Jawad Ahmad and Adam Slivka

BACKGROUND

Primary sclerosing cholangitis (PSC) is a chronic inflammatory disease of the biliary tree. It is characterized by stricturing and dilation of the intrahepatic and/or extrahepatic bile ducts, with concentric obliterative fibrosis of intrahepatic biliary radicles. PSC is closely associated with inflammatory bowel disease, particularly ulcerative colitis, which is found in approximately two-thirds of northern European PSC patients.[1,2] The disease leads to chronic cholestasis, but patients can be asymptomatic at presentation and diagnosed by abnormal liver enzymes, particularly elevation of alkaline phosphatase. Patients may also present with pruritus, fatigue, right-upper-quadrant pain, and jaundice. As the disease progresses, symptoms of cirrhosis can be manifested. PSC is associated with an unpredictable risk of developing cholangiocarcinoma (CCA) in up to 10% to 20% of patients.[3] The etiology and pathogenesis of PSC are unclear, but it is likely an immune-mediated disease involving an exaggerated cell-mediated immune response leading to chronic inflammation of the biliary epithelium. Like other autoimmune diseases, the incidence of PSC may be rising in the Western world.[4]

PSC is diagnosed by radiographic imaging of the biliary tree (Fig. 48.1). This has traditionally been performed using endoscopic retrograde cholangiopancreatography (ERCP), but magnetic resonance cholangiopancreatography (MRCP) is thought to be as sensitive as ERCP in the diagnosis of PSC, although both are equipment dependent and operator dependent[5] (Fig. 48.2). The latter can be improved by the use of certain contrast agents, such as Gadoxetic acid, a gadolinium-based MRI contrast agent.[6]

Liver biopsy has a limited role in diagnosis but is a useful adjunct to determine the stage of the disease. Histology can range from normal to frank biliary cirrhosis, with the typical appearances being portal inflammation, concentric "onion skin" periductal fibrosis, and periportal fibrosis developing into septal and bridging necrosis.

The endoscopist's role in PSC involves diagnostic cholangiography; therapeutic intervention of strictures in the bile duct, including dilation and stenting; managing bile duct stones that can complicate PSC; and differentiating between benign and malignant strictures.

DIAGNOSIS AND NATURAL HISTORY

Introduction and Scientific Basis

The role of ERCP in the diagnosis of PSC has become more controversial with the availability of high-quality MRCP (Box 48.1). The latter has the benefit of being noninvasive, but is operator dependent and machine dependent and does not allow therapeutic intervention or cytologic sampling. Furthermore, subtle intrahepatic strictures as the only manifestation of PSC can be missed by MRCP. ERCP is still considered the gold standard and allows sampling and intervention, although it is

Video for this chapter can be found online at www.expertconsult.com.

also dependent on the machine (i.e., the quality of the radiographic equipment) and the operator. In addition, ERCP provides endoscopic staging of portal hypertension through assessment of varices and portal hypertensive gastropathy.

Several studies have compared ERCP and MRCP in patients with clinical or biochemical evidence of cholestasis. MRCP has a comparable diagnostic accuracy of over 90% and a specificity of 99%.[5] However, many patients also require therapeutic intervention.[7]

Description of Technique

The technique for ERCP in PSC does not differ from the standard approach to biliary cannulation and is described elsewhere (see Chapter 14). In certain cases, particularly in the setting of prior biliary sphincterotomy and also in the presence of an intact gallbladder, an occlusion cholangiogram is required to fill the intrahepatic ducts, using a stone-extraction balloon to prevent drainage of contrast from the biliary tree or filling of the gallbladder (after passing the balloon above the takeoff of the cystic duct). However, care should be taken to avoid filling of segments of the intrahepatic ducts that subsequently cannot be drained, which increases the risk of infection (cholangitis). The American Society for Gastrointestinal Endoscopy recommends prophylactic antibiotics in cases in which there exists the possibility of opacifying but not draining an obstructed bile duct. This scenario exists for all PSC patients, and we administer antibiotics to all patients immediately before and continue for several days after ERCP.

Indications/Contraindications

Any patient with a clinical picture consistent with cholestasis is a candidate for imaging of the biliary tree. This is especially true for patients with underlying inflammatory bowel disease. The use of ERCP or MRCP will be affected by several factors, as described in preceding sections. If therapy is potentially indicated, then ERCP has the advantage of treating a stricture without the need for an additional test, although MRCP may help in planning a therapeutic intervention.

Secondary causes of biliary sclerosis need to be excluded before a diagnosis of PSC can be confidently made. Biliary surgery, calculi and neoplasms, hepatic artery injury, hepatic arterial chemotherapy, and AIDS can lead to strictures in the biliary tree. Fig. 48.3 illustrates the cholangiogram of a patient several months after intra-arterial chemotherapy with floxuridine (FUDR) with resultant toxic cholangiopathy.

Several processes can mimic PSC on a cholangiogram. IgG4-mediated autoimmune cholangiopathy, hepatic malignancies, polycystic liver disease, infiltrative liver disease, and inflammatory pseudotumors need to be considered. Abdominal computed tomography scan or ultrasonography can differentiate many of these disease entities from PSC.

Complications

The adverse events (AEs) of ERCP in the setting of PSC are typical of those for any other indication and are described in Chapter 8. There appears to be an increased risk of cholangitis despite the use of prophylactic antibiotics. A recent study examined 294 patients with PSC and 657 ERCPs in a single center over 14 years and noted an overall AE rate of 4.3%, with a 2.4% rate of cholangitis. Performing a biliary sphincterotomy had a fivefold increased risk of adverse events.[8] Comparing 168 patients with PSC and 981 non-PSC patients undergoing ERCP over a 1-year period, Bangarulingam et al. noted no difference in the overall AE rate but a 4% incidence of cholangitis in PSC patients (compared with 0.2% in the non-PSC group), which correlated with the length of the procedure.[9] In comparison to patients with biliary strictures from other diseases, ERCP in PSC patients appears to carry the same overall AE rate in elective cases (13%), but this can increase in cases with an acute indication (29%).[10] In a large Swedish registry study the risk of post-ERCP pancreatitis was doubled in PSC patients compared with non-PSC patients undergoing ERCP.[11]

Relative Cost

Studies examining the relative cost of MRCP versus ERCP in the diagnosis of PSC have been conflicting and are affected by the prevalence of disease and the quality of imaging. One study suggested that the average cost per correct diagnosis by MRCP or ERCP as the initial testing strategy in 73 patients with clinically suspected biliary disease was $724 and $793, respectively. MRCP had a sensitivity of 82% and a specificity of 98%. MRCP thus resulted in cost savings when used as the initial test strategy for diagnosing PSC, particularly as there are essentially no procedure-related adverse events. However, this was in a cohort of patients with a 32% prevalence of PSC and with a very high specificity of MRCP. With a lower MRCP specificity (<85%) and a higher prevalence of PSC (>45%), ERCP becomes more cost-effective, suggesting that ERCP should be used when the suspicion of PSC is high, when local MRCP is suboptimal,[12] and when MRCP is nondiagnostic. The same study illustrated the high cost of dealing with ERCP-related AEs in

BOX 48.1   Diagnosis of Primary Sclerosing Cholangitis

Endoscopic Retrograde Cholangiopancreatography	Magnetic Resonance Cholangiopancreatography
Invasive	Noninvasive
Operator dependent	Operator dependent
Gold standard	Accuracy <100%
Therapeutic	Nontherapeutic
Tissue sampling	No sampling
Stage portal hypertension	Less expensive
	No complications

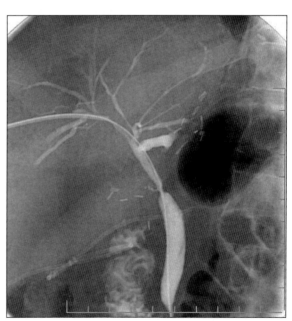

FIG 48.3 Cholangiogram demonstrating the effects of intra-arterial chemotherapy using floxuridine (FUDR). Note the discrete area of narrowing in the extrahepatic duct that otherwise looks normal, and the areas of diffuse structuring in the intrahepatics.

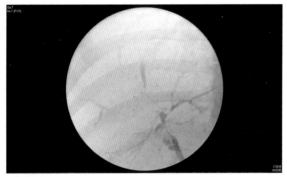

FIG 48.1 Typical endoscopic retrograde cholangiogram of the intrahepatic biliary tree in a patient, with primary sclerosing cholangitis. The disease is in a relatively early stage, with areas of stricturing and beading of the intrahepatic biliary tree but little attenuation.

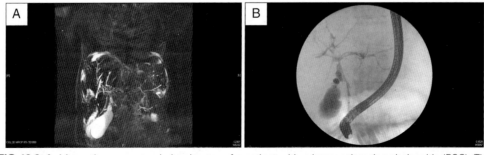

FIG 48.2 A, Magnetic resonance cholangiogram of a patient with primary sclerosing cholangitis (PSC). The biliary radicles appear to be greater in diameter more peripherally and several discrete strictures are seen centrally. Both the left and right systems are involved but the extrahepatic duct is not well seen. The gallbladder is seen in the bottom left of the image. B, Endoscopic retrograde cholangiogram of the same patient with PSC as seen in (A).

PSC patients. The average cost of managing post–ERCP-related AEs was $2902, with a range of $1915 to $5032.

A cost-effectiveness analysis suggested that in patients with suspected PSC, an initial negative MRCP followed by ERCP is the most cost-effective method in the workup of these patients.[13]

ENDOSCOPIC TREATMENT

Introduction and Scientific Basis

Interpreting the results of endoscopic therapy trials for PSC is limited by the small sample sizes and the variety of endoscopic techniques used. In addition, most series reporting therapy involve dilation or stenting of a *dominant* stricture—a term for which there is no consensus definition. The most commonly used definition is a stenosis of <1.5 mm in the extrahepatic bile duct, or <1 mm in the right or left common hepatic duct. The status of the upstream bile duct is not considered in this definition and is critically important in determining the impact of an intervention.

Repeated endoscopy to maintain biliary patency may improve the survival of patients with PSC.[14] Gluck and colleagues compared the survival of 84 patients with PSC who underwent therapeutic ERCP (primarily treatment of dominant biliary strictures) with the predicted 3-year or 4-year survival using the Mayo Clinic survival model for PSC, over a mean 8-year follow-up period.[14] Significantly improved survival in the treated patients ($p = 0.021$) was seen. However, the Mayo risk score weighs bilirubin very heavily in its formula and therefore will be profoundly affected by stenting of a stricture with resultant *rapid* decrease in serum bilirubin. It was not intended to assess the small subgroup of PSC patients with acute obstruction. This raises the question of whether the Mayo risk model is appropriate for assessing the outcome of therapy in highly selected jaundiced PSC patients, which was designed to assess slow longitudinal decompensation as a comparison for a control group after acute endoscopic interventions in these patients. Indeed, at least one study has found no change in cholestatic laboratory values in patients with and without dominant strictures after therapeutic ERCP.[15]

The paucity of controlled data indicates that it is unclear whether endoscopic therapy alters the long-term natural history of PSC, but it is certainly effective for treating acute symptomatic obstruction in patients with a dominant stricture (Box 48.2).

Description of Technique

Once biliary cannulation has been achieved, a variety of instruments can be used to perform stricture dilation (see Chapter 43). Wire access across strictures is the first step in therapy, and soft-tip wires with diameters of 0.018 to 0.035 inches must be used to avoid perforation of the biliary tree. Push catheters have a tapered tip, and the maximal

---

BOX 48.2   Key Points: Endoscopic Therapy in Primary Sclerosing Cholangitis

- Dominant strictures in primary sclerosing cholangitis can be treated at ERCP.
- More important than the stricture is the state of the prestenotic biliary tree.
- Tissue sampling of dominant strictures and use of antibiotics pre-ERCP and post-ERCP are suggested.
- Reserve treatment for patients with symptomatic jaundice.
- Concomitant dilation with stenting may improve results compared with either alone.
- Balloon dilation and short-term (10 to 14 days) stenting preferable.
- Avoid sphincterotomy, if possible.
- Higher adverse event rate than diagnostic ERCP.
- No convincing data that endoscopic therapy alters long-term natural history.

---

diameter of the dilating catheter is typically 7 to 10 Fr in diameter. They are wire guided, but because of their limited diameter and radial force, they are seldom used alone in PSC. More commonly, dilation balloons are employed. These are also wire guided but come in a variety of diameters (up to 10 mm) and have a greater radial force. They are difficult to use if the stricture is tortuous. In cases of refractory strictures in which only a wire can be passed and catheters will not follow, a screw catheter (e.g., Soehendra stent extractor; Cook Endoscopy, Winston-Salem, NC) can be used to increase the stricture diameter; there are no controlled data on its efficacy.

A temporary plastic stent can be placed after dilation, or in some cases can be placed without dilation. Dominant strictures should be sampled to assess for CCA. We perform brush cytology and/or intraductal forceps biopsy, with tissue sent for cytology/histology and molecular analysis.

Many endoscopists perform biliary sphincterotomy before dilation or stent insertion, but we do not advocate this as there are no reliable data that this is required and the AE rate may be higher. However, in patients for whom recurrent interventions are anticipated, it may reduce the risk of post-ERCP pancreatitis because of the ease of subsequent cannulation and lack of manipulation of the pancreas.

Published data on endoscopic therapy of dominant strictures in PSC patients are hampered by the lack of a standardized technique. Van Milligen de Wit and colleagues demonstrated technical success in 21 of 25 PSC patients with a dominant stricture who underwent endoscopic stent therapy.[16] Of these 25 patients, 18 had a biliary sphincterotomy and 9 underwent dilation before stent insertion with either a balloon or dilating catheter. Stents were exchanged electively every 2 to 3 months or if they became occluded. After a median follow-up of 29 months, 16 of the 21 patients had improved or stable liver test results. The same group demonstrated similar effectiveness using short-term stenting (mean of 11 days), with the benefit extending for several years. Improvements in symptoms and cholestasis were seen in all patients, and these improvements were maintained for several years, with 80% of patients intervention-free at 1 year and 60% at 3 years. There were 7 transient procedure-related AEs out of 45 procedures; all but one were managed conservatively.[17]

The addition of ursodeoxycholic acid (UDCA) to endoscopic therapy has been examined in a prospective trial by Stiehl et al. in 106 PSC patients followed for up to 13 years, with improvement in overall survival rates compared with the Mayo PSC survival model.[18] However, the use of high-dose UDCA (at 28 to 30 mg/kg) has been shown to increase the risk of AEs in PSC patients, including death and the development of colorectal neoplasia, and hence is not routinely recommended.[19,20]

Our approach to PSC patients is to perform therapeutic ERCP in those with a dominant stricture who have prestenotic biliary dilation and an elevated serum bilirubin or severe symptomatic cholestasis. We use balloon dilation over a guidewire, ensuring that the diameter of the balloon is no greater than the smallest diameter of the duct either proximal or distal to the stricture. The balloon is inflated with contrast until the waist has disappeared or when the maximum pressure for the specific balloon (per package insert) is reached. We then leave a 10-Fr plastic stent across the stricture for 2 to 3 weeks, followed by repeat ERCP, and provide further therapy if indicated. Prophylactic antibiotics are administered for all procedures and oral antibiotics are continued for several days after the procedure to minimize the risk of cholangitis. Figs. 48.4 and 48.5 illustrate dilation and stent therapy in patients with a dominant stricture.

Indications/Contraindications

Endoscopic therapy is indicated in PSC patients if there is clinical or biochemical evidence of cholangitis or if a dominant stricture is suspected.

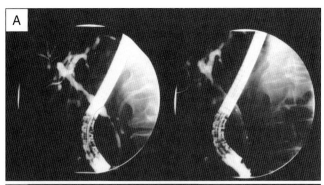

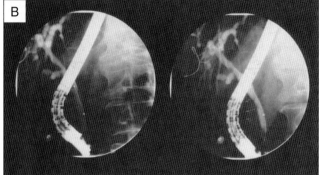

FIG 48.4 A, Balloon dilation of a dominant stricture in a patient with primary sclerosing cholangitis (PSC). The cholangiogram on the left demonstrates intrahepatic and extrahepatic PSC. The extrahepatic duct has a dominant stricture (just below the scope) with prestenotic dilation. Retained contrast in the pancreatic duct is seen. The cholangiogram on the right shows a deflated balloon introduced into the extrahepatic duct over a wire. Note the radiopaque markers on the proximal and distal ends of the balloon. **B,** Balloon dilation of a dominant stricture in a patient with PSC. The cholangiogram on the left demonstrates the balloon inflated across the stricture. There is no waist to the balloon. Typically the balloon is inflated to 12 atmospheres for 30 to 45 seconds. This can lead to pain and additional sedation may need to be given. The postdilation appearance is shown on the right. Note the marked improvement.

However, because of the lack of controlled data, it is unclear whether treatment alters the natural history of the disease. Occasionally bile duct calculi are encountered in patients with PSC and can be removed using standard techniques (see Chapter 19), although stones proximal to a stricture can be challenging. We typically do not perform stricture therapy in asymptomatic patients who are not clinically jaundiced, as there is a definite AE rate and the potential benefit is questionable.

Adverse Events and Their Management

AEs after therapeutic procedures in PSC patients are more frequent than after diagnostic ERCP.

Alkhatib et al. reviewed a total of 185 ERCPs performed in 75 PSC patients over a 10-year period at several academic institutions and noted that performing biliary sphincterotomy, dilating a stricture, presence of comorbid conditions (cirrhosis, Crohn's disease, autoimmune hepatitis), and low endoscopist ERCP volume were associated with an increased risk of AEs. However, stent placement or the presence of a dominant stricture did not predict AEs.[21]

The most common AE after therapeutic ERCP in PSC patients appears to be cholangitis, and the risk increases in emergent situations and correlates with the length of the procedure.[8–11] Cholangitis can occur despite the use of prophylactic antibiotics but is typically treated easily

with intravenous antibiotics in the hospital setting, although liver abscesses and septic shock have been reported. Prolonged stent therapy is associated with cholangitis or jaundice because of stent occlusion, which can be successfully treated with stent exchange or removal. Studies using short-term stent therapy indicate a similar early AE rate but with less frequent cholangitis.[17]

Relative Cost

There are no cost-effectiveness data available in studies of therapeutic endoscopy in PSC patients. Although balloon dilators are more expensive than push dilators, the likely increased efficacy of the former may translate into fewer follow-up procedures and hence reduced cost. We typically always deploy a stent after dilation, and this necessitates a repeat procedure for removal several weeks later, which adds to the cost of treatment. Because of the lack of controlled trials in PSC patients undergoing therapeutic ERCP, it is unclear whether dilation therapy alone is sufficient. Reducing the number of subsequent procedures without affecting long-term outcomes would improve the cost-effectiveness of endoscopic treatment.

CHOLANGIOCARCINOMA

Introduction and Scientific Basis

CCA will develop in up to 10% to 20% of patients with PSC, with a lifetime risk of 10% to 15%.[3] Investigators from the Mayo Clinic determined the incidence of and risk factors for CCA in 161 patients with PSC who were monitored for a median of 11.5 years. CCA developed in 11 patients (6.8%) at a rate of approximately 0.6% per year.[22] This equated to a relative risk of CCA of 1560 compared with that in the general population. No association was found between the duration of PSC and the incidence of CCA. Similarly, in a Swedish cohort of 604 PSC patients followed for many years, the frequency of CCA was 13% and the incidence rate of CCA after the first year of diagnosis was 1.5% per year.[23]

Early diagnosis of CCA may improve patient survival, as it may permit curative surgical resection or liver transplant in selected cases and in selected centers, but it is hampered by the absence of sufficiently accurate and noninvasive diagnostic tests. Diagnosing CCA in PSC patients is even more challenging because of the presence of multiple nonneoplastic strictures.

Description of Technique
Diagnosis

Several endoscopic methods have been employed to diagnose CCA in PSC patients. Brush cytology, fine-needle aspiration, and forceps biopsy have been used, but all have low sensitivity and high specificity. In addition, the tumor markers carbohydrate antigen 19-9 (CA19-9) and carcinoembryonic antigen (CEA) have been examined alone or in various combinations.

Brush cytology involves gaining access to the biliary tree and then inserting a wire into the intrahepatic ducts. The sheathed cytology brush is then advanced over the wire into the area of the stricture to be brushed and then passed out of the sheath and vigorously pushed in a to-and-fro motion across the stricture to increase the cellular yield. Occasionally, push or balloon dilation of the stricture is required to enable passage of the cytology brush. The brush is then withdrawn into the sheath while still inside the duct and removed through the endoscope. The cellular specimen can be sent to cytology on preprepared slides or the entire brush placed in saline and sent to cytology. If slides are prepared in the endoscopy suite, it is important for the nurse or endoscopy technician to prepare the cytology slides quickly to prevent excessive drying, which can cause artifacts that affect interpretation.

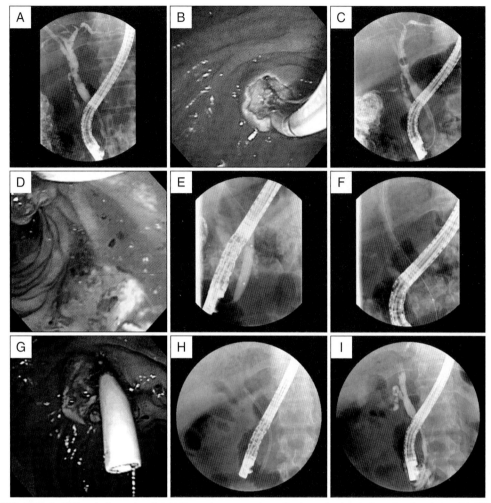

FIG 48.5 A, Diffusely irregular distal bile and common hepatic ducts in deeply jaundiced patient with PSC and pigment stones in the biliary tree. Note intrahepatic duct changes. After biliary sphincterotomy and stone extraction (**B–D**), the strictures are balloon dilated (**E**), brushed for cytology (**F**), and stented with a 10-Fr biliary stent (**G**). **H** and **I,** Note persistent but improved stenosis at time of stent retrieval 4 weeks later.

The overall sensitivity of cytology in the diagnosis of CCA in PSC is around 50%. Adding K-ras or p53 mutational analysis of brush samples does not appear to increase the sensitivity, although repeated brushing on two or three occasions appears to increase the sensitivity significantly. Brush cytology may also be able to identify a subset of patients with high-grade dysplasia who may be candidates for aggressive resection or liver transplantation.[24–26]

The increased cellular load obtained by an intraductal biopsy also appears to increase the sensitivity. The technique involves cannulating directly with the biopsy forceps (sometimes made easier by passing alongside an indwelling guidewire). The biopsies are obtained under fluoroscopic guidance. Alternatively, biopsies are obtained using a small-caliber forceps passed through the working channel of a cholangioscope under direct endoscopic visualization. Fig. 48.6 illustrates a biopsy being taken in a patient with a suspicious stricture.

The combination of a CEA level of >5.2 ng/mL and a CA19-9 of >180 U/mL leads to 70% sensitivity, and combined with brush cytology a sensitivity of close to 90% can be achieved in diagnosing CCA in PSC.[27] Similarly, combining brush cytology, DNA analysis by flow cytometry, CA19-9, and CEA, diagnostic sensitivity of 88% and specificity of 80% can be expected. Interestingly, measurement of CA19-9 or CEA in bile has no diagnostic significance.[28]

Screening patients with PSC for CCA with CA19-9 and CEA would appear to be reasonable, but the ideal interval at which to obtain these tests and the cost-effectiveness remain to be determined.

There is increasing interest in using several genetic techniques to try to differentiate benign from malignant disease in PSC. Quantifying nuclear DNA content from a stricture using digital image analysis, analyzing tumor suppressor gene–linked microsatellite marker loss of heterozygosity and K-ras mutations, and detecting aberrant DNA methylation of brush cytology specimens have all been shown to improve the diagnostic yield compared with brush cytology alone.[29–31]

The majority of studies have examined fluorescence in situ hybridization (FISH) of brush cytology specimens. Commercially available DNA probes for CCA look for alterations (aneuploidy) in chromosomes 3, 7, 9, and 17, which are associated with malignancy. Aneuploidy can be further categorized into trisomy (10 cells or more with 3 copies of chromosome 7 and fewer than 3 copies of the others), tetrasomy (10 cells or more with 4 copies of all chromosomes), or polysomy (5 cells or more with an increase of 2 or more of all 4 chromosomes). FISH polysomy indicates chromosomal instability, a marker of cancer, and is associated with CCA. A recent study of 371 PSC patients demonstrated that polysomy in multiple areas of the biliary tree was the strongest predictor of CCA, with a hazard ratio of 82, compared with polysomy

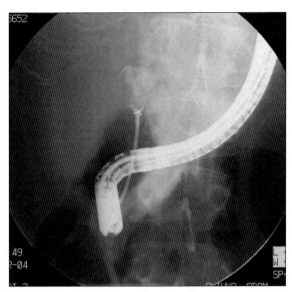

FIG 48.6 Intraductal biopsy in a patient with primary sclerosing cholangitis (PSC) and a dominant stricture. The scope is in a short position and the forceps have been placed into the bile duct. The bile duct proximal to the stricture is irregular and dilated. This technique enables a biopsy of the stricture such that tissue can be obtained for pathology rather than cytology, improving the diagnostic yield.

in a single area (hazard ratio of 13).[32] Probes to chromosomes 3, 7, 9, and 17 were originally used to detect bladder cancer, and better sensitivity can be achieved by using probes to chromosomes 1, 7, 8, and 9, as validated in a study of patients with pancreaticobiliary malignancy, two-thirds of whom had PSC.[33] FISH testing is superior to digital image analysis or routine cytology for the diagnosis of malignancy in indeterminate biliary strictures.[34] However, analysis of a cohort of 235 PSC patients followed longitudinally found that 120 patients (51%) tested positively for FISH but only 40 of those patients actually had CCA, highlighting that FISH should not be used as a routine screening test in PSC.[35] In patients with persistently positive FISH testing (specifically polysomy on serial ERCP brushings), there is a high likelihood of developing CCA compared with patients with an isolated positive result, which can even predate the diagnosis of CCA by conventional methods (imaging or pathology) by up to 2.7 years.[36] Adding K-ras mutational analysis to FISH testing appears to increase the malignancy detection rate in pancreaticobiliary strictures,[37] as does adding CA19-9 >129 U/mL to FISH polysomy in PSC.[38]

There are a number of mutations associated with CCA that elude detection by FISH. Recently, large panels of such mutations have been studied by next-generation sequencing (NGS) and applied to samples obtained at ERCP. These techniques are lower cost, less complex, and not subject to human interpretation and thus have distinct advantages over FISH. One study compared NGS to FISH in detecting CCA on ERCP brush samples and found superior performance with NGS.[39] A similar study found that dominant IgG4 + B-cell receptor clones determined by NGS can distinguish IgG4 cholangitis from PSC and biliary/pancreatic malignancies with 94% sensitivity and 99% specificity.[40]

Direct cholangioscopy has been used in PSC patients and has some advantages over cholangiography, but its role needs to be better defined. Initial studies have suggested an improvement in sensitivity and specificity in diagnosing malignancy compared with brush cytology,[41] but consensus on malignant features is lacking and interobserver agreement poor. Adding narrow-band imaging to cholangioscopy does not increase the detection of dysplasia in PSC.[42]

Probe-based confocal laser endomicroscopy (pCLE) may prove to be a promising tool in the detection of malignancy compared with standard histopathology. Irregular vessels, large black bands (>20 μm), and aggregates of cellular structures were seen in malignant strictures and were absent in benign disease.

Two large prospective studies have shown that pCLE is able to diagnose CCA more often than tissue sampling during ERCP. However, false positives remain problematic and PSC patients were excluded from these studies.[43,44] An international registry studying PSC using pCLE is currently in progress.

Treatment and Palliation

Until the emergence of ERCP, patients who presented with jaundice in the setting of malignant biliary obstruction underwent percutaneous drainage, or surgical biliary bypass if fit enough for surgery. Smith and colleagues demonstrated the efficacy of endoscopic stent insertion compared with surgical biliary bypass in a randomized prospective controlled trial of 204 patients with malignant low bile duct obstruction.[45] Technical success was achieved in 94 surgical and 95 stented patients, with functional biliary decompression obtained in 92 patients in both groups. The overall survival between the two groups did not differ (median survival: surgical 26 weeks, stented 21 weeks). The authors concluded that endoscopic stenting and surgery were both effective palliative treatments, with the former having fewer early treatment-related complications and the latter fewer late complications. However, these results cannot be extrapolated directly to patients with PSC

For patients with unresectable disease, an expandable metal stent can be deployed for palliation (see Chapter 23). In a prospective randomized trial, Davids et al. demonstrated that metal stents resulted in significantly prolonged patency compared with polyethylene stents in 105 patients with unresectable distal bile-duct malignancy.[46] Median patency of the metal stent was 273 days compared with 126 days for a plastic stent. Tumor ingrowth typically led to occlusion in metal stents, whereas sludge deposition caused occlusion with plastic stents. However, the overall median survival was 149 days and did not differ significantly between patients with metal or plastic stents. Metal stents may be appropriate in PSC patients with distal CCA and upstream dilation but should not be placed if the proximal end of the stent will be deployed in a narrow diseased segment. The use of metal stents in PSC patients with more proximal malignancies should generally be avoided and reserved for case-by-case consideration at tertiary centers.

Stenting with adjuvant chemotherapy has been tried without much success, but the addition of photodynamic therapy (PDT) to stent therapy in nonresectable proximal CCA (involving the hilum) provides a survival benefit.[47] The technique requires initial placement of plastic stents (see Chapter 22) into both the left and right intrahepatics so that biliary drainage is achieved. Patients receiving PDT then are treated with Photofrin at a dose of 2 mg/kg intravenously 48 hours before laser activation. The plastic stents are then removed during a repeat ERCP and intraluminal photoactivation is performed, after which the plastic stents are redeployed. Patients are kept in a darkened room for 3 to 4 days after the procedure. In this randomized study, PDT and stenting resulted in a median survival of 493 days compared with 98 days with stenting alone. In addition, jaundice and quality of life were also significantly improved. The only adverse event seen in the PDT group was photosensitivity in 10% of the patients. This procedure should be performed only by experienced endoscopists and in facilities with PDT capability. The costs may also be prohibitive.

Indications/Contraindications

Any patient with PSC who has an unexpected rise in cholestatic enzymes or bilirubin should be investigated for the development of CCA. In addition, a sudden rise in serum CA19-9 or CEA should prompt a cholangiogram to detect underlying CCA. We do not advocate routine surveillance ERCP in asymptomatic patients with PSC. Diagnosing CCA at an early stage is not usually helpful in PSC patients, as resection is usually contraindicated because of the presence of cirrhosis, its multifocal location, and involvement of the hilum, and liver transplant for selected CCA cases is seldom possible. The diagnosis should ideally be made in a premalignant stage, but as yet this is not possible. The timing of liver transplant in patients with PSC is therefore difficult, as many patients will have preserved liver synthetic function and are early for transplant but are still at risk of developing a tumor that will then likely preclude transplant.

Adverse Events and Their Management

The AEs and management of metal or plastic stent insertion for patients with CCA in the setting of PSC are as described elsewhere (see Chapters 8 and 24).

Comparing stent insertion to surgical bypass in CCA, Smith et al. demonstrated lower procedure-related mortality (3% vs 14%) and major complication (11% vs 29%) rates and median total hospital stay (20 vs 26 days) in stented patients compared with surgery. However, late complications, including recurrent jaundice and late gastric outlet obstruction, were more frequent in stented patients.[45] The increasing use of direct cholangioscopy in patients with PSC to aid in the diagnosis of CCA may be associated with an increased risk of AEs. Sethi et al. demonstrated a significant increase in cholangitis (1.0% vs 0.2%) in patients undergoing ERCP with cholangioscopy.[48] It remains to be seen whether this occurs in patients with PSC.

Relative Cost

For diagnostic purposes, CEA and CA19-9 measurements are relatively inexpensive but their low sensitivity means that cytology is required. The cost-effectiveness of these tumor markers and the newer DNA-based tests remains to be seen.

In terms of providing palliation, metal stents are more cost-effective than plastic stents, because the longer patency compared with plastic

---

BOX 48.3   Key Points: Diagnosing Cholangiocarcinoma in Primary Sclerosing Cholangitis

- Cholangiocarcinoma may develop in 10–20% patients with primary sclerosing cholangitis (PSC).
- No proven screening method exists for detecting cholangiocarcinoma in PSC.
- Brush cytology has only 50% sensitivity for detecting cholangiocarcinoma.
- Combining tumor markers with cytology may increase sensitivity.
- DNA and molecular techniques such as fluorescence in situ hybridization and next-generation sequencing increase sensitivity.
- Premalignant diagnosis would allow liver transplant before development of cholangiocarcinoma in selected centers.

---

stents translates into fewer follow-up procedures. Although there are no formal studies looking at risks and benefits of plastic versus metal stents in PSC patients who develop CCA, Davids et al., using an incremental cost-effectiveness analysis, showed that initial placement of a metal stent resulted in a 28% decrease in subsequent endoscopic procedures in patients with distal malignant obstructive jaundice.[46] However, in patients with a life expectancy of less than 3 months, a plastic stent may be adequate palliation, as a follow-up procedure is unlikely to be required. Again, patients with PSC may have obstruction at the level of the bifurcation and need bilateral stents, and the presence of nondilated ducts even in the face of obstruction makes their insertion difficult. There are no studies comparing plastic and metal stents for palliation of malignant obstruction in PSC patients.

The high initial cost of surgical palliation compared with endoscopic therapy means that the former has very limited application (Box 48.3).

The complete reference list for this chapter can be found online at www.experconsult.com.

49

Tropical Parasitic Infestations

D. Nageshwar Reddy, G. Venkat Rao, and Rupa Banerjee

Parasitic infestation of the biliary tract is a common cause of hepatobiliary disease in developing countries and in rural areas of developed countries. With increasing international travel and immigration, clinicians in developed countries will likely encounter these conditions with increasing frequency. Ascariasis, hydatid liver disease, clonorchiasis, opisthorchiasis, and fascioliasis are the commonly encountered parasitic infestations of the biliary tract. They may present with cholestasis, obstructive jaundice, biliary colic, acute cholangitis, and, less commonly, pancreatitis. In developing countries, biliary parasitoses often mimic biliary stone disease. Transabdominal ultrasonography facilitates the diagnosis in most cases. Although medical therapy remains the mainstay of treatment, endoscopic retrograde cholangiopancreatography (ERCP) and endoscopic sphincterotomy with bile duct clearance are essential when biliary complications occur.[1] In contrast to ascariasis and hydatid disease, in which the radiologic assessment usually supports a diagnosis of ascariasis, the diagnosis of clonorchiasis, opisthorchiasis, or fascioliasis requires astute clinical suspicion in nonendemic areas.

ASCARIS LUMBRICOIDES

The roundworm *Ascaris lumbricoides* is the most common helminthic infestation in the world, infecting over 1 billion people.[2] Cases have been reported from nonendemic areas in both developing and developed countries.[3–5]

The infestation is usually asymptomatic. *A. lumbricoides* organisms normally reside in the jejunum but are actively motile and can invade the papilla, migrating into the bile duct and causing biliary obstruction, with a variety of hepatobiliary complications, including biliary colic, pancreatitis, cholecystitis, postcholecystectomy syndrome, hepatic abscess, and hepatolithiasis.[2] Ascariasis has also been reported to cause obstruction of a biliary self-expandable metal stent.[6] Identification of parasite DNA in biliary stones suggests that *Clonorchis sinensis* and *A. lumbricoides* may predispose to biliary stone formation and recurrent pyogenic cholangitis (RPC). Over 5% cases of hepatobiliary ascariasis develop RPC and 10% of patients with RPC have definite evidence of ascariasis.[7]

Biliary-pancreatic ascariasis is commonly reported in high-endemic regions such as the Kashmir valley in India. In a study of 500 patients with hepatobiliary and pancreatic ascariasis, Khuroo et al.[8] reported biliary colic in 56%, acute cholangitis in 24%, acute cholecystitis in 13%, acute pancreatitis in 6%, and hepatic abscess in less than 1%. Biliary-pancreatic ascariasis should be suspected in patients from an endemic area presenting with biliary symptoms.[8]

In this setting, identification of eggs, larva, or the adult worm from bile or feces is strongly suggestive of the disease. Ultrasonography is the imaging modality of choice for diagnosis and follow-up of patients with hepatobiliary ascariasis. Characteristic sonographic findings include thick echoic stripe with a central, longitudinal anechoic tube (gastrointestinal tract of the worm; inner tube sign), thin nonshadowing strip without an inner tube (strip sign), overlapping longitudinal interfaces in the main bile duct (spaghetti sign), and the characteristic movement of these long echogenic structures within the bile duct.[9]

In cases where ultrasonography is nondiagnostic, endoscopic ultrasonography (EUS) and magnetic resonance cholangiopancreatography (MRCP) may be performed. By EUS, worms appear as a long linear hyperechoic structure without acoustic shadowing ("single-tube" sign) or with central hypoechoic tube ("double-tube" sign).[10]

ERCP and Endotherapy for Hepatobiliary Ascariasis

Endotherapy is indicated if there is no clinical improvement after intensive medical management is administered and if the worm is known to persist in the ductal lumen up to 3 weeks after therapy.[2] During endoscopy, worms can be seen in the duodenum and are often seen protruding from the ampulla of Vater. During ERCP, cholangiographic features of the *Ascaris* worm include the presence of long, smooth, linear filling defects with tapering ends (Fig. 49.1); smooth, parallel filling defects; curves and loops crossing the hepatic ducts transversely; and dilatation of bile ducts (usually the common bile duct). With the recent availability of the SpyGlass direct visualization system (Boston Scientific, Marlborough, MA), the worm can also be visualized directly within the bile duct. Endoscopy is the mainstay of treatment for biliary ascariasis.[1,11–14]

Worm extraction is easy when the worm protrudes out of the ampulla of Vater (Fig. 49.2). The worm can be held with a grasping forceps and slowly brought out by withdrawing the endoscope out of the patient. A Dormia basket can also be used to maneuver the outer end of the worm into the strings of the basket and gently hold it before it is extracted.[12]

It is best to avoid using a polypectomy snare for a protruding worm, as it tends to cut the worm. Remnant worms can lead to stone formation, and all efforts must be made to ensure complete removal.[1] Worms within the common bile duct occasionally protrude out of the papilla after contrast injection. Alternatively, they can be extracted using a Dormia basket or a biliary occlusion balloon.[1]

It has been postulated that endoscopic sphincterotomy should be avoided in endemic areas, in view of the high reinfestation rates and easy entry of worms into postsphincterotomy bile ducts. In a study including more than 300 patients, Sandouk et al. suggested that pancreaticobiliary ascariasis was more common in patients with prior cholecystectomy or sphincterotomy.[14] On the other hand, Alam et al. needed a wide sphincterotomy in 94.8% of the 77 patients with pancreaticobiliary ascariasis in their study but did not report any major adverse event or recurrence after sphincterotomy.[15]

Similarly, Bektas et al. did not report any recurrence of biliary ascariasis in their patients after sphincterotomy.[16] Ascariasis may coexist with biliary calculi or strictures. In these situations, endoscopic balloon dilation of the biliary sphincter (sphincteroplasty) is an alternative to

---

Video for this chapter can be found online at www.expertconsult.com.

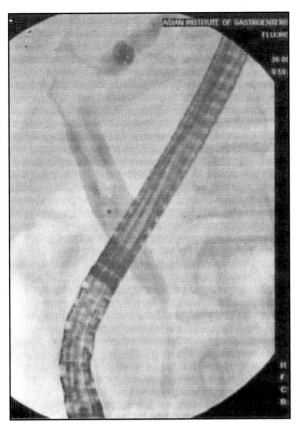

FIG 49.1 Linear filling defect within the opacified common bile duct in a case of biliary ascariasis. The worm was eventually removed with a Dormia basket after endoscopic biliary sphincterotomy.

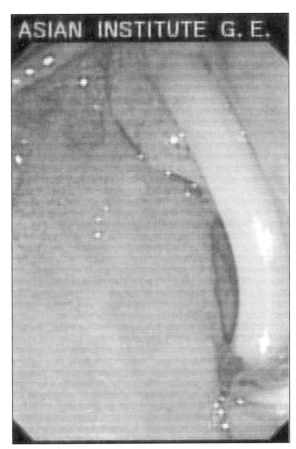

FIG 49.2 Ascaris protruding from the ampulla of Vater. Held with a grasping forceps, the worm can be brought out by withdrawing the endoscope out of the patient.

sphincterotomy to retrieve the parasite and associated calculi.[17] In endemic areas, pregnant women are prone to develop biliary ascariasis. Endoscopic intervention in such cases requires special precautions, including lead shielding of the fetus and limitation of total fluoroscopic exposure (see Chapter 3). Failure of endoscopic extraction may require surgical extraction, which has increased risks of fetal wastage and premature labor.[18]

Extraction of the culprit worm is usually associated with rapid symptom relief and is successful in more than 80% of patients.[12,14]

However, infection may be associated with calculi or strictures, which can usually be dealt with endoscopically.[11] After endoscopic therapy, all patients should receive antihelminthic therapy to eradicate remaining worms. A single dose of albendazole (400 mg) is highly effective against ascariasis.[19] In endemic areas, periodic deworming may have a role in preventing recurrences.

ECHINOCOCCUS GRANULOSUS

The "domestic" strain of Echinococcus granulosus is the main cause of human hydatid disease. Infections are found worldwide and remain endemic in sheep-raising areas. The life cycle involves two hosts: the adult tapeworm is usually found in dogs (definitive host), whereas sheep (intermediate host) are the usual host for the larval stages. Human exposure is via the oral–fecal route with food or water contaminated by the feces of the infected definitive host, usually a dog.[20]

Embryonated eggs hatch in the small intestine and liberate oncospheres that migrate to distant sites. The right lobe of the liver is the most common site for hydatid cyst formation. The majority of patients remain asymptomatic. In symptomatic patients, abdominal ultrasonographic and serologic studies usually establish the diagnosis.

In approximately one-fourth of cases, hydatid cysts rupture into the biliary tree, causing obstructive jaundice.[21]

Contents of the cyst (the scolices and daughter cysts) draining into the biliary ducts cause intermittent or complete obstruction of the bile duct, resulting in obstructive jaundice, cholangitis, and sometimes cholangitic abscesses. Rarely, acute pancreatitis complicates intrabiliary rupture of a hydatid cyst.[22]

Cysto-biliary communication is common, occurring in 10% to 42% of patients,[23,24] and is often recognized at surgery when cysts are stained with bile. Unrecognized cysto-biliary communication may present in the postoperative period as a persistent biliary fistula, resulting in prolonged hospitalization, and can increase morbidity.

Hydatid cyst involving the pancreatic head and body has been rarely reported.[25] These cysts can enlarge and may manifest as acute pancreatitis, chronic pancreatitis, or obstructive jaundice, and easily confused with pancreatic pseudocysts, tumors, or other congenital pancreatic cysts.[26] Surgical intervention is generally required for management.

Management

The treatment options for hepatic hydatid disease include antihelminthic therapy (albendazole), either alone or in combination with surgery, or puncture, aspiration, injection of a scolicidal agent, and reaspiration (PAIR). The classification of hydatid cysts by Gharbi and the World Health Organization (WHO) into active (CE1, CE2), inactive (CE4,

CE5), and transitional (CE3a, CE3b) cysts has important implications for management.[27] The candidates for medical treatment include those with small cysts (<5 cm), WHO class CE1/CE3a, and ruptured cysts.

Albendazole is typically used at a dose of 10 to 15 mg/kg/day for 3 to 6 months. Alternatively, mebendazole and praziquantel may also be used.[27]

Endotherapy

Endoscopic intervention plays an important role (1) when intrabiliary rupture of the hydatid cyst occurs and (2) in the management of biliary complications after surgery.[28]

Intrabiliary Rupture of a Hydatid Cyst

Intrabiliary rupture is a common and serious complication of hepatic hydatid cyst. The incidence ranges from 1% to 25%[29] and it is usually because of high pressure in the cyst, often up to 80 cm H_2O. In their series of 120 patients, Sharma et al. found biliary fistulae in 28 patients.[30] ERCP is indicated when intrabiliary rupture is suspected clinically (because of jaundice), biochemically (because of cholestasis), or sonographically (a dilated biliary ductal system in association with hydatid cysts in the liver).[31–33]

Duodenoscopy sometimes shows whitish, glistening membranes lying in the duodenum or protruding from the papilla of Vater. On cholangiography, the hydatid cyst remnants appear as (1) filiform, linear, wavy material in the common bile duct representing the laminated hydatid membranes; (2) round or oval lucent filling defects representing daughter cysts floating in the common bile duct; or (3) brown, thick, amorphous debris.[33]

Cholangiography often reveals minor communications, particularly with peripheral ducts, which are of unclear clinical significance.

In patients presenting with obstructive jaundice or cholangitis, endoscopic biliary sphincterotomy facilitates extraction of the cysts and membranes using a Dormia basket (Fig. 49.3) or a biliary occlusion balloon.[34,35] Saline irrigation of the bile duct may be necessary to flush out the hydatid sand and small daughter cysts. Life-threatening episodes of acute cholangitis can be temporized by nasobiliary drainage, followed by extraction of hydatid cysts and membranes with or without sphincterotomy.[30] The nasobiliary drain output can be examined for hydatid hooklets or membranes. Endoscopic management of acute biliary complications allows for definitive surgery to be performed electively. Rarely, rupture with complete drainage may be treated endoscopically alone.[36]

In the presence of a hydatid cyst frankly communicating with the biliary ductal system, a hydrophilic guidewire can be negotiated into the cyst; a nasobiliary catheter is then inserted to facilitate emptying of the cyst contents. Irrigating the cyst using hypertonic saline solution through the nasobiliary catheter ensures sterilization of the germinal layers and the remaining daughter cysts.[37] In the presence of extensive disease with multiple communications with the bile ducts, this method should not be used for fear of causing biliary strictures by seepage of the hypertonic saline solution into the bile ducts.[38,39]

There have been only a handful of case reports of successful nonsurgical treatment of complicated hydatid disease with ERCP and medical therapy.[40]

Biliary Adverse Events After Surgery

Biliary adverse events occur in up to 16% of patients after surgery.[23,41]

Early postoperative complications include persistent biliary fistula and obstructive jaundice. Sclerosing cholangitis and sphincter of Oddi stenosis are late postoperative complications.

Persistent biliary fistula is the commonest postoperative complication, occurring in 50% to 63% of patients after surgery.[24,41] Unrecognized

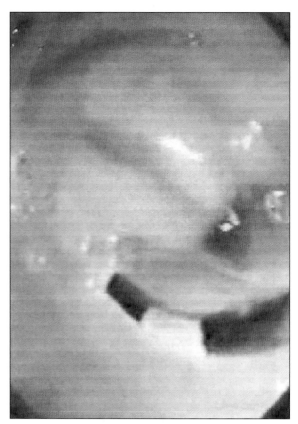

FIG 49.3 Hydatid membranes protruding from the ampulla of Vater in a case of hydatid disease of the liver with intrabiliary rupture. Endoscopic biliary sphincterotomy facilitates extraction of the cysts and membranes using a Dormia basket.

cysto-biliary communications manifest as persistent biliary drainage through the T-tube or an external biliary fistula in the postoperative period. Low-output fistulae (<300 mL/day) close spontaneously after a mean duration of 4 weeks. Patients with high-output fistulae require endoscopic intervention.[23]

Endoscopic biliary sphincterotomy and ductal clearance followed by internal biliary stenting for approximately 4 to 8 weeks is usually sufficient to achieve fistula closure. Sphincterotomy alone may also be effective.[32] Occasionally, fistulous communication may develop between the hepatic hydatid cyst and the bronchi, leading to the development of a bronchobiliary fistula either de novo or after surgery. Endoscopic biliary sphincterotomy and nasobiliary drainage or stenting are effective at closing these fistulae.[42]

Obstructive jaundice occurs in up to 2% of patients after surgical resection of hydatid cyst. This typically presents within 2 to 4 weeks of surgery.[31–34,43]

Obstructive jaundice results from common bile duct obstruction by echinococcal remnants in the presence of cysto-biliary communications. As such, endoscopic biliary sphincterotomy and ductal clearance followed by internal stenting are required for approximately 4 to 8 weeks to achieve fistula closure.

Sclerosing cholangitis and sphincter of Oddi stenosis can occur after formalin is used to sterilize the cysts during surgery. Seepage of formalin into bile ducts through minor communications results in early inflammatory changes and late stricture formation. Almost all scolicidal agents are associated clinically or experimentally with this complication. Among the various scolicidal agents available, hypertonic saline (20%) may be preferred.[44,45] These complications can be treated endoscopically by sphincterotomy and stenting with or without balloon dilatation of the stricture.

CLONORCHIS SINENSIS

Clonorchis sinensis, also known as the Chinese liver fluke, is common in East Asia as a result of consuming raw freshwater fish.[46] It is estimated that about 35 million people are infected globally, of whom approximately 15 million are in China.[47] It is harbored in the biliary tract of humans and other fish-eating animals. Liver flukes have a lifespan of 10 to 30 years; this creates a problem for Asian immigrants who develop clinical symptoms many years after leaving the endemic area.[48]

Opisthorchis felineus and *Opisthorchis viverrini* also cause similar clinical manifestations.

Clonorchiasis is acquired from eating infested raw freshwater fish (carp and salmon group). The infective metacercariae adhere to the common bile duct and migrate along the epithelial lining of the duct into the intrahepatic ducts, where they mature into flat, elongated, 10-mm-long to 23-mm-long adult worms. The smaller branches of the left lobe of the liver are commonly involved, where the adult form attains maturity in about 1 month and begins to lay eggs. The migration of the immature flukes causes trauma, ulceration, and desquamation of the bile duct epithelium. Adenomatous hyperplasia and goblet cell metaplasia develop as a result of epithelial injury and may lead to encapsulating fibrosis of the bile duct.

Whereas a single exposure to the parasite is of little significance, repeated exposures provoke diffuse involvement of the biliary tree, including the large bile ducts and gallbladder. The average infection leads to harboring of about 20 to 200 adult flukes, which can increase to 20,000 flukes during a heavy infection. Dilated subcapsular bile ducts, adenomatous ductal hyperplasia with or without periductal fibrosis, and eosinophilic infiltration are seen in early infections. Cirrhosis may develop in patients with repeated infections during the later phases. The endemic areas of *Clonorchiasis* and *Opisthorchiasis* coincide with the geographic distribution of liver tumors in Southeast Asia, notably that of cholangiocarcinoma.[49] Recent studies reveal that liver flukes cause distinct patterns of genomic and transcriptional alterations leading to cholangiocarcinoma, which may have diagnostic, preventive, and therapeutic implications.[50,51]

The clinical presentation of biliary clonorchiasis is protean. Most patients with low parasite loads remain asymptomatic. Patients with large parasite loads present with cholangitis, cholangiohepatitis, or intrahepatic calculi. The liver fluke causes mechanical obstruction of bile flow; subsequent bile stasis predisposes to cholangitis that results in the death of the fluke. Paroxysms of colicky upper abdominal pain caused by cholangitis may be confused with gallstone disease. Biliary calculi may coexist, as the eggs can act as a nidus for stone formation. Chronic infection is associated with the development of cholangiocarcinoma.

Chonorchiasis should be suspected in any patient who has lived in or traveled to an endemic region and consumed raw freshwater fish, and subsequently developed clinical signs consistent with a biliary or hepatic disease.

Endotherapy

In patients presenting with acute cholangitis, emergency biliary decompression with sphincterotomy is the treatment of choice.[52] Aspirated bile may show adult worms and ova. On cholangiography, characteristic features include a mulberry-like appearance, caused by multiple saccular or cystic dilatations of the intrahepatic bile ducts; the "arrowhead" sign, caused by rapid tapering of the intrahepatic bile ducts toward the periphery; and a decrease in the number of intrahepatic radicles because of portal and periportal fibrosis. Ductal irregularities are caused by adenomatous hyperplasia and vary from small indentations to hemispherical filling defects. A scalloped appearance is seen as filamentous, wavy, and elliptical filling defects.

Endoscopic biopsy or brush cytology is indicated whenever cholangiocarcinoma is suspected. Surgical intervention is indicated in patients with hepatolithiasis complicated by multiple biliary strictures.

All patients with biliary clonorchiasis should receive praziquantel (75 mg/kg per day in 3 divided doses for 2 days) to eradicate the infection. Tribendimidine was also shown to have good efficacy in preliminary studies.[46] Biliary ductal abnormalities usually persist even after successful drug therapy.[53]

FASCIOLA HEPATICA

Fascioliasis is caused by *Fasciola hepatica*, the sheep liver fluke. The most important definitive hosts are sheep, in which it remains an important veterinary disease. A wide variety of mammalian ruminants, particularly goats, cattle, horses, camels, hogs, rabbits, and deer, are commonly infected. Intermediate hosts include numerous species of snail, both amphibious and aquatic. Because of the wide range of definitive and intermediate hosts, the disease is geographically widespread and occurs worldwide. Physicians should therefore be aware of the possibility of infection in all geographic areas. Peru and Bolivia (La Paz, Lake Titicaca) are areas of highest endemicity.[54]

Fascioliasis occurs where watercress (water plant) is eaten; it is epidemiologically related to the distribution of the intermediate snail host populations in freshwater areas. Human infection occurs after ingestion of watercress that is infested with metacercariae, the infective form of the fluke. These larvae pass through the duodenal wall into the abdominal cavity and migrate toward the liver.

The disease occurs in two stages. The acute or hepatic phase of the illness occurs when the organism penetrates the liver capsule and migrates through the liver parenchyma toward the biliary system. Patients in the acute phase usually present with dyspepsia, followed by an acute onset of fever and abdominal pain, especially in the right hypochondrium or in the right upper quadrant. Urticaria and eosinophilia may be present. These symptoms result from the destruction and inflammatory response caused by the migrating larvae. In approximately 50% of such cases, the infection remains subclinical. The acute phase usually lasts for 3 months after ingestion of the metacercariae.

The second, chronic or biliary, phase occurs when the parasite enters the bile canaliculi 3 to 4 months after ingesting the contaminated meal. Patients typically present with jaundice, fever, and right-upper-quadrant pain and rarely with acalculous cholecystitis, severe hemobilia, and acute pancreatitis.[55,56]

During the chronic stage, motile flukes may be visualized in the gallbladder.[57]

Liver function tests reflect a cholestatic picture. Serologic tests (FAST-ELISA/Falcon assay screening test or dot blot ELISA) are highly sensitive (95% to 100%) and specific (97%), thus aiding in diagnosis.[58]

Inflammation caused by toxic metabolites and mechanical effects of the larvae in the bile ducts leads to epithelial necrosis and adenomatous changes, eventually leading to biliary fibrosis. These changes further evolve into cystic dilatation, total or partial obstruction of bile ducts, and periportal fibrosis and cirrhosis. Although the fibrotic changes are likely to persist despite successful therapy, some of the ductal changes are reversible.[56]

The adult form has a lifespan of approximately 9 to 13 years. Eggs or dead parasites can form a nidus for calculus formation, potentially leading to intrahepatic or extrahepatic biliary calculi.

Treatment

Oral drug therapy is the standard treatment for hepatic fascioliasis. Triclabendazole (10 mg/kg as a single dose) is the drug of choice. For severe or persistent infections, 2 doses of 10 mg/kg administered 12 to 24 hours apart are recommended.[58] Alternatives include bithionol (30 to 50 mg/kg on alternate days for 10 to 15 doses), chloroquine, mebendazole, albendazole, and praziquantel, which have been used with variable success. Patients should be advised regarding expected biliary colic caused by expulsion of parasites or parasite fragments, which usually occurs 2 to 7 days after commencing drug therapy.

Role of ERCP and Endoscopic Ultrasonography

Endoscopic therapy is required (1) when biliary complications occur or medical therapy fails and (2) in the management of severe infection with multiple worms. During ERCP, *Fasciola* appear as small, radiolucent, linear or crescent-like shadows with jagged, irregular margins in the gallbladder or in dilated bile ducts. Biliary fasciolosis has also been diagnosed on EUS and cholangioscopy, which shows a dilated common bile duct with a floating, linear structure within it.[59,60]

The worms can be extracted by using a balloon catheter or Dormia basket after biliary sphincterotomy (Fig. 49.4). Patients usually harbor a single *Fasciola* worm in the bile duct, with an occasional one in the gallbladder. When worms are present in the gallbladder or in the intrahepatic biliary radicles, where they are not amenable to mechanical extraction, irrigating the biliary system with 20 mL of 2.5% povidone iodine solution (5 mL of 10% povidone iodine plus 15 mL of contrast material) during ERCP is helpful.[61] Bile aspirated may be examined for parasite eggs. It is essential to achieve adequate drainage, particularly in patients with acute cholangitis.

The management of "massive" forms of biliary fascioliasis, where dozens or hundreds of mature parasites reside in the intrahepatic and extrahepatic ducts, has been successfully described.[62] Initial extraction of parasites with a basket or balloon catheter is performed. This is

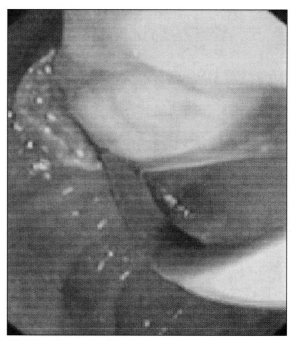

FIG 49.4 Fasciola hepatica extracted using a balloon catheter after biliary sphincterotomy.

followed by 10-minute instillation of 20 mL of 2.5% povidone iodine solution (5 mL of 10% povidone iodine plus 15 mL of contrast material) with balloon occlusion of the common hepatic duct. The ducts are then washed with saline solution and the dead parasites are removed with instruments. Repeat treatment session may be required for complete parasite clearance. In cases with cholangitis and liver abscesses, nasobiliary drainage with iodine treatment repeated three times under direct fluoroscopic control may be done.

SUMMARY

Biliary parasitosis will remain a problem infrequently encountered by practicing endoscopists in nonendemic areas. Ascariasis and hydatid disease are clinically and radiologically evident: *Fasciola, Clonorchis,* and *Opisthorchis* infections require astute clinical suspicion and awareness for early diagnosis and appropriate management.

The complete reference list for this chapter can be found online at www.expertconsult.com.

50

Recurrent Pyogenic Cholangitis

Tae Jun Song, Dong Wan Seo, and Khean-Lee Goh

INTRODUCTION AND SCIENTIFIC BASIS

Recurrent pyogenic cholangitis (RPC) is a condition characterized by repeated attacks of bacterial infection of the biliary tract. It is believed that the initiating event is the entry of enteric flora into the biliary tree, which causes infection, inflammation, and the formation of primary biliary stones through bacterial deconjugation of bilirubin diglucuronide.[1,2] Persistent inflammation results in biliary strictures and stasis of bile in the biliary tree, which encourages further stone formation, leading to a vicious cycle of repeated or persistent inflammation and infection. There have been reports linking helminthiasis to RPC—*Ascaris lumbricoides* and *Clonorchis sinensis* worms have been identified in the biliary tracts of patients with RPC.[2] RPC has been most commonly reported in countries in the Asia-Pacific region, including China, Taiwan, Japan, South Korea, and the Southeast Asian countries; however, it is rapidly declining in this region and is distinctly uncommon in the Western world.[3] Many patients are now elderly and present with complications of RPC such as cholangiocarcinoma.

The hallmark of RPC is the presence of stones and strictures, which can be both intrahepatic and extrahepatic in location (Fig. 50.1 and Video 50.1). The treatment of RPC is difficult and requires a multimodal approach encompassing endoscopy, radiologic techniques, and surgery. Successful treatment of RPC depends on the success of clearing stones, dilating strictures, and maintaining patency of the stenosed ducts. Specific management aims at accurate localization of the pathology, application of specific techniques of removing stones, and dilation of strictures. It serves to eliminate bile stasis and achieve control of cholangitis. Among the endoscopic techniques used are standard endoscopic retrograde cholangiopancreatography (ERCP) with or without peroral cholangioscopy, percutaneous transhepatic cholangioscopy (PTCS), and postoperative cholangioscopy through a T-tube tract.

Surgery is an important treatment modality in RPC and will be discussed briefly at the end of the chapter to place it in the overall scheme of management.

INITIAL MANAGEMENT OF PATIENTS WITH CHOLANGITIS

Patients with RPC often present with acute ascending cholangitis. Acute cholangitis may be the initial attack or a recurrent episode. Patients may develop septic shock quite rapidly. Initial management includes intravenous fluid replacement and institution of intravenous potent broad-spectrum antibiotics. Emergency surgical decompression may be necessary in some patients but carries high postoperative morbidity and mortality rates.

Nonsurgical biliary drainage procedures provide an important alternative treatment option in these patients, especially those with concomitant common bile duct stones.[4] Urgent ERCP with placement of an indwelling stent or a nasobiliary catheter has reduced the mortality rate compared with emergent surgery (Fig. 50.2). Percutaneous transhepatic biliary drainage (PTBD) may be necessary in patients with cholangitis associated with intrahepatic stones.[5]

SPECIFIC TREATMENT OF INTRAHEPATIC STONES

Description of Techniques

Standard ERCP and Peroral Cholangioscopy

Stones that are found in the extrahepatic bile duct and the main intrahepatic ducts can often be dealt with using conventional ERCP techniques of sphincterotomy and basket and/or balloon extraction (see Chapter 19). Strictures in the common bile duct or in the right and left hepatic ducts can be balloon dilated from 4 to 10 mm, depending on upstream ductal diameter, (Quantum TTC balloon [Cook Endoscopy, Winston-Salem, NC] and MaxForce Hurricane [Boston Scientific, Marlborough, MA]) to facilitate passage of a retrieval basket for stone extraction. The use of a "through the scope" mechanical lithotripter (Olympus Optical Company, Tokyo, Japan; MTW, Wessel, Germany; Trapezoid RX, Boston Scientific) is helpful in crushing large stones. However, use of these devices is limited by the often-difficult access into intrahepatic ducts because of angulated bile ducts, tight strictures, and impacted stones.

Peroral cholangioscopy can be used at the time of ERCP. There are several different approaches to the insertion of thin-caliber cholangioscopes into the biliary tree (see Chapter 27). Use of mother-baby scope systems requires two endoscopists, one for the mother scope and one for the baby scope. Single-operator peroral cholangioscopes are also available, with the newer digital image superior to the prior fiberoptic image, and are now comparable to other types of cholangioscopes. An ultraslim upper endoscope can be introduced directly into the biliary tree for direct peroral cholangioscopy (Video 50.2, courtesy of Prof. Jong Ho Moon, South Korea).[6] These endoscopes offer excellent image quality and the possibility of narrow-band imaging. Additionally, the larger working channels compared with dedicated cholangioscopes allow endoscopic-directed biopsy and other therapeutic procedures (Video 50.3, courtesy of Prof. Jong Ho Moon, South Korea).

Lithotripsy using an electrohydraulic lithotripsy (EHL) or a laser probe passed through a mother–baby scope setup can be performed to fragment main intrahepatic duct stones and allow further passage of Dormia baskets and balloons. Stone location, severity of strictures, and duct angulation are limiting factors.

Endoscopic Ultrasonography–Guided Therapy

Recent reports of endoscopic ultrasonography (EUS)–guided therapy for intrahepatic stones have emerged (see Chapters 32 and 33).

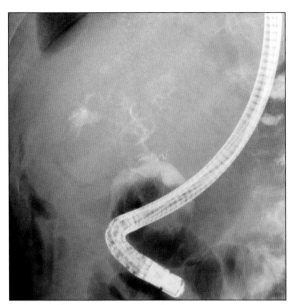

FIG 50.1 Endoscopic retrograde cholangiogram from a patient presenting with acute ascending cholangitis showing intrahepatic and extrahepatic strictures with stones.

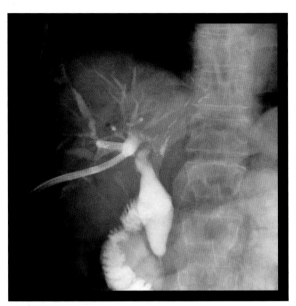

FIG 50.3 Acute angulation caused by inappropriate selection of percutaneous transhepatic biliary drainage site.

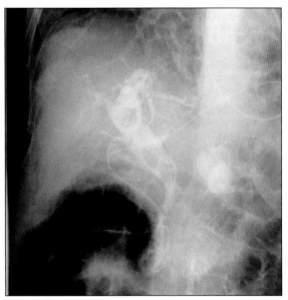

FIG 50.2 Extrahepatic stones and strictures. A nasobiliary tube has been placed via ERCP to relieve cholangitis.

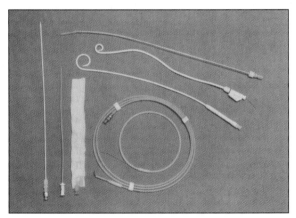

FIG 50.4 Percutaneous transhepatic biliary drainage kit. A complete kit includes Chiba needles for puncture, guidewires, a dilator, and pigtail drainage catheters.

Transgastric and transhepatic approaches with or without percutaneous approaches have been used.[7–9]

Percutaneous Transhepatic Cholangioscopy

PTCS requires a percutaneous transhepatic tract and three steps: percutaneous transhepatic biliary drainage, dilation of the tract, and cholangioscopic examination.

Percutaneous transhepatic biliary drainage. The technique, PTBD, is used to relieve obstructive jaundice and drain infected bile and to prevent or control cholangitis and sepsis. It is an initial step in creating a percutaneous tract and can be performed under fluoroscopic or ultrasonographic guidance. For PTCS, the site of PTBD is very important. If the puncture site is incorrectly placed, an acute angulation may be

created and prevent access to the target lesion (Fig. 50.3). This is an important factor in PTCS failure. Before selecting a PTBD site, the cholangioscopist or interventional radiologist should be familiar with the anatomy of the biliary tree. The ideal PTBD site is selected after meticulous review of all available imaging studies, such as ultrasonography, CT scan, endoscopic retrograde cholangiography, and magnetic resonance cholangiography (MRCP) (see Chapter 34).[10–12] A PTBD kit is composed of puncture needles, guidewire, dilators, and pigtail drainage tubes (Fig. 50.4). The usual diameter of an initial PTBD tube is 6 to 8.5 Fr. For the initial puncture, the selection of a peripheral duct is important because direct insertion of a PTBD tube into the central duct carries a significant risk of bleeding. Ultrasonography-guided puncture or fluoroscopy-guided puncture techniques are commonly adopted for initial peripheral duct selection. After selective puncture of a peripheral duct, a guidewire is inserted and a bougienage dilator is advanced over the guidewire. After dilation of the tract, a pigtail catheter is introduced into the biliary tree (Fig. 50.5). In cases of nondilated intrahepatic ducts, PTBD carries a high risk of bleeding and biliary leakage. To prevent these adverse events, insertion of an endoscopic nasobiliary drainage tube before PTBD allows cholangiography to be

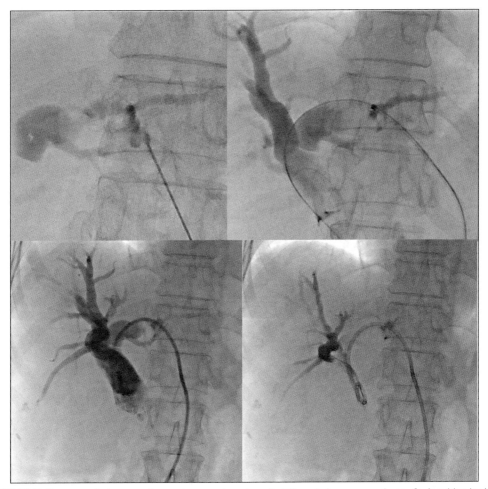

FIG 50.5 Fluoroscopic images of percutaneous transhepatic biliary drainage procedures. **A,** A guidewire is inserted into the left intrahepatic duct after selection of S3 segmental duct by needle puncture. **B,** The tract is dilated up to 8 Fr. **C,** A 7.5-Fr pigtail drainage catheter is inserted into the dilated tract. **D,** Previously injected contrast material is well drained through the pigtail catheter.

performed during PTBD and is helpful to accurately target the desired intrahepatic duct.

Tract dilation. For cholangioscopic examination of the biliary tree, the diameter of the percutaneous transhepatic tract should be larger than that of the cholangioscope (e.g., CHF-P20; Olympus Optical Company, Tokyo, Japan). The cholangioscope diameter ranges from 3.0 to 5.2 mm. Therefore the diameter of the percutaneous tract should be dilated to at least 11 to 12 Fr when an 11-Fr cholangioscope is used. In most centers, the tract is dilated to 16 to 18 Fr, because a cholangioscope with an outer diameter of 16 Fr is commonly used for therapeutic purposes. This dilation procedure can be performed with the aid of a specialized dilation kit (Nipro, Tokyo, Japan) (Fig. 50.6). The dilation process can be accomplished by "multistage" dilation or by "one-stage" dilation. Multistage dilation entails reaching the fully dilated diameter of the percutaneous tract through several repeated dilations. The diameter of the PTBD tube is around 6 to 8.5 Fr at the first attempt. The tract can be dilated in stages every 2 to 4 days: to 10 to 12 Fr, then up to 14 to 16 Fr, and finally up to more than 18 Fr. In the one-stage dilation protocol, the PTBD tract is dilated up to 16 or 18 Fr in a single session, performed 2 to 4 days after initial PTBD.

There are advantages and disadvantages of each method. The main advantage of multistage dilation is that the dilation process is less painful and less traumatic. Gradual dilation with repeated procedures can reduce

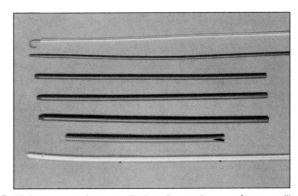

FIG 50.6 Nipro set for tract dilation. A complete set for tract dilation is composed of a guidewire, a tapered-tip catheter, variable-sized bougienage tubes, and a percutaneous transhepatic cholangioscopy catheter.

the risk of severe pain or the chance of significant bleeding after dilation. However, multistage dilation is time-consuming, requires several procedures until satisfactory dilation is achieved, and is costlier. The one-stage dilation protocol saves time and cost compared with the multistage dilation protocol but can cause significant pain and bleeding

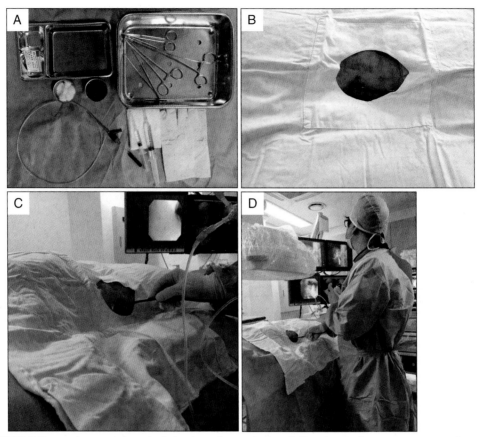

FIG 50.7 Percutaneous transhepatic cholangioscopic examination. **A,** Dressing set for percutaneous transhepatic cholangioscopy (PTCS). **B,** Draping was done before cholangioscopic examination. An 18-Fr PTCS catheter is visible and the tube is tied to the skin to prevent migration. **C,** Assessment of light source and saline flow before insertion of the cholangioscope into the body. **D,** Insertion of cholangioscope. After insertion of the tip of the cholangioscope into the tract, the cholangioscopist monitors the videoscopic view and guides the cholangioscope tip to maintain a view of the bile duct lumen.

during the procedure. For the one-stage dilation protocol, it is mandatory to provide adequate analgesia.

Percutaneous transhepatic cholangioscopic examination. After full dilation of the percutaneous transhepatic tract, 10 to 14 days are usually required for maturation of the sinus tract, at which time the cholangioscopic examination can be safely performed (Fig. 50.7). The patient is positioned in the supine position on the fluoroscopy table. The position of the cholangioscopist can be changed according to the site of PTBD. For example, when PTBD is performed on a right intrahepatic duct, the right side of the patient is the preferred position; when PTBD is done on a left intrahepatic duct, the left side of the patient is the preferred position. The video monitor and fluoroscopic monitor should be positioned accordingly for the cholangioscopist. Premedication using a combination of meperidine and midazolam or diazepam is required to relieve pain and anxiety. The insertion of a cholangioscope into a fully dilated tract is not difficult. However, if the waiting period between tract dilation and cholangioscopic examination is short, cholangioscope insertion can be difficult and sometimes traumatic. The tract may collapse after removal of the dilation tube, especially during the first cholangioscopic examination. A guidewire, which is inserted before removal of the dilation tube, is used to smoothly guide the cholangioscope into the biliary tree.

PTCS offers several advantages. The percutaneous approach allows evaluation of both the intrahepatic ducts and the common bile duct, and it is the shortest distance to the biliary tree. The handling and angulation maneuvers of the tip of the percutaneous cholangioscope are easier compared with those for peroral cholangioscopy. The application of various techniques, such as biopsy, suction, and dye spraying, during cholangioscopic examination is also technically easy. Insertion of a balloon or a catheter under cholangioscopic guidance and application of biopsy forceps or EHL are also much easier than with the peroral approach. The only drawback compared with the peroral route is the necessity of creating a percutaneous tract, which is an invasive process, and uncomfortable for the patient.

During cholangioscopic evaluation of the biliary tree, irrigation is required to obtain an optimal view of the biliary ducts. Pus, sludge, and blood can obscure the endoscopic view. Thick bile may also "coat" the bile duct wall. To obtain a clear view of the bile duct, continuous saline irrigation is recommended and is usually achieved by suspending a bottle of normal saline and allowing it to flow continuously into the instrumental channel of the cholangioscope to "wash" the bile duct (Fig. 50.8).

Postoperative Cholangioscopy

Although ERCP and laparoscopic cholecystectomy are commonly performed in patients with gallbladder and common bile duct stones, patients may still undergo open cholecystectomy with common bile duct exploration followed by T-tube placement in the common bile duct. Postoperative cholangioscopy can be performed in these patients after maturation of the T-tube tract.

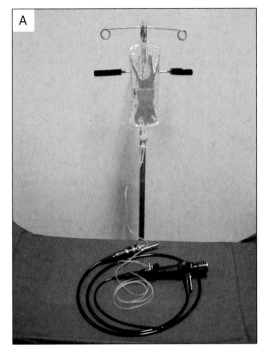

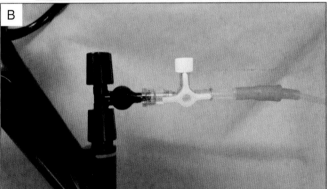

FIG 50.8 Normal saline irrigation by gravity. **A,** A bottle of normal saline is connected to the cholangioscope. Gravity provides a continuous flow of normal saline into the bile duct during cholangioscopic examination. **B,** The flow can be controlled by on-and-off switching of a two-way stopcock.

Compared with a percutaneous transhepatic tract, the T-tube tract is a relatively long tract and traverses a longer length of free peritoneal space before reaching the common bile duct. When percutaneous transhepatic cholangioscopy is employed, the distance of free space between parietal peritoneum and liver capsule is usually less than 1 cm, whereas the T-tube tract has a free space between parietal peritoneum and common bile duct, which is usually longer than 4 to 5 cm. Because of this difference, maturation of the T-tube tract usually takes a longer period, normally at least 4 weeks after T-tube insertion.

An ideal T-tube tract should run a straight course from the skin to the insertion point in the bile duct. If this tract meets the common bile duct at a right angle, cholangioscopic examination of the common bile duct and intrahepatic ducts is not difficult (Fig. 50.9). The technique of bile duct examination is basically similar to that of percutaneous transhepatic cholangioscopy. However, there are also limitations of postoperative cholangioscopy. In addition to having to wait a longer period until full maturation of the tract, insertion of the cholangioscope may not be easy, because the T-tube tract may be angulated (Fig. 50.10). Angulation makes cholangioscopic examination very difficult, and

disruption (perforation) of the T-tube tract during cholangioscope insertion can occur.

Techniques for Cholangioscopic Stone Removal
Basket Removal

Biliary stones can be found in a straight duct and/or an angulated duct. Cholangioscopic removal of stones requires an experienced operator in order to make an otherwise laborious procedure less time-consuming and safer. The basic steps for cholangioscopic removal of stones are as follows: first, the basket is inserted into the biliary tract; second, the basket is opened just beyond the stones; third, the stone is engaged by withdrawing the opened basket; fourth, stones are grasped firmly by withdrawing the basket further; finally, the stone is removed by simultaneous removal of the cholangioscope and basket (Fig. 50.11).

For removal of stones, a Dormia-type basket is used. The ideal position of the basket tip before opening is just beyond the stones, and they can be captured only by gentle withdrawal of the opened basket (Fig. 50.12). If a basket is opened proximal to a stone, there is a possibility that the stone will be pushed into a peripheral duct. The basket may be opened just before the stone or at the exact site of the stone; the stone can be captured by advancing the opened basket or by moving the basket back and forth. However, these maneuvers can cause deformity of the basket. Gentle withdrawal and closure of the basket to engage the stones is recommended.

Stone Fragmentation

Large stones often cannot be extracted directly from the biliary tree and need to be fragmented. The easiest way to fragment large stones is to crush them by tightening or closing the basket. Softer brown-pigment stones can be broken into several pieces by this simple maneuver. EHL or laser lithotripsy[13,14] is needed to fragment harder stones. The mechanism of EHL fragmentation is generation of compression waves (shock waves). The shock waves are generated at the tip of the probe directly in front of the stones by an explosive spark discharged in a liquid medium (Fig. 50.13 and Video 50.4). Adjustment of power and frequency modes permits adaptation to various fields of application and sites. Higher energy with high frequency is effective at fragmenting hard stones but can easily damage the bile duct wall. To avoid tissue damage, lower energy levels are preferable. For best results, the probe is placed directly on the stone. The EHL shock wave can be generated only in an aqueous medium, and therefore an electrolyte solution such as physiologic saline (0.9% NaCl) is used for irrigation.

EHL can be used not only to fragment large and hard stones but also to fragment smaller stones that are impacted in peripheral ducts or within a strictured segment. It may not be possible to remove impacted stones using only a basket because of inadequate space to open the basket and grasp the stones. When EHL is used, only a small aperture is needed and the tip of the probe can then come into contact with the stone. Once the tip of the EHL probe is directed at the stone, electrohydraulic shock wave can be generated in an aqueous medium and the force applied to the stone (Fig. 50.14). After fragmentation of large stones into small pieces, a basket can be introduced beyond the strictured segment and they can be extracted or flushed out using forceful saline irrigation. Occasionally extracorporeal shock wave lithotripsy (ESWL) is also used, followed by percutaneous cholangioscopic management.[15]

Stricture Dilation

Intrahepatic stones frequently occur upstream of a strictured segment of the bile duct. For cholangioscopic removal of these stones, stricture dilation is required (see Chapter 43). A balloon dilator or dilating catheter can be used for this purpose.

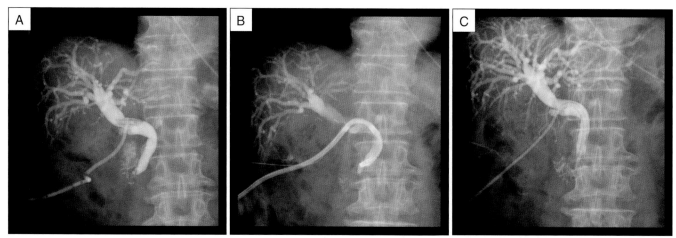

FIG 50.9 Ideal course of T-tube tract. **A,** A successful cholangioscopic examination is dependent on the straightness of the tract. The ideal T-tube tract for postoperative cholangioscopy should be straight and the insertion angle into the common bile duct (CBD) is a right angle. **B** and **C,** In the setting of a right angle, insertion of the cholangioscope into intrahepatic duct or distal CBD is possible with the aid of flexion or extension movement of the cholangioscope tip.

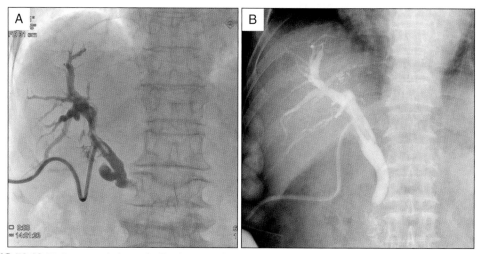

FIG 50.10 Various angulations of a T-tube tract. **A** and **B,** During operative insertion of T-tube into the bile duct, various angulations can be made at the sinus tract, and this is an important factor that limits successful cholangioscopy. The surgeon should be cautious to prevent these types of angulations.

When balloon dilation is performed, a balloon and pressure gauge are required. There are several types of balloons that can be used for dilation of strictures. The ideal balloon has a small shaft diameter and the balloon should be strong enough to endure the pressure applied during dilation. The balloon must be long enough to cover the strictured segment. For balloon dilation, a guidewire is inserted across the strictured segment under cholangioscopic and fluoroscopic guidance. The balloon is advanced though the strictured segment over the guidewire and positioned under fluoroscopy. It is important to keep the guidewire straight during advancement of the balloon catheter. The optimal location of the balloon is usually obtained when the midportion of the balloon (also known as the waist, where the expansile force is greatest) is located at the stricture. If the balloon is not placed centrally over the stricture as described, there is a tendency for the balloon to slip in or out of the stricture during inflation. Contrast media or distilled water mixed with radiopaque contrast material is used to inflate the balloon and allow visualization of the dilating balloon under fluoroscopy. Radiopaque contrast material acts as an indicator

of the degree of dilation (Fig. 50.15) by demonstrating the waist of the balloon at the site of the stricture; obliteration of the waist occurs with successful dilation (Fig. 50.16). The dilation pressure should be monitored to achieve and maintain the optimum inflation pressure of 6 to 10 atmospheres.

Dilation of the bile duct can also be achieved with catheters. There are two types of catheters according to the shape of the tips: a tapered-tip catheter (Akita Sumitomo; Bakelite Company, Akita, Japan) and a straight-tip catheter (Cook Medical, Bloomington, IN) (Fig. 50.17). The main advantage of the tapered-tip catheter is ease of passage into and across the strictured segment. However, a catheter with tapered tip has a tendency to slip away from the lesion when the strictured segment is tight, whereas a straight-tip catheter does not. The main disadvantage of a straight-tip catheter is that insertion of this catheter can be traumatic and may cause severe pain or bleeding because of its blunt end.

For insertion of a catheter into the strictured segment, a guidewire is passed through the strictured portion. The catheter is pushed

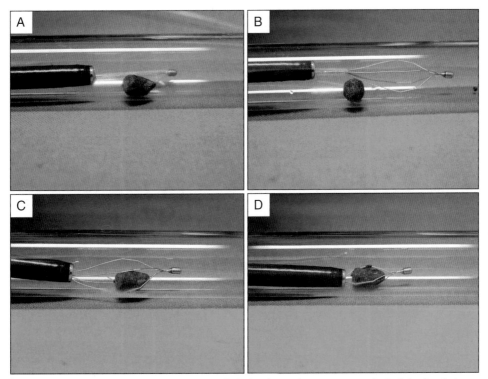

FIG 50.11 Illustration of the four basic steps of cholangioscopic stone removal. **A,** A basket is inserted through the cholangioscope and the basket tip is positioned beyond the stone. **B,** The basket is opened just beyond the stone to grasp. **C,** Gentle withdrawal of the opened basket is usually adequate to engage intraluminal stones. To facilitate this step, the basket should keep its original shape when it is opened within the lumen. **D,** Further closure of the basket in which the stone is engaged allows the stone to be grasped tightly; removal of the stone is usually achieved by gentle simultaneous withdrawal of the cholangioscope and the stone basket.

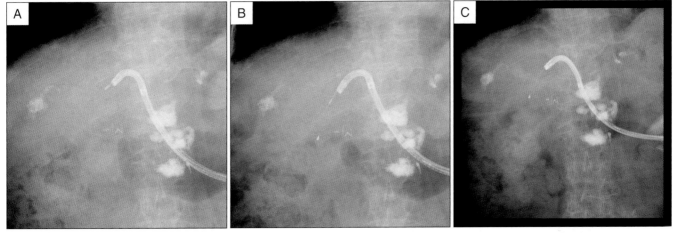

FIG 50.12 Cholangiography during basket stone removal. **A,** The cholangioscope is positioned immediately in front of an intrahepatic stone and the basket tip is located just beyond the stone before opening. **B,** The basket is opened beyond the stone. **C,** By withdrawing the opened basket, a small stone is engaged within the basket.

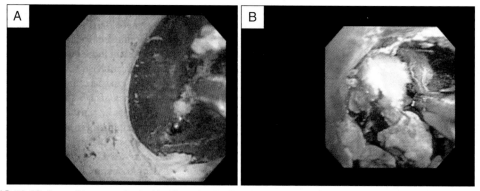

FIG 50.13 Stone fragmentation using electrohydraulic lithotripsy (EHL). **A,** The tip of the EHL probe is placed on the surface of a pigmented stone. **B,** After EHL, the inner core is exposed. Layered structure of inner core is visible after destruction of outer shell.

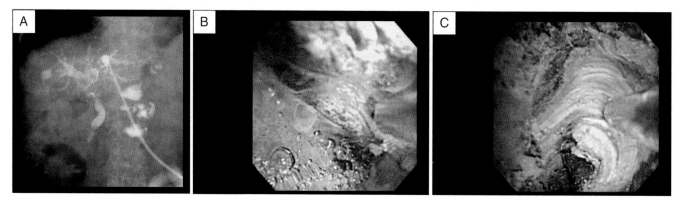

FIG 50.14 Application of electrohydraulic lithotripsy (EHL) for treatment of an impacted stone. **A,** Cholangiogram shows multiple large stones impacted in the intrahepatic and extrahepatic bile ducts. There is no space to permit introduction of a stone basket. **B,** Cholangioscopic view reveals only small anterior surface of the impacted large stone. The tip of the EHL probe is positioned at the surface of the stone. **C,** Stones are fragmented by EHL.

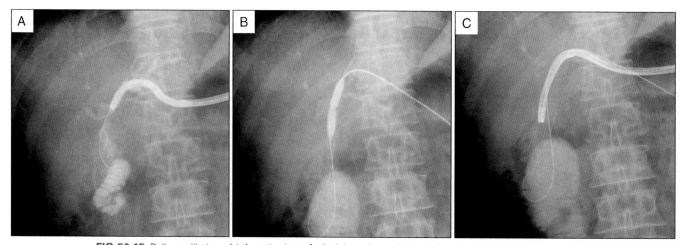

FIG 50.15 Balloon dilation of left main duct. **A,** A tight stricture in the left main duct with upstream duct dilation is seen. Under cholangioscopic and fluoroscopic guidance, a guidewire is passed into the stricture segment. **B,** A balloon is inserted over the guidewire and centered across the strictured segment (the two radiopaque markers of the balloon are seen). The balloon is inflated with contrast material. **C,** After successful dilation, the cholangioscope can pass the strictured segment.

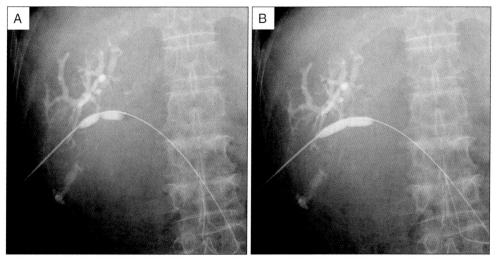

FIG 50.16 Waist formation and disappearance during balloon dilation. **A,** A waist in the balloon is seen during inflation. **B,** When the pressure exceeds the strength of the stricture, the waist disappears. Once this occurs, the inflation pressure should not be increased.

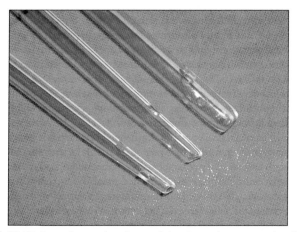

FIG 50.17 According to the shape of the tip, catheters are classified into two types: tapered (lower two catheters) and straight (uppermost catheter).

though the strictured segment over the guidewire. If there is an acute angulation during the course of passage, catheter insertion frequently fails. To overcome difficult angulations, two or more guidewires can be used simultaneously to guide the tip of the dilating catheter (Fig. 50.18). Balloon dilation and catheter dilation can be used in combination. In case of a tight stricture, balloon dilation followed by catheter placement into the stricture segment allows for an effective dilation.

To allow efficient bile drainage from other intrahepatic ducts at the same time, the catheters should have side holes. The side holes can be made just before catheter insertion (Fig. 50.19). The number, location, and size of side holes are important to ensure adequate drainage through the catheter and to prevent bile leakage. Before making side holes, the cholangioscopist should measure the length of catheter that will be inserted into the bile duct. This can be done by measuring the length of the cholangioscope inserted into the target lesion or the length of a guidewire inserted into the strictured segment. Side holes should not be located at the portion of the catheter at the sinus tract because this can cause bile leakage.

Results of Cholangioscopic Stone Removal

The cholangioscopic approach is useful for treatment of intrahepatic stones, especially when there are multiple and bilateral stones. Complete stone removal can usually be achieved after several cholangioscopic sessions (Fig. 50.20). However, it is difficult in the presence of multiple strictures and angulations. Complete stone clearance can be achieved in 80% of patients and is significantly lower in patients with severe intrahepatic strictures than those without strictures. Patients with severe intrahepatic strictures also show a higher recurrence rate than those with mild or no strictures. In addition, the stone recurrence rate is different according to the hepatic functional reserve. The recurrence rate is significantly higher in patients with advanced biliary cirrhosis, such as Child class B or C, than those with mild cirrhosis, such as Child class A or no cirrhotic change.

INDICATIONS AND CONTRAINDICATIONS

Standard ERCP is important and indicated in the initial evaluation of a patient presenting with acute cholangitis. A good-quality cholangiogram can be obtained with ERCP. However, with tight strictures and impacted stones, the biliary anatomy upstream of the pathology may not be adequately demonstrated. Extrahepatic stones and stones with strictures in the main intrahepatic ducts can be treated using conventional ERCP techniques with retrieval baskets and balloons and balloon dilation of strictures. ERCP can provide acute, although temporary, relief of biliary obstruction and cholangitis with the placement of plastic stents or nasobiliary drains.

PTCS is indicated in patients with peripheral intrahepatic stones, multiple bilateral intrahepatic stones, or stones located upstream of tight intrahepatic strictures. It allows better access to the affected intrahepatic ducts with a cholangioscope. It is also indicated when providing biliary drainage with a PTBD.

Apart from the general contraindications to ERCP, there are no specific contraindications in the setting of RPC. PTCS is contraindicated in patients with bleeding diathesis. The risk of bleeding is high in patients with concomitant advanced cirrhosis. The presence of ascites makes establishing a mature percutaneous tract difficult, and special precautions are needed, including the use of sheaths. For patients with a history of allergy to contrast media, prophylactic corticosteroids should be

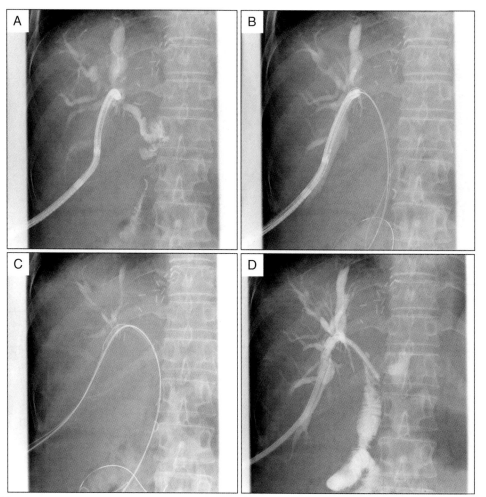

FIG 50.18 Catheter insertion using double guidewires. **A,** Cholangiogram shows anastomotic stricture. **B,** Two guidewires are inserted across the anastomosis. **C,** A 16-Fr percutaneous transhepatic cholangioscopy (PTCS) catheter is inserted. After several negotiations, it was possible for the catheter to pass the angulated area. **D,** Cholangiogram shows the PTCS catheter tip located in the distal common bile duct.

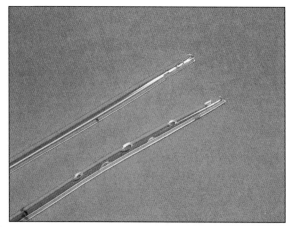

FIG 50.19 Percutaneous transhepatic cholangioscopy (PTCS) catheters before (*above*) and after (*below*) making side holes.

administered or, alternatively, nonionic contrast media used. Patients must be cooperative and adequately sedated for both ERCP and PTCS. These procedures are relatively high risk and sophisticated, and those for patients with other indications experienced endoscopists and assistants are needed.

ADVERSE EVENTS AND THEIR MANAGEMENT

Adverse events (AEs) of ERCP in patients with RPC are similar to those for patients with other indications (see Chapter 8). Cholangitis may be a particularly difficult problem, especially when contrast is injected into intrahepatic ducts that cannot be drained and/or after insertion of catheters and manipulation of the biliary tree. Percutaneous drainage of the appropriate undrained ducts should be carried out. Preprocedural intravenous antibiotics are administered and continued postprocedurally.

The main AEs from PTCS are related to transhepatic catheter placement and dilation of the cutaneous hepatic fistula. Hemobilia caused by biliovenous fistula is a commonly encountered problem. Bleeding may not be apparent when the percutaneous catheter is in place, as the catheter provides a tamponade effect and bleeding occurs when the catheter is removed.

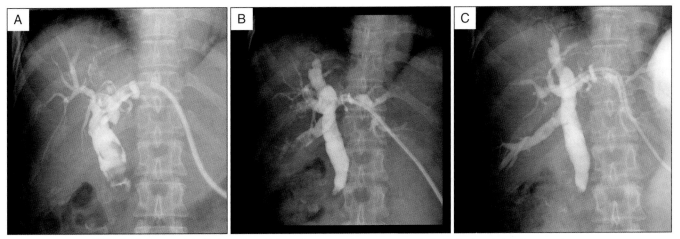

FIG 50.20 Sequential dilation of multiple strictures and stone removal. **A,** Catheter cholangiogram shows that many right intrahepatic ducts are missing. Several right intrahepatic stones are faintly delineated. **B,** After several sessions of stricture dilation using balloons and percutaneous transhepatic cholangioscopy (PTCS) catheters, cholangiography reveals multiple stones in the right superior and inferior branch ducts. **C,** After full dilation of multiple segmental ducts and cholangioscopic stone removal, many right intrahepatic ducts are visualized.

AEs with the use of the cholangioscope are usually minor. Bleeding is reported in about 10% of cases, but major bleeding requiring transfusion or therapeutic intervention occurs in 1% to 2%. Perforation of the intrahepatic bile ducts occurs in 1.7%.

Cholangitis after PTCS occurs after vigorous manipulation of the biliary tree, and there may be an inability to completely drain the bile ducts where "lakes" of contrast-filled intrahepatic ducts are present.

If a sinus or T-tube tract is not mature enough, partial or complete disruption of the catheter tract causes bile leakage and bile peritonitis, which is a serious AE. The risk of percutaneous tube dislocation is reduced if the distal end of the tube is placed in the common bile duct or through the papilla into the duodenum. When dislocation of the tube occurs, immediate replacement of the tube along the same tract is required, although this may not be possible.

LONG-TERM MANAGEMENT OF RPC

As complete dilation of intrahepatic strictures is rarely successful, one of the biggest problems in RPC is persistent infection and recurrent stone formation. When percutaneous access has already been created for cholangioscopy, access can be maintained with placement of a Yamakawa-type transhepatic tube, which can be occluded at the skin level.[16] Repeat cholangioscopy with extraction of newly formed stones or further dilation of strictures can then be performed.

One of the long-term sequelae of RPC is liver cirrhosis, and preservation of hepatic functional reserve is very important. Once liver function deteriorates, subsequent stone removal becomes more difficult and recurrent cholangitis can aggravate the deterioration of hepatic functional reserve. Cholangiocarcinoma is one of the most dreadful long-term sequelae of RPC. Elevated serum CA 19-9 levels in patients with intrahepatic stones may be an indicator of underlying cholangiocarcinoma.[17] Bile duct stones and/or repeated cholangitis can cause postinflammatory ductal changes. Strictures, dilation, and ductal deformities are commonly seen after stone removal in patients with intrahepatic stones (Video 50.5). Ductal mucosa can also be altered.

Benign mucosal hyperplasia or papillary projections are often identified by cholangioscopy after stone removal (Video 50.6). Surgical resection can be performed to avoid the development of cholangiocarcinoma from abnormal mucosa; however, surgery does not completely abolish the risk of cholangiocarcinoma.[18]

SURGERY

Nonsurgical approaches to the treatment of RPC have often proven to be difficult, as persistent or recurrent cholangitis occurs. Another concern in patients with RPC is the development of cholangiocarcinoma. Hepatectomy, when feasible, can provide definitive treatment for hepatolithiasis,[19,20] as it removes not only the stones but also the strictured bile ducts and eliminates the possibility of recurrent stone formation and the risk of cholangiocarcinoma in the segments resected.[21] Recently, laparoscopic hepatectomy has been performed in patients with RPC.[22,23] Intrahepatic stones that are confined to one lobe allow removal of the affected lobe with cure of the disease. In most cases there is a predilection for stones to be confined to the left lobe of the liver. Bilobar stone disease poses a therapeutic dilemma.[24] Aggressive surgeons resect the more severely affected lobe and fashion a hepaticocutaneous jejunostomy from the remaining lobe to allow access for further percutaneous cholangioscopic treatments.

RELATIVE COST

Surgery, although incurring the highest initial cost, offers definitive treatment when feasible and is probably the most cost-effective approach. PTCS requires repeated procedures and consumes the time of both endoscopists and radiologists. Cost of treatment using these approaches increases over time, because repeated sessions are required.

The complete reference list for this chapter can be found online at www.expertconsult.com.

51

Cystic Lesions of the Pancreas

Omer Basar and William R. Brugge

Pancreatic cystic lesions comprise a spectrum ranging from benign to premalignant to invasive malignancies. Pancreatic cystic neoplasms (PCNs) are relatively rare, accounting for less than 10% of all pancreatic neoplasms.[1] Their diagnostic frequency increases with age and has noticeably increased with widespread availability of cross-sectional imaging. Although most cystic lesions are detected incidentally in patients who undergo abdominal imaging for an unrelated reason, large or invasive lesions may produce sufficient symptoms to cause the patient to seek medical attention.

After detection of a cyst within the pancreas, the first step in management is to exclude pancreatic pseudocyst. Peripancreatic inflammatory fluid collections may mimic PCNs both clinically and morphologically. Furthermore, patients with PCNs may present with pancreatitis and patients with pseudocysts may have subclinical mild pancreatitis.

The type of epithelial lining typically categorizes PCNs into mucinous and nonmucinous neoplasms (Table 51.1).[1] The type of epithelial lining determines the malignant potential and therefore management. Mucinous cysts have malignant potential, whereas serous cystic neoplasms (SCNs) are predominantly benign. Mucinous lesions include intraductal papillary mucinous neoplasms (IPMNs) and mucinous cystic neoplasms (MCNs). The nonmucinous lesions include SCNs, solid pseudopapillary neoplasms (SPNs), cystic pancreatic neuroendocrine tumors (cPNETs), and other rare lesions.

PREVALENCE

The prevalence of pancreatic cysts in adults as examined in autopsy series and a Japanese study was 24.3% in 300 cases (186 lesions in 73 cases) of patients without known pancreatic disease. The prevalence increased with age, and pathologic examination of cysts showed that the cystic epithelium displayed a spectrum of dysplastic changes in which invasive cancer arose.[2] Several studies have reported high malignancy risk for PCNs (38% to 68% for mixed-duct IPMNs [MD-IPMNs], 12% to 47% for branch-duct IPMNs [BD-IPMNs], 10% to 17% for MCNs, 8% to 20% for SPNs, and 6% to 31% for cPNETs).[3–18]

The prevalence of pancreatic cysts ranges from 2% to 19% in cross-sectional imaging studies, and in patients older than 70 years, the cumulative prevalence increased to 40%.[19] A study including 24,039 computed tomography (CT) and magnetic resonance imaging (MRI) scans at one institution revealed that 290 (1.2%) patients had pancreatic cysts without signs of pancreatitis and those cyst were likely (60%) to be PCNs in patients older than 70 years old.[20]

CLINICAL EPIDEMIOLOGY

IPMNs, MCNs, and SCNs account for approximately 85% of primary PCNs. A population-based study in the Western Hemisphere revealed

that MCNs account for 10% to 45%, SNCs for 32% to 39%, IPMNs for 21% to 33%, and SPNs for less than 10% of cases. On the other hand, in a nationwide Korean survey, IPMN was found in 41%, MCN in 25.2%, SPN in 18.3%, and SCN in 15.2%.[21] In a retrospective study including 851 patients undergoing surgery for PCN, IPMNs accounted for 38%, MCNs for 23%, SCNs for 16%, and SPNs for 3%.[22]

IPMNs are an intraductal proliferation of mucin-producing cells arising in pancreatic neoplastic ductal epithelium. The main pancreatic duct and/or branch ducts may be involved.[23] IPMNs predominantly affect men at a mean age of 65 years, which is why they tend to occur in an older age group than MCNs.[23]

MCNs are the second type of mucinous lesion that more commonly affect women (20:1 ratio).[24] The mean age at diagnosis is 55 years, slightly younger than patients with IPMNs.[1] They are predominantly located in the tail of the pancreas.

SCNs are considered benign; although malignant SCNs (i.e., serous cystadenocarcinomas) occur, they are extremely rare.[25] The majority of patients with SCNs are female, with a median age in the seventh decade. SCNs are slow-growing tumors[26] that are almost always incidentally detected on abdominal imaging or during surgery.[27,28]

SPNs consist of solid and cystic components. SPNs occur predominantly in women[29] in their twenties or thirties[30,31] and are generally considered a low-grade malignancy.

CNETs of the pancreas are indolent tumors that are reported to account for less than 10% of all PCNs[1,32] and 1% to 2% of all pancreatic tumors.[33] They are composed of neuroendocrine tissue and have variable malignant potential. Both sexes are equally affected, and the mean age at diagnosis is between the fifth and sixth decade.[34,35] It is rare for CNETs to produce sufficient hormones to be clinically active.[34,36] CNETs are usually sporadic but may be seen in association with von Hippel–Lindau (VHL) syndrome, neurofibromatosis type 1, multiple endocrine neoplasia type 1, and tuberous sclerosis.[34,37]

RISK FACTORS FOR CYSTIC LESIONS

In the vast majority of patients with a cystic lesion, no risk factor is apparent. The VHL syndrome is the best-described inherited disorder associated with pancreatic cystic lesions. In the largest series to date, pancreatic involvement was observed in 122 of 158 patients (77.2%) and included true cysts (91.1%), serous cystadenomas (12.3%), neuroendocrine tumors (12.3%), and combined lesions (11.5%).[38]

PATHOGENESIS

The pathogenesis of cystic neoplasms of the pancreas is poorly understood. IPMNs share several molecular changes with pancreatic adenocarcinoma; however, some newly found mutations are not observed in patients with pancreatic cancer and the incidence of similar mutations

Video for this chapter can be found online at www.expertconsult.com.

TABLE 51.1 Features of Pancreatic Cystic Neoplasms

Tumor Type	Gender	Age	Morphology	Type of Epithelium	Risk of Malignancy
Intraductal papillary mucinous neoplasm	Mixed	Elderly	Unilocular, septated, associated dilated ducts	Papillary mucinous	High
Mucinous cystic neoplasm	Female	Middle-aged	Unilocular	Mucinous	High
Serous cystic neoplasm	Female	Middle-aged	Microcystic	Serous (PAS positive for glycogen)	Low
Solid-pseudopapillary neoplasm	Female	Young	Mixed solid and cystic	Endocrine-like	Low
Cystic neuroendocrine neoplasm	Mixed	Middle-aged	Associated mass	Endocrine	Low

PAS, Periodic acid-Schiff.

differs in both entities. The frequency of *KRAS* mutations is reported to increase with increasing dysplasia in patients with IPMN[23,24] and MCN.[39] Additionally, the *p53* mutation is reported in MCN patients with high-grade dysplasia and cancer.[39] Loss of *DPC4* is also reported in malignant MCN but not in benign cases, suggesting a role in malignant transformation.[40] The frequency of *KRAS* mutations in IPMN ranges from 38% to 100%. Loss of *p16*, whose frequency increases with increasing dysplasia, is found in 78% of IPMNs.[41] Similar to MCNs, *p53* mutations are seen in 50% of IPMNs,[41] especially in patients with high-grade dysplasia.[42] An atypical mutation, such as *PIK3CA*, is only seen in 11% of IPMNs.[43] *GNAS* mutations are reported in up to 66% of patients, whereas *RNF43* is reported in some IPMN patients; however, these genes are exclusively mutated in IPMNs but not in MCNs.[44] The *STK11/LKB1* gene is inactivated in 25% of sporadic IPMNs and in almost all IPMNs occurring in the background of Peutz-Jeghers syndrome.[45]

The pathogenesis of SCNs is likely to be very different from that of mucinous cysts, because *KRAS* mutations are not seen in SCN.[46] The *VHL* gene, which is located on chromosome 3p25, seems to play an important role.[46,47] In one study, 70% of sporadic SCNs demonstrated loss of heterozygosity at 3p25 with a *VHL* gene mutation in the remaining allele.[48]

PATHOLOGY

Intraductal Papillary Mucinous Neoplasms

IPMNs originate from pancreatic ductal epithelium, secrete mucin, and are characterized by papillary projections from the ductal surface into pancreatic lumen. IPMNs are classified as main-duct–type IPMN, branch-duct–type IPMN, or combined-type IPMN, depending on the pancreatic ductal system involved.[49] According to the grade of dysplasia, the 2010 World Health Organization classification separates IPMNs as IPMN with low-grade or intermediate-grade dysplasia, IPMN with high-grade dysplasia (carcinoma in situ), and IPMN with an associated invasive carcinoma. The intraluminal growth of papillary neoplasm and obstructing mucus causes the upstream pancreatic duct to dilate.[23] The degree of ductal ectasia varies with the degree of mucin production, but ductal dilation seen on imaging studies or gross pathologic examination is a diagnostic feature. Mucin production may be so excessive that it may be seen to spontaneously excret from the ampulla.[50] IPMNs are premalignant lesions, and within a single tumor the lining of the epithelium may exhibit areas ranging from low-grade dysplasia to carcinoma. Foci of early malignancy may be evident by the presence of mural nodules.[51] Solid malignancies that arise from IPMNs are more likely to have papillary features compared with typical pancreatic adenocarcinoma that arises from the main pancreatic duct.[52]

Based on the predominant histologic architectural and epithelial cell differentiation, four subtypes of IPMNs have been determined that predict biologic behavior:

1. Gastric foveolar type: a common low-grade lesion that is predominant in BD-IPMNs.[53,54]

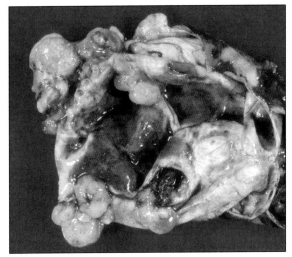

FIG 51.1 Gross mucinous cystic neoplasm.

2. Intestinal type: intermediate-grade to high-grade dysplasia, which is predominantly seen in MD-IPMNs. Colloid-type adenocarcinoma commonly develops in association with intestinal type.[55]
3. Pancreatobiliary type, often tubular type: invasive cancers developing from this type have a worse prognosis than colloid type.
4. Intraductal oncocytic papillary cancer type: extremely rare and accepted as identical to pancreatic ductal adenocarcinoma.[56,57]

The best prognosis is seen in patients with gastric-type IPMNs and the worst prognosis is with pancreatobiliary-type IPMNs.[56,58]

Mucinous Cystic Neoplasms

MCNs usually consist of solitary locules with varying diameters that do not communicate with the pancreatic ductal system and are located in the tail of pancreas (Fig. 51.1).[22,59] MCNs often contain translucent viscous fluid. Mucin-producing cells in a columnar epithelium line MCNs with an underlying ovarian-type stroma. This highly thick cellular layer usually contains estrogen and progesterone receptors and variably stains for these receptors. This may help differentiate MCN from BD-IPMN. Although MCNs with ovarian stroma can be observed in postmenopausal women and male patients, the stroma usually occurs in younger women. Mucinous transitional epithelium is the source of almost all MCN-associated malignancies. The clinical spectrum of MCNs ranges from obviously benign to frankly malignant. Based on the maximal degree of epithelial dysplasia, the current pathologic classification distinguishes MCNs as (1) mucinous cystadenoma (benign), (2) mucinous cystic tumor (borderline), or (3) mucinous cystadenocarcinoma (malignant).[60,61]

Serous Cystic Neoplasms

SCNs (Table 51.2) are typically benign solitary tumors that arise from centroacinar cells located throughout the entire pancreas. According

TABLE 51.2 **Use of FNA Samples: Prioritizing the Use of Samples**

Type of Lesion	First Priority	Second Priority	Third Priority	Experimental
Serous	CEA	Imaging	Fluid cytology	*VHL* gene testing
Mucinous	CEA	Cytology	Subjective assessment of viscosity	*GNAS* mutation analysis
Malignant	Tissue cytology	Fluid cytology	CEA	*GNAS* mutation analysis

CEA, Carcinoembryonic antigen; *FNA*, fine-needle aspiration.

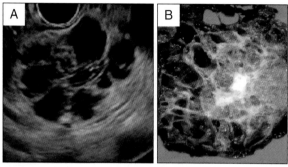

FIG 51.2 A, Endoscopic ultrasonography image of serous cystadenoma. **B,** Gross serous cystadenoma.

to the degree of dysplasia, they are classified as serous cystadenoma or serous cystadenocarcinoma, but the latter is extremely rare.[25] SCN has a thin wall composed of cuboidal glycogen-rich epithelial cells that stain positively with PAS. The wall surrounds a thin amount of bloody fluid and is hypervascular. SCNs contain a prominent fibrous stroma, glycogen-rich epithelial cells, and endothelial and smooth muscle cells.[47] Ultrastructurally, the fibrocollagenous stroma is composed of myofibroblasts and endothelial cells embedded in thick collagen bundles. Estrogen and progesterone receptors are not present.[62]

Although the majority of serous cystadenomas are microcystic, there are four histologic variants: (1) macrocystic serous cystadenoma, (2) solid serous adenoma, (3) VHL-associated SCN, and (4) mixed serous neuroendocrine neoplasm.[25] Classical cross-sectional and endoscopic ultrasonography (EUS) imaging of "microcystic" serous cystadenomas (Fig. 51.2) shows a cluster of small thin-walled cysts resembling a honeycomb-like appearance. Microcystic serous cystadenomas are slow-growing lesions that may achieve large diameters. The large lesions often have a more solid spongiform central core "stellate-shaped" scar. Macrocystic serous cystadenomas are composed of far fewer cysts and the diameter of each cyst varies from subcentimeters to large cavities.[63] The large separate cystic appearance can be indistinguishable from unifocal BD-IPMNs, MCNs, or pseudocysts; however, the cystic fluid is thin and may contain blood as a result of the vascular nature of the lesions.[64] Despite the solid gross appearance, solid serous adenomas share cytologic and immunohistologic features of classic SCN. VHL-associated SCNs consist of multiple SCNs that affect patients with VHL syndrome. Mixed serous neuroendocrine neoplasms are rare and highly suggestive of VHL syndrome.[25]

Solid Pseudopapillary Neoplasms

SPNs are low-grade malignant neoplasms that do not demonstrate histologic criteria for malignancy, such as perineural and vascular invasion or parenchymal infiltration with metastasis. They are composed of poorly cohesive monomorphic epithelial cells that form solid and pseudopapillary structures. Microscopically they are a combination of solid (solid pseudopapillary) and cystic (hemorrhagic-necrotic, pseudocystic) components. SPNs frequently undergo hemorrhagic-cystic

degeneration.[29] Mucin is absent and glycogen is lacking.[29] SPNs form single, round, large, and frequently fluctuant masses.

Cystic Pancreatic Neuroendocrine Tumors

cPNETs arise from endocrine and nervous system cells. Although mild cystic change is common in solid pancreatic neuroendocrine neoplasms, marked cystic alteration is rare. They may be unilocular or multilocular, varying from small to large size, well circumscribed, and surrounded by a thick fibrous capsule, and they usually do not communicate with the pancreatic duct. The cyst portion contains clear serosanguineous fluid[65] and may be hemorrhagic in large cysts. The pathophysiology of cPNETs is controversial. In general, infarction and necrosis within a solid pancreatic neuroendocrine tumor are thought to result in a cystic neuroendocrine neoplasm with similar biologic behavior and malignant potential.[66,67] Some advocate that cPNET is a different tumor type from its solid counterparts.[34] The classic cPNET is populated with a characteristic small granular population of cells that are stainable for immunoreactive hormones, chromogranin, and synaptophysin.[34,67]

CLINICAL PRESENTATION

Patients with pancreatic cysts are usually asymptomatic or have non-specific abdominal symptoms. The cysts are usually found during cross-sectional imaging obtained for the evaluation of another condition. A cystic lesion causes pancreatitis when it involves the main duct, when an obstructing mucus plug is present, or when the cyst compresses the pancreatic duct.[1] Abdominal pain, nausea, and vomiting are common symptoms. Patients with cystic malignancy may have pain, weight loss, and jaundice as presenting symptoms.[68]

Most patients with IPMNs are asymptomatic, although some of these patients have symptoms related to acute recurrent pancreatitis or chronic pancreatitis. Patients with MCNs may present with abdominal pain, gastric outlet obstruction, and a palpable mass.[69] Most SCN patients are asymptomatic and only become symptomatic as a result of cyst enlargement and space occupation[70,71] (especially when >4 cm in size).[72] Common symptoms include pain, a palpable mass, pancreaticobiliary ductal obstruction, and gastric outlet obstruction.[69] SPN patients may present with pain, nausea and vomiting, and weight loss.[73]

DIFFERENTIAL DIAGNOSIS

In the past, the majority of pancreatic cysts were believed to be pseudocysts. Pseudocysts may arise after an episode of acute pancreatitis or insidiously in the setting of chronic pancreatitis and are associated with chronic abdominal pain. In the absence of clinical symptoms and a history of pancreatitis, the incidental finding of a cyst on cross-sectional imaging is common. Because management of a pancreatic cyst and a pseudocyst is dramatically different, they must be differentiated. Patients with pseudocysts usually present with preceding symptoms and a history of pancreatitis, but some patients may present after only a mild episode of pancreatitis, which may not be clinically overt. Furthermore, pancreatic cysts may also cause pancreatitis. Abdominal imaging may demonstrate inflammatory changes suggestive of a pseudocyst.[74] However, in the initial setting of mild pancreatitis, it may be difficult to differentiate between a cystic neoplasm that has caused pancreatitis and a small pseudocyst that has formed as a result of pancreatitis.[75] If a cystic lesion has been present for many years, it is highly likely that the lesion represents a cystic neoplasm. Congenital cysts of the pancreas are rare.[76]

Once the clinical diagnosis of pseudocyst has been excluded, the evaluation should focus on identifying the type of cystic neoplasm and determining whether surgery is required for treatment. Because mucinous cysts have premalignant potential, the principal differentiation is between mucinous and serous lesions. Serous lesions may be confidently diagnosed on initial imaging because of their classical microcystic appearance; the lesion should be followed for growth by surveillance imaging (except for lesions >4 cm and symptomatic cysts, which are surgically managed). In contrast, tumors with malignant potential include mucinous cysts (MCNs and IPMNs), SPNs, and pNETs, which require surgical resection or careful surveillance.

DIAGNOSTIC METHODS

Although multidetector CT (MDCT) is the current preferred method of imaging, most pancreatic cysts are incidentally detected on conventional imaging, including CT and MRI with contrast enhancement.[77,78] Furthermore, the combination of MRI with MDCT was found to be superior to each tool alone.[79] For tissue sampling and clinical guidance, EUS-guided fine-needle aspiration (EUS-FNA) is preferred. Analysis of aspirated cystic fluid (either biochemical, cytologic, molecular, or a combination) helps differentiate among benign, premalignant, and malignant cystic neoplasms. Positron emission tomography–CT may also predict a malignant cyst and present an argument for resection, but a negative scan cannot exclude malignancy.[80]

A CT or MRI demonstrating a central scar with characteristic calcification surrounded by numerous tiny cysts is highly diagnostic of a serous cystadenoma, although only seen in up to 30%.[26] In contrast, MCNs and BD-IPMNs have similar morphologic appearance and are difficult to differentiate from macrocystic (oligocystic) serous cystadenomas on cross-sectional imaging.[63,81] Conversely, pancreatic pseudocysts seen with chronic pancreatitis are unilocular cysts associated with the presence of pancreatic calcifications and parenchymal atrophy. The presence of multiple small, thin-walled cysts is suggestive of VHL syndrome.[82] MCNs are classically solitary, macrocystic, thinly septated lesions, occasionally with peripheral calcification (specific for MCNs) on cross-sectional imaging (Fig. 51.3).[83–85] Peripheral calcifications (so-called eggshell calcifications) are lamellated and contrast the central calcification of SCNs. A thick wall, peripheral calcifications, and thickened septations on MRI are highly suggestive of carcinoma. Typically MCNs and SCNs do not communicate with the pancreatic duct on magnetic resonance cholangiopancreatography (MRCP). SPNs are well-demarcated, thick-walled lesions that consist of varying areas of nonseptated soft tissue and necrotic foci on cross-sectional imaging.[86]

IPMNs may involve the main pancreatic duct exclusively, a branch duct, or both. Endoscopic examination of the papilla using a side-viewing or oblique endoscope may demonstrate a "fish mouth" papilla (patulous and mucin-filled pancreatic orifice).[50] Formal pancreatography as a diagnostic tool is no longer commonly used and MRCP is superior to ERCP at showing mural nodules, pancreatic duct dilation, and cystic communication with the pancreatic duct (Fig. 51.4).[87] ERCP can demonstrate mucin extrusion, intraductal filling defects, and cystic side branches of IPMN in 70% to 90% of patients (Fig. 51.5).[88,89] MRCP is more sensitive for detecting side-branch lesions of IPMN.[90]

EUS is the current preferred method to diagnose cystic lesions of the pancreas and allow FNA to be performed.[91] The detailed imaging

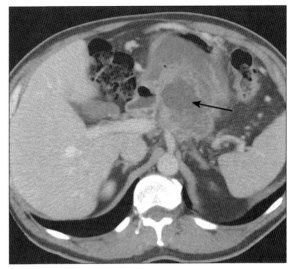

FIG 51.3 Computed tomography scan of a mucinous cystadenocarcinoma (*arrow*).

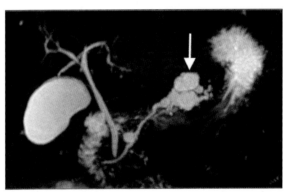

FIG 51.4 Magnetic resonance cholangiopancreatography of a branch-duct–type intraductal papillary mucinous neoplasm at the pancreatic tail (*arrow*).

features of cystic neoplasms by EUS do not appear to be sufficiently accurate to differentiate between benign and malignant, unless there is evidence of a solid mass or invasive tumor[92] (the accuracy ranges from 40% to 90%).[27] EUS is also very sensitive for detecting IPMNs that demonstrate papillary projections, septations, wall thickening, mural nodules, and debris.[93–97] The strength of EUS is its ability to detect and facilitate aspiration of small cystic lesions.[98] EUS can also be used to survey IPMN lesions, by evaluating increases in the cyst size and the main pancreatic duct diameter.[99] The macrocystic variant serous cystadenoma can be diagnosed using a combination of EUS imaging of a thick cyst wall, the presence of microcysts, and detection of low cyst-fluid carcinoembryonic antigen (CEA) (Fig. 51.6).[100] Peroral pancreatoscopy can be used in patients with IPMN to assess the locations of pancreatic ductal lesions and allow biopsy confirmation (see Chapter 26).[101]

The fluid contents of pancreatic cysts are often analyzed for cytology, biochemistry, and molecular genetics.[102] Macroscopically, highly mucoid, viscous, thick fluid is suggestive of mucinous cysts. The diagnostic yield of cytology is often low, because cyst fluid is of low cellularity. The presence of inflammatory cells suggests the presence of a pseudocyst.[103] The presence of granulocytes reflects acute infection, epithelial cells suggest neoplastic cysts rather than pseudocysts,[103] and small cuboidal cells are diagnostic for SCNs. MCNs may have large secretory epithelial cells with evidence of mucin secretion or atypia,[104] and cyst fluid is

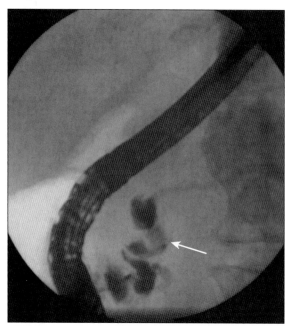

FIG 51.5 ERCP of an intraductal papillary mucinous neoplasm. Note the dilated and tortuous main pancreatic duct (*arrow*).

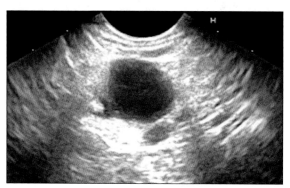

FIG 51.6 Endoscopic ultrasonography image of a cystic pancreatic neuroendocrine tumor.

highly cellular in SPNs. Malignant cytology is 100% specific for mucinous cysts,[105] and high-grade dysplasia in cytology is 80% accurate at predicting malignancy.[106]

A variety of tumor markers have been studied to help differentiate between the major types of cystic neoplasms. CEA has better accuracy at diagnosing mucinous cysts among the tumor markers, including CA19-9, CA125, CA72-4, and CA15-3. A cyst-fluid CEA level <5 ng/mL is highly diagnostic of serous cystadenomas.[107] Increasing the cutoff values of cyst-fluid CEA level will increase the specificity, at the cost of sensitivity for the diagnosis of mucinous lesions,[108] and the cutoff value of 192 ng/mL was found to be the best predictor of a mucinous cyst.[109] In general, cyst-fluid amylase level is high in IPMNs and low in MCNs and SCNs.

Initial molecular studies of cyst-fluid DNA have revealed that *KRAS* mutations are highly specific for mucinous cysts.[110] Subsequent studies have shown them to be able to differentiate between benign and malignant cysts.[111] The cyst fluid is often positive for *KRAS* in patients with IPMN and MCN, but *GNAS* mutation seems specific for IPMN. Furthermore, SCNs are negative for both *KRAS* and *GNAS* mutations but positive for VHL mutations.[39,40,112]

Recently, needle-based confocal endomicroscopy has been developed, which enables real-time optical biopsies. This provides in vivo histopathologic assessment during EUS-FNA. SCNs demonstrate a superficial vascular network, and IPMNs demonstrate papillary projections with an epithelial border and vascular core. However, its role in the diagnosis of pancreatic cysts is not yet established.[113,114]

More recently, a microforceps has been developed for tissue acquisition from pancreatic cystic lesions. During EUS-FNA, the microforceps is introduced through a 19G needle and pinch biopsies are obtained from the cyst wall, septations and nodules, or adjacent masses. In a preliminary study, the tissue acquisition yield was 90% and microforceps histology was superior to EUS-FNA cytology, especially for providing a specific pancreatic cyst diagnosis.[115]

DIAGNOSTIC EVALUATION

Pancreatic cysts are usually incidental findings on cross-sectional imaging, and a history of pancreatitis strongly suggests a pseudocyst. The majority of pancreatic cysts are nonmalignant. When cross-sectional imaging demonstrates a diagnostic finding such as pancreatitis with a fluid collection, a malignant cystic mass, or the classical appearance of a microcystic SCN, further evaluation is not necessary. If a neoplastic lesion is suspected, the next step is to distinguish a mucinous from a nonmucinous cyst. A young woman presenting with a unilocular solitary cystic lesion in the tail of the pancreas is more likely to have an MCN and should be evaluated for surgical resection. Indeterminate lesions should be assessed via EUS-FNA. Aspirated cyst fluid should undergo biochemical analysis with assessment of at least amylase and CEA content. Amylase is generally high in pseudocysts and IPMNs, because there is a connection with the pancreatic duct; CEA is one of the best markers to differentiate a mucinous cyst. Fluid should be sent for cytology, especially in malignant-appearing cysts. Molecular analyses for *KRAS* and *GNAS* mutations can also be obtained. At least 0.3 mL of aspirated fluid is needed for each of these analyses. If fluid volume is inadequate, the decision as to what to analyze in the fluid is individualized according to the patient. For example, when there is a concern for malignancy, cytology should be the first choice. For differentiation of cyst types, cyst-fluid CEA level may be more helpful. EUS-FNA or fine-needle biopsy is helpful not only for aspirating cystic fluid but also for obtaining tissue from mural nodules, thickened septations, and adjacent masses, if present.

TREATMENT

Although most PCNs can be monitored with surveillance using cross-sectional imaging or EUS-FNA, surgical resection is the treatment of choice for symptomatic patients, documented malignant cysts by cytology, and premalignant cystic neoplasms, including MCNs, MD-IPMNs, and SPNs. The decision to resect a lesion, however, should take into account the surgical risk of the patient. Patients at high risk for surgery with low-grade cystic neoplasms may be followed up with surveillance imaging.[116] Alternatively, EUS-guided cyst ablation with absolute alcohol or a combination of alcohol and chemotherapeutic agents can be offered to selected patients in selected centers.[117,118]

Cysts located in the head of the pancreas require pancreaticoduodenectomy (Whipple resection), whereas cysts in the body or tail require distal pancreatectomy. Surgery is not indicated for serous cystadenomas unless symptomatic because of large size.[119] As IPMNs invade the pancreas along ductal structures, it is important that frozen section histology be done during surgery to assure negative margins.[120,121] Furthermore, intraoperative pancreatoscopy combined with intraductal biopsies can help define the area of resection, and in one study modified the operative strategy in 25% of patients.[122] Distal pancreatectomy is favored for patients with solitary cysts in the tail of the pancreas because of relatively low surgical mortality and elimination of malignant potential. Patients with SPNs or cystic neuroendocrine neoplasms should also be offered surgery. Surgical resection is recommended for MCNs and MD-IPMNs, whereas patients with BD-IPMNs are directed to surgery based on the presence of enhancing nodules, MPD ≥10 mm, and obstructive jaundice or cytology suspicious/positive for malignancy, or cysts >3 cm in young surgically fit patients.[7] On the other hand, MCNs occur in young women who have a projected long life expectancy and who would require extended surveillance. Thus, because there is a concern for the development of cancer and because resection is curative, surgical resection is recommended when located in the body or tail of the pancreas.

PROGNOSIS

Cystic neoplasms are slow growing and 19% will demonstrate an increased diameter at 16 months.[20] The prognosis of noninvasive IPMNs is excellent, with postresection 5-year survival of 90% to 100%.[123,124] The prognosis for patients with invasive IPMN is poor but better than that for pancreatic adenocarcinoma, with postresection 5-year survival of 60% and 36%, respectively.[3,121,125,126] The overall postoperative recurrence rate ranges from 7% to 43%, which consists of either local or distant metastases and occurs more commonly in invasive IPMNs.[121] Similarly, after resection, noninvasive MCNs exhibit excellent prognosis; however, prognosis is poor for *in situ* carcinoma and invasive MCNs. Five-year survival for invasive and noninvasive IPMNs is reported to be 57% to 83% and 95% to 100%, respectively.[14,126] The postoperative recurrence at 5 years is 0% for noninvasive MCNs and 40% after 33 months for invasive MCNs.[14,128] The prognosis for SCNs is excellent.[25] There are reports of long-term survival after resection even in the rare cases of serous cystadenocarcinoma.[127,129] After complete surgical resection, 85% to 95% of SPN patients experience long-term survival[29] even with metastases, local invasion, or recurrence.[30,130,131] The prognosis for CNETs is comparable to that for solid neuroendocrine neoplasms, with the 5-year survival rate of resected patients ranging from 87% to 100%.[34–36]

The complete reference list for this chapter can be found online at www.expertconsult.com.

52

Unexplained Acute Pancreatitis and Acute Recurrent Pancreatitis

Ihab I. El Hajj and Stuart Sherman

Determining the cause of acute pancreatitis (AP) is usually not difficult. AP results most commonly from alcohol abuse or gallstone disease. These etiologies account for 60% to 90% of the cases (Box 52.1).

Alcoholism is diagnosed by patient history, and gallstones by a combination of demographic characteristics, laboratory findings, and radiographic imaging studies. Other causes of AP include hypertriglyceridemia, hypercalcemia, drug reactions, trauma, surgery, and endoscopic retrograde cholangiopancreatography (ERCP). In these cases the relationship of the episode of pancreatitis to the cause is usually clear. However, despite a careful analysis of patient history, physical examination, laboratory testing, and radiologic evaluation, the cause of AP will not be identified in 10% to 30% of patients.[1] These patients are conventionally classified as having unexplained or idiopathic acute pancreatitis (IAP).[2,3]

Idiopathic acute recurrent pancreatitis (IARP) is defined as the occurrence of two or more episodes of AP with complete resolution of symptoms between episodes and without concurrent clinical or imaging evidence supportive of chronic pancreatitis (CP).[2-7] Smoldering pancreatitis refers to a syndrome in which patients recovering from AP experience unremitting abdominal pain, persistently elevated pancreas enzymes, and inflammatory changes in and around the pancreas on imaging studies in the absence of systemic or local complications.[8]

Evaluation and therapy are important because a high percentage of untreated patients with IARP experience recurrent episodes that may lead to CP. In a recent meta-analysis of 14 studies, 10% of patients with a first episode of AP and 36% of patients with ARP developed CP.[9] The risk is higher among smokers, alcoholics, men, and patients with severe first-time AP.[10,11]

PATHOPHYSIOLOGY AND ROLE OF ERCP, EUS, AND MRCP

Data suggest that the pathophysiologic process of AP might consist of three phases. The initial phase involves triggering events that are, for the most part, extrapancreatic in origin. Clinically, the most important of these appears to be either passage of a biliary tract stone or ingestion of ethanol. Other events, such as exposure to pancreatotoxins, pancreatic ischemia, and infection, may also be capable of triggering AP. The second phase involves a series of events that occur within the acinar cells of the pancreas. Finally, a third phase consisting of both acinar cell and nonacinar cell events occurs, which determines the ultimate severity of an attack of pancreatitis. There are two key points with these events that are important with regard to endoscopic intervention: (1) pancreatic ductal (PD) obstruction leads to ductal hypertension that is exacerbated by pancreatic secretion, and (2) ductal hypertension causes inhibition of enzyme secretion, resulting in colocalization of inactive pancreatic enzymes and lysosomal hydrolases with subsequent acinar cell injury and the clinical sequelae of AP.[12] Several factors play an etiologic role in ARP; in fact, any cause of AP can lead to recurrent episodes if not corrected. Thus the role of ERCP, EUS, and MRCP in patients with IAP and IARP is to identify causes of triggering events that led to the PD obstruction, with the therapeutic goal of relieving the obstruction. It is assumed that relief of the obstruction will prevent further episodes of pancreatitis. The obstructive theory of IAP also assumes that ductal obstruction is intermittent or that a second risk factor predisposes patients with impaired ductal drainage.[13]

DIAGNOSTIC FINDINGS AND TIMING OF ERCP, EUS, AND MRCP

There are two major concerns that prompt physicians to do a more intensive evaluation of the patient with IAP. The first is that the patient may have an underlying disease that will predispose to further attacks of AP unless the cause is identified and adequately treated. AP is likely to recur in 33% to 67% of patients with biliary tract disease when not diagnosed and treated.[14] Similarly, other anatomic or functional disorders of the pancreaticobiliary tree may predispose patients to recurrent episodes of pancreatitis. The second concern is that the pancreatitis may be related to a tumor. As a result, ERCP, EUS, and MRCP now play a central role in the evaluation and therapy of patients with IAP.

In the past, when EUS and MRCP were not widely available, ERCP was considered a reasonable option to investigate IAP and IARP as it was both diagnostic and offered therapeutic options. There are a number of potential causes of IAP that can be diagnosed and potentially treated by ERCP and ancillary techniques. These include occult gallstones, abnormalities and anomalies of the PD and bile duct, sphincter of Oddi dysfunction (SOD), and ampullary and pancreatic neoplasms. The techniques applied at ERCP to diagnose the cause of IAP are shown in Box 52.2.

Although there are potential gains in performing ERCP (identifying and treating the cause and preventing another episode of AP), there are potential downsides for the patient and the health care system as a whole (inappropriate performance of the procedure and its adverse events).[15] The timing of ERCP in patients with IAP is controversial. Ballinger and colleagues reported that only 1 of 27 patients with one unexplained episode of pancreatitis with a gallbladder (GB) in situ had a second episode of pancreatitis during a 3-year follow-up period.[2] They felt that the risks of ERCP were greater than the risks of a second episode of AP and advised against its use. On the other hand, Trapnell and Duncan reported that 35 of 148 patients (24%) with IAP suffered a recurrence, but if gallstones were present, the rate increased to 38%.[16] Using an actuarial method, the authors found that 10% of patients with IAP were likely to have a first recurrence within 1 year of the initial attack, 17% within 2 years, and 25% within 6 years. Patients

Video for this chapter can be found online at www.expertconsult.com.

BOX 52.1   Etiologies of Acute Pancreatitis

- Alcohol
- Autoimmune pancreatitis
- Biliary calculous disease
  - Macrolithiasis (bile duct stone)
  - Microlithiasis (biliary crystals)
- Biliary cystic disease
  - Choledochal cyst
  - Choledochocele/duplication cyst
- Congenital anomaly
  - Annular pancreas
  - Anomalous pancreaticobiliary junction
  - Pancreas divisum
- Chronic pancreatitis
- Duodenal obstruction
  - Afferent limb obstructed (Billroth II)
  - Atresia
  - Crohn disease
  - Diverticulum
- Drugs
- Genetic
  - Alpha 1-antitrypsin deficiency
  - Cystic fibrosis
  - Hereditary pancreatitis
- Iatrogenic
  - ERCP
  - Abdominal surgery
- Idiopathic
- Infection
  - Bacterial
  - Parasites/worms
  - Viral
- Metabolic
  - Hypercalcemia
  - Hyperlipidemia
  - Inborn errors of metabolism
- Neoplasm
  - Duodenal
  - Ampullary
  - Pancreatic
  - Biliary
- Renal disease
  - Chronic renal failure
  - Dialysis related
- Sphincter of Oddi dysfunction
- Toxin
  - Organophosphate insecticides
- Scorpion bite
- Trauma
- Tropical
- Vasculitis
  - Polyarteritis nodosa
  - Systemic lupus erythematosus

BOX 52.2   Techniques Applied at ERCP to Diagnose the Cause of Idiopathic Acute Pancreatitis

- Screening endoscopy
  - Ampullary and intraductal papillary mucinous neoplasms
- Ductography/intraductal ultrasonography
  - Bile duct stones
  - Anomalies/abnormalities of the pancreatic duct and bile duct
  - Chronic pancreatitis
  - Tumors
- Sphincter of Oddi manometry
  - Sphincter of Oddi dysfunction
- Aspiration of bile for crystals
  - Microlithiasis

TABLE 52.1   Idiopathic Acute Pancreatitis: Yield of ERCP With or Without Sphincter of Oddi Manometry and With or Without Bile Microscopy Correlated With Age (n = 225)

Diagnosis	<20 yr (n = 15)	20–40 yr (n = 53)	40–60 yr (n = 95)	>60 yr (n = 62)
Pancreatic cancer (%)	0	0	2	2
Ampullary Ca/adenoma (%)	0	2	2	0
Mucinous tumor (%)	0	2	17	23
SOD (%)	47	43	35	26
Pancreas divisum (%)	13	15	19	23
Chronic pancreatitis (%)	27	11	9	3
Miscellaneous (%)	7	9	9	3
Normal (%)	7	21	6	11

From Choudari et al.[20]
Ca, Cancer; *ERCP,* endoscopic retrograde cholangiopancreatography; *SOD,* sphincter of Oddi dysfunction.

EUS [S-EUS]) and MRCP (secretin-enhanced MRCP [S-MRCP]) has further improved the diagnostic yield for identifying underlying structural etiologies for IAP.[18,19] The results of EUS and MRCP can direct an alternative therapy (e.g., cholecystectomy for microlithiasis) and obviate more invasive ERCP. The limitations to these two diagnostic modalities are that they have no therapeutic options and a separate procedure may have to be carried out for treatment. ERCP is now used primarily as a therapeutic option directed by the results of EUS and MRCP, unless the EUS and/or MRCP is negative. In such a setting, sphincter of Oddi manometry (SOM) is usually combined with ERCP.

Our approach to evaluating patients with IAP and IARP has evolved over the years as mounting evidence supported a central role of EUS and MRCP in this setting. Traditionally, for young patients with a negative standard evaluation, we would recommend no further evaluation unless a second episode occurred. In contrast, for patients age 40 years and older in whom findings are negative or inconclusive on standard evaluation, we would then proceed with ERCP (usually with SOM and bile microscopy with a GB in situ if not already done after their first episode of AP). This is based on the findings of Choudari and colleagues.[20] In this study, 21% of patients 40 to 60 years of age and 25% of patients older than 60 years had a neoplastic process as the cause for their pancreatitis, in contrast to only 3% younger than 40 years (Table 52.1).

In a similar series of 1241 patients with idiopathic pancreatitis reported by Fischer and colleagues, the incidence of malignancy and premalignant conditions was 4.7% (58 of 1241).[21] Analysis of a subgroup of patients with intraductal papillary mucinous neoplasm (IPMN), which accounted for 52 of 58 of the malignant and premalignant conditions, showed an increasing trend with age, ranging from 1.3% in patients <40 years to 13% in patients older than 70 years (Fig. 52.1).

Based on these studies, which show an increasing incidence of a neoplastic process with age, and given the critical diagnostic role of EUS and S-MRCP, our current approach is to evaluate patients 40 years and older with EUS and/or S-MRCP after their first episode of IAP to assess for a tumor or other structural cause of the pancreatitis.

The roles of ERCP, EUS, and MRCP in relation to diagnosis and outcomes of therapy for each disease identified will be discussed

who had one recurrence were likely to have a second. In a cost-utility analysis, Gregor and colleagues found that performing ERCP on all patients after a first episode of IAP was neither of great benefit nor particularly costly.[15] However, it was of substantial benefit and cost-effective in a subgroup of patients with greater probability of having an occult stone.

EUS and MRCP have assumed a central role in the evaluation of patients with IAP and IARP because of their high diagnostic accuracy and low morbidity.[17] The use of secretin in both EUS (secretin-enhanced

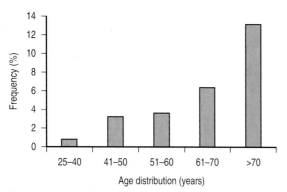

FIG 52.1 Frequency of intraductal papillary mucinous neoplasms by age.

individually, and a recommended algorithm for the workup of patients with IAP and IARP will be presented.

OCCULT GALLSTONE DISEASE

Although microlithiasis and biliary sludge are technically different, the terms are often used interchangeably. Microlithiasis most commonly refers to stones <3 mm in diameter and biliary sludge is considered to be a suspension of crystals, mucin, glycoproteins, cellular debris, and proteinaceous material within bile.[22] The crystals are made of cholesterol monohydrate, calcium bilirubinate, or calcium carbonate. Microlithiasis and biliary sludge can be found within the GB or bile ducts and might not be detected by standard GB imaging techniques, such as ultrasonography or computed tomography (CT) scan.

Microlithiasis of the GB has been implicated as a common cause of IAP. Two prospective studies found that approximately two-thirds to three-fourths of patients with IAP harbored occult gallstones in the GB.[7,23] The diagnosis was based on microscopic examination of bile for crystals and usually confirmed on evaluation of the resected GB or follow-up GB ultrasonography showing gallstones and/or sludge. On multivariate analysis, the finding of biliary crystals in bile is a strong predictor of small stones or sludge in the GB ($p < 0.001$).[23] Moreover, the finding of crystals in bile had a sensitivity of 86%, specificity of 86%, and positive predictive value of 92% for the diagnosis of gallstone disease as the missed cause of IAP. In contrast to the results of Lee and colleagues and Ros and colleagues, some investigators have detected microlithiasis in less than 10% of patients with IAP.[5,7,23,24] Bile may be collected at the time of ERCP from the duodenum or bile duct after GB stimulation with cholecystokinin or by direct cannulation of the GB.

In patients with IAP, EUS may help identify those with underlying microlithiasis when conventional transcutaneous ultrasonography is normal.[25–27] Frossard and colleagues reported that EUS identified a biliary cause of IAP in 103 of 168 patients (61%). Of those 103 patients, 52 (50%) had gallstones or microlithiasis, 12 (12%) had GB sludge, 10 (10%) had common bile duct stones, and 29 (28%) had a combination of these findings.[28] Yusoff and colleagues compared the diagnostic yield of EUS in 201 patients with a single episode of IAP with that of 169 patients with recurrent episodes. Biliary tract disease (46 of 246 [18.7%]) was the most common positive finding in the patients with GB in situ. In postcholecystectomy patients, 4 of 124 (3.2%) had evidence of stones in the bile duct.[29] Morris-Stiff and colleagues showed that in 42 patients with idiopathic pancreatitis and a normal MRCP, EUS detected cholelithiasis or microlithiasis alone in 9 (21.4%), cholelithiasis and choledocholithiasis in 6 (14.3%), and choledocholithiasis alone in 1 (2.4%).[30] In another series of 44 patients with IAP, EUS found cholelithiasis in

3 (6.8%), microlithiasis in 20 (45.5%), and choledocholithiasis in 2 (4.5%).[31] Ardengh and colleagues found GB microlithiasis in 27 of 36 patients with IAP (75%). Compared with the final surgical resection specimen, the sensitivity, specificity, and positive and negative predictive values for EUS identification of GB microlithiasis were 92.6% (74.2% to 98.7%), 55.6% (22.7% to 84.7%), 86.2% (67.4% to 95.5%), and 71.4% (30.3% to 94.9%), respectively. Overall EUS accuracy was 83.2%.[32]

Intraductal ultrasonography (IDUS) has also been shown to be useful in detecting occult biliary stones, microlithiasis, and sludge.[33–36] In a study by Kim and colleagues[36] of 31 patients with IARP and negative findings on ERCP, IDUS revealed small bile duct stones (≤3 mm) in 5 patients (16.1%) and sludge in 3 patients (9.7%).

The role of MRCP in detecting choledocholithiasis is well established.[35,37] Its role in detecting microlithiasis or sludge of the GB has been extensively studied. Calvo and colleagues evaluated 80 patients undergoing both transabdominal ultrasonography and MRCP for suspected gallstones; the sensitivity of MRCP in diagnosing GB stones (43 patients [97.7%]) was comparable to that of transabdominal ultrasonography (44 patients). MRCP diagnosed biliary sludge or microlithiasis in 13 patients, versus 5 using ultrasonography. The authors concluded that MRCP is a good technique for diagnosing cholelithiasis and biliary sludge. However, high cost, contraindications, and the need for patient cooperation limit MRI for routine GB evaluation.[38]

Treatment of microlithiasis can significantly reduce the incidence of recurrent pancreatitis.[7,23] There are several therapeutic options for managing patients with pancreatitis caused by microlithiasis. Laparoscopic cholecystectomy should be considered the procedure of choice as it is almost always curative. Ros and colleagues reported no further episodes of pancreatitis in 17 of 18 patients followed for 3 years after cholecystectomy.[23] Endoscopic biliary sphincterotomy is an excellent alternative for elderly and high-risk surgical patients.[14] Dissolution therapy with ursodeoxycholic acid has also been shown to prevent recurrent pancreatitis.[14] However, maintenance therapy is expensive and necessary to prevent recurrent stone formation.

Given the high prevalence of occult microlithiasis in some series, some authors advocate empiric cholecystectomy as a first-line therapy, particularly in patients with recurrent attacks.[39,40]

SPHINCTER OF ODDI DYSFUNCTION (SEE CHAPTER 47)

SOD refers to the abnormality of sphincter of Oddi contractility that is manifested clinically by pancreaticobiliary pain, pancreatitis, or deranged liver function tests. SOM is considered by most authorities to be the gold-standard test for diagnosing SOD.[41–45] It is most commonly performed at the time of ERCP but can also be done percutaneously or during surgery. SOM uses a water-perfused catheter that is inserted into the common bile duct, pancreatic duct, or both to measure sphincter pressure. The diagnosis of SOD is established when the basal pressure is ≥40 mm Hg.[43]

Because SOM is difficult to perform, invasive, not widely available, and associated with a high adverse event rate, several noninvasive and provocative tests have been designed in an attempt to identify patients with SOD. The currently available data suggest that these tests lack the sensitivity and specificity to replace SOM.[42,46]

The role of S-MRCP in diagnosing SOD is still debatable. Mariani and colleagues reported that S-MRCP and SOM were concordant in 13 of 15 patients (86.7%).[47] However, subsequent larger studies did not show this high concordance. Pereira and colleagues showed diagnostic accuracy of S-MRCP for SOD type II and III at 73% and 46%, respectively.[48] Aisen and colleagues also showed that there was no difference in the magnitude of the increase of pancreatic duct diameter between

TABLE 52.2 **Manometrically Documented Sphincter of Oddi Dysfunction Causing Idiopathic Acute Pancreatitis**

Author (Year)	Frequency (%)
Toouli et al. (1985)[51]	16/26 (62)
Guelrud et al. (1986)[53]	17/42 (40)
Gregg et al. (1989)[54]	38/125 (30)
Venu et al. (1989)[5]	17/116 (15)
Raddawi et al. (1991)[55]	7/24 (29)
Sherman et al. (1993)[56]	18/55 (33)
Toouli et al. (1996)[52]	24/33 (73)
Choudari et al. (1998)[20]	79/225 (35)
Testoni et al. (2000)[57]	14/40 (35)
Coyle et al. (2002)[58]	28/90 (31)
Kaw and Brodmerkel (2002)[59]	67/126 (53)
Fischer et al. (2010)[21]	418/952 (44)
Total	**743/1854 (40)**

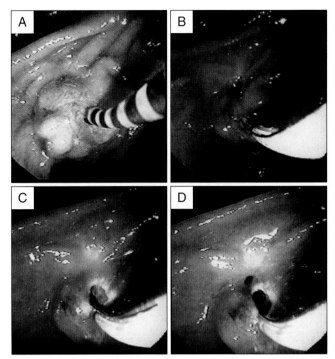

FIG 52.2 Patient with idiopathic acute recurrent pancreatitis that reoccurred after biliary sphincterotomy. **A,** Pancreatic manometry being performed. **B–D,** Pancreatic sphincterotomy being performed.

patients with elevated basal sphincter pressure and normal basal sphincter pressure.[49]

Siddiqui et al. reported a low but significant yield of EUS in 143 patients with suspected SOD type 3 with previous normal endoscopies and imaging studies.[50] The role of S-EUS in diagnosing SOD in idiopathic pancreatitis is unclear. The study by Mariani and colleagues labeled 2 patients with SOD because there was persistent main pancreatic duct dilation 15 minutes after secretin injection. There was no recurrent pancreatitis in these patients 18 months after sphincterotomy was performed.[18]

SOD is a frequent cause of IAP. It has been manometrically documented in 15% to 73% of such patients (Table 52.2).[5,20,21,51–59]

The role of SOM and sphincter ablation for IARP patients is controversial, though a recent survey of American Society for Gastrointestinal Endoscopy members showed considerable variation in approaches to managing patients with SOD and IARP.[60]

Many authorities recommend performing pancreatic SOM in patients with IARP, particularly those with normal biliary manometry and those who have recurrent attacks after a biliary sphincterotomy. Isolated pancreatic sphincter hypertension is commonly found among patients with IARP.[10,55]

Historically, pancreatic sphincter ablation has been done surgically.[61,62] However, with the endoscopic sphincterotomy has become the treatment of choice. Studies evaluating the role of SOM and sphincter ablation for patients with IARP began to appear in the late 1980s. The value of ERCP, SOM, and sphincter ablation therapy was studied in 51 patients with IARP.[63] Twenty-four patients (47.1%) had an elevated basal sphincter pressure. Thirty were treated by biliary endoscopic sphincterotomy (BES; $n = 20$) or surgical sphincteroplasty with septoplasty ($n = 10$). Fifteen of 18 patients (83%) with an elevated basal sphincter pressure had long-term benefit (mean follow-up, 38 months) from sphincter ablation therapy (including 10 of 11 treated by BES) in contrast to only 4 of 12 (33.3% $p < 0.05$) with a normal basal sphincter pressure (including 4 of 9 treated by BES). The results of this study suggested that SOM was predictive of outcome from sphincter ablation in patients with IARP and that BES could prevent recurrent pancreatitis. In the early 1990s, BES became the standard of care for patients with IARP found to have SOD. However, Guelrud and colleagues found that severing the pancreatic sphincter was necessary to resolve pancreatitis (Fig. 52.2).[64]

In this series, 69 patients with IARP caused by SOD underwent treatment by standard BES ($n = 18$), BES with pancreatic sphincter balloon dilation ($n = 24$), BES followed by pancreatic endoscopic sphincterotomy (PES) in separate sessions ($n = 13$), or dual-endoscopic sphincterotomy (DES) ($n = 14$). Eighty-one percent of patients undergoing DES had resolution of pancreatitis compared with 28% of patients undergoing BES alone ($p < 0.005$). Sherman and colleagues reported that only 44% of SOD patients with IARP had no further attacks during a 5-year follow-up interval after BES.[56] These data are consistent with the theory that many such patients who benefit from BES alone may have subtle gallstone pancreatitis or perhaps follow-up that has not been long enough to detect another attack of pancreatitis. Wehrmann[65] attempted to help clarify the issue by studying patients with a longer follow-up (11.5 ± 1.6 years) after endoscopic therapy for SOD with IARP. In this study, 5 of 37 (14%) had recurrent pancreatitis over a mean duration of 32.4 months (range 24 to 53 months) and this increased to 19 of 37 (51%) at 11.5 years. The frequency of pancreatitis episodes was, however, lower than that before endoscopic therapy. The authors suggest that endoscopic sphincter ablation may slow the progress of the natural course of the disease.[65]

The results of Guelrud and colleagues also support the anatomic findings of separate biliary and pancreatic sphincters, in addition to manometric findings of residual pancreatic sphincter hypertension, in more than 50% of persistently symptomatic patients who undergo BES alone.[64] Kaw and Brodmerkel reported that among patients with idiopathic pancreatitis secondary to SOD, 78% had persistent manometric evidence of pancreatic sphincter hypertension despite biliary sphincterotomy.[59] Toouli and colleagues demonstrated the importance of pancreatic and biliary sphincter ablation in patients with idiopathic recurrent pancreatitis.[52] In this series, 23 of 26 patients (88%) undergoing surgical ablation of both the biliary and pancreatic sphincters were either asymptomatic or had minimal symptoms at a median follow-up of 24 months (range 9 to 105 months). In contrast, only 43% of patients treated conservatively ($n = 7$) and 29% treated by BES alone ($n = 7$) had no further episodes of pancreatitis. Okolo and colleagues retrospectively evaluated the long-term results of PES in 55 patients with manometrically documented or presumed pancreatic sphincter hypertension (presumption based on recurrent pancreatitis along with PD dilation and contrast medium drainage time from the PD greater than 10 minutes).[66] During a median follow-up of 16 months (range 3 to 52 months), 34 patients (62%) reported significant pain improvement. Patients with normal pancreatography were more likely to respond to therapy than those with pancreatographic evidence of CP (73% vs 58%). Jacob and colleagues postulated that SOD might cause recurrent episodes of pancreatitis even though SOM was normal and that pancreatic stent placement might prevent further attacks.[67] In a randomized study, 34 patients with IARP, normal pancreatic duct SOM, ERCP, secretin testing, and without biliary crystals (probably best considered "true" IARP) were treated with pancreatic stents (n = 19; 5 to 7 Fr; with stents exchanged 3 times over a 1-year period) or conservative therapy (n = 15). During a 3-year follow-up, pancreatitis recurred in 53% of patients in the control group and only 11% of the stented patients (p < 0.02). This study suggests that SOM may be an imperfect test, as patients may have SOD that is not detected at the time of SOM. However, long-term studies are needed to evaluate the outcome after removal of stents, and concerns remain regarding stent-induced ductal and parenchymal changes.[68,69] Because of the concern of stent-induced injury to the pancreas, trial PD stenting to predict the outcome from PES is not routinely recommended.[57]

Thus the therapeutic landscape had changed. Initial recommendations for BES alone were replaced with dual pancreatic and biliary sphincterotomy for those with SOD. However, no randomized trials were performed with long-term follow-up to support this approach. At present, controversy persists as to the appropriateness of performing SOM in patients with IAP and IARP.[70] In an editorial by Tan and Sherman,[71] it was stated that although the aforementioned studies suggest that endoscopic therapy may benefit a majority of patients with IARP caused by SOD, there are many limitations that need to be emphasized: (1) the majority of published studies are retrospective (except for one study) and suffer from incomplete follow-up, lack homogeneity of patient selection for therapy, and are not blinded or compared with an untreated group; (2) uncontrolled prospective studies are prone to bias; (3) length of follow-up of most studies is less than 3 years; and (4) short follow-up may result in an underestimate of the true recurrence rates.

DIFFERENCES IN DEFINING STUDY OUTCOMES

Authors have used different outcomes, including documented recurrent pancreatitis, the need for reintervention, or a grading system of no relief, good relief, or complete relief of symptoms. The lack of a homogeneous population of IARP patients treated is also a problem. Other issues that decrease the robustness of the studies include variable interventions used, with different studies performing BES, PES, or DES with undefined reasons as to why the particular management strategy was chosen. Completeness of sphincter ablation was also often not determined. In the absence of further randomized trials and long-term follow-up, many authorities consider the benefits of sphincter ablation therapy to be currently unproven.[71–73]

Coté et al. performed a randomized controlled trial (RCT) of ERCP with SOM for patients with IARP and no morphologic evidence of CP.[74] Patients with pancreatic SOD (n = 69) were randomly assigned to undergo either a BES (standard of care at the inception of the study) alone or DES; patients with normal SOM (n = 20) were randomly assigned to BES or a sham sphincterotomy (no therapy was the standard of care at the inception of the study). The median follow-up after the intervention was 7 years. Among patients with pancreatic SOD, BES and

DES had similar effects in preventing recurrent pancreatitis (48.5% vs 47.2%; p = 1). For patients with normal SOM, BES was associated with a higher rate (but not statistically significant) of recurrent pancreatitis than sham sphincterotomy (27.3% vs 11.1%; p = 0.59). Overall, 16.9% of subjects developed CP during a median follow-up period of 7 years. The odds of recurrent pancreatitis during follow-up evaluation were significantly greater among patients with SOD than those with normal SOM. Specifically, there was a 4.3 times greater chance of recurrent pancreatitis in patients with SOD than normal SOM (p < 0.02), and that remained so after adjusting for potential confounders. The authors concluded that pancreatic SOD is an independent prognostic factor, identifying patients at higher risk for recurrent pancreatitis. Other predictors for developing recurrent pancreatitis included the development of CP (odds ratio [OR] 3.5; p < 0.02), post-ERCP pancreatitis (OR 5.8; p < 0.001), and the number of episodes of pancreatitis before enrollment (OR 1.1; p < 0.05). The authors concluded the following:

1. In patients with pancreatic SOD, pancreatic sphincterotomy had no incremental benefit over BES alone in reducing the incidence of recurrent pancreatitis. The reason for this is uncertain, but it suggests that pancreatic SOD is not the cause of the AP but perhaps the consequence. Alternatively, endoscopic pancreatic sphincterotomy is an inadequate therapy to ablate the pancreatic sphincter.
2. Pancreatic SOD predicts an aggressive phenotype.
3. There is a significant incidence of CP during long-term follow-up.
4. The benefit of BES alone in IARP regardless of SOM results is unclear. In a post hoc analysis with long-term follow-up of this RCT, the relative rate of ARP decreased after endoscopic sphincterotomy for patients regardless of the presence of SOD.[75] IARP patients with SOD had a higher baseline rate of AP, which translates into higher rates of AP after ES. In SOD patients, DES does not offer significant efficacy over BES in decreasing the rate of recurrent pancreatitis. Based on these results, one can consider recommending BES for patients with IARP, normal pancreatic duct anatomy, and no evidence of CP. The authors also found that any AP and a higher rate of recurrent pancreatitis after ES are associated with progression to CP and indicative of an aggressive phenotype.

Characteristics of studies of endoscopic therapy for SOD associated with recurrent AP are summarized in Table 52.3.

PANCREAS DIVISUM

Pancreas divisum is the most common congenital variant of PD anatomy. It occurs when the dorsal and ventral ducts fail to fuse during the second month of gestation.[76] With nonunion of the ducts, the major portion of the pancreatic exocrine juice drains into the duodenum via the dorsal duct (DD) and minor papilla. It has been proposed that relative obstruction of pancreatic exocrine juice through the minor papilla with resultant pancreatic duct hypertension could precipitate recurrent pancreatitis in a subpopulation of pancreas divisum patients.[77–79] In a study by Bertin et al. evaluating the frequency of pancreas divisum in patients with ARP or CP, pancreas divisum was noted more commonly in patients with genetic mutations of the PRSS1, SPINK 1, and CFTR genes (16%, 16%, and 47%, respectively).[80] There was no difference in frequency of pancreas divisum in patients with IAP and no gene mutations (5%), control group (7%), and alcohol-induced pancreatitis (7%). The authors suggested that pancreatitis may be a cumulative effect of two cofactors rather than from pancreas divisum alone.[80] Whereas a few epidemiologic studies dispute the relation of pancreas divisum to pancreatitis, three lines of evidence favor this association: (1) histologic studies and pancreatography have demonstrated features of CP isolated to the DD; (2) numerous studies have shown a statistically significant

TABLE 52.3 Characteristics of Studies of Endoscopic Therapy for Sphincter of Oddi Dysfunction Associated With Acute Recurrent Pancreatitis

Author (Year)	Study Type	N	Endoscopic Therapy	Follow-up (mo)	% Improved
Kaw and Brodmerkel (2002)[59]	P	37	BES and/or PES	29	78
Wehrmann (2011)[65]	P	37	BES and/or PES with PD stent	32	86
	R			140	49
Coté et al. (2012)[74]	RCT, p-SOD	69	BES vs DES	78	52 vs 53
	RCT, nl-SOM	20	BES vs sham		73 vs 89

BES, Biliary endoscopic sphincterotomy; *DES,* dual-endoscopic sphincterotomy; *nl,* normal; *p,* pancreatic; *P,* prospective; *PD,* pancreatic ductal; *PES,* pancreatic endoscopic sphincterotomy; *R,* retrospective; *RCT,* randomized controlled trial; *SOM,* sphincter of Oddi manometry.

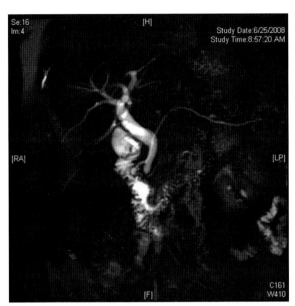

FIG 52.3 Secretin-enhanced magnetic resonance cholangiopancreatography showing pancreas divisum. Note the dorsal duct crossing the biliary tree and the small ventral duct entering the major papilla.

higher prevalence of pancreas divisum; and (3) numerous studies indicated symptom resolution by facilitating DD decompression endoscopically or surgically.[76,81–83]

The diagnosis of pancreas divisum is suspected at ERCP when only a small ventral duct system is visualized after contrast injection of the major papilla. It is confirmed when the remainder of the PD system (DD) is visualized by injecting contrast into the minor papilla and there is no communication between the two ductal systems. The clinical presentation and response to therapy for incomplete pancreas divisum, where there is a small filamentous communication between the ventral and DDs, appear to be similar to those of complete pancreas divisum.[3,84]

S-MRCP is frequently used in the setting of IAP. Previous studies have reported sensitivity and specificity of MRCP for detecting pancreas divisum (Fig. 52.3) of up to 100% (range 36% to 100%).[85–89] To assess the accuracy of MRCP in detecting pancreas divisum, Mosler and colleagues studied 146 patients undergoing MRCP with and without secretin followed by ERP. Nineteen patients had pancreas divisum.[90] The results showed that when S-MRCP was compared with ERP, the overall sensitivity and specificity were 73% and 97%, respectively. The sensitivity and specificity improved to 83% and 99% in the subgroup of patients without CP. The authors concluded that S-MRCP had high specificity but only modest sensitivity for pancreas divisum detection.[90] In the setting of IARP, Mariani and colleagues showed that S-MRCP

and ERP had similar detection rates of pancreas divisum in 8/44 (18.2%) and 7/43 (16.3%) patients.[18]

There are limited data on the role of EUS in diagnosing pancreas divisum.[91,92] In the setting of IARP, Mariani and colleagues showed that S-EUS and ERP had similar detection rates of pancreas divisum in 6/44 (13.6%) and 7/43 (16.3%) patients.[18]

The aim of endoscopic therapy in symptomatic pancreas divisum patients is to alleviate the outflow of obstruction at the level of the minor papilla. The available endoscopic options include dilation, long-term DD stenting, minor papilla endoscopic sphincterotomy (MiES), or a combination of therapies. Table 52.4 shows the outcomes of endoscopic therapy in selected series.[93–107] Overall, 78% of 316 patients had no further episodes of pancreatitis during a mean follow-up interval of 30 months.

It must be appreciated that AP is an episodic illness. A follow-up duration as short as 20 months after intervention would not be long enough to conclude that a patient is "cured."[70] Moreover, the necessary randomized trials proving the efficacy of endoscopic intervention are lacking.

There is only one randomized study evaluating the role of endoscopic therapy of pancreas divisum in the setting of IARP. Lans and colleagues reported the results of an RCT of long-term (12 months) stenting of the minor papilla in patients with at least two prior episodes of unexplained pancreatitis (n = 19).[95] The mean follow-up interval was 2.5 years and all stented patients were followed for at least 12 months after stent removal. Stented patients had statistically significant fewer hospitalizations and episodes of pancreatitis (p < 0.05) and were more frequently judged to be improved (90% vs 11% for controls, p < 0.05). These promising results certainly support the role of endoscopic therapy in patients with pancreas divisum having IARP. However, long-term stenting requires repeated procedures for stent change, each with an associated risk. Moreover, pancreatic stenting is associated with ductal and parenchymal changes that may be irreversible.[68,69] Finally, an unanswered question is whether stenting for 1 year permanently alleviates the obstruction at the level of the minor papilla. We prefer performing MiES for "more permanent" enlargement of the minor papilla orifice (Fig. 52.4).[76]

In summary, patients with IARP found to have pancreas divisum are good candidates for minor papilla therapy. However, long-term outcome studies (at least 5 to 10 years of follow-up), preferably as randomized trials, are necessary to prove the safety and efficacy of endoscopic therapy not only in the setting of pancreas divisum, but also in other settings where a cause for the IARP has been uncovered.

CHOLEDOCHOCELE

Choledochocele, or type III choledochal cyst using the Todani et al. classification system, refers to a cystic dilation of the terminal

TABLE 52.4	Endoscopic Therapy of Acute Pancreatitis Caused by Pancreas Divisum					
Author (Year)	**Study Type**	**N**	**Endoscopic Therapy**	**Follow-up (mo)**	**% Improved**
Liguory et al. (1986)[93]	R	8	MiES	24	63
McCarthy et al. (1988)[94]	P	19	Stent	14	89
Lans et al. (1992)[95]	RCT	10	Stent	30	90
Lehman et al. (1993)[96]	R	17	MiES	20	76
Coleman et al. (1994)[97]	R	9	MiES/stent	23	78
Kozarek et al. (1995)[98]	R	15	MiES/stent	20	86
Jacob et al. (1999)[99]	R	10	MiES/stent/dilation	16	60
Ertan (2000)[100]	P	25	Stent	24	83
Heyries et al. (2002)[101]	R	24	MiES/stent	39	92
Kwan et al. (2008)[102]	R	21	MiES	38	62
Chacko et al. (2008)[103]	R	27	MiES/stent	20	76
Borak et al. (2009)[104]	R	62	MiES/stent/dilation	48	71
Romagnuolo et al. (2013)[105]	P	40	MiES/stent	6	90
Mariani et al. (2014)[106]	R	33	MiES/stent	54	74
Zator et al. (2016)[107]	R	41	MiES/stent	53	81
Total		**316**		**30**	**78**

MiES, Minor papilla endoscopic sphincterotomy; *P,* prospective; *R,* retrospective; *RCT,* randomized controlled trial.

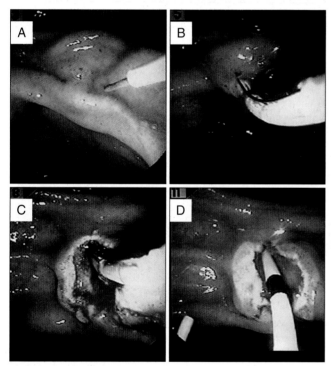

FIG 52.4 Minor papilla sphincterotomy. **A,** A normal minor papilla. A highly tapered catheter and guidewire used to cannulate the dorsal duct are in view. **B,** A sphincterotome in the minor papilla. **C,** Completed minor papilla sphincterotomy. **D,** A dorsal pancreatic duct stent was placed for pancreatitis prophylaxis.

common bile duct usually involving the intramural segment.[108] IAP has been reported in 30% to 70% of patients found to have a choledochocele.[109] Although choledochoceles commonly present with pancreatitis, they are an uncommon cause of IAP because of their low prevalence.

Choledochoceles are most commonly diagnosed at the time of ERCP. Endoscopically, the papilla has a "bulging" appearance but is soft (pillow sign) when probed with a catheter tip. A rounded cystic structure can

be demonstrated at the terminal end of the common bile duct after contrast injection into the biliary tree, with associated progressive enlargement or "ballooning" of the papilla.[110,111]

There are limited published series reporting the value of EUS in detecting choledochoceles. A few case reports have suggested that EUS is helpful in diagnosing choledochoceles in the setting of a dilated common bile duct.[112,113]

The role of MRCP in detecting choledochoceles in adults has been reported in the literature.[114,115] In a study of 72 patients using ERCP as the gold standard, Park and colleagues showed that the sensitivity, specificity, and accuracy of MRCP for detecting choledochal ductal anomalies were 83%, 90%, and 86%, respectively. Specifically looking at type III choledochal cysts, sensitivity was 8/11 (73%), specificity 61/61 (100%), positive predictive value 8/8 (100%), and negative predictive value 61/64 (95%). The authors suggested that MRCP may supersede the diagnostic role of ERCP for patients with choledochal cysts. However, MRCP showed limited capacity to detect minor ductal anomalies or small choledochoceles.[116]

Surgical therapy, either by excision or by sphincteroplasty, was the traditional approach to choledochoceles.[109] There are limited data to support endoscopic therapy as a safe and effective alternative to surgery (Table 52.5), though there is certainly no reason that it should not be. Table 52.5 presents the results of five selected series reporting the outcome of endoscopic therapy. Thirteen of 14 patients treated had no further episodes of pancreatitis during the follow-up period.[110,117,118] The endoscopic approach is to unroof the cyst and perform a biliary sphincterotomy (Fig. 52.5).

TUMORS

Five to seven percent of patients with benign or malignant pancreaticobiliary and ampullary tumors have IAP.[3] These tumors should be considered in patients age 40 years or older who have their first episode of pancreatitis.[20,21] Patients with hereditary conditions such as familial adenomatous polyposis may have ampullary involvement and suffer from IAP at a younger age. The most common tumors reported in IARP series are IPMNs and mucinous cystic neoplasms, ampullary (papillary) tumors, pancreatic adenocarcinoma, and islet cell tumors. Ampullary tumors and IPMN deserve special mention because they are commonly

TABLE 52.5 **Endoscopic Therapy of Choledochoceles in Patients With Idiopathic Pancreatitis**

Author (Year)	N	Pancreatitis (n)	Improved (n)/With IARP Treated at ERCP (n)
Venu et al. (1984)[110]	8	5	2/3
Martin et al. (1992)[118]	10	7	7/7
Ladas et al. (1995)[117]	15	1	1/1
Akkiz et al. (1997)[119]	1	1	1/1
Jang et al. (2010)[120]	2	2	2/2
Total	**36**	**16 (44%)**	**13/14 (93%)**

ERCP, Endoscopic retrograde cholangiopancreatography; *IARP,* idiopathic acute recurrent pancreatitis.

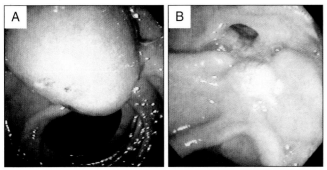

FIG 52.5 A, Endoscopic view of a choledochocele. **B,** Six weeks after endoscopic unroofing of the choledochocele and biliary sphincterotomy.

missed on standard abdominal imaging tests and identified at the time of ERCP.[10]

There are a wide variety of benign tumors that arise at the major papilla, including adenoma, lipoma, fibroma, lymphangioma, leiomyoma, and hamartoma with adenoma being the most common.[121] All have the potential to cause AP by obstructing pancreatic flow. Endoscopy is the most sensitive and specific method for diagnosing papillary tumors, as it accurately localizes the lesion and provides biopsy confirmation. Although there is uniform agreement that papillary adenomas should be resected, there is controversy as to the optimal method of excision. Regardless of the method of resection, complete removal is mandatory.[121] The trend in management of papillary adenomas has been toward increased use of endoscopic therapy, perhaps because of more widespread use and experience with endoscopic mucosal resection in other parts of the gastrointestinal tract (Fig. 52.6). Evidence is accumulating to indicate that endoscopic resection ("snare papillectomy"), thermal ablation, or a combination of the two is the treatment of choice for most papillary adenomas.[121–127] Ampullectomy and papillectomy are discussed in detail in Chapter 25.

Primary malignant tumors of the major papilla include carcinoma, lymphoma, and neuroendocrine tumors.[128] Metastatic tumors include malignant melanoma, renal cell carcinoma, and lymphoma.[121] Although most patients with malignant tumors of the papilla have obstructive jaundice, there are occasional patients who develop pancreatitis as their first sign of the disease. ERCP is used to confirm the diagnosis and offer palliative stenting in nonresectable patients.

IPMNs are premalignant lesions with varying malignant potential based on their location with respect to the pancreatic duct. Patients with main-duct IPMN (MD-IPMN) have a 35% to 80% incidence of invasive pancreatic cancer at the time of surgical resection, in contrast to patients with side-branch disease, who have a 0% to 31% incidence.[129] It is not uncommon to find patients with IPMN having recurrent pancreatitis for many years before the diagnosis is made.[130] Endoscopy and ERCP are essential to the diagnosis. Before the widespread availability of MRCP and EUS, ERCP was considered the standard for evaluation and diagnosis.[131,132] In patients with MD-IPMN, pancreatography typically reveals a dilated main pancreas duct (MPD) with cast-like filling defects representing mucin (Fig. 52.7).[131]

A patulous pancreatic orifice exuding mucin is seen in up to 60% to 80% of patients with MD-IPMN (Fig. 52.8).[131]

However, pancreatographic findings may be much more subtle and can be misinterpreted as normal when a small cast-like filling defect is missed or a filling defect is labeled as a pancreatic stone or air bubble. A missed diagnosis often comes in the setting of a normal pancreatic duct diameter (Fig. 52.9).

Finally, IPMN may be misinterpreted as CP. A high index of suspicion by the endoscopist is therefore critical, particularly in patients older than 40 years. During pancreatography, early radiographic films should be obtained and the fluoroscopic image should be carefully observed so that small filling defects are not missed. At ERCP, it is also possible to obtain cytologic specimens by aspiration or brushings, guided forceps biopsy specimens for histology, and tissue and pancreatic juice for tumor markers. Pancreatoscopy (see Chapter 26) and IDUS are ancillary techniques used at the time of ERCP to help localize the tumor, differentiate benign from malignant disease, and aid in the differential diagnosis of amorphous filling defects in the PD.[133–135] IDUS has also been useful in detecting distant, smaller, not previously detected IPMNs along the main duct and in guiding the extent of surgical resection.[136,137] IPMN is discussed in detail in Chapter 51.

There appears to be little to no role for endoscopic therapy in IPMN (except when biliary obstruction occurs). However, the value of PES in assisting with the passage of mucin in high-risk surgical patients has not been evaluated. Given the fact that many of these patients already have gaping pancreatic orifices, it is unlikely to be of significant long-term benefit.

EUS has an important role in identifying IMPNs and other tumors in patients with IAP and IARP.[28,138] In the setting of IPMNs, the rate of AP is highly variable, with published rates in surgical series from 12% to 67%.[139] Many studies have found EUS to have the highest sensitivity for identifying pancreatic neoplasms relative to other imaging modalities, especially for tumors smaller than 2 to 3 cm in diameter.[3,140,141] In a series of 90 patients with an undetermined cause of acute or recurrent pancreatitis, EUS identified a benign or malignant pancreatic tumor in 8 patients that was not previously detected on CT scan.[58] In a study comparing the performance characteristics of EUS and ERCP for diagnosing IPMN, EUS had a sensitivity of 86% and specificity of 99%.[142] AP was reported to occur more often in patients with IPMN than in those with usual pancreatic adenocarcinoma.[143] One possible explanation proposed was that obstruction of the main pancreatic duct or branch duct by abundant mucus secretion caused AP and/or pain more frequently than obstruction caused by a solid tumor.[144] The ability of EUS to safely guide fine-needle aspiration (FNA) of fluid and tissue makes it a powerful tool in determining the nature of a fluid collection. Thus, by aspirating fluid from a cyst for cytology, DNA characteristics, tumor markers, and pancreatic enzymes, one can usually distinguish a benign (e.g., pseudocyst) from a premalignant process. The cooperative pancreatic cyst study showed that using EUS-FNA with cyst fluid analysis is helpful in differentiating mucinous versus nonmucinous cystic lesions when carcinoembryonic antigen (CEA) is >192 ng/mL.[145] However, the absolute value of CEA is not predictive of malignancy. Pais and colleagues studied 74 patients with IPMN who underwent surgery and found that older

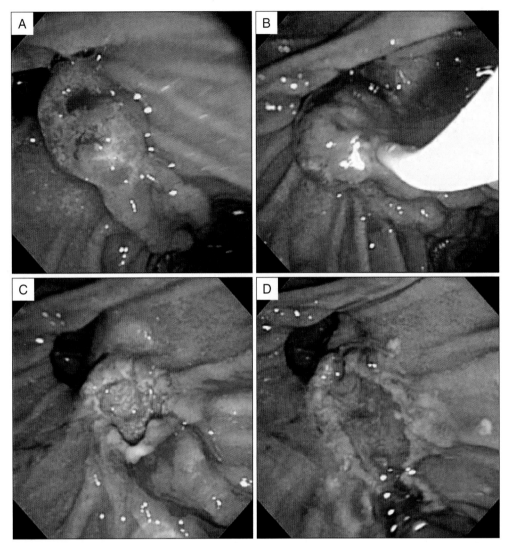

FIG 52.6 A, Endoscopic view of a tubulovillous adenoma involving the papilla and extending caudally down the duodenal wall. **B,** The papilla was snared and electrocautery applied. **C,** Appearance of the ampullary segment after snare resection of the papilla. **D,** The tumor involving the duodenal wall was resected and a biliary sphincterotomy was done (patient has pancreas divisum, and thus a pancreatic stent was not placed in the ventral pancreatic duct). This endoscopic picture shows the area of the resected tumor.

age, jaundice and weight loss, and EUS features of a solid lesion, dilated MPD, ductal filling defects, and thickened septa are predictive of malignancy in these patients. EUS-FNA cytology was helpful, but cyst fluid CEA and CA19-9 were of limited value in differentiating malignant from benign IPMNs.[146] Other comparative studies have also indicated that EUS is the most accurate imaging study for diagnosing malignancy in the setting of IPMN.[147–150] Thus, in the setting of IAP and IARP, EUS seems to be a reasonable test to perform, particularly in patients older than 40 years, when other radiologic imaging tests are negative, indeterminate cystic lesions of the pancreas are present after resolution of pancreatitis, or malignancy is suspected in a background of IPMN (Fig. 52.10).

MRCP has been shown to be superior at detecting IPMN compared with ERCP[151,152] (Figs. 52.11 and 52.12).

The reason MRCP is better than ERCP at depicting dilated MPD and side-branch cystic lesions is that mucinous fluid produced by the tumor or the tumor itself inhibits adequate inflow of ERCP contrast material into the MPD or the cystic dilated branches.[153] In a study by Waters and colleagues of 18 patients undergoing surgery for IPMN,

MRCP was found to be superior to CT scan at detecting a ductal connection, estimating main duct involvement, and identifying small branch-duct cysts.[154] A ductal connection was detected on 73% of MRCPs and only 18% of CT scans. IPMN type was classified differently in 7 (39%), 4 (22%) of which were read on CT as having main duct involvement, which was not appreciated on MRCP or surgical pathology. MRCP showed multifocal disease in 13 (72%) versus only 9 (50%) on CT. Finally, 101 branch lesions were identified on MRCP compared with 46 on CT. This study demonstrated that MRCP better characterized the type, location, and extent of IPMN compared with CT. However, in another study by Sahani and colleagues of 25 patients undergoing surgery for IPMN, multidetector-row CT (MDCT) with 2D curved reformations showed results similar to MRCP. Cyst communication was seen in 20 and 21 of 24 branch-duct IPMNs with CT and MRCP, respectively. Sensitivity, specificity, and accuracy for detection of malignancy were 70%, 87%, and 76% for CT and 70%, 92%, and 80% for MRCP. Interobserver agreement was good to perfect for both readers in all comparisons (overall, kappa = 0.70 to 1.00).[155] Yoon and colleagues showed that 3D MRCP provided better image quality, offered superior

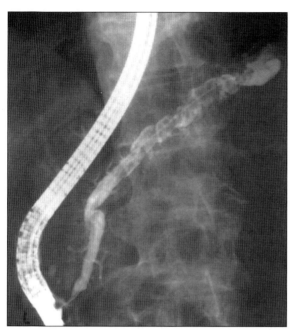

FIG 52.7 Intraductal papillary mucinous neoplasm (IPMN). Endoscopic retrograde pancreatogram showing a markedly dilated pancreatic duct containing filling defects in the body and tail consistent with mucus.

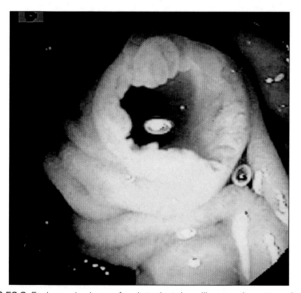

FIG 52.8 Endoscopic views of an intraductal papillary mucinous neoplasm (IPMN). The patulous pancreatic orifice is exuding mucin.

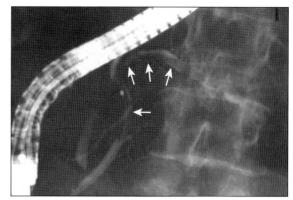

FIG 52.9 Intraductal papillary mucinous neoplasm (IPMN). In this case the castlike filling defect (*arrows*) is present in a normal-diameter pancreatic duct.

evaluation of the PD and morphologic details of IPMN compared with 2D MRCP, and was preferred for surgical planning.[156] Thus, in the evaluation of IARP when small pancreatic tumors or IPMNs may have been missed on initial imaging, MRCP (2D or 3D) or MDCT with 2D curved reformations is noninvasive, with little to no risk, and should be considered before performing ERCP.[151–156]

OTHER ANATOMIC CAUSES

There are a number of nonneoplastic structural lesions that can cause AP. These can be evaluated with EUS, MRCP, or ERCP. PD strictures, which result in upstream ductal hypertension, are usually the result of

prior trauma or develop after healing of a pseudocyst or pancreatic necrosis.[10] Duodenal diverticula are rarely associated with pancreatitis.[157] Anomalous pancreaticobiliary duct junction is a rare congenital malformation in which the union of the PD and bile duct occurs outside the duodenal wall. As a result, the sphincter of Oddi is unable to prevent reciprocal regurgitation of pancreatic enzymes and bile into the alternate biliary and pancreatic ducts. Such a union may occur in isolation or be associated with choledochal cyst disease. Pancreatitis may be a complication of this anomaly. Samavedy and colleagues suggested that endoscopic sphincterotomy eliminates or reduces the frequency of recurrent pancreatitis and would be a logical first step in the management of most symptomatic patients.[158] Annular pancreas is another congenital anomaly associated with pancreatitis that manifests as a band of pancreatic tissue partially or completely encircling the duodenum. ERCP typically identifies the duct of the annulus. Pancreas divisum is present in about one-third of these patients.[76,159] EUS has also been shown to be useful in aiding the diagnosis of annular pancreas.[160,161] MRI/MRCP can also diagnose this condition.[162–164] Duodenal duplication cysts, also a distinctly rare congenital anomaly, may present with pancreatitis. A potential role of endoscopic therapy in the treatment of such cysts has been described.[165] Finally, CP can be diagnosed at ERCP when main-duct and/or side-branch changes are present. However, EUS is perhaps the most sensitive technique to detect early-stage disease. In a series of 90 patients with IAP and IARP, 44% had CP by EUS and ERCP criteria.[58] Fischer and colleagues showed that CP was diagnosed on ERCP in 17% of patients with one episode of IAP and 35% of patients with IARP.[21]

GENETIC MUTATIONS

The literature is now replete with evidence showing that patients with IAP and IARP may have various genetic mutations. Poddar et al. reported a genetic predisposition in almost 45% of children with IAP and 33% of children with IARP.[166]

Cystic fibrosis transmembrane conductance regulator (*CFTR*) gene mutation represents the most common inherited disease of the exocrine pancreas. Some phenotypic *CFTR* gene mutations occur in about 5% of the Caucasian European and North American populations. However, the true incidence of *CFTR* gene mutations is probably underestimated. Cationic trypsinogen (*PRSS1*) gene mutations have been found in patients with hereditary pancreatitis and predispose individuals to recurrent bouts of pancreatitis in childhood and frequent progression to CP. Serine protease inhibitor Kazal type 1 (SPINK-1) mutation has been detected in 16% to 23% of patients with apparent idiopathic

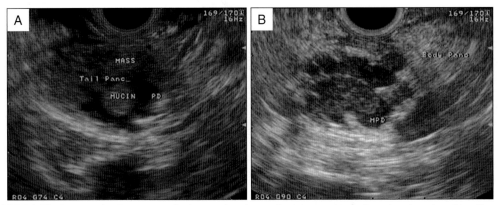

FIG 52.10 Endoscopic ultrasonography image showing malignant transformation of an intraductal papillary mucinous neoplasm. Note the solid component.

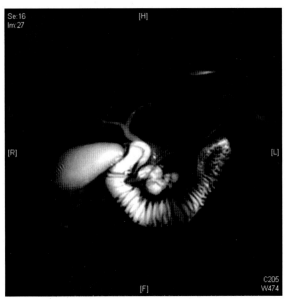

FIG 52.11 Secretin-enhanced magnetic resonance cholangiopancreatography demonstrating a large side-branch intraductal papillary mucinous neoplasm in the pancreatic head.

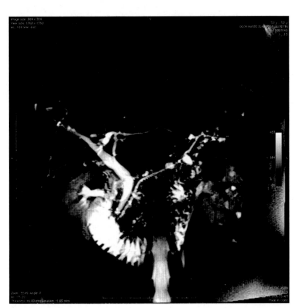

FIG 52.12 Secretin-enhanced magnetic resonance cholangiopancreatography demonstrating a multifocal side-branch intraductal papillary mucinous neoplasm.

pancreatitis, compared with only about 2% of healthy controls.[167] Ariza et al. identified two novel mutations in the glycosylphosphatidylinositol-anchored high-density lipoprotein–binding protein 1 (GPIHBP1) in patients with recurrent pancreatitis.[168]

A lack of long-term follow-up studies hinders proper understanding of the role of genetic factors. Moreover, data have shown that patients with IAP and IARP may have different genetic backgrounds.[169,170] Thus, genetic testing is mostly beneficial in patients with recurrent pancreatitis of younger age. Although it may help in planning treatment, it can help in establishing a cause-effect relationship and provide prognosis for the development of CP or pancreatic adenocarcinoma.[171,172]

AUTOIMMUNE PANCREATITIS

Autoimmune pancreatitis (AIP) is an uncommon cause of IAP and IARP.[173] AIP is characterized radiographically by diffuse or segmental irregular narrowing of the main pancreatic duct and diffused enlargement of the pancreas, laboratory evidence of elevated levels of serum IgG (particularly the IgG4 subtype), and the presence of autoantibodies, and histopathologically by fibrotic changes with lymphoplasmacytic

infiltration of the pancreas.[173] Various diagnostic criteria have been proposed from different countries to make the diagnosis of AIP.[174–176] An international consensus on diagnosis has been proposed, further subdividing AIP into type 1 and type 2.[177,178] An international multicenter survey showed that obstructive jaundice was a more frequent presentation in type 1 than in type 2 (75% vs 47%, $p < 0.001$), whereas abdominal pain (41% vs 68%, $p < 0.001$) and AP (5% vs 34%, $p < 0.001$) were more frequent in type 2 patients.[179] In contrast to other forms of CP, AIP responds dramatically to corticosteroid therapy. Thus laboratory screening with serum immunoglobulin IgG subtypes and core biopsies of the pancreas should be considered in selected IAP patients with clinical or radiologic features suggestive of AIP.[39,180]

YIELD OF ERCP, MRCP, AND EUS FOR IAP AND IARP

Table 52.6 summarizes the results of four selected series that used ERCP, SOM, and bile microscopy in the assessment of patients with IAP and IARP.[5,20,56,59] Overall, 73% of patients were found to have a cause of pancreatitis, with SOD being the most common diagnosis.

In a prospective study by Kim et al., in 31 IARP patients with negative findings on ERCP, IDUS performed during ERCP identified a possible cause in 42% of patients (microlithiasis 16.1%, biliary sludge 9.7%, CP 9.7%, and distal PD lesions 6.5%).[36] In a prospective study of 44 consecutive IARP patients with nondilated pancreatic ducts, the diagnostic yield of S-EUS was 13.6% and 16.7% higher than S-MRCP and ERCP, respectively (which both gave similar diagnostic yields).[15] The combined use of S-EUS and S-MRCP documented findings that could have explained the cause of AP in 63.3% of cases. The authors concluded that S-MRCP and S-EUS should both be used in the diagnostic workup of IARP as complementary first-line techniques instead of ERCP.

Many patients with IARP have findings of CP by EUS, MRCP, or ERCP, or may develop evidence of CP in follow-up, thereby indicating that these patients might have subtle evidence of CP from the onset and may develop CP as a result of repeated insults to the pancreas. Endoscopic pancreas function testing (e-PFT) allows accurate evaluation of pancreas exocrine function and early detection of CP. Duodenal aspirates are typically collected at timed intervals after intravenous injection of secretin for determination of bicarbonate concentration. Testing is performed using a standard end-viewing or side-viewing endoscope or a linear or radial echoendoscope.[181,182] The combination of EUS with PFT has been shown to increase test sensitivity for diagnosis to 100%.[183] The pancreatic duct cell bicarbonate secretion can be affected by several variables, thus affecting the specificity of e-PFT. In a retrospective study of 131 subjects undergoing e-PFT, cigarette smoking was found to be independently associated with impaired pancreatic duct cell secretory function regardless of age, gender, alcohol intake, and the presence of CP.[184]

OUTCOMES OF ENDOSCOPIC THERAPY IN IARP

Unfortunately there is a paucity of controlled data regarding outcomes in patients undergoing endoscopic therapy for previously diagnosed IARP. In fact, only three RCTs have been reported.[67,74,95] It is also difficult to interpret the data that are available because of loosely defined outcome measures, inhomogeneous clinical characteristics, generally short-term follow-up, and varied treatment techniques.[10,71] Also, as emphasized earlier, because recurrent pancreatitis is an episodic illness, long-term follow-up (at least 5 to 10 years) after therapy is necessary before concluding that therapy was effective.[71,185]

The outcomes of endoscopic therapy are detailed in the preceding sections. The prospective study by Kaw and Brodmerkel should be highlighted.[59] One hundred and twenty-six patients with IARP underwent ERCP, SOM, and biliary crystal analysis. Patients had a mean of 3.2 episodes of pancreatitis (mean interval between recurrent attacks was 3.8 months). A cause for pancreatitis was identified in 100 patients (79%) and included SOD or papillary stenosis with or without crystals in 67 (53%), microcrystals alone in 12 (9.5%), pancreas divisum in 9 (7.1%), common duct stones in 6 (4.8%), malignancy in 2 (1.6%), CP with a PD stricture in 2 (1.6%), and choledochocele in 2 (1.6%). Endoscopic therapy was performed in 95 patients, and 3 patients underwent surgery. The outcome of therapy is shown in Table 52.7. During a mean follow-up of 30 months, 81% of patients were asymptomatic. Twenty-four patients had procedure-related adverse events; 20 had pancreatitis.

CONCLUSIONS

IAP and IARP are challenging clinical problems for the physician and often frustrating for the patient. ERCP with ancillary techniques can identify a probable cause for the pancreatitis in about 75% of patients. The majority of the diseases uncovered appear to be treatable by endoscopic or surgical techniques. EUS and MRI/MRCP have assumed a more central role in the evaluation of patients with IAP and IARP. When these studies identify the cause of the pancreatitis, appropriate targeted treatment is recommended. In this setting, ERCP should be used for therapy when appropriate. S-EUS and S-MRCP appear to

TABLE 52.6 Idiopathic Acute Recurrent Pancreatitis: Diagnostic Yield of ERCP, Sphincter of Oddi Manometry, and Bile Microscopy (Four Selected Series of 522 Patients)

Diagnosis	Abnormal, *n* (%)
Sphincter of Oddi dysfunction	179 (34)
Pancreas divisum	70 (13)
Pancreatic or papillary tumor	46 (9)
Gallbladder or duct stones	37 (7)
Pancreatic duct stricture/chronic pancreatitis	37 (7)
Choledochocele	12 (2)
Total abnormal	**381 (73)**

Data from Venu et al.,[5] Choudari et al.,[20] Sherman et al.,[56] and Kaw and Brodmerkel.[59]
ERCP, Endoscopic retrograde cholangiopancreatography.

TABLE 52.7 Outcome of Endoscopic Therapy in 100 Patients Found to Have a Cause of Idiopathic Acute Recurrent Pancreatitis

Diagnosis	Patients (*n*)	Treated at ERCP (*n*)	Follow-up (mo)	Asymptomatic (%)
Sphincter of Oddi dysfunction	67	67	33	79
Gallbladder or duct stones	18	16*	31	89
Pancreas divisum	9	8†	24	89
Tumor	2	0‡	28	50
Choledochocele	2	2	18	100
Pancreatic duct stricture	2	2	31	50
Total	**100**	**95**	**30**	**81**

From Kaw and Brodmerkel.[59]
ERCP, Endoscopic retrograde cholangiopancreatography.
*Two treated with cholecystectomy.
†One had unsuccessful minor papilla sphincterotomy.
‡One treated with Whipple, one with unresectable adenocarcinoma.

BOX 52.3   **Step-by-Step Management of Idiopathic Acute Recurrent Pancreatitis**

1. EUS with or without bile microscopy
2. Secretin-stimulated imaging (EUS or MRCP)
3. Consider genetic testing (*PRSS1, CFTR,* and *SPINK-1*)
4. Laparoscopic cholecystectomy versus ERCP
5. ERCP with sphincter of Oddi manometry with or without IDUS

CFTR, Conductance regulatory gene; *ERCP,* endoscopic retrograde cholangiopancreatography; *EUS,* endoscopic ultrasonography; *IDUS,* intraductal ultrasonography; *MRCP,* magnetic resonance cholangiopancreatography; *PRSS1,* cationic trypsinogen gene; *SPINK1,* trypsin inhibitor gene.

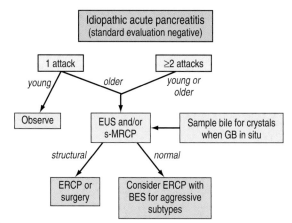

FIG 52.13 Algorithm for workup of patient with idiopathic acute pancreatitis.

increase the diagnostic capability of these two modalities. Each diagnostic modality has both strengths and weaknesses in diagnosing certain etiologies, and both modalities are complementary in the workup for IAP and IARP.

Based on these factors and the risks associated with ERCP, we would recommend EUS and MRCP as the first diagnostic imaging tests to identify the cause of the pancreatitis and direct appropriate targeted treatment. ERCP should be used for therapy when appropriate after EUS and MRCP. ERCP with ancillary endoscopic techniques should be considered when EUS, MRI/MRCP, bile microscopy, appropriate genetic testing, and autoimmune serology fail to identify a cause of IAP or IARP and the patient has an aggressive course of repeated attacks. Papachristou and Topazian suggested a stepwise approach to IARP in order to minimize risk and cost to the patient (Box 52.3).[186] Empiric cholecystectomy has also been shown to significantly reduce the risk

of acute idiopathic pancreatitis and should also be considered in select patients who otherwise have IARP.[187]

Our recommended algorithm used currently in our unit is shown in Fig. 52.13. Further investigation is necessary to develop the best algorithm that will provide the most cost-effective approach for these patients. Patients with IAP and IARP are best evaluated in centers where specialized expertise and equipment are available when advanced endoscopic methods are required.

The complete reference list for this chapter can be found online at www.expertconsult.com.

53

Biliary Intervention in Acute Gallstone Pancreatitis

Andrew Korman and David L. Carr-Locke

Gallstones are the most common cause of acute pancreatitis (AP), accounting for approximately 35% of cases in the United States and Europe[1,2] and up to 65% of cases in Asia.[3] The majority of patients with acute gallstone pancreatitis (AGP) will follow a benign clinical course. However, up to 25% will progress to severe acute pancreatitis (SAP), which causes a significant increase in morbidity and mortality.[4] Although the exact mechanism by which gallstones cause AP remains elusive, the correlation between gallstones and AP is well documented. Gallstones are found in the stool of approximately 90% of patients with recent AGP, whereas they are found in only 10% of patients with cholelithiasis without AP.[5] In addition, persistent obstruction of the ampulla by a common bile duct (CBD) stone is believed to result in more severe pancreatic injury.[6] Endoscopic retrograde cholangiopancreatography (ERCP) and endoscopic sphincterotomy (ES) are effective tools for removal of such obstructing stones and reestablishment of biliary drainage,[3,7,8] with success rates exceeding 90%. However, performing ERCP is not without risk of adverse events, especially if performed in patients with AP in less-than-ideal circumstances. Determining who requires emergent ERCP is therefore of paramount importance.

DIAGNOSIS OF ACUTE GALLSTONE PANCREATITIS

The effective use of ERCP intervention for the management of AGP necessitates differentiating AGP from other causes of AP. As with all examples of diagnostic investigation, this requires a combination of accurate history taking, physical examination, and interpretation of laboratory values and imaging. A history of cholelithiasis or symptoms consistent with biliary pain is suggestive, but not diagnostic, of a biliary etiology. The physical examination is not specific in distinguishing AGP from other causes. However, concurrent cholecystitis producing Murphy's sign and/or signs of cholangitis are findings that can increase the likelihood that gallstones are the etiology of a patient's pancreatitis. Much of the published literature involves the use of biochemical values and imaging studies for predicting a biliary etiology of AP.

Serum amylase levels have been shown to be higher in patients with AGP than in those with alcohol-related AP, and authors have postulated that a serum amylase level >1000 U/L indicates a biliary cause of AP.[9,10] The presence of elevated liver chemistries has been studied and a meta-analysis demonstrated that elevations of alanine aminotransferase (ALT) levels >3 times normal at the time of presentation are suggestive of AGP.[11] This study also found that total bilirubin and alkaline phosphatase levels were not useful and aspartate aminotransferase (AST) was no more useful than ALT in diagnosing AGP. In addition, once AGP is established, patients with rising serum pancreatic enzymes or liver tests have a four times greater risk of persistent CBD stones and approximately

three times greater risk of complications compared with patients with stable or declining laboratory values.[12]

Demonstration of cholelithiasis by imaging can further support the diagnosis of AGP. Abdominal ultrasonography is the preferred initial imaging study, given its high sensitivity and specificity for gallstones.[13] In the setting of AP, however, this sensitivity can be reduced by the presence of overlying air-filled loops of bowel.[14] A recent study found that abdominal ultrasonography in the setting of AP remains a very sensitive test (86%) and, when combined with an elevation of ALT >80 IU/L, is 98% sensitive and 100% specific for a biliary etiology.[15] The lack of biliary dilatation on ultrasonography does not exclude choledocholithiasis in the setting of AP, especially in the first 48 hours of an attack.

The attendant risks of ERCP and the gold standard for detecting choledocholithiasis have prompted the study of magnetic resonance cholangiopancreatography (MRCP) and endoscopic ultrasonography (EUS) as alternative, safer diagnostic modalities. MRCP has high sensitivity (84% to 95%) and high specificity (96% to 100%) for the diagnosis of common duct stones.[16–18] The most common cause of a false-negative MRCP is gallstone size <5 mm.[17] A prospective study comparing multiple imaging modalities (abdominal ultrasonography, computed tomography [CT], MRCP, ERCP, and intraductal ultrasonography) showed an 80% sensitivity for MRCP at detecting choledocholithiasis with 90.6% agreement between ERCP and MRCP.[19] EUS demonstrates equivalent accuracy to MRCP for the detection of choledocholithiasis.[18] EUS can detect choledocholithiasis at a sensitivity of 98% with 99% specificity. In a recent analysis, the results of EUS were helpful in identifying a biliary cause for AP in half of the patients with unknown etiology and negative imaging.[20]

The exact role of each of these modalities in the diagnosis of AGP and the patient groups to which they should be individually applied must be clarified in future studies and is inevitably dependent on local availability and logistics.

PREDICTION OF COMMON BILE DUCT STONES

Many scoring systems and prognostic factors are available to assess the likelihood of a CBD stone in AP. Although no single prediction model has been validated as better than another, the American Society for Gastrointestinal Endoscopy (ASGE) published guidelines in 2010 to help risk stratify patients based on an algorithm created by Maple et al. (Box 53.1).[21] Patients are categorized as low risk, intermediate risk, or high risk for choledocholithiasis. Those who are high risk should go directly to ERCP and then cholecystectomy. Intermediate-risk patients should be further evaluated with EUS or MRCP. Low-risk patients are considered to have <10% probability of having a CBD stone. If imaging shows sludge or gallstones in the gallbladder and the patient is a good surgical candidate, he or she should proceed directly to cholecystectomy. Ultimately, a CBD stone found on imaging is the best marker for choledocholithiasis.

Video for this chapter can be found online at www.expertconsult.com.

BOX 53.1 Predictors of Choledocholithiasis

Very Strong

CBD stone on transabdominal ultrasonography

Clinical cholangitis

Bilirubin >4 mg/dL

Strong

Dilated CBD on ultrasonography (>6 mm with gallbladder in situ)

Bilirubin 1.8–4 mg/dL

Moderate

Abnormal liver chemistries other than bilirubin

Age >55 years

Clinical gallstone pancreatitis

Assigning a Likelihood of Choledocholithiasis Based on Predictors

Presence of any very strong predictor: high

Presence of any strong predictor: high

No predictors present: low

All other patients: intermediate

CBD, Common bile duct.
From ASGE Standards of Practice Committee. The role of endoscopy in the evaluation of suspected choledocholithiasis. *Gastrointest Endosc.* 2010;71:1–9.

ASSESSMENT OF SEVERITY OF ACUTE PANCREATITIS

Early recognition of patients with SAP is crucial, as these patients will require intensive care management and will likely benefit from early endoscopic intervention.[3,8,22] Several clinical and radiographic parameters have been used to create scoring systems that help predict the severity of AP (Table 53.1). Organ failure, the presence of local complications such as pancreatic necrosis, and acute fluid collections by cross-sectional imaging are just a few included in these prognostic indices. Using these parameters, the Atlanta Classification of 1992 categorized AP as mild or severe, with the latter defined as local complications and/or organ failure. In 2013 this system was revised to delineate moderate SAP from SAP based on the presence or absence of organ failure at <48 hours or >48 hours, respectively.[23]

Furthermore, it standardized the definition of SAP as the presence of local complications and/or organ failure (see Table 53.1) or an Acute Physiology and Chronic Health Evaluation II (APACHE II) (Table 53.2) score greater than 8 or greater than three Ranson's criteria.[24]

Over the past 2 decades the Atlanta Classification of 1993 and its revision in 2013 have come under significant criticism as the understanding of the pathophysiology of the disease process and therapeutic options improved. This classification lacked differentiation between transient and persistent organ failure and definitions of local complications (e.g., fluid collections, necrosis, and pseudocysts), which led to inconsistent use.[25] A recent review of 447 studies showed significant variations in the use of the classification system in both research and clinical settings.[26] This has led the Acute Pancreatitis Classification Working Group to formulate a new set of tools for assessment and definition of severity of AP incorporating scoring systems such as the Marshall scoring system and the sequential organ failure assessment (SOFA) score. However, the revised criteria have not been validated and consensus needs to be established between radiologists and clinicians before using them.

Organ failure, particularly persistent or worsening organ failure, is a strong determinant of mortality in patients with SAP.[27,28] Although

TABLE 53.1 Definition of Severe Complications Requiring Intensive Care Unit Monitoring and Treatment

System	Complication
Pulmonary	Mechanical ventilation; pneumonia with hypoxemia (PaO_2 ≤60 mm Hg); and hypoxemia (PaO_2 ≤60 mm Hg) or dyspnea requiring frequent assessment of need for intubation
Cardiovascular	Hypotension requiring pressor support; ischemia or acute myocardial infarction noted on electrocardiogram or cardiac enzymes; and new onset arrhythmia other than sinus tachycardia
Infectious	Sepsis of any origin
Renal	New onset oliguric or nonoliguric renal failure or new onset dialysis
Hematologic	Disseminated intravascular coagulation and platelet counts <50 × 10^9/L
Neurologic	Glasgow Coma Scale score ≤9 and diminished responsiveness or agitation (requiring significant sedation) with need for frequent airway monitoring
Gastrointestinal	Stress ulcer with hematemesis or melena tract (requiring >2 U of blood per 24 hours

Reproduced with permission from Meek K, Toosie K, Stabile BE, et al. Simplified admission criterion for predicting severe complications of gallstone pancreatitis. *Arch Surg.* 2000;135:1048–1052.

TABLE 53.2 The APACHE II Scoring System*

Physiologic Variable	Reference Range
Rectal temperature, °C	36–38.4
Mean arterial pressure, mm Hg	70–109
Heart rate (ventricular response), beats/min	70–109
Respiratory rate, breaths/min	12–24
Oxygenation, mm Hg	$PaO_2 – PaO_2$ <200 or PO_2 >70
Arterial pH	7.33–7.49
Serum sodium level, mmol/L	130–149
Serum potassium level, mmol/L	3.5–5.4
Serum creatinine level, µmol/L or mg/dL (double point score for acute renal failure)	0.6–1.4 (53–123)
Hematocrit	0.30–0.46
Leukocyte count, ×10^9/L	0.003–0.015
Glasgow Coma Scale (GCS) score	15—actual GCS score

*To calculate the Acute Physiology and Chronic Health Evaluation II (APACHE II) score, the 12 physiologic variables are assigned points between 0 and 4, with 0 being normal and 4 being the most abnormal. The sum of these values is added to a point weighting for patient age (≤44 years = 0; 45–54 years = 2; 55–64 years = 3; 65–74 years = 5; ≥75 years = 6) and a point weighting for chronic health problems. $PaO_2 – PaO_2$ indicates alveolar–arterial difference in partial pressure of oxygen.
Reproduced with permission from Meek K, Toosie K, Stabile BE, et al. Simplified admission criterion for predicting severe complications of gallstone pancreatitis. *Arch Surg.* 2000;135:1048–1052.

TABLE 53.3　Summary of Randomized Controlled Trials of ERCP in AGP

Study	No. of Treated Patients	No. of Control Patients	Study Design	Outcomes
Neoptolemos et al.[8]	59	62	Single center	Significant morbidity reduction in severe AGP
			Consecutive patients with suspected AGP	Significant length of stay reduction in severe AGP
Fan et al.[3]	97	98	Single center	Significant morbidity reduction in AGP
			Consecutive patients with AP, regardless of etiology	Significant reduction in biliary sepsis in severe AGP
			AGP analyzed separately	
Fölsch et al.[7]	126	112	Multicenter	Similar morbidity rates between study groups
			Patients with suspected AGP, excluding those with bilirubin >5 mg/dL	Significantly higher incidence of respiratory insufficiency in ERCP group
Oria et al.[43]	51	52	Single center	Similar morbidity and mortality
			Consecutive patients with suspected AGP	No benefit of performing early endoscopic therapy

AGP, Acute gallstone pancreatitis; *AP,* acute pancreatitis; *ERCP,* endoscopic retrograde cholangiopancreatography.

many definitions of organ failure have been used, more recent studies use the multiple organ dysfunction syndrome (MODS) score or the systemic inflammatory response syndrome (SIRS) score to ensure that findings can be generalized.[29,30] Mortality in the setting of AP with organ failure can range from 20% to as high as 50% and is dependent on the duration, severity, and number of organ systems in failure.[23,24,31] Prognostic indices have been formulated to predict which patients are more likely to develop severe AGP and to direct appropriate care to that group. These include Ranson's criteria (biliary version), modified Glasgow criteria, Bedside Index of Severity in Acute Pancreatitis (BISAP), Harmless Acute Pancreatitis Score (HAPS), blood urea nitrogen levels, and APACHE II score.[32–34] Radiologic scores, such as the Balthazar score and the modified CT severity index, are based on the extent of pancreatic necrosis and fluid collections and have been shown to correlate with mortality.[35,36] Several biochemical markers of inflammation have been studied to predict SAP, but serum C-reactive protein level >150 mg/L at 48 to 72 hours after symptom onset remains the standard.[37] Recent data suggest that a genetic polymorphism that confers an enhanced chemokine response to an inflammatory stimulus is a risk factor for progression to SAP.[38] The search continues for an easily measurable biochemical marker in the first 24 hours of AP that reliably predicts progression to severe disease.

TREATMENT OF ACUTE GALLSTONE PANCREATITIS

The mainstay of initial therapy for all forms of AP remains supportive care, including aggressive hydration, adequate nutritional support, pain control, and often placement in an intensive care unit (ICU) for patients with SAP.[39] Persistent biliary obstruction or stone impaction at the ampulla was once thought to be the only mechanism worsening the course of pancreatitis. For this reason, in the 1980s, early surgery and biliary decompression were advocated as the treatment of choice in patients with AGP.[40] However, clinical trials showed that morbidity and mortality were increased in patients with severe AGP who underwent early surgery.[41,42] During the last 30 years, ERCP has provided a less invasive approach to biliary diseases and numerous publications have evaluated the role of ERCP in early biliary pancreatitis.

Endoscopic Therapy for Acute Gallstone Pancreatitis

Patients diagnosed with AP can be categorized for severity and further divided into patients with or without concurrent cholangitis, based on physical examination, laboratory studies, and imaging. This distinction is important in terms of initial management with urgent endoscopic therapy. There has been much debate on the benefit of performing early endoscopic therapy for AGP.

Early ERCP With or Without Endoscopic Sphincterotomy

Multiple studies have been published in the past 3 decades, including randomized controlled trials (RCTs) pertaining to early ERCP-guided therapy for AGP. Of note are four RCTs, two meta-analyses, and a Cochrane review to define the role of early ERCP and ES.[3,7,8,43–46] These studies differ on the assessment of pancreatitis severity, timing of ERCP, exclusion criteria, and possibly endoscopic expertise. The four RCTs, designed to assess the safety and benefit of early ERCP in AGP, are described below and summarized in Table 53.3.

In 1988, Neoptolemos et al. published a landmark study comparing early ERCP and ES to conservative management of AGP.[8] This study was performed from 1983 to 1987. The investigators randomized 121 of 146 consecutive patients who presented to a single institution with suspected AGP to receive either conservative management or early ERCP within 72 hours of admission. The diagnosis of AGP was established by ultrasonography and laboratory data. The severity of pancreatitis was predicted within 48 hours of admission using the modified Glasgow criteria.[47] If choledocholithiasis was found on ERCP, an ES with stone extraction was performed. Outcome measures included mortality, length of stay, local complications, and organ failure. Predicted severe AP was present in 44% of all patients enrolled (25 of 59 in the ERCP group and 28 of 62 in the conservative management group). ERCP was successful in 94% of mild disease and 80% of severe disease. One ERCP-related adverse event occurred, a case of vertebral osteomyelitis. There were no cases of ERCP-related hemorrhage, cholangitis, or perforation.

The overall mortality was not significantly different between the two patient groups (2% in the ERCP group vs 8% in the conservative management group; $p = 0.23$). However, the overall morbidity was significantly lower in the group that underwent ERCP within 72 hours of admission (17% vs 34%; $p = 0.03$). Subgroup analysis demonstrated that the morbidity difference was limited to the group of patients with predicted SAP in whom the overall complication rate was 24%, in comparison to 61% in patients with predicted SAP managed conservatively ($p < 0.01$). Accordingly, the length of hospitalization was shorter for the patients with SAP who underwent urgent ERCP (9.5 days vs 17 days; $p < 0.035$). This study demonstrated that not only was it safe to perform ERCP in patients with AGP admitted to an expert center, but also early ERCP was associated with significantly decreased morbidity and reduced hospital stay for patients with predicted severe AGP compared to conservative management.

Even then investigators acknowledged a concern that the benefit of early ERCP ± ES might be a result of treating cholangitis and not pancreatitis. They controlled for this possible confounding factor post hoc, by excluding patients who presented with cholangitis and analyzing the remaining patients separately. The complication rate remained significantly lower in the group of patients without cholangitis who underwent urgent ERCP (11% vs 33%; $p = 0.02$). Again, the majority of this difference occurred in the subgroup of patients with predicted SAP. Another criticism of the study was that patients were included from time of enrollment rather than onset of symptoms, which may have led to some patients not being identified early in the course of pancreatitis.

In 1993, Fan and colleagues published a trial randomizing 195 patients with AP of any etiology to undergo urgent ERCP within 24 hours of hospital admission or conservative management followed by selective ERCP for clinical deterioration.[3] The authors used this approach of selecting all patients with pancreatitis in order to minimize selection bias. Analysis of the subgroup of patients with AGP revealed that 127 of the 195 randomized patients (65%) had biliary stones. Sixty-four of the 97 patients randomized to early ERCP were found to have biliary stones and 38 of these required ES for CBD or ampullary stones. Of the 98 patients in the conservative therapy group, 63 had biliary stones and 27 of these patients required ERCP for clinical deterioration. Ten of these patients were found to have CBD or ampullary stones. Cholangitis remained a significant confounding factor in the study population.

The severity of pancreatitis was graded by serum urea concentration and plasma glucose concentration and Ranson's score. Patients were categorized as having SAP when admission serum urea concentration was >45 mg/dL or when plasma glucose concentration was >198 mg/dL. Predicted SAP was diagnosed in 41.5% of the patient population, distributed evenly between the treatment groups. The overall morbidity (18% in the urgent ERCP group vs 29% in the conservative management group; $p = 0.07$) and mortality (5% vs 9%; $p = 0.4$) were not significantly different in the two patient groups. When considering only those patients with confirmed biliary stones (66%), the morbidity rate in the urgent ERCP group was significantly lower than that in the conservative management group (16% vs 33%, $p = 0.03$) and there was a trend toward lower mortality (2% vs 8%; $p = 0.09$). These findings were driven by the significant morbidity advantage of urgent ERCP in the subgroup of patients with predicted SAP. In particular, the incidence of biliary sepsis among those patients predicted to have SAP was significantly lower in the urgent ERCP group than in the conservative management group (0% vs 20%; $p = 0.008$). In contrast, among patients with mild pancreatitis, there was no difference in the incidence of biliary sepsis between the two study groups.

In summary, Fan and colleagues demonstrated a morbidity benefit in patients with predicted severe AGP who underwent urgent ERCP ± ES compared with those managed conservatively. Despite the high prevalence of cholelithiasis in the study population, this trial corroborates the findings of an earlier study from the United Kingdom.

In 1997, the German Study Group on Acute Biliary Pancreatitis conducted a prospective multicenter study. In this study, Fölsch et al. randomized 126 patients with AGP to early ERCP within 72 hours of symptom onset and 112 patients with AGP to conservative management.[7] The inclusion criteria in this study were distinct from the previous studies in that patients with obstructive jaundice (total bilirubin >5 mg/dL) were excluded. In doing so, the investigators sought to determine the effect of early ERCP on AGP independent of its known benefit in patients with cholangitis.[48] In these patients with AP, the diagnosis of AGP was made if gallstones were seen on imaging or if twoo of three serum liver chemistry values (ALT, alkaline phosphatase, and/or total bilirubin) were abnormal. The severity of pancreatitis was predicted by the modified Glasgow criteria. Early ERCP was successful in 96% of the treatment group, and 46% of patients in this group were found to have choledocholithiasis. Elective ERCP was required in 20% of the conservative treatment group, and 59% of those patients were found to have bile duct stones.

Predicted SAP was seen in 19.3% of patients overall and similarly distributed between the treatment groups. Adverse events directly attributable to ERCP were minimal, with postsphincterotomy hemorrhage seen in 2.8% and no duodenal wall perforations reported. Overall adverse events were similar in the early ERCP and control groups (46% vs 51%) and mortality rates were also similar (11% vs 6%; $p = 0.10$). Stratification of patients by predicted severity of pancreatitis did not alter these findings. Although systemic complications overall were not significantly different, the patients in the early ERCP group had a higher rate of respiratory insufficiency, as defined by pO_2 <60 mm Hg despite use of an oxygen mask (12% vs 4%; $p = 0.03$).

Several critiques of this study have been put forth in the literature. In this multicenter trial involving 22 institutions, the majority of patients were enrolled by three centers. This brings into question the level of experience and frequency of patients with AGP at a number of the study centers. Also, the excessive rate of respiratory insufficiency in the treatment group was not seen in any of the other trials addressing this subject.

The investigators, apart from highlighting the invasive nature of performing ERCP, concluded that early ERCP in patients with AGP without biliary obstruction or sepsis does not confer a mortality or morbidity benefit and may result in a higher rate of respiratory insufficiency compared with conservative management.

In 2007, Oria et al.[43] published a randomized clinical trial testing the hypothesis that early endoscopic intervention performed on patients with AGP and biliary obstruction reduces systemic and local inflammation. This was a single-center, randomized clinical trial performed in Argentina between 2001 and 2005. Consecutive patients presenting to the emergency room within 48 hours after onset of AGP were enrolled. The diagnosis was made based on presence of abdominal pain, elevated serum amylase to ≥3 times the upper limits of normal, choledocholithiasis on ultrasonography, CT evidence of pancreatitis, and absence of other causes of AP. Included patients had a bile duct diameter of ≥8 mm on ultrasound and a bilirubin of ≥1.2 mg/dL on admission. Patients were excluded if they could not undergo endoscopy or if they had acute cholangitis. Patients who met these criteria were randomized to receive either early endoscopic intervention ($N = 51$) or conservative management ($N = 52$). All patients received antibiotics. Severity of attack was predicted using the APACHE II scale. The primary outcome of the study was to determine whether early endoscopic therapy could reduce organ failure scores during the first week after admission and limit the extension of pancreatic and peripancreatic lesions. Organ Failure Assessment score was also calculated. CT findings were graded using the CT severity index.

The incidence of bile duct stones was similar in the endoscopy group according to predicted mild (72%) or severe pancreatitis (73%). The organ failure scores, CT severity index, overall morbidity and mortality, and local and systemic complications were not significantly different between the early endoscopy group and the conservative management group.

The authors concluded that despite the presence of biliary obstruction, there was no benefit to performing ERCP with or without ES early in the course of the disease.

The belief that early ERCP (within 24 to 72 hours of symptom onset) can reduce the progression of AP to severe pancreatitis has been widely investigated. The outcomes of many clinical trials and meta-analyses have shown conflicting reports. To study the ideal interval time to ERCP and classification of SAP, Acosta et al. performed a randomized trial of early ERCP + ES in a more narrowly defined group of patients.[49] The investigators randomized 61 consecutive patients with AGP and presumed persistent ampullary obstruction to undergo ERCP ± ES between 24 and 48 hours after the onset of symptoms (study group, $n = 30$) or conservative management followed by selective ERCP ± ES if jaundice or cholangitis were present 48 hours after the onset of symptoms (control group, $n = 31$). Persistent ampullary obstruction was defined by a previously validated method.[50] This method used three clinical findings to detect ampullary obstruction: severe and continuous epigastric pain, bile-free gastric aspirate, and elevated serum bilirubin (followed serially every 6 hours). Ranson or Acosta criteria were used to predict severity of pancreatitis, and only 10% of patients had severe disease.

The majority of patients experienced spontaneous relief of biliary obstruction within 48 hours of the onset of symptoms (71% of control group and 53% of study group). Fourteen patients in the study group underwent ERCP within 48 hours of symptom onset; impacted stones were found in 11 (79%) of these patients. There were no deaths in either group and no adverse events attributable to ERCP or ES. The study group had a significantly lower incidence of immediate adverse events (3% vs 26%; $p = 0.026$) and overall adverse events (7% vs 29%; $p = 0.043$). The incidence of severe AGP (10%) was relatively low in this study. The two groups did not differ in length of hospitalization or time to cholecystectomy. Collective analysis of both the study and control groups demonstrated that ampullary obstruction of <48 hours was associated with fewer complications ($p < 0.001$), shorter time interval to cholecystectomy ($p = 0.018$), and shorter hospitalization ($p = 0.003$).

In 2012, Tse et al. analyzed seven randomized clinical trials in an effort to identify the clinical effectiveness of performing early routine ERCP versus conservative management with or without delayed ERCP in AGP.[51] Subgroups of patients who may have benefited from early ERCP were investigated as well. Outcomes in mortality were defined by the Atlanta Classification. Among 644 participants included in 5 RCTs for mortality analysis, statistical heterogeneity was evident among the trials. Trials that included patients with cholangitis showed that early, routine ERCP significantly reduced mortality (relative risk [RR] 0.20, 95% confidence interval [CI] 0.06 to 0.68) and local and systemic complications as defined by the Atlanta Classification (RR 0.45 and 95% CI 0.20 to 0.99, and RR 0.37 and 95% CI 0.18 to 0.78, respectively). Trials that included patients with biliary obstruction showed that early, routine ERCP was associated with a nonsignificant reduction of local and systemic complications as defined by the Atlanta Classification (RR 0.53 and 95% CI 0.26 to 1.07, and RR 0.56 and 95% CI 0.30 to 1.02, respectively).

The authors concluded that early, routine ERCP should not be based on the severity of pancreatitis but rather the presence or absence of cholangitis.

Early ERCP With or Without ES in AGP: Systematic Reviews

Any attempt to create a unified recommendation for the care of patients with AGP based on these trials is hindered by their distinct study methods.

In 1999, Sharma and Howden sought to estimate the overall effect of ERCP for AGP.[44] They performed a pooled analysis of four trials, including Neoptolemos et al. (1988),[8] Fan et al. (1993),[3] and Fölsch et al. (1997),[7] and assessed 460 treated patients and 374 controls. In analyzing complications and mortality, they found that the number of patients with AGP needed to treat (NNT) with ERCP + ES for avoidance of complications was 7.6 and the NNT for avoidance of death was 25.6. Subgroup analysis by severity of AGP was not possible because of

unavailable data. The authors concluded that ERCP + ES reduces mortality and morbidity in patients with AGP. These results must be viewed with caution, as this was a pooled data analysis and the largest contribution to the pool of patients came from a study only available in abstract form.

More recently, a meta-analysis was published by Moretti and colleagues in 2008,[45] which included five trials: Neoptolemos et al. (1988),[8] Fan et al. (1993),[3] Fölsch et al. (1997),[7] and Oria et al. (2007),[43] along with another published by Zhou (2002).[51a] The authors wanted to compare early ERCP-guided therapy with conservative management of AGP. A total of 702 patients were selected; 353 of them were randomized to early ERCP and 349 to conservative management and eventually elective ERCP if required. There was a significant reduction in the complication rate in the early ERCP group (NNT = 12), but no difference in mortality was observed. On subgroup analysis, patients with severe AGP benefited the most, with a reduction in the complication rate of almost 40% (NNT = 3).

The 2004 Cochrane Database systematic review of this subject by Ayub and colleagues included only the studies by Neoptolemos et al., Fan et al., and Fölsch et al. discussed in the preceding paragraphs.[46] The authors sought to assess the value of ERCP ± ES versus conservative therapy in patients with AGP. In particular, this review sought to address the effect of confounding by indication by controlling for associated acute cholangitis and stratifying according to disease severity. To this end, the investigators of the Fölsch trial provided additional data regarding the severity of pancreatitis in each patient group. The authors concluded that ERCP ± ES was associated with a significant reduction in morbidity in patients with predicted severe AGP (odds ratio [OR] = 0.27, 95% CI = 0.14 to 0.53). However, there was no significant difference in morbidity in patients with predicted mild AGP. In addition, no significant difference in mortality was found, regardless of predicted disease severity. Fig. 53.1 demonstrates their findings, comparing ERCP ± ES versus conservative management stratified by severity of AGP.

Early ERCP With or Without ES in AGP: Summary

In light of current data, if pancreatitis is determined to be mild, early endoscopic therapy with ERCP + ES can be avoided unless the patient develops signs of worsening disease or biliary sepsis, depending on the urgency of cholecystectomy and bile duct stone clearance. If, however, the patient has predicted severe AGP, it would be prudent to consider therapeutic ERCP, especially if the patient has evidence of cholangitis. It is also important to remember that there may not be a beneficial effect on overall mortality. Most endoscopists prefer empiric biliary sphincterotomy and duct sweeping with balloon or basket even if a stone is not seen on cholangiography, as stones can be missed, and it prevents pancreatitis if another stone passes during the time the patient is awaiting cholecystectomy. It also can allow patient discharge and elective outpatient cholecystectomy or obviate the need for cholecystectomy in poor surgical candidates.[52] Nonetheless, biliary sphincterotomy alone may not be completely protective of further attacks of gallstone pancreatitis in patients with an intact gallbladder,[53,54] and small-caliber stent placement (7 Fr) may be useful in nonoperative candidates and while awaiting cholecystectomy.

ROLE OF MRCP VERSUS ENDOSCOPIC ULTRASONOGRAPHY

As per published guidelines by the ASGE on the role of endoscopy in the management of suspected choledocholithiasis, a less invasive imaging study, such as EUS, or noninvasive study, such as MRCP, should be performed in patients with AGP. The decision as to which modality to use and the timing has been argued.

Review: Endoscopic retrograde cholangiopancreatography in gallstone-associated acute pancreatitis
Comparison: 01 Early ERCP+/– ES versus Conservative Mx
Outcome: 02 Adverse events stratified by severity of AGP

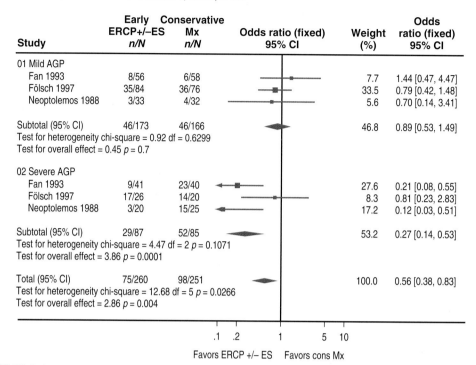

Study	Early ERCP+/–ES n/N	Conservative Mx n/N	Odds ratio (fixed) 95% CI	Weight (%)	Odds ratio (fixed) 95% CI
01 Mild AGP					
Fan 1993	8/56	6/58		7.7	1.44 [0.47, 4.47]
Fölsch 1997	35/84	36/76		33.5	0.79 [0.42, 1.48]
Neoptolemos 1988	3/33	4/32		5.6	0.70 [0.14, 3.41]
Subtotal (95% CI)	46/173	46/166		46.8	0.89 [0.53, 1.49]

Test for heterogeneity chi-square = 0.92 df = 0.6299
Test for overall effect = 0.45 p = 0.7

02 Severe AGP					
Fan 1993	9/41	23/40		27.6	0.21 [0.08, 0.55]
Fölsch 1997	17/26	14/20		8.3	0.81 [0.23, 2.83]
Neoptolemos 1988	3/20	15/25		17.2	0.12 [0.03, 0.51]
Subtotal (95% CI)	29/87	52/85		53.2	0.27 [0.14, 0.53]

Test for heterogeneity chi-square = 4.47 df = 2 p = 0.1071
Test for overall effect = 3.86 p = 0.0001

Total (95% CI)	75/260	98/251		100.0	0.56 [0.38, 0.83]

Test for heterogeneity chi-square = 12.68 df = 5 p = 0.0266
Test for overall effect = 2.86 p = 0.004

.1 .2   1   5 10

Favors ERCP +/– ES   Favors cons Mx

FIG 53.1 Cochrane Database systematic review. (From Ayub K, Imada R, Slavin J. Endoscopic retrograde cholangiopancreatography in gallstone-associated acute pancreatitis. *Cochrane Database Syst Rev.* 2004;(4):CD003630.)

Both MRCP and EUS are sensitive and specific for diagnosing choledocholithiasis. MRCP is a reliable noninvasive test that requires radiologic expertise for interpretation but is accessible in most medical centers. The sensitivity of MRCP for detecting CBD stones decreases according to stone size: 67% to 100% for stones >10 mm, 89% to 94% for stones 6 to 10 mm, and 33% to 71% for bile duct stones <6 mm.[55] EUS has a sensitivity of 95%, specificity of 98%, and accuracy of 96%. EUS has the additional benefit of being superior in detection of stones <5 mm compared with MRCP.[55] Both MRCP and EUS are operator dependent, and the former is also dependent on the image quality of the scanner.

Anderloni et al.[56] conducted a single-center prospective study investigating the clinical usefulness of early EUS (within ≤48 hours of admission) in patients with AGP. Between January 2010 and December 2012, patients presenting with acute abdominal pain with biochemical and/or radiologic findings consistent with possible AGP were evaluated. Patients were classified as having a low, moderate, or high probability of a CBD stone based on the following risk criteria: low risk was defined as a bilirubin level <2 mg/dL and nondilated CBD; high risk was defined as bilirubin level >4 mg/dL or >2 mg/dL with concomitant CBD dilation; moderate-risk was any other combination. In total, 71 patients were included. All were considered as having mild AGP as per the Glasgow criteria. The probability of finding CBD stones was considered low in 21 cases (29%), moderate in 26 (37%), and high in 24 (34%). The authors identified that 20% of patients in the low-probability group indeed had CBD stones on EUS, thus avoiding delay of definitive treatment and potentially further damage to the pancreas. In the high-risk group, 50% of patients did not have CBD stones, thus avoiding an unnecessary ERCP, whereas 20% of patients with a normal gallbladder on ultrasonography were found to have microlithiasis, which is important in the investigation of patients with "idiopathic pancreatitis."

EUS has also been shown to detect stones in patients with gallstone pancreatitis and bile duct stones not imaged by multidetector CT.[57]

Biliary Microlithiasis

Small-diameter biliary stones, measuring <5 mm, are known as microlithiasis, biliary sludge, or biliary sand. These have been implicated as a cause of "idiopathic" and recurrent AP (see Chapter 52) and other biliary complications.[58] In practice, microlithiasis can be diagnosed by transabdominal ultrasonography and is seen as mobile echogenic material that layers with gravity and does not produce shadows.[59] EUS has also been shown to be effective at detecting microlithiasis, particularly in the setting of typical biliary pain and normal abdominal ultrasonography.[60] The gold standard for the detection of biliary microlithiasis is microscopic analysis, which documents cholesterol monohydrate crystals or calcium bilirubinate granules in up to 80% of patients with AP of presumed biliary origin in whom gallstones could not be documented on imaging.[61] Although no prospective RCTs have been performed to establish the role of ERCP in patients with AGP caused by microlithiasis, uncontrolled studies have suggested that these patients benefit from intervention.[62,63]

EMERGING EVIDENCE: PANCREATIC DUCT STENT PLACEMENT

Pancreatic injury in the setting of AGP arises from a number of postulated mechanisms. Pancreatic duct obstruction may occur after stone obstruction or sphincter of Oddi spasm.[64] The ability to minimize the severity of pancreatitis and progression to necrosis is critical. Recent studies evaluated pancreatic drainage procedures during urgent ERCP in AGP.

Dubravcsik et al.[65] prospectively investigated outcomes in patients with AGP who received pancreatic duct stenting and biliary sphincterotomy versus sphincterotomy alone during ERCP (within 72 hours of symptom onset), and 71/141 nonalcoholic patients received a temporary pancreatic stent (5 Fr, 3 to 5 cm long). All stents were removed within 10 days of the index procedure. Although mortality rates were not significantly different between the two groups, adverse event rates between the two were: 10% in the stent group versus 31% in the nonstent group. Guoqian et al.[66] found similar results in a study of patients with AGP and difficult biliary sphincterotomy who were randomized to receive a pancreatic stent. The stents had internal flanges and measured 3 Fr to 5 Fr and 5 to 7 cm long. All stents were removed after 1 to 2 weeks. Patients who received pancreatic stents had an overall lower adverse event rate compared with the nonstent group (7.7% vs 31.9%). Again, there was no difference in overall mortality between the two.

Although there is a good rationale for pancreatic duct stenting in AGP, the patients in these studies also had difficult biliary cannulation and/or sphincterotomy and thus had another reason to receive a pancreatic duct stent. Moreover, for patients with severe necrotizing pancreatitis, there is a concern that pancreatic duct stenting may lead to infection.

Cholecystectomy After AGP

Once a patient stabilizes from an episode of mild AGP, laparoscopic cholecystectomy should be performed before discharge from the hospital.[67] Delay in cholecystectomy is associated with a 20% risk of recurrent biliary complications, including AGP, cholangitis, and cholecystitis, and a near 50% recurrence rate of any biliary symptoms.[68,69]

A recent prospective study of 178 Chinese patients over the age of 60 years demonstrated that those patients randomized to early cholecystectomy after ES and bile duct clearance had a significantly lower rate of biliary events compared with those randomized to conservative management after ES (7% vs 24%; $p = 0.001$). A recent randomized prospective study from California studied the effect on hospital length of stay in patients with mild gallstone pancreatitis who underwent early (within 48 hours irrespective of resolution of abdominal pain or laboratory values) versus delayed cholecystectomy. There was a statistically significant decrease in the length of hospital stay from a mean of 5.8 days in the delayed group to 3.5 days in the early group. There was, however, no difference in the technical difficulty or perioperative adverse event rate between the two groups.[70] In patients who are unable to undergo surgery, ES does confer some degree of protection from subsequent biliary events.[71]

In the case of severe AGP, cholecystectomy should be delayed until the systemic inflammatory response has subsided. In cases with significant pancreatic necrosis or pancreatic fluid collection, cholecystectomy should be delayed for 3 to 6 weeks because of an increased risk of infection and surgical adverse events.[72,73] If necessary and indicated, cholecystectomy can be combined with drainage procedures for pancreatic fluid collection or debridement of pancreatic necrosis.

ALGORITHM FOR THE MANAGEMENT OF ACUTE GALLSTONE PANCREATITIS

The studies presented here provide a framework within which to manage patients with AGP (Fig. 53.2). We advocate ERCP ± ES, when available, in patients with severe AGP, defined by Ranson's criteria, APACHE II,

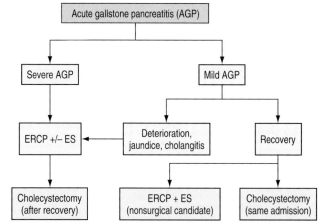

FIG 53.2 Algorithm for the management of acute gallstone pancreatitis.

or the modified CT severity index, as soon as that diagnosis is made. Additional indications for ERCP include concurrent cholangitis or jaundice from biliary obstruction, persistent ampullary obstruction, and clinical deterioration in a patient who initially presented with mild disease. Once selection criteria are met for ERCP, ES should be performed in those patients with confirmed choledocholithiasis or ampullary edema causing obstruction. In patients who cannot undergo cholecystectomy because of medical comorbidities, ES is protective against further bouts of AGP but may not protect against other biliary complications. The fear that ERCP with or without ES can exacerbate existing AP is not warranted based on either the literature or our clinical experience.

MISCELLANEOUS ISSUES

It is important to understand that ERCP in the setting of AP can be technically difficult depending on the severity of pancreatitis. In the setting of clinically severe pancreatitis, edema in the duodenum and periampullary area can make endoscopic identification of the papilla difficult, if not impossible. Additionally, the edema can narrow the duodenum, which decreases the amount of working space and often distorts the anatomy.

Several days to a week after the onset of AP, edema in the pancreatic head can result in bile duct compression and jaundice because of biliary obstruction. In the presence of an ongoing systemic inflammatory process from pancreatitis and rising bilirubin, it can be clinically difficult to distinguish if this represents cholangitis from an obstructing stone. In this scenario, ERCP with cannulation is often performed and can be technically difficult, but when achieved, a smooth distal biliary stricture may be identified. Biliary stent placement is mandatory to prevent post-ERCP cholangitis from instrumentation of an otherwise sterile biliary tree if left undrained. Placement of a 7-Fr stent can be performed without sphincterotomy and may be preferable when the landmarks to allow safe sphincterotomy are distorted by edema; this also prevents additional bouts of pancreatitis caused by stone passage. The stent is subsequently removed after the pancreatitis has resolved and cholecystectomy has been performed.

The complete reference list for this chapter can be found online at www.expertconsult.com.

54

Pancreatic Interventions in Acute Pancreatitis: Ascites, Fistulae, Leaks, and Other Disruptions

Michael Larsen and Richard A. Kozarek

BACKGROUND

Over time, the role of endoscopic retrograde cholangiopancreatography (ERCP) in the setting of acute pancreatitis has evolved.[1] Previously, ERCP was commonly used after resolution of an acute attack, or more commonly multiple attacks, in an attempt to define pancreatic ductal anatomy and determine an etiology for unexplained pancreatitis. Congenital variants, including duodenal duplication, anomalous pancreaticobiliary union, annular pancreas, and pancreas divisum, can be diagnosed, as can other anatomic causes of pancreatitis, such as ampullary adenoma or surreptitious stone disease. For the most part, less invasive approaches to imaging the pancreatic duct (PD), such as endoscopic ultrasonography (EUS), magnetic resonance imaging (MRI), and magnetic resonance cholangiopancreatography (MRCP), have supplanted the need for ERCP (see Chapter 34), a procedure that can actually cause the disease for which it is being applied (see Chapter 52).[2]

As advanced imaging has nearly eliminated the need for diagnostic ERCP, the role of ERCP has become primarily therapeutic. The main role of ERCP in the acute setting is in the treatment of acute biliary pancreatitis.[3,4] This subject is covered in detail in Chapter 53. However, selective use of ERCP in patients with presumed biliary pancreatitis who have high suspicion for choledocholithiasis or biliary sepsis is common clinical practice.

Another situation where ERCP can provide therapy is in patients with "idiopathic" relapsing acute pancreatitis. Most series suggest that sphincter of Oddi dysfunction is the most common etiology when other diagnostic studies have been exhausted (see Chapter 47). As such, there remains a significant role for ERCP in conjunction with sphincter of Oddi manometry (SOM) (see Chapter 16) in such patients (Box 54.1).

In addition to its application in conjunction with SOM in patients with acute relapsing pancreatitis and its selective application in biliary pancreatitis, ERCP has been used as a means to provide pancreatic endotherapy in the setting of ductal disruptions caused by acute pancreatitis.[5-8] PD leaks can manifest in various ways, including smoldering pancreatitis, pseudocysts, fistulae, pancreatic ascites, and high amylase pleural effusions. The mainstay of treatment for these conditions is the placement of a PD stent to bridge the area of disruption (when possible) during ERCP. Disconnected duct syndrome represents the most severe form of a PD disruption that commonly occurs in the setting of severe acute pancreatitis, but the role of ERCP in this setting is limited. Management of this condition is covered in Chapter 55. This chapter will focus on the role of ERCP in the management of ductal disruptions.

Video for this chapter can be found online at www.expertconsult.com.

Ductal disruptions are seen in a background of chronic and acute pancreatitis.

EPIDEMIOLOGY OF DUCTAL DISRUPTION

The majority of cases of ductal disruption in the setting of acute pancreatitis are likely secondary effects of damage to the ductular epithelium from the underlying inflammation rather than the initial cause of the pancreatitis.[5,9] However, acute sphincter obstruction in the setting of a common bile duct stone may increase intraductal pressure, leading to side branch or acinar leak with resultant pancreatitis. Likewise, any other downstream obstruction may increase upstream duct pressure, leading to PD blowout and perpetuation or exacerbation of pancreatitis.[10,11] In patients with acute pancreatitis this is most commonly caused by severe edema, whereas in chronic pancreatitis, disruptions are usually the consequence of a downstream stricture or stone and resultant upstream ductal hypertension. In the setting of severe pancreatic necrosis, ductal disruption is almost invariable, although whether the ductal disruption is the cause or the consequence of the necrosis remains unclear.[11,12] The presence of a peripancreatic fluid collection does not imply a significant ongoing leak in all instances. Whereas up to 40% of patients with acute pancreatitis develop acute fluid collections, less than 5% of these patients develop a pseudocyst.[13]

CLASSIFICATION

PD leaks are typically defined anatomically by the location of the ductal disruption within the pancreas. The location, in conjunction with the size of the leak and the presence or absence of concomitant necrosis, often determines the clinical manifestations (Fig. 54.1). Low-grade leaks will typically result in intrapancreatic fluid collections that can result in smoldering pancreatitis or remain asymptomatic. Larger leaks are more likely to result in significant pancreatic or peripancreatic necrosis and can cause abdominal fluid collections, high-amylase pleural effusions, pancreatic ascites, and even mediastinal involvement.[9,13,14]

A large leak of the PD tail may cause an acute perisplenic fluid collection with or without a high-amylase left-pleural effusion. Alternatively, pancreatic juice may follow anatomic pathways around the left kidney and even into the pelvis, with resultant scrotal or labial edema. In some situations, fluid collections from pancreatic tail leaks can fistulize to either the small bowel near the ligament of Treitz or to the descending colon.

Ductal disruptions in the head of the pancreas have a variety of different manifestations depending on the body's ability to contain the output. Often this results in organized fluid collections in the right upper quadrant, which may be associated with C-loop edema and gastric outlet obstruction with biliary compression, or even with pancreaticobiliary fistulization. In larger leaks the fluid can track more remotely and result in right perinephric fluid accumulation and dissection into the pelvis or perihilar area.

Central disruptions typically result in fluid collections within the lesser sac and are commonly seen in the setting of severe acute pancreatitis with walled-off pancreatic necrosis (WOPN) and often result in a permanently disconnected duct/gland syndrome.[14] Leaks in this area can also result in dissection into the mediastinum or pericardium, or pancreatic ascites. Patients with pancreatic ascites will experience abdominal pain with abdominal distension and occasionally develop bacterial peritonitis.

In addition to being classified by the location of origin, PD leaks (fistulae) are also typically classified as either internal or external. External leaks represent pancreatocutaneous or pancreaticocutanous fistulae and are most typically a consequence of trauma, surgery, or interventional radiologic drainage procedures.[15–19] Internal fistulae, in turn, classically have included pseudocysts, pancreatic ascites, high-amylase pleural effusions, and erosion of pancreatic fluid collections into contiguous organs, resulting in pancreaticoenteric, gastric, colonic, or biliary fistulae.[20–24] They also include evolving pancreatic necrosis, in which variable amounts of high-amylase fluid collect, usually in the context of central pancreatic necrosis. Anatomic classifications based on the presence of an acute or chronic PD leak are outlined in Box 54.2.

Although this chapter focuses on PD leaks and their endoscopic treatment, Box 54.3 summarizes some of the other pancreatitis-related endoscopically amenable lesions that endoscopists see in a busy ERCP practice. They include bile duct obstruction from stones, edema within

---

CT, Computed tomography; *ERCP,* endoscopic retrograde cholangiopancreatography; *EUS,* endoscopic ultrasonography; *MRCP,* magnetic resonance cholangiopancreatography; *MRI,* magnetic resonance imaging.

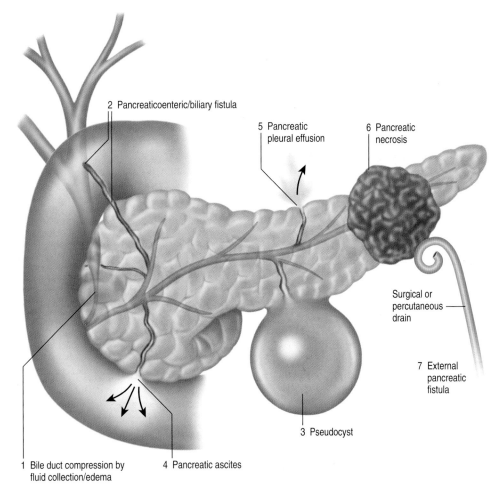

FIG 54.1 Consequences of pancreatic duct leak. *(1)* Bile duct compression by fluid collection/edema. *(2)* Pancreaticoenteric/biliary fistula. *(3)* Pseudocyst. *(4)* Pancreatic ascites. *(5)* Pancreatic pleural effusion. *(6)* Pancreatic necrosis. *(7)* External pancreatic fistula.

the head of the pancreas, and neoplasms that occasionally present with pancreatitis. From a pancreatic standpoint, they include neoplastic obstruction of the papilla or duct, edema or spasm of the sphincter mechanism, and an inflammatory PD stenosis.

MANAGEMENT STRATEGIES (BOX 54.4)

Diagnosis

The diagnosis of external pancreatic fistulae is typically straightforward compared with internal fistulae, as diagnostic imaging is usually not needed. A pancreaticocutaneous fistula should be considered in patients with persistent output of clear pancreatic juice after percutaneous drainage of a pseudocyst or peripancreatic fluid collection (Box 54.5).[1]

Similarly, persistent output from a Jackson-Pratt (JP) drain after pancreatic resection, decompression, or peripancreatic surgery (e.g., splenectomy, left nephrectomy, right hemicolectomy, or gastrectomy) is another manifestation of an external PD leak.[25] More troublesome, however, may be the patient who sustains a penetrating abdominal injury, such as a knife or gunshot wound, in whom the external fistula is overlooked because of concern for other injuries. Pancreatic injury should be considered in all cases of severe abdominal trauma.

The diagnosis of internal fistulae is outlined in Box 54.5. In essence, noninvasive imaging, particularly pancreas protocol computed tomography (CT), remains the best initial diagnostic test in patients with smoldering or severe pancreatitis or in patients with underlying chronic pancreatitis and an acute exacerbation of symptoms.[14] Not only will CT define the consequences of pancreatitis (fluid collections, necrosis, effusions, ascites),[26] but it can also be used to define the potential etiology (e.g., stones or strictures) and follow the subsequent evolution of pancreatitis. CT remains an imperfect tool, however, in that biliary stone disease is underestimated, the fluid component associated with evolving pancreatic necrosis is overestimated, and leaks are implied rather than defined.[27] Further confirmation of a ductal disruption may require sequential scans demonstrating an enlarging fluid collection, aspiration of that fluid collection with measurement of amylase or lipase, an ERCP demonstrating the presence and location of the leak, or secretin-enhanced MRCP (S-MRCP). The latter study has been shown to be predictive of ongoing ductal disruption and clearly minimizes potential ERCP adverse events, such as exacerbation of pancreatitis and iatrogenic infection of an undrained fluid collection.[28–30] It may also demonstrate patients with a complete ductal disruption and a disconnected gland syndrome in whom leak closure by ERCP alone is unlikely to be successful. Finally, use of S-MRCP before ERCP may help to define subsequent endoscopic management comparable to its use in hilar neoplasms of the liver. ERCP, in turn, is usually definitive in showing not only the site of the ductal disruption (if persistent) but also the proximate cause or reason for persistence (PD stones, inflammatory or fibrotic structure).[14,31] For the most part, however, diagnostic pancreatography adds an unnecessary risk to the care of acutely or chronically ill patients with presumptive leak, unless endoscopic, percutaneous, or surgical therapy is contemplated.[32]

MANAGEMENT (BOX 54.6)

Indications for Endoscopic Treatment

The presence of a presumptive pancreatic fistula alone is not a reason to undertake endotherapy. Important considerations include whether the patient has acute or underlying chronic pancreatitis, whether pancreatic necrosis is present, whether there is superinfection of a fluid collection, whether the presumptive leak is accessible to endoscopic control, and whether the leak is controlled at the time of presentation. For instance, the vast majority of low-volume leaks after pancreatic resection are controlled by a surgically placed JP drain and spontaneously close with or without concomitant octreotide over days or several weeks.[33,34] On the other hand, a patient may have rapidly increasing ascites or pleural effusion or concomitant jaundice or cholestasis that demands urgent attention.

In general, the following are relative indications for initiation of endoscopic therapy in a patient with a presumed PD leak:

1. An enlarging pancreatic fluid collection (pseudocyst, pancreatic ascites, high-amylase pleural effusion) despite conservative management
2. A symptomatic fluid collection
3. Persistence of an external fistula
4. Inability to refeed the patient without development of recurring pain or pancreatitis[14]

A fifth indication may be the question of concomitant biliary tract disease. Although the latter may occasionally be a concern for a retained stone in the setting of biliary pancreatitis, it is more commonly seen in patients with jaundice or cholangitis from pancreatic head edema or pseudocyst.

Perhaps as important as indications for study are contraindications. Aside from medical instability precluding endoscopy, possibly the most important contraindication to an attempt at endoscopic therapy for a PD leak is the inability to render therapy if a ductal disruption is demonstrated. In this setting the diagnosis of a leak may result in iatrogenic infection of a concomitant fluid collection or necrosis, which ultimately may result in the need for endoscopic, percutaneous, or even surgical drainage. Given the potential for "therapeutic misadventure" and the complexity of patients with pancreatic fistulae, careful planning with the use of high-quality cross-sectional imaging and a multidisciplinary approach to management are essential.

Pancreatic Fluid Collections

The endoscopic and nonendoscopic management of pancreatic pseudocysts[35–39] and evolving pancreatic necrosis[40–45] is covered in Chapter 56. Treatment invariably requires treatment of the underlying ductal disruption, if anatomically feasible, as well as the consequences of that disruption. Thus surgical decompression, percutaneous decompression, and endoscopic decompression of fluid collections have all been variously described.

Pancreatic Ascites and High-Amylase Pleural Effusions

Historically, pancreatic ascites and pleural effusions were treated with gut rest and total parenteral nutrition to minimize pancreatic juice stimulation. Diuretics, large-volume thoracentesis and paracentesis, and octreotide have all been used for weeks or months in an attempt to preclude the need for surgical resection or bypass. Successful in less than 50% of these patients, "salvage-type" surgery, usually defined by ERCP preoperatively, consisted of partial pancreatectomy or Roux-en-Y cystojejunostomy in the subset of patients with concomitant pancreatic pseudocysts. Surgical attempts were associated with high morbidity, periprocedural mortality of 8% to 15%, and recurrence rates of 15% to 20%.[14]

Our group was the first to describe transpapillary stent placement beyond the site of ductal disruption, in conjunction with large-volume paracentesis, as a successful treatment for patients with pancreatic ascites (Fig. 54.2).[46] Since our initial publication a number of series have confirmed our findings.[47–52] The available literature to date suggests that endoscopic transpapillary stent placement across the site of ductal disruption is successful in resolving pancreatic ascites and pleural effusions in more than 90% of patients and is associated with minimal procedure-related morbidity and close to zero mortality.

One of the largest series was published by Telford et al. of 43 patients with PD disruption and a variety of clinical manifestations.[53] The etiology was acute pancreatitis in 24 patients, chronic pancreatitis in 9, operative injury in 7, and trauma in 3. Stent placement was successful in resolution of the disruption in 25 patients, unsuccessful in 16 patients, and indeterminate in 2 patients. On univariate analyses, bridging of the ductal disruption and duration of stenting were associated with a statistically significant successful outcome, whereas female gender and acute pancreatitis were negative predictive factors of success. With multivariate analysis, only bridging of the disruption remained statistically significant as a predictor of success (Figs. 54.3, 54.4, and 54.5). Other studies have confirmed the importance of bridging the site of the leak for successful treatment of pancreatic fistulae.[54] A similar retrospective series was recently published with data from two tertiary referral centers' experience with pancreatic leaks of various presentations and etiologies. In this series PD stent placement was successful in 103/107 (96%) of patients, and resolution of the leak was successful in 80 (75%).[55]

The effectiveness of transpapillary stenting is likely due to a change in the ductal drainage gradient and making the duodenum the path of least resistance to flow. Potential areas of downstream obstruction that are bypassed include the sphincter, possible stones, and the inflammatory or fibrotic stricture frequently associated with a leak (Fig. 54.6). This approach does not work in the setting of a disconnected gland syndrome, in which the bulk of the pancreatic juice that enters the thoracic or abdominal cavity comes from a disconnected PD tail that cannot be reached transpapillarily.[14,52]

Pancreaticoenteric Fistulae and Acute Pancreatic Trauma

Until now, our group has treated more than 30 patients with pancreaticoenteric or biliary fistulae. Although these patients may present with

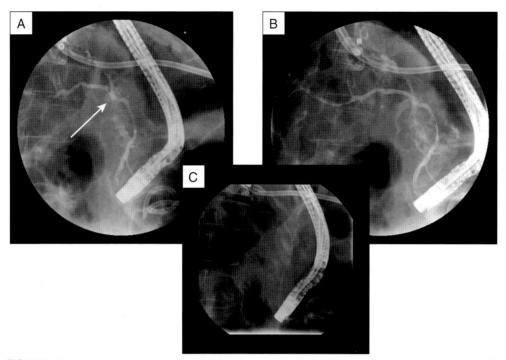

FIG 54.2 **A,** A pancreatogram of a patient with high-amylase ascites demonstrating a ductal disruption in the midbody *(arrow).* A wire guide is placed across the disruption **(B),** followed by a bridging pancreatic endoprosthesis **(C).**

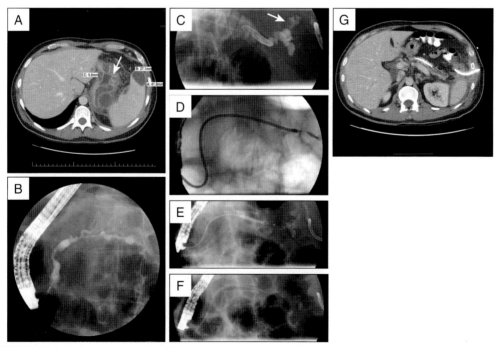

FIG 54.3 Computed tomography (CT) demonstrates perisplenic fluid collection **(A)** and markedly thickened gastric wall *(arrow)* in a patient with hereditary pancreatitis. Endoscopic retrograde cholangiopancreatography (ERCP) demonstrates severe chronic pancreatitis **(B)** with dilated tail and ductal disruption **(C)** requiring percutaneous drainage. The stricture is "dilated" with a Soehendra stent extractor **(D),** followed by balloon dilation **(E)** and 7-Fr stent placement beyond the ductal disruption **(F).** Note the improvement on CT scan and persistent dilation of the pancreatic duct tail **(G).**

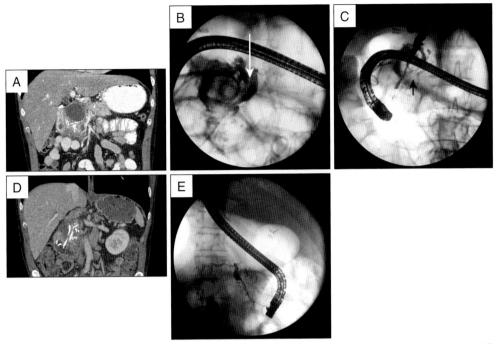

FIG 54.4 **A,** A large internal fistula (pseudocyst) in the head of the pancreas in a patient with chronic calcific pancreatitis. **B,** A pancreatogram demonstrates a ductal disruption *(arrow)* secondary to a high-grade pancreatic duct stricture. **C,** A pancreatic endoprosthesis is placed across the stenosis and leak *(arrowhead)*. **D,** A computed tomography scan 6 weeks later demonstrates complete resolution of the pseudocyst after endoscopically placed transduodenal double-pigtail stents. **E,** A pancreatogram reveals changes of chronic pancreatitis but the leak has resolved.

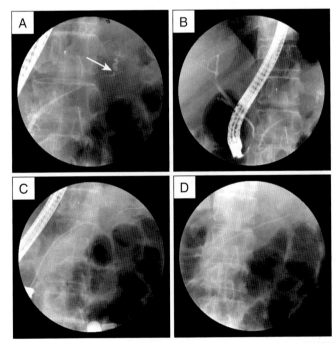

FIG 54.5 Endoscopic retrograde cholangiopancreatography (ERCP) demonstrates pancreatic duct disruption at junction of body and tail **(A** and **B)** in a patient with severe left-upper-quadrant/flank pain and splenic vein thrombosis. Pain and ductal disruption are resolved with prosthesis placement **(C** and **D)**. Disruption recurred 1 year later, requiring distal pancreatectomy/splenectomy.

spontaneous and rapid resolution of a fluid collection for which no treatment is required, a stenosis at the site of ductal disruption may result in relapsing attacks of pancreatitis. Alternatively, fistulization into the bile duct (Fig. 54.7) or colon may result in cholestasis or cholangitis, or recurrent sepsis, respectively.[56] In our initial series of eight patients with pancreaticoenteric fistulae, three resolved with downsizing or removing an external drain that had eroded into a contiguous loop of bowel, three resolved with transpapillary stent placement, and two ultimately required surgical resection.[57] In the case of pancreaticocolonic fistulae, diverting ileostomy may be necessary to close the fistulae and reduce bacterial translocation and ongoing sepsis.[58] Fistulization into the bile duct, in turn, is almost invariably treated successfully by concomitant biliary and PD stenting, assuming that the fistula is not from the upstream disconnected portion of the pancreas (Figs. 54.8 and 54.9).[59]

In addition to pancreaticoenteric or biliary fistulae that usually occur in the setting of pancreatic necrosis or chronic pancreatitis, ERCP has also been used to treat internal fistulae as a consequence of acute pancreatic trauma. For example, Kim et al. diagnosed normal pancreatograms in 14 of 23 patients with acute abdominal trauma.[19] In eight of these patients a leak from the main PD into the parenchyma resolved spontaneously, whereas three had a main PD leak that resolved after bridging with a transpapillary stent. Although the authors of this study suggested that early ERCP was believed to be advantageous in projecting the need for medical, surgical, or endoscopic therapy, it is possible that S-MRCP may evolve to play a diagnostic role, selecting patients who have the greatest potential to benefit from transpapillary therapy.[18]

External Fistulae

As previously discussed, with the exception of penetrating abdominal trauma, the vast majority of external fistulae are iatrogenic. They may occasionally follow partial pancreatic resection or bypass in the setting

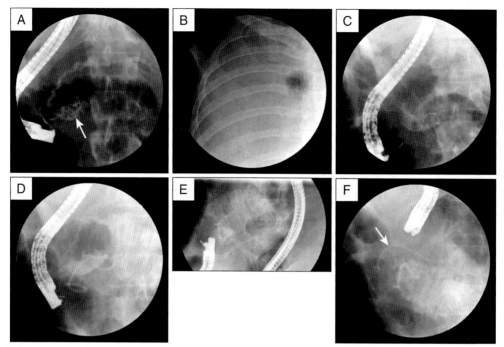

FIG 54.6 Endoscopic retrograde cholangiopancreatography (ERCP) demonstrates ductal disruption in the pancreatic head **(A)** in a patient with huge high-amylase effusion of the right lung **(B)**. The patient is treated with a transpapillary pigtail stent into the fluid collection **(C)** as well as stenting of the minor papilla to decompress the upstream pancreatic duct **(D–F)**.

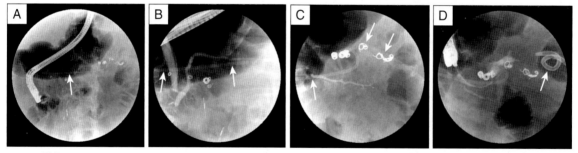

FIG 54.7 Endoscopic retrograde cholangiopancreatography (ERCP) demonstrates transgastric pigtail stent (*arrows*, **A** and **B**) in a patient with severe necrotizing pancreatitis, portal vein thrombosis, and disconnected pancreatic duct. Note the embolized coils for previous splenic artery aneurysm (*arrows,* **C**) and the Jackson-Pratt (JP) drain for persistent colonic fistula into the pancreatic head **(D)**.

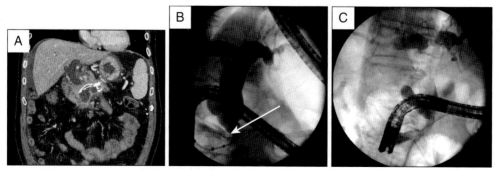

FIG 54.8 A, Computed tomography scan demonstrating a dilated bile duct and transduodenal pigtail stents into a peripancreatic fluid collection. **B,** Cholangiogram demonstrating a communication *(arrow)* between the bile duct and the pancreatic fluid collection. **C,** A fully covered metal bile duct stent is placed to seal the fistula.

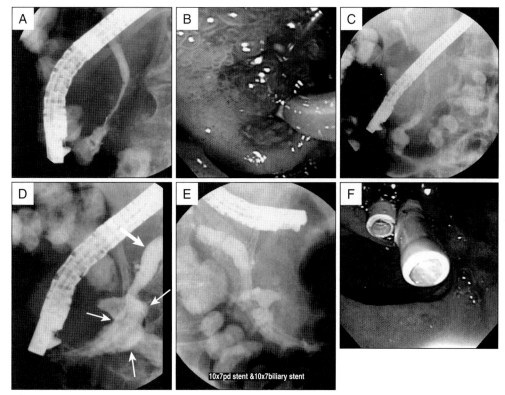

FIG 54.9 High-grade bile duct stricture in a patient with pancreatic necrosis and intramural pancreatic ductal disruption. Note contrast in colon **(A)**, deformed edematous papilla **(B)**, and biliary stent placement **(C)**. *Small arrows* demonstrate intraduodenal abscess and the *large arrow* demonstrates dilated pancreatic duct **(D)**. Note the dual-stent placement **(E and F)**, which resolved jaundice and concomitant PD disruption and obstruction.

of a downstream stricture. Most, however, are a consequence of a disconnected gland after percutaneous or surgical drainage of a pancreatic fluid collection or necrosis.[14] Our group initially reported a series of patients undergoing transpapillary stenting for amenable external fistulae more than a decade ago.[60] Since that time, multiple additional series have been published or abstracted.[14,61,62] By way of summarizing the available series, 86% of patients (50 of 58) could be successfully stented and 46 of those patients (92%) had resolution of their fistulae. Procedural adverse events were limited to mild flares of pancreatitis, although there were two deaths in the series by Costamagna et al.,[61] neither related to the fistula or its endoscopic treatment. No recurrences were reported in patients undergoing successful fistula closure at follow-up ranging from 12 to 36 months.

Our approach to endotherapy of pancreaticocutaneous fistulae has evolved over the past decade. Whereas endoscopic therapy was initially reserved for postoperative or percutaneously drained patients whose external fistulae did not respond to several weeks of clear liquids, total parenteral nutrition, and octreotide, our current practice is to study patients with high-volume fistulae with S-MRCP if they have a marginal decrease in fistula volume after several days of somatostatin analog. ERCP and transpapillary stent placement are undertaken unless imaging documents a disconnected gland syndrome (Fig. 54.10; see also Fig. 54.7).

Disconnected Pancreatic Duct Syndrome

Our experience has taught us that prevention of disconnected PD syndrome (DPDS) is paramount, because treatment is complex. It is clear that a significant number of patients who have WOPN treated

with percutaneous drainage alone will develop pancreaticocutaneous fistulae secondary to disconnected duct syndrome. Our group has devised a treatment for WOPN, which is termed "dual-modality drainage," in order to prevent such fistulae from developing. This technique involves the placement of both a percutaneous drain and endoscopic transluminal stents into areas of WOPN, with subsequent removal of the percutaneous drain once the necrosis resolves.[63] If it is determined that there is no DPDS, the transluminal drains are also removed. However, if the patient has DPDS, the transmural stents are left in place indefinitely to prevent recurrent fluid collections. This combined approach has reduced our cutaneous fistula rate to zero when treating WOPN.[64,65]

Historically, patients with disconnected gland syndrome and pancreaticocutaneous fistulae have required distal pancreatectomy.[14] More recently, less invasive approaches have been described, with varying levels of success.[66]

Interventional radiologist–administered cyanoacrylate injection into the disconnected tail has been described. This requires guidewire placement into the PD tail through the fistulous tract, placement of a microcatheter over the wire, and injection of the entire disconnected portion of the duct to include side branches. Mild postprocedural pancreatitis has been noted in approximately 50% of patients, and recurrent fistulae may occur unless the entire duct and its side branches are sealed. This procedure works best when there is only 3 to 4 cm of disconnected gland and is less likely to be successful when the glandular disconnection is at the genu, which requires a significant portion of the gland to be glued shut.

In addition to the percutaneous approach to the disconnected gland, as well as the surgical approach using glue injection to minimize

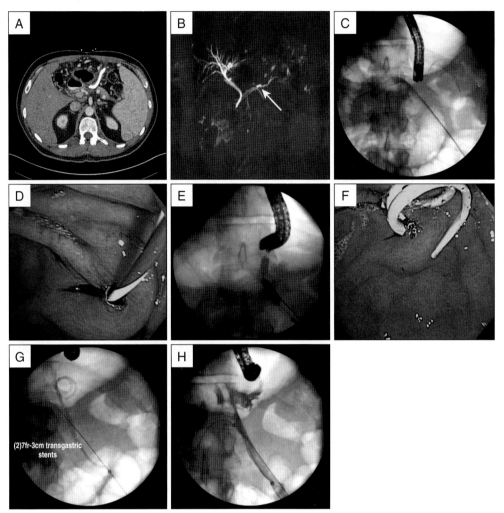

FIG 54.10 A, Computed tomography scan demonstrating a percutaneous drain adjacent to the body of the pancreas in a patient with a history of severe acute pancreatitis and central gland necrosis. The drain had a high output of amylase-rich fluid on a daily basis. **B,** Magnetic resonance cholangiopancreatography demonstrates a dilated pancreatic duct in the tail *(arrow)* with no communication with the head of the gland, suggesting disconnected pancreatic duct syndrome. **C,** The fistula tract is accessed percutaneously using a TIPS needle, which is directed across the gastric wall. **D,** Wire guides are placed through the needle and grasped using an endoscopic snare. **E,** Dilation across the gastric wall is performed using a controlled radial expansion balloon dilator followed by the placement of two double-pigtail stents **(F** and **G).** Injection of contrast through the fistula tract opacifies the stomach, thus demonstrating an alternate route for the flow of pancreatic juice from the fistula tract **(H).** *TIPS,* transjugular intrahepatic portosystemic shunt.

postpancreatectomy leak,[67] Soehendra's group has used transpapillary injection of methyl-butyl cyanoacrylate into the distal duct at the site of glandular disruption.[68] Eight of 11 patients in their series had resolved disruptions without recurrence, although all had concomitant PD stents or drains and endoscopic transmural drainage of associated fluid collections. This group also used glue injection as an adjunct in patients with severe pancreatic necrosis undergoing aggressive endoscopic drainage using EUS-directed lavage or debridement.[69]

Our group has also devised a combined endoscopic and percutaneous rendezvous approach to internalization of chronic pancreaticocutaneous fistulae in patients with disconnected gland syndrome (see Fig. 54.8). This technique involves an interventional radiologist initially accessing the fistula tract using a transjugular intrahepatic portosystemic shunt (TIPS) needle. The needle is then passed under fluoroscopic and endoscopic control into the stomach. The tract is then dilated using an 8-Fr microcatheter, and two guidewires are passed through the catheter, grasped using an endoscopic

snare, and pulled through the endoscope. Further dilation of the tract is then performed using a controlled radial expansion balloon dilator, subsequent to which two double-pigtail stents are placed across the gastric wall into the fistula tract. The resultant "redirection" of pancreatic juice into the stomach has been used to close fistulae in 15 patients treated at our institution. During long-term follow-up, recurrent pancreatic fluid collections developed in two patients because of migrated stents and were treated with endoscopic cystgastrostomy.[70]

Despite the success with glue injection and the combined approach described above, these are small case series performed at centers with significant experience in managing patients with complicated pancreatitis. The widespread application of these nonsurgical techniques requires additional critical assessment before widespread adoption can be advocated. However, they do provide "proof-of-principle" that viable alternatives to long-term drain placement and surgery are very much on the horizon.

ADVERSE EVENTS (BOX 54.7) (SEE CHAPTER 8)

Immediate Adverse Events

The immediate adverse events of transpapillary stent placement are those of diagnostic ERCP and include drug reaction, aspiration, cardiopulmonary events, pancreatitis from contrast injection or sphincter manipulation, and cholangitis in patients with underlying endoscopically untreated concomitant biliary stenosis. Bleeding and iatrogenic perforation can occasionally be seen if sphincterotomy is performed to facilitate stent placement.[71] Pancreatitis flare approximates 10% in normal ducts and is uncommon in patients who have ductal changes of chronic pancreatitis. It may approach 50% in the setting of unsuccessful stenting when multiple accessories and guidewires have been placed into the PD to facilitate bridging the area of the leak. This pancreatitis is usually attenuated, however, if a short transpapillary stent is left to preclude ductal obstruction by an edematous papilla or traumatized sphincter.[72] Pancreatitis is more common in the setting of an improperly sized prosthesis for the duct, even if the disruption can be bridged. Examples include placement of a 7-Fr stent into a 5-Fr-diameter duct or placement of a 12-cm prosthesis to bridge a ductal leak 3 cm from the papilla.

Subacute Adverse Events

Subacute adverse events are usually infectious and result from iatrogenic introduction of bacteria into a fluid collection or necrotic debris at the time of ERCP. As such, all patients with a presumptive internal fistula should receive a broad-spectrum antibiotic before undergoing diagnostic ERCP and may require more prolonged treatment afterward, particularly in the setting of pancreatic necrosis. Moreover, clearly contaminated fluid collections should be considered for concomitant endoscopic or percutaneous drainage of necrosis, as described in Chapter 53. Note that our group has previously demonstrated that bacterial contamination within the PD is invariable in patients with indwelling stents and that stent occlusion is a necessary but not sufficient cause of pancreatic sepsis.[73] Stent occlusion may also be associated with obstructive pancreatitis, and it is for this reason, as well as fear of iatrogenic duct injury,[74] that indwelling stents should be retrieved quickly after external fistula closure and after 4 to 6 weeks of treating an internal PD fistula.[14]

Chronic Adverse Events

Although iatrogenic ductal injury is listed under chronic adverse events, PD prostheses (other than short-term prophylactic for prevention of post-ERCP pancreatitis) never belong in the pancreas, particularly in patients with otherwise normal PDs. A number of procedural and stent modifications have decreased trauma to the major PD and minimized side-branch occlusion over the past several years. These modifications include use of 3-Fr-diameter to 4-Fr-diameter stents, elimination of internal stent flanges, and recognition that stents that apply significant pressure proximally (toward the tail), especially when in an angulated position, may cause duct ulceration and subsequent fibrosis.[74,75] Despite this, 3-Fr unflanged pigtail stents almost always spontaneously migrate within a week or two and are probably appropriate only in the patient in whom bridging of the disruption was unsuccessful, and then only to prevent or ameliorate post-ERCP pancreatitis. Iatrogenic ductitis should be anticipated and minimized by selecting a prosthesis that has a smaller diameter than the PD downstream from the leak, is the appropriate length to bridge the disruption without an inordinate stent length beyond the site of the leak, and avoids upstream impaction or angulation on the ductal wall.

SUMMARY

1. Pancreatic duct leaks are a consequence of acute inflammation with duct disruption, downstream obstruction, or both.
2. Minor leaks in the setting of acute pancreatitis or necrosis are probably common and respond to conservative therapy.
3. The consequences of major ductal disruptions include internal fistulae (pseudocysts, necrosis, pancreatic ascites, pancreatic pleural effusions, pancreaticoenteric or biliary communication) and external fistulae.
4. Treatment of internal fistulae requires treatment of the leak and/or the sequelae/consequences of the leak.

5. Bridging the site of ductal disruption with a transpapillary prosthesis is more likely to result in resolution of the disruption unless there is disconnected gland syndrome.
6. The complexity of most pancreatic leaks requires management by a multidisciplinary team with expertise in pancreatic diseases. This is particularly true in the setting of DPDS.

The complete reference list for this chapter can be found online at www.expertconsult.com.

55

Chronic Pancreatitis: Stones and Strictures

Jacques Devière, Todd H. Baron, and Richard A. Kozarek

Chronic pancreatitis (CP) is a rare disease in Western countries (incidence 2 to 10/100,000 per year). It ultimately leads to irreversible damage of the pancreas, with exocrine and endocrine insufficiency. In the majority of cases pain is the major clinical symptom and present early in the course of the disease.[1,2] With the exception of tropical and hereditary CP, the etiology of CP has not yet been clearly elucidated. Chronic alcoholism is a precipitating factor and dramatically increases the probability of CP development; however, the disease can also develop in nonalcoholic patients without an obvious genetic background and is then referred to as "idiopathic" CP (see Chapter 52). Cigarette smoking plays a major role in the progression of alcoholic pancreatitis.[3]

The pathophysiology of CP is still debated. Adherents of the "stone" theory believe that the initiating event is protein plug formation caused by a congenital lack of lithostatin,[3] but this theory is becoming obsolete. Proponents of the "necrosis-fibrosis" theory, on the other hand, ascribe fibrosis and ductal stricture to focal inflammation and necrosis.[1]

Pain associated with CP is multifactorial and includes increased interstitial and intraductal pressures, closed compartment syndrome, neural infiltration, ongoing acute pancreatitis, and presence of pseudocyst(s) and/or biliary obstruction. Elevated intraductal pressure caused by the presence of stones and/or stricture is one of the primary mechanisms leading to pain in CP.[4–6] Because of lack of compliance of the pancreatic gland already present at the early stages of CP, elevated intraductal pressure is quickly associated with increased parenchymal pressure that impairs blood flow,[6] leading to hypoxia, release of oxygen-derived free radicals, and further stimulation of inflammation with subsequent fibrosis. Surgical decompression of the main pancreatic duct (MPD) has been shown to be associated with pain relief in many patients and is associated with a decrease in intraductal and interstitial pressures, a similar mechanism being considered for endoscopic drainage of the MPD.[7]

Another characteristic of pain in CP is its heterogeneous pattern, from relapsing episodic to persistent pain of varying intensity, which cannot be predicted by pancreatic morphology. The initial episodes of acute recurrent abdominal pain or acute pancreatitis often increase and may evolve into a continuous pain syndrome requiring narcotics. During the natural history of CP, pain may disappear after several years, and this is associated with the development of endocrine and/or exocrine insufficiency.[8] This heterogeneous pain pattern is very often associated with the difficulties faced when interpreting results of clinical studies reporting the effectiveness of surgical or endoscopic drainage for pain relief in CP. In addition, ongoing smoking has a dose-dependent effect on pain relief, even after surgical treatment of CP.[9]

Video for this chapter can be found online at www.expertconsult.com.

ENDOSCOPIC TREATMENT: DUCTAL DECOMPRESSION BY MANAGING STONES AND STRICTURES

The goal of endotherapy (ET) in severe CP is to decompress the MPD by removing stones and bypassing strictures. Another goal when undertaking MPD drainage is to reduce or delay the development of steatorrhea by increasing the flow of pancreatic juice to the duodenum. Significant pancreatic function improvement related to ET has not been demonstrated, although ET seems to postpone the occurrence of de novo steatorrhea for up to 10 years.[10,11]

Endoscopic relief of MPD obstruction can be achieved in several ways, including endoscopic pancreatic sphincterotomy, stone removal with and without the aid of extracorporeal shock wave lithotripsy (ESWL), stricture dilation, insertion of pancreatic stents, transmural drainage of collections communicating with the MPD (see Chapter 56), and even direct transmural drainage of the MPD.

Planning of Endoscopic Therapy

In addition to standard laboratory testing and plain abdominal radiographs of the pancreatic area or abdominal computed tomography (CT) scan without contrast injection for detection of pancreatic calcifications, magnetic resonance imaging (MRI) is currently the best modality for selection of patients who may benefit from endoscopic treatment and for planning endoscopic therapy (Fig. 55.1).

Secretin-stimulated magnetic resonance cholangiopancreatography (S-MRCP) provides information about pancreatic ductal anatomy, presence of peripancreatic fluid collection, and presence of biliary obstruction. Moreover, S-MRCP can be used to quantify pancreatic exocrine function and evaluate the short-term and long-term effects of pancreatic ductal drainage procedures[12,13] (Fig. 55.2).

MPD Cannulation and Endoscopic Pancreatic Sphincterotomy

MPD cannulation and endoscopic pancreatic sphincterotomy are the first steps of pancreatic ET (see Chapters 14 and 20) and provide improved access to the MPD. Minor papilla sphincterotomy (see Chapter 21) may be needed in up to 20% of patients in the setting of dominant dorsal duct anatomy (complete or incomplete pancreas divisum, ansa pancreatica). In a small subset of patients, endoscopic pancreatic sphincterotomy itself may resolve papillary stenosis and allow the removal of small floating MPD stones. Indeed, in some patients with MPD obstruction in the head and absence of divisum, the minor papilla can be used to bypass the obstruction and provide pain relief with sphincterotomy and stent placement.[14]

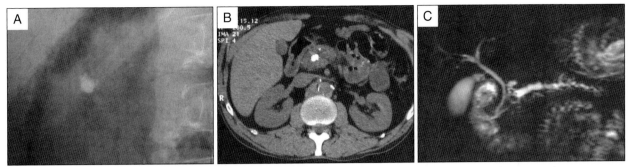

FIG 55.1 Example of planning endoscopic therapy in a patient with chronic pancreatitis and severe pain. The plain film **(A)** shows a dense calcification, which is even more clearly visible on an unenhanced computed tomography scan **(B)**, whereas the dynamic magnetic resonance cholangiopancreatography after secretin injection shows an impacted stone at the level of the genu of the pancreas, with upstream dilation, and the main pancreatic duct in the head has a normal size **(C)**. In this patient, extracorporeal shock wave lithotripsy was performed before endoscopic intervention.

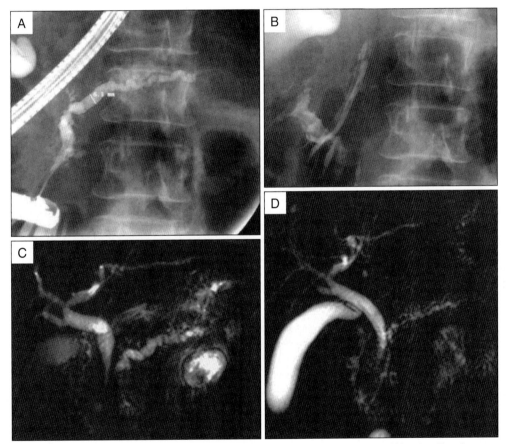

FIG 55.2 Patient with a residual prepapillary stricture after stone fragments extraction **(A)**, treated by placement of two 8.5-Fr stents side-by-side **(B)**. A comparison of secretin-stimulated magnetic resonance cholangiopancreatography performed before **(C)** and after **(D)** drainage shows a decrease in main pancreatic duct diameter and the earlier duodenal filling by pancreatic secretions.

In Western countries, calcifications in the head of the pancreas seen on routine radiographic images often imply that MPD stones are deeply impacted in the ductal wall and will be difficult to remove. In this case, ESWL should be performed before consideration of endoscopic intervention and, as will be discussed later, may be the only intervention required in selected patients.[15]

Biliary sphincterotomy is performed before endoscopic pancreatic sphincterotomy in the setting of cholangitis, obstructive jaundice, or associated cholestasis, or when it is technically necessary to facilitate access to the MPD. If a biliary sphincterotomy is performed, the MPD orifice is located between the 3 and 6 o'clock positions on the right margin of the sphincterotomy. After pancreatic opacification, a hydrophilic guide wire (Terumo Inc. [Tokyo, Japan]; Glidewire [Olympus Corp., Center Valley, PA]) can be maneuvered through the stricture or alongside the stones, using a torque device under radiologic guidance (Fig. 55.3). Pancreatic sphincterotomy is then performed over the

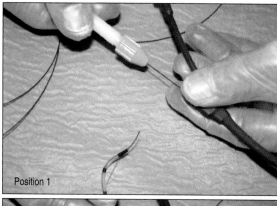

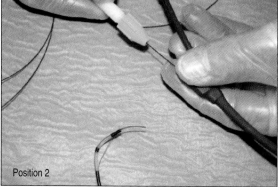

FIG 55.3 The use of a minitome (Cook Endoscopy, Winston-Salem, NC) with a 0.018 J-tip Terumo guidewire manipulated by the assistant with a torque device offers the best performance for cannulating difficult and tortuous strictures under fluoroscopic guidance.

guidewire after deep cannulation with a standard or tapered pull-type sphincterotome. We prefer to use pure cutting current, extending the incision to the duodenal wall. The same technique can be used for minor papilla sphincterotomy. Alternatively, a stent can be inserted into the MPD and sphincterotomy performed using a needle knife over the stent.

Extracorporeal Shock Wave Lithotripsy

In tertiary referral centers that specialize in endoscopic management of severe pancreatitis, ESWL is often performed before endoscopic therapy is undertaken.[16] Its role was clarified in recent European Society for Gastrointestinal Endoscopy guidelines[15]: "ESWL consistently provides stone fragmentation in 90% of patients (Evidence level 1+); it facilitates endoscopic extraction of MPD stones (Evidence level 2+). Spontaneous elimination of stone fragments following ESWL occurs in approximately 80% of patients. ESWL alone is more cost-effective than routinely combining ESWL with ERCP (Evidence level 1+)."

A recent meta-analysis[17] (27 studies, including 6 prospective; 3189 patients) reported pancreatic ESWL to be safe and effective for the treatment of patients who have MPD stones larger than 5 mm, and do not experience pain relief after conservative management.

Technically, it is important to use a lithotriptor with a bidimensional x-ray focusing system and a high-power generator. Ultrasonic localization of pancreatic stones lacks precision. When performed under general anesthesia or deep sedation, 3000 to 6000 shock waves can be applied at an intensity of 0.33 to 0.54 mJ/mm^2, which provides complete fragmentation of the stones after a median of 1 session, though in our experience up to 5 sessions are rarely needed.[18] Intravenous administration of secretin during ESWL may facilitate subsequent endoscopic extraction.[19]

With the patient in the prone position, the shock wave generator is placed to the patient's right side when stones are located in the head of the pancreas, and to the patient's left side when stones are located in the body or tail of the pancreas. ESWL is much more effective for fragmentation of calcium carbonate pancreatic stones than for biliary stones. Stones fragmented into millimeter size can usually be easily removed during endoscopic retrograde cholangiopancreatography (ERCP) (Figs. 55.4 and 55.5). When the lithotriptor is located within or close to the endoscopy unit, ESWL and therapeutic ERCP may be performed consecutively during one general anesthetic session.[18,20]

Intraductal Lithotripsy

Mechanical intraductal lithotripsy (IL) implies capture of stone(s) within a basket, which is often impossible with impacted calcified stones. IL can be performed using pancreatoscopy-guided electrohydraulic lithotripsy (EHL) (Cholangiopancreatoscope [Olympus, Tokyo, Japan] or Spyglass [Boston Scientific, Marlborough, MA]) (see Chapter 26) electrohydraulic lithotripsy (EHL) or pulsed dye-laser lithotriptor. Although first described 25 years ago,[21] there are limited studies available on the use of intraductal laser or electrohydraulic lithotripsy.[22–24] The largest series reported on 46 patients with 74% clinical success; adverse events occurred in 10%. Pancreatoscopy allows direct visual control of the fiber, though laser or EHL fibers can also be directly applied under fluoroscopic control. The technical challenges observed during IL include difficult access to impacted pancreatic stones and the presence of strictures. This might be improved with the maneuverability of the new Spyglass catheter but remains challenging in the majority of cases. There are no comparative studies between ESWL and IL, and they are used in a few centers with considerable expertise and/or limited access to ESWL.

Stone Extraction and Dilation

After ESWL, minute stone fragments can be visualized within the MPD or passing spontaneously through the papilla. If located upstream to a stricture, the stricture is dilated using a 4-mm to 6-mm balloon (Hurricane; Boston Scientific) to facilitate stone removal. We prefer to use a small Dormia basket to remove stone fragments (see Figs. 55.4 and 55.5). When stones are visible on fluoroscopy, a useful maneuver is to introduce a guidewire into the MPD and then pass the Dormia basket alongside using minimal or no contrast injection, because residual radiopaque fragments become isodense and are not visible when contrast is injected. The basket is then manipulated to trap the stones. Most often, the basket is left opened in the duct, turning on its axis, while the duct is gently irrigated with saline. A slightly inflated balloon catheter may be used in some cases but is of limited value because pancreatic duct stones and fragments are sharp and frequently rupture the balloon. Tight strictures are often present and, although balloon dilation is used most frequently, bougies (Soehendra dilators; Cook Endoscopy, Winston-Salem, NC) may be necessary. In case of strictures for which catheter passage proves impossible, a Soehendra stent retriever with a screw tip (8.5 Fr) can usually be rotated through the stricture to allow subsequent passage of a dilation balloon (Fig. 55.6).

If multiple sessions of endoscopy are necessary for fragmentation and removal of stones, a nasopancreatic catheter (NPC) is left in place for drainage between sessions. This may decrease the risk of acute pancreatitis caused by fragment impaction.[25] NPC placement can also be used to predict the need for pancreatic stenting; if saline infusion through the NPC is well tolerated and does not produce pain, an underlying significant MPD stricture is unlikely and stent placement may be avoided. In contrast, if saline infusion is painful, the catheter should be placed to facilitate gravity drainage and further stone extraction or stent placement performed.

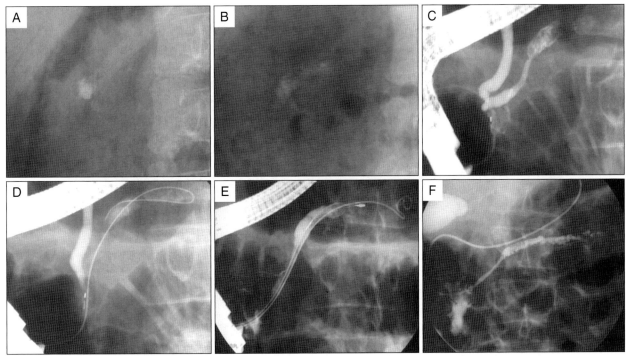

FIG 55.4 Same patient as in Fig. 55.1. Successful fragmentation (**A** vs **B**) after extracorporeal shock wave lithotripsy is illustrated by a decrease in radiologic density, an increase in the stone surface area, and heterogeneity of the stones (powder-like material). After fragmentation, a pancreatic sphincterotomy is performed (**C**), a guidewire is inserted into the pancreatic duct (**D**), and a small Dormia basket (**E**) is maneuvered alongside the guidewire to remove the stone fragments. At the end of the procedure, a nasobiliary catheter is left in place (**F**).

Stenting

When an obstructive MPD stricture is present, adequate outflow from the pancreas to the duodenum must be achieved by MPD plastic stent placement. In contrast to stent placement to prevent post-ERCP pancreatitis in high-risk patients, multiple 7-Fr to 10-Fr plastic stents are placed. Stent lengths are selected based on pancreatic duct anatomy and stricture location. Our policy is to replace plastic stents every 6 months or "on demand" when symptoms recur, for a total duration of 2 years. The stents are removed without replacement and additional treatment is based on clinical course. Stent placement has evolved from single to multiple side-by-side stents. Two 8.5-Fr stents usually can be placed after dilation to 6 mm. The number of stents can be further increased over successive exchanges, depending on the degree of upstream ductal dilation (see Fig. 55.2). This approach has been used to reduce the duration of stenting and to prolong symptom relief.[26] Multiple stent placement is facilitated by placement of two guidewires across the stricture, followed by successive stent placement. This technique avoids the need to recannulate the MPD and negotiate a guidewire across a tight stricture alongside an indwelling stent.

Use of the Fusion system (Cook Endoscopy) allows intraductal exchange and placement of multiple side-by-side stents without losing access and using only one guidewire. This has become our preferred technique for placement of multiple 8.5-Fr plastic pancreatic stents.

Placement of fully covered self-expandable stents (FCSEMS) into the MPD (Fig. 55.7) might be an alternative to multiple plastic stent placement or in cases of strictures refractory to plastic stent therapy. One study of 32 patients with chronic painful pancreatitis and dominant ductal strictures who underwent placement of a specially designed FCSEMS showed promising results 3 months after removal.[27] However,

these were small series without comparison to plastic stent therapy. In addition, eligible patients must have dilated ducts large enough to accommodate the stent (often 8 to 10 mm), and it should only be long enough to bridge the stricture so as to prevent occlusion of side branches upstream to the stricture. SEMS placement can facilitate endoscopic removal of stones upstream to a stricture. Use of SEMS for benign pancreatic duct therapy is off-label.

Overall, results using FCSEMS are mixed and their use should be considered in the setting of clinical trials.[15] The major adverse events reported with the use of FCSEMS include pain, migration, and development of iatrogenic strictures.[28,29]

Another route for draining the MPD is through the gastric or duodenal wall in case of an associated pancreatic fluid collection (PFC) that is in communication with the pancreatic duct (see Chapter 56). In such cases, transmural drainage should be performed without attempting transpapillary MPD drainage, which has no additional effect on pain relief and treatment outcomes and negatively affects long-term recurrence of PFC.[30]

Technical Results

The majority of patients with severe painful calcifying CP require ESWL for stone removal. In our experience, ESWL is required in two-thirds of patients referred for treatment. In a multicenter study of more than 1000 patients, pancreatic obstruction was caused by the presence of obstructive stones alone in 17%, MPD stricture in 47%, and both stones and stricture in 32%.[10] Numerous reports have shown that ESWL is a low-risk procedure with a rate of fragmentation up to 100%. Nevertheless, complete stone clearance of the MPD is achieved in only 44% to 75% of cases (Table 55.1). A meta-analysis[31] showed that the use of ESWL was significantly associated with ductal clearance and pain relief. A

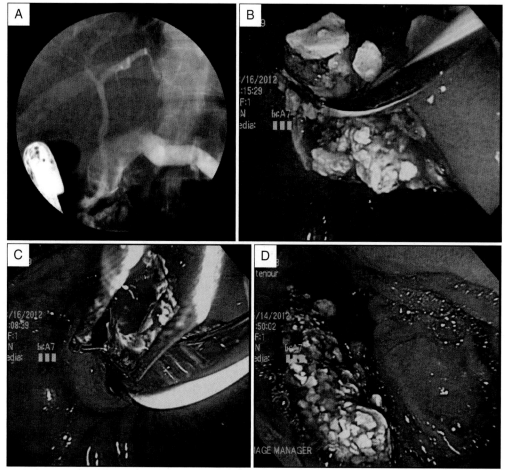

FIG 55.5 Extracorporeal shock wave lithotripsy (ESWL) followed by ERCP. **A,** Pancreatogram after ESWL shows large, amorphous filling defect. Note that there is no focal stone and dispersion of prior stone consistent with successful ESWL. **B,** Endoscopic view of guidewire placement into main pancreatic duct (MPD) with stone fragments passing out of prior pancreatic sphincterotomy. **C,** Endoscopic view of basket passed alongside guidewire placed into MPD with removal of stone fragments. **D,** Endoscopic view of stone fragments in the duodenum after complete endoscopic clearance.

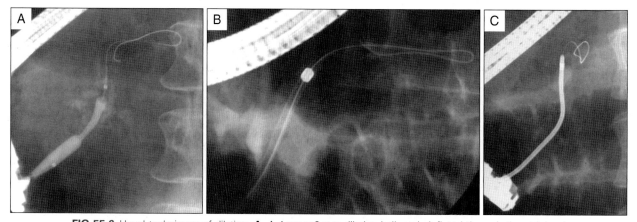

FIG 55.6 Usual techniques of dilation. **A,** A 4-cm × 6-mm dilating balloon is inflated through the stricture, of which the waist is visible early in the inflation period. **B,** A biliary bougie is passed over a guidewire. **C,** In an extremely tight stricture, an 8.5-Fr Soehendra stent retriever is rotated through the stricture in order to create room necessary for insertion of a dilating balloon. In this case, after dilation, the stent retriever is removed while rotating anticlockwise in order to avoid losing the guidewire.

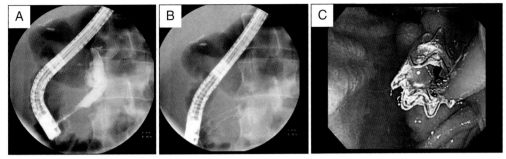

FIG 55.7 Fully covered self-expandable stent placement in a patient with chronic pancreatitis, pain, and refractory stricture in the pancreatic head. **A,** Pancreatogram showing stricture present after prior plastic stent therapy with upstream ductal dilation. **B,** Radiograph showing stent immediately after placement. **C,** Endoscopic photograph of stent exiting the papilla.

TABLE 55.1   Results of Extracorporeal Shock Wave Lithotripsy and Endotherapy for Chronic Calcific Pancreatitis

Study	Year	No. of Patients	Fragmentation (%)	Complete Clearance (%)	Complete or Partial Pain Relief (%)	Need for Surgery (%)	Mean Follow-up (mo)
ESWL and Endotherapy							
Delhaye et al.[18]	1992	123	99	59	85	8	14
Schneider et al.[33]	1994	50	86	60	62	12	20
Costamagna et al.[36]	1997	35	100	74	72	3	27
Adamek et al.[37]	1999	80	54	ND	76	10	40
Brand et al.[38]	2000	48	60	44	82	4	7
Farnbacher et al.[35]	2002	125	85	64	48*	13	29
Kozarek et al.[39]	2002	40	100	ND	80	20	30
Inui et al.[20]	2005	470	92	73	69*	4	44
Tandan et al.[40]	2010	1006	100	ND	84	ND	6
Seven et al.[41]	2012	120	100	ND	85	16	52
Tandan et al.[32]	2013	632	100	77	93	ND	60
Hu et al.[42]	2016	214	87	72	95	ND	19
ESWL Alone							
Ohara et al.[43]	1996	32	100	75	86	3	44

ND, Not determined.
*Patients with complete pain relief during follow-up.

recent meta-analysis of ESWL and ET for pain management in CP[17] reported pain reduction in 89% of the patients, with complete pain relief in 50%. The largest single-center series so far had a 93% success rate of stone fragmentation and clearance in 1006 patients undergoing ESWL.[32] Technical success of endoscopic ductal drainage, however, is generally defined as a decrease in the diameter of the MPD with or without complete ductal stone clearance.[11] Success using this definition was obtained in 54% to 99% of cases in the largest series published to date.[11,18,20,33–43] Dumonceau et al.[34] identified ESWL as the only independent factor associated with technical success. In most reports, successful fragmentation and stone clearance have not been correlated with the initial size and number of MPD stones.

Clinical Results

Early pain relief after endoscopic drainage of the MPD is experienced in 82% to 94% of patients and can be expected when drainage of the MPD is adequate.[3,15,17,32,34] Medium-term clinical improvement has been observed in 48% to 84% of patients after a mean follow-up period of 2 to 5 years. Predictors of pain relapse during follow-up include high frequency of pain attacks,[34,39] long duration of disease before treatment,[34,41] and presence of MPD stenosis[30,44] (Table 55.2). In our series

with the longest follow-up to date (14.4 years), a good clinical outcome was observed in two-thirds of patients and associated with a short duration of disease before treatment and cessation of smoking.[11]

Notably, cessation of smoking was the single clinical factor associated with long-term pain relief in another study.[41] This confirms the role of ongoing smoking in pain relief reported in CP patients after surgery.[9]

Overall, it appears that ESWL and/or endoscopic therapy should be initiated as early as possible in the course of CP because it increases the probability of long-term benefit, and that patients should be encouraged to quit both alcohol intake and smoking.

In most series, recurrent pain attacks during follow-up were related to impaction of stone fragments; recurrent, progressive MPD stricturing; and pancreatic stent obstruction or dislodgment. Retreatment is usually easier than initial treatment and remains very effective at controlling pain.[34,47] This is in contrast to surgery, which has increased morbidity when repeated.

Pain recurrence does not necessarily relate to stone recurrence. For instance, in the largest single-center study to date,[32] 59% of patients in the 2-year to 5-year follow-up group and 56% of patients in the >5-year follow-up group who had pain recurrence did not have stone recurrence. This reiterates that there are multiple mechanisms contributing to pain

TABLE 55.2 **Predictive Factors of Technical and Clinical Success in Published Series of More Than 50 Chronic Pancreatitis Patients Treated by ESWL and Endoscopic Pancreatic Ductal Drainage**

Series	Number of Patients	Technical Success (%)	Associated Factor	Clinical Success (%)	Associated Factor
Short-term follow-up <2 y[18]	123	90	None	85	Decrease in MPD diameter
Medium-term follow-up 2–5 y[11,36–42,44–46]	53–996	54–99	Availability of ESWL Single stone	48–84	Short duration of disease Low frequency of pain Absence of MPD stricture
Total	1557	86		65	
Long-term follow-up >5 y[11]	56	86	None	66	Short duration of disease
Long-term follow-up >4 y[41]	120	100	None	85	No current smoking Ongoing smoking

ESWL, Extracorporeal shock wave lithotripsy; *MPD,* main pancreatic duct.

in patients with CP, which may not be improved by ductal clearance using ET or surgical drainage.

Dominant strictures of the MPD are often the main indication for insertion of pancreatic duct stents. These are required, in addition to pancreatic sphincterotoy and stone management, in 50% to 60% of patients with severe CP.[10,11] The problem with stent placement is stent occlusion, which results in recurrent symptoms. Stents can be exchanged on a regular basis or on demand (in patients with recurrent pain and recurrent MPD dilation).

In patients with multiple side-by-side stents in place, we prefer the "on demand" exchange strategy. In such cases, stent replacement is required at a mean period of 8 to 12 months,[47] likely because occluded stents may serve as wicks, allowing pancreatic juice to flow into the duodenum. Short-term stent placement[48] (6 months) is usually not adequate to provide sufficient stricture calibration and long-term pain relief. However, because the presence of a stent is associated with the need for repeat endoscopy, two large studies have assessed long-term outcomes in patients with severe CP after pancreatic stent removal. In one study[41] stents could be removed from 49/93 patients (52%) after a mean stent duration of 16 months, and 73% of these patients remained pain-free without a stent during a mean follow-up of 3.8 years. In a second study,[47] 62% of patients maintained satisfactory pain control after a median stent duration of 23 months without the need for pancreatic stent replacement during a median follow-up of 27 months. The only significant predictive factor of the need for pancreatic stent replacement within 1 year of stent removal was the presence of pancreas divisum. Notably, the majority of patients who experienced pain recurrence did so during the first year after stent removal. Therefore, if a patient remains clinically well during the first year after stent removal, subsequent relapse and need for repeat stent placement are unlikely. Importantly, patients who have frequent pain relapses caused by stent occlusion but achieve pain control with a patent stent have a good outcome after surgical decompression (pancreaticojejunostomy). This further reinforces the idea that ET should be performed using a multidisciplinary approach. In addition, pancreatic ET does not complicate subsequent surgical procedures.[49]

In an attempt to decrease stent duration, Costamagna's group[26] was the first to propose placement of multiple MPD stents for a duration of 6 to 12 months. Their approach is to insert as many stents as possible (median of 3), contingent upon the severity of the MPD stricture and the upstream ductal diameter. After stent removal, 16/19 patients remained asymptomatic after a mean follow-up of 38 months. The majority of these patients were found to have occluded stents at time of removal yet did not experience pain relapse. This reinforces the concept that pancreatic juice can still flow between the stents and that

a more aggressive approach to the treatment of dominant pancreatic strictures may decrease the stent duration required to provide long-term pain relief.

Another area needing further investigation in patients with pancreatic head strictures and associated communicating pseudocyst is the long-term efficacy when an iatrogenic pancreaticoduodenal or pancreaticogastric fistula is created during transmural drainage of a PFC and direct transmural ductal drainage using EUS. The fistula can be maintained by placement of one or two stents.[50] This technique also can be applied to patients with complete MPD obstruction and has the potential advantage of creating a true pancreaticoduodenal fistula that may not be dependent on stent patency. The fistula would act more as a wick, comparable to the communication created after drainage of a pancreatic pseudocyst associated with a disconnected MPD. In case of transmural drainage of a communicating pseudocyst in the setting of severe CP, ductal decompression can be achieved with this therapy and transpapillary access is both unnecessary and not recommended.[30]

Another endoscopic option for patients with PD stones is to initiate treatment using only ESWL.[51] Indeed, ESWL produces millimeter stone fragments that can pass through the papilla in the absence of a pancreatic sphincterotomy, resulting in ductal clearance without the need for endoscopic intervention. This approach is best reserved for patients without biliary stenosis or the presence of pseudocyst(s) and with short MPD strictures located in the head of the pancreas. The ESWL-only approach was prospectively studied in a multicenter randomized controlled trial of 55 patients (Table 55.3) with a mean follow-up of more than 4 years and had similar long-term pain relief compared with combined ESWL and ET, with a decrease in hospital stay, cost, and need for additional procedures. We have adopted this strategy for pain management in selected patients.

Adverse Events

The main adverse event after stone fragmentation and pancreatic ET is acute pancreatitis. Fortunately the rate of severe pancreatitis after pancreatic manipulations in patients with calcific CP is low. In a review of 572 endoscopic pancreatic sphincterotomies performed in patients with pancreatic disease, 12% of patients developed pancreatitis (none severe). By multivariate analysis, significant factors that decreased the risk of acute pancreatitis after sphincterotomy were the presence of pancreatic ductal stones, performance of only major papilla sphincterotomy, and adequate duct drainage. Although the use of rectally administered nonsteroidal antiinflammatory drugs (NSAIDs) to prevent post-ERCP pancreatitis (see Chapter 8) has not been studied specifically in patients with CP, we recommend it after endoscopic pancreatic interventions.

TABLE 55.3 ESWL Versus ESWL and Endotherapy as Initial Treatment for Chronic Pancreatitis With Obstructive Stones, No Large Pseudocyst, and No Biliary Stenosis

	ESWL (n = 26)	ESWL and Endotherapy (n = 29)
Initial hospital stay (days)	2	7*
Morbidity	0%	3%
At least 1 pain relapse over 51 months	42%	45%
Patients requiring additional ERCP/ESWL	8 (31%)	18 (62%)*

From Dumonceau JM, Costamagna G, Tringali A, et al. Treatment for painful calcified chronic pancreatitis: extracorporeal shock wave lithotripsy versus endoscopic treatment: a randomized controlled trial. *Gut.* 2007;56:545–552.
ERCP, Endoscopic retrograde cholangiopancreatography; *ESWL,* extracorporeal shock wave lithotripsy.
$*p < 0.05$.

In a recent meta-analysis covering 27 studies (3189 patients undergoing ESWL and ET), there was a 4.2% rate of acute pancreatitis related to the procedures and no mortality. ESWL alone is associated with very few adverse events.[52] Indeed, the use of EWSL in the presence of a pancreatic pseudocyst is also safe.[53] Post-ESWL pancreatitis is observed in <1% of cases, even without previous sphincterotomy. Minor gastric and/or duodenal erosions are commonly seen. We administer proton pump inhibitors after ESWL for 2 weeks.

Impact of Pancreatic Duct Drainage on Pancreatic Endocrine and Exocrine Functions

In contrast with the multicenter study published by Rosch et al.,[10] our long-term results[11] suggest that endoscopic ductal drainage including ESWL can delay the development of clinical steatorrhea by about 10 years compared with untreated patients with CP.[8] A recent meta-analysis reported increased or maintained weight in 82% of patients treated by ET and ESWL.[17]

The risk of new-onset steatorrhea was higher in alcoholic patients and also significantly associated with long duration of symptomatic ductal obstruction before treatment, suggesting that early ductal decompression in the course of the disease may be beneficial. However, in the setting of painless steatorrhea, ET cannot currently be recommended.

Moreover, previous studies[11,34,54] showed that the development of diabetes mellitus was not prevented by pancreatic duct drainage. Rather it appeared to be a consequence of ongoing alcohol abuse. This suggests that only exocrine pancreatic function may be dependent on early relief of ductal obstruction.

Use of Endoscopic Ultrasonography

In patients with CP and impassable strictures and/or stones, EUS-guided rendezvous or pancreaticogastrostomy can be used to provide drainage with stent placement. These procedures are discussed further in Chapter 33.

Biliary Strictures

Biliary strictures in the setting of severe CP are not uncommon. Such strictures are located distally, in the intrapancreatic portion of the biliary tree. Endoscopic management consists of placement of multiple large-bore (10 to 11.5 Fr) plastic stents or a single fully covered SEMS. In case of failure, surgical bypass or resection of the pancreatic head is undertaken, depending on whether only the bile duct obstruction needs to be addressed (with or without pancreatic drainage [lateral pancreaticojejunostomy]) or concomitant pancreatic head resection (Whipple) is performed, respectively. The role of endoscopy in the management of strictures is discussed in Chapter 43.

SUMMARY

Multiple large series with long duration of follow-up demonstrate the effectiveness of pancreatic ET for painful CP and support ET as a viable first-line intervention. However, criticisms of ET remain.

One criticism is the absence of sham-controlled trials, which are difficult to perform in referral centers where patients with severe pain are referred for surgical treatment. Over a 3-year period, we were able to enroll only eight patients in such a trial at our institution. This number represents only 5% of new patients. In a recent publication of pancreatic ET in patients with continuous pain and a dilated duct,[55] complete pain relief occurred in all patients and allowed for analgesic discontinuation. This suggests that in this subset of patients MPD drainage is better than placebo.

Whether ET is an alternative to surgery for the treatment of pain remains debatable. The first randomized trial comparing ET with surgery showed similar short-term pain relief, though surgery was better for medium-term pain control.[56]

Of note, surgery included resection in 80% of patients, which is not comparable to ductal drainage alone. Moreover, ESWL was not available for endoscopic treatment, which in our experience would prevent successful treatment in 44% of cases. Additionally, repeat ET was not performed when symptoms recurred. Multiple previous studies have demonstrated the need for such retreatment during the early period after endoscopic decompression.[11,34] In another trial,[57] surgery resulted in superior pain relief compared with ET at 2 years (75% vs 32%). However, in this study, stents remained in place for treatment of strictures for a median of 6 months, which is ineffective for long-term pain relief.[45] The vast majority of patients had severe MPD strictures. Moreover, the endoscopic group included patients with obstructive CP, biliary strictures, and pseudocysts. The same study[58] reported the 6-year follow-up of these patients. Significantly fewer patients in the endoscopic group (6/16) had partial or complete pain relief compared with the surgical group (12/15). However, overall pain scores, quality of life, total hospital stay, and costs were similar. Interestingly, nine patients in the endoscopic group underwent surgery and only two had subsequent pain relief. Although the authors suggested that delayed surgery using ET was the cause of poor response after surgery, it may reflect the heterogeneity of the endoscopic group, which included patients who needed more than pancreatic ductal drainage, such as resection. These randomized trials are helpful to establish the optimal approach to the treatment of patients with CP.

Moreover, standardization of the endoscopic approach (ESWL, duration of stent placement, treatment in multidisciplinary units) is required to allow meaningful interpretation of outcomes and comparison of outcomes among centers.

Measurement of outcomes is also important, as most pain relapses after ET occur within 1 year after initial treatment.[11] In contrast, relapse after surgery commonly occurs after a median of 6 to 7 years.[7]

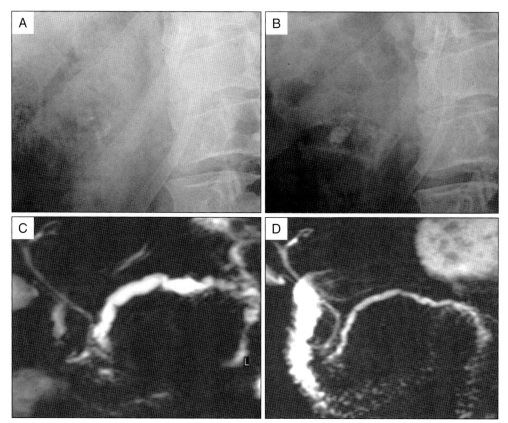

FIG 55.8 Patient with chronic pancreatitis and daily pain. **A** and **C,** Plain film and secretin-stimulated magnetic resonance cholangiopancreatography at admission, showing a single impacted stone in the head of the pancreas with upstream main pancreatic duct (MPD) dilatation. **B** and **D,** After a single session of ESWL, without endoscopic therapy, the majority of the stone has disappeared **(B),** the size of the MPD has decreased **(D),** and duodenal filling, at the same time point after secretin injection, is much more obvious.

A final issue is to define whether or not an excessive number of procedures are being performed in these patients. Studies from Japan show that ESWL alone results in pain relief for many patients.[43,44] This is likely a consequence of minute fragmentation of calcium carbonate stones, especially in patients with solitary stones located in the pancreatic head.

As previously mentioned, a randomized control trial[45] in this particular group of patients compared ESWL as an initial treatment to ESWL plus ET and showed that the less invasive initial approach of ESWL alone was as effective as the combination of ESWL and ET. Only 31% of patients from the "ESWL alone" group required additional ET over a median 4-year follow-up (Fig. 55.8). This also supports the use of ESWL as a cornerstone in the management of these patients. ESWL alone has now become our initial interventional approach to pain management in patients with obstructive stones. If additional therapy is needed, ET or surgery is performed. Surgery is preferred in patients with associated strictures in whom PD stricture improvement is not obtained after 1 year of stent therapy (preferably using two 8.5-Fr stents implanted side-by-side).

However, endoscopic management of patients with CP should be performed as part of a multidisciplinary approach by clinicians with experience in both surgical and endoscopic approaches.

The complete reference list for this chapter can be found online at www.expertconsult.com.

56

Endoscopic Drainage of Pancreatic Pseudocysts, Abscesses, and Walled-Off (Organized) Necrosis

Ryan Law and Todd H. Baron

Pancreatic pseudocysts, abscesses, and walled-off necrosis (WON) are types of pancreatic fluid collections (PFCs) that arise as a consequence of pancreatic injury. These sequelae of pancreatic injury result from a disruption of the main pancreatic duct (PD) and/or side branches. Ductal disruption can occur secondary to acute pancreatic injury (i.e., acute pancreatitis, trauma, surgical resection, or inadvertent damage to the pancreas during abdominal surgery) or chronic injury (i.e., chronic pancreatitis, autoimmune pancreatitis). Ductal injury subsequently leads to formation of a collection of fluid with or without solid debris.

Endoscopic therapy is directed at drainage of fluid and solid components using a transmural approach, treatment of PD disruption or stricture using a transpapillary approach, or a combination of both techniques in select patients. Treatment of PD disruption is believed to decrease the long-term recurrence rate and improve the outcome after successful resolution of a collection. This chapter discusses endoscopic approaches to PFCs.

SPECIFIC TYPES OF FLUID COLLECTIONS

Classification systems for defining types of PFCs are useful for understanding mechanisms of formation and allowing comparisons of therapies between and among disciplines. Since the previous edition of this text, the classification and nomenclature of PFCs have been revised,[1] and they will likely continue to evolve.

When intervention is indicated, the therapeutic approach can be simplified by addressing three questions: (1) Is the collection a result of pancreatitis or does it represent a cystic neoplasm (see Chapter 51)? (2) Is the collection composed primarily of liquid or does it contain significant solid debris? (3) What is the PD anatomy? Using these three basic questions, the short-term and long-term approaches to the patient with a PFC can be formulated. The approach to collections that are composed primarily of fluid is different from the approach to those containing significant solid debris, because liquefied collections can be managed with placement of small-diameter stents via a transpapillary or transmural approach alone, whereas those with solid debris may require direct endoscopic necrosectomy, placement of large-bore self-expandable metal stents (SEMS), adjuvant percutaneous catheters, and direct removal of necrotic debris from the collection with or without placement of irrigation catheters.

COLLECTIONS COMPOSED ENTIRELY OR PREDOMINANTLY OF LIQUID

1. *Acute fluid collections.* Acute fluid collections arise early in the course of acute pancreatitis and are usually peripancreatic in location. These collections usually resolve without sequelae but may evolve into pancreatic pseudocysts.[1,2]

2. Pancreatic pseudocysts.
   a. *Acute pancreatic pseudocysts.* Acute pseudocysts arise as sequelae of acute pancreatitis, require at least 4 weeks to encapsulate, and are devoid of significant solid debris. Acute pancreatic pseudocysts usually form as a result of limited pancreatic necrosis in conjunction with a PD leak (Fig. 56.1). Alternatively, areas of pancreatic and peripancreatic fat necrosis may completely liquefy over time and become a pseudocyst. Despite the requirement of at least 4 weeks for a pseudocyst to mature, this time period does not define the collection as a pancreatic pseudocyst. Significant pancreatic necrosis (≥30%) may evolve into a collection that resembles a pseudocyst radiographically but has been present for more than 4 weeks (see the Walled-Off Necrosis section of this chapter). By definition, collections that contain significant solid debris are not pseudocysts, and endoscopic treatment of these collections by pseudocyst drainage methods alone often results in infection of the remaining unremoved solid debris.
   b. *Chronic pseudocysts.* A chronic pseudocyst arises as a sequela of chronic pancreatitis because of downstream pancreatic obstruction from fibrotic strictures and/or stones. This results in a pancreatic ductal disruption, blowout, or leak and accumulation of pancreatic fluid. These collections do not contain solid debris and usually do not arise as a result of acute inflammatory processes (Fig. 56.2).

Pancreatic pseudocysts can be subdivided into sterile and infected (the latter is referred to as pancreatic abscess in some nomenclature systems).

3. *Pancreatic abscesses.* True pancreatic abscesses are rare and are not synonymous with infected pancreatic pseudocysts.[1] However, for the purposes of this chapter and based on pending revisions of the existing nomenclature, an abscess will be considered as an infected PFC that contains little to no solid debris (as opposed to infected pancreatic necrosis, which is described later). The authors believe that when this definition is used, abscesses can be drained through modest-sized catheters without an absolute need for irrigation or debridement.

INDICATIONS FOR DRAINAGE OF LIQUEFIED COLLECTIONS

In general, the indications for drainage of a liquefied PFC are driven by symptoms and/or signs of infection and not merely by the presence of a collection on cross-sectional imaging. Symptoms related to sterile pancreatic collections include abdominal pain, often exacerbated by

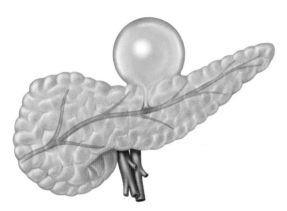

FIG 56.1 Illustration of the mechanism of formation of an acute pancreatic pseudocyst. Limited necrosis of the main pancreatic duct produces a ductal leak with accumulation of amylase-rich fluid.

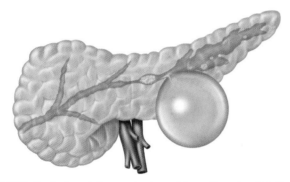

FIG 56.2 Illustration of the mechanism of formation of a chronic pancreatic pseudocyst. Obstruction of the main pancreatic duct by stones and/or stricture produces a duct blowout with accumulation of amylase-rich fluid.

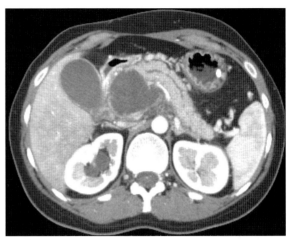

FIG 56.3 Metastatic malignant fibrous histiocytoma detected in a woman with abdominal pain and "pancreatitis" mimicking a pancreatic pseudocyst. She had a previous known primary lesion. The lesion was diagnosed by endoscopic ultrasonography–fine-needle aspiration and resected for palliation.

BOX 56.1 Masqueraders of Pancreatic Fluid Collections

- Cystic pancreatic neoplasm
- Duplication cyst
- True pancreatic cyst
- Pseudoaneurysm
- Solid necrotic neoplasm (e.g., retroperitoneal sarcoma)
- Lymphocele
- Gallbladder

eating, weight loss, gastric outlet obstruction (nausea and vomiting), obstructive jaundice, and ongoing PD leaks. PD leaks can manifest as pancreatic ascites or high-amylase pleural effusion and pancreatic fistulae and are discussed in Chapter 54. Infection is considered an absolute indication for drainage.

For many years a size cutoff of 6 cm and persistence of a collection were used as criteria for drainage. However, patients may remain asymptomatic with collections ≥6 cm with little risk of adverse events such as rupture, infection, or bleeding, whereas endoscopic intervention is associated with a finite (as well as potentially higher) risk of adverse events. Progressive enlargement of a collection is one exception that is cited as an indication for drainage, although even then such patients potentially can be followed until they become symptomatic.

PREDRAINAGE EVALUATION

Before undertaking drainage of a liquefied pancreatic collection, a predrainage evaluation should be performed that includes the following:

1. Establish whether or not the collection represents a PFC or a "masquerader" of a PFC such as a cystic neoplasm or other entity (Box 56.1; Fig. 56.3). If the patient does not have a well-documented history of acute or chronic pancreatitis, the endoscopist should be concerned that the collection does not represent a pseudocyst or other inflammatory collection. Endoscopic ultrasonography (EUS) allows for diagnosis of cystic neoplasms, as discussed in Chapter 51. Clinical presentation and cross-sectional imaging with CT and magnetic resonance imaging (MRI) can also be useful in making the differentiation between cystic neoplasms and inflammatory PFCs (see Chapter 34).

2. Establish whether the collection is predominantly liquid or contains a significant amount of solid debris.

3. Establish the relationship of the collection to surrounding luminal and vascular structures.

4. Consider underlying etiologies of true pancreatic pseudocyst that have implications for alternative or adjuvant therapies, such as pancreatic cancer, autoimmune pancreatitis, and intraductal pancreatic mucinous neoplasms (IPMNs).

In addition to a complete history and physical examination, the following evaluation should be undertaken before endoscopic drainage:

1. Coagulation profile in patients with a suspicion of coagulopathy and/or liver disease, especially when transmural drainage is considered. Management of antithrombotic agents, as appropriate for high-risk bleeding procedures (see Chapter 10).

2. Contrast-enhanced abdominal computed tomography (CT). This allows assessment of the precise location of the collection in relation to the stomach and duodenum in anticipation of possible transmural drainage. Additionally, the relationship of the collection to potential intervening vascular structures can be assessed. Surrounding varices from splenic vein or portal vein thrombosis also may be visualized. The finding of inhomogeneity within the collection suggests the presence of underlying solid debris and/or blood (Fig. 56.4).

Consideration should be given to the following additional studies:

1. *Endoscopic ultrasonography.* EUS can be used before drainage to allow assessment of the presence of significant solid debris that may alter the management strategy. In addition, if there is uncertainty as to whether the collection represents a true pseudocyst or other noninflammatory cystic lesion, EUS allows a definitive diagnosis to be achieved by using ultrasonographic features, aspiration and analysis of cyst contents, biopsy of the cyst wall, and even confocal imaging with a probe passed through a fine-needle aspiration (FNA) needle (see Chapter 28). Once the endoscopist is certain that the lesion in question is a PFC and the decision has been made to proceed with endoscopic drainage, EUS is used to guide transmural drainage, as discussed in the next section.

2. *MRI with or without magnetic resonance cholangiopancreatography.* MRI also allows detection of the presence of solid debris, and so plans for removal and/or alternative drainage strategies can be chosen depending on local expertise and necrosis drainage preferences. Magnetic resonance cholangiopancreatography (MRCP) can define the ductal anatomy and be augmented by secretin stimulation. Secretin-enhanced MRCP (S-MRCP) may demonstrate the presence or absence of an ongoing ductal disruption.

DRAINAGE TECHNIQUES

Liquefied PFCs may be drained using a transpapillary approach, transmural approach, or a combination of these.[3,4] The decision to use one approach over the other depends on the size of the collection, its proximity to the stomach or duodenum, and the ability to enter the PD and/or reach the area of disruption. For example, although the intended approach to draining a pseudocyst that formed from an obstructing PD stone may be transpapillary (Fig. 56.5, *A* and *B*), failure to negotiate a guidewire beyond the obstructing ductal stone may require transmural drainage. Assessment and treatment of the ductal stone at a later date by other techniques, such as extracorporeal shock wave lithotripsy (ESWL), can then be performed (Fig. 56.5, *C* to *E*).

Transpapillary Drainage

If the collection communicates with the main PD, placement of a pancreatic endoprosthesis (stent) with or without pancreatic sphincterotomy is an approach that is useful, especially for collections measuring ≤6 cm that are not otherwise approachable transmurally.[5,6] The upstream end of the stent (toward the pancreatic tail) may enter the collection directly or bridge the area of leak into the PD upstream from the leak (Fig. 56.6). The latter is the preferred approach (Fig. 56.7) because it restores ductal continuity. In patients with chronic pseudocysts, it is important that the stent bridge any obstructive process (stricture or stone) between the duodenum and the leak site. The diameter of pancreatic stent used is dependent on the pancreatic ductal diameter (see Chapters 22 and 55), although 7-Fr stents are most frequently used. In patients with chronic pancreatitis, endoscopic therapy of underlying PD strictures and pancreatic stones may reduce the recurrence rate of pancreatic pseudocysts.[7]

The advantage of a transpapillary approach compared with a transmural approach is avoidance of bleeding (because pancreatic sphincterotomy is not mandatory during stent placement) and a decrease

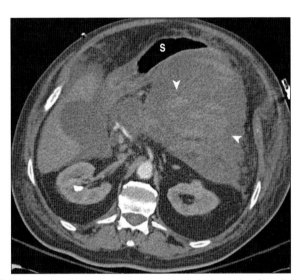

FIG 56.4 Computed tomography scan obtained 4 weeks after clinically severe gallstone pancreatitis. Note the large homogeneous fluid collection posterior to the stomach (*S*) with inhomogeneous density (*arrowheads*) suggesting solid debris.

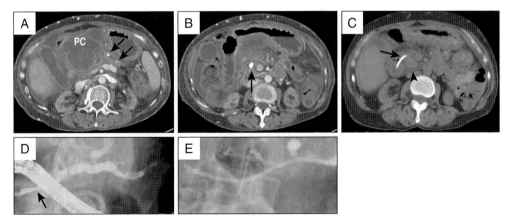

FIG 56.5 A patient with a pseudocyst caused by chronic pancreatitis. **A,** The pseudocyst (*PC*) is seen compressing the duodenum; calcifications are present near the tail (*arrows*). **B,** Lower cuts of the same patient. A large stone (*arrow*) is obstructing the main pancreatic duct. **C,** Follow-up computed tomography after transmural drainage and extracorporeal shock wave lithotripsy. Transduodenal stents can be seen (*arrow*). The prior stone has been fragmented (*arrowhead*). **D,** At the time of duodenal stent removal, pancreatography shows a stricture in the head (*arrow*). **E,** Stone fragments were removed, the stricture was balloon dilated, and a pancreatic duct stent was placed.

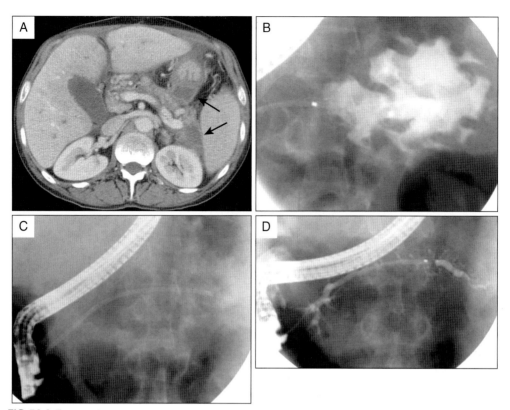

FIG 56.6 Transpapillary drainage of a pancreatic pseudocyst. **A,** Computed tomography scan. Collections are seen (*arrows*). **B,** Pancreatogram shows leakage at the tail. **C,** Transpapillary stent placed to tail. **D,** Follow-up pancreatogram shows no leak.

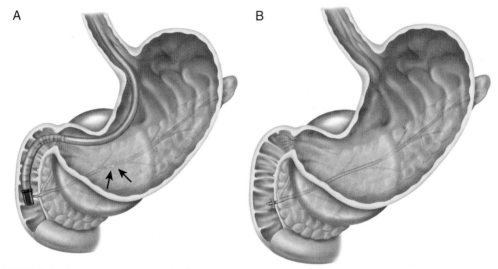

FIG 56.7 A, Schematic of pancreatic duct leak. **B,** Illustration of ideal position of pancreatic duct stent placement across a leak site.

in the risk of perforation. The disadvantage of transpapillary drainage is the potential for pancreatic stent-induced ductal injury in patients whose PD is otherwise normal. Examples include patients with acute pseudocysts and small side-branch disruption and patients with ductal leaks after distal (tail) pancreatectomy (see Chapter 45).

Transmural Drainage

It has become increasingly clear that transmural drainage of PFCs using EUS-guided drainage is superior to the unguided (blind) passage of needle

catheters and electrosurgical catheters (needle knife or cystoenterostomy needle knife), formerly done by using endoscopic landmarks (visible extrinsic compression) and fluoroscopy. An older randomized trial of EUS-guided and non–EUS-guided drainage found non–EUS-guided drainage to be an acceptable first-line therapy in patients with bulging collections.[8] EUS imaging reduces adverse events related to transmural entry of PFCs. Localization of the collection using EUS can be followed by a second non–EUS-guided endoscopic puncture,[9] although this requires an additional endoscope and exchange and may be less accurate.

Devices used to perform transmural puncture of a collection can be divided into electrosurgical and nonelectrosurgical. Electrosurgical devices include standard diathermy wires (e.g., needle knife) and specialized cystoenterostomy devices (Cystotome, CST-10; Cook Endoscopy, Winston-Salem, NC). In addition, a novel lumen-apposing metal stent (LAMS) with a dedicated cautery-enhanced tip is available (AXIOS-EC; Boston Scientific, Marlborough, MA) (Fig. 56.8).

Nonelectrosurgical devices include EUS-FNA needles and other miscellaneous aspiration needles (Marcon-Haber variceal injector needle MHI-21; Cook Medical, Winston-Salem, NC). EUS-guided puncture and drainage are described in detail in Chapters 32 and 33. Using a linear echoendoscope (oblique or forward), successful entry and one-step drainage can be achieved in at least 95% of patients, with a low rate of adverse events, including those without an endoscopically visible extrinsic compression.[9,10] Doppler capabilities reduce the risk of puncture of large vessels.

If a non–EUS-guided drainage approach is undertaken, the collection is entered at a point of endoscopically visible extrinsic compression using electrosurgery with or without prelocalization using a needle (Fig. 56.9). An alternative is localization and entry into the collection using a needle that accepts a guidewire without the use of electrocautery using the Seldinger technique. Entry is confirmed by aspiration of fluid and/or injection of radiopaque contrast (Fig. 56.10, *A* to *C*; Video 56.1). ▶ Nonelectrosurgical puncture may be safer than cautery puncture for non–EUS-guided entry. In this setting, if unsuccessful entry occurs, the needle is withdrawn. Similarly, if bleeding occurs upon needle entry, if gross blood is aspirated, or if a visible hematoma develops, the needle is withdrawn to allow the vessel to tamponade. Another transmural entry site may be subsequently chosen during the same endoscopic session. Using this technique, successful non–EUS-guided transmural entry has been reported in 94 of 97 patients (97%) in lesions as small as 3 cm and without endoscopically visible extrinsic compression, though these were performed by one endoscopist with lengthy experience in non–EUS-guided drainage.[11]

Drainage of collections containing fluid only (acute fluid collections and pseudocysts) successfully resolves with transmural placement of two 10-Fr double-pigtail plastic stents or one fully covered biliary SEMS.[12]

Stent placement across the transmural track requires balloon dilation with a standard endoscopic retrograde cholangiopancreatography (ERCP) dilating balloon of 8-mm to 10-mm diameter (Fig. 56.10, *D*) to allow placement of one or two 7-Fr to 10-Fr plastic stents (Fig. 56.10, *E*; see Video 56.1). If a biliary SEMS is used, the tract does not need to ▶ be dilated more than 4 mm to allow passage of the delivery system. It is important to secure an ample length of guidewire into the collection with at least one complete loop of wire (Fig. 56.10, *D*). The practice of enlarging the transmural tract using electrosurgery is now infrequently performed because of the increased risk of bleeding at the entry site.

The type of plastic stents used for transmural drainage may be straight or pigtail. Double-pigtail stents are recommended for at least two reasons. First, they are less prone to migrate into or out of the collection. Second, straight stents can cause delayed bleeding from impaction of the stent against the contralateral wall of the collection or stomach as the collection resolves. We routinely place one or two short-length (3 to 5 cm) 10-Fr double-pigtail stents during transmural drainage. Stents are available from several companies. We prefer to use "standard" 10-Fr double-pigtail stents (Zimmon stent; Cook Medical), although one end is tapered and does not allow passage of an inner guiding catheter. One must be careful when placing double-pigtail stents not to push the entire stent into the collection. This can be avoided by

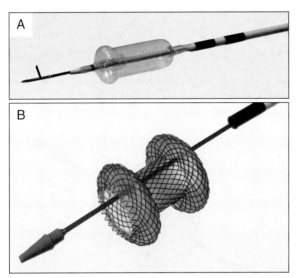

FIG 56.8 **A,** NAVIX Access Device. **B,** AXIOS stent deployed while still on delivery system (Xlumena, Mountain View, CA).

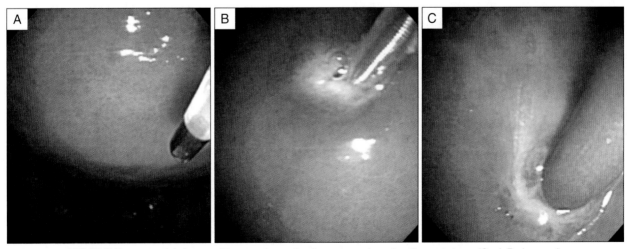

FIG 56.9 Transmural drainage without endoscopic ultrasonography using the cystotome (Cook Endoscopy). **A,** Extrinsic compression with the cystotome in view. **B,** Initial entry is made with the inner, smaller-sized cautery device. **C,** The outer, larger (10 Fr) cautery portion is passed over the smaller one and through the wall of the collection.

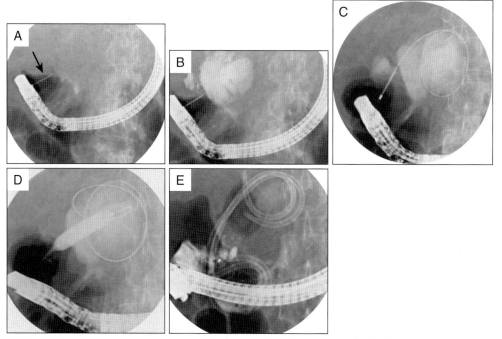

FIG 56.10 Transmural drainage using the Seldinger technique (same patient as in Fig. 56.5). **A,** A needle is passed transduodenally through the duodenal wall. **B,** Contrast is injected and fills the pseudocyst. **C,** A guidewire is coiled within the collection. **D,** The duodenal wall is balloon dilated using a 10-mm biliary dilating balloon. **E,** Two double-pigtail stents are placed.

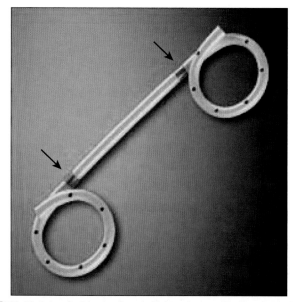

FIG 56.11 Solus double-pigtail stent. The markers are both endoscopically and radiographically visible (*arrows*).

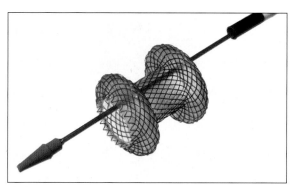

FIG 56.12 Self-expandable metal stent (AXIOS stent; Xlumena, Mountain View, CA) designed for transmural pseudocyst drainage.

passing no more than 50% of the stent into the collection. An indelible marker can be placed at the midpoint of the stent if radiopaque markers are not already present. When the midpoint of the stent is at the gastric or duodenal wall, the endoscope is drawn away from the collection while simultaneously pushing the stent out of the endoscope channel (see Video 56.1). Softer, more pliable stents (Hobbs Medical Inc., Stafford Springs, CT, and the Solus stent, Cook Medical) are also available. The Solus stent has an inner guiding catheter and endoscopic and radiopaque markers (Fig. 56.11), and spontaneous dislodgment before or with resolution of the fluid collection is common (see Chapter 22).

Fully covered biliary SEMS and specially designed short stents (Fig. 56.12) have been used to drain liquefied contents.[13] A double-pigtail stent placed through or alongside the metal stent lumen may help to prevent migration (see figures in Chapter 42).[14,15] More recently, the introduction of LAMS (AXIOS; Boston Scientific) has mitigated many of the limitations of traditional drainage options. These stents have an overall stent length of ~1 cm and are available with midbody luminal diameters of 10 and 15 mm and external flange diameters of 21 and 24 mm, respectively. Two AXIOS stent delivery systems are available: one requires placement via the standard cadence (i.e., 1, puncture; 2, guidewire placement; 3, tract dilation; 4, stent deployment), and the other is fitted with an electrosurgical tip designed for simultaneous puncture and tract dilation followed by stent deployment, without the need for guidewire placement in select circumstances. Many endoscopists place one double-pigtail plastic stent within the LAMS to maintain stent patency as the cavity resolves. As can be seen, traditional transmural approaches using plastic or metal biliary SEMS require needle puncture, application of electrosurgery, dilation, and several device exchanges.

The use of a cautery-enhanced LAMS has greatly simplified the approach as one-step placement of a 10-mm or 15-mm stent without the need for exchange. This benefit is somewhat offset by the high cost of the device.

PANCREATIC NECROSIS

Pancreatic necrosis is defined as nonviable pancreatic parenchyma usually with associated peripancreatic fat necrosis. In the earliest form this is detected radiographically on contrast-enhanced CT by the presence of nonenhancing pancreatic parenchyma (Fig. 56.13). Pancreatic necrosis is frequently accompanied by major pancreatic ductal disruptions. Over the course of several weeks, the collection continues to evolve and expand the initial area of necrosis. This collection contains both liquid and solid debris (Fig. 56.14) and was originally termed "organized pancreatic necrosis" to differentiate this process from the early (acute) phase of pancreatic necrosis. This entity is now referred to as WON (Fig. 56.15).[1] The CT appearance of WON may be similar to that of an acute pseudocyst because the underlying solid debris is frequently indistinguishable by CT, often appearing homogeneous. This may lead one to embark on standard pseudocyst drainage methods that do not adequately remove the underlying solid material, potentially exposing the patient to serious infection.

The distinction between an acute pseudocyst and WON may be made on clinical, temporal, radiologic, and endoscopic findings at the time of drainage. Clinically, most patients with WON have suffered a severe or complicated course of acute pancreatitis. Several radiographic features can indicate the presence of underlying solid material within a collection. A contrast-enhanced CT scan after the initial episode of pancreatitis often demonstrates significant glandular necrosis. The evolution by CT scan can trace the original pancreatic necrosis to the present collection. CT findings that distinguish pseudocysts from WON include larger size, extension to a paracolic space, irregular wall definition, the presence of fat attenuation debris, and pancreatic deformity or discontinuity.[16] A follow-up CT scan after endoscopic drainage will depict solid material once the liquid component has been evacuated (Fig. 56.16). Endoscopic findings at the time of drainage that indicate the presence of necrotic debris include endoscopically visible solid material, the presence of chocolate brown or extremely turbid fluid (in the absence of clinical infection), and the finding of complete main PD disruption (Fig. 56.17). During contrast injection through the main PD or transmurally, large filling defects within the collection correspond to the solid material. EUS findings of WON can also be seen as hyperechoic areas within the collection, which can consist of free-floating debris or focal areas of

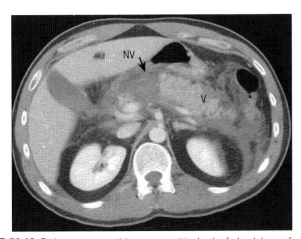

FIG 56.13 Early acute necrotizing pancreatitis. Lack of glandular perfusion of nonviable pancreatic parenchyma (*NV*) is seen in the neck of the pancreas. The viable parenchyma (*V*) is seen in the body and tail.

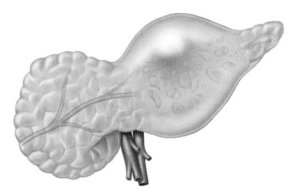

FIG 56.15 Illustration depicting organized pancreatic necrosis (walled-off necrosis). Note that viable pancreatic head and tail typically occurs and is the mechanism of pancreatic duct disconnection.

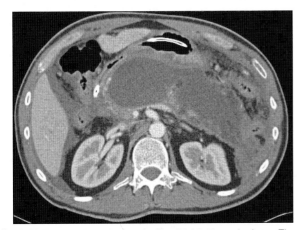

FIG 56.14 The same patient as in Fig. 56.13, 5 weeks later. There is now a large collection occupying the area of the pancreatic bed consistent with walled-off necrosis (organized pancreatic necrosis).

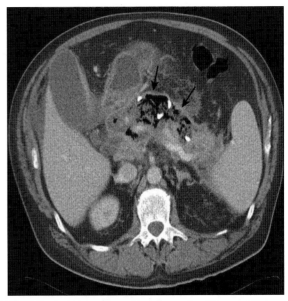

FIG 56.16 Typical appearance after intervention in pancreatic necrosis. The collection (*arrows*) contains nondependent air and debris.

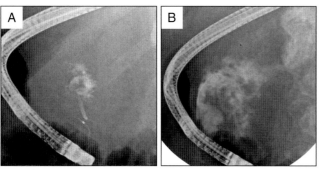

FIG 56.17 Severe pancreatic duct disruption identified at the time of endoscopic drainage of pancreatic necrosis. **A,** Initial injection shows short normal pancreatic duct that then disrupts into the necrotic cavity **(B).**

solid material. These can range from a small percentage to nearly the entire collection (i.e., minimal liquid component). If any or all of the above is recognized, appropriate steps must be taken to evacuate the underlying solid debris to prevent secondary infection. Overall, one should consider the evolution of a pancreatic collection from the early phase of acute pancreatic necrosis toward a pseudocyst as a spectrum, with WON as an intermediate stage, realizing that some collections will never completely liquefy even after a prolonged period.

The indications for and the timing of drainage of sterile pancreatic necrosis are controversial. Pancreatic necrosis is not amenable to endoscopic drainage until the process becomes organized, which usually occurs 4 to 6 weeks after the inciting event. By definition, WON does not form until 4 weeks. Before this it is referred to as an acute necrotic collection. If the process remains sterile, the general indications for drainage are similar to those encountered in liquefied collections (i.e., refractory abdominal pain, gastric outlet or biliary obstruction, or failure to thrive [i.e., continued systemic illness, anorexia, and weight loss]) at 4 or more weeks from the onset of acute pancreatitis. The severity of CT scan findings alone is not an indication for drainage. Endoscopic drainage of WON carries a higher rate of adverse events than for pseudocysts and tends to involve a more severely ill patient population. Thus the decision to intervene endoscopically in patients with sterile pancreatic necrosis must be carefully considered. Alternative management options to endoscopic drainage include parenteral or enteral nutritional support and percutaneous or surgical drainage (which should include minimally invasive approaches, such as laparoscopic and video-assisted retroperitoneal debridement). Management is usually based on local expertise and the severity of comorbid medical illnesses. Ideally, these patients are best managed by a multidisciplinary approach at a tertiary center.

Infected pancreatic necrosis is considered an indication for drainage. Clinically, infected necrosis may not be distinguishable from sterile necrosis based on the presence of leukocytosis and fever. In the past, percutaneous FNA was often used to determine the bacteriologic status of the necrosis when the decision to intervene was predicated on infection. Open surgical therapy is no longer considered the gold standard[17] and has largely been replaced by less invasive approaches[18,19] using flexible-endoscopic, rigid-endoscopic,[20] percutaneous, and laparoscopic techniques, either alone or in combination.[21]

Endoscopic Drainage of Walled-Off Necrosis

Because of the need to evacuate solid material, the endoscopic approach to WON differs from drainage of other (liquefied) PFCs. In general, the transpapillary approach is inadequate for removing solid debris. Therefore transmural drainage remains the preferred approach,

mimicking the technique described earlier for liquefied collections. When plastic stents are used, the gastric or duodenal wall is balloon dilated to a diameter ≥15 mm (Fig. 56.18, *A;* Video 56.2). This allows immediate egress of liquefied contents and facilitates endoscopic removal of necrotic debris. Several approaches, alone or in combination, can be used to evacuate solid debris. One option is to employ an irrigation system to lavage the solid debris. This can be achieved by placing a 7-Fr nasoirrigation tube (standard nasobiliary tube) into the collection alongside the transmural stents[22] (Fig. 56.18, *B* and *C*) using one or more transmural sites.[23] Up to 200 mL of normal saline is forcefully and rapidly infused via the tube every 2 to 4 hours initially. In patients who are intolerant of nasocystic irrigation tubes and/or for whom it is anticipated that irrigation may be required for many weeks, an alternative to nasocystic lavage is placement of a percutaneous endoscopic gastrostomy tube with placement of a "jejunal" extension tube into the collection (Fig. 56.19; see Video 56.2). The gastric port may then be used for supplementing nutritional needs. A "dual-modality" approach has also been described in which a transmural puncture and percutaneous puncture into the WON are performed on the same day as the initial intervention (Fig. 56.20).[24] Irrigation via the percutaneous catheter is then done to debride necrotic tissue.

An alternative endoscopic approach is physical removal of necrotic debris. Endoscopic debridement can be performed by transmural passage of catheters into the collection to irrigate and remove debris with stone retrieval baskets, balloons, and retrieval nets under fluoroscopic guidance. Direct endoscopic necrosectomy (DEN) is performed by passing a forward-viewing or side-viewing endoscope transmurally into the collection (Fig. 56.21). Baskets, grasping forceps, and snares are used to remove solid debris (Fig. 56.22; Videos 56.3 and 56.4). Transmural placement of large-diameter covered (esophageal) SEMS or LAMS (as described earlier) can both obviate and facilitate direct necrosectomy and completely avoids the need for repeated balloon dilation before debridement.[25] LAMS are ideal for DEN (Fig. 56.23), as the 15-mm stent diameter can accommodate the repeated endoscope entry and exit necessary for adequate debridement, and the wide flanges provide stable apposition between the gastric wall and cavity wall.[26,27] A 20-mm LAMS has been FDA approved for WON but at the time of this writing is not yet commercially available. Additionally, these larger-caliber metal stents may allow for egress of necrotic tissue between DEN procedures. As mentioned earlier, a single double-pigtail plastic stent can be placed within the SEMS or LAMS to maintain stent patency as the cavity resolves and possibly prevent migration. Regardless of the approach, repeat procedures are often required. These procedures may be scheduled or performed "on demand" based on clinical status and/or CT scan findings.

Paracolic gutter extensions can be accessed percutaneously for irrigation or to allow subsequent placement of large-bore (20-mm to 25-mm diameter) fully covered SEMS to perform DEN using a flexible endoscope via the percutaneous tract (Video 56.5).[28] Fistulization to the colon wall, often near the distal transverse colon or splenic flexure, may permit endoscopic debridement during colonoscopy.

Patients undergoing endoscopic drainage of sterile, organized pancreatic necrosis are given antibiotics (i.e., a carbapenem, extended spectrum penicillin agent, or fluoroquinolone). Patients with infected necrosis continue antibiotic therapy, either empirically or based on culture data obtained during drainage and/or debridement.

Outpatients may require hospitalization postprocedurally for observation and teaching of irrigation catheter care (if placed). Patients are discharged home after they are able to tolerate oral intake and care for their irrigation tube(s). Postprocedural oral antibiotics are administered and irrigation is continued (if used) until the collection has resolved, as documented by follow-up CT. CT scans are generally obtained every

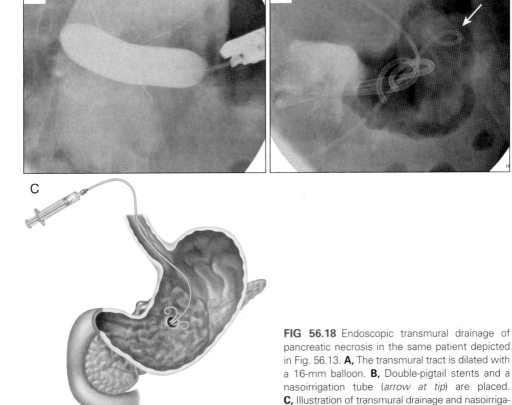

FIG 56.18 Endoscopic transmural drainage of pancreatic necrosis in the same patient depicted in Fig. 56.13. **A,** The transmural tract is dilated with a 16-mm balloon. **B,** Double-pigtail stents and a nasoirrigation tube (*arrow at tip*) are placed. **C,** Illustration of transmural drainage and nasoirrigation catheter.

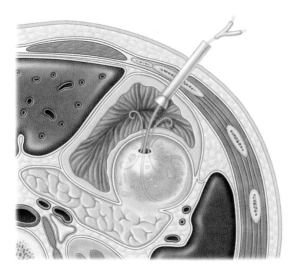

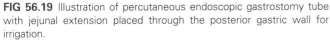

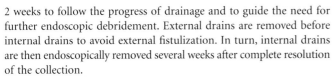

FIG 56.19 Illustration of percutaneous endoscopic gastrostomy tube with jejunal extension placed through the posterior gastric wall for irrigation.

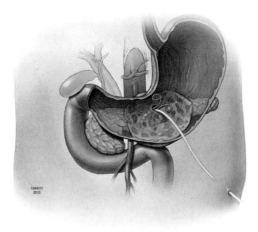

FIG 56.20 Illustration of dual-modality drainage that combines transmural drainage and percutaneous irrigation into the same collection.

2 weeks to follow the progress of drainage and to guide the need for further endoscopic debridement. External drains are removed before internal drains to avoid external fistulization. In turn, internal drains are then endoscopically removed several weeks after complete resolution of the collection.

Recently we have changed our strategy for the management of WON. We place large-diameter LAMS with an internal 10-Fr double-pigtail through the stent. The latter (1) allows egress of fluid in the event that necrotic material impacts within the stent lumen; (2) protects the inner wall of the collection from contact-related delayed bleeding; (3) allows retrieval of buried LAMS, should it occur; and (4) creates space if long-term double-pigtail stents are placed to manage disconnected duct syndrome. We ensure that patients are not on acid suppression therapy to allow acid-induced debridement. We do not routinely perform DEN and reserve it for failure to improve or in the event of clinical deterioration. Nasoirrigation tubes are no longer routinely placed.[29] After

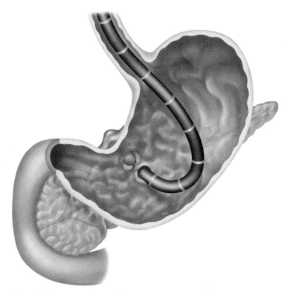

FIG 56.21 Illustration of direct endoscopic debridement using a forward-viewing endoscope.

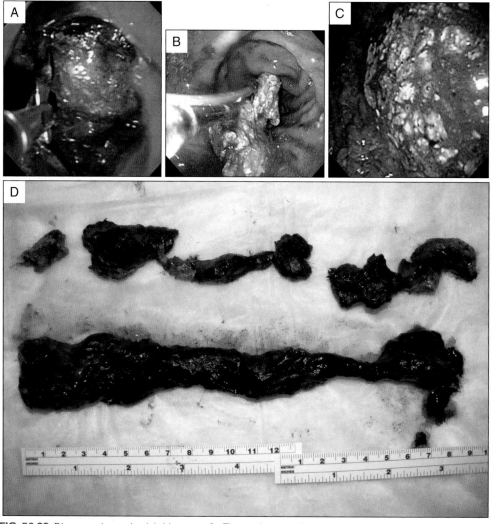

FIG 56.22 Direct endoscopic debridement. **A,** The endoscope is just within the cavity through a large transmural tract. A pelican forceps can be seen grasping the solid material. **B,** The necrotic material is withdrawn and deposited into the antrum. **C,** A large amount of necrotic debris is seen in the stomach at the end of the procedure. **D,** A large amount of necrotic debris removed in one session during direct endoscopic necrosectomy.

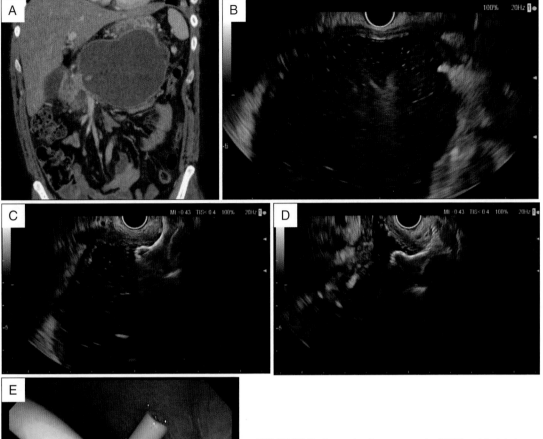

FIG 56.23 Endoscopic ultrasonography (EUS)–guided drainage of walled-off necrosis. **A,** Coronal computed tomography scan obtained 4 weeks after severe pancreatitis shows a large fluid collection compressing the stomach. **B,** EUS image from the stomach shows the collection containing solid debris. **C,** EUS image of distal flare of lumen-apposing metal stent (LAMS) deployed across the gastric wall into the collection. **D,** EUS image of LAMS deployed across the gastric wall into the collection. **E,** Endoscopic image of proximal flange of LAMS deployed in the stomach. A 10-Fr pigtail stent can be seen within the LAMS lumen.

resolution of the cavity, the LAMS can be traction removed using either a standard polypectomy snare or grasping forceps. The timing of LAMS removal should be determined on a case-by-case basis, with a goal to retrieve the stent at the earliest practical time point, because of concern for delayed bleeding that may occur in the setting of longer dwell times.

RESULTS OF ENDOSCOPIC THERAPY OF PANCREATIC FLUID COLLECTIONS

Pancreatic Pseudocysts

In the past, rates of success, recurrence, and adverse events after endoscopic drainage of pancreatic pseudocysts were variable. This can be attributed to heterogeneity in patient populations and interventions across series; for example, transpapillary drainage methods were included with transmural drainage methods. Recent studies have used more uniform nomenclature and techniques. A large multicenter study recently demonstrated no additional benefit when transpapillary drainage was performed in addition to EUS-guided transmural drainage.[30] Moreover, transpapillary drainage was negatively associated with long-term radiologic resolution. Successful drainage of liquefied collections is achieved in approximately 90% of patients, with adverse event rates from 5% to 10% and recurrence rates of 5% to 20%. The results of endoscopic drainage compare favorably to surgery.[31–33] Although percutaneous drainage of pancreatic pseudocysts has a high clinical success rate, it can lead to pancreaticocutaneous fistulae, as pseudocysts often communicate with the main PD.

There may be a slightly lower pseudocyst recurrence rate after transduodenal drainage compared with transgastric drainage, though this has not been proven. This may be because of prolonged patency of transduodenal fistulae that allows long-term drainage of the main PD.

Pancreatic Abscesses

When a broad definition of pancreatic abscess is taken to include infected pseudocysts and other infected liquefied collections without necrosis, success rates after endoscopic drainage are high, although there are few series and small patient numbers.

Walled-Off Necrosis

There is an increasing number of series showing that endoscopic treatment of WON is successful at achieving nonsurgical resolution in a majority of patients.[34,35] Two systematic reviews have shown complete resolution of WON in >80% of patients using traditional endoscopic drainage techniques alone, with a mean of four procedures necessary for resolution.[36,37] Outcomes regarding the use of esophageal SEMS and LAMS to facilitate DEN have recently emerged. Early cohort data suggest a high degree of resolution (~90%) with a low risk for adverse events (~5%).[38–40]

Paracolic gutter extension is considered a poor predictor of endoscopic therapy alone,[22] although in some cases the endoscope can be passed into these pelvic collections transmurally (Video 56.6) or managed with adjuvant percutaneous drains. Fistulization to the colon may occur in the setting of paracolic extensions, potentially allowing for transmural drainage and/or DEN through the colon wall.[41]

OUTCOME DIFFERENCES AFTER ENDOSCOPIC DRAINAGE OF PANCREATIC FLUID COLLECTIONS

Significant differences in success rates using endoscopic drainage have been noted between patients with pseudocysts and patients with pancreatic necrosis.[7,42] Adverse events occur more commonly in patients with pancreatic necrosis than in those with pseudocysts. Likewise, hospital stay is shorter for patients with pseudocysts than for those with WON. Recurrent collections occur more often in patients with pancreatic necrosis and chronic pancreatic pseudocysts. The differences in rates of success, adverse events, and recurrence and length of hospital stay are explained by differences in pathology, pathophysiology, and severity of illness between the groups. Patients with pancreatic necrosis tend to be more severely ill, and endoscopic evacuation of solid debris is less efficient than evacuation of liquid. Patients with acute pseudocysts tend to have less severe ductal abnormalities and less recurrence, whereas patients with chronic pancreatitis have underlying ductal abnormalities, such as strictures and stones, that may lead to recurrences, especially if unrecognized and untreated and after transgastric drainage.[43] In terms of recurrence rates, acute pancreatic ductal disruptions in patients with necrosis frequently lead to either severe stricturing or a completely disconnected main PD, whereby the head and tail of the pancreas are not in communication (Figs. 56.24 and 56.25). Recurrent collections may arise from the undrained viable pancreatic tail. We recommend aggressive endoscopic intervention to correct underlying ductal abnormalities, if possible, in all types of PFCs so that recurrent collections or symptoms can be avoided (Fig. 56.5, D and E).

Management of the disconnected duct after acute necrotizing pancreatitis has not been standardized. Some authors recommend leaving pigtail stents in place at the transmural site when a disconnected duct is identified preprocedurally or postprocedurally by any modality (pancreatography, CT, MRI). Others prefer to remove all stents and follow the patient for symptoms (disconnected duct syndrome). Such symptoms include acute recurrent pancreatitis in the disconnected tail, recurrent PFCs (pseudocysts), or pancreatic fistula (pleural effusions, ascites). Transpapillary drainage is not feasible in these patients, and EUS-guided techniques and surgery may be required.

ROLE OF ENDOSCOPIC EXPERIENCE

Endoscopic therapy of PFCs requires a high skill level. Operator experience may play a role in the outcome of these patients, as there appears to be a learning curve associated with drainage of PFCs. Animal training

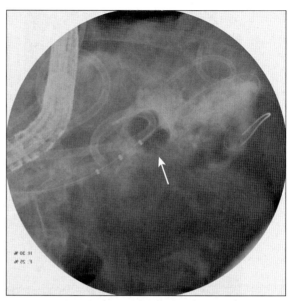

FIG 56.24 Indirect endoscopic debridement of the same patient as in Fig. 56.13. A stone retrieval balloon (*arrow*) was inflated inside the cavity and solid debris was swept out of the transmural site.

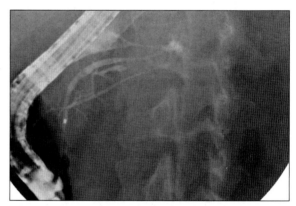

FIG 56.25 Final pancreatogram of the same patient in Fig. 56.13. The necrotic cavity resolved, as documented by computed tomography. Extravasation of contrast is seen from the pancreatic duct back into the duodenum at the transmural entry site. There is no communication with the tail.

models for learning pseudocyst drainage techniques have been described and may be helpful in acquiring these skills.[44]

ADVERSE EVENTS OF ENDOSCOPIC THERAPY OF PANCREATIC FLUID COLLECTIONS

Life-threatening adverse events may arise after attempted endoscopic drainage of PFCs, and these are listed in Box 56.2. It is recommended that endoscopic drainage of PFCs be performed with the availability of surgical and interventional radiology (IR) support. The most feared adverse events of transmural drainage are bleeding and perforation. Bleeding after transmural drainage can be managed supportively, endoscopically, surgically, or with IR-guided angiographic embolization. If perforation occurs during attempted transgastric drainage and is limited to the gastric wall (does not involve the collection), it can be successfully managed nonsurgically, assuming that an endoprosthesis is not inadvertently placed through the perforation into the peritoneal

---

BOX 56.2 Adverse Events of Endoscopic Therapy of Pancreatic Fluid Collections

- Bleeding
- Perforation
- Infection
- Pancreatitis
- Sedation-related adverse events
- Aspiration
- Stent migration or occlusion
- Pancreatic duct damage
- Air embolism (transmural approach)

---

space. If egress of gastric contents is prevented, the gastric wall rapidly closes with conservative treatment consisting of nasogastric suction and antibiotics. Large-diameter (esophageal) SEMS can be used to seal perforations[45] and in some cases tamponade bleeding. Some believe that transduodenal perforation may be managed conservatively because the perforation is within the retroperitoneum. Infectious adverse events usually occur from inadequate drainage of fluid and/or solid debris. If transpapillary drainage is performed on a liquefied collection, stent exchange and/or upsizing of the stent may resolve the infection. If solid material is present, placement of irrigation tubes or changing to transmural drainage (if transpapillary drainage was initially performed) may resolve the infection. Occasionally some patients will require adjuvant placement of percutaneous drainage and/or irrigation catheters to manage infectious adverse events, particularly when the necrosis extends to paracolic gutters.[22] Stent migration into the collection through the gastric or duodenal wall may occur during or after endoscopic stent placement. Endoscopic retrieval is possible if the collection has not completely collapsed and the transmural tract remains patent. The use of new LAMS may mitigate stent migration, as these include large (i.e., >20 mm) proximal and distal flanges. Fatal air embolism has been reported after both drainage of pseudocysts (without entering the collection with the endoscope)[46] and DEN.[47] This has prompted the use of carbon dioxide rather than air insufflation during PFC drainage.

Endoscopic therapy may be associated with adverse events and/or failures that require surgical management. It is possible that the outcome of surgical therapy may be adversely altered compared with those patients undergoing primary surgical therapy.

The complete reference list for this chapter can be found online at www.expertconsult.com.

Page number followed by f indicates figure; by t table; and by b box.